Oxford Textbook of

Children's Sport and Exercise Medicine

Oxford Textbook of Children's Sport and Exercise Medicine

Edited by

Neil Armstrong
Professor of Paediatric Physiology, Founding Director of the Children's Health and Exercise Research Centre, and Formerly Provost of the University of Exeter, United Kingdom

and

Willem van Mechelen
Professor of Occupational and Sports Medicine, Director of the Amsterdam Public Health research institute, VU University Medical Centre Amsterdam, the Netherlands

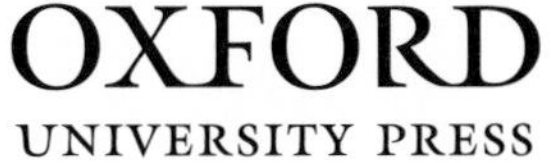

OXFORD
UNIVERSITY PRESS

Great Clarendon Street, Oxford, OX2 6DP,
United Kingdom

Oxford University Press is a department of the University of Oxford.
It furthers the University's objective of excellence in research, scholarship,
and education by publishing worldwide. Oxford is a registered trade mark of
Oxford University Press in the UK and in certain other countries

Second Edition Published in 2008
Impression: 1

Published in the United States of America by Oxford University Press
198 Madison Avenue, New York, NY 10016, United States of America

British Library Cataloguing in Publication Data
Data available

Library of Congress Control Number: 2016954555

ISBN 978–0–19–875767–2

Printed in Great Britain by
Bell & Bain Ltd., Glasgow

Contents

PART 2
Exercise medicine

Foreword

Physical inactivity is one of the biggest public health problems of the 21st century. Modern society has been busy engineering human energy expenditure out of life for decades. It is possible for many people to spend most of their time sitting and living at a very low-energy expenditure. Most people spend far fewer calories in household maintenance, at work, during leisure time, and in most other lifestyle activities than people did several decades ago. To address this serious problem we need initiatives in many sectors of society, including worksites, education, environmental planning, and governmental initiatives. Clinical medicine is an area where much more attention must be given to encouraging more physical activity for patients. There is a major initiative called Exercise Is Medicine, which was started in 2007 by the American Medical Association and the American College of Sports Medicine. Many other scientific and clinical organizations have joined the effort, and the programme now exists in dozens of countries around the world. Much of the early efforts have focused on getting physicians to do more patient counselling about exercise. Most of the effort has been for adults, but clearly children and adolescents are also susceptible to the aspects of modern society that have made it easier and more attractive to sit, rather than move.

Professors Armstrong and van Mechelen have not only focused on incorporating exercise into medical counselling in paediatric settings, but also on providing a comprehensive resource for clinicians and scientists teaching and researching in paediatric exercise science and sport medicine. The first two editions of their book have been very informative and influential, have received excellent reviews, and have been widely used. The new edition includes 17 new chapters on emerging topics of importance to the understanding of exercise and health in young people. The prior chapters in the book have been completely rewritten, and include the latest information on the wide variety of topics. The editors have retained a great majority of the international experts who wrote chapters in the previous editions, and there also are several new authors who have made numerous contributions to the various scientific areas on which they focus. I am extremely impressed with the overall expertise of the authors, who are an outstanding group of top-quality scientists in the multiple topics addressed in the book. I do not think it would be possible to assemble a more high-quality group of experts on these topics. They present the latest evidence-based research on a wide variety of issues.

Professors Armstrong and van Mechelen are exceptional scientists who have made many important contributions to physical activity and exercise science and medicine. They have addressed a wide variety of topics investigated by their research groups, and have publication records that are matched by few exercise scientists.

The chapters in this edition of *Children's Sport and Exercise Medicine* are all up to date and supported by strong evidence-based research. There are extensive important references in each chapter, and each chapter ends with a bulleted summary of the key points.

Dr Steve Blair
Professor (Retired)
Arnold School of Public Health
University of South Carolina

Preface

The first two editions of Paediatric Exercise Science and Medicine were welcomed by international reviewers as volumes which offered 'state of the art', evidence-based coverage of the topic by recognized leaders in the field. In the Preface to the first edition we referred to 'this emerging discipline' and in the Preface to the second edition we commented on the 'dramatic increase in published research focusing on the exercising child and adolescent'. Since publication of the second edition, experimental techniques initially pioneered with adults and new non-invasive technologies have been successfully developed and modified for use with children. The recent emergence of molecular exercise physiology has unlocked new avenues of research and knowledge in paediatric exercise science and medicine. The discipline is now well-established internationally, numerous professorial appointments have been made in international universities, postgraduate and postdoctoral research activity is flourishing, and publications in the field are growing at an ever-increasing rate. The material presented in the second edition is approaching the 10 years mark, and in a rapidly developing discipline it requires regular updating, refreshing, and re-appraising in the light of recent developments.

This edition has retained the ethos of previous editions. Each comprehensively referenced chapter critically analyses the research literature, establishes what we know, and identifies gaps in our knowledge. Where appropriate, chapters examine how recently developed experimental techniques, technologies, and methods of interpreting data have provided new insights into understanding the physically active child and adolescent. Contributors are internationally recognized experts in their field and they draw upon their own research to enrich the text and to inform and challenge readers. Chapters are cross-referenced to promote access to complementary material and each chapter ends with a bulleted summary and extensive reference list to support the rapid identification and further study of key issues.

Millions of young people enjoy and benefit from physical activity and sport participation and it is estimated that in England ~80% of youth partake in competitive sport each year. International organizations, such as the International Olympic Committee (IOC), are devoting resources to support the optimum development of the young athlete, as evidenced by the initiation of the Youth Olympics and the IOC investment in a series of Consensus Statements on youth athlete development, health of the youth athlete, and training elite young athletes. However, winning margins in elite-level sport competitions are small, and financial and other rewards for success are extremely large. Therefore, there is a concerted effort by some National Governing Bodies of sport, clubs, agents, coaches, and other interested parties to identify talented children and train them intensively from a young age to compete at an elite level. This is exemplified by English Premier League football clubs investing heavily in youth academies and comprehensive scouting networks to actively recruit and contract children still in primary schools. This activity has led to a plethora of concerns about the current and future health and well-being of young athletes.

The mass participation of children and adolescents in community sport programmes and the challenges faced by elite young athletes have resulted in a surge of research into youth sport and the development of the elite young athlete. This is reflected in the current edition, which retains its comprehensive coverage of paediatric exercise science and medicine but offers more extensive coverage of sport science and sport medicine than in previous editions. As a result the book has been retitled the *Oxford Textbook of Children's Sport and Exercise Medicine* to better describe its content.

Chapters on 17 new topics have been added to this edition, and even where chapter titles remain the same or similar to the second edition, the content has been comprehensively updated and rewritten, often by new contributors who have emerged as leading researchers in their field since the publication of the previous edition. Twenty-eight scientists and clinicians from the first edition and 45 from the second edition once again contribute to this edition, with 39 new authors from 17 countries enhancing the content.

The primary aims of the *Oxford Textbook of Children's Sport and Exercise Medicine* are to provide an up-to-date, comprehensive reference work with a sound scientific evidence-based foundation to support and challenge scientists, medical practitioners, professionals allied to medicine, senior coaches, physical educators, and students involved in youth physical activity, sport, and/or paediatric exercise science and medicine. If the book stimulates the initiation of innovative research programmes, informs best practice in children's sport and exercise medicine, and thereby contributes to the promotion of young people's personal development, health, well-being, and enjoyment of physical activity and sport, it will have served its purpose.

Neil Armstrong
Willem van Mechelen

Contributors

Neil Armstrong, PhD, DSc, Professor, Children's Health and Exercise Research Centre, St Luke's Campus, University of Exeter, Exeter, EX1 2LU, England

Willem van Mechelen, PhD, MD, Professor, Department of Public and Occupational Health, Amsterdam Public Health research institute, VU University Medical Center Amsterdam, van der Boechorststraat 7, 1081 BT, Amsterdam, The Netherlands

Frank JG Backx, MD, PhD, Professor, Department of Rehabilitation, Physical Therapy Science and Sports, University Medical Center Utrecht, Huispostnummer W01.121, Postbus 85500, 3508 GA, Utrecht, The Netherlands

Astrid CJ Balemans, PhD, Department of Rehabilitation Medicine, VU University Medical Center Amsterdam, PO Box 7057, 1007 MB, Amsterdam and Brain Center Rudolf Magnus and Center of Excellence for Rehabilitation Medicine, University Medical Center Utrecht and De Hoogstraat Rehabilitation, Rembrandtkade 10, 3585 TM, Utrecht, The Netherlands

Saulo Delfino Barboza, Department of Public and Occupational Health, EMGO+ Institute for Health and Care Research, VU University Medical Center Amsterdam, van der Boechorststraat 7, 1081 BT, Amsterdam, The Netherlands

Alan R Barker, PhD, Children's Health and Exercise Research Centre, St Luke's Campus, University of Exeter, Exeter, EX1 2LU, England

Meike Bartels, PhD, Professor, Department of Biological Psychology, Amsterdam Public Health research institute, VU University and VU University Medical Center Amsterdam, van der Boechorststraat 1, 1081 BT, Amsterdam, The Netherlands

Adam DG Baxter-Jones, PhD, Professor, College of Kinesiology, University of Saskatchewan, 87 Campus Drive, Saskatoon, Saskatchewan, S7N 5B2, Canada

Roselien Buys, PhD, Department of Rehabilitation Sciences, KU Leuven, Tervuursevest 101, Bus 1501, 3001 Leuven, Belgium

Nuala M Byrne, PhD, Professor, School of Health Sciences, University of Tasmania, Launceston, Tasmania, Australia 7250

Robert C Cantu, MD, Professor, Neurosurgery Service, Service of Sports Medicine, Emerson Hospital, Concord, MA 01742, USA

Robert V Cantu, MD, Orthopaedic Surgery, Dartmouth-Hitchcock Medical Center, One Medical Center Drive, Lebanon, NH 03756, USA

Akin Cil, MD, Division of Shoulder, Elbow and Sports Medicine, Department of Orthopaedics, University of Missouri-Kansas City, Kansas City, MO, USA

Dorine CM Collard, PhD, Mulier Instituut Centre for Research on Sports in Society, Postbus 85445, 3508 AK Utrecht, The Netherlands

Sean P Cumming, PhD, Department for Health, University of Bath, Bath, BA2 7AY, England

Annet J Dallmeijer, PhD, Department of Rehabilitation Medicine, Amsterdam Public Health research institute, VU University Medical Center Amsterdam, PO Box 7057, 1007 MB, Amsterdam, The Netherlands

Eco JC de Geus, PhD, Professor, Department of Biological Psychology, Amsterdam Public Health research institute, VU University and VU University Medical Center Amsterdam, van der Boechorststraat 1, 1081 BT, Amsterdam, The Netherlands

Mark BA De Ste Croix, PhD, Professor, Exercise and Sport Research Centre, Oxstalls Campus, Oxstalls Lane, University of Gloucestershire, Gloucester, GL2 9HW, England

Raffy Dotan, Faculty of Applied Health Sciences, Brock University, St Catharines, Ontario, LS2 3A1, Canada

Ulf Ekelund, PhD, Professor, Department of Sport Medicine, Norwegian School of Sport Sciences, PO Box 4014, 0806 Ulleval Stadion, Oslo, Norway

Alon Eliakim, MD, Professor, Pediatric Department, Meir Medical Center, Sackler School of Medicine, Tel-Aviv University, Israel

Roger G Eston, DPE, Professor, Alliance for Research in Exercise, Nutrition and Activity, Sansom Institute for Health Research, School of Health Sciences, University of South Australia, Adelaide, Australia

Avery D Faigenbaum, EdD, Professor, Department of Health and Exercise Science, The College of New Jersey, Ewing, NJ 08628, USA

Bareket Falk, PhD, Professor, Department of Kinesiology, Faculty of Applied Health Sciences, Brock University, St Catharines, Ontario, LS2 3A1, Canada

Rômulo A Fernandes, PhD, Department of Physical Education, School of Science and Technology, Sao Paulo State University (UNESP), Roberto Simonsen 305, 19060-900, Presidente Prudente, Brazil

Isabel Ferreira, PhD, Division of Epidemiology and Biostatistics, School of Public Health, University of Queensland, Public Health Building, Herston Road, Herston 4006, Brisbane, Queensland, Australia

David Gerrard, MD, Emeritus Professor, Dunedin School of Medicine, University of Otago, PO Box 56, Dunedin 9054, New Zealand

Marc Gewillig, PhD, MD, Professor, Cardiovascular Developmental Biology, University Hospitals Leuven, Herestraat 49—box 7003 64, 3000 Leuven, Belgium

Helge Hebestreit, PhD, MD, Professor, Paediatric Department, Julius-Maximilians University of Würzburg, Josef-Schneider Strasse 2, 97080 Würzburg, Germany

Luiz Carlos Hespanhol Junior, Department of Public and Occupational Health, Amsterdam Public Health research institute, VU University Medical Center Amsterdam, van der Boechorststraat 7, 1081 BT, Amsterdam, The Netherlands

Maria Hildebrand, Department of Sport Medicine, Norwegian School of Sport Sciences, PO Box 4014, 0806 Ulleval Stadion, Oslo, Norway

Andrew P Hills, PhD, Professor, Sports and Exercise Science, School of Health Sciences, Faculty of Health, University of Tasmania, Building C, Room C114, Locked Bag 1322, Newnham Drive, Launceston TAS 7250, Australia

Barbara Joschtel, School of Human Movement and Nutrition Sciences, University of Queensland, Brisbane QLD 4072, Australia

Jaak Jürimäe, PhD, Professor, Institute of Sport Sciences and Physiotherapy, University of Tartu, 18 Ulikooli Street, Tartu, 50090, Estonia

Han CG Kemper, PhD, Professor Emeritus, Department of Public and Occupational Health, Amsterdam Public Health research institute, VU University Medical Center Amsterdam, van der Boechorststraat 7, 1081 BT, Amsterdam, The Netherlands

Sandi Kirby, Professor Emerita, University of Winnipeg, 515 Portage Avenue, Winnipeg, Manitoba, Canada R3B 2E9

Stef Kremers, PhD, Professor, Department of Health Promotion, NUTRIM School of Nutrition and Translational Research in Metabolism, Maastricht University Medical Centre, P. Debyeplein 1, 6200 MD Maastricht, The Netherlands

Susi Kriemler, MD, Professor, Epidemiology, Biostatistics and Prevention Institute, University of Zürich, Hirschengraben 84, 8001 Zürich, Switzerland

Kevin L Lamb, PhD, Professor, Department of Sport and Exercise Sciences, Parkgate Road, University of Chester, Chester, CH1 4BJ, England

Rhodri S Lloyd, PhD, Cardiff Metropolitan University, Cardiff School of Sport, Cyncoed Campus, Cyncoed Road, Cardiff, CF23 6XD, Wales

Umile Giuseppe Longo, PhD, MD, Department of Trauma and Orthopaedic Surgery, Campus Bio-Medico University, Via Álvaro Del Portillo 200, 00128 Trigoria, Rome, Italy

Nicola Maffulli, PhD, MD, Professor, Centre for Sports and Exercise Medicine, Queen Mary University, London E1 4DG, England, and Department of Trauma and Orthopaedic Surgery, Faculty of Medicine and Surgery, University of Salerno, Italy

Per Bo Mahler, MD, Service de Santé de l'Enfance et de la Jeunesse, Canton de Genève, and La Tour Sport Medicine SOMC, Hôpital de La Tour, Meyrin, Switzerland

Robert M Malina, PhD, Professor Emeritus, Department of Kinesiology and Health Education, University of Texas at Austin, Austin, TX, USA

Ronald J Maughan, PhD, School of Medicine, University of St Andrews, North Haugh, St. Andrews, KY16 9TF, Scotland

Alison M McManus, PhD, Centre for Heart, Lung and Vascular Health, School of Health and Exercise Sciences, University of British Columbia, 1147 Research Road—ART 360, Kelowna, British Columbia, V1V 1V7, Canada

Melitta A McNarry, PhD, Applied Sports, Exercise, Technology and Medicine Research Centre, Bay Campus, Swansea University, Swansea, SA1 8EN, Wales

Ree M Meertens, Department of Health Promotion, P.O. Box 616, 6200 MD Maastricht, The Netherlands. Visiting address: P. Debijeplein 1, 6229 HA Maastricht, The Netherlands

Lyle J Micheli, MD, Professor, Children's Hospital, Boston and Harvard Medical School, 319 Longwood Avenue, Boston, MA 02115, USA

Margo Mountjoy, PhD, MD, IOC Medical Commission Games Group and Michael G DeGroote School of Medicine, McMaster University Hamilton, Ontario, Canada

Shareef F Mustapha, MD, Department of Pediatrics and Child Health, University of Manitoba, A8025-409 Tache Avenue, Winnipeg, Manitoba, R2H 2A6, Canada

Joske Nauta, PhD, Department of Public and Occupational Health, Amsterdam Public Health research institute, VU University Medical Center Amsterdam, van der Boechorststraat 7, 1081 BT Amsterdam, The Netherlands

Dan Nemet, MD, Professor, Child Health and Sports Center, Meir Medical Center, Sackler School of Medicine, Tel-Aviv University, Tel-Aviv, Israel

Jon L Oliver, PhD, Cardiff Metropolitan University, Cardiff School of Sport, Cyncoed Campus, Cyncoed Road, Cardiff, CF23 6XD, Wales

Gaynor Parfitt, PhD, Alliance for Research in Exercise, Nutrition and Activity, Sansom Institute for Health Research, School of Health Sciences, University of South Australia, Adelaide, Australia

Thomas Radtke, PhD, Epidemiology, Biostatistics and Prevention Institute, University of Zürich, Hirschengraben 84, 8001 Zürich, Switzerland

Sébastien Ratel, PhD, Université Clermont Auvergne, Université Blaise Pascal, EA 3533, Laboratoire des Adaptations Métaboliques à l'Exercice en conditions Physiologiques et Pathologiques (AME2P), BP 80026, F-63171 Aubière, Cedex, France

Tony Reybrouck, PhD, Emeritus Professor, Department of Rehabilitation Sciences, KU Leuven, Tervuursevest 101, Bus 1501, 3001 Leuven, Belgium

Thomas W Rowland, MD, Professor, Tufts University School of Medicine, Boston, MA, and Pediatric Cardiologist, Baystate Medical Center, Springfield, MA, USA

Robert AC Ruiter, PhD, Professor, Department of Work and Social Psychology, Faculty of Psychology and Neuroscience, Maastricht University, 6200 MD Maastricht, The Netherlands

Nienke M Schutte, Department of Biological Psychology, EMGO+ Institute for Health and Care Research, VU University and VU University Medical Center Amsterdam, van der Boechorststraat 1, 1081 BT, Amsterdam, The Netherlands

Christopher M Shaw, MD, Division of Shoulder, Elbow and Sports Medicine, Department of Orthopaedics, University of Missouri-Kansas City, 2301 Holmes Street, Kansas City, MO, 64108, USA

Lauren B Sherar, PhD, School of Sport, Exercise and Health Sciences, Loughborough University, Epinal Way, Loughborough, Leicestershire LE11 3TU, England

Susan M Shirreffs, PhD, School of Medicine, University of St Andrews, North Haugh, St. Andrews, KY16 9TF, Scotland

James W Smallcombe, School of Sport, Exercise and Health Sciences, Loughborough University, Loughborough, Leicestershire, LE11 3TU, England

Jonathon Smith, School of Medical Sciences, University of Aberdeen, Aberdeen AB25 2ZD, Scotland

Helen Soucie, PhD, #103, 100 rue Marcel-R.-Bergeron, Bromont, Québec, J2L 0L2, Canada

Steven J Street, PhD, School of Health Sciences, University of Tasmania, Launceston, Tasmania, Australia 7250

David Sugden, PhD, Professor, School of Education, University of Leeds, Leeds, LS2 9JT, England

Christine Sundgot-Borgen, Department of Sport Medicine, Norwegian School of Sport Sciences, PO Box 4014, 0806 Ulleval Stadion, Oslo, Norway

Jorunn Sundgot-Borgen, PhD, Professor, Department of Sport Medicine, Norwegian School of Sport Sciences, PO Box 4014, 0806 Ulleval Stadion, Oslo, Norway

Anne Tiivas, National Society for the Prevention of Cruelty for Children (NSPCC), Child Protection in Sport Unit. c/o NSPCC National Training Centre, 3, Gilmour Close, Beaumont Leys, Leicester LE4 1EZ, England

Keith Tolfrey, PhD, School of Sport, Exercise and Health Sciences, Loughborough University, Epinal Way, Loughborough, Leicestershire, LE11 3TU, England

Stewart G Trost, PhD, Professor, Institute of Health and Biomedical Innovation, Queensland University of Technology, 60 Musk Ave, Kelvin Grove QLD 4059, Australia

Jos WR Twisk, PhD, Professor, Department of Epidemiology and Biostatistics, Amsterdam Public Health research institute, VU University Medical Center Amsterdam, van der Boechorststraat 7, 1081 BT, Amsterdam, The Netherlands

Edgar GAH van Mil, PhD, MD, Department of Paediatrics, Jeroen Bosch Hospital, Henri Dunantstraat 1, 5223 GZ,'s-Hertogenbosch, The Netherlands

Evert ALM Verhagen, PhD, Department of Public and Occupational Health, Amsterdam Public Health research institute, VU University Medical Center Amsterdam, van der Boechorststraat 7, 1081 BT, Amsterdam, The Netherlands

Alan Vernec, MD, World Anti-Doping Agency, 800 Place Victoria, Bureau 1700, Montreal, Quebec H4Z 1B7, Canada

Olaf Verschuren, PhD, Brain Center Rudolf Magnus and Center of Excellence for Rehabilitation Medicine, University Medical Center Utrecht and De Hoogstraat Rehabilitation, Rembrandtkade 10, 3585 TM, Utrecht, The Netherlands

Henning Wackerhage, PhD, Professor, Technical University of Munich, Uptown München-Campus D, Georg-Brauchle-Ring 60, D-80992 München, Germany

James Watkins, PhD, Emeritus Professor, College of Engineering, Swansea University, Bay Campus, Fabian Way, Swansea, SA1 8EN, Wales

Craig A Williams, PhD, Professor, Children's Health and Exercise Research Centre, St Luke's Campus, University of Exeter, Exeter, EX1 2LU, England

Richard J Winsley, PhD, Children's Health and Exercise Research Centre, St Luke's Campus, University of Exeter, Exeter, EX1 2LU, England

Darren Wisneiwski, School of Medical Sciences, University of Aberdeen, Aberdeen AB25 2ZD, Scotland

Merrilee Zetaruk, MD, Department of Pediatrics and Child Health, University of Manitoba, Section of Pediatric Sport and Exercise Medicine, 14-160 Meadowood Drive, Winnipeg, Manitoba, R2M 5L6, Canada

Introduction

Children and adolescents are not mini-adults. They are growing and maturing at their own rate, and the assessment and interpretation of their responses to exercise are complex as they progress through childhood and adolescence into adult life.

Historically, research with healthy young people has been constrained to measuring variables such as power output or the examination of blood and respiratory gas markers of exercise performance, as ethical considerations have restricted more informative research at the level of the myocyte. The development of non-invasive technologies such as ^{31}P magnetic resonance spectroscopy, near infra-red spectroscopy, and stable isotope tracers; the application of appropriate mathematical modelling techniques to interpret physical and physiological variables during growth and maturation; and the emergence of molecular exercise physiology have provided new avenues of research and novel insights which have greatly enhanced the knowledge base and research potential in children's sport and exercise medicine.

The *Oxford Textbook of Children's Sport and Exercise Medicine* provides the most comprehensive and in-depth coverage of the topic to date. It is presented in four sections, namely exercise science, exercise medicine, sport science, and sport medicine, which between them systematically address the science and medicine underpinning sport, health, and exercise during childhood and adolescence. Fifty innovative chapters are extensively referenced to promote further study and are cross-referenced across sections where appropriate to enable interested readers to easily access complementary information.

Current knowledge in exercise science is discussed in the first section of the book. As growth and biological maturation are fundamental to understanding paediatric exercise science, the book opens with a critique of methods of assessing maturation, followed by a review of the processes of growth and maturation. The next two chapters focus on developmental biomechanics and motor development. Subsequent chapters rigorously examine muscle strength and aerobic and anaerobic metabolism during exercise, and focus on 'what we know' and 'what we need to know'. The physiological responses of the muscular, pulmonary, and cardiovascular systems to exercise of various types, intensities, and durations in relation to chronological aging, biological maturation, and sex are critically reviewed. The exercise science section ends with chapters which analyse young people's kinetic responses at the onset of exercise, scrutinize their responses to exercise during thermal stress, and evaluate how the sensations arising from physical exertion are detected and interpreted during youth. Noteworthy additions to this edition include chapters devoted to peripheral and central neuromuscular fatigue and to the responses of hormones to exercise.

The beneficial effects of appropriate physical activity during adult life are well-documented, but the potential of physical activity to confer health benefits during childhood and adolescence is controversial and has not been explored fully. There is widespread concern about the prevalence of childhood physical inactivity and the supposed decline of physical activity over the last two decades, but it is difficult to determine what is fact and what is fiction. How much exercise is necessary to promote children's health and well-being? Do we know? The tremendous success of the Paralympic Games has stimulated interest in sport and exercise for youth with physical or intellectual disabilities, but evidence-based literature is sparse. Similarly, knowledge of the therapeutic role of exercise with young people with chronic diseases is growing, but much remains to be researched and, importantly, disseminated.

These health-related issues are addressed in the section on exercise medicine, which critically reviews the extant literature and explores young people's health behaviours and the role of physical activity and physical fitness in the promotion of health and well-being. The opening chapter provides a foundation by overviewing the relationship between physical activity, physical fitness, and health. Subsequent chapters are dedicated to the effects of physical activity and physical fitness on cardiovascular health, bone health, health behaviours, diabetes mellitus, asthma, cerebral palsy, eating and weight disorders, cystic fibrosis, congenital heart disease, and physical and intellectual disabilities. The assessment and systematic promotion of physical activity are addressed and a notable addition to this section is a chapter on the genetics of physical activity and physical fitness.

Participation in youth sport provides a positive environment for the promotion of enjoyment, health, and personal development, but evidence is accumulating that youth sport also presents risks to health and well-being. The growing participation of children in organized sport and intensive training (~30+ h per week) from a young age (~5–8 years); concerns over the (mis)use of nutritional supplements; the use of performance-enhancing drugs; the effect of training on normal growth and maturation; the prevalence of disordered eating and eating disorders, overtraining syndrome, child abuse in sport, and sport-related injuries; the role and potential influence of genetic factors in youth sport; and the premature involvement of youth athletes in senior international competition have brought new challenges as sport becomes ever more pressurized, professionalized, and politicized. These issues are addressed in the sections devoted to sport science and sport medicine.

The sport science section, which consists of ten completely new chapters, begins with a review of the development of the young athlete which also serves as an introduction to the sport science and sport medicine sections. The chapter initially discusses the interaction of chronological aging, biological maturation, and sport performance in youth before identifying some of the key challenges facing the young athlete. The next chapter introduces molecular exercise physiology and examines its current and potential application to youth sport. The influence of training on growth and maturation and hormonal adaptations to training are addressed in the following chapters. Subsequent chapters evaluate the evidence underpinning current training regimens during youth and analyse aerobic, high-intensity, resistance, speed, and agility training. The penultimate chapter in the sport science section examines the prevalence, causes, and prevention of the overtraining syndrome. The final chapter in this section focuses on the rationale, ethics, development, and implementation of a physiological monitoring programme for elite young athletes.

In the European Union there are ~1.3 million annual cases of sports-related injuries requiring hospitalization for children younger than 15 years of age. Data from the American Academy of Orthopedic Surgeons show ~3.5 million annual youth sport-related injuries in the US require a medical visit. The aetiology, prevention, and treatment of sport injuries and the management of the long-term health of young athletes provide major challenges for medical practitioners, sport scientists, physiotherapists, coaches, and others supporting youth sport.

The sport medicine section opens with an insightful overview of the epidemiology and prevention of sports injuries. Subsequent chapters address the topic with specific reference to physical education, contact sports, and non-contact sports. These chapters are followed by three chapters that focus on the diagnosis and management of sport injuries to the upper extremity and trunk, the lower limbs, and the head and cervical spine. The sport medicine section concludes with four intriguing new chapters which address current concerns in youth sport about disordered eating and eating disorders, dietary supplementation, performance-enhancing drugs, and the medical management and protection of child athletes.

Overall, the *Oxford Textbook of Children's Sport and Exercise Medicine* is a comprehensive, evidence-based text in which internationally recognized scientists and clinicians enrich their contributions with their own research and practical experience and present complex scientific material in an accessible and understandable manner. The book is designed to inform, challenge, and support research scientists, medical practitioners, professionals allied to medicine, physical educators, teachers, students, and coaches. It will be of interest to all involved in the study of the exercising child and adolescent, the promotion of young people's health and well-being, youth sport, and the optimum development of young athletes.

Neil Armstrong
Willem van Mechelen

List of Abbreviations

1 RM	one repetition maximum
^{31}PMRS	^{31}P magnetic resonance spectroscopy
AAI	atlantoaxial instability
AAP	American Academy of Pediatrics
AAS	androgenic anabolic steroids
ABC	Airway, Breathing, and Circulation
ABP	Athlete Biological Passport
ABQ	Athlete Burnout Questionnaire
ACE	angiotensin-converting enzyme
ACL	anterior cruciate ligament
ACSA	anthropometric cross-sectional area
ACSM	American College of Sports Medicine
ACTH	adrenocoticotrophin
ADA	American Diabetes Association
ADHD	attention-deficit-hyperactivity disorder
ADI	atlanto-dens interval
ADO	anti-doping organization
ADP	adenosine diphosphate
ADRV	anti-doping rule violation
AGHLS	Amsterdam Growth and Health Longitudinal Study
AIIS	anterior inferior iliac spine
AIS	abbreviated injury scale
AK	adenylate kinase
AMP	adenosine monophosphate
AN	anorexia nervosa
ANGELO	ANalysis Grid for Environments Linked to Obesity
AOI	atlantooccipital instability
AP	anteroposterior
APA	American Psychological Association
ASD	autism spectrum disorder
ASD	atrial septal defect
ASIS	anterior superior iliac spine
ATLS	advanced trauma life support
ATP	adenosine triphosphate
a-vO_2 diff	arteriovenous oxygen difference
B	breasts
BABE	Bug and Bag Effort
BALCO	Bay Area Laboratory Co-Operative
BASES	British Association of Sport and Exercise Sciences
BD	body dissatisfaction
BED	binge eating disorder
BF	body fat
BIA	bioelectrical impedance analysis
BMAD	bone mineral apparent density
BMC	bone mineral content
BMD	bone mineral density
BMI	Body mass index
BMR	basal metabolic rate
BN	bulimia nervosa
BP	blood pressure
BSA	body surface area
BUA	broadband ultrasound attenuation
BW	body weight
C1-2 injury	axial spine injury
C3-7 injury	sub-axial spine injury
CA	chronological age
Ca^{2+}	calcium
CALER	Cart and Load Effort Rating
CAT	carnitine acyltransferase
CBF	cerebral blood flow
CCT	continuous cycling training
CERT	Children's Effort Rating Table
CF	cystic fibrosis
CFRDM	cystic fibrosis-related insulin-dependent diabetes mellitus
CFTR	Cystic Fibrosis Transmembrane Conductance Regulator
CG	centre of gravity
CGM	continuous glucose monitoring
CHOexo	^{13}C-labelled enriched carbohydrate
CHOs	carbohydrates
CI	confidence interval
CIET	constant-intensity exercise training
CK	creatine kinase
CMJ	countermovement jump test
CNS	central nervous system
CO_2	carbon dioxide
CON	habitual control
CP	cerebral palsy
CPo	critical power
CPET	cardiopulmonary exercise testing
CPP	cycling peak power output
CPR	cardiopulmonary resuscitation

CPT	carnitine palmitoyl-transferase
Cr	creatine
CR 10	Category-Ratio 10 scale
CRF	cardiorespiratory fitness
CRH	corticotropine-releasing hormone
CSF	cerebrospinal fluid
CT	computerized tomography
CTE	chronic traumatic encephalopathy
CVC	cutaneous vascular conductance
CVD	cardiovascular disease
D2	dopamine-2 receptor
DAI	diffuse axonal injury
DCCT	Diabetes Control and Complications Trial
DCD	developmental coordination disorder
DE	disordered eating
DEXA	dual energy X-ray absorptiometry
DHEA	dehydroepiandrosterone
DILIN	Drug-Induced Liver Injury Network
DIP	distal interphalangeal
DISI	dorsal intercalated segment instability
DIT	diet-induced thermogenesis
DJ	drop jump
DLW	doubly labelled water
DMAA	Methylhexanamine, or 1,3-dimethylamylamine
DNA	deoxyribonucleic acid
DNMT	DNA methyltransferase
DOMS	delayed onset muscle soreness
DPA	dual photon absorptiometry
DS	Down syndrome
DSHEA	US Dietary Supplements Health and Education Act 1994
DSM-5	Diagnostic and Statistical Manual of Mental Disorders, 5th Edition
DT	drive for thinness
DZ	dizygotic
EA	energy availability
EAR	estimated average requirement
ECG	electrocardiogram
ECSS	European College of Sport Science
ED	eating disorder
EEE	energy expended in exercise
EELV	end-expiratory lung volume
EG	Prohibited List Expert Group
EI	energy intake
EIA	exercise-induced asthma
EILV	end-inspiratory lung volume
EMD	electromechanical delay
EMG	electromyography
EnRG	environmental research framework for weight gain prevention
EP	effector proteins
E-P	Eston-Parfitt
EPO	erythropoietin
ERV	expiratory reserve volume
ESA	Erythropoietin Stimulating Agent
ET	endurance training
EYHS	European Youth Heart Study
FDA	US Food and Drug Administration
FDHO	force driven harmonic oscillator
FDP	flexor digitorum profundus
FEV_1	forced expiratory volume in 1 s
FFAs	free fatty acids
FFM	Fat-free mass
FI	fatigue index
FIFA	Federation Internationale de Football Associations
FM	Fat mass
FMD	flow mediated dilation
fMRI	functional magnetic resonance imaging
FMS	fundamental movement skill
FN	femoral neck
F_{opt}	optimal force
FOR	functional overreaching
f_R	respiratory frequency
FRC	functional reserve capacity
FRV	functional residual volume
FSA	UK Food Standards Agency
FSH	follicle-stimulating hormone
F-V	force-velocity
FVC	forced vital capacity
G	genitalia (penis, scrotum, testes)
Gb	DNA base pair
GCS	Glasgow Coma Scale
GDR	German Democratic Republic
GET	gas exchange threshold
GH	growth hormone (somatotrophin)
GHBP	GH binding protein
GHRH	growth hormone-releasing hormone
GlobalDRO	Global Drug Reference Online
GLUT	glucose transporter
GM	general movements
GMFCS	Gross Motor Function Classification System
GnRH	gonadotropin-releasing hormone
GP	Greulich-Pyle
GRAV	gravitational moment
GWAS	genome-wide association studies
HAT	histone acetyltransferase
HDAC	histone deacetylase
HDL	high-density lipoprotein
HDL-C	high-density lipoprotein cholesterol
HHb	deoxygenated haemoglobin and myoglobin
HIIT	high-intensity interval training
HIT	high-intensity training
HLA	human leukocyte antigen
HOMA-IR	homeostatic model assessment for insulin resistance
HPG	hypothalamic-pituitary-gonadal axis
HR	heart rate
HRmax	maximum heart rate
HRQoL	health-related quality of life
HRR	heart rate reserve
HRV	heart rate variability
HS	heel strike
hs-CRP	high-sensitivity C-reactive protein
HTO	high take-off
HVT	high-volume training
Hz	hertz
IAAF	International Association of Athletic Federations
IBSA	International Blind Sports Association
IBU	International Biathlon Union

IC	inspiratory capacity
ICDH	isocitrate dehydrogenase
IGFBP	IGF-I binding protein
IGF-I	insulin-like growth factor 1
IL-6	interleukin 6
IM	Intervention Mapping
IMT	intima-media thickness
IOC	International Olympic Committee
IPC	International Paralympic Committee
IPS	information processing systems
iPSC	induced pluripotent stem cells
IQ	intelligence quotient
IRMS	isotope ratio mass spectrometry
IRV	inspiratory reserve volume
ISCD	International Society for Clinical Densitometry
ISTUE	International Standard for Therapeutic Use Exemptions
ISU	International Skating Union
ITs	intercellular thresholds
J	joule(s)
kcal	kilocalorie(s)
KDH	α-ketoglutarate dehydrogenase
KTS	Knowledge Transfer Scheme
L	litre(s)
LCL	lateral collateral ligament
LDH	lactate dehydrogenase
LDL-C	low-density lipoprotein cholesterol
LEA	low energy availability
LEN	Ligue Européenne de Natation
LGBT	lesbian, gay, bisexual, and transgender
LH	luteinizing hormone
LHRH	luteinizing-hormone-releasing hormone
LL	leg length
LLV	lean leg volume
LMPA	light-to-moderate physical activity
LogMAR	Logarithm of the Minimal Angle of Resolution
LS	lumbar spine
LTM	lean tissue mass
LTO	low take-off
LTV	lean thigh volume
LV	left ventricular
$m\dot{V}O_2$	muscle oxygen uptake
MAC	Medications Advisory Committee
MAS	maximal aerobic speed
MCL	medial cruciate ligament
MCP-ulnar	metacarpophalangeal-ulnar
mCSA	muscle cross-sectional area
MCT	moderate-intensity continuous training
MDM	motion dependant moment
MEFV	maximal expiratory flow-volume
MetS	metabolic syndrome
MHC	major histocompatibility complex
min	minute(s)
mL	millilitre(s)
MLSS	maximal lactate steady state
MODY	Maturity Onset Diabetes of the Young
MP	mean power output
MPA	moderate physical activity
MPST	Muscle Power Sprint Test
MRC	Medical Research Council
MRI	magnetic resonance imaging
MRS	magnetic resonance spectroscopy
MRT	mean response time
MTU	muscle tendon unit
MUS	generalized muscle moment
MVC	maximal voluntary contraction
MVPA	moderate-to-vigorous physical activity
MVV	maximal voluntary ventilation
MyoD	muscle-making transcription factor
MZ	monozygotic
NaCl	sodium chloride
NAD	nicotinamide adenine dinucleotide
NADO	national anti-doping organization
$NADP^+$	nicotinamide adenine dinucleotide phosphate
NBA	National Basketball Association
NET	net joint moment
NFL	National Football League
NFOR	non-functional overreaching
NGB	National Governing Body
NHANES	US National Health and Nutrition Examination Survey
NHIS	US National Health Interview Survey
NIRS	near-infrared spectroscopy
NMT	non-motorized treadmill
NPH	Neutral Protamine Hagedorn
NSAID	non-steroidal anti-inflammatory drug
NSPCC-CPSU	National Society for the Protection of Cruelty to Children—Child Protection in Sport Unit
NYHA	New York Heart Association
O_2	oxygen
OCD	osteochondritis dissecans
OGDH	2-oxoglutarate dehydrogenase
OPP	optimized peak power
ORIF	open reduction and internal fixation
OSA	obstructive sleep apnoea
OSFED	other specified feeding or eating disorder
OTS	overtraining syndrome
OUES	oxygen uptake efficiency slope
$p\dot{V}O_2$	pulmonary oxygen uptake
PA	physical activity
PaO_2	partial pressure of arterial oxygen
$PaCO_2$	partial pressure of arterial carbon dioxide
PAEE	physical activity energy expenditure
PAI	physical activity intensity
PAL	physical activity level
PBMD	peak bone mineral density
PCERT	Pictorial Children's Effort Rating Table
PCr	phosphocreatine
PCSA	physiological cross-sectional area
PDAY	Pathobiological Determinants of Atherosclerosis in Youth
PDH	pyruvate dehydrogenase
PE	physical education
PED	performance-enhancing drug
PEFR	peak expiratory flow rate
$P_{ET}CO_2$	end tidal carbon dioxide
PFK	phosphofructokinase
PH	pubic hair
PHV	peak height velocity
Pi	inorganic phosphate

PIP proximal interphalangeal
PK pyruvate kinase
P_{max} maximal power
PMV peak muscle mass velocity
PP peak power output
PSF preferred step frequency
PSV peak strength velocity
PWV pulse wave velocity
$\dot{Q}$ cardiac output
$\dot{Q}_{CAP}$ capillary blood flow
QCT quantitative computed tomography
R respiratory exchange ratio
RAE relative age effect
RCT randomized controlled trial
RDI recommended daily intake
RED relative energy deficiency
RED-S Relative Energy Deficiency in Sport
REE resting energy expenditure
REST-Q Recovery Stress Questionnaire
RH relative humidity
rhEPO recombinant human erythropoietin
RM repetition maximum
RNA ribonucleic acid
RPE rate of perceived exertion
RQ respiratory quotient
RSI reactive strength index
RV residual volume
RWT Roche-Wainer-Thissen method
s second(s)
SA skeletal age
SaO_2 oxygen saturation
SAR serious adverse reaction
SARM Selective Androgen Receptor Modulator
SBJ standing broad (long) jump
SBP systolic blood pressure
SCD sudden cardiac death
Scx scleraxis gene symbol
SD standard deviation
SDH succinic dehydrogenase
SDT self-determination theory
SIS second-impact syndrome
SIT sprint interval training
SJ squat jump
SLI specific language impairment
SMS somatostatin
SNP single nucleotide polymorphism, or snip
SOS speed of sound
SP signal transduction proteins
SPA single photon absorptiometry
SPECT single photon emission computed tomography
SRT Shuttle Run Test
SV stroke volume
τ time constant (tau)
T:C testosterone:cortisol ratio
T:E testosterone:epitestosterone ratio
T1DM type 1 diabetes mellitus
T_2 transverse relaxation time
T2DM type 2 diabetes mellitus
TAG triacylglycerol
T_{body} body temperature
TC total cholesterol
TCA tricarboxylic acid
TD typically developing
TDI tissue Doppler imaging
TEE total energy expenditure
TEF thermic effect of feeding
TFCC triangular fibrocartilage complex
TGA transposition of the great arteries
T_{LAC} lactate threshold
TLC total lung capacity
TMW total mechanical work
T*n* thyroid hormone (e.g. T3)
ToF Tetralogy of Fallot
TOYA Training of Young Athletes study
T_{re} rectal temperature
TRIPP Translation Research into Injury Prevention Practice
TSH thyroid stimulating hormone (thyrotrophin)
T_{sk} skin temperature
TT time trial
TUE Therapeutic Use Exemption
TUE EG Therapeutic Use Exemption Expert Group
TUEC Therapeutic Use Exemption Committee
T_{VENT} ventilatory threshold
TW Tanner-Whitehouse
TW2 Tanner-Whitehouse method edition two
TW3 Tanner-Whitehouse method edition three
UCI Union Cycliste Internationale
UNICEF United Nations International Children's Emergency Fund
URTI upper respiratory tract infection
USADA United States Anti-Doping Agency
UUS unexplained underperformance syndrome
$\dot{V}_A$ alveolar ventilation
$\dot{V}CO_2$ carbon dioxide output
$\dot{V}_E$ pulmonary ventilation
$\dot{V}O_2$ oxygen uptake
$\dot{V}O_2$ max maximal oxygen uptake
VA voluntary activation
VC vital capacity
V_D physiologic dead space
VISI volar intercalated segment instability
VJ vertical jump
VLDL very low-density lipoprotein
V_{opt} optimal pedalling velocity
VPA vigorous physical activity
VSD ventricular septal defect
V_T tidal volume
VTI velocity-time integral
W watt(s)
WADA World Anti-Doping Agency
WAnT Wingate anaerobic test
WHO World Health Organization
y year(s)
YPDM Youth Physical Development Model
YRBS Youth Risk Behaviour Survey

PART 1

Exercise science

CHAPTER 1

Assessment of biological maturation

Robert M Malina

Introduction

The focus of this chapter is on the assessment of biological maturation of children and adolescents. Maturation refers to progress towards the biologically mature state, which varies among tissues, organs, and systems of the body. Tempo or rate of maturation varies considerably among systems of the body and among and within individuals. Outcomes of the underlying biological processes of maturation are observed, assessed, and/or measured to provide an indication of progress towards the mature state (maturity).

It is difficult to separate maturation from growth. Growth refers to the increase in the size of the body as a whole and of its parts as the child progresses from birth to adulthood (of course, allowing for prenatal growth). The processes of growth and maturation occur concurrently and are related. Moreover, indicators of growth are used in deriving estimates of maturation.

Selected methods and issues in the measurement of growth status and estimated rate are initially considered. Methods for the assessment of biological maturity status and timing, and several non-invasive estimates of status and timing are subsequently considered.

Chronological age and age groups

Chronological age (CA) is the basic reference in studies of growth and maturation. Chronological age is calculated as the difference between date of measurement and date of birth, and is ordinarily expressed as a decimal of the whole year. Children and adolescents are commonly sorted into single year CA groups, which vary depending on the method of grouping. For example, 9 years can include children between 9.0 through 9.99 years, so that the midpoint of the age group is 9.5 years, or can include children 8.50 through 9.49 years, so that the midpoint of the age group is 9.0 years. The method of grouping should be specified. Depending on the purpose of a study and sample sizes, half-year age groups can also be used.

It is common in studies of youth athletes that participants are separated into competitive age groups which often span 2 years, for example, under 12 (U12), where participants are not yet 13 years of age. The age groups are defined by age at a specific date, e.g. 1 January of the competitive year. In the context of issues related to growth and maturation, athletes are often measured at different points of the year and as such the CAs of some athletes may exceed the upper limit of the competitive age group.

Brief overview of methods for the assessment of growth

Growth status

Growth status refers to the size attained at the date of observation. Height and weight are the primary indicators of growth status. The pattern of growth and associated variation in height and weight are well documented. Height, or more appropriately standing height, is the distance from the standing surface to the top of the skull (vertex). Sitting height, the distance from the flat sitting surface to the top of the skull, is often measured and provides information on upper body segment length. Standing height minus sitting height provides an estimate of leg or lower body length. The ratio of sitting height to height provides an indication of relative body proportions, i.e. relative trunk or relative leg length.

Weight is a measure of body mass which is heterogeneous in composition. Body mass is often partitioned into fat-free mass (FFM) and its two major components, lean tissue mass (LTM) and bone mineral content (BMC), and fat mass (FM).

Standard methods for the measurement of weight, standing height, and sitting height are described elsewhere.[1–3] Measurements should be made by trained individuals using standard techniques. Quality control is essential, i.e. accuracy and reliability of measurements, and measurement variability within and between technicians.[2,4]

Methods for the assessment and quantification of body composition have been driven by technology and have advanced considerably.[5,6] Descriptions are beyond the scope of this discussion. Dual energy X-ray absorptiometry (DEXA) and bioelectrical impedance analysis (BIA) are often used in paediatric sports medicine and science. It is essential that underlying assumptions and limitations of both technologies and others as applied to youth be recognized.

Height and weight increase gradually through childhood, increase at an accelerated rate during adolescence (growth spurt), and then slowly increase into late adolescence. Growth in height stops in the late teens or early twenties, whereas weight often continues to increase. Fat free mass, LTM, and BMC have a growth pattern like height and weight and each has an adolescent spurt, while FM increases more gradually with CA. Relative fatness (% fat) increases during childhood but declines during adolescence in males and continues to increase at a slower pace in females during adolescence. The decline in % fat in males is due to the rapid growth in FFM.[2]

The body mass index ([weight (kg)/ height (m^2)], BMI), is commonly used to classify youth as overweight or obese, i.e. excess weight-for-height, although at the other extreme, low weight-for-height is a concern in some sports. The BMI has limitations as an indicator of adiposity. It is significantly correlated with both FFM and FM in normal weight youth[7] and is perhaps more closely associated with LTM rather than FM among relatively thin youth.[8] The latter applies to elite youth female artistic gymnasts among whom the BMI was more closely correlated with the FFM index (DEXA FFM adjusted for height) than the FM index (FM adjusted for height); the association with the FFM index was also stronger among gymnasts in the lower half of the BMI distribution (Malina, unpublished).

Growth rate

The increment in height or other dimensions between two observations provides an estimate of growth rate, or tempo of growth. Measurements are not always taken at prescribed dates or intervals; as such, observed increments need to be adjusted for the actual interval between measurements. Increments are influenced by technical errors of measurement at each observation, and, in the case of estimated leg length, are influenced by measurement error in both height and sitting height. Diurnal and seasonal variation affects increments, especially estimates over shorter durations, e.g. 3–6 months. Height and especially sitting height show significant diurnal variation, while seasonal variation in height occurs in some parts of the world. Height measurements taken after a period of physical activity or training (running, jumping, etc.) are less than those taken after a period of rest. The recommendation of the Long Term Athlete Development model[9] for quarterly height measurements to estimate velocities and monitor the velocity curve in the context of the adolescent spurt thus has major limitations.[10]

Growth rates decline with increasing CA during childhood, reach a nadir at the onset of the spurt (take-off), increase to a maximum (peak height velocity, PHV) and then decline until growth ceases.[2] Distributions of increments vary within CA intervals and also tend to be skewed.[11] Annual or semi-annual height increments have been used in studies of youth athletes to estimate growth rates relative to a reference for non-athletes,[12–14] and at times to estimate the potential influence of training on growth rate.[15] Reference values for estimated growth rates have been reported.[10,11,16,17]

Assessment of maturity status

Maturity status refers to the level or state of maturation at the CA of observation. Indicators of skeletal and pubertal maturation are used most often. Dental maturation is another indicator, although it generally proceeds independently of other indicators.[2] If longitudinal data during childhood and adolescence and a measure of adult height are available, expressing height attained at a specific CA as a percentage of adult height can be used as an indicator of maturity status. This indicator is discussed in more detail later in this chapter in the section entitled, Percentage of predicted adult height.

Skeletal age

Skeletal maturation is estimated as skeletal age (SA) derived from evaluation of the bones of the hand and wrist viewed on a standard radiograph. Each bone goes through a series of changes from initial ossification, which begins prenatally in some bones, to the adult state. The changes in each bone are used to mark progress from immaturity to maturity and are the basis for assessing SA of the hand-wrist. The process is based on the assumption that specific features of each bone as noted on a radiograph occur regularly and in an irreversible order, and as such provide a record of the progress of each bone towards maturity. Other parts of the skeleton, e.g. knee and foot and ankle, have also been used to derive estimates of SA.[2]

Three methods are commonly used to estimate SA of the hand-wrist. Each method calls for the hand-wrist radiograph of a child to be compared to specific criteria; ratings are subsequently converted to a SA specific to the method. Indicators of maturity defined for specific bones in each method are somewhat arbitrary and suggest discrete steps in a continuous process.[2,18–21]

Greulich-Pyle method

The Greulich-Pyle method (GP)[22] is an extension of the method initially described by Todd.[23] It is sometimes called the atlas method and was developed on well-off American white children from Cleveland, Ohio. The method calls for each individual bone of the hand-wrist to be rated relative to sex-specific standard plates representing specific SAs from infancy through adolescence; plate descriptions note variation in SAs of individual bones. The method may require interpolation between the standard plates. An SA is assigned to each bone and the median of the SAs is the estimate of SA for the child. In practice, however, the GP method is most often applied by comparing the radiograph as a whole to the pictorial standards, and assigning the SA of the standard to which the radiograph most closely matches. As such, variation in level of maturity among individual bones is overlooked.

Tanner-Whitehouse method

The Tanner-Whitehouse (TW)[24–27] method was developed on British children. The method specifies criteria and associated maturity scores for 20 bones: the radius, ulna, metacarpals and phalanges of the first, third, and fifth digits (long bones), and for the carpals except the pisiform.[24,25] The scores for the 20 bones are summed into a skeletal maturity score; the 7 carpals and 13 long bones each contribute 50% to the skeletal maturity score. The maturity score is converted to a SA. Potential problems in assigning age equivalents to maturity point scores have been noted.[18,28] The first revision of the TW method (TW2)[26] did not change the criteria for maturity indicators and scores, and provided SAs based on 20 bones (TW2 20 Bone SA), for the carpals (TW2 Carpal SA), and for the radius, ulna, and short bones (TW2 RUS SA). British children were the reference for the first two versions of the TW method.

The most recent version, TW3,[27] eliminated the 20 Bone SA and retained the RUS (TW3 RUS) and Carpal (TW3 Carpal) SAs. The tables for the conversion of RUS maturity scores to SAs were modified, while those for Carpal scores were not. Reference values for TW3 RUS SA were based on a composite of the original British series, and Belgian (Flemish), Italian, Spanish, Argentine, Japanese, and American children and adolescents surveyed in the late 1960s through mid-1990s; the American sample was from a well-off area in the Houston, Texas region. The reference for TW3 Carpal SA was the original British series. Ages at attaining skeletal maturity with the RUS protocol were lowered from 18.2 to 16.5 years in boys and from 16.0 to 15.0 years in girls.

Fels method

The Fels method was based on participants in the Fels Longitudinal Growth Study of children from middle-class families in south-central Ohio.[29] The method specifies criteria for the radius, ulna, carpals, and metacarpals and phalanges of the first, third, and fifth rays. Grades are assigned to each bone depending on CA and sex. Ratios of linear measurements of the widths of the epiphysis and metaphysis of the long bones are also used, and the presence (ossification) or absence of the pisiform and adductor sesamoid is noted. Grades assigned to the individual bones and width measurements are entered into a programme that calculates SA and standard error; the latter provides an estimate of the error of the assigned SA, which is not available with the other methods. The computational procedures weight the contributions of specific indicators depending on CA and sex in the derivation of a SA; as such, the method is to some extent calibrated relative to CA.

Skeletal age

The SA assigned to the radiograph of an individual represents the CA at which a specific level of maturity of the hand-wrist bones was attained by the reference sample, upon which the method of assessment was developed. It is an indicator of biological maturity status, i.e. the level of maturity of the bones of the hand and wrist at the CA of observation. An individual who has attained skeletal maturity is simply noted as skeletally mature; an SA is not assigned. Skeletal age has meaning when expressed relative to CA. Is it equivalent? Is it advanced? Is it delayed? The difference between SA and CA (SA minus CA) and the ratio of SA to CA (SA/CA) are often used in studies.

Skeletal ages derived with each of the three methods, though related, are not equivalent as criteria, methods, and references differ among methods. Skeletal ages based on the GP and Fels methods, and the revisions of the TW method (TW2 20 Bone, TW2 RUS, TW3 RUS) in a sample of German boys[30–32] are summarized in Table 1.1. Heights of the boys matched, on average, the medians of current US reference data. Standard deviations for SA are three to four times larger than those for CA. Mean SAs with each method vary and overlap within each CA group, except for the lower SAs with the most recent TW revision. Beginning at 9–10 years, TW3 RUS SAs are consistently lower than TW2 RUS SAs.

Although not indicated in Table 1.1, a number of boys were skeletally mature, especially with the TW method (1 each at 14 and 15 years, 5 at 16 years) compared to the GP (2 at 16 years) and Fels (1 at 16 years). Numbers of skeletally mature boys were larger at 17 years (GP 9, Fels 11, TW 17). The discrepancy between the TW and both the GP and Fels methods likely relates to criteria for the radius and ulna. The final stage with the TW method is as follows 'fusion of the epiphysis and metaphysis has begun'.[27(pp.63,65)] Time between onset and completion of union of the radius and ulna is not considered. Many youth are thus classified as skeletally mature although the epiphysis and diaphysis of each bone are still in the process of fusing. The GP and Fels methods both consider beginning through complete fusion of the distal radius and ulna.

Skeletal maturation varies considerably among individuals of the same CA and fluctuates above and below 1 year (Table 1.1). This is consistent with other studies.[20] Normal variation in SA within CA groups is generally accepted as plus and minus three standard deviations except as maturity is approached.

The difference between SA and CA (SA minus CA) is often used to classify youth into contrasting maturity groups using a band of ± 1.0 year which approximates standard deviations for SAs within specific CA groups. Use of narrower bands is affected by errors associated with assessments. Skeletal maturity sets a ceiling effect which may limit some maturity groupings. This is relevant in studies of male athletes where many have attained skeletal maturity at 15, 16, and 17 years; the number attaining maturity is greater with TW RUS.[20]

Overview of skeletal age

Skeletal age can be used throughout the postnatal maturation period in contrast to other maturity assessment methods, which are limited to puberty and adolescence. Estimates of SA by each method are reasonably precise and reliable, although inter- and intra-observer variability should be reported. The use of SA is often criticized because specific training is required to learn the protocol(s). This is a shallow criticism as anthropometry, body

Table 1.1 Skeletal ages with five different methods of assessment in boys.

	Skeletal Ages, years											
	CA, years		GP		Fels		TW2 20 Bone		TW2 RUS		TW3 RUS	
N	M	SD	M	SD	M	SD	M	SD	M	SD	M	SD
26	8.4	0.3	8.3	0.9	8.1	0.9	8.3	0.9	8.0	1.0	8.0	0.9
23	9.5	0.3	10.1	1.0	9.6	1.0	9.8	0.9	9.8	1.2	9.4	0.9
22	10.5	0.3	10.2	1.0	9.7	1.0	10.1	1.2	9.9	1.1	9.5	0.8
20	11.5	0.2	11.0	0.8	10.7	1.2	11.2	0.9	11.3	1.2	10.5	0.9
31	12.4	0.3	12.1	1.0	12.2	1.5	12.6	1.5	12.6	1.6	11.6	1.3
22	13.5	0.3	12.8	1.0	13.0	1.4	13.5	1.4	13.5	1.6	12.3	1.5
23	14.3	0.3	13.8	1.0	14.2	1.1	14.8	1.1	14.9	1.3	13.8	1.0
20	15.4	0.3	14.9	0.8	15.4	0.9	15.8	0.8	15.9	0.9	14.9	1.0
10	16.5	0.3	15.8	0.8	16.5	0.8	16.8	0.8	17.0	0.8	16.0	0.8

Source data from Kujawa KI. Skeletal maturation in boys: Comparison of methods and relationships to anthropometry and strength. Doctoral dissertation, University of Texas at Austin; 1977.

composition assessment, and more specific laboratory protocols also need specific training.

Major limitations of SA are expenses associated with the radiographs per se, the need for qualified individuals to take them, and radiation exposure. With modern technology, exposure to radiation presents minimal risk, 0.001 millisievert, which is less than natural background radiation and radiation exposure associated with the equivalent of 3 h·day^{-1} television viewing.[33,34] The lack of qualified individuals knowledgeable of the different assessment protocols and interpretations is a major limitation in the sport sciences.

Methods for assessing and assigning SA are based on samples of European ancestry. Applications of the GP and TW protocols have shown ethnic variation.[35–41] Applications of the Fels method to youth of different ethnic groups are not available. It is relevant to note that ethnic identification of youth in some countries is not permitted.

Other protocols

Other protocols for the assessment of skeletal maturity of the hand-wrist are available and have been used primarily in the clinical setting. However, application and validation of these and perhaps other protocols in the context of the sport sciences are limited.

Skeletal age based on ultrasound assessment of the maturity status of the distal radius and ulna, scaled relative to the GP method, has been proposed,[42,43] but its validity has been questioned.[44] Use of DEXA scans of the hand-wrist for the assessment of SA have also been proposed.[45–47] Automated methods for the assessment of SA are increasingly available.[27,48–50] The procedures are generally based upon the GP and TW methods and are largely designed for clinical use. The BoneXpert method[49] is unique in that it derives an 'intrinsic' bone age based on the bone borders (shapes) and wavelet texture on images of 15 bones: radius, ulna, the 5 metacarpals, and the 8 phalanges in the first, third, and fifth rays of Danish children. The 'intrinsic' bone ages are subsequently calibrated to GP and TW RUS SAs.

Secondary sex characteristics

Secondary sex characteristics are limited to the pubertal years. Characteristics in males include pubic hair (PH), genitalia (G, penis, scrotum, testes), testicular volume, voice change, and facial and axillary hair. Characteristics in females include PH, breasts (B), axillary hair, and menarche.[2,21] Facial hair and voice change in boys and axillary hair in both sexes generally develop late during puberty and are not widely used.

Pubertal stages

The five stages of PH, G, and B described by Tanner[51] are commonly used to assess pubertal status. Stages are labelled PH1 through PH5, B1 through B5, and G1 through G5. Stage 1 of each characteristic indicates the prepubertal state—absence of overt development, although hormonal changes that trigger puberty may already be under way. Stage 2 marks the overt development of each characteristic; B2 and G2 are typically the first overt sign of the transition into puberty, but PH2 may precede B2 and G2 in a minority of youth. Stages 3 and 4 mark progress in pubertal maturation; the respective stages are sometimes labelled as mid- and late-puberty. Stage 5 indicates the mature state.

The stages are specific to the respective characteristics in each sex and are not equivalent, i.e. B3 ≠ PH3, G3 ≠ PH3, B3 ≠ G3, PH3 in girls ≠ PH3 in boys, and so on. The term 'Tanner stages' is often used in the literature without indicating which characteristic was assessed. The characteristic(s) assessed should be specified.

Stages are discrete categories superimposed on the continuous process of sexual maturation. A youngster is either in a stage or not in a stage at the time of assessment; there are no intermediate stages. Stage at time of assessment provides no information on when the youngster entered the stage (timing) or how long he/she has been in the stage.

Maturation of the neuroendocrine system involving the hypothalamic-pituitary-gonadal-adrenal axes drives the overt development of the characteristics. Gonadal hormones drive the initial development of B and G, while adrenal hormones drive the initial development of PH in both sexes.[52]

Direct assessments of stage of pubertal development are made at clinical examination. Self-assessments are often used in non-clinical settings; they require privacy, good quality photographs of the stages, simplified descriptions, and a mirror to assist in process. Some self-assessment scales include pictures or drawings of the stages, and questions regarding facial and axillary hair in males and axillary hair and menarcheal status in girls.[2]

There is need for quality control, including intra- and inter-observer reliability in assessment of stages, and concordance between self-assessments and those of experienced assessors. Overall reproducibility by experienced assessors is generally good, about 80% of agreement in assigning stages, but lower percentages have been reported.[2] Of relevance, a recent study has concluded that '... preoperative Tanner staging performed by orthopedic surgeons is unreliable'.[53(p.1229)]

Accuracy of self-assessments is a concern, but opinions vary depending upon purpose of study. Based on self-assessments of pubertal status in three annual visits of girls between 11 and 14 years and assessments by trained examiners, it was concluded that '... self-assessment can substitute for examiner evaluation only when crude estimates of maturation are needed'.[54(p.197)] On the other hand, agreement to within one stage was suggested as potentially useful in epidemiological surveys of youth,[55] even though concordance between self- and physician-assessments indicated limited accuracy. Concordance between and among self-assessment scales currently in use needs further evaluation.

Testicular volume

Testicular volume provides a more direct estimate of genital maturity in boys. The method requires palpation of the testes in order to match their size with a series of models of known volume (Prader orchidometer).[56,57] The ellipsoid models have the shape of the testes and range from 1 to 25 mL; a volume above 4 mL marks the beginning of puberty. The method is used primarily in the clinical setting. Sonography can also be used to estimate testicular volume.[58]

Menarcheal Status

Although age at menarche is an indicator of maturity timing, menarcheal status (pre or post) is an indicator of maturity status. It is specifically useful in single year CA groups. Among girls spanning several years, classifications by menarcheal status are confounded by CA per se, i.e. an 11-year-old premenarcheal girl is quite different physically and behaviorally from a 14-year-old premenarcheal girl.

Analytical concerns

Stages of PH, B, and G are variably reported. Ratings for individuals are periodically combined into a mean of B and PH, or of G and PH; there is no such thing as a mean stage. The stages are not equivalent and should be considered separately. Stages are also reported 3+or 4+. A youngster is either in a stage or not in a stage; there are no intermediate stages. Studies often report means stages of PH, B, or G by CA at observation; although potentially of interest in showing trends, distributions of stages within each CA group would be more informative.

It is common to group youngsters by stage of puberty independent of CA. This presents problems associated with variation by stage within a CA group and by CA within a stage. For example, within single year CA groups of soccer players 11–14 years of age, boys in less advanced stages of PH tend to be younger, shorter, and lighter, on average, than players in more advanced stages who are older, taller, and heavier. Additionally, among players grouped by stage of PH, younger boys tend to be, on average, shorter and lighter than older boys who are taller and heavier.[59] Classifications of girls by stages of PH, B, or menarcheal status within single year CA groups 13–17 years of age would likely yield similar results.

Overview of secondary sex characteristics

Secondary sex characteristics are limited to the interval of puberty and reflect changes in several hormonal axes of the neuroendocrine system. Stages are somewhat arbitrary and discrete, and direct assessment is often considered invasive, especially outside the clinical setting. Cultural sanctions may limit or prohibit assessment of secondary sex characteristics in some groups. Concordance of clinical and self-assessments is variable and needs further study. Stages of puberty are also variably reported and present analytical concerns.

Assessment of maturity timing

Maturity timing refers to the CA at which specific maturational events occur. The two most commonly used indicators of timing are age at PHV and age at menarche. Both are limited to the adolescent period and require longitudinal data for estimation.

Age at peak height velocity

Age at PHV is the estimated CA at the maximum rate of growth in height during the adolescent spurt. Onset of the spurt occurs when growth velocity in height reaches its minimum in late childhood (age at take-off), followed by acceleration to a maximum rate (PHV), and then by deceleration until growth in height terminates in the late teens/early twenties. Age at PHV is ordinarily estimated from serial height measurements of individuals taken annually or semi-annually from late childhood through adolescence. Historically, growth rates from individual height records were graphically plotted to identify take-off, peak, and eventual cessation of growth. Mathematical modeling or fitting of individual height records is currently used and a variety of methods are available.[60] Estimated ages at PHV vary somewhat among methods but are generally more uniform for age at PHV than for peak velocity of growth in height ($cm \cdot year^{-1}$). Allowing for normal variation, mean ages at PHV are reasonably similar in longitudinal studies of European and North American youth.[2,61,62] Variation in age at PHV among individuals is considerable. In longitudinal samples of British, Swiss, Polish, Belgian, Canadian, and American youth, estimated ages at PHV ranged from 9.0–15.0 years in individual girls and 11.1–17.3 years in individual boys.[2,63–66]

Age at menarche

Age at menarche refers to the timing of the first menstrual flow. At each regularly scheduled visit/observation in longitudinal studies (usually 3–6 months, but annually in some studies), girls and/or their mothers are interviewed whether or not menarche has occurred. If menarche occurred between visits, further questions pinpoint the specific date/age when the first menstrual flow occurred. This is labeled the prospective method. Prospectively recorded ages at menarche in longitudinal studies of American[65] and Polish[63,64] girls ranged from 10.77–15.25 years and 10.49–16.30 years, respectively.

Longitudinal studies generally follow subjects across adolescence so that early and late maturing girls are included. Depending on ages at which short-term longitudinal studies start and finish, there is potential risk that early and late maturing girls may be excluded.

Ages at menarche based on the prospective method are sometimes confused with estimates based on the *status quo* method. The method requires two bits of information in a cross-sectional sample spanning 9 through 17 years: CA, and whether or not menarche has occurred (yes/no). The data are subsequently analyzed with probits or logits to derive a median age at menarche for the sample. The *status quo* method is used in surveys, including a limited number of surveys of youth athletes.[59]

Ages at menarche can also be obtained retrospectively from late adolescents and adults who are asked to recall when they experienced their first menstruation. The method relies on memory, i.e. recall of the age when first menstrual flow occurred. In addition to potential errors with memory per se, reported ages are influenced by recall bias (the shorter the recall interval, the more accurate the recall, and vice versa) and a tendency to report whole years, typically age at the birthday before menarche.[2]

Estimates of age at menarche using the retrospective method with samples of young adolescents are biased. Girls who have not yet attained menarche are excluded from the estimates. Some late maturing girls may not attain menarche until 15 or 16 years, or perhaps later. In a nationally representative sample of American girls, 90% attained menarche by 13.75 years,[67] but 10% of girls attained menarche after this age.

Other indicators of timing and interrelationships

Assuming longitudinal data are available, other potential maturity indicators can be estimated, e.g. age at take-off, ages at peak velocity for body weight, estimated leg length or sitting height, and ages at attaining specific SAs, stages of pubertal development, or specific percentages of adult height. A summary of mean ages at take-off and at PHV, and mean ages of onset for selected stages of sexual maturation noted in European and American longitudinal studies have been summarized.[2,21]

Although data are not extensive, the differential timing of growth spurts in body dimensions other than height, components of body composition, and functional performances relative to age at PHV are of interest in the sport sciences. Available data suggest the following trends in estimated mean ages at peak velocities of several dimensions, tissues, and functions occur relative to age at PHV: leg length—before PHV (both sexes); peak $\dot{V}O_2$—same time as PHV (both sexes); weight, sitting height, LTM, BMC, FM, static strength (both sexes), and power (boys)—after PHV.[2,62,68–70]

Analyses of ages at attaining several different maturity indicators in two longitudinal series highlight interrelationships among maturity timing during adolescence.[71–73] Common indicators in the two longitudinal series included ages at PHV and menarche, ages at attaining stages of pubertal development, ages at attaining specific SAs, and percentages of adult height. The analyses indicated a general maturity factor in both sexes underlying the timing of maturity indicators during the interval of the adolescent spurt. The analyses for boys indicated a second factor which loaded on ages at attaining SAs of 11 and 12 years, 80% of adult height, and early stages of pubic hair and genital development. These indicators are characteristic of early puberty or early adolescence, and suggest a degree of independence of ages at attaining (i.e. timing) several maturity markers characteristic of late pre-puberty or early puberty.[73] The preceding observations are based on ages at attaining specific maturity indicators. Longitudinal data for 30 boys indicated considerable variation in SA at the time of pubertal onset (serum testosterone ≥30 ng · DL^{-1}).[74]

Tempo of maturation

Tempo refers to the rate at which maturation progresses. Data are limited. Estimated increments in GP SAs in a longitudinal sample of American children approximated 1 year; variation was considerable and was associated in part with maturity status, i.e. early versus late.[75,76] In a mixed longitudinal sample of American white and black girls 6–12 years, mean single year velocities for TW2 20 Bone SAs varied between 0.66–1.14 years per year and standard deviations varied between 0.33–0.52; corresponding mean single year velocities for boys varied between 0.75–1.27 years per year and standard deviations ranged from 0.32–0.60 years.[36] Single year rates of maturation expressed as maturity points per year of the American children[35] overlapped the mean rates and ranges for British children.[28] Observations in a longitudinal series of 34 boys suggested that annual increments (years per year) in TW2 SAs (presumably 20 bone) increased during the interval of puberty and the growth spurt; increments appeared to reach a peak near PHV.[77] Allowing for limited data, it is important to ask whether a skeletal year equals a chronological year.

Similar questions can be asked of the tempo of transition from one pubertal stage to the next, but data for the time between stages are not extensive. Evidence from the Zurich Longitudinal Study indicated the following trends. The intervals (means ± standard deviations) between B2 and B3 and between PH2 and PH3 in Swiss girls were, respectively, 1.4 ± 0.8 years, and 1.8 ± 1.0 years, while intervals between G2 and G3 and between PH2 and PH3 in Swiss boys were, respectively, 1.7 ± 1.0 years and 1.3 ± 0.9 years.[78,79] The intervals between the transition into puberty (B2, G2, PH2) and the mature state (B5, G5, PH5) were, on average, 2.2 ± 1.1 years for breast and 2.7 ± 1.1 years for pubic hair development in Swiss girls, and 3.5 ± 1.1 years for genital and 2.7 ± 1.0 years for pubic hair development in Swiss boys.[78,79] The standard deviations for the transition through puberty for each characteristic approximated 1 year and highlighted the variation in tempo of maturation of secondary sex characteristics within and among individuals.

Non-invasive estimates of maturity status and timing

Given logistical difficulties in conducting longitudinal studies spanning adolescence, concern for minimal radiation exposure with hand-wrist X-rays, and cultural perceptions of the assessment of secondary characteristics, there is considerable current interest in the sport sciences in non-invasive estimates of biological maturation. Two estimates are currently used. Percentage of predicted adult height attained at the time of observation provides an estimate of maturity status, while predicted maturity offset or time before age at PHV provides an estimate of maturity timing.

Percentage of predicted adult height

Although age at attaining specific percentages of adult height has been used in analyses of longitudinal data, the use of percentage of predicted adult height at a given age as a maturity indicator was apparently proposed by Roche and colleagues.[80] Given two youngsters of the same CA, the one closer to adult height is advanced in maturity compared to a youth further removed from adult height. Percentage of predicted adult height at a given age provides an estimate of maturity status.

Height prediction is standard practice in many clinical settings, but the commonly used clinical protocols require an estimate of SA.[2] A commonly used general clinical guide without SA is mid-parent target height, based on the average of the heights of both parents.[81] The protocol has a large associated error of ~9 cm. The protocol developed in the Fels Longitudinal Growth Study[82] predicts adult height from CA, height, and weight of the child and mid-parent height in children and adolescents 4–17 years.

Percentage of predicted adult height based upon the Khamis-Roche equations[82] has been used as an indicator of maturity status in studies of physical activity and of youth athletes.[83] Maturity status based on percentage of predicted adult height had moderate concordance with classifications of maturity status based on SA in youth American football[84] and soccer[85] players. The protocol requires further validation. The prediction equations were developed on samples of European ancestry, which probably limits their utility among youth of non-European ancestry.

Equations developed on youth 13–16 years of age from the Leuven Longitudinal Study of Belgian Boys use CA, current height, sitting height, and the subscapular and triceps skinfolds.[86] The protocol has been validated in an independent sample of boys 13–16 years of age from the Madeira Growth Study,[87] but apparently has not been used in studies of physical activity and youth athletes.

Predicted maturity offset/age at peak height velocity

Equations for the prediction of maturity offset, time before or after PHV, have been developed.[66] Predicted age at PHV is estimated as CA minus maturity offset. The sex-specific equations incorporate CA, height, weight, sitting height, and estimated leg length (height minus sitting height). Predicted offset was suggested as a categorical variable, pre- or post-PHV, i.e. an indicator of maturity status, but has been used to estimate maturity status and timing.[83]

Results of validation studies in longitudinal samples of Polish children from the Wrocław Growth Study[63,64] and American children from the Fels Longitudinal Study[65] from 8 to 18 years highlight several limitations of the maturity offset prediction protocol:

First, within the age range of the two longitudinal studies, intra-individual variation in predicted offset and ages at PHV was considerable.

Second, predicted maturity offset and in turn predicted age at PHV were dependent upon CA at prediction and probably age-associated variation in body size. Predicted maturity offset decreased and estimated age at PHV increased, on average, with CA at prediction.

Third, standard deviations of mean predicted ages at PHV indicated reduced ranges of variation which increased from 8 to 16 years, 0.29–0.47 years in girls and 0.26–0.68 years in boys. Standard errors (SE = SD/√n) of the prediction equations were 0.59 for boys and 0.57 for girls.[66]

Fourth, predictions of maturity offset and age at PHV were affected by individual differences in observed ages of PHV as evident in comparisons of youth of contrasting maturity status. Among early maturing boys and girls classified by observed ages at PHV, predicted ages at PHV were later than observed ages at PHV, while among late maturing boys and girls classified by observed ages at PHV, predicted ages were earlier than observed ages at PHV. Trends were similar for contrasting maturity groups of girls based on ages at menarche. Observations for a longitudinal sample of 13 female artistic gymnasts were consistent with those for late maturing girls.[88]

Fifth, predicted age at PHV appears to be useful close to the time of actual age at PHV in average (on time) maturing boys within a narrow age range, 13.00–15.00 years; this range includes the standard deviation around mean age at PHV in average maturing boys. The protocol appears to overestimate age at PHV more so in girls than in boys; nevertheless, predicted age at PHV may be useful among some average and late maturing girls.[65]

Application of the maturity offset prediction equations depends, of course, on the purpose of a specific study, and the limitations of predicted values should be recognized. Revised equations have been reported.[89] Chronological age and sitting height in boys and CA and height in girls are the predictors, although an alternative equation for boys using CA and height is reported. The new equations require validation in independent samples and also in samples of athletes.

Conclusions

Though related, indicators of maturity status and timing are not equivalent. Currently used predictors of maturity status and timing have limitations and require further validation and care in application.

Summary

- The processes of growth and maturation occur concurrently and are related.
- Growth status—size attained at the time (chronological age [CA]) of observation, and growth rate—increment between observations, are basic to the assessment of growth. Indicators of growth are also used in deriving estimates of maturation.
- Maturity status refers to the state of maturation at the time of observation. Indicators of skeletal and pubertal maturity status are used most often.
- Maturity timing refers to the CA at which specific maturational events occur. Chronological age at peak height velocity (PHV) and CA at menarche are used most often.
- Skeletal age is the only maturity indicator that spans childhood through adolescence; other indicators (pubertal status, CA at PHV, CA at menarche) are limited to the interval of puberty and the growth spurt.
- Tempo refers to the rate at which maturation progresses. Data are limited.
- There is increasing interest in the application of non-invasive indicators of maturation. Percentage of predicted adult height attained at the time of observation provides an estimate of maturity status, while predicted maturity offset or time before age at PHV provides an estimate of maturity timing. Both have limitations and require further validation and care in application.

References

1. Lohman TG, Roche AF, Martorell R, eds. *Anthropometric standardization reference manual*. Champaign: Human Kinetics; 1988.
2. Malina RM, Bouchard C, Bar-Or O. *Growth, maturation, and physical activity*, 2nd ed. Champaign, IL: Human Kinetics; 2004.
3. Cameron N. The measurement of human growth. In: Cameron N, Bogin B (eds.) *Human growth and development*, 2nd ed. London: Academic Press; 2012. p. 487–513.
4. Malina RM. Anthropometry. In: PJ Maud, C Foster (eds.) *Physiological assessment of human fitness*. Champaign, IL: Human Kinetics; 1995. p. 205–219.
5. Heymsfield SB, Lohman TG, Wang Z, Going SB, (eds.) *Human body composition*, 2nd ed. Champaign, IL: Human Kinetics; 2005.
6. Zemel B. Body composition during growth and development. In: Cameron N, Bogin B (eds.) *Human growth and development*, 2nd ed. London: Academic Press; 2012. p. 461–486.
7. Malina RM, Katzmarzyk PT. Validity of the body mass index as an indicator of the risk and presence of overweight in adolescents. *Am J Clin Nutr*. 1999; 70(Suppl): 131S–136S.
8. Freedman DS, Wang J, Maynard LM, Thornton JC, Mei Z, Pierson RN, *et al.* Relation of BMI to fat and fat-free mass among children and adolescents. *Int J Obes*. 2005; 29: 1–8.
9. Balyi I, Way R. *The role of monitoring growth in long-term athlete development*. Canadian Sport Centres/Centres Canadiens Multisports: Canadian Sport for Life; 2009. Available at http://canadiansportforlife.ca/sites/default/files/resources/MonitoringGrowth%281%29.pdf
10. Marshall WA. Evaluation of growth rate in height over periods of less than one year. *Arch Dis Child*. 1971; 46: 414–420.
11. Baumgartner RN, Roche AF, Himes JH. Incremental growth tables: supplementary to previously published charts. *Am J Clin Nutr*. 1986; 43: 711–722.
12. Eisenmann JC, Malina RM. Growth status and estimated growth rate of young distance runners. *Int J Sports Med*. 2002; 23:168–173
13. Malina RM. Attained size and growth rate of female volleyball players between 9 and 13 years of age. *Pediatr Exerc Sci*. 1994; 6: 257–266.
14. Malina RM, Eveld DJ, Woynarowska B. Growth and sexual maturation of active Polish children 11–14 years of age. *Hermes, Tijdschrift van het Intituut voor Lichamelijke Opleiding* [Journal of the Institute of Physical Education, Catholic University of Leuven, Belgium]. 1990; 21: 341–353.
15. Daly RM, Caine D, Bass SL, Pieter W, Broekhoff J. Growth of highly versus moderately trained competitive female artistic gymnasts. *Med Sci Sports Exerc*. 2005; 37: 1053–1060.
16. Roche AF, Himes JH. Incremental growth charts. *Am J Clin Nutr*. 1980; 33: 2041–2052.
17. Kelly A, Winer KK, Kalkwarf H, *et al.* Age-based reference ranges for annual height velocity in US children. *J Clin Endocrinol Metab*. 2014; 99: 2104–2112.

18. Acheson RM. Maturation of the skeleton. In: Falkner F (ed.) *Human development*. Philadelphia: Saunders; 1966. p. 465–502.
19. Malina RM. A consideration of factors underlying the selection of methods in the assessment of skeletal maturity. *Am J Phys Anthropol.* 1971; 35: 341–346.
20. Malina RM. Skeletal age and age verification in youth sport. *Sports Med.* 2011; 41: 925–947.
21. Beunen GP, Rogol AD, Malina RM. Indicators of biological maturation and secular changes in biological maturation. *Food Nutr Bull.* 2006; 27 (suppl): S244–S256.
22. Greulich WW, Pyle SI. *Radiographic atlas of skeletal development of the hand and wrist*, 2nd ed. Stanford, CA: Stanford University Press; 1959.
23. Todd TW. *Atlas of skeletal maturation. Part 1. The hand.* St. Louis: Mosby; 1937.
24. Tanner JM, Whitehouse RH, Healy MJR. *A new system for estimating skeletal maturity from the hand and wrist, with standards derived from a study of 2,600 healthy British children.* Paris: International Children's Centre; 1962.
25. Tanner JM, Whitehouse RH, Marshall WA, Healy MJR, Goldstein H. *Assessment of skeletal maturity and prediction of adult height (TW2 method).* New York: Academic Press; 1975.
26. Tanner JM, Whitehouse RH, Cameron N, Marshall WA, Healy MJR, Goldstein H. *Assessment of skeletal maturity and prediction of adult height*, 2nd ed. New York: Academic Press; 1983.
27. Tanner JM, Healy MJR, Goldstein H, Cameron N. *Assessment of skeletal maturity and prediction of adult height (TW3 method)*, 3rd ed. London: Saunders; 2001.
28. Marshall WA. Individual variation in rate of maturation. *Nature.* 1969; 221 (5175): 91.
29. Roche AF, Chumlea WC, Thissen D. *Assessing the skeletal maturity of the hand-wrist: Fels method.* Springfield, IL: CC Thomas; 1988.
30. Bouchard C, Hollman W, Herkenrath G. Relations entre le niveau de maturité biologique, la participation à l'activité physique et certaines structures morphologiques et organiques chez des garçons de huit a dix-huit ans. *Biometrie Humaine.* 1968; 3: 101–139.
31. Bouchard C, Malina RM, Hollman W, Leblanc C. Relationships between skeletal maturity and submaximal working capacity in boys 8 to 18 years. *Med Sci Sports.* 1976; 8: 186–190.
32. Kujawa KI. *Skeletal maturation in boys: Comparison of methods and relationships to anthropometry and strength.* Doctoral dissertation, University of Texas at Austin; 1977.
33. US Department of Energy. *Radiation safety: Americans' average radiation exposure.* US Department of Energy, Office of Civilian Radioactive Waste Management, DOE/YMP-0337. Available at URL: www.ymp.gov [Accessed 2010 Jan 2].
34. Radiological Society of North America. *Safety: Radiation exposure in X-ray examinations.* 2009. Available at URL: www.radiologyinfo.org [Accessed 2010 Jan 2].
35. Malina RM. Skeletal maturation rate in North American Negro and White children. *Nature.* 1969; 223: 1075.
36. Malina RM. Skeletal maturation studied longitudinally over one year in American Whites and Negroes 6 through 13 years of age. *Hum Biol.* 1970; 42: 377–390.
37. Roche AF, Roberts J, Hamill PVV. Skeletal maturity of youths 12–17 years: Racial, geographic area, and socioeconomic differences. *Vital and Health Statistics*, Series 11, no 167. Hyattsville, MD: Department of Health Education and Welfare, National Center for Health Statistics, DHEW publication, (PHS); 79–1654.
38. Zhen O, Baolin L. Skeletal maturity of the hand and wrist in Chinese school children in Harbin assessed by the TW2 method. *Ann Hum Biol.* 1986; 13: 183–187.
39. Ontel FK, Ivanovic M, Ablin DS, Barlow TW. Bone age in children of diverse ethnicity. *Am J Roentgenol.* 1996; *167*: 1395–1398.
40. Ashizawa K, Asami T, Anzo M, *et al.* Standard RUS skeletal maturation of Tokyo children. *Ann Hum Biol.* 1996; 23: 457–469.
41. Cole TJ, Rousham EK, Hawley NL, Cameron N, Norris SA, Pettifor JM. Ethnic and sex differences in skeletal maturation among the Birth to Twenty cohort in South Africa. *Arch Dis Child.* 2015; 100: 138–143.
42. Mentzel H-J, Vilser C, Eulenstein M, *et al.* Assessment of skeletal age at the wrist in children with a new ultrasound device. *Pediatr Radiol.* 2005; 35: 429–433.
43. Mentzel H-J, Vogt S, Vilser C, *et al.* Abschätzung des Knochenalters mit einer neuen Ultraschallmethode. *Fortschr Röntgenstr.* 2005; 177: 1699–1705.
44. Khan KM, Miller BS, Hoggard E, Somani A, Sarafoglou K. Application of ultrasound for bone age estimation in clinical practice. *J Pediatr.* 2009; 154: 243–247.
45. Płudowski P, Lebiedowski M, Lorenc RS. Evaluation of the possibility to assess bone age on the basis of DXA derived hand scans—preliminary results. *Osteoporos Int.* 2004; 15: 317–322.
46. Płudowski P, Lebiedowski M, Lorenc RS. Evaluation of practical use of bone age assessments based on DXA-derived hand scans in diagnosis of skeletal status in healthy and diseased children. *J Clin Densitom.* 2005; 8: 48–60.
47. Heppe DHM, Taal HR, Ernst GDS, *et al.* Bone age assessment by dual-energy X-ray absorptiometry in children: An alternative for X-ray? *Br J Radiol.* 2012; 85: 114–120.
48. Gertych A, Zhang A, Sayre J, Pospiech-Kurkowska S, Huang HK. Bone age assessment using a digital hand atlas. *Computer Med Imag Graph.* 2007; 31: 322–331.
49. Thodberg HH, Kreilborg, S., Juul A, Pedersen KD. The boneXpert method for automated determination of skeletal maturity. *IEEE Trans Med Imag.* 2009; 28: 52–66.
50. van Rijn RR, Thodberg HH. Bone age assessment: Automated techniques coming of age? *Acta Radiol.* 2013; 54: 1024–1029.
51. Tanner JM. *Growth at adolescence*, 2nd ed. Oxford: Blackwell; 1962.
52. Malina RM, Rogol AD. Sport training and the growth and pubertal maturation of young athletes. *Pediatr Endoc Rev.* 2011; 9: 441–455.
53. Slough JM, Hennrikus W, Chang Y. Reliability of Tanner staging performed by orthopedic sports medicine surgeons. *Med Sci Sports Exerc.* 2013; 45: 1229–1234.
54. Wu Y, Schreiber GB, Klementowicz V, Biro F, Wright D. Racial differences in accuracy of self-assessment of sexual maturation among young Black and White girls. *J Adol Hlth.* 2001; 28: 197–203.
55. Taylor SJC, Whincup PH, Hindmarsh PC, Lampe F, Odoki K, Cook DG. Performance of a new pubertal self-assessment questionnaire: A preliminary study. *Paediatr Prenat Epidemiol.* 2001; 15: 88–94.
56. Prader A. Testicular size: assessment and clinical importance. *Triangle.* 1966; 7: 240–243.
57. Zachman M, Prader A, Kind HP, Hafliger H, Budliger H. Testicular volume during adolescence: Cross-sectional and longitudinal studies. *Helveta Paediatr Acta.* 1974; 29: 61–72.
58. Goede J, Hack WWM, Sijstermans K, *et al.* Normative values for testicular volume measured by ultrasonography in a normal population from infancy to adolescence. *Horm Res Paediatr.* 2011; 76: 55–64.
59. Malina RM, Rogol AD, Cumming SP, Coelho e Silva MJ, Figueiredo AJ. Biological maturation of youth athletes: Assessment and implications. *Br J Sports Med.* 2015; 49: 852–859.
60. Hauspie RC, Cameron N, Molinari L (eds.) *Methods in human growth research.* Cambridge: Cambridge University Press; 2004.
61. Malina RM, Bouchard C, Beunen G. Human growth: selected aspects of current research on well-nourished children. *Ann Rev Anthrop.* 1988; 17: 187–219.
62. Beunen G, Malina RM. Growth and physical performance relative to the timing of the adolescent spurt. *Exerc Sport Sci Rev.* 1988; 16: 503–540.
63. Malina RM, Kozieł SM. Validation of maturity offset in a longitudinal sample of Polish boys. *J Sports Sci.* 2014; 32: 424–437.
64. Malina RM, Kozieł SM. Validation of maturity offset in a longitudinal sample of Polish girls. *J Sports Sci.* 2014; 32: 1374–1382.
65. Malina RM, Chow AC, Czerwinski SA, Chumlea WC. Validation of maturity offset in the Fels Longitudinal Study. *Pediatr Exerc Sci.* 2016; 28: 439–455.
66. Mirwald RL, Baxter-Jones ADG, Bailey DA, Beunen GP. An assessment of maturity from anthropometric measurements. *Med Sci Sports Exerc* 2002; 34: 689–694.

67. Chumlea WC, Schubert CM, Roche AF, *et al.* Age at menarche and racial comparisons in US girls. *Pediatrics.* 2003; 111: 110–113.
68. Mirwald RL, Bailey DA. *Maximal aerobic power: A longitudinal analysis.* London, ON: Sports Dynamics; 1986.
69. Iuliano-Burns S, Mirwald RL, Bailey DA. The timing and magnitude of peak height velocity and peak tissue velocities for early, average and late maturing boys and girls. *Am J Hum Biol.* 2001; 13: 1–8.
70. Geithner CA, Satake T, Woynarowska B, Malina RM. Adolescent spurts in body dimensions: Average and modal sequences. *Am J Hum Biol.* 1999; 11: 287–295.
71. Nicolson AB, Hanley C. Indices of physiological maturity: deviation and interrelationships. *Child Dev.* 1953; 24: 3–38.
72. Bielicki T. Interrelationships between various measures of maturation rate in girls during adolescence. *Stud Phys Anthrop.* (Wrocław). 1975; 1: 51–64.
73. Bielicki T, Koniarek J, Malina RM. Interrelationships among certain measures of growth and maturation rate in boys during adolescence. *Ann Hum Biol.* 1984; 11: 201–210.
74. Flor-Cisneros A, Roemmich JN, Rogol AD, Baron J. Bone age and onset of puberty in normal boys. *Mol Cell Endocrinol.* 2006. 254–255: 202–206.
75. Johnston FE. Individual variation in the rate of skeletal maturation between five and eighteen years. *Child Dev.* 1964; 35: 75–80.
76. Johnston FE. The use of the Greulich-Pyle method in a longitudinal growth study. *Am J Phys Anthrop.* 1971; 35: 353–358.
77. Buckler JMH. Skeletal age changes in puberty. *Arch Dis Child.* 1984. 59: 115–119.
78. Largo RH, Prader A. Pubertal development in Swiss boys. *Helv Paediatr Acta.* 1983; 38: 211–228.
79. Largo RH, Prader A. Pubertal development in Swiss girls. *Helv Paediatr Acta.* 1983; 38: 229–243.
80. Roche AF, Tyleshevski F, Rogers E. Non-invasive measurement of physical maturity in children. *Res Q Exerc Sport.* 1983; 54: 364–371.
81. Tanner JM, Goldstein H, Whitehouse RH. Standards for children's height at ages 2-9 years allowing for height of parents. *Arch Dis Child.* 1970; 45: 755–762.
82. Khamis HJ, Roche AF. Predicting adult stature without using skeletal age: The Khamis-Roche method. *Pediatrics.* 1994; 94: 504–507 (*Pediatrics.* 1995; 95:457, for the corrected version of the tables).
83. Malina RM. Top 10 research questions related to growth and maturation of relevance to physical activity, performance, and fitness. *Res Q Exerc Sport.* 2014; 85: 157–173.
84. Malina RM, Dompier TP, Powell JW, Barron MJ, Moore MT. Validation of a noninvasive maturity estimate relative to skeletal age in youth football players. *Clin J Sports Med.* 2007; 17: 362–368.
85. Malina RM, Coelho e Silva MJ, Figueiredo AJ, Carling C, Beunen GP. Interrelationships among invasive and non-invasive indicators of biological maturation in adolescent male soccer players. *J Sports Sci.* 2012; 30: 1705–1717.
86. Beunen GP, Malina RM, Lefevre J, Claessens AL, Renson R, Simons J. Prediction of adult stature and non-invasive assessment of biological maturation. *Med Sci Sports Exer.* 1997; 29: 225–230.
87. Beunen GP, Malina RM, Freitas DI, *et al.* Cross-validation of the Beunen-Malina method to predict adult height. *Ann Hum Biol.* 2010; 37: 593–597.
88. Malina RM, Claessens AL, Van Aken K, *et al.* Maturity offset in gymnasts: Application of a prediction equation. *Med Sci Sports Exerc.* 2006; 38: 1342–1347.
89. Moore SA, McKay HA, Macdonald H, *et al.* Enhancing a somatic maturity prediction model. *Med Sci Sports Exerc.* 2015; 47: 1755–1764.

CHAPTER 2

Growth and maturation

Adam DG Baxter-Jones

Introduction

The concepts of a child's growth and maturation are central to all studies related to paediatric exercise science. It is therefore imperative that any studies recording the acute and chronic responses of the child and adolescent to both exercise and physical activity (PA) take into consideration the growth and maturity status of the participant. Morphological parameters and physiological functions such as heart volume, lung function, aerobic power, and muscular strength develop with increasing age and body size. Furthermore, physical fitness parameters (e.g. muscular, motor, and cardiorespiratory) also change with growth and maturation. Thus the effects of growth and maturation may mask or be greater than both the exercise and PA effects under investigation.

Interest in the effect that both PA and exercise has on a child's growth and maturation has a long history. At the beginning of the 20th century D'arcy Thompson wrote his classic treatise *On Growth and Form*, and suggested that exercise was a direct stimulus to growth.[1] In 1964, James Tanner published *The Physique of the Olympic Athlete*, in which he concluded that 'the basic body structure must be present for the possibility of being an athlete to arise'.[2] Other authors who have subsequently measured the growth and development of young athletes concurred with Tanner, and concluded that body size is likely genotypic and probably reflects selection at a relatively young age for the size demands of the sport.[3] However, a number of studies have suggested that when heavy training regimens are started at a young age, especially with aesthetic sports like gymnastics, the growth and maturation of the child may be adversely effected.[4] Thus the nature versus nurture debate continues (see Chapter 31 and Chapter 32).[5]

Concern about a child's size does not just pertain to childhood; the importance of size and measuring growth itself begins much earlier, even before birth. It has now been shown that both the size of a foetus and the child's growth in the first year after birth can determine their lifelong health status.[6] It should be emphasized that regular exercise for the pregnant mother and pre-school child is only one of many factors that may influence an individual's growth and maturation. Growth and maturation are maintained primarily by genes, hormones, energy, and nutrients which not only interact among themselves but also with the environment in which the individual lives, both inter-and intra-uterine. Since the process by which genes interact with the environment develops through time is non-linear, it is important to realize that the same genes will be expressed differently when exposed to different environmental conditions.[7] To fully understand the potential of exercise or PA on a child's growth, a sound understanding of the general principles of human growth and maturation, i.e. auxology, are required.

Growth refers to changes in size of an individual, as a whole or in parts. As children grow, they become taller and heavier, they increase their lean and fat tissues, and their organs increase in size. Changes in size are a result of three cellular processes: i) an increase in cell numbers, i.e. hyperplasia, ii) an increase in cell size, i.e. hypertrophy, and iii) an increase in inter-cellular substances, i.e. accretion. All three occur during growth, but the predominance of one process over another varies both with chronological age as well as the tissue involved.[8]

Maturation is the progressive achievement of adult status and comprises a subset of developmental changes that include morphology, function, and complexity. The acquisition of secondary sexual characteristics, such as breast development in girls and facial hair in boys, are common examples of maturation during adolescence. Size and morphological changes can also be scaled relative to achievement of adult status and can be used as a continuous scale of maturation; e.g. percentage of adult height attained.[9] The major distinction between size per se and maturation is that all children eventually achieve the same adult maturity, whereas adult size and body dimensions vary considerably. It is therefore important to remember that growth and maturation occur simultaneously and interact, although they may not follow the same time line. A young person could appear to be tall for their age but could also be delayed in biological maturation, or vice versa.

The process of maturing has two components: timing and tempo. The former refers to when specific maturational events occur (e.g. age when menarche is attained, age at the beginning of breast development, age at the appearance of pubic hair, or age at maximum growth in height during the adolescent growth spurt, known as peak height velocity, or PHV). Tempo refers to the rate at which maturation progresses (i.e. how quickly or slowly an individual passes from the initial stages of sexual maturation to the mature state). Maturation occurs in all biological systems in the body but at different rates. Furthermore, the timing and tempo of maturity vary considerably among individuals, with children of the same chronological age differing dramatically in their degree of biological maturity.

The terms 'growth' and 'maturation' are used broadly to include all developmental processes, for example, cognitive growth and social maturation.[10] However, this chapter uses a stricter definition and limits its focus to physical aspects, primarily the growth at the organism level, i.e. the level of the whole child. In the growth and maturity literature, life leading up to maturity is split into three stages: the prenatal period, childhood, and adolescence.

Prenatal to postnatal growth

The period of prenatal life is vitally important to the child's wellbeing,[11] as is the transition from prenatal to postnatal life. There is now compelling evidence that the origins of many chronic diseases occur prenatally and are related to the trajectory of a child's growth.[6] The current particular concern is the accrual of adipose tissue. During pregnancy certain lifestyle factors, including but not limited to, PA promote healthy growth of the foetus. After birth the neonate has to make adjustments from the limited intrauterine environment to the rich and varied extrauterine world. The newborn infant must successfully make the transition from a regulatory system that was largely dependent on characteristics of the mother to one based on the infant's own genetic and homeostatic mechanisms (see Chapter 31).

Growth in uterine is particularly important. In the last 30 years, the foetal programming hypothesis has received much attention.[6] This hypothesis suggests that undernutrition, and thus restricted growth, during foetal life causes long-term changes to the structure and function of the body, and that these changes predispose it to the development of many chronic diseases in later life. As already indicated, growth is defined as the increase or decrease in some measurable quantity of tissue. Infants triple in weight during their first year, with the most notable change occurring during the first month of life. The most overt signs of growth are the changes in somatic growth, which are measured by the techniques of anthropometry. The number of measurements that can be made on the body are almost limitless. However, the most common dimensions of child growth cluster along the longitudinal axis of the body, and tend to be limited to dimensions that reflect skeletal growth at the metaphysis of endochondrally formed bones. Size is often measured in terms of body breadth. Two of the most frequently used are the biacromal breadth of the shoulders and the bicristal breadth of the hip. These measures reflect the complex internal changes in architecture of the shoulder and hip regions, including associated development of musculature and adipose tissue. However, the most commonly taken measure of somatic growth is stature. Other dimensions, for example sitting height, are of equal importance. It is important to remember that humans generally grow proportionately and it is the interrelationships between various measurements that provide important information about the growth process. For example, the ratio of sitting height to stature assists in diagnosing particular types of growth failure.

Body size and composition at birth reflect foetal growth. Postnatal growth velocities are highest immediately after birth, falling off sharply by 12 months. During the same time period, hip and shoulder breadths increase by about 55%. At birth skinfold thickness at the triceps and subscapular vary considerably and reflect the roles of prenatal growth and gestation. After birth these skinfold thicknesses rise markedly, peak at around 6–9 months before starting to decline. As the newborn infant makes the transition from growth controlled by maternal influences to their own influences, growth becomes more regularized and predictive of future growth; this is called canalization. Canalization reflects the adherence of individuals to specific patterns of growth. Figure 2.1 shows the growth of one individual's stature over time. To assess whether this depicts the normal range of height for age, individual age points can be compared with growth charts that consist of normal ranges in heights bound by centile limits. Although individuals during times of rapid growth may leave their centile, they return to the same centile position in adulthood. Thus in a healthy environment children exhibit patterns of growth that more or less parallel a particular centile or fall within some imaginary 'canal'. It is very likely that such patterns

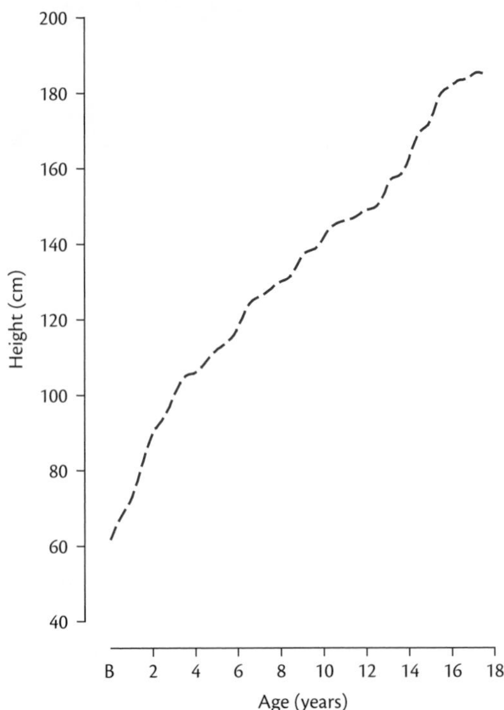

Figure 2.1 The growth in height of de Montbeillard's son 1759–1777: distance curve.

Source data from Scammon RE. The first seriatim study of human growth. Am J Phys Anthrop. 1927; 10: 329–336.

of growth are genetically predetermined. This suggests that individuals seek a target height and progress in a proportional manner to this target. Because of maternal influences, body size during the first year of life is poorly correlated with final adult size, at birth representing ~30% of final adult height. However, by 2 years of age growth has stabilized to an extent that, in well-nourished populations, the correlation between an individual's size and adult height is about 0.8, representing 50% of final adult stature. At PHV an individual is 92% of their final adult height.

Statural growth

One of the most famous records of human statural growth is that of a boy known simply as De Montbeillard's son. Between 1759 and 1770, Count Philibert Gueneau De Montbeillard successively measured his son at approximately 6-month intervals. Although initially published in 1778 using the French units of the time, in 1927 the measurements were translated into centimetres and plotted in the form of a chart by RE Scammon[12] (Figure 2.1). This is known as a height distance or height-for-age curve.

If growth can be thought of as a journey, then the curve describes the distance travelled from birth to 18 years of age; therefore, a child's height at any particular age is a reflection of how far that child has progressed towards the mature adult state or their target height. The pattern of the growth curve, to a large extent, is related to the frequency of data collection. If only two data points had been collected, e.g. birth and 18 years of age, the line between these two points would be linear. However, in this case, data were collected approximately every 6 months, and it clearly illustrates that growth is not a linear process, i.e. individuals do not gain the same amount of height during each calendar year. Figure 2.1 also

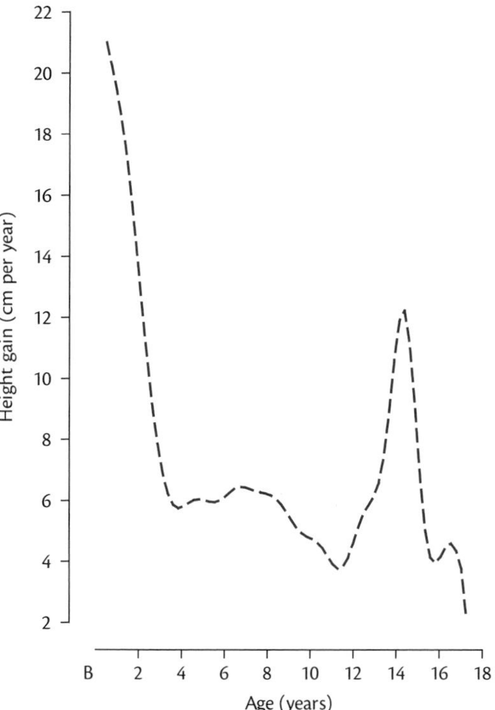

Figure 2.2 The growth in height of de Montbeillard's son 1759–1777: velocity curve.

Source data from Scammon RE. The first seriatim study of human growth. Am J Phys Anthrop. 1927; 10: 329–336.

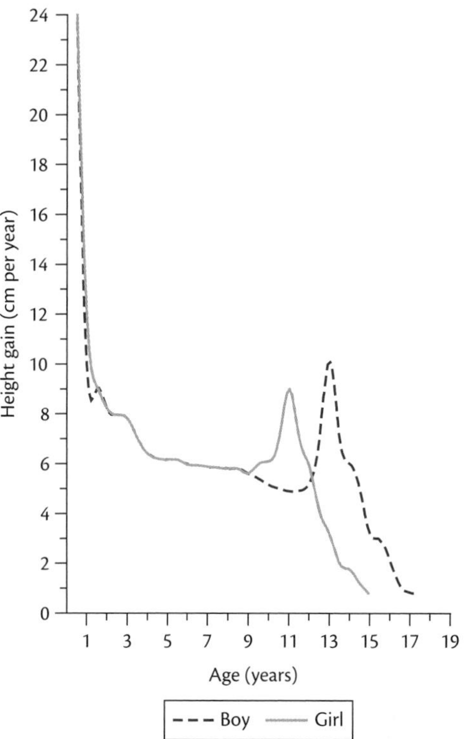

Figure 2.3 Typical-individual height velocity curves for boys and girls, representing the velocity of the typical boy and girl at any given instance.

Source data from Malina RM, Bouchard C, Bar- Or O. Growth, maturation, and physical activity. 2nd ed. Champaign, IL: Human Kinetics: 2004.

illustrates the fact that between birth and 18 years of age, the distance curve comprises a number of differently shaped curves with different slopes. Relatively rapid growth is observed in infancy, which gradually declines by 5 years of age, and thereafter, the slope of the line decreases. Steady growth in childhood (between 5 and 10 years of age) and then rapid growth during adolescence (between 10 and 16 years of age) is then observed. During adolescence an S-shaped, or sigmoid curve, is observed. Finally, very slow growth is observed as the individual approaches an asymptote at 18 years of age. Although the data come from a boy measured in the 18th century, it is significant because the pattern of growth seen then is the same as that seen in children today.

This distance curve shows the continuous rate of magnitude of change in stature with age. However, in terms of the journey it only tells the observer where the individual is at any particular point in time. No information is provided as to how the individual reached this point; therefore, the distance point is largely dependent on how much the child has grown in all proceeding years.

What is therefore required is a measure of growth that describes the speed of the journey at any one point in time. To get an idea of speed, the data have to be expressed in terms of a rate of growth (e.g. $cm \cdot year^{-1}$) (see Figure 2.2).[12] Velocity of growth is a better reflection of the child's state at any particular time than the distance achieved. This is important to the paediatric exercise scientist because substances whose amounts change with age, such as metabolites concentrations in blood, or tissue physiology, will likely show similar patterns of growth to the velocity rather than the distance curve.

The curve in Figure 2.2 shows that, following birth, two distinct increases in growth rates occur. The first of these is the juvenile or mid-growth spurt which occurs between 6 and 8 years of age. The second increase, which is more dramatic, occurs between 11 and 18 years and is called the adolescent growth spurt. While the juvenile growth spurt varies in magnitude between individuals, it occurs at roughly the same age both within and between genders. The adolescent growth spurt, however, varies in both magnitude and timing within and between the genders. Males enter their adolescent growth spurt almost 2 years later than females and have a slightly greater magnitude of height gain (Figure 2.3).[8] The extra 2 years of growth prior to adolescence, in combination with a greater magnitude of growth during adolescence, explains in part the increased final adult height observed in males. At the same time other skeletal changes occur that result in gender differences in adulthood, such as wider shoulders in males and wider hips in females. Males also demonstrate rapid increases in muscle mass while females accumulate greater amounts of fat, and therefore, as a result of natural biological development, by the end of adolescence males are stronger. The increase in size also results in other physiological advantages in males over females, such as increased lung capacity.

Types of growth data

When describing a growth curve it is important to distinguish between a curve fitted to a single individual's data (longitudinal data) and curves of yearly averages derived from different children measured only once (cross-sectional data), as each of these curves will have a different shape.[13] Cross-sectional studies are attractive as they can be carried out quickly and include larger numbers of children. Unfortunately, although cross-sectional studies provide information about a static picture of the population variation in growth variables (e.g. growth reference charts and the distance curve), they provide little information about individual growth rates or the timing of particular phases of growth. The individual differences, timing, and tempo, in growth velocity are important in clarifying the genetic control of growth and the correlation of growth with physical development. Most of seminal growth research has been longitudinal in design. Longitudinally measuring the same subjects over time provides information on a part or the entire growth pattern of an individual. A pure longitudinal design is where a cohort of children born within the same year is followed continuously and assessed on at least three separate occasions. In practice, it is virtually impossible to measure exactly the same group of children every year for a prolonged period; inevitably some children leave the study, others may join, and others may be measured sporadically. This type of study is called a mixed-longitudinal study and is a compromise between cross-sectional and longitudinal design. The mixed-longitudinal design consists of a number of relatively short longitudinal studies that interlock and cover a whole age range (e.g. 8–10 years, 9–11 years, 10–13 years, etc.). Mixed-longitudinal studies provide information on status and rate of growth, however sophisticated statistical techniques are required to accurately interpret the data.[14] The advantage of longitudinal over cross-sectional designs is that in longitudinal design, individual variance can be obtained and therefore the timing and tempo of an individual's pattern of growth can be identified. When conducting longitudinal research it is important to remember that two measures separated by a time period do not constitute longitudinal data; true longitudinal data have at least three measures and thus two velocities. Unfortunately, longitudinal research is often impractical for paediatric exercise research as the process is laborious, expensive, and time consuming for both the participants and the investigators. This means that most knowledge in paediatric exercise science is based on cross-sectional research. Although valuable in itself for describing distance curves, cross-sectional data can, in some respects, be misleading. Because of the large variation observed in the timing and tempo of growth, average velocity data inevitably produce growth curves that are smoothed or flattened and distance curves that are distorted because they do not rise sufficiently in periods of rapid growth, such as adolescence.[13]

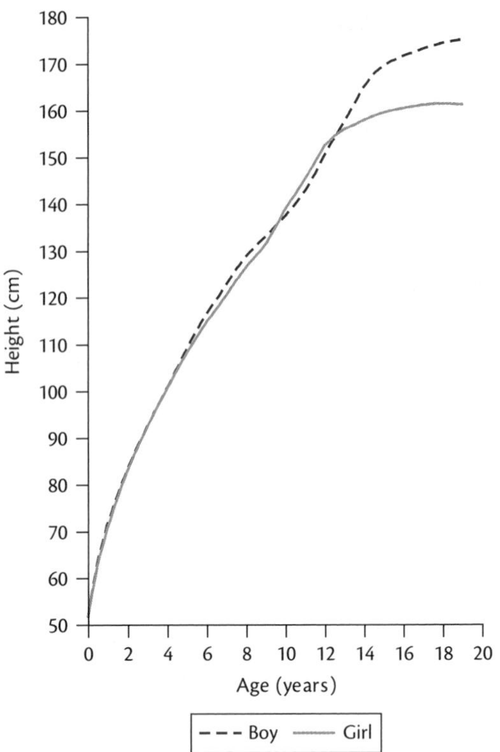

Figure 2.4 Typical-individual distance curves for boys and girls.
Source data from Malina RM, Bouchard C, Bar- Or O. Growth, maturation, and physical activity. 2nd ed. Champaign, IL: Human Kinetics: 2004.

Growth in stature

Stature is made up of sitting height (distance from the sitting surface to the top of the head) and leg length, or subischial length (distance between the hip joint and the floor). It can be difficult to locate the exact landmark of the hip joint, so leg length is most often calculated by subtracting sitting height from standing height. Stature varies during the course of the day and readings decrease throughout the day. Shrinkage during the day occurs as the intervertebral disks become compressed due to weight bearing, and therefore the diurnal variation may be as much as 1 cm or more.[8]

During the first year of life, infants grow quickly at approximately 25 cm·year^{-1}, and during the first 6 months of life the velocity may be even faster at around 30 cm·year^{-1}. During the second year of life there is growth of another 12–13 cm in stature. This accelerated growth means that by 2 years of age boys have attained approximately 50% of their adult stature. Girls, even at birth, are always closer to their mature status than boys, and reach 50% of their final adult stature by 18 months of age (Figure 2.3).[8] From then on there is a steady deceleration in growth, dropping to a rate of about 5–6 cm·year^{-1} before the initiation of the adolescent growth spurt. Between 6.5 and 8.5 years, there is a small but distinct increase in growth rate, known as the juvenile or mid-growth spurt. During adolescence the maximum velocity of growth is known as PHV. Girls, on average, attain PHV approximately 2 years earlier than boys, with PHV occurring between 8.2 and 10.3 years (Figure 2.4).[8] On average, PHV is reached between 11.3 and 12.2 years. Corresponding ages for boys are 10.0–12.1 years and 13.3–14.4 years.[13] As already mentioned, by PHV individuals have attained 92% of their adult height.

Upon reaching final adult height males are, on average, 13 cm taller than females, although up until the initiation of PHV the sex differences in height are small (Figure 2.4).[8] Therefore, boys achieve their height advantage during the adolescent period. On average, boys experience about 2 years more of preadolescent growth—approximately 5 cm·year^{-1}—than girls. This is roughly 10 cm of growth that girls do not experience. Boys also achieve a slightly greater (on average 2 cm) magnitude of height at PHV. Both of these growth differences cause males, on average, to have a greater adult stature. Girls stop growing in stature by ~16 years of age and boys by ~18 or 19 years of age. However, these ages may be spuriously young as many growth studies stop measuring youth at 17 or 18 years of age, and it is known that many youth continue to grow into their early- to mid-twenties.

The curves of growth of stature depicted (Figure 2.4) reflect the growth patterns found in all healthy children who live in a normal environment. As discussed, individuals will differ in absolute height (i.e. adult height) and in the timing of the adolescent growth spurt; however, to reach their final height target each individual will go through a similar pattern of growth.

Patterns of growth

Statural growth, as demonstrated in Figure 2.4,[8] shows only one of several patterns of growth found within the human body. Different parts of the body grow at different rates and at different times.[15] It has been proposed that all tissues and systems follow four patterns of growth: i) neurological (e.g. brain and head), ii) reproductive (e.g. reproductive organs), iii) lymphoid (e.g. lymph glands, tonsils, and appendix) and iv) general (e.g. stature and heart size).[15] Brain and head growth (neural tissue) exhibit the most rapid early growth. At birth a child's head is roughly half its adult size. From birth there is steady growth until 7 years of age, and by 8 years of age neural tissue growth is almost complete. In contrast, reproductive tissue does not really start to increase in size until 12–14 years of age. The reproductive curve includes primary sex characteristics (e.g. uterus, vagina, fallopian tubes in females; prostate and seminal vesicles in males) and secondary sex characteristics (e.g. breasts in females, facial hair in males, and axillary and pubic hair in both genders). The reproductive curve shows some growth during infancy followed by reduced growth during childhood; by 10–12 years of age reproductive organs are only 10% of their adult size. During adolescence (puberty) there is a rapid growth in genital tissues. The lymphoid tissues, which act as a circulatory system for tissue fluid, are involved with the immunological capacities of the child and show a different growth curve from the rest of the body. There is a remarkable increase in size of lymphoid tissue until the early adolescent years (~11–13 years). The relative size of lymphoid tissue then steeply declines during puberty, probably as a result of the up-regulation of sex hormones during this period. The general curve of growth also includes skeletal tissue, the respiratory system, and the digestive system. As illustrated by the shape of stature shown in Figure 2.4, the general curve follows a sigmoid curve of growth and reflects a rapid growth during infancy and early childhood, steady growth during mid-childhood, rapid growth during early adolescence, and asymptotes in late adolescence.[15]

Growth in body mass

Body mass is made up of a composite of tissues, including fat, lean, and bone tissue, that accrue at different rates and times. Significant changes in body composition occur during growth and maturation, especially during infancy and puberty. Importantly, this indicates why body composition assessment in children is far more challenging than in adults.[16] Changes in body mass are a result of changes in fat or fat-free mass as well as changes in body water concentrations (dehydration or over- hydration). The relative proportions and distributions of fat and fat-free components depend on age, sex, and other environmental and genetic factors. Body mass is very sensitive and fluctuates potentially changing from day to day due to minor alterations in body composition. Furthermore, body mass, like stature, also shows diurnal variation. An individual is lightest in the morning, upon voiding the bladder.[17] Throughout the day body mass increases and is affected by diet and PA. In menstruating adolescent girls the phase of the menstrual cycle can also affect body mass.[8]

As seen with the development of height, body mass follows a four-phase growth pattern: rapid growth in infancy and early childhood, rather steady gain during mid-childhood, rapid gain during adolescence, and usually a slower increase into adulthood. The water content of the foetus is high and represents about 75% of body weight at birth. Much of this weight is lost during the first few days of life, declining to 45%. By puberty, water represents approximately 19% of total body weight. Additionally, at birth the brain represents 13% of body weight, compared to 2% in adulthood. Thus the brain, along with other organ tissue, makes a greater contribution to body weight and lean body mass during infancy. During the first year of life body mass doubles and by the end of the second year it has quadrupled. Most children show the lowest annual increment in body mass around 2–3 years of age; from this point to the onset of adolescence body mass increases, but at a slower rate. At the onset of adolescence there is a rapid gain in the velocity of body mass development. The precise timing of the adolescent growth spurt in body mass is generally less clear than it is for height. It has been estimated that peak velocity in body mass normally occurs 0.2–0.4 years after PHV in boys and 0.3–0.9 years after PHV in girls.[18]

Boys and girls follow the same pattern in body mass development. Before the adolescent growth spurt boys are slightly heavier than girls. Girls experience a growth spurt earlier than boys and thus for a short time are heavier. However, when boys experience their adolescent growth spurt they then become and remain heavier than girls. Importantly, there is a normal range of individual variation in body mass resulting in some girls being heavier than most boys at virtually all ages.

In boys, the growth spurt in body mass is primarily due to gains in muscle mass and skeletal tissue; fat mass remains fairly stable. However, girls experience a less dramatic rise in muscle mass and skeletal tissue but experience a continuous rise in fat mass during adolescence. Specifically, before adolescence boys have a slightly larger lean body mass than girls, although during the adolescent growth spurt the magnitude of the velocity of change is greater and more prolonged. A consequence of this growth pattern is that by young adulthood males have 50% more lean body mass than females. Although sex differences in skeletal tissue may be present during infancy and childhood,[19] they become far more pronounced during adolescence.[20] Approximately 40% of peak bone mass (the maximum amount of bone in the body) is attained during adolescence. This is due to the growth and expansion of the skeleton; the density of bones also changes. When aligned by chronological age no sex differences are observed until 14 years of age. After age 14, boys have approximately 10% more bone mineralization. When the confounders of body size and lean mass are controlled, boys have significantly greater bone mineralization at all ages during adolescence, suggesting that much of this difference between the sexes is due to boys' greater stature and lean mass.[21]

With regards to fat mass development in mid-foetal life, body fat is 1% of total body weight. Subcutaneous fat begins to be laid down in the foetus at about 34 weeks and increases continuously thereafter, so that by birth, fat represents 15% of total body weight, 25% at 6 months, and 30% at 1 year of age. Skinfold thickness, an index of subcutaneous fat, peaks about 6–9 months after birth, and then decreases until between ages 6 to 8 years, when they again begin to rise. This pattern of flow, ebb, and flow is called the adiposity rebound.[22] The rebound occurs earlier in children at higher percentiles for fatness and there is a tendency for children with an early rebound to have higher fatness at the end of growth. In general, girls have greater skinfold thicknesses than boys, even at birth, but the divergence becomes marked by 8 years of age. Both boys and girls experience a prepubescent adipose tissue gain, but girls more than boys. Girls' skinfolds continue to increase through adolescence. In contrast, during mid-puberty, boys' skinfolds decrease, particularly at the triceps and to a lesser extent at the subscapular. During childhood the ratio of trunk and extremities skinfolds is relatively stable, but at adolescence both genders gain proportionally more on the trunk. The gain is less in girls, and boys experience a decrease at the extremity sites resulting in boys having relatively more subcutaneous adipose tissue on the trunk by the end of adolescence.[23]

While the timing and magnitude of peak velocity of the different tissues differ between the sexes, the pattern of growth of the different tissues is consistent. Peak lean velocity is attained first—approximately 0.3 years after PHV—followed by peak fat and peak bone mineralization. Because total body mass represents the composite of lean, fat, and bone, peak body mass occurs after lean and fat mass peaks but before the peak in bone mass.[18]

Development of shape

In contrast to changes in size, which just shows a child's progression in terms of a percentage of adult status, the concept of change in shape reflects the changes in proportionality of body segments from infancy to adulthood. From these changes in proportionality, growth gradients can be identified. As discussed, head size increases twofold from birth to maturity, although other segments show different patterns. The trunk increases threefold, the arms fourfold, and the legs at maturity are five times their birth length. These changes illustrate a head-trunk-legs gradient. In early foetal growth the head grows fastest, in infancy trunk growth accelerates, and in childhood leg growth accelerates. However, within the trunk itself no cephalocaudad gradients are found, as findings indicate abdominal growth proceeds growth in the thorax, and the second to seventh thoracic are the last vertebral epiphyses to fuse. Since change in shape is difficult to measure, ratios are often used to characterize physiological age, e.g. volume of trunk to the volume of head and volume of trunk to the length of limbs. Since the increase in these physical parameters occurs at different times and tempos, these ratios thus increase with increasing age and can be used to measure shape maturity. Other gradients of growth are also observed; during childhood and adolescence, limb growth occurs distal to proximal. For example, the hand and feet experience accelerated growth first, then the calf and the forearm, the hips and the chest, and finally the shoulders. Thus, during childhood there may be a period where children appear to have large hands and feet in relation to the rest of their body. Once the adolescent growth spurt has ended, hands and feet are a little smaller in proportion to arms, legs, and stature. Most body dimensions follow a growth pattern similar to that of stature with the exception of subcutaneous adipose tissue and the dimensions of the head and face. However, there are wide variations in the timing of growth spurts. From childhood to adolescence, the lower extremities grow faster than the trunk. This results in sitting height contributing less to stature as age progresses. During the adolescent growth spurt, the legs experience a growth spurt earlier than the trunk. Thus, for a period during early adolescence a youth will have relatively long legs, but the appearance of long-leggedness disappears with the later increase in trunk length. Sex differences in leg length and sitting height are small during childhood. For a short time during the early part of adolescence, girls generally have slightly longer legs than boys, who experience the adolescent growth spurt approximately 2 years later. By about 12 years of age, boys' leg length exceeds girls', but boys do not catch up in sitting height until about 14 years of age. The longer period of preadolescent growth in boys is largely responsible for the fact that mens' legs are longer than womens' in relation to trunk length.[13]

Other gender shape differences also occur during adolescence. Where boys experience a broadening of the shoulders relative to the hips, girls experience a broadening of the hips. These differences are evident during childhood but become accentuated during adolescence. During the adolescent growth spurt boys gain more in shoulder (biacromial) breadth (about 2.3 cm), whereas girls gain slightly more in hip (bicristal) breadth (about 1.2 cm).[8] Boys catch up to girls in bicristal breadth in late adolescence. The timing and speed of these changes in body dimensions may have a dramatic effect on several aspects of physical performance. An increase in shoulder width can result in increased muscle mass in the upper body in boys. This is one reason why sex differences in strength are much greater in the upper compared to the lower body. Furthermore, this greater upper body muscle, combined with longer arms, may explain why older boys are better at throwing, racquet sports, and rowing than older girls. Girls tend to have a lower centre of gravity, due to the relative broadening of the hips, which may contribute to their better sense of balance.[24]

Adolescence and puberty

As discussed, maturation is the progressive achievement of adult status. Adolescence or puberty refers to the time period of adult reproductive capacity onset. The terms adolescence and puberty are used frequently in the paediatric literature to explain the later period of growth and maturity, often with no clear distinction in their definitions. Some authors refer to adolescence when talking about psychosocial changes and puberty when talking about the physical changes. However, most of the literature uses these terms interchangeably.

Adolescence is a dramatic period involving rapid transformation of anatomy, physiology, and behaviour.[25] The progressive acquisition of secondary sexual characteristics are common examples of maturation during adolescence. In these examples, the progress of sexual maturation is determined by attainment of stages, a qualitative term.[26,27] In contrast, size and morphological variables can be scaled continuously, e.g. percentage of adult height attained, or age of attainment of PHV. Growth at adolescence is characterized by the presence of the adolescent or pubertal growth spurt and is a time of greatest sex differentiation since the early intrauterine months. There is wide variation among populations, individuals, and the two sexes as to the timing of the adolescent growth spurt, its magnitude, and the age at which mature size is reached. When large numbers of individuals' velocity curves are compared it soon becomes apparent that some children reach PHV earlier than others. In 1930, Boas[28] coined the expression *tempo of growth* drawing an analogy with classical music: some children are marked *allegro* (fast), others *lento* (slow). The empirical findings from this study were that adult height, in general, did not differ, indicating there are two independent patterns of growth: size and maturation.

Often within paediatric exercise physiology there is an interest in examining the trainability of the child, or the association between PA and health outcomes. However, interpretation of these outcomes must consider the process of normal growth and maturation, particularly during adolescence, before any definitive conclusion can be reached. Unless body size and biological maturity indicators are considered, the independent effects of PA or training on the outcome cannot be definitively identified. (Interested readers are referred to Chapter 32 for a detailed discussion of the effects of PA and training on growth and maturation).

Regulation of growth and maturation

The regulation of growth and maturation involves the complex and continuous interaction of genes, hormones, nutrients, and the physical environment. A genotype is the group of genes making up an individual. Simply, an individual's genotype can be thought of as a potential for growth and maturation.[7] Whether a child achieves that potential, however, depends on the conditions (i.e. environment) into which the child is born and subsequently raised. An individual's phenotype is the observed physical or physiological characteristics and traits that are produced by the genotype in conjunction with the environment[7] (see Chapter 31 for further discussion). General health and well-being of the child is paramount to normal growth, and in turn normal growth is a strong indicator of the overall good health of the child. Adequate levels of several hormones are essential to normal growth and development. Hormones are therefore essential for a child to reach full genetic potential.

A large number of hormones are of particular importance in the initiation and regulation of pubertal events (i.e. maturation of secondary sex characteristics, attainment of reproduction function, and PHV). Recent scientific advances in endocrinology have shed light on the mechanisms, actions, and interactions among hormones and highlight the complexity of these processes. Some of the most prominent hormones involved in the regulation of growth and maturation include testosterone (primarily from the leydig cells of the testes and also the adrenal cortex), oestrogen (primarily from the ovarian follicle and also the adrenal cortex), thyroxine (from the thyroid gland), cortisol and adrenal androgens (from the adrenal cortex), insulin (from the β-cells of the Islets of Langerhans of the pancreas), and a series of hormones from the pituitary glands. The pituitary hormones include but are not limited to adrenocoticotrophin (ACTH), follicle-stimulating hormones (FSH), growth hormone (GH) (or somatotrophin), leutenizing hormone (LH), and thyrotrophin (TSH, or thyroid stimulating hormone). There are many other hormones, growth factors, and cytokines that are also actively involved in the regulation of growth and maturation, and these are beyond the scope of this chapter.

Postnatal growth is a result of GH secretion and the final component of post-natal growth, i.e. puberty, when GH interacts with gonadal steroids.[29] Growth hormone and thyroid hormones are the primary hormones for growth prepubertally. Growth hormone is secreted in a pulsatile fashion from the somatotrophins in the anterior pituitary gland. Growth hormone is regulated by growth-hormone-releasing hormone, which causes release and synthesis of GH, and somatostatin, which inhibits GH release. In humans there is a dose-dependent relationship between the amount of GH secreted over a 24-h period and the growth rate of an individual. Although GH has direct effects on some cells, many of its effects are mediated by the local generation of insulin-like growth factor I (IGF-I).[29] Prepubertal growth is therefore largely dependent on the thyroid hormones and the GH/IGF–1 axis. Insulin-like growth factor-I plays an important role in muscle tissue growth through the stimulation of glycogen accumulation and the transfer of amino acids into cells for protein synthesis. Insulin-like growth factor-I also promotes connective tissue, cartilage, and bone growth through the stimulation of cartilage growth and the formation of collagen.[30]

During the final component of post-natal growth, i.e. pubertal, sex steroids modulate growth. Since puberty is a process integrating the antecedent and development of immaturity and adulthood, it is quite difficult to clearly identify its beginning and its end.[27] What is observed is a rapid and profound trajectory of change from the immature to mature state. The central feature of puberty is the maturation of the primary reproductive endocrine axis. This is comprised of the hypothalamus, pituitary gland, and gonads. This three-part system is known as the hypothalamic-pituitary-gonadal (HPG) axis. The secondary features of puberty include the development of secondary sexual characteristics, the development of sexual dimorphic anatomical features, and the acceleration and cessation of linear growth. Virtually all these secondary changes of puberty are downstream consequences of the maturation of the HPG axis.

The central features of the HPG axis are shown in Figure 2.5,[25] although it should be noted that the details are far more complex than is shown. Hormone signals flow between the components of the HPG axis. The hypothalamus serves as the main enabling centre, and its primary signal is a hormone known as gonadotropin-releasing hormone (GnRH) or luteinizing-hormone-releasing hormone (LHRH) that is released in a pulsatile fashion.[31] Conceptually the hypothalamus is seen as the primary on-off switch controlling reproductive function and is thought to be influenced by a vast range of stimuli. The effect of GnRH release is to simulate production and release of two gonadotropins from the pituitary, FSH and LH.[32,33] In the ovary LH stimulates testosterone production and FSH stimulates the conversion of testosterone to oestradiol. At the same time, inhibin is secreted which has a suppressive effect on FSH. After ovulation, progesterone is secreted. The combined effect of these steroids and inhibin is to inhibit the pituitary.[34] In the testis, LH stimulates testosterone production and FSH inhibin secretion, which act as feedback controls on the pituitary. Gonadal function is also regulated by a number of metabolites including insulin, cortisol, GH, and IGF-I.[35]

Circulating levels of FSH are much higher in girls compared to boys during infancy, whereas no sex differences are noted in LH. During childhood the levels of FSH and LH remain stable, with girls maintaining slightly higher levels of FSH than boys. In late childhood, the hypothalamus stimulates the anterior pituitary gland to release FSH and LH, causing the blood levels to increase substantially. Thus, one of the first detectable signs of biological maturity, related to a change in HPG axis activity, is the appearance of sleep-associated increased LH pulse amplitude. On average LH concentrations will rise first in girls at about 8–9 years of age, reflecting their earlier onset of puberty, and then in boys 1–2 years later.[36]

Elevations of gonadotropins are associated with gonadal maturation, as evidenced by testicular volume increase. The resultant rising testosterone levels stimulate a host of other pubertal changes, including the appearance of pubic, axillary, and facial hair, voice changes, accelerated linear growth, and increase in muscle mass. In girls, increased LH stimulation leads to increases in ovarian steroid production with oestradiol levels approaching those characteristic of women in the follicular phase. As a result, pubic and

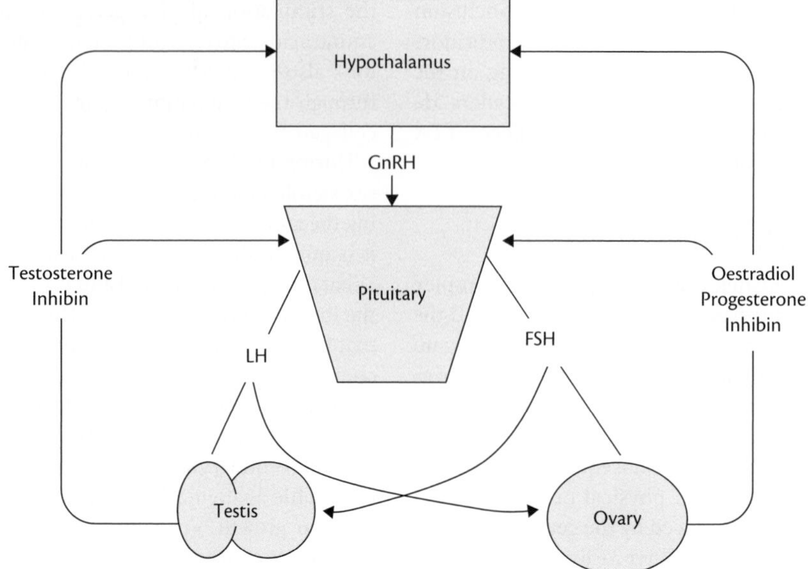

Figure 2.5 The hypothalamic-pituitary-gonadal axis and its principal hormones.
Source data from Ellison PT. Puberty. In: Cameron (ed.) Human growth and development. San Deigo: Academic Press; 2002. p. 65–84.

axillary hair develop, breasts enlarge, linear growth accelerates, the pelvis remodels, there is an increase in adiposity, and menarche occurs.

In late puberty, the secretion of FSH and LH becomes cyclic in females. In boys LH stimulates testosterone production and FSH stimulates growth of tubules and sperm production. In contrast to the cyclic secretion of FSH and LH in females with the attainment of sexual maturity, in males FSH and LH secretions remain constant. Blood levels of gonadatrophins increase with puberty in both males and females. On average, girls experience a threefold increase in the secretion of FSH and LH by stage 4 of breast and pubic hair development. On average, boys experience a sixfold increase by stage 5 of genital and pubic hair development (i.e. attainment of sexual maturity).[8]

Oestradiol is produced in the ovaries and is the most potent oestrogen in females. Testosterone is also present in females, but in smaller amounts than in boys. In males testosterone is synthesized in the testes. Although testosterone is the most abundant androgen in males, the most potent androgen is dihydrotestosterone, which is derived from testosterone. Circulating androgens are also converted to oestrogens in the peripheral tissues of males.

Levels of testosterone and oestradiol differ considerably during infancy, childhood, and puberty. During infancy boys demonstrate higher levels of testosterone than girls. Compared to infancy, levels of testosterone and oestradiol are reduced during childhood, with no marked sex differences. During the prepubertal years oestradiol increases gradually with a rapid spurt at the onset of sexual maturation (puberty). In addition to oestrogen, other less potent oestrogenic hormones are produced that also contribute to sexual maturation. Similar to the production of gonadatrophic hormones, in females oestrogen production also becomes cyclic during late puberty. Similarly, in pubescent boys, circulating testosterone increases steadily. The sex differences in hormones are accentuated during puberty (i.e. increased oestradiol levels in girls and increased testosterone levels in boys).

Both oestradiol and testosterone affect GH production by augmenting GH pulse amplitude. Increases in IGF-I, the major mediator of GH action on skeletal growth, are correlated with secondary sex stages of pubertal development and gonadal steroid levels. GH and IGF-I also have stimulatory effects on gonadal steroid production, and gonadal steroids have independent effects on skeletal growth not mediated by the somatotropic axis.[37,38] Thus, the somatotropic axis and the HPG axis function synergistically in promoting the adolescent growth spurt. However it must be remembered that the initial stimulation comes from the maturation of the HPG axis.[25]

Oestrogens and androgens increase anabolism through nitrogen retention. Androgens, however, are much more potent anabolic hormones than oestrogen and likely contribute to the sex differences in body size that occur during puberty. During puberty, males experience a dramatic growth spurt in muscle and fat-free mass, primarily due to the rise in circulating levels of testosterone. The more modest gain of muscle mass during puberty in females is primarily caused by the lower levels of adrenal androgens produced. The increase in fat disposition in females during puberty is due to the rising levels of oestrogens at this time.

As discussed, androgens and oestrogens also promote bone growth and skeletal maturation. Androgens stimulate longitudinal growth and increased thickness of bones. Greater growth is experienced during puberty in boys and is primarily due to the actions of testosterone. While oestrogen has little effect on linear growth, it plays an important role in bone formation and maturation. Oestrogens stimulate the production of bone matrix and act to maintain a positive calcium balance. Most importantly, oestrogens are responsible for the final stage of skeletal maturation (i.e. epiphyseal closure).

The causes and correlates of HPG axis maturation are still debatable. However, what is known is that changes in hypothalamic function are responsible for pubertal activation of the HPG axis and that puberty is not limited by the maturational status of either the pituitary or the gonad. What is uncertain is the process that leads to the establishment of the mature pattern of GnRH release. It has been suggested that at puberty the hypothalamus becomes less sensitive to the gonadotropins' and steroids' negative feedback effects,[39] although this hypothesis has been questioned.[40] The alternative hypothesis is that there is a positive stimulation of gonadotropin production. Unfortunately, neither of these hypotheses resolves the question as to what causes the maturational changes of the hypothalamus. However, what is important is that when considering this question, the researcher adequately distinguishes potential causes of HPG axis maturation, such as training, from correlated and consequent events, such as menarche. Readers interested in the effect of exercise and training on hormones are referred to Chapter 5 and Chapter 33 respectively.

Biological maturity

There is wide variation among children both within and between genders as to the exact timing and tempo of maturation. Therefore, to adequately distinguish the effects of PA or exercise on a group of children, biological maturity needs to be controlled. Firstly, when considering how to assess biological maturation it is important to understand that 1 year of chronological time does not equal 1 year of maturational time. While every individual passes through the same stages of maturity, each does so at a different rate, so children of the same chronological age often differ in their degree of maturity. Certainly, in very general terms, size is associated with maturity, in that a bigger individual is likely to be chronologically older, and thus more mature than a smaller individual. However, it is well recognized that size does not play a part in the assessment of maturity.

To adequately control for maturity, a maturity indicator needs to be incorporated into the research methodology. The maturity indicator chosen should be any definable and sequential change in any part of the body that is characteristic of the progression of the body from immaturity to maturity.[42] The most commonly used methods to assess maturity or pubertal events are: skeletal maturity, sexual maturity, biochemical and hormonal maturity, somatic or morphological maturity, and dental maturity.[9,43,44] Figure 2.6 illustrates how a number of pubertal events occur at the same time, all under the control of various endocrine systems and ultimately controlled by genetic expression. However, the timing of pubertal events varies between individuals of the same sex. As well as individual variation there is also a marked sex difference in the timing of somatic and sexual maturation. The maturity technique of choice varies with the study design.[45] Each method, with its associated limitations, is described in detail in Chapter 1. Correlations between the timing of maturity indicators are generally moderate to high, suggesting that there is a general maturity factor underlying the tempo of growth and maturation during adolescence in both boys and girls. However, there is sufficient variation to suggest that no single system (i.e. sexual, skeletal, or somatic) provides a complete description of the tempo of maturation during adolescence.

Furthermore, although sexual maturation and skeletal development are associated, an individual in one stage of secondary sexual development cannot be assumed to be in a set stage of skeletal development.[9] The apparent discord among these maturation indicators reflects individual variation in the timing and tempo of sexual and somatic maturity, and the methodological concerns in the assessment of maturity.

Relationship of maturity to body size and function

It is clear that a child's maturity status will influence measures of growth and performance. Early maturing individuals of both sexes are taller and heavier than those of the same chronological age who mature at an average or late rate. If a child's height is expressed as a percentage of their adult height, individuals maturing early sould be closest to their adult height at all ages during adolescence. Early maturing individuals also have a greater weight for height at each age. The height advantage of the early maturing individual is primarily due to an earlier attainment of PHV as well as a greater magnitude of peak height gain. Studies have repeatedly shown little or no correlation between the timing of the adolescent growth spurt (i.e. maturity status) and adult stature, suggesting that early, average, and late maturing children reach, on average, the same adult height. This is not the same for weight. Early maturing individuals have, on average, greater body weights as young adults. Early maturing individuals and late maturing individuals also vary in body shape. Late maturers tend to have relatively longer legs (i.e. legs account for a greater percentage of adult stature) than early maturers. Furthermore, early maturing girls and boys tend to have relatively wider hips and relatively narrower shoulders. In contrast, late maturing individuals tend to have relatively narrower hips and relatively wider shoulders.

The average age at which the velocity in growth of lean mass and fat mass peak occurs is earliest in early maturers, later in average maturers, and latest in late maturers.[16] In both sexes early maturing youngsters have, on average, larger measurements of muscle and fat. The differences between children of contrasting maturity groups are primarily due to size differences, because early maturers are taller and heavier than late maturers of the same chronological age. When muscle widths are expressed relative to height, the differences between maturity groups are often eliminated. However, there is some evidence that during the later adolescent years early maturing boys have larger muscle widths even after taking into account height differences. On the other hand, early maturing individuals of both sexes appear to have greater fat widths at all ages through adolescence, even when height differences are controlled.[8] In summary, at any given chronological age during adolescence, early maturing boys and girls are on average taller, heavier, have greater fat-free mass (especially in boys), total body fat, and percent body fat (especially in girls) than their less mature peers. The maturity-associated differences in body size and body composition are especially marked during adolescence and influence strength and aerobic power.

Increases in strength during adolescence are associated with the natural development in lean mass, and generally reach a peak at the same time as PHV in girls and a year after PHV in boys. Studies have shown that early maturing boys are stronger than late maturing boys during adolescence. Early maturing girls tend to be slightly stronger than late maturing girls early in adolescence (11 through 13 years of age), but as adolescence continues the difference between maturity groups disappears. When strength is expressed relative to height, the difference among maturity groups persists in boys, probably due to the early maturers' rapid growth in muscle mass. On the other hand, when strength is expressed relative to height, in girls the differences between maturity groups disappear (see Chapter 7).

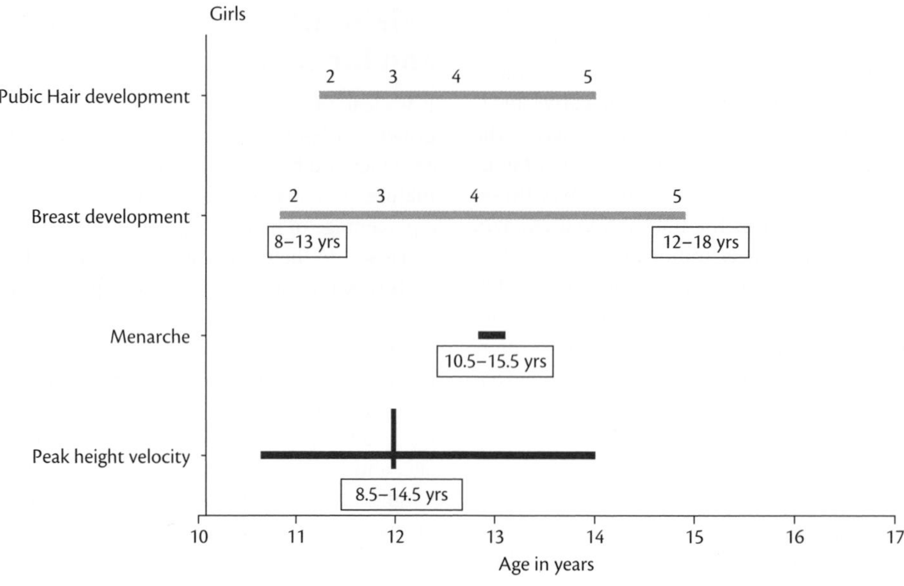

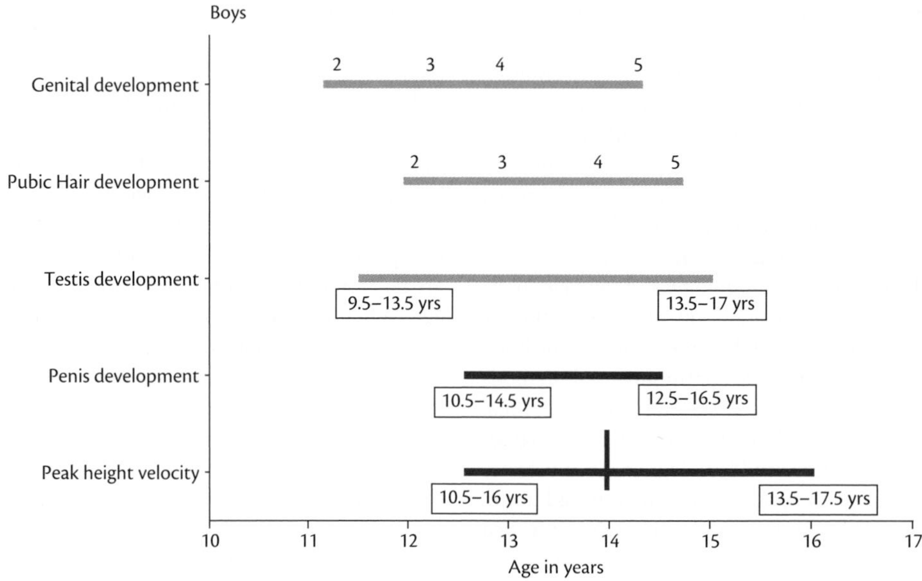

Figure 2.6 Diagram of sequence of events at puberty in girls and boys.
Source data from Marshall WA, Tanner JM (1969). Variations in the pattern of pubertal changes in girls. Arch Dis Child, 44, 291–303 and Marshall WA, Tanner JM (1970). Variations in the pattern of pubertal changes in boys. Arch Dis Child, 45, 13–23.

It has been shown that early maturing individuals, when compared to late maturing individuals of the same chronological age, have a higher absolute maximal oxygen uptake ($\dot{V}O_2$ max). Although the size advantage of the early maturing individual is reflected in a greater $\dot{V}O_2$ max, a maturity affect independent of body size, has been demonstrated. This difference in $\dot{V}O_2$ max between contrasting maturity groups is more pronounced in males than in females, which may be due to males developing greater muscle mass, red blood cells, haemoglobin, lung capacity, pulmonary ventilation, and oxygen uptake than females during adolescence[44] (see Chapter 12). When both early and late maturers are fully grown and have achieved the same stature, the differences in $\dot{V}O_2$ max disappear.

Conclusions

Paediatric exercise science examines the acute and chronic responses of the child and adolescent to both exercise and PA. Of primary interest are the physiological changes, PA, and health-related outcomes during childhood and adolescence, and the differences of the aforementioned between sexes, and between children and adults. It is important to understand that the prenatal and infant environment influence long-term trajectories of growth as well as disease status later in life. The time period that shows greatest differences in growth is at the onset of pubertal development. Because children of the same age do not all follow the same tempo and timing of biological maturity (i.e. there are early, average, and late maturers), it is essential to consider growth and maturity confounders when studying paediatric exercise physiology. For example, many studies have found that participation in PA decreases during adolescence and that the decline in PA is more pronounced in girls than in boys.[46–49] However, when aligned by biological age (years from PHV), PA measured either subjectively[48] or objectively[49] (see Chapter 21) is not significantly different at any biological age between the sexes. This highlights the importance of understanding the difference between chronological and biological ages.

Summary

- The process of growth and maturation is continuous throughout childhood and adolescence, with girls, on average, experiencing the onset of puberty about 2 years before of boys.
- Although all young people follow the same pattern of growth from birth into full maturity, there is considerable variation both between and within sexes in the timing and magnitude of these changes.
- During adolescence boys become considerably larger and acquire broader shoulders, whereas girls enlarge their pelvic diameter and have increased deposits of fat in various places like the breast.
- Adolescent males lay down a considerably greater amount of lean tissue compared to girls, and this increase in skeletal size and muscle mass leads to increased strength in males.
- Within an age group, early maturers are, on average, taller, heavier, and have a larger fat-free mass (especially boys) and fat mass (especially girls) than late maturers.
- The effects of a child's maturation, in a biological context, may mask or be greater than the effects associated with exposure to physical activity or exercise, and the paediatric exercise scientist must therefore include an assessment of biological age in their study design.
- Indicators of skeletal, sexual, and somatic maturation are moderately to highly correlated during adolescence, although no single indicator provides a complete description of the tempo of growth and maturation.
- It is suggested that for sex specific comparisons, any of the discussed methods are appropriate. However, for studies that make sex comparisons, either skeletal age or one of the somatic indices should be used.

References

1. Thompson D'AW. *On growth and form*. Cambridge: Cambridge University Press; 1942.
2. Tanner JM. *The physique of the Olympic athlete*. London: George Allen and Unwin Ltd; 1964.
3. Malina RM. Physical growth and biological maturation of young athletes. *Exerc Sport Sci Rev*. 1994; 22: 389–434.
4. Caine D, Bass SL, Daly R. Does elite competition inhibit growth and delay maturation in some gymnasts? Quite possibly. *Pediatr Exerc Sci*. 2003; 15: 360–372.
5. Malina RM, Baxter-Jones ADG, Armstrong N, Beunen GP, Caine D, Daly RM, Lewis RD, Rogol AD, Russell K. Role of intensive training on growth and maturation in artistic gymnasts. *Sports Med*. 2013; 43: 783–802.
6. Barker DJB. *Fetal and infant origins of adult disease*. London: BMJ Publishing Group; 1992.
7. Thomis MA, Towne B. Genetic determinants of prepubertal and pubertal growth and development. *Food Nutr Bull*. 2006; 27 (suppl.): S257–S79.
8. Malina RM, Bouchard C, Bar-Or O. *Growth, maturation, and physical activity*, 2nd ed. Champaign, IL: Human Kinetics; 2004.
9. Baxter-Jones ADG, Eisenmann JC, Sherar LB. Controlling for maturation in pediatric exercise science. *Pediatr Exerc Sci*. 2005; 17: 18–30.
10. Salkind NJ. *Child development*. New York: Macmillan; 2002.
11. Cameron N, Demerath EW. Critical periods in human growth and their relationship to disease of aging. *Yearbook Phys Anthrop*. 2002; 45: 159–84.
12. Scammon RE. The first seriatim study of human growth. *Am J Phys Anthrop*. 1927; 10: 329–36.
13. Tanner JM. *Foetus into man*. London: Castlemead Publications; 1978.
14. Baxter-Jones A, Mirwald R. Multilevel modelling. In: Hauspie RC, Cameron N, Molinari L (eds.) *Methods in Human Growth Research*. Cambridge: Cambridge University Press; 2004. p. 306–330.
15. Scammon RE. The measurement of the body in childhood. In: Harris JA, Jackson CM, Paterson DG, Scammon RE (eds.) *The measurement of man*. Minneapolis: University of Minnesota Press; 1930. p. 173–215.
16. Zemel B, Barden E. Measuring body composition. In: Hauspie RC, Cameron N, Molinari L (eds.) *Methods in human growth research*. Cambridge: Cambridge University Press; 2004. p. 141–178.
17. Jones PRM, Norgan NG. Anthropometry and the assessment of body composition. In: Harries M, Williams C, Stanish WD, Micheli LJ (eds.) *Oxford textbook of sports medicine*. Oxford: Oxford University Press; 1994. p. 149–160.
18. Iuliano-Burnes S, Mirwald RL, Bailey DA. Timing and magnitude of peak height velicity and peak tissue velocities for early, average, and late maturing boys and girls. *Am J Hum Biol*. 2001; 13: 1–8.
19. Rupich RC, Specker BL, Lieuw AF, Ho M. (1996). Gender and race differences in bone mass during infancy. *Calc Tiss Int*. 1996; 58: 395–397.
20. Maynard LM, Guo SS, Chumlea WC, *et al*. Total-body and regional bone mineral content and areal bone mineral density in children aged 8–18 y: the Fels Longitudinal Study. *Am J Clin Nutr*. 1998; 68: 1111–1117.
21. Baxter-Jones ADG, Mirwald RL, McKay HA, Bailey DA. A longitudinal analysis of sex differences in bone mineral accrual in healthy 8- to 19-year-old boys and girls. *Ann Hum Biol*. 2003; 30: 160–175.
22. Rolland-Cachera M-F. Adiposity rebound and prediction of adult fatness. In: Ulijaszek SJ, Johnston FE, Preece MA (eds.) *The Cambridge encyclopedia of human growth and development*. Cambridge: Cambridge University Press; 1998. p. 51–53.
23. Norgan NG. Body composition. In: Ulijaszek SJ, Johnston FE, Preece MA (eds.) *The Cambridge encyclopedia of human growth and development*. Cambridge: Cambridge University Press; 1998. p. 212–215.
24. Armstrong N, Welsman J. *Young people and physical activity*. Oxford: Oxford University Press; 1997.
25. Ellison PT. Puberty. In: Cameron N (ed.) *Human growth and development*. San Deigo: Academic Press; 2002. p. 65–84.
26. Reynolds EL, Wines JV. Physical changes associated with adolescence in boys. *Am J Dis Child*. 1951; 82: 529–547.
27. Tanner JM. *Growth at adolescence*, 2nd ed. Oxford: Blackwell Scientific Publications; 1962.
28. Boas F. Observations on the growth of children. *Science*. 1930; 72: 44–48.
29. Hindmarsh P. Endocrinological regulation of post-natal growth. In: Ulijaszek SJ, Johnston FE, Preece MA (eds.) *The Cambridge encyclopedia of human growth and development*. Cambridge: Cambridge University Press; 1998. p. 212–215.
30. Rogol AD, Roemmich JN, Clark PA. Growth at puberty. *J Adolesc Health*. 2002; 31: 192–200.

31. Matsuo H, Babba Y, Nair RMG, Arimura A, Schaly AV. Structure of the porcine LH- and FSH-releasing hormone. *Biochem Biophy Res Commun*. 1971; 43: 1334–1339.
32. Carmel PW, Araki S, Ferin M. Pituitary stalk portal blood collection in rhesus monkeys: Evidence for pulsatile release of GnRH. *Endocrinol.* 1976; 99: 243–248.
33. Beil JD, Patton JM, Dailey RA, Tsou RC, Tindall GT. Luteinizing hormone releasing hormone (LHRH) in pituitary portal blood of rhesus monkeys: Relationship to level of LH release. *Endocrinol.* 1977; 101: 430–434.
34. Yen SSC. The human menstrual cycle: Neuroendocrine regulation. In: Yen SSC, Jaffe RB (eds.) *Reproductive endocrinology*, 3rd ed. Philadelphia: Saunders; 1991. p. 273–308.
35. Hall PF. Testicular steroid synthesis: organization and regulation. In: Knobil E, Neill JD (eds.) *The physiology of reproduction*. New York: Raven Press; 1998. p. 975–998.
36. Boyar RM. Control of the onset of puberty. *Ann Rev Med.* 1978; 29: 509–520.
37. Libanti C, Baylink DJ, Lois-Wenzel E, Srinvasan N, Mohan S. Studies on the potential mediators of skeletal changes occurring during puberty in girls. *J Clin Endocrinol Metab*. 1999; 84: 2807–2814.
38. Lackey BR, Gray SL, Henricks DM. The insulin-like growth factor (IGF) system and gonadotropin regulation: Actions and interactions. *Cytokine Growth Factor Rev*. 1999; 10: 201–217.
39. Kulin HE, Grumbach MM, Kaplan SL. Changing sesnsitivity of the pubertal gonadal hypothalamic feedback mechanism in man. *Science*. 1969; 166: 1012–1013.
40. Plant TM. Puberty in primates. In: Knobil E, Neill JD (eds.) *The physiology of reproduction*. New York: Raven Press; 1988. p. 1763–1788.
41. Mirwald RL. Saskatchewan growth and development study. In: Ostyn M, Beunen G, Simons J (eds.) *Kinanthropometry II*. Baltimore: University Park Press; 1978. p. 289–305.
42. Cameron N. Assessment of maturation. In: Cameron N (ed.) *Human growth and development*. San Deigo: Academic Press; 2002. p. 65–84.
43. Marshall WA, Tanner JM (1969). Variations in the pattern of pubertal changes in girls. *Arch Dis Child*, 44, 291–303.
44. Marshall WA, Tanner JM (1970). Variations in the pattern of pubertal changes in boys. *Arch Dis Child*, 45, 13–23.
45. Kemper HC, Verschuur R. Maximal aerobic power in 13- and 14-year-old teenagers in relation to biologic age. *Int J Sports Med.* 1981; 2: 97–100.
46. Riddoch CJ, Andersen LB, Wedderkopp N, *et al.* Physical activity levels and patterns of 9- and 15-yr-old European children. *Med Sci Sports Exerc*. 2004; 36: 86–92.
47. Trost SG, Pate RR, Sallis JF, *et al.* Age and gender differences in objectively measured physical activity in youth. *Med Sci Sports Exerc*. 2002; 34: 350–355.
48. Thompson AM, Baxter-Jones AD, Mirwald RL, Bailey DA. Comparison of physical activity in male and female children: does maturation matter? *Med Sci Sports Exerc*. 2003; 35: 1684–1690.
49. Sherar LB, Esliger DW, Baxter-Jones ADG, Tremblay MS. Age and gender related differences in childhood physical activity: Does physical maturity matter? *Med Sci Sports Exerc*. 2007; 39: 830–835.

CHAPTER 3

Developmental biodynamics

The development of coordination

James Watkins

Introduction

Human movement is brought about by the musculoskeletal system under the control of the nervous system. The skeletal muscles pull on the bones to control the movements of the joints and, in doing so, control the movement of the body as a whole. By coordination of the various muscle groups, the forces generated by the muscles are transmitted by the bones and joints to enable the application of forces to the external environment, usually via the hands and feet, so that humans can adopt upright postures (counteract the constant tendency of body weight to collapse the body), transport the body, and manipulate objects, often simultaneously.[1] The forces generated and transmitted by the musculoskeletal system are referred to as internal forces. Body weight and the forces that are applied to the external environment are referred to as external forces. At any point in time body weight cannot be changed, and as such body weight is a passive external force. The external forces that are actively generated are active external forces. The magnitude, duration, and timing of the active external forces are determined by the magnitude, duration, and timing of the internal forces. Biomechanics is the study of the forces that act on and within living organisms and the effect of the forces on the size, shape, structure, and movement of the organisms.[2]

The brain coordinates and controls movement via muscular activity.[3] Coordination refers to the timing of relative motion between body segments and control refers to the optimization of relative motion between body segments, i.e. the extent to which the kinematics of segmental motion and, consequently, the motion of the whole body centre of gravity (CG), matches the demands of the task.[4] For example, the mature form of coordination of the leg action in a countermovement vertical jump, as shown in Figure 3.1, is characterized by simultaneous flexion of the hips, knees, and ankles in the countermovement phase (Figure 3.1a–c), followed by simultaneous extension of the hips, knees, and ankles in the propulsion phase (Figure 3.1c–e). This pattern of coordination normally occurs between 3 and 4 years of age.[4] However, whereas most mature individuals exhibit similar coordination in the countermovement vertical jump (and other whole body movements), there are considerable differences in the extent to which individuals can control the movement, that is, optimize the relative motion of the body segments in order to match the task demands.[4]

If the objective in performing a countermovement vertical jump is to maximize height jumped (upward vertical displacement of the whole body CG measured from the floor) then control of the movement is concerned with maximizing the height of the CG at take-off (h_1) and maximizing the upward vertical displacement of the CG after take-off (h_2) (Figure 3.1e and f). The height of the CG at take-off (h_1) is determined by body position which, in turn, is determined by the range of motion in the joints and the extent to which the available range of motion is used. The upward vertical displacement of the CG after take-off (h_2) is determined by the vertical velocity of the CG at take-off, and therefore the greater the vertical component of take-off velocity, the greater h_2. The vertical component of take-off velocity is determined by the impulse of the vertical component of the resultant ground reaction force (the force exerted between the feet and the floor) prior to take-off, so the larger the impulse the greater the velocity. The impulse $F \cdot t$ of the vertical component of the resultant ground reaction force F is determined by the magnitude of F and its duration t; the larger the force and the longer its duration the larger the impulse. The magnitude of F will depend upon the strength of the jumper's muscles, especially the extensor muscles of the hips, knees, and ankles. The duration of F will depend upon the ranges of motion in the jumper's hips, knees, and ankles and the extent to which the available ranges of motion are used. Clearly, restricted ranges of motion in any of the joints, especially hips, knees, and ankles, and lack of strength in any of the muscles, especially the extensor muscles of the hips, knees, and ankles, will adversely affect the jumper's ability to control the movement and, consequently, result in less-than-optimal performance.

There are numerous studies of jumping performance in adults, especially elite athletes.[5,6] However, there are relatively few studies on the development of coordination and control of jumping in young children. Jensen *et al.*[4] investigated coordination and control in the countermovement vertical jump in two groups of young children (mean ± standard deviation (SD) age = 3.4 ± 0.5 years) and a group of skilled adults. The two groups of children ($n_1 = n_2 = 9$) were selected from a larger group ($n = 32$) on the basis of their take-off angle (angle of velocity vector of the whole body CG at take-off) into a high take-off group (HT0) and low take-off group (LT0). Take-off angle is a key control variable, since to maximize vertical displacement after take-off, the take-off angle should be 90° (with respect to the horizontal). The criterion for inclusion in the HT0 and LT0 groups was a take-off angle at least 1 SD greater or less than the total group mean, respectively. All jumps were performed on a force platform to measure the ground reaction force. To encourage maximum effort, a suspended ball, just out of reach, was used as a visual target. Coordination was assessed by examining the timing of reversals (between the countermovement and propulsion phases

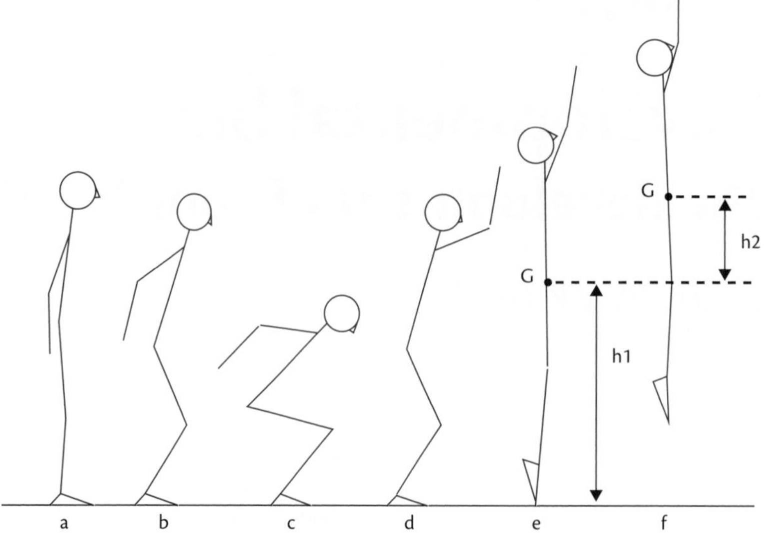

Figure 3.1 Stick figure sequence of a countermovement vertical jump from a standing position.
a = standing position.
a to c = countermovement or dip phase.
c to e = propulsion phases.
G = whole body centre of gravity.
h1 = height of G above the floor.
h2 = upward vertical displacement fo G after take-off.

of the jump) of the hip, knee, and ankle joints and the timing of the peak extension velocities of the hip, knee, and ankle joints. Control was assessed by examining the body position (hip, knee, and ankle joint angles) at three events during the jump; the time of maximum acceleration downward (minimum vertical ground reaction force), the time of maximum acceleration upward (maximum vertical ground reaction force), and take-off.

No significant differences were found between the three groups with regard to the coordination variables. This finding is consistent with the results of a study by Clark *et al.*[7] of 3, 4, 7, and 9-year-old children involving the same task and methodology. The mean take-off angles for the adults, HT0, and LT0 groups—91.8° ± 3.8°, 82.0° ± 3.5°, and 61.2° ± 5.6° respectively—were significantly different from each other and the mean of the adult group was closest to the theoretically desired angle of 90°. There were also significant differences between the groups in some of the other control variables (hip, knee, and ankle angles) at one or more of the three events, in particular, the ankle angle between adults and both child groups at take-off and the knee angle between all three groups at take-off. The small mean angle of take-off of the LT0 group was found to be associated with a large (relative to the adults and HT0 groups) forward displacement of the CG during the countermovement and propulsion phases, that is, the trajectory of the CG was V-shaped, downward and forward then upward and forward. In contrast, the trajectory of the CG of the adults was U-shaped, downward, and very slightly forward then upward and very slightly forward. The trajectory of the CG of the HT0 group was in between those of the adult and LT0 groups. In general, the smaller the forward displacement of the CG, the greater the take-off angle and vice versa. Whereas the HT0 and LT0 groups had smaller take-off angles than the adult group, the HT0 and LT0 groups still accomplished a clearly recognizable vertical jump, although the jumps were simply not optimized for maximum vertical displacement of the CG. Jensen *et al.*[4] concluded that the performances of the children were coordinated but poorly controlled, due perhaps to inadequate strength of the leg extensor muscles, especially during the braking period of the countermovement phase (the period when the downward velocity of the CG is reduced to zero).

Development of coordination and control

The human neuromusculoskeletal system consists of approximately 10^{11} neurons, 10^3 muscles, and 10^2 moveable joints.[3,8] The way that the nervous system organizes movement in the face of such complexity has been viewed historically from two viewpoints: the neuromaturational perspective and the information-processing perspective.[8]

The neuromaturational perspective has been used primarily to explain motor development in infants and children. The neuromaturational perspective arose from the work of Gesell and Thompson,[9] and McGraw[10] who observed and described the gradual and sequential development of motor skills in infants from apparently unintentional reflex movements through the development of intentional movements like crawling, sitting, standing, and walking. The legacy of Gesell and McGraw was twofold: first, the assumption that motor development was sequential and inevitable, and, second, that progress directly reflected the gradual maturation of the nervous system.[11] This view became widely held and the age norms for the emergence of motor skills in infants and children produced by Gesell and McGraw became, and still are, widely used.[11] Whereas neuromaturation is undeniably a major determinant of motor development in infants and children, it does not explain skill acquisition in adults where the nervous system is considered to be fully mature.[12]

Traditionally, the information-processing perspective has dominated theories of skill acquisition in adults.[13] From the information-processing perspective, the brain is regarded rather like a computer with a very large number of motor programmes which can be executed at will to match the specific demands of each movement task as defined by the available sensory information. However, similar to the neuromaturational perspective, the information-processing perspective does not account for the great flexibility demonstrated by individuals in accommodating rapidly changing task demands, especially in the context of sports.[14]

The deficiencies of the neuromaturational and information-processing perspectives were pointed out by Bernstein.[15] He argued that the complexity of the neuromusculoskeletal system was such that a one-to-one relationship between activity in the nervous system and actual movements was not possible, i.e. that the nervous system cannot simultaneously directly control the activity of every nerve cell. Consequently, it then cannot simultaneously directly control the activity of every muscle cell. He also pointed out that a particular set of muscular contractions is not always associated with the same movement pattern, and that not all movements are controlled by the nervous system. For example, if you raise your arm to the side by using the shoulder abductor muscles and then relax the muscles, the arm will fall down under its own weight without any involvement of the nervous system. Similarly, if you hold your arm with the upper arm horizontal, the lower arm vertical, and the wrist relaxed, and then alternately slightly flex and extend the elbow fairly rapidly, the hand will flail about the wrist due to its own inertia and the force exerted on the hand at the wrist by the movement of the lower arm; again this happens without any involvement of the nervous system. At any particular point in time each body segment may be acted on by five kinds of forces, which can be classified in two ways[16]; internal (muscle, articular, inertial) and external (gravitational, contact) forces, and active (muscle) and passive (articular, inertial, gravitational, contact) forces. Muscle forces are the forces exerted by active muscles. Articular forces arise from passive deformations of inactive muscles, tendons, ligaments and other connective tissues. Inertial forces are the forces exerted on one segment arising from the motion of other segments linked to it. Gravitational force is the weight of the segment. Contact forces are forces acting on the segment that result from contact of the segment with the physical environment, such as the floor.

Reference axes and degrees of freedom

It is useful to refer to three mutually perpendicular axes—anteroposterior, transverse, and vertical—when describing the movement of a joint (Figure 3.2). With respect to the three reference axes there are six possible directions, called degrees of freedom, in which a joint, depending upon its structure, may be able to move. The six directions consist of three linear directions (along the axes) and three angular directions (around the axes). Most of the joints in the body have between one and three degrees of freedom. Most movements of the body involve simultaneous movement in a number of joints, and the degrees of freedom of the whole segmental chain is the sum of the degrees of freedom of the individual joints in the chain. For example, if the wrist (comprised of eight small irregular shaped bones) is regarded as a single joint with two degrees of freedom (flexion-extension and abduction-adduction) then the arm has approximately 25 joints (joints of the shoulder, elbow, wrist, and fingers) and approximately 35 degrees of freedom.

Coordination and degrees of freedom

Bernstein[15] pointed out that in any motor skill (purposeful task-oriented movement) that involves a part of or the whole body, like reaching with an arm from a seated position, the total number of

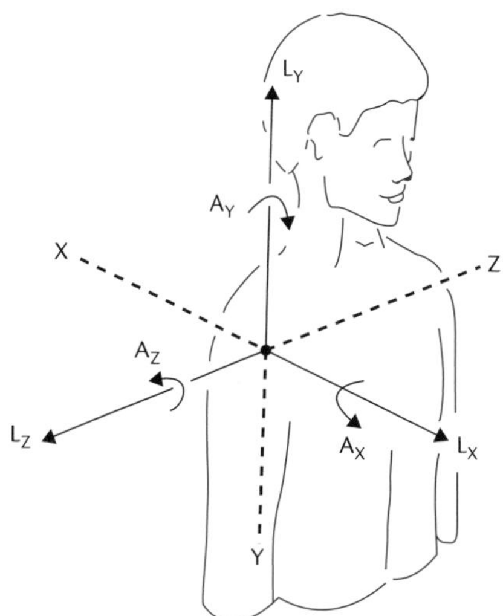

Figure 3.2 Linear and angular degrees of freedom with respect to the shoulder joint.
X = anteroposterior axis.
Y = vertical axis.
Z = Transverse axis.
L_x = linear motion along X axis.
L_y = linear motion along Y axis.
L_z = linear motion along Z axis.
A_x = angular motion about X axis.
A_y = linear motion along Y axis.
A_z = linear motion along Z axis.

degrees of freedom of the joints involved normally greatly exceeds the number of degrees of freedom that are minimally necessary to accomplish the task. Consequently, when learning a new or unfamiliar motor skill, Bernstein described the problem for the learner as 'the process of mastering redundant degrees of freedom'[15(p.127)], i.e. reducing the number of degrees of freedom to a manageable number. He suggested that there are essentially three stages in the development of motor skill. In the first stage, the influence of the many degrees of freedom is restricted by i) minimizing the ranges of motion in the joints and ii) forming temporary strong couplings between the joints e.g. moving multiple joints in close phase relations. The latter is likely to compress the many degrees of freedom into a much smaller number of virtual degrees of freedom which, in turn, is likely to simplify neuromuscular control. The second stage is characterized by the establishment of relatively stable phase relations between the movements of the joints, in association with changes in joint kinematics (ranges of motion and angular velocities). The notion of a functional assembly of relatively stable phase relations has been referred to as a 'coordinative structure'[17] and a 'coordinative mode'.[18] The third stage is characterized by an increase in economy of movement (reduction in energy expenditure) by exploitation of the passive forces in a manner that minimizes the active forces i.e. the work done by muscles, and maximizes mechanical energy conservation i.e. facilitating mechanical energy exchanges, potential to kinetic and vice-versa, and energy transfer between segments.

Most of the muscles (muscle-tendon units) of the body cross over more than one joint. These muscles, such as the rectus femoris and hamstrings, are usually referred to as biarticular muscles, since muscles which cross over more than two joints function in the same way as muscles that cross over just two joints.[19] Biarticular muscles are too short to fully flex or fully extend all the joints that

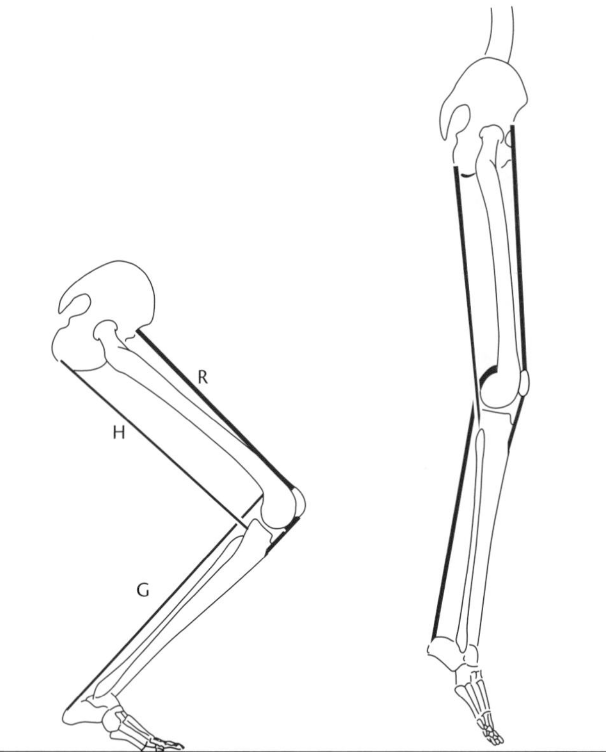

Figure 3.3 Coupling of the trunk, upper leg and lower leg by the rectus femoris, hamstrings and gastrocnemius.

The trunk is linked to the lower leg by the hamstrings (H) and the rectus femoris (R) and the upper leg is linked to the foot by the gastrocnemius (G). If the length of H, R and G are approximately set, hip extension will result in simultaneous knee extension and ankle plantar flexion.

Adapted from Ingen Schenau GJV. From translation to rotation: constraints on multijoint movements and the unique action of biarticular muscles. Hum Mov Sci. 1989; 8: 301–337.

they cross over simultaneously. For example, the hamstrings are too short to fully extend the hip and fully flex the knee at the same time; indeed, hip extension is usually associated with knee extension and hip flexion is usually associated with knee flexion, as in a countermovement vertical jump[20,21] (Figure 3.3). Consequently, anatomical constraints, like biarticular muscles, tend to reduce the range of movements that are possible in a segmental chain such that the apparent degrees of freedom in the segmental chain may be lower than initially appears. For example, Valero-Cuevas[22] demonstrated that biarticular muscles and their specialized aponeuroses in the human hand couple the degrees of freedom of the corresponding joints and constrain possible patterns of use. Such contraints are likely to simplify neuromuscular control.

Bernstein's three stages of motor skill development are now generally accepted[23,24] and supported by an increasing volume of empirical data.[25,26,27,28] Recent technological improvements, including multi-camera systems allied to subject-mounted wireless accelerometers, have facilitated more ecological (real-world) studies of the biomechanics of coordination.[29,30] However, there still appear to be few studies which have clearly related kinematics to kinetics, investigated the effects of practice, or involved children.

Kinematics of coordination

Whereas control of movement is essential to maximize performance, the development of coordination is a necessary precursor to the development of control. This was demonstrated by Anderson and Sidaway[26] in a study of the effects of practice on performance in kicking. A novice group of right foot dominant subjects, five males and one female (mean age 20.3 years, age range 18–22 years) was selected on the basis of no previous experience of organized soccer or soccer training. An expert group of three males (mean age 25.2 years, age range 22–30 years), each with more than 10 years experience of organized soccer, was included in the study in order to determine whether the coordination of the three experts was similar, and to compare the pre- and post-practice coordination of the novices with the experts. The task to be learned (only the novice group took part in the practice sessions) was a right-footed instep drive at a 2 m^2 target placed 5 m from the ball following a two step approach. The primary goal was to maximize the velocity of the ball while trying to hit the target. The subjects practised twice a week for 10 weeks and had between 15 and 20 trials during each session. Prior to and after the practice period, three trials of each subject were videotaped with a single camera placed perpendicular to the plane of motion on the right side of the subject. By using markers on the right shoulder, right hip, right knee, right ankle, and right small toe (Figure 3.4), the angular displacement and angular velocity of the hip and knee and linear velocity of the foot (toe) was found for each subject at 60 Hz throughout each trial. From the linear and angular velocity data and the angular displacement data, three velocity measures, three timing measures, and two ranges of motion were derived for each subject in each trial (see Table 3.1). As each subject exhibited a high degree of consistency with regard to the eight variables, the data were averaged across the three trials.

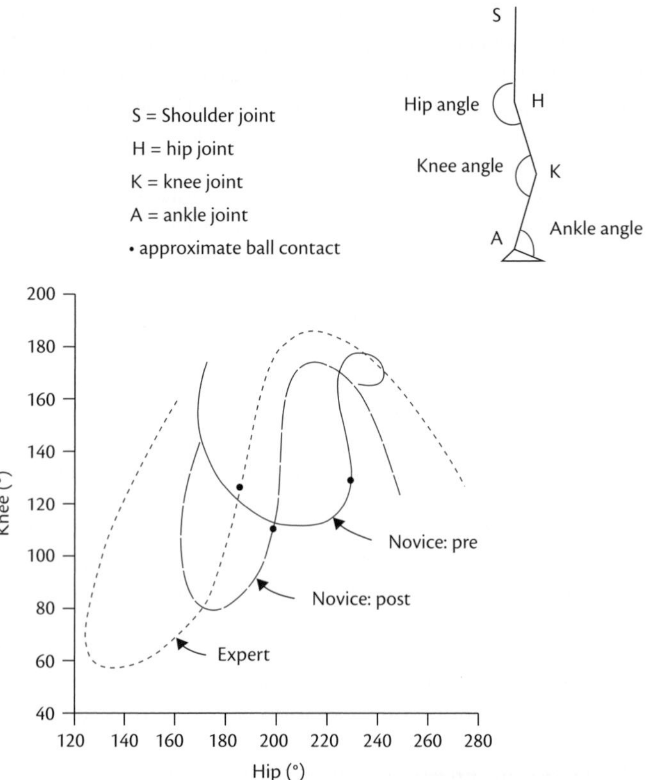

Figure 3.4 Kicking a soccer ball: hip angle-knee angle diagrams for one representative novice's performance, pre and postpractice, and one representative expert's performance.

Adapted from Anderson DI, Sidaway B. Coordination changes associated with practice of a soccer kick. Res Q Exerc Sport. 1994; 65: 93–99.

Table 3.1 Kicking a soccer ball: means, standard deviations, and comparative data for foot linear velocity, hip and knee angular velocity, timing*, and hip joint and knee joint ranges of motion for novice and expert subjects.

NoviceExpert									
Pre-practice	**Post-practice**								
	Mean	**SD**	**%E**	**Mean**	**SD**	**%E**	**%pp**	**Mean**	**SD**
MFLV ($m \cdot s^{-1}$)	14.9	1.7	58	21.9	1.5	85	47	25.6	1.1
MHAV ($deg \cdot s^{-1}$)	671	77	78	685	168	79	2.1	864	49
MKAV ($deg \cdot s^{-1}$)	1146	213	77	1287	251	86	12.3	1494	115
SKE/IMHAV	1.02	0.06	117	0.89	0.05	102	−13	0.87	0.03
IMHAV/IMKAV	0.61	0.1	77	0.69	0.03	87	13	0.79	0.01
IMKAV/IMFLV	1.14	0.06	109	1.04	0.05	100	−8.7	1.04	0.03
Hip ROM (deg)	86	14	64	103	21	77	19.8	135	9.5
Knee ROM (deg)	90	16	75	104	13	86	14.5	121	5.7

MFLV: maximum foot linear velocity; MHAV: maximum hip angular velocity; MKAV: maximum knee angular velocity; SKE: start of knee extension; I: Instant of; %E: percent of expert value; %pp: percent difference between pre- and post-practice.

* The ratios of the durations of the events (SKE, IMHAV, IMKAV, IMFLV) measured from the start of the backswing of the right leg. A ratio greater than 1.0 indicates that the numerator event occurred after the denominator event, and vice-versa.

Source data from Anderson DI, Sidaway B. Coordination changes associated with practice of a soccer kick. Res Q Exerc Sport. 1994; 65: 93–99.

Table 3.1 shows the group means and standard deviations for the eight variables for the novices, pre- and post-practice, and the experts, together with percentage changes pre- and post-practice for the novices, and percentage comparison of the novices, pre- and post-practice, with the experts. It is clear that the performance of the novices, in terms of maximum foot linear velocity (which reflects ball velocity) improved considerably with practice (47%) but was still well below that of the experts (85%) post-practice. However, the 47% increase in maximum foot linear velocity was associated with much smaller increases in maximum hip angular velocity (2.1%), maximum knee angular velocity (12.3%), hip range of motion (19.8%), and knee range of motion (14.5%). These changes, especially the angular velocity changes, suggest that improvement in performance resulted largely from a change in coordination rather than from an increase in the speed of execution of the pre-practice movement pattern. This interpretation is supported by the change in the timing variables which were much closer to those of the experts post-practice than pre-practice (see Table 3.1). It is also supported by the change in relative motion of the thigh and lower leg as reflected in the representative knee angle—hip angle diagrams shown in Figure 3.4. The post-practice pattern was similar to that of the experts, which suggests that the novices had developed coordination. However, comparison of the novice post-practice and expert linear and angular velocities and ranges of motion in Table 3.1 indicates that control was less than optimal. The results of the study provide support for Bernstein's theory of motor skill acquisition, i.e. development of coordination (establishment of a coordinative structure) followed by development of control (changes in joint kinematics).

Kinetics of coordination

A kinematic analysis describes the way an object moves, that is, the changes in linear and/or angular displacement, velocity, and acceleration of the object with respect to time. To understand why an object moves the way that it does, it is necessary to carry out a kinetic analysis, i.e. an analysis of the impulses and timing of the impulses of the forces acting on the object during the movement. With regard to human movement this involves analysis of the active and passive forces acting on each body segment.

Modelling

Each body segment is comprised of hard and soft tissues. Whereas the segment may deform to a certain extent during movement, the amount of deformation is usually very small and, as such, for the purpose of biomechanical analysis, the body segments may be regarded as rigid.[31] Consequently, the human body may be regarded as a system of rigid segments with the main segments (head, trunk, upper arms, forearms, hands, thighs, lower legs, and feet) linked by freely moveable joints.

Free body diagram

Kamm *et al.*[32] carried out kinetic analyses of spontaneous leg movements in infants while reclined at 45°, as shown in Figure 3.5a. Figures 3.5b and 3.5c show free body diagrams of the thigh and the combined lower leg and foot of the right leg, that is, sketches of the segments showing all of the forces acting on them. It is assumed that the movement of the legs takes place in the sagittal plane (X-Y plane with respect to Figure 3.5). There are no contact forces acting on the segments and, as such, the only forces shown are the weights of the segments acting at the segmental CGs, and the force distributions around the hip and knee joints. It can be shown that any force distribution is equivalent to the resultant force R acting at an arbitrary point P together with a couple C equal to the resultant moment of the force distribution about P.[31] The combination of R (acting at P) and C is referred to as the equipollent of the force distribution. In a kinetic analysis of human movement, it is usual to show the force distribution around a joint as the equipollent with respect to the joint centre. In Figures 3.5b and 3.5c, the equipollent of the force distribution around the hip joint (IF_H) is shown as F_H and M_H, and the equipollent of the force distribution around the knee joint is (IF_K) shown as F_K and M_K. In Figures 3.5d and 3.5e, the resultant forces through the hip and knee joint centres are replaced by their horizontal (F_{HX}, F_{KX}) and vertical (F_{HY}, F_{KY}) components.

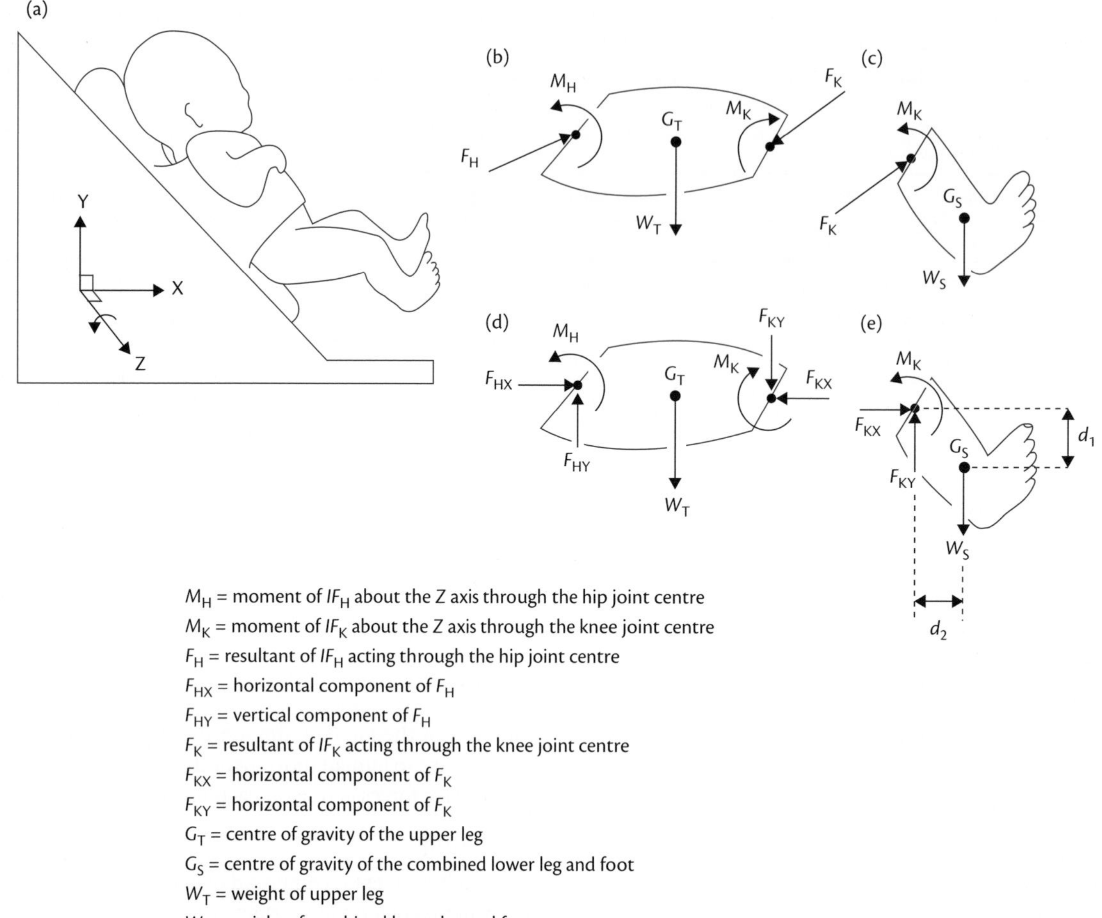

Figure 3.5 Free body diagrams of the thigh and combined lower leg and foot of the right leg of a 3 month old infant inclined at 45°.
(a) Infant inclined at 45°; (b) free body diagram of right upper leg; (c) free body diagram of combined right lower leg and foot; (d) free body diagram of right upper leg with resultant joint forces replaced by horizontal and vertical components; (e) free body diagram of combined right lower leg and foot with resultant joint forces replaced by horizontal and vertical components.

Components of net joint moment

Each segment will move in accordance with Newton's laws of motion. Consequently, with respect to the lower leg and foot segment:

$$F_X = ma_x \quad (3.1)$$

$$F_Y = ma_y \quad (3.2)$$

$$M_Z = I\alpha \quad (3.3)$$

where F_X = resultant of horizontal forces acting on the segment; F_Y = resultant of vertical forces acting on the segment; m = mass of the lower leg and foot; a_x = horizontal component of the linear acceleration of the CG of the segment; a_y = vertical component of the linear acceleration of the CG of the segment; M_Z = resultant moment about the Z axis through the CG of the segment; I = moment of inertia of the segment about the Z axis through the CG of the segment; α = angular acceleration of the segment about the Z axis through the CG of the segment.

From Equations (3.1), (3.2), and (3.3) it follows that:

$$F_{KX} = ma_x \quad (3.4)$$

$$F_{KY} - W_S = ma_y \quad (3.5)$$

$$M_K - F_{KX}d_1 - F_{KY}d_2 = I\alpha \quad (3.6)$$

From equation (3.5),

$$F_{KY} = ma_y + W_S \quad (3.7)$$

By substitution of F_{KX} from Eqn (3.4) and F_{KY} from Eqn (3.7) into Eqn (3.6),

$$M_K - ma_xd_1 - (ma_y + W_S)d_2 = I\alpha$$

$$M_K - ma_xd_1 - ma_yd_2 - W_Sd_2 = I\alpha$$

$$M_K - (ma_xd_1 + ma_yd_2) - W_Sd_2 = I\alpha$$

M_K = Generalized Muscle Moment (*MUS*): the moment arising from active muscles and passive deformations of inactive muscles, tendons, ligaments, and other connective tissues about the Z axis through the knee joint centre, that is, the moment exerted by active muscles and articular forces about the joint. $(ma_xd_1 + ma_yd_2)$ = Motion Dependent Moment (*MDM*) (also referred to as the inertial moment): the moment acting on the segment as a result of the motion of adjacent segments, that is, the thigh. $W_S d_2$ = Gravitational Moment (*GRAV*): the moment acting on the segment due to its weight. $I\alpha$ = Net Joint Moment (*NET*): the resultant of *MUS*, *MDM*, and *GRAV* moments acting on the segment.

In this example, there is no external contact force, such as the ground reaction force in walking or running acting on the lower leg and foot segment. However, when there are contact forces, these must be included in the analysis of the components of joint moment. Consequently, the general equation relating the components of joint moment may be expressed as:

$$NET = MUS + GRAV + MDM + EXT \qquad (3.8)$$

EXT represents the moments about the joint exerted by one or more contact forces. The *NET* moment is the joint moment required to accomplish the task; it is clear from Eqn (3.8) that the *NET* moment may be influenced by each of the four component moments. The actual signs of the components in Eqn (3.8) would depend upon the directions of the components. The relationship between *MUS, GRAV, MDM*, and *EXT* is usually referred to as the biodynamics of joint movement.[15]

Bernstein[15] referred to the *MDM* component as 'reactive phenomena' when stating that,

> The secret of coordination lies not only in not wasting superfluous force on extinguishing reactive phenomena but, on the contrary, in employing the latter in such a way as to employ active muscle forces only in the capacity of complementary forces. In this case the same movement (in the final analysis) demands less expenditure of active force.[15(p.109)]

With current technology it is not possible to directly measure the forces which contribute to *MUS* or, therefore, to measure the separate contributions of muscle and articular forces to the *MUS*. However, since the *MUS* includes the only active (muscle) component of the *NET*, the *MUS* is particularly important for understanding coordination. Whereas *MUS* cannot be measured directly, it can be determined indirectly, i.e. $MUS = NET - MDM - GRAV - EXT$. *EXT* can usually be measured. For example, ground reaction force can be measured by a force platform. *NET, MDM*, and *GRAV* can be calculated directly by kinematic analysis of the movement of the body segments. This indirect method of determining *MUS* is referred to as indirect dynamics or inverse dynamics.[33] The converse of indirect dynamics, that is, determination of kinematics from directly measured kinetic (forces and moments of force) data is referred to as direct dynamics.[33]

In the study by Kamm *et al.*[32] of spontaneous leg movements in children reclined at 45°, it was found that the infants naturally produced kicks of varying degrees of vigour and range of motion. In general, the infants exhibited a consistent pattern of relative motion between trunk, thigh, and lower leg segments, suggesting a high level of coordination. The relationship between the *MUS, MDM*, and *GRAV* profiles was similar at the hip and knee joints. At slow speeds of movement the *MDM* were very small and the *MUS* served mainly to counteract the *GRAV* (Figure 3.6a). The *GRAV* profile, as expected, was similar at all kicking speeds. However, at fast speeds the *MUS* and *MDM* profiles were sinusoidal and out of phase by approximately 180°, suggesting that as speed of movement increased the main function of the *MUS* was to counteract the *MDM* (Figure 3.6b). The *MUS* profile was also found to be approximately 180° out of phase with the change in joint angle, i.e. the peaks of the *MUS* profile corresponded to changes in direction of movement of the segment. Since change in direction of movement is associated with eccentric muscle activity during the deceleration phase, the correspondence between the profiles of joint angle, *MUS*, and *MDM* suggest that coordinated movement tends to exploit the capacity of muscle-tendon units to store energy (in the elastic components during eccentric contractions) which, in turn, is likely to enhance energy conservation and reduce the energy expenditure

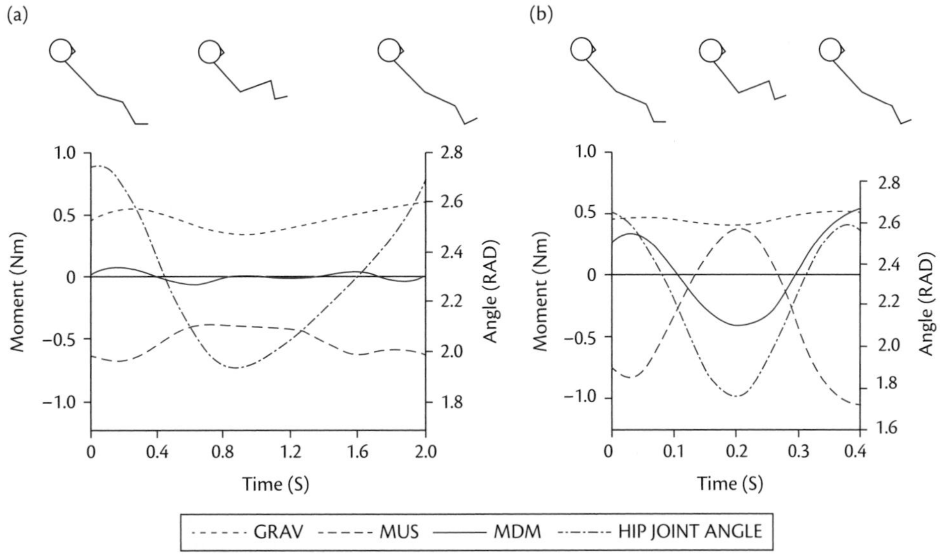

Figure 3.6 Profiles of generalized muscle moments (*MUS*), motion dependent moments (*MDM*), and gravitational moments (*GRAV*) about the hip joint in relation to hip joint angle for an infant performing a spontaneous nonvigorous kick (a) and a vigorous kick (b).

Adapted from Kamm K, Thelen E, Jensen J L. A dynamical systems approach to motor development. Phys Ther. 1990; 70: 763–775.

of the muscles. Schneider *et al.*[34] found similar correspondence between the profiles of joint angle (shoulder, elbow, and wrist), *MUS*, and *MDM* in adults performing a rapid reciprocal precision hand-placement task. The studies by Kamm *et al.*[32] and Schneider *et al.*[34] support the now generally-held view that the development of coordination and control involves a process of optimization of the passive and active components of joint moment around each joint in order to maximize the use of passive moments. This, in turn, decreases the contribution of active moments and, therefore, decreases energy expenditure. Lockman and Thelen[35] introduced the term 'developmental biodynamics' to describe the development of coordination and control in infants, or how infants learn to coordinate joint biodynamics.

Dynamical systems approach to development of coordination

Studies of spontaneous kicking,[32] reaching,[36] and stepping[37,38] clearly indicate that infants have a high level of coordination in spontaneous (non-task oriented, non-intentional) multi-joint limb movements, which suggests an intrinsic ability of the body segments to self-organize their relative motion.[39] Self-organization is a key feature of complex dynamical systems which, like the human body, have many degrees of freedom and are subject to a range of constraints.[40] Dynamical systems theory was developed nearly a century ago as an attempt to explain the way physical systems change over time.[8] Dynamical systems theory was first applied to coordination of human movement by Kugler *et al.*,[41] and since then concepts from dynamical systems have been increasingly used to explain the development of coordination.[42,43]

Self-organization and constraints

From a neuromaturational perspective, motor development in children is considered to result directly from the gradual maturation of the nervous system; the more mature the nervous system, the higher the level of motor skill displayed. Similarly, from an information-processing perspective, motor learning in adults is assumed to result from the triggering of established motor programmes. In contrast to these two perspectives, from a dynamical systems perspective, motor learning at any age (in humans and in all other animals) is regarded as a dynamic process whereby motor ability (the ability to perform motor skills) emerges from the intrinsic self-organizing properties of the dynamical system consisting of the individual, the task, and the environment.[7,44,45]

Self-organization refers to the spontaneous integration of the dynamical properties of the subsystems that comprise a system and results in the spontaneous establishment of a pattern of activity.[46] The actual pattern that emerges is dependent upon the constraints on the system. With regard to human movement, a constraint is any influence that serves to decrease the number of degrees of freedom that need to be controlled, that is, the constraints acting on the system limit the types of movement that can emerge.[18,22,47] Constraints can be broadly classified into three groups: individual, task, and environmental.[48]

Individual constraints, also referred to as organismic constraints, refer to the limitations imposed by the current status of the individual in terms of all aspects of physical, cognitive, and affective functions. There are essentially two types of task constraints: extrinsic and intrinsic.[47] Extrinsic task constraints refer to the mechanical requirements of the task which may include, for example, the speed (e.g. running for a bus) and/or precision (e.g. threading a needle) needed to successfully complete the task. Intrinsic task constraints refer to the individual's perception of the potential costs (e.g. energy expenditure and risk of injury) of particular types of movement that could be used to complete the task. There is clear evidence that individuals normally move in ways that tend to minimize energy expenditure (e.g. walk rather than run) and risk of injury (e.g. walk slowly rather than quickly on a slippery surface). Environmental constraints arise from the physical and socio-cultural environment.[8] Physical environmental constraints include, for example, weather conditions, conditions of light and heat, surface conditions, and the availability of protective clothing (e.g. in industry and sport). Socio-cultural environmental constraints include peer pressure and the pressure to behave in culturally acceptable ways.

All organisms within a species share a common gene pool (the sum total of all the genes in a species).[49] However, the genome of each individual organism (the genes and assembly of genes) is slightly different to all of the other organisms within the species. The genome determines ontogenesis, which is the innate process of development of the individual from zygote to maturity.[50] Ontogenesis is similar for all organisms within a species, but not identical because ontogenesis imposes individual constraints on development. Development is simultaneously influenced by environmental constraints; different environments tend to result in different rates of development.[42] Consequently, the actual development of an organism, referred to as epigenesis,[50] is the result of the interaction of individual and environmental constraints (see Chapter 32).

A main feature of the ontogeny of motor development is the propensity of infants to develop those behaviours that enable them to explore and interact with the environment (locomotion and manipulation skills).[42,51] Most normally developing infants experience similar motor development outcomes in terms of the timing and types of motor skills that emerge. From a dynamical systems perspective, these predictable early milestones emerge as the result of species-similar constraints.[7,42] From this perspective, the maturational status of the nervous system is regarded as a major individual constraint, but only one of many individual constraints that, together with task and environmental constraints, determine the form of movement that emerges. For example, while infants normally learn to crawl and then stand before walking,[51] there is no pre-determined programme for crawling. Crawling emerges as the best available solution to a particular motor problem (to travel in a particular direction), which is later replaced by the more effective and efficient solution of walking, which comes about as a result of changes in individual constraints.[42,51] Furthermore, as the constraints are continually changing, the system as a whole is in a constant state of flux. Therefore, no two movements are exactly the same.

The appropriateness of the dynamical systems approach to understanding motor development was clearly shown by Thelen and her colleagues in a series of studies on infant locomotion.[52–57] Thelen monitored the spontaneous behaviours of infants and found that certain behaviours appeared, disappeared and then re-appeared some time later.[53] For example, she found that infants exhibit from birth kicking movements when lying on their backs and stepping movements when they are held upright. She also observed that stepping disappeared within the first 3 months, only to re-appear a few weeks later, while kicking continued and increased in frequency over the same period. She also observed that infants who gained weight fastest were the first to stop stepping. Thelen reasoned that if the appearance and disappearance of stepping was due solely to nervous system maturation, then changing the prevailing environmental constraints, such as the effect of gravity, should not affect the behaviour. She tested the hypothesis by artificially increasing and decreasing the weight of the legs of the infants. She found that stepping behaviour disappeared when the weight of the infants' legs was increased by attaching small weights to the ankles; conversely, removing the weights restored the stepping behaviour. Furthermore, she found that the stepping behaviour could also be restored by submerging the infants' legs in water. The buoyancy provided by the water artificially reduced the weight of the infants' legs which, in turn, increases the strength: weight ratio of the leg to a level that restores the stepping behaviour. These observations clearly indicate that the strength:weight ratio is an important individual constraint that influences the motor behaviour of infants (see Chapter 4).

Most researchers agree that the development of strength and postural control are major influences on infants' rate of development of walking, and that body growth, neural maturation, and practice of walking determine strength and postural control.[58] However, there is less agreement and little empirical research on the relative importance of body growth, neural maturation, and walking practice on the development of strength and postural control. The lack of empirical research would appear to be due, at least in part, to methodological difficulties associated with assessing neural development and practice and in separating out the effects of body growth, neural maturation, and walking practice, which are all constantly changing. Adolph *et al.*[59] investigated the relative contribution to improvements in walking skill of body growth (height, weight, leg length, head circumference, crown-rump length, and ponderal index), neural maturation (assumed to be reflected in chronological age), and practice in walking (assumed to be reflected in the number of days since the onset of walking, defined as the first day that the infant could walk at least 3 m independently) in a part-longitudinal and part cross-sectional study. The subjects were 210 infants (101 girls, 109 boys) aged 9–17 months and, for comparison, 15 children (eight girls, seven boys) aged 5–6 years and 13 adults (ten women, three men). Walking skill was assessed by changes in step length, step width, foot angle (toe-in or toe-out), and dynamic base (the angle formed by three consecutive steps). Using robust statistical methods based on hierarchical regression analyses, the results showed that body growth did not explain improvements in walking skill independent of neural maturation and walking practice. Similarly, neural maturation did not explain improvements in walking skill independent of body growth and walking practice. In contrast, walking practice played the single most important role in the improvements in walking skill. It was concluded that the magnitude, distributed nature, and variability of infants' walking experience facilitate exploration of passive forces and differentiation of perceptual information which, in turn, promote the development of strength and postural control.

In a subsequent study, Adolph *et al.*[60] quantified the amount of walking practice engaged in by infants by analysing video tapes of infants playing freely under caregivers' supervision in a laboratory playroom. To simulate the infants' home environments while eliminating differences in their home environments, the laboratory playroom was equipped with furniture, varied ground surfaces, and a variety of large and small toys.

Fifteen to 60 min of continuous spontaneous activity was recorded for each of 151 infants aged 12–19 months. The results showed that the infants took an average of 2368 steps $\cdot$ h^{-1}, travelled an average distance of 701 m $\cdot$ h^{-1}, and fell an average of 17 times $\cdot$ h^{-1}. Based on these data, and assuming a walking infant is active for 6 h $\cdot$ day^{-1} (approximately half of an infant's waking day), walking infants may complete approximately 14 000 steps $\cdot$ day^{-1} and travel approximately 4200 m $\cdot$ day^{-1} (2.61 miles). Adolph *et al.*[60] suggest that such a large amount of walking practice (involving forward, backward, and sideways steps) reflects the difficulty of learning to walk (maintenance of an asymmetric upright posture while moving forward, backward, and sideways) and is comparable to the amount of daily practice required by concert musicians and athletes to achieve expert performance. The transition from crawling to walking results in a greater number of falls, but the cost of this intrinsic task constraint would appear to be outweighed by the ability of the learner to cover more space more quickly, experience more varied visual input, access and play with more distant objects, and interact in qualitatively new ways with caregivers.[51]

In accordance with the dynamical systems approach, Clark[8] pointed out that motor skill acquisition takes place throughout the whole of the life of the individual and that the process underlying the emergence of new skills is basically the same at any age. Consequently, to describe the process of children learning to walk as motor development and that of adults learning a new sports technique as motor learning is to make an unnecessary artificial distinction between the way that children and adults learn new motor skills (see Chapter 4).

Coordinative structures, control parameters, and order parameters

According to the principles of dynamical systems, the movement pattern of the human body that emerges in response to the need to solve a particular movement task, such as reaching, pointing, walking, running, hopping, skipping, jumping, and landing, is the result of self-organization of the individual constraints in relation to the task and environmental constraints on the system. For a particular movement task, self-organization assembles the muscles/joints of the body into functional groups (referred to by Bernstein[15] as functional synergies) that together form a coordinate structure for the whole body[41] (Figure 3.7). The muscles/joints in each functional group move together (e.g. extend simultaneously or flex simultaneously) which reduces the number of degrees of freedom within the functional group and, in turn, reduces the number of degrees of freedom in the coordinate structure. The smaller the number of degrees of freedom in the coordinate structure, the lower the demand on the nervous system. The coordinate structure sets the timing (relative phasing) of the movements of the body segments.

Different task constraints give rise to different coordinative structures. For example, for speeds of locomotion up to about 2.0 m $\cdot$ s^{-1} most humans naturally adopt a walking pattern (bipedal alternate right-left-right-left stepping) rather than another form of locomotion such as running or hopping. The coordinate structure for walking is characterized by two double support phases (both feet in contact with the ground at the same time) and separate single support and swing phases of each leg during each stride. Different forms of locomotion, such as walking, running, hopping, skipping,

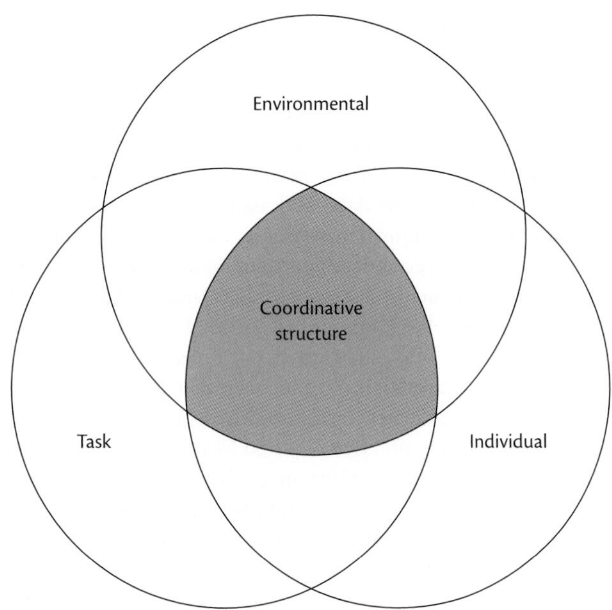

Figure 3.7 The emergence of a coordinate structure from self-organization of the individual, task, and environmental constraints.

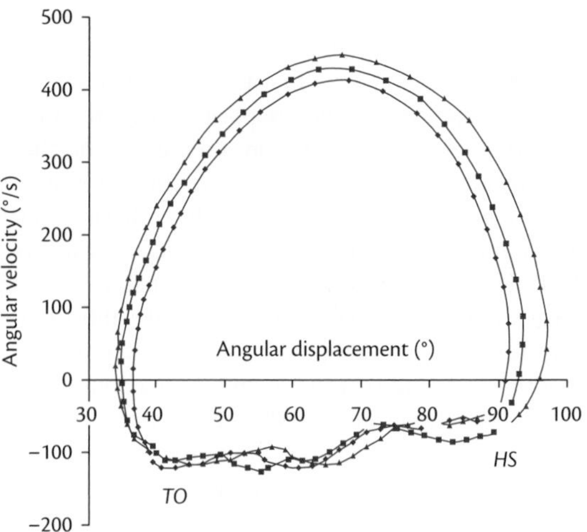

Figure 3.8 Phase plane of the sagittal plane movement of the shank in three successive stride cycles of an infant 4 weeks after starting to walk.
HS: heel strike, TO: toe off.
Adapted from Clark JE, Phillips SJ. A longitudinal study of intralimb coordination in the first year of independent walking: a dynamical systems analysis. Child Dev. 1993; 64: 1143–1157.

and jumping have different coordinative structures. A coordinative structure is stable over particular ranges (or scaling) of certain constraints (referred to as control parameters) so that the observed movement pattern may change qualitatively (reflected in changes in order parameters) while the coordinate structure remains the same.[61] For example, as walking speed (control parameter) increases up to about 2.0 $m \cdot s^{-1}$, the movement pattern changes qualitatively (change in the order parameters of stride length and stride frequency), but the coordinative structure (walking) remains the same. However, as the speed of walking increases above 2 $m \cdot s^{-1}$, the walking pattern becomes increasingly unstable, reflected in increasing variability of the relative phasing of the body segments and increasing asymmetry between the movements of the left and right sides of the body. At about 2.3 $m \cdot s^{-1}$ there is an abrupt change from walking to running, which is a new coordinative structure characterized by two flight phases (instead of two double support phases as in walking) and separate single support and swing phases of each leg during each stride. This coordinate structure remains stable over most of the 2.3 $m \cdot s^{-1}$ to maximum speed range.

The abrupt change from walking to running illustrates a major characteristic of dynamical systems. Changes in coordinative structure are triggered by instability resulting from a change in the scaling of one or more control parameters.[42] In the case of bipedal locomotion, speed is a control parameter that determines the most appropriate coordinative structure, either walking or running, for a given speed.

Patterns, attractors, and stability

Coordinate structures result in stable patterns of activity which are likely to be reflected in the activity of the system as a whole and/or in the activity of the subsystems. In human movement, the pattern of activity resulting from a particular coordinative structure is likely to be manifest in a very wide range of kinematic (e.g. the movement of each body segment), kinetic (e.g. peak force at heel strike, rate of loading during the passive phase of ground contact), physiological (e.g. tidal volume, breathing rate, stroke volume, heart rate, and rate of oxygen consumption), and neuromusculoskeletal (e.g. intensity and duration of contractions of individual muscles) indicators. Kinematic indicators are likely to show highly repeatable whole body movement patterns (movement of the CG), highly repeatable movement patterns of individual body segments, and low variability in the relative phasing (coordination) of the movement of body segments.

The stability of a movement pattern can be illustrated and quantified in a number of ways.[62] One of the most frequently used dynamical systems techniques for illustrating the stability of the movement pattern of a body segment is the phase plane (also referred to as phase portrait, phase plane trajectory, and parametric phase plot). A phase plane captures the space-time pattern of the movement of the segment by plotting the velocity (linear or angular) of the segment as a function of the displacement of the segment.[63] For example, Figure 3.8 shows a phase plane of the movement of the shank of an infant in the sagittal plane 4 weeks after starting to walk.[64] It shows the angular velocity-angular displacement trajectory of the shank in three successive stride cycles. It is clear that there is some overlap between the trajectories, but no direct mapping of one trajectory onto the next. In dynamical systems terminology, the phase plane exhibited by the shank occupies a region in the state space.[65] The state space encompasses all possible trajectories of the shank in the state space. The state space is defined by the relevant state variables. In this example, the state variables are the angular velocity and angular displacement of the shank which define a two-dimensional state space.

The trajectories of the shank define a region in the state space referred to as the attractor, which is the region of the state space in which the movement of the shank is most stable. The stability of the phase plane of the shank from cycle to cycle is reflected in the bandwidth of the attractor. The narrower the bandwidth, the more stable the attractor. The standard deviation of the length of the angular velocity-angular displacement vectors, which are determined at the same frequency as the data used to plot the phase plane, over a

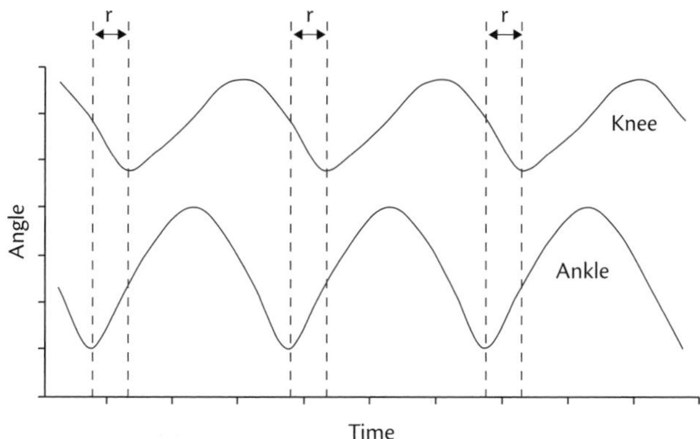

Figure 3.9 Determination of the relative phase (*r*) between peak knee flexion and peak ankle dorsi-flexion during the ground contact phase in running.
Source data from Holt KG, Hamill J, Andres RO. Predicting the minimal energy costs of human walking. Med Sci Sport Exerc. 1991; 23: 491–498.

number of cycles provides an estimate of the bandwidth; the lower the standard deviation, the more stable the attractor.

Another frequently used dynamical systems technique for estimating the stability of a movement pattern is the variability of the relative phase between two events in the movement pattern over a number of trials or cycles. For example, in running, the relative phasing of the movement of the knee and ankle joints of each leg could be determined by the time difference between peak knee flexion and peak ankle dorsi-flexion during the ground contact phase expressed as a proportion of ground contact time (Figure 3.9). A similar measure of relative phase could be obtained for any pair of joints in the same leg during each ground contact phase (hip/knee, knee/ankle, and hip/ankle) or for corresponding joints in the left and right legs during each stride (left hip/right hip, left knee/right knee, and left ankle/right ankle). The stability of each measure of relative phase is reflected in the standard deviation of the relative phase over a number of cycles; the smaller the standard deviation, the more closely coupled is the movement of the two joints and, therefore, the more stable is the movement pattern.

Cyclicity in biological systems

The dynamical systems approach emphasizes the thermodynamic nature (patterns of changes in energy) of biological systems and how thermodynamic laws guide behaviour.[63] Biological systems obey the second law of thermodynamics, which is that all systems tend toward instability and disorder. In the case of a living organism, this culminates in death. However, during life a biological system can maintain an ordered state by a cyclical process of generation, transformation, and dissipation of energy which occurs at all levels of the system. These include circadian rhythms, cardiac rhythms, respiratory rhythms, and locomotion.[66] It is believed that the oscillatory nature of biological systems is analogous to inanimate self-organizing oscillatory systems.[40,67] This viewpoint has led to the application of the physics of pendulums to such systems.[40]

Any object that is free to oscillate about a horizontal axis is a pendulum. For example, a pendulum in a clock usually consists of a long light bar or rod that supports a small dense mass. The idealized form of this type of pendulum, referred to as a simple pendulum, consists of a mass-less rod of length L that supports a point mass m. As the rod has no mass, the centre of mass of a simple pendulum is at the centre of mass of the point mass. Consequently, the distance D from the axis of rotation to the centre of mass of the pendulum is equal to L. The moment of inertia I of the pendulum about the axis of rotation through its point of support is given by $I = mL^2$ where L = the radius of gyration of the pendulum about the axis of rotation. A real pendulum is usually referred to as a compound pendulum. In a compound pendulum, L is always longer than D.

If a pendulum (simple or compound) is displaced from its vertical resting position and then released, it will oscillate about the vertical rest position with a constant period, which means that the duration of each cycle of movement will be constant even though the amplitude of movement will gradually decrease. This decrease is due to friction around its axis of rotation and, to a lesser extent, air resistance. The period τ of a simple pendulum is given by $\tau = 2\pi(L/g)^{½}$.[68] An oscillator that has a constant period, like a swinging pendulum, is referred to as a harmonic oscillator.[68]

The period (seconds per cycle) of a pendulum is entirely determined by its physical properties, in particular the distribution of the mass of the pendulum. For a given mass, a change in the distribution of mass will result in a change in the moment of inertia of the pendulum with respect to its axis of rotation. In other words, a change in L, will result in a change in the period. The reciprocal of the period is the frequency of oscillation (cycles per second). As the period of a pendulum is constant, its frequency of oscillation is referred to as natural frequency or resonant frequency.[68]

If there was no friction around the axis of rotation of a pendulum and no air resistance, the pendulum would oscillate with constant amplitude and the energy of the system would be entirely conserved at the level it had at the point of release. In practice, there would be some friction around the axis of rotation and some air resistance such that a certain amount of energy would be dissipated (lost to the pendulum in the form of heat and movement of the air) during each oscillation. Consequently, the amplitude of oscillation would gradually decrease and the pendulum would eventually come to rest and hang vertically. A pendulum is a very simple example of a dynamical system. The movement of the system after release is self-organized (amplitude and frequency of oscillation), entirely predictable, and energy is conserved (to a level determined by friction and air resistance). Similarly, if a metal spring is stretched or compressed and then released, the spring will oscillate in a predictable manner and come to rest at its equilibrium position; there is no brain controlling its movement, which is instead determined completely by its physical properties of stiffness and damping. Just as the physical properties of a pendulum and a spring determine their movement when allowed to oscillate freely, it is reasonable to infer that the movement of the arms and legs might be determined in a similar manner in certain movements. For example, in walking, if the stiffness and damping levels of the legs are set by the muscles that control the hips, knees, and ankles, the oscillation of the legs will be determined to a certain extent by their physical properties, which is likely to simplify neural control of the movement.[40]

Force-driven harmonic oscillators

If a child's swing is set in motion, its swing amplitude will gradually decrease due to friction around its axis of rotation and to air resistance. In order to maintain a constant swing amplitude, the swing must receive a brief push at the start of each swing to replace the energy lost due to friction and air resistance in the preceding swing. A harmonic oscillator that requires energy input at the start of each oscillation in order to maintain a constant amplitude of oscillation, which is like a child's swing, is referred to as a force driven harmonic oscillator (FDHO).[69]

The motion of the legs in constant speed walking is quasi-periodic (alternate oscillation of the legs with similar swing time and similar swing amplitude). However, the body as a whole loses energy in each step due to damping, where kinetic energy transformed into strain energy during the period of double support as a result of eccentric muscle contraction is partially dissipated as heat. Unless replenished, the loss of energy during each step would quickly bring the body to rest. The continued oscillation of the legs is maintained by a burst of muscular activity just prior to the start of each leg swing (to replace the energy lost in the previous step). Consequently, the motion of the legs in constant speed walking is similar to that of an FDHO.[69]

In an FDHO, there is a particular frequency, referred to as the resonant frequency, which requires minimal impulse (intensity of force multiplied by the duration of the force) to maintain oscillations. In human movement, muscle forces (intensity, duration, and frequency of muscular activity) determine energy expenditure. There is considerable evidence that adults and children naturally adopt a step frequency and step length in walking that minimizes energy expenditure and maximizes stability.[69–73] Furthermore, the preferred step frequency can be predicted from the resonant frequency of an FDHO model of the leg swing[69,71] where the period $\tau = 2\pi(L/2g)^{½}$.[40] Similarly, Ledebt and Breniere[74] found that in 4- to 8-year-old children, gait initiation (from the start of movement to maximum horizontal velocity in the first step) can be closely predicted from the resonant frequency of an FDHO model of the movement of the body over the grounded foot. Even very young children appear to adopt movement patterns at resonant frequency in certain situations. For example, Goldfield *et al.*[75] showed that infants bouncing up and down in a jumper device tend to adopt resonant frequency as modelled by an FDHO mass-spring system.

Self-optimization of coordinative structures

The observation that cyclic human movement like walking tends to be performed at resonant frequency has led to the suggestion that coordination is self-optimized in relation to so-called optimality criteria to which the individual is sensitive in adopting a particular movement pattern.[69,70] The optimality criteria reflect the prevailing intrinsic task constraints and result in movement patterns that minimize the 'costs' to the system.[47] The main optimality criterion would appear to be energy expenditure, but others have been suggested, including stability, bilateral symmetry, and shock absorption at foot-strike.[71,76] For example, at a particular walking speed, minimal expenditure usually occurs at preferred step frequency in children and adults and is usually associated with high stability and high bilateral symmetry.[70,71]

With regard to symmetry, Clark *et al.*[72] investigated coordination in walking in a cross-sectional study involving seven groups of subjects: new walkers (capable of three consecutive steps) with support, new walkers without support, children who had been walking for 2 weeks, 1 month, 3 months, and 6 months, and a group of adults. There were five subjects in each group. The average age of onset of walking in the infant subjects was 11.2 months. Interlimb coordination, at preferred speed of walking, was assessed by measuring the step time:stride time ratio (temporal phase) and the step length:stride length ratio (distance phase). It was expected that in a mature walking gait, the temporal phase and the distance phase would be close to 50% and that a low variability (measured as the standard deviation of each phase) would indicate a stable coordinative structure. The results showed that there was no significant difference in mean temporal phase or mean distance phase (all close to 50%) across all age groups. Additionally, variability decreased with age with no significant difference in variability between the 3 months, 6 months, and adult groups. The variability of the supported new walkers (two-handed support by a parent) was not significantly different from the 2 weeks, 1 month, and 3 months groups in temporal phase and not significantly different from the 3 months and 6 months groups in distance phase. Clark *et al.*[72] concluded that i) the coordinative structure for interlimb coordination used by new walkers is similar to, but not as tightly coupled as, that used by adults, and ii) the practice of walking increases postural stability which, in turn, increases the stability of the coordinative structure. The results of the study suggested that bilateral symmetry is a feature of coordination in walking.

Jeng *et al.*[71] investigated energy expenditure, stability, and symmetry in walking in 3- to 12-year-old children and adults. There were six groups of subjects with nine subjects in each group: 3–4 years, 5–6 years, 7–8 years, 9–10 years, 11–12 years, and 20–21 years. The subjects were carefully selected to represent the full range of body sizes in each age group. After familiarization, each subject was required to walk for 8 min on a treadmill at preferred walking speed (established in overground walking) at three different step frequencies in time with a metronome: preferred step frequency (PSF), PSF—25% and PSF + 25%. Energy expenditure during steady-state walking was assessed at each step frequency by the physiological cost index (in beats $\cdot$ m^{-1}), which is the difference between resting heart rate and walking heart rate (in beats $\cdot$ min^{-1}) divided by walking speed (in m $\cdot$ min^{-1}).

Coordination was assessed at each step frequency via symmetry and relative phase. Bilateral symmetry was assessed by the ratio of the durations of the stance phases of each leg in each stride, the ratio of the durations of the swing phases of each leg in each stride, and the ratio of the duration of the right step to the stride duration in each stride. The mean of each ratio was calculated over ten consecutive stride cycles during steady-state walking. The relative phase (time difference between the occurrences of the maximum angles of each pair of joints in each stride as a percentage of stride time) was determined for the hip/knee, knee/ankle, and hip/ankle joint couplings. The mean of each relative phase was calculated over ten consecutive stride cycles during steady-state walking. Stability was assessed as the standard deviation of each of the symmetry and relative phase measures.

The results clearly indicated that energy expenditure, symmetry, and stability were all optimal at preferred step frequency for all age groups and that preferred step frequency was consistent with resonant frequency as predicted by an FDHO model of the leg swing.[40] Seven of the 3- to 4-year-olds and four of the 5- to 6-year-olds had difficulty in modulating their step frequency at the non-preferred step frequencies. All of the other subjects were able to modulate their step frequency at the non-preferred step frequencies. Jeng *et al.*[77] concluded that the ability to self-optimize walking appears to be established by 7 years of age and seems to involve three stages. Stage 1 (1–4 years of age) is characterized by early sensitivity to resonance and difficulty in modulating step frequency to non-preferred frequencies. Stage

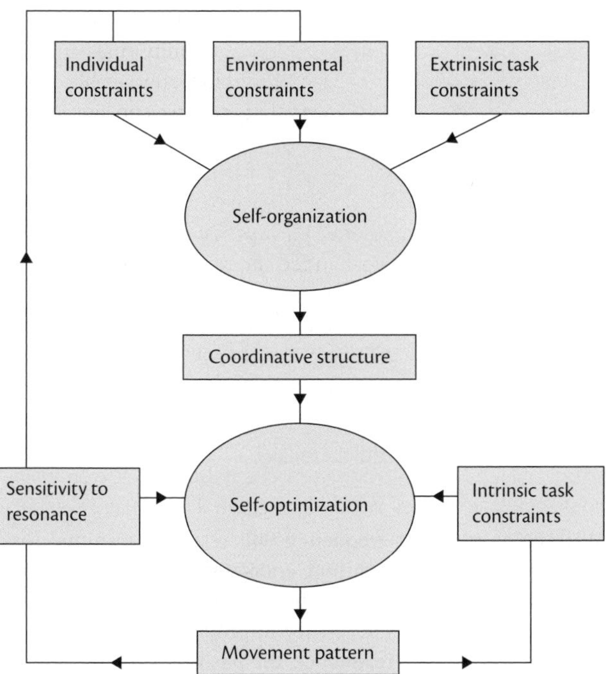

Figure 3.10 A dynamical systems-based model of motor learning.

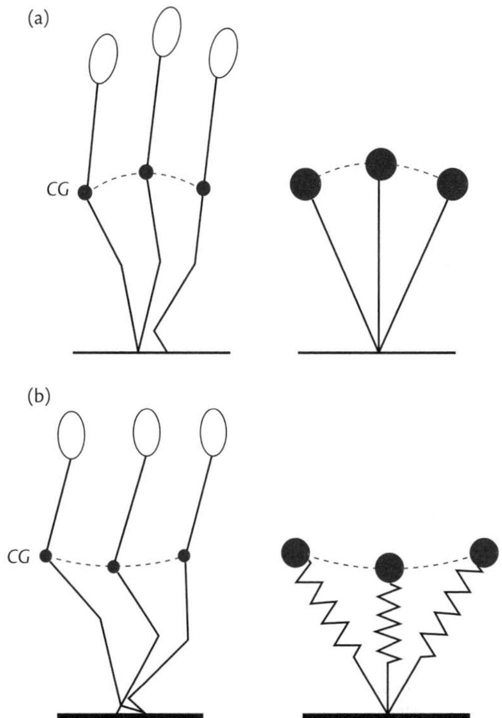

Figure 3.11 Pendulum dynamics (a) is the predominant form of energy conservation in walking. Spring dynamics (b) is the predominant form of energy conservation in running.

CG: whole body centre of gravity.

Adapted from Farley CT, Ferris DP. Biomechanics of walking and running: Center of mass movements to muscle action. Exerc Sport Sci Rev. 1998; 26: 253–285.

2 (4–6 years of age) is characterized by a progressive increase in the ability to modulate step frequency and a decrease in stability which may be due to the need to adapt to marked changes in body composition that are characteristic of this period. Stage 3 (6–7 years of age) is characterized by the ability to consistently modulate step frequency.

Jeng *et al.*[77] suggested that sensitivity to resonance (an awareness of how to minimize energy expenditure by maximizing energy conservation in energy exchanges between and within body segments) may be a mechanism underlying the development of self-optimization in walking. They also suggested that sensitivity to resonance is a function of the individual's sensitivity to the physical properties of her/his body and to the environment. Sensitivity to personal physical properties would suggest awareness of the anthropometric (size and shape), inertial (mass and distribution of mass), viscoelastic (stiffness and damping), and gravitational (weight) properties of body segments and combinations of body segments. Sensitivity to the environment would suggest awareness of what movements are possible in a given environment, for example, negotiating an obstacle or moving through a confined space. Awareness of the possibilities afforded by a particular environment has been referred to by Gibson[78] as affordance. Figure 3.10 presents a model of the emergence of motor behaviour based on the dynamical systems approach.

Dynamic resources

As shown by Adolph *et al.*,[59,60] the rapid improvement in walking ability in the first month following the onset of walking would appear to be largely due to the effects of practice. According to Fonseca *et al.*[79] and Holt *et al.*,[80] the practice of walking enables toddlers to explore the sources of energy available to them to maintain upright posture and forward progression. These dynamic resources available may be categorized as i) energy generation by concentric muscle contractions, ii) conservation of energy in soft tissues, which is the potential to store and then release strain energy in muscle-tendon units (spring dynamics) and iii) conservation of energy by interchange of kinetic energy and gravitational potential energy within and between body segments (pendulum dynamics).[80] The gait (walking movement pattern) that emerges will reflect the relative contribution of the three sources of energy.

There are potentially a number of ways of using these resources to maintain upright posture and forward progression. For example, pendulum dynamics is more evident in walking than in running and spring dynamics is more evident in running than in walking[81,82] (Figure 3.11).

Figure 3.12 shows a picture sequence of a young boy walking at preferred speed from just after heel-strike of the right foot to just after heel-strike of the left foot. From toe-off of the left foot (TO_L) to heel-strike of the left foot (HS_L) (single support phase of the right leg, approximately 40% of the stride cycle) the body rotates forward over the right foot similar to an inverted pendulum (Figure 3.11a and Figure 3.12a–e). During the period TO_L to mid-stance (Figure 3.12a–c), kinetic energy is converted to gravitational potential energy (as the CG moves upward) and during the period from mid-stance to HS_L (Figure 3.12c–e), gravitational potential energy is converted to kinetic energy (as the CG moves downward). There will be some loss of energy during these phases due to damping in soft tissues (dissipated as heat inside the body and then to the surrounding air), but energy will be largely conserved due to pendulum dynamics.[83]

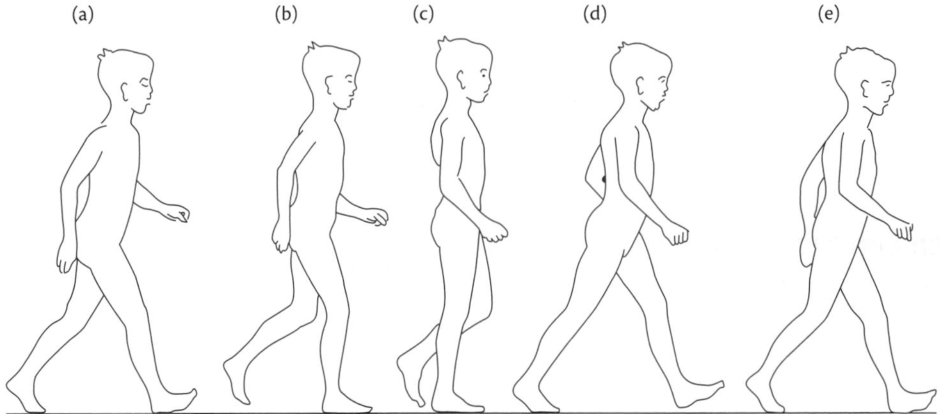

Figure 3.12 A young boy walking at preferred speed from just after heel-strike of the right foot to just after heel-strike of the left foot.

During the period HS_R to TO_L (Figure 3.12a and b) (double support phase prior to left swing phase, approximately 10% of the stride cycle), kinetic energy is converted to strain energy in the right leg (i.e. the leg is compressed like a spring). Most of the strain energy will be immediately returned as kinetic energy and gravitational potential energy, but some of the strain energy will be lost due to damping in the soft tissues. Simultaneous to the storage and release of strain energy in the right leg, active plantar flexion of the left ankle (the push-off of the left foot) generates new energy (kinetic and gravitational). To maintain forward progression, the new energy generated by the push-off must be sufficient to replace the energy that was lost due to damping in soft tissues.[83] The energy changes between HS and TO of each foot are illustrated in Figure 3.13.

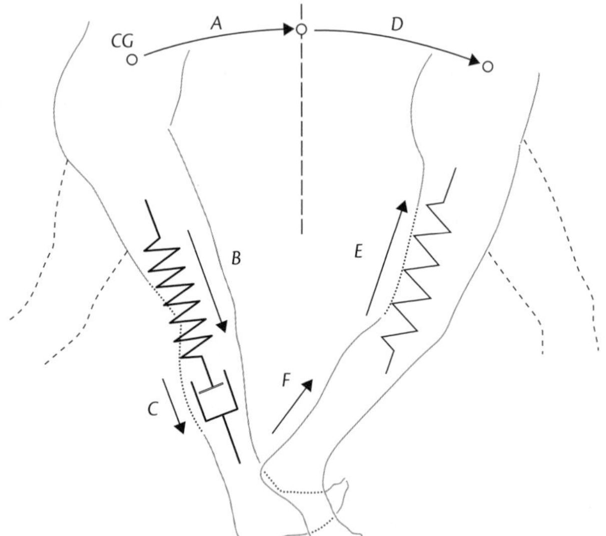

Figure 3.13 The energy changes between heel strike and toe-off of each foot during walking.

A: conversion of kinetic energy to gravitational potential energy; B: storage of strain energy in the muscle-tendon units and other soft tissues; C: loss of some strain energy as heat; D: conversion of gravitational potential energy to kinetic energy; E: release of strain energy; F: push-off; CG: whole body centre of gravity.

Adapted from Holt KG, Obusek JP, Fonseca ST. Constraints on disordered locomotion: a dynamical systems perspective on spastic cerebral palsy. Hum Mov Sci. 1996; 15: 177–202.

Walking at resonant frequency will result in minimal loss of energy and therefore minimal energy expenditure. As in any FDHO, correct timing of the push-off (referred to by Holt *et al.*[80] as the escapement force) is necessary to produce resonant frequency in walking. To produce resonance, the push-off should begin as, or just before, the landing foot strikes the ground at the start of the double support phase, which means that the period of generation of new energy should correspond to the period when energy is lost due to compression of the lead leg.[83]

Holt *et al.*[80] investigated the use of pendulum dynamics and spring dynamics in new walkers. The subjects were seven infants who were encouraged to walk on a walkway in a laboratory while being video-taped from the side. The infants were video-taped on seven visits to the laboratory at 1-month intervals. The first video-taping of each infant occurred as soon as possible after the infant could perform three to six independent steps. The mean age of the infants was 11 months at the first visit and 17 months at the last visit. The timing of the push-off (referred to as escapement timing) was assessed in terms of the time difference (t_c–t_a) between foot-strike (t_c) and peak forward acceleration of the whole body centre of gravity (t_a). A negative escapement time indicates that t_a occurs after t_c, which means that it occurs during double support when the push-off would be most effective (correspondence between the new energy generation phase of the rear leg and the energy loss phase of the lead leg). However, a positive escapement time indicates that t_a occurs before t_c, indicating lack of correspondence between the energy generation phase and the energy loss phase of the lead leg. At visit one, mean escapement time was positive with high variability. At visit two, mean escapement time was negative with high variability. In visits three to seven, the mean escapement time was consistently negative with much lower variability than in visits one and two. Consequently, in contrast to visit one, escapement time in visits two to seven was consistent with resonant frequency.

The changes in the effectiveness of escapement over visits one to seven were reflected in changes in walking speed, step length, and step frequency. There were significant increases in speed of walking (0.18 $m \cdot s^{-1}$ to 0.59 $m \cdot s^{-1}$), step length (0.10 m to 0.21 m), and step frequency (1.83 to 2.87 Hz) between visits one and two, but no significant changes in any of the three variables over visits two to seven. There were no significant differences in weight, standing height, or sitting height of the subjects between visits one and two, but there were significant increases in all three variables over visits two to seven. The results suggested that in the early stages of walking (within the first month after the onset of walking) infants rapidly learn to provide active force (via appropriate escapement timing) in a way that is consistent with the utilization of pendulum and spring dynamics to optimize energy expenditure.

A dynamical systems perspective of walking in children with cerebral palsy

The major task constraints in walking are the maintenance of an upright posture and continued oscillation of the legs despite energy losses.[79] As a result of weakness in the calf muscles (ankle plantar-flexors), children with spastic diplegia, a condition of cerebral palsy, are unable to generate the same amount of new energy during push-off in walking as normally-developing children. The reduced new energy available from the push-off makes the use of a pendulum gait pattern almost impossible.[79] As energy generation (concentric muscle contractions), pendulum dynamics, and spring dynamics are the only dynamic resources that are potentially available, and energy generation and pendulum dynamics are severely restricted, it follows that forward progression can only be maintained by increasing the amount of energy available from spring dynamics. Consequently, it should be no surprise that children with spastic diplegia tend to adopt a gait that is more similar to running (a bouncing pattern) than walking as spring dynamics are predominant in running whereas pendulum dynamics are predominant in walking.

The increase in energy available via spring dynamics is the result of increased stiffness of the legs due to co-contraction of the flexors and extensors of the hips, knees, and ankles and an equinus foot position (plantar flexed ankles). The increase in energy available via spring dynamics is the result of the body being projected upwards following each bounce which increases the amount of gravitational potential energy available at mid-stance (relative to normal walking) and, even allowing for loss of strain energy as heat during the subsequent compression phase of the lead leg, results in sufficient energy being returned to maintain forward progression. The bouncing gait requires a higher level of energy expenditure than normal walking, but it is reasonable to assume that such a gait is optimal in relation to the dynamic resources available. There is evidence that the efficiency of the bouncing gait is increased over time by adaptive morphological changes that increase the tendon length:muscle length ratio in the leg extensor muscles which, in turn, increases the resilience of the muscle-tendon units and, therefore, reduces the amount of energy that is lost.[84]

Traditional therapy for such gait abnormalities has been directed at normalizing the abnormal kinematics. For example, attempts have been made to reduce the equinus foot position in children with spastic diplegia by electrical stimulation of the tibialis anterior (to dorsiflex the ankle), but such intervention has been largely unsuccessful.[44,85] From a dynamical systems perspective, the lack of success of traditional therapy is not surprising; all of the abnormal joint movements in an abnormal gait will be the result of a particular coordinative structure and, consequently, all of the abnormal joint movements will be symptoms of the abnormal individual constraints in the form of abnormal dynamic resources. The corollary is that therapy directed at normalizing the abnormal dynamic resources is likely to be more effective than therapy directed at normalizing the abnormal kinematics. There is evidence in support of this view. For example, electrical stimulation of the gastrocnemius-soleus group to improve the push-off in children with spastic diplegia (which might have been expected to worsen the equinus gait) has been shown to result in a more normal gait that included a normal heel strike.[86,87] The implication of these findings is that normalizing the dynamic resources results in a more normal coordinative structure which, in turn, produces a more normal gait.

Conclusions

From a dynamical systems perspective, coordination of human movement emerges from the intrinsic self-organizing properties of the dynamical system consisting of the individual, the task, and the environment. Self-organization refers to the spontaneous integration of the dynamical properties of the subsystems (individual, task, and environment) and results in the spontaneous establishment of a coordinative structure, which is a relatively stable pattern of phase relations and joint kinematics when performing the task. There is considerable evidence that coordinative structures are self-optimized in relation to optimality criteria to which the individual is sensitive. The main optimality criterion would appear to be a propensity to minimize energy expenditure in such a way that a well-practised pattern of movement that appears abnormal is likely to be optimal in relation to the dynamic (energy) resources available to the individual. Consequently, therapy directed at normalizing the abnormal dynamic resources is likely to be more effective than therapy directed at normalizing joint kinematics.

Summary

- The brain coordinates and controls movement via muscular activity. Coordination refers to the timing of relative motion between body segments, and control refers to the optimization of relative motion between body segments.
- The development of coordination has been viewed historically from two viewpoints: the neuromaturational perspective (in relation to motor development in children) and the information-processing perspective (in relation to motor learning in adults). However, these approaches fail to account for the great flexibility demonstrated by individuals in accommodating rapidly changing task demands.
- The deficiencies of the neuromaturational and information-processing perspectives were highlighted by Bernstein.[15] He pointed out that all joint movements are the result of active (muscle) and passive (motion dependent, gravitational, and external) components of joint moments (collectively referred to as joint biodynamics), and that coordination results in utilization of the passive components to minimize energy expenditure.
- Bernstein's biodynamical approach was a major influence on the increasingly widely held dynamical systems view of the development of coordination. From a dynamical systems perspective, coordination of human movement emerges from the intrinsic self-organizing properties of the dynamical system consisting of the individual, the environment, and the task.
- Self-organization refers to the spontaneous integration of the dynamical properties of the subsystems (individual, environment, and task) and results in the spontaneous establishment of a coordinative structure within and between the subsystems.

This, in turn, results in a pattern of movement. The actual pattern of movement that emerges depends upon the state of the subsystems that impose constraints on the types of movement that may emerge; the constraints arise from the anthropometry and functional ability of the individual (individual constraints), the requirements of the task (task constraints), and the prevailing environmental conditions (environmental constraints). Each type of constraint influences the movement pattern that emerges by encouraging certain types of movement and discouraging others.

- There is considerable evidence that coordination is self-optimized in relation to optimality criteria to which the individual is sensitive. The main optimality criteria would appear to be energy expenditure and injury risk, but there is clear evidence of others, including, for example, stability, bilateral symmetry, and shock absorption at foot-strike in walking.
- Traditional therapy for gait abnormalities has been directed at normalizing the abnormal kinematics. However, such intervention has been largely unsuccessful. From a dynamical systems perspective, the lack of success of traditional therapy is not surprising; all of the abnormal joint movements in an abnormal gait will be the result of a particular coordinative structure and, consequently, all of the abnormal joint movements will be symptoms of the underlying cause, that is, abnormal individual constraints in the form of abnormal dynamic resources. The corollary is that therapy directed at normalizing the abnormal dynamic resources is likely to be more effective than therapy directed at normalizing the abnormal kinematics. There is increasing evidence in support of this view.

References

1. Watkins J. *Structure and function of the musculoskeletal system*, 2nd ed. Champaign, : Human Kinetics; 2010.
2. Watkins J. *Fundamental biomechanics of sport and exercise*. Oxford: Routledge; 2014.
3. Turvey MT. Coordination. *Am Psychol*. 1990; 45: 938–953.
4. Jensen JL, Phillips SJ, Clark JE. For young jumpers, differences are in movement's control, not in coordination. *Res Q Exerc Sport*. 1994; 65: 258–268.
5. Bobbert MF, Ingen Schenau, GJV. Coordination in vertical jump. *J Biomech*. 1988; 21: 249–262.
6. Hay JG. Citius, altius, longius (faster, higher, longer): the biomechanics of jumping for distance. *J Biomech*. 1993; 26 (suppl 1: 7–21.
7. Clark JE, Phillips SJ, Petersen R. Developmental stability in jumping. *Dev Psychol*. 1989; 25: 929–935.
8. Clark JE. On becoming skillful: patterns and constraints. *Res Q Exerc Sport*. 1995; 66: 173–183.
9. Gesell A, Thompson H. *The psychology of early growth including norms of infant behavior and a method of genetic analysis*. New York: Macmillan; 1938.
10. McGraw MG. *The neuromaturation of the human infant*. New York: Columbia University Press; 1943.
11. Thelen E. Motor development: a new synthesis. *Am Psychol*. 1995; 50: 79–85.
12. Kamm K, Thelen E, Jensen JL. A dynamical systems approach to motor development. *Phys Ther*. 1990; 70: 763–775.
13. Handford C, Davids K, Bennett S, Button C. Skill acquisition in sport: some implications of an evolving practice ecology. *J Sports Sci*. 1997; 15: 621–640.
14. Newell KM. Motor skill acquisition. *Ann Rev Psychol*. 1991; 42: 213–237.
15. Bernstein N. *The coordination and regulation of movements*. London: Pergamon; 1967.
16. Zernicke RF, Schneider K. Biomechanics and developmental neuromotor control. *Child Devel*. 1993; 64: 982–1004.
17. Fitch F, Tuller B, Turvey MT. The Bernstein perspective III. Tuning of coordinative structures with special reference to perception. In: Kelso JAS (ed.) *Understanding human motor control*. Champaign, IL: Human Kinetics: 1982. p. 271–278.
18. Sparrow WA, Newell KM. Metabolic energy expenditure and the regulation of movement economy. *Psychon Bull Rev*. 1998; 5: 173–196.
19. Lieber RL. *Skeletal muscle structure and function*. Baltimore: Williams and Wilkins; 1992.
20. van Ingen Schenau GJ. From translation to rotation: constraints on multijoint movements and the unique action of biarticular muscles. *Hum Mov Sci*. 1989; 8: 301–337.
21. van Ingen Schenau GJ, Pratt CA, Macpherson JM. Differential use and control of mono- and biarticular muscles. *Hum Mov Sci*. 1994; 13: 495–517.
22. Valero-Cuevas FJ. A mathematical approach to the mechanical capabilities of limbs and fingers. *Adv Exp Med Biol*. 2009; 629: 619–633.
23. Turvey MT. Action and perception at the level of synergies. *Hum Mov Sci*. 2007; 26: 657–697.
24. Chow JY, Davids K, Button C, Koh M. Coordination changes in a discrete multi-articular action as a function of practice. *Acta Psychol*. 2008; 127: 163–176.
25. Vereijken B, van Emmerik REA, Whiting HTA, Newell KM. Free(z)ing degrees of freedom in skill acquisition. *J Mot Behav*. 1992; 24: 133–142.
26. Anderson DI, Sidaway B. Coordination changes associated with practice of a soccer kick. *Res Q Exerc Sport*. 1994; 65: 93–99.
27. Cignetti F, Schena F, Zanone PG. Dynamics of coordination in cross country skiing. *Hum Mov Sci*. 2009; 28: 204–217.
28. Quinzi F, Sbriccoli P, Alderson J, Di Mario A, Camomilla V. Intra-limb coordination in karate kicking: effect of impacting or not impacting a target. *Hum Mov Sci*. 2014; 33: 108–119.
29. Dumas G, Laroche J, Lehmann A. Your body, my body, our coupling moves our bodies. *Front Hum Neurosci*. doi: 10.3389/fnhum.4014.01004.
30. Asmussen MJ, Przysucha EP, Dounskaia N. Intersegmental dynamics shape joint coordination during catching in typically developing children but not in children with developmental coordination disorder. *J Neurophysiol*, 2014; 111: 1417–1428.
31. Andrews JG. Biomechanical analysis of human motion. In: Hay JG (ed.) *Kinesiology IV*. Reston, VA: American Alliance for Health, Physical Education and Recreation; 1974. p. 32–42.
32. Kamm K, Thelen E, Jensen J L. A dynamical systems approach to motor development. *PhysTher*, 1990; 70: 763–775.
33. Winter DA. *Biomechanics and motor control of human movement*. New York: John Wiley; 1990.
34. Schneider K, Zernicke RF, Schmidt RA, Hart TJ. Changes in limb dynamics during the practice of rapid arm movements. *J Biomech*. 1989; 22: 805–817.
35. Lockman JJ, Thelen E. Developmental biodynamics: brain, body and behavior connections. *Child Dev*. 1993; 64: 953–959.
36. Thelen E, Corbetta D, Kamm K, Spencer J, Schneider K, Zernicke RF. The transition to reaching: mapping intention and intrinsic dynamics. *Child Dev*, 1993; 64: 1058–1098.
37. Dominici N, Ivanenko YP, Cappellini G, *et al*. Locomotor primitives in newborn babies and their development. *Science*. 2011; 334: 997–999.
38. Ivanenko YP, Dominici N, Cappellini G, *et al*. Changes in the spinal segmental motor output for stepping during development from infant to adult. *J Neurosci*. 2013; 33: 3025–3036.
39. Jensen JL, Thelen E, Ulrich BD. Constraints on multi-joint movements: from spontaneity of infancy to the skill of adults. *Hum Mov Sci*. 1989; 8: 393–402.
40. Kugler PN, Turvey MT. *Natural law, and the self-assembly of rhythmic movement*. New York: Erlbaum, Hillside; 1987.

41. Kugler PN, Kelso JAS, Turvey MT. On the concept of coordinative structures as dissipative structures: I. Theoretical lines of convergence. In: Stelmach GE, Requin J (eds.) *Tutorials on motor behavior.* New York: North Holland; 1980. p. 3–47.
42. Smith LB, Thelen E. Development as a dynamic system. *Trends Cogn Sci.* 2003; 7: 343–348.
43. Davids K, Glazier P, Araujo D, Bartlett R. Movement systems as dynamical systems: the functional role of variability and its implications for sports medicine. *Sports Med.* 2003; 33: 245–260.
44. Holt KG, Obusek JP, Fonseca ST. Constraints on disordered locomotion: a dynamical systems perspective on spastic cerebral palsy. *Hum Mov Sci.* 1996; 15: 177–202.
45. Dickinson MH, Farley CT, Full RJ, Koehl MAR, Kram R, Lehman S. How animals move: an integrative view. *Science.* 2000; 288(5463): 100–106.
46. Madore BF, Freedman WL. Self-organizing structures. *Am Sci.* 1987; 75: 252–259.
47. Holt KG. Constraints in the emergence of preferred locomotory patterns. In: Rosenbaum DA, Collyer CE (eds.) *Timing of behavior: neural, psychological, and computational perspectives.* Cambridge, MA: MIT Press; 1998. p. 261–291.
48. Newell KM. Constraints on the development of coordination. In: Wade MG, Whiting HTA (eds.) *Motor development in children: aspects of coordination and control.* Dordrecht: Martinus Nijhoff; 1986. p. 341–360.
49. Clugston MJ. *The new penguin dictionary of science.* London: Penguin; 1998.
50. Sipper M, Sanchez E, Mange D, Tomassini M, Perez-Uribe A, Stauffer A. A phylogenetic, ontogenetic, and epigenetic view of bio-inspired hardware systems. *IEEE Transactions on Evolutionary Computation.* 1997; 1: 83–97.
51. Adolph KE, Tamis-LeMonda CS. The costs and benefits of development: the transition from crawling to walking. *Child Dev Perspect.* 2014; 8: 187–192.
52. Thelen E. Kicking, rocking and waving: contextual analysis of stereotyped behaviour in normal infants. *Anim Behav.* 1981; 29: 3–11.
53. Thelen E, Fisher DM. Newborn stepping: an explanation for a 'disappearing reflex'. *Dev Psychobiol.* 1982; 18: 760–775.
54. Thelen E. Developmental origins of motor coordination: leg movements in human infants. *Dev Psychobiol.* 1985; 18: 1–22.
55. Thelen E. Treadmill-elicited stepping in seven-month-old infants. *Child Dev.* 1986; 57: 1498–1506.
56. Thelen E. Motor development. *Am Psychol.* 1995; 50: 79–95.
57. Spencer JP, Corbetta D, Buchanan P, Clearfield M, Ulrich B, Schoner G. Moving toward a grand theory of development: in memory of Esther Thelen. *Child Dev.* 2006; 77: 1521–1538.
58. Adolph KE. Learning to keep balance. In: Kail R (ed.) *Advances in child development and behavior*, 30. Amsterdam: Elsevier Science; 2002. p. 1–40.
59. Adolph KE, Vereijken B, Shrout PE. What changes in infant walking and why. *Child Dev.* 2003; 74: 475–497.
60. Adolph KE, Cole WG, Komati M, *et al.* How do you learn to walk? Thousands of steps and dozens of falls per day. *Psych Sci.* 2012; 23: 1387–1994.
61. Kelso JAS, Holt KG, Kugler PN, Turvey MT. On the concept of coordinative structures as dissipative structures: II. Empirical lines of convergence. In: Stelmach GE, Requin J (eds.) *Tutorials on motor behavior.* New York: North Holland; 1980. p. 49–70.
62. Hamill J, Haddad JM, McDermott WJ. Issues in quantifying variability from a dynamical systems perspective. *J Appl Biomech.* 2000; 16: 407–418.
63. Holt KG, Jeng S-F. Advances in biomechanical analysis of the physically challenged child: cerebral palsy. *Pediatr Exerc Sci.* 1992; 4: 213–235.
64. Clark JE, Phillips SJ. A longitudinal study of intralimb coordination in the first year of independent walking: a dynamical systems analysis. *Child Dev.* 1993; 64: 1143–1157.
65. van Emmerik REA, van Wegen EEH. On variability and stability in human movement. *J Appl Biomech.* 2000; 16: 394–406.
66. Morowitz HJ. *Foundations of bioenergetics.* New York: Academic Press; 1978.
67. Beek PJ, Wieringen PCWV. Perspectives on the relation between information and dynamics: an epilogue. *Hum Mov Sci.* 1994; 13: 519–533.
68. Nelkon M, Parker P. *Advanced level physics*, London: Heinemann Educational; 1964.
69. Holt KG, Hamill J, Andres RO. The force driven harmonic oscillator as a model for human walking. *Hum Mov Sci.* 1990; 9: 55–68.
70. Holt KG, Hamill J, Andres RO. Predicting the minimal energy costs of human walking. *Med Sci Sport Exerc.* 1991; 23: 491–498.
71. Jeng SF, Liao HF, Lai JS, Hou JW. Optimization of walking in children. *Med Sci Sport Exerc.* 1997; 29: 370–376.
72. Clark JE, Whitall J, Phillips SJ. Human interlimb coordination: the first 6 months of independent walking. *Dev Psychobiol.* 1988; 21: 445–456.
73. Holt KG, Jeng SF, Ratcliffe RJ, Hamill J. Energetic cost and stability during human walking at the preferred stride frequency. *J Mot Behav.* 1995; 27: 164–178.
74. Ledebt A, Breniere Y. Dynamical implication of anatomical and mechanical parameters in gait initiation process in children. *Hum Mov Sci.* 1994; 13: 801–815.
75. Goldfield EC, Kay BA, Warren WH. Infant bouncing: the assembly and tuning of action systems. *Child Dev.* 1993; 64: 1128–1142.
76. Ratcliffe RJ, Holt KG. Low frequency shock absorption in human walking. *Gait Posture.* 1997; 5: 93–100.
77. Jeng SF, Holt KG, Fetters L, Certo C. Self-optimization of walking in nondisabled children and children with spastic hemiplegic cerebral palsy. *J Mot Behav.* 1996; 28: 15–27.
78. Gibson EJ. The concept of affordances in perceptual development: the renascence of functionalism. In: Collins WA (ed.) *Minnesota symposia on child psychology*, 15. Hillsdale, NJ: Erlbaum; 1982. p. 55–80.
79. Fonseca ST, Holt KG, Fetters L, Saltzman E. Dynamic resources used in ambulation by children with spastic hemiplegic cerebral palsy: relationship to kinematics, energetics, and asymmetries. *Phy Ther.* 2004; 84: 344–354.
80. Holt KG, Saltzman E, Ho CL, Kubo M, Ulrich BD. Discovery of the pendulum and spring dynamics in the early stages of walking. *J Mot Behav.* 2006; 38: 206–218.
81. Alexander RM. Energy-saving mechanisms in walking and running. *J Exp Biol.* 1991; 160: 55–69.
82. Farley CT, Ferris DP. Biomechanics of walking and running: Center of mass movements to muscle action. *Exerc Sport Sci Rev.* 1998; 26: 253–285.
83. Kuo AD, Donelan JM. Dynamic principles of gait and their clinical implications. *Phys Ther.* 2012; 90: 157–176.
84. Holt KG, Fonseca ST, LaFiandra ME. The dynamics of gait in children with spastic hemiplegic cerebral palsy: theoretical and clinical implications. *Hum Mov Sci.* 2000; 19: 375–405.
85. Holt KG, Wagenaar RO, Saltzman E. A dynamic systems/constraints approach to rehabilitation. *Braz J Phys Ther.* 2010; 14: 446–463.
86. Carmick J. Clinical use of neuromuscular electrical stimulation in children with cerebral palsy. *Phys Ther.* 1993; 73: 505–513.
87. Comeaux P, Patterson N, Rubin M, Meiner R. Effect of neuromuscular electrical stimulation during gait in children with cerebral palsy. *Pediatr Phys Ther.* 1998; 9: 103–109.

CHAPTER 4

Motor development

David Sugden and Helen Soucie

Introduction

Movement is probably the most observable trait that we note from infancy through to adulthood. Movement usually progresses, and this progression is known as motor development, which is an adaptive change towards motor competence. Movement is involved in many aspects of living, and participating in activities that do not involve movement is difficult to envision; perhaps thinking, or types of meditation, may fall into this category. However, it is through movement that humans are able to interact with other living things and the environment. How children develop the motor skills that allow them to smoothly and competently participate, and interact, as part of their daily lives, presents multiple opportunities to explain these phenomena.

Thinking on motor development has progressed through quite significant stages. In the early twentieth century, most observational studies investigated the ages and stages children went through from birth to maturity. Classic studies, like those of Gesell[1] and McGraw[2] have provided excellent descriptions of how children progress in motor development and include some early explanations of this progress. More recently, these noted progressions have involved further explanatory studies that look at how and why the changes take place. Since the Second World War, the majority of these explanations have emerged from an information processing field giving computer analogies, schemas, motor programmes, and cognitive rationales. The work of Schmidt,[3] Adams,[4] and others in the adult motor learning domain has provided useable development models that offer greater scope for progress than the purely maturational theories. More recently, a different perspective suggesting dynamical explanations has been mooted. It considers the tri-directional influences of child resources, environmental contexts, and manner of presentation, all of which contribute through a self-organizing system to influence motor development. This work originated with Bernstein[5] and Gibson[6,7] and has been taken forward by Turvey and others[8–11] who differentiate the self-organizing system from the agent-task-environment system. This dynamical explanation has permeated the developmental field with the work of Adolph *et al.*,[12–17] but has yet to make a substantial impact on the atypical development field; however, studies are progressing.

This chapter begins with a traditional description of children's motor development and proceeds through the explanations from maturational and information processing research, of which there is an abundance. Development from a dynamic perspective is presented using research involving detailed studies on coordination, rather than on cognitive 'in the head' explanations. Paradoxically, there is an emerging field entitled 'embodied cognition'. Instead of explaining motor development through cognitive processes, it refers to motor development as the driver and underpinning influence on the development of the cognitive processes. Finally, atypical motor development is analysed through research work on children diagnosed with Developmental Coordination Disorder (DCD). By examining children with atypical motor development, not only is information about and support for these specific children identified, but data are also able to provide insight into the processes in typically developing children.

General description of change

The motoric changes that children make in their progression from birth through to maturity are well documented (see Sugden and Wade[18] for summary). The first 2 years of life see dramatic changes, followed by periods of stability, with further major changes occurring during the pubertal period. For example, locomotion is not present at birth, but during the first year of life the child gains postural control, develops turning over and changing positions, creeping and crawling, and finally at around 12 months of age, walking is accomplished. By age two, the child is performing rudimentary jumps and attempting running. By the time a typically developing child is 6 or 7 years of age, all the fundamental gross motor skills are observable, albeit in a rudimentary manner. These fundamental gross motor skills include running, jumping, hopping, skipping, climbing, throwing, catching, and galloping. After age seven, gross motor skills are further honed by using them in more challenging environments, refining them, modifying them, and using them in a series of other activities like playing games, recreation, and leisure activities. The acquisition of these fundamental skills during this period makes a strong argument for skilled teaching during this period. In children with difficulties, e.g. those on the autistic spectrum, current studies suggest that these fundamental skills contribute to overall development.[19,20]

A similar pattern is seen in manual skills. The newborn and young infant has crude but goal-directed manual skills involving manipulation, reaching, and grasping. Classic studies by Connolly and Elliott[21] describe how finger and thumb opposition occurs early in life. The very young infant grasps an object using the palm and ulna side of the hands. During the first year of life this changes to the more radial and distal location, and eventually the grasp becomes a combination of the thumb and index finger in true opposition. As the child develops, more complex manual skills are evident in activities like writing and drawing. At 18 months the first random scribbling is evident and between the ages of 3 to 5 years, the child acquires drawing of lines and circles, copying a square, and sometimes a triangle. Considering that, at these ages, a child can copy a figure using matchsticks before he/she can draw it suggests that the issue is more one of motor control rather than a perceptual one. Activities of daily living, like the use of feeding utensils, also develop during this early period. Again, by age six or seven, the child is competent in performing most manuals skills. With development and learning, children refine manual skills, augment the speed of performance, and use skills flexibly in increasingly demanding environmental situations. Description of change is provided in many sources of motor development.[18,22–24]

Explanation of change

What accounts for the changes that take place from birth through to maturity? Explanations come from a number of different sources. On the one hand, the developmental literature has been strongly influenced by general theories of development that are not necessarily devoted to the motor domain and that are mainly cognitive in nature. An early source of these theories is the neuro-maturational literature, which usually involves descriptive studies of the abilities 'unfolding' in some predetermined manner. In addition, the motor control and motor learning literature that has looked mainly at adult performance and learning has strongly influenced developmental thinking.

Traditional maturational explanations

The work of Myrtle McGraw[25] typified traditional maturational explanations in her descriptions of the twin males Johnny and Jimmy. Together with Arnold Gesell[1] they noted the changes through the first 6 or 7 years of life, calling them 'motor milestones'. They concluded that this seemingly orderly progression was a result of neuro-maturational development and that this controlled both the emergence and timing of actions. This was exemplified by McGraw's description and explanation of the four-stage progression from reflexive to voluntary behaviour. As an example she used the development of palmar grasp:

i) Reflex from pressure on the palm.

ii) At 3–4 months inhibition of palm pressure producing extension of fingers and thumb.

iii) Palmar grasp occurs without palmar pressure when, for example, reaching to grasp an object.

iv) Flexibility in producing a variety of grasps to accommodate the environmental context.

This example typified the approach of the time, as did similar reports from Piaget describing his sensorimotor period.

Since then, maturational theories have been elaborated upon and extended. This early period provided the basis for an approach inferring that development emerges solely in the brain, and that it flows in a hierarchical manner through the central nervous system. The process involves a gradual unfolding of predetermined patterns with cortical control taking over from lower brain stem and spinal reflexes. A number of arguments have been proffered against this view. Ulrich,[26] for example, notes that some maturationists maintain that, because people pass through similar sequences, a programme is prepared in advance and is genetically determined. Ulrich argues that this would be such a cumbersome process for humans to deal with: assigning neurons for the development of movement patterns is not a economical way of dealing with the complex issue of evolving development. However, this maturational line of research did provide some classic information on children's motor development. It established milestones and expectancies for motor development, giving great insight through these researchers' meticulous observations into the changes that take place. It is not that neural development has no part to play in the evolving motor development of the child, but rather that it is not the whole story.

Information processing and cognitive explanations

It is paradoxical that explanations from a cognitive perspective have dominated the field of motor development and often appear under the usual heading of Information Processing Systems (IPS). There exists a similar debate in language development about the relationship between language and cognition. There are many variations of IPS but they all usually have a number of characteristics in common, most commonly that information is taken into the system and flows through various transformations to a motor output. The field of motor development has moved on from its initial ideas and now encompasses different concepts, but information transformation is still the central tenet.

Memory has always been a prominent feature of most processing models. This concept also developed from early studies like Tulving,[27] developmental models from Brown,[28] and more recently to those using new technologies like brain imaging or functional magnetic resonance imaging (fMRI), which can show actual structural parts of the brain that are active, rather than having to infer processes.[29,30] Information entering the processing system is usually either visual or kinaesthetic and is purported to be held in a working memory store so that it may be used for a plan of action. This plan is often labeled as a programme and contains such parameters as force, timing, and spatial characteristics, as well as other variables that may influence the movement outcome.

An important and related concept comes directly from the motor learning field and involves Schmidt's[3] schema theory of a generalized motor programme containing rules about the relationships between the various parameters pertaining to a particular task. Accordingly, a given task will have force, spatial, and speed variables attached to it and after several trials on related but slightly different task conditions, a schema is developed from four sources of information. These are i) the initial conditions prior to the movement; ii) the response specifications for the motor programme; iii) the sensory consequences of the movement; and iv) the movement outcome. A schema involving both recognition and recall is built up from these sources. This thinking led to the influential proposition that variability of experience, or practice, will lead to a stronger schema with improved learning, leaving the learner in a more advantaged position, able to respond flexibly to a changing environmental context. However, later studies have revised some of the recommendations of schema theory.[31–33]

More recent theoretical concepts have emerged from the motor control area with an examination as to how the neuromotor system produces movement. Work on computational explanations, e.g. Wolpert *et al.*,[34] Wolpert and Flanagan,[35] and Karniel,[36] examine how the neuromotor system produces movement, and often employs Baysian decision-making theory. These explanations have resulted in much progress, but as Sugden and Wade[18] note, 'the problem of simulating natural biological control remains a challenge … … (and) while progress has been made, the successes remain more robotic than human'.[18(p.57)]

Some promising work is being done by Peter Wilson and his colleagues in Australia on internal modeling both in typically developing children and children with DCD. Wilson's current work explores the ability of children to make rapid online (or in-flight) adjustments to their movements, as well as the mediation of frontal executive control on these systems.[37] Further work in this area may lead to more specific information about neurological functions during motor actions.

The past history of these processing models and ideas to account for motor development in children has shown consistent results but, as yet, do not fulfill all the criteria for explanation. Work with children on memory, attention, capacity allocation, processing speed (including reaction and movement time), and feedback and knowledge of results has provided quite consistent results. As children develop, they become more efficient, effective, and more flexible in task performance.[38–50] These studies from the early days of information processing describe how children become more proficient with age on various types of tasks. With development, children react and move faster, have improved memory use, and are more effective at using different types of feedback. Since the 1960s the studies from this theoretical processing perspective have provided the base of much of the motor learning and developmental research. Additionally, the paradigms have also shown that children with atypical resources perform more poorly than their peers on motor tasks. However, while this perspective has provided better, deeper, and different descriptions, it has not provided explanations as to how the changes in motor control take place.[26] There are areas in neuropsychology that are exploring this area, but all have the fundamental premise that information is transformed by the brain in some way. Much of the work on processing systems has mirrored work on cognition without paying particular attention to the most distinctive feature of motor behavior, which is the control of movement itself. To look for alternative explanations it is important to examine different theoretical perspectives involving ecological psychology and dynamical systems theories. Much of the theoretical ideas for these two related areas come from the work of James Gibson,[6] an ecological psychologist, and the Russian neurophysiologist Nicolai Bernstein.[5]

Ecological psychology and dynamic systems

Gibson: direct perception

For James Gibson, rather than having to transform information coming into the system through various indirect perceptual processes, perception and action are viewed as directly linked without any complicated intermediary processing operations. There is no need for any internal representation of the world. In Gibson's view, when a person sees an object in the environment, he/she is sensitive to the inherent opportunities for action. Gibson termed these opportunities 'affordances'. A spoon may afford picking up an object, an approaching ball may afford catching, and no action can occur effectively without consideration of both the person doing the action and the environmental context in which it takes place.

The perception action links proposed by Gibson play a major role in the control of movements through the repeated cycle of exploration-perception-action, where the child is an active participant in the process that affords change. As humans perceive the environment, the activity of seeing creates an optical flow field providing space and time information. For example, the rate of expansion given by light hitting the retina offers direct information about incoming objects. Gibson suggests that this information, via the rate of expansion, offers direct perception of approaching or colliding objects as well as the timing of interceptions without the need for higher cortical calculations and transformations. In experiments with a visual cliff, Gibson and Walk[51] demonstrated the use of direct perception and the relationships in the environment with personal affordances in the control of movements from an early age. This perception/action link is one of the integrated branches of an ecological perspective on motor development.

Bernstein: dynamic systems

Bernstein questioned how a human body with approximately 1000 muscles, 100 bones, and associated linkages is organized to produce the simplest of movements. He examined the notion that the central nervous system (CNS) alone was responsible for controlling the degrees of freedom. The potential degrees of freedom resulting from the interconnectivity of these muscles, bones, and linkages refer to the many possibilities a person may have in their movements by the fixing, or the releasing, of the limb joints. The grouping of the degrees of freedom is referred to as synergies, or coordinative structures, and defined as a group of muscles and joints constrained to act as a single unit. They are constrained, but not totally controlled by the CNS. However the CNS is one of many internal and external constraints on the system. Bernstein's idea promotes a more dynamic view of motor control as a self-organizing system influenced by the context, rather than reliant on motor programmes. Movements are described as being 'softly assembled', with the CNS playing a part, but not with rigid predetermined programmes. Thus the resources the child brings, the contextual situation, and the task results in movement outcome.[52,53] Newell *et al.* provide compelling evidence[54] in their hand-grasping study. The study investigates how the type of grasp, either one or two hands, depended on the size of the cup to be grasped, with the hand width grasp formed by the thumb and index finger being scaled to the size of the cup. This is similar to the action analysis in Newell's[52] constraint paper and the concept that body-scaled responses to the environmental context are logical. More recently, Lopresti-Goodman and Frank[11] seemingly confirm Newell's earlier work in their study on the decision, when presented with differently sized items, to use one or two hands to grasp an object. Hand span was found to be part of the perceived affordance (a body-scaled response) as well as the presentation sequence of the differently sized objects (environmental context).

The notion of softly assembled coordinative structures, or synergies, has important developmental implications. The development of synergies to accomplish a task does not solely demand the use of higher cortical processed instructions, but rather can rely on the physical properties of the dynamic system as the individual self-organizes, e.g. the spring-like properties of muscles, the task, and the environmental context. As the infant or young child explores his/her environment, the movements used are changed from simply exploratory to more refined and purposeful ones; this results in greater efficiency. The movements that developing children use are seen to change the degrees of freedom while they adapt the synergies to suit the task in hand as well as their changing resources. The self-assembly of the synergies required to meet the demands of the task in the case of the developing child is dependent on the child's own resources, like postural control, muscular strength, and the attractiveness of the task. This particular approach to the explanation of motor control and change examines development from a multi-causal perspective showing how a complex, dynamic, and evolving system supports the performance of a task or skill.

The neuronal group selection theory from Sporns and Edelman[55] also challenges the idea that development evolves solely from genetic instructions, and they propose that through periods of instability (where many options to solve a motor problem are experienced) and stability (where fewer options are used to solve a motor problem), individuals select solutions that strengthen (through use) certain connections within groups of neurons. They note that the evidence points to the plasticity of the brain being moulded by experience and that coordinated movements are tied to both brain development and the biomechanical context. A coordinated response is the result of reciprocal signals from many areas of the brain integrating messages in order to produce coordinated responses. Thelen[56] has referred to this as a kind of mapping of maps, with neural diversity and cross entries of sensory information allowing the CNS to recognize and categorize signals thorough a dynamic and self-organizing system. Experience has a major part to play in brain development, with this development being a self-organizing process. Sporns and Edelman[55] provide a relatively intermediate position between traditional processing theories and more dynamical perception action positions. They provide an important role for the CNS but their research does not label it as the overall controller.

Studies from the ecological perspective involving both direct perception and dynamical theories emphasize the notion of active learning from a multidisciplinary, multicausal position. They also offer a model for change throughout the lifespan, not just for young infants. If experience and resources afford adaptation, if exploration leads to selection, and further exploration develops into retention of preferred actions, the same model can be applied to the acquisition of new or adapted skills learned by adults. If young children alter and adapt the degrees of freedom used to accomplish a task as they experiment with the nature of the task and their own constraints, then it is reasonable to suggest that this may be applied to the older child or adult when they are learning a new task.

It is clear from these different theoretical perspectives that the brain plays a significant role in coordinated motor activity. However, many question whether the brain is solely responsible for this control. Both maturational and information processing approaches have provided better descriptions at deeper and more complex levels. The ecological viewpoint and dynamical systems approach are having a major impact on explanations of development and change and how they are linked to development of other facilities like perception and cognition.

Early movement development

The time from birth to 24 months represents a significant period in a baby's life with a transition from a state of minimal control of their arms, legs, and posture, to one of good postural control, walking, and to a certain degree, the ability to reach, grasp, and manipulate a variety of objects. The ability to react to fast moving objects or changing environments is still developing, but the developmental trajectory over the first 2 years is remarkable.

Spontaneous movements and reflexes

Prechtl[57] reported on a series of studies looking at movements in utero and for 30 weeks post-term. He describes three classes of movements: writhing movements, fidgety movements, and voluntary movements, all developing from the tenth week in utero to the 20th week post-term. He notes that these observations of movements are good predictors of neurological dysfunction in young children. This position was taken further by Hadders-Algra,[58] who followed these movement classifications up to 18 months post-term. Both researchers provide slightly different views to the early maturationists such as Gesell and McGraw, but both still emphasize a neural explanation.

A more dynamic explanation of development was initiated by Thelen[59] who looked at rhythmical movement stereotypies in the young infant. After extensive observations of infants in the first year of life she reported a total of 47 different stereotypies, identifying 11 as the most frequent. These movements did not seem to have a particular goal and involved total body, or parts of the body, movement at regular short intervals. These movements were combined into logical groups, such as those associated with kicking, looking at age of onset and age of peak activity level. These spontaneous movements were not considered reflexes or involuntary movements, but instead were viewed as possible precursors to later voluntary actions. Thelen's work considers the relationship between some of these rhythmic kicking actions, the stepping reflex, and later walking. The spontaneous movement seen in young babies was measured, and the kinematics of the spontaneous kicking movements was noted to resemble the spatial and temporal components of mature walking patterns.

The early reflexes found in babies are related to infant survival and are nourishment-seeking as well as protective actions. These subcortically controlled reflex movements are present in newborn babies, and the rate and strength at which they appear and disappear are considered as indicators of healthy development or early indicators of CNS disorders. Although it has been postulated that reflex behaviours and later crawling, swimming, and stepping are related, there is a gap between the disappearance of the reflex and the emergence of the later voluntary movement. However, in the case of spontaneous leg movements there is no disappearance of the movements before the onset of locomotion. The reflexive movements seen in the stepping reflex disappear with time, but the spontaneous kicking of a child on his/her back remains.

The stepping reflex occurs when a young infant is held upright with their feet on a support surface and they perform alternating step like movements. Traditionally the disappearance of this stepping reflex was attributed to the maturation of the voluntary cortical centres which inhibited reflexive movements and later facilitated the movements under a different and higher level of control. This was a long-held theory explaining the onset of the stepping reflex, its disappearance, and reappearance as a voluntary movement towards the end of the child's first year. Thelen proposed different explanations for this disappearance and subsequent reappearance, suggesting it is multi-causality of action rather than its dependence solely on maturation.

Taking this multi-causality view, Thelen and Fisher[61] noted that supine infants' random, spontaneous kicking actions had similar movement patterns to the stepping reflex, but unlike the reflex, these spontaneous kicks did not disappear after a few months. This observation led Thelen to assert that the reflex stepping and spontaneous kicking were the same movements performed in two different postures. The question then arises as to why the stepping reflex is suppressed, and spontaneous kicking continues. Thelen and Fisher[61] posit that the answer lies not solely in the maturational system but rather in the total dynamics of the infant's task demands. Thus as the stepping reflex disappears, infants simultaneously experience a rapid gain in mass, most of which is subcutaneous fat rather than muscle tissue. Thelen and Fisher[61] propose that in order for the infant to move their legs in a stepping manner he/she requires postural support from a prone or supine position as the legs have become too heavy for the infants to move while in an upright position. To test this theory, they submerged infants in warm water that offered support, or added weights to either restore or inhibit the stepping reflex. The relationship between gravity and weight bearing was seen to afford, or not afford, the stepping action from different support positions. Other studies corroborate this position: Goldfield *et al.*,[62] found children adjusted their kicking in a baby bouncer to get optimal bounce, and kinematic analysis showed that 'infants assemble and tune a periodic kicking system akin to a mass spring, homing in on its resonant frequency'. [62(p.1137)]

This work involving infants performing basic movements illustrates the complexity of how voluntary control evolves from earlier movements like reflexes and spontaneous movement stereotypies. Thelen *et al.*'s classic work shows that maturation alone does not totally explain the emergence and disappearance of these various movements. In a similar vein, it is highly unlikely that an explanation can be found from an information-processing, cognitive perspective; it suggests transformation and elaboration of input through various stages through to a motor programme, and finally movement. A multifaceted answer is more likely, as proposed by those supporting a dynamic systems explanation, with many components being self-organized to produce the required action. This becomes evident when considering the constraints as noted by Newell[52] and Thelen and Smith,[63] who observed affordances, with the so-called walking reflex. In this case, the internal constraint to the child is fat content, and the external affordance being the use of water as support.

Environmental affordances

A similar situation arises when considering how information enters the system and is analysed. There is a given difference between indirect perception (information processing systems), and Gibsonian direct perception involving affordances in the environment.

Again the developing infant offers some clues. Gibson and Walk's[51] groundbreaking study from 1960 examined infant perception and action. Infants aged 6 to 14 months were presented with a perceived visual cliff made using a glass-topped table with a chequer board pattern underneath. The infants were then placed on the table top and encouraged to crawl to their mothers at the other side. Even coaxing from their mothers would not induce the infants to crawl over the 'cliff', suggesting that even at ages 6–14 months, the infants exhibited depth perception.

Adolph *et al.*[12] studied toddlers aged 14 months to examine their perceived affordances when presented with ascending or descending sloping walkways of different angles. The action of walking is adapted to suit the terrain and children, relatively new to locomotion, were studied to observe their adaption to different contextual situations. The toddlers, all able to walk on the flat for 3 m, were beckoned by their parents to walk towards them on an inclined or declined surface. All toddlers perceived the affordances, all overestimated their ability on the ascending slopes, and all showed different ways to descend, for example, by sliding. Additionally, all asked for help on the declining slopes. There were few falls and all toddlers actively explored different ways of achieving the task, which demonstrated their ability to perceive affordances. Adolph *et al.*[64–66] have more recently reported further studies of infants' perceived affordances, presenting the infants a bridge to cross, or a choice between a step or a cliff, and analyzing how perceived affordances are linked to posture. When presented with a cliff or a step, experienced crawling infants refused to negotiate the cliff, while novice walkers went ahead with the task. However, experienced walkers would not walk over the cliff, and rather chose to use another form of locomotion to achieve the task. Of note was that the experienced crawlers had learned to avoid a cliff situation, but their previous crawling experience did not teach the novice walkers to be wary of the cliff. It was only when an infant became an experienced walker that he/she learned to negotiate the cliff. Thus, crawling experiences taught crawling affordances, and walking experiences taught walking affordances. This notion of visual perception linked to postural development was also observed when infants were asked to cross a bridge that varied in width and in height of drop off. The width of the bridge determined the likelihood of a fall while the extent of the drop off determined the severity of the fall. Experienced crawlers and experienced walkers adapted their locomotion to cross the bridge according to the width, but interestingly, they did not consider the severity of the potential fall in their decision making. Experience for both crawlers and walkers led to accurate perceived affordances, but the risk of a severe fall was not taken into consideration. Kretch *et al.*[66] believe that locomotion affordances for infants are directly related to their postural development, which influences their visual field. Crawling infants perceive their affordances more from looking at the floor, although they will use their necks to look up, or stop and sit to attain a different perspective. Walkers who look straight ahead are able to see the walls and their caregivers more easily. However, this does not mean that walkers are universally advantaged, as crawlers can see their limbs more readily than walkers, which can be a positive aspect when perceiving some affordances.

Other studies complement these results. Stoffregen *et al.*[67] examined whether young infants with only a few weeks' standing experience were able to maintain and adapt their standing posture to the constraints placed upon them by different support surfaces. The children used complex movements, including movements of the hips (not thought previously to occur until ages 3–4 years of age), the ankles, and use of hands and arms, to maintain postural control. In related but different studies, Thelen[68] found that 3- to 4-month-old infants can learn patterns of interlimb coordination on a novel task. Thelen observed them moving an overhead mobile with their ankles tethered to soft elastic straps and the mobile. These studies demonstrate that learning processes are at work early in life and that patterns of movement are not simply driven by autonomous maturational brain processes. The infants in these studies demonstrated an awareness of their environment, environmental constraints, and an ability to link their perceptions with their actions, and subsequently to develop solutions. The children's motor activities provided the means to explore their environment and the opportunity to learn about its properties. As each new solution was gained, it provided opportunities for further perceptual motor exploration; the children built upon their knowledge from the demands of the task. This perspective of motor development disputes the notion of inevitable stages in motor development, and instead stresses the dynamic changing and ecological nature of development.

Vision and visual perception development

How information is taken into the system has a profound effect on future actions and movements. While most human senses affect the resulting actions, the primary source for action early in life, and the best understood, is vision. Vision specifies the context in which the body moves, it controls movements through the use of feedback, it helps with preplanning movement, and it provides information about the results of the movement. Vision also provides spatial information in the form of location, distance, and size, and provides temporal information about moving things, both alive and inanimate, in relation to the self.

At birth the visual structures are present but immature. Myelinization has occurred to a certain extent, but the optic nerve develops rapidly up to around 4 months. Newborn acuity is lower than that at maturity, but by 2 months of age, vision has developed enough for the infant to recognize faces. Object perception is not truly developed at birth. Infants have difficulty seeing space between objects, although object constancy develops early and provides information for the infant showing that objects are the same from any angle, and how objects are portrayed as retinal images. Depth perception enables the brain to judge distances for both near and far, like reaching for a mobile, or throwing a ball to someone. Infants at around 4 months of age are relatively accurate in reaching and contacting slow-moving objects; they clearly perceive the movement and any inaccuracy in reaching and grasping comes about as a result of a lack of motor control rather than inaccurate perception.[69]

Both binocular parallax, the ability to integrate the input from both eyes, and motion parallax, when the retinal image is displaced when the head is moved, are important developments for the infant. Binocular parallax is present by 5 months of age, while motion parallax is present at around 2 months, subsequently becoming more accurate during the first year of life.[70,71]

How infants use vision is the topic of several important studies involving approaching objects, control of stance, and reaching and grasping.[72–75] Many of these studies using 'moving' rooms, showing how vision not only allows seeing, but also that it provides proprioception, for example, in stance control. These studies, and others such as the von Hofsten[76] study, have moved away from the notion of vision and kinaesthesis as separate systems working on their own. Perception is now regarded as a more global concept and that with age, children become more efficient at integrating visual information into a holistic unit as they develop though experience. More recently, Corbetta *et al.*[77] have revealed how the role of vision in infants' reaching and grasping is part of an embodied process wherein the child learns how to direct his/her limbs and correct the directional aspect of movements via vision. In other words, the infants explore limb movements using proprioceptive and haptic feedback, followed by a 'mapping' via the visual tracking of reaching and grasping. Corbetta *et al.*[77] suggest that this early visuomotor mapping of reaching and grasping is the crux for future visually elicited motor control but that haptic and proprioceptive feedback gained from the infant's environment is the basis of reaching and grasping control; vision itself plays a 'mapping' role. It is almost a reversal of previous work suggesting that an infant's reaching is guided by vision, with Corbetta *et al*'s[77] findings showing that infants align their look to where they reach. This idea concurs with Thelen's notion of spontaneous movements being the foundation of future exploration, which leads to directed actions once the mapping, either visual or haptic, has confirmed the relationships between the intended action and the results.

Motor development 2–7 years of age

At 2 years of age, children are capable of a number of basic skills, including walking, running, climbing, releasing objects, a bit of scribbling, some self-care, and, in general, using motor skills to independently enjoy and explore their environment. In Campos *et al.*'s[78] classic paper '*Travel Broadens the Mind*', locomotion brings with it the enhancement of a new set of related behaviours. By ages 6–7 years, the child will have developed most of the fundamental skills that they are likely to acquire. From then on, children play with these skills, adapt to differing environmental contexts, and start to show maximum performance measures.

When examining the explanations for changes in walking and stair climbing, for example, maturational explanations have been proposed by Hamilton[79] and by Hirschfeld and Forssberg,[80] who clearly show that maturation does play a part. However, the focus of this chapter is on dynamical systems explanations that focus on more multicausal factors. Adolph *et al.*[14] looked at walking in infants aged 1–2 years and young children aged 5–6 years by analysing a number of variables in the walking process. These variables included neural maturation and various morphological measures such as height, weight, and leg length, plus practice calculated from the number of days from a child's first step. The conclusion was that practice was the most important variable and neither maturation, nor morphological variables, could solely account for the improvement in walking skill. This line of thought was similar to that of Cesari *et al.*,[81] who looked at stair climbing in children. This study revealed that children perceive environmental invariants, such as the size of the stair riser and their body-scale size, with their climbing actions. Thus it appears that these early actions are developed and improved by a number of both internal and external constraints, including body scaling, perceptual factors, emerging coordinative structures, and practice, and are not simply dependent on maturational variables.

The children in these studies demonstrated an awareness of their environment, its constraints, and an ability to link their perceptions with their actions and develop solutions. Their motor activities provided the means to explore their environment and the opportunity to learn about its properties. As each new solution was gained, it opened up opportunities for further perceptual exploration as the children built upon their knowledge from the demands of the task. This again disputes the notion of inevitable stages in motor development, while emphasizing the dynamic and ecological notion of development.

As the young child's resources increase to perceive affordances, so do the biomechanical features of any movement. If the action of throwing is examined, the constraints limit the child in the early stages to freezing, or reducing, the degrees of freedom in the action. In the younger child the throwing action is mainly from the elbow with little rotary movement. The child's body mass is not transferred into the throw and the feet tend to remain stationary. The degrees of freedom are kept to a minimum as releasing them would result in an uncontrolled movement. This self-organizing system demonstrates the resource the child has at this moment and how he/she adapts to the internal and external constraints placed upon them.

As the child develops, these degrees of freedom are released to give greater flexibility and more adaptive movements. Eventually, the throwing action becomes more dynamic, the arm and body movements more extensive, and the throw becomes more efficient in a variety of contexts. The child's constantly evolving resources results in the refinement of his or her movements. This is a dynamic situation according to task demands, for example, a 6-year-old child reverting to freezing degrees of freedom when throwing a ball on the run.

Motor development in later childhood

Between age 6 years and puberty, a number of developmental changes take place in the child. First, he/she starts to refine the already accomplished skills and becomes more constant and less variable in his/her performances, i.e. the child consistently produces an effective movement. Paradoxically at the same time, they become more flexible, or more variable, in their performances, which allows them to adapt to the spatial and temporal requirements of the environment, and to move in response to non-stationary others and objects.[82] This development has been constant through the years between 6 and puberty, but at puberty, more complex environmental demands become prevalent in a child's life. Another development is an extension of this flexibility where the child engages in play-game activities for which normative comparisons in maximum performances are made.

If a simple task is examined, like reaching and grasping, it is notable that children have a relatively mature reach and grasp by age 7, but from 7 onwards, children are able to exploit reaching in more complex contexts. Kuhtz-Buschbeck *et al.*[83] examined children aged 4–12 years of age. They monitored the trajectory of the reach and the shaping of the hand as it approached a cylindrical object. In the first experiment, object size and distance were kept constant and the object was scaled to each individual. In the second, object sizes and distance were varied to examine adaptability. Trials were carried out with and without the hands visible to the children. With age, the kinematics of hand transport improved with smoother bell-shaped velocity profiles. On repetitive trials the variability decreased with age although all children showed appropriate movement velocity scaling when distance was varied. Grip anticipation was present in all children with the younger children 'playing safe' with a wider grip at the start. This grip formation became more stable with age and showed a consistent pattern of single peak in synchrony with the deceleration of hand transport. When analysing visual control, all children scaled their hand transport to the distance to travel even in non-visual mode, but the younger children often missed the target and took longer. The data showed younger children relying more on vision, with big improvements occuring between ages 4 to 7, and further progressive changes occurring up to 12 years of age.

An interceptive task involves prediction, anticipation, and coincidence. Everyday tasks such as walking on a busy pavement or riding a bicycle are typical interceptive tasks. Research groups in the Netherlands have been using the concept of the bearing angle to look at changes in interceptive tasks.[84–86] In these tasks, the constant bearing angle involves adults using the head as the angle centre with the angular position of the ball remaining constant with respect to an interception point. By keeping this bearing angle constant, the mover needs only one piece of information to aid interception. In adults, this angle remains constant during locomotion, but it breaks down at the point of interception and the bearing angle of the wrist takes over. Chohan *et al.*[86] required two groups of children, 5- to 7-year-olds and 10- to 12-year-olds, to walk and intercept a tennis ball while moving on a platform. Light-emitting devices were placed on the children and monitored by a motion analysis system. Both groups showed fluent movement with appropriate acceleration and deceleration, but the older children showed more stability and consistent strategy regardless of the speed of the ball. The younger children reacted more, and deviated more, from a constant bearing angle strategy, which occurred when the velocity of the ball was high. In all probability, the younger children required more time. With the slower ball speeds the younger children deviated earlier, unlike the older children, who behaved like adults, and who kept the bearing angle irrespective of the speed of the ball.

In situations that require anticipation, prediction, and interception, it is clear even in everyday tasks that children improve between the ages of 6 and 10, up to age 12 years. Laboratory experiments have confirmed these improvements, which continue to around 14 years of age, but at a slower rate, when mean performance probably approximates that of adults.[18]

Maximum performance

Between the ages of 6 years and puberty and onwards, maximum performance on a number of measures increases greatly. Examples include standing long jump improving in males from 46 inches (1.17 m) at 7 to over 80 inches (2.03 m) at 16 years; for girls this moves from 45 inches (1.14 m) at 7 to ~60 inches (1.52 m) at 16 years, with a plateau at 13 years, which suggests a motivational rather than physiological effect. In running speed, for the same cohort, boys move from 15 feet$\cdot$s^{-1} (4.57 m$\cdot$s^{-1}) at 7 to 22 feet$\cdot$s^{-1} (6.71 m$\cdot$s^{-1}) at 16 years, while speeds for girls are 15 feet$\cdot$s^{-1} (4.57 m$\cdot$s^{-1}) and 18 feet$\cdot$s^{-1} (5.49 m$\cdot$s^{-1}) respectively. Throwing for distance shows similar graphs with similar gender differences. When one examines balance in tasks such as beam walking, there is a steady increase in performance from 7 to 14 years of age, but with no gender differences. The same trend appears in manual movements, like speed of peg placement, where 15-year-olds tend to be almost two times faster than 7-year-olds. Other maximum performance measures show similar results: reaction time drops from 350 ms at 6 to 240 ms at 12 years; movement time is lower in older children, particularly in difficult movements where there is a higher task demand. Smits-Engelsman[87] suggests that younger children's slower movement speed is the result of their impaired ability to use open loop control. (see Sugden and Wade[18] for summary).

By age 7, children have developed a full range of motor facilities involving either total body or simple manual skills. From then on, their lives become more complex and increasing demands are made on them; their motor skills improve to accommodate these demands in three ways. First, children older than 7 years show more consistency and less variability in the performances of tasks that are repeated in a similar manner. Secondly, children become more variable and flexible, by being able and proficient in dealing with unpredictable environmental contexts like moving objects or persons. They improve greatly in prediction and anticipation between the ages of 6 to 7 years, and 12–13 years, with adult-like performances seen at the latter ages. Thirdly, in terms of maximum performance, children improve greatly between the ages of 6 and 7 years to post-puberty with less improvement after that time. These are all transactional factors impinging on each other in a manner that is self-organizing. Thus, children become quicker and more adept at recognizing affordances for action, which leaves them more time to anticipate and intercept moving objects and others in the environment. The changes that take place at puberty allow movers to use their increased strength, speed, and endurance to increase their performance on a wide a variety of tasks.

Embodied cognition

The term embodied cognition is used to describe the idea that intelligence, or cognition, emerges in the early years as an interaction between the sensorimotor actions of a baby with his/her environmental context. In other words, cognition is grounded in sensorimotor coupling[88] and is organized through actions and sensorimotor processing.[89] Embodied cognition, as an explanatory theory of human behaviour, rejects the causal primacy of neural processes and structures as the basis for both developing and learned behaviours, including motor development. The proponents of embodied cognition propose an all-embracing notion of development and learning that comprises dynamical systems theory, social behaviour theory, and the concept of self-organizing processes.[90] Sensorimotor interactions, or couplings, that occur on a daily basis between the child and the child's environment, including the affordances and the constraints of both the child and environment at any given moment in time, are the foundations for motor development that will support the cognitive and the language development of the infant.[91]

This is not a new idea. Piaget[92] made similar assertions, but researchers have taken these further with the rationale appearing in a number of areas. These studies note, and encourage, that children make contact with the physical world through multiple senses, creating redundancy such that the loss of one sensory component does not affect the overall function. Multiple sensory inputs, such as touch and sight reinforce the whole experience of an event, for example, picking up a toy. The two, or more, systems start to map on to each other, reinforce, and enable higher processes to evolve. In this way, when a physical object is visually perceived, the tactile sensation associated with the object are automatically evoked, and vice versa. Through vision and hearing, for example, a child perceives the spatial structure of the environment and through his/her own actions, they change that spatial structure. These ongoing cycles of perception/action couplings are the self-organizing processes for cognition or understanding.[93] These multimodal interactions change over time, so a baby of 4 months of age will have a different sensory motor experience than a 1-year-old, and that difference, in turn, will affect the developmental outcome. For example, self-locomotion changes the nature of the type of visual, tactile, and auditory inputs for the infant, which in turn have a profound effect on cognition. For example, when babies are able to self-locomote, they do not make the same errors of conservation of place of objects that occurs when they are stationary.[92]

Random exploration is also a way by which babies learn about their world and reciprocally develop actions. For example, in reaching and grasping there is a continuous process of arousal to an object, with exploration by the hand and arms leading to different solutions. This then leads to new tasks and challenges being attempted and consequently new solutions being derived. Smith and Gasser[93] noted that young mammals move in a variety of ways often for no apparent reason; these movements, often called play, are ways of exploring new avenues which are essential to the building of intelligence and cognitive operations. Thelen[68] demonstrated, as noted earlier, how spontaneous kicking actions of a baby, with their ankles linked to an overhead mobile toy, can result in intended actions to prolong the satisfying movement of an overhead mobile. More recently, exploration linked to the attainment of certain motor milestones has been found to predict the development of spatial cognition and spatial language.[91] Once children have the possibility to move around, i.e. roll, crawl, walk, or change their postural position from lying to sitting or standing, their attention changes, their perception alters, and their spatial skills develop. Exploration has a mediating role in developing spatial processing. Longitudinal studies, as well as later academic and intellectual measures, examining motor exploration in 5-month-old infants found that infants with greater competence for movement, balance, locomotion, and exploratory activity were more successful intellectually and academically at 4, 10, and 14 years of age.[94] What is suggested here is that greater opportunities for movement and exploration benefit cognitive development.

Thirdly, infant and mother interaction gaze, imitation, and the progressive action and transaction between mother and child are other areas whereby the development of context affects development. Parents and children look at each other, parents introduce a toy to a child, and the toy is moved and waved and named. This range of modality in a social setting helps to establish the concept of the object in the world. Finally, action and language are linked in ways similar to action, sensory, and social areas. In a study of manual skills and cognitive abilities in children ages 3–6, it was observed that fine motor hand skills related not only to a child's visual-spatial ability, but also to his/her vocabulary level. The earlier the manual skill was acquired, the stronger the association with cognitive tasks.[95] Young infants possess multiple sensory and action systems that develop as the infant explores the environmental context and interacts with others. Intelligence and cognition emerge from these interactions; more accurately, these transactions continually affect each other. This intelligence is embedded in these multiple systems and develops in a dynamic manner where all of the components change and interact. Wilson and colleagues[96–98] have proposed the idea of off-line embodied cognition as a powerful force in the development of cognition. Off-line cognition involves those activities where the sensorimotor activity is simulated in the cognitive action. For example, all forms of imagery provide good examples of simulating external events, and recent work with children having coordination difficulties shows interesting ways forward for possible interventions. In off-line embodied cognition, episodic memory involving the visual, kinaesthetic, and motor impressions is linked to the body's experiences with the world; other examples are available in the area of problem solving and reasoning.

Atypical motor development

Because movement is essential in daily life, any deviation, delay or pathology may interfere with daily functioning. In addition, movement also plays a part in other aspects of children's lives; it is a critical component when identifying difficulties that children may have across a spectrum of abilities. Thus, movement may be a predictor of later difficulties, and of children with developmental coordination problems.

Movements as early indicators of later difficulties

Developmental disorders such as attention-deficit-hyperactivity disorder (ADHD) and constitutional motor disorders such as cerebral palsy are difficult to diagnose early. This difficulty is reflected in the diversity of methods used to try and assess the brain at an early age. These methods include functional neurological examinations using little or no equipment, to technical assessments using a variety of sophisticated machinery, including various forms of brain imaging. The task of predicting is made more difficult by the fact that the brain is constantly developing, most likely in a non-linear and highly plastic way, and does not reach full maturity until far past childhood. The varying consequences of these changes and attributes require age-specific neurological assessment.

Because of these challenges, any predictions with high validity would be greatly valued, not least for early identification of difficulties, which can then lead to early intervention. Work on early general movements has provided promising results in this area.[99–101] General movements (GM) are a series of gross movements involving all parts of the body, but which do not have the usual sequences seen in coordinated movements. GM emerge in utero from about 28 weeks, before isolated limb movements, and they show great variation in speed and amplitude. From 36–38 weeks, the initial GM are replaced by more forceful, writhing movements. A second change takes place around 6 to 8 weeks post-term, when the writhing movements become highly fidgety in character.

Four different types of GM have been identified: two forms of normal GM, normal optimal and subnormal optimal; and two forms of abnormal GM, mildly abnormal and definitely abnormal. Hadders-Algra and Groothius[100] have made some interesting links between GM and a range of subsequent behaviours and difficulties in later childhood. They found that definitely abnormal GM at the fidgety stage (between 2 and 4 months post-term) were associated with a high risk of the children developing cerebral palsy; those with mildly abnormal GM had an association with the development of minor neurological disorders such as ADHD and aggressive behavior between the ages of 4 and 9 years. Groen *et al.*[99] confirmed that these predictions held true for older children aged 9–12 years, with the quality of GM being related to the types and severity of neurological outcome.

Research on GM and embodied cognition is indicative of the different approaches and rationale to studying motor development. It is employing the knowledge available about motor behaviour in the developing child and applying it to related and relevant fields. In doing this, two advances in the field are being promoted. First, it is becoming apparent that the motoric development of the child has implications beyond the motor domain. Second, by closely examining the implications and relationships there is more in depth analysis of motor development itself.

Children with developmental coordination disorder

Most children develop their motor skills in a typical manner and reach motor milestones within reasonable limits. They may vary in the manner in which they do this, but by school age, the vast majority will show competent skills for the demands of everyday living. There are however, a small number of children whose motor development does not progress in the expected manner. These children, like those with cerebral palsy, usually have a constitutional aetiology for their condition and display both delayed and atypical movements according to their classification. However, there also exists a less-well-known group who display delayed motor milestones, and have delayed everyday skills. This group has had numerous labels,[102,103] including minimal brain damage, clumsy children, developmental dyspraxia, but the international term of Developmental Coordination Disorder (DCD) as noted by the American Psychiatric Association since 1987[104] and registered in their current Diagnostic Statistic manual (DSM-5) in 2013,[105] seems most appropriate, and its use is logically explained by Henderson and Henderson.[103] These children have no outward signs of physical disability and rarely show movements that are pathological, e.g. jerkiness or continuous motion often seen in cerebral palsy, yet their motor skills are poor, they lag behind their peers, and this negatively interferes with their daily lives.

The DSM-5[105] provides the four criteria needed to complete a diagnosis of DCD: a) the acquisition and performance of motor skills is substantially below what is expected, given age and opportunity; b) that the motor deficit interferes with either activities of daily living or academic/vocational/ leisure activities; c) the onset of the symptoms occurs in the developmental period; and d) that the deficits are not attributable to intellectual disability, visual impairment, or a neurological condition affecting movement.

DSM 5[105] reports that the prevalence of this developmental condition is 5–6% in children ages 5–11 years, with estimates varying according to measurement instruments and cut-offs from 1.8% for severe cases, to more at-risk children around 4%.[106–108] Males tend to show a higher prevalence, ranging from 2.1% to 7.1% according to tests and criteria.[105,108,109]

Descriptions of children with DCD change as they develop. In the younger years, there are parent reports of the children having great difficulties dressing in the morning, and being disorganized in eating/washing activities.[110] At school they are often poor and slow at handwriting[111–113] and in the playground they are reluctant to engage in normal playground activities.[114] They are poor in these everyday skills and participate less, thus increasing any skill gap through lack of practice.[115,116] As they enter middle childhood, such social activities as bicycle riding present difficulties and, often writing problems continue. There is also strong evidence that shows the difficulties continue into emerging adulthood with the incumbent social consequences of motor problems. Specifically, driving is a challenging issue.[117,118]

In the last 30 years there has been a huge interest in these children. The diagnosis has formal recognition by both the American Psychological Association (APA) and the World Health Organization (WHO). There have been 11 world conferences between 1993 and 2015, with over 300 participants from over 30 countries. Frequently, motor difficulties, or DCD, co-occur with other developmental disorders such as ADHD, autism spectrum disorder (ASD), specific language impairment (SLI), and dyslexia. Indeed the 2015 World DCD Conference featured 'comorbidity' as its theme. In early research, the emphasis was on the age range 5–11 years, but now both preschool children and adults are the foci of many investigations (see Sugden and Wade[18]). This increase in interest has also led to a search for underlying neural substrates through fMRI studies,[119–121] which paradoxically, if found, will challenge the fourth criterion in the DSM-5, which notes that the difficulties are not due to a neurological condition.

Children diagnosed with DCD do not form a homogenous group, as some have severe difficulties while others only show mild symptoms.[116] In addition, the nature of the disorder is not constant: some children have problems in all activities, while others' problems involve handwriting and other manual skills.[116] There have been a few studies examining the intragroup characteristics of children with DCD by analysing sub-groups using factor and cluster analysis techniques. These studies have generally found that children with DCD do have different profiles,[122,123] but currently there are not strong enough data to precisely determine the subtypes.

Like many developmental conditions, DCD usually does not occur in a vacuum. It is often associated with other developmental disorders and conditions.[116] This can be interpreted in two ways. First, a group of children with DCD, upon examination, will exhibit a prevalence of co-occurring characteristics over and above what one would expect from a typically developing group. For example, Kadesjo and Gillberg[109] identified ADHD in around 50% of the children diagnosed with DCD; Green and Baird[124] found 53% of children with DCD were reported by their parents to have activity and attention problems. More recently, Goulardins *et al.*[125] have suggested that 50% of children with ADHD and/or DCD in fact have separate disorders and that these disorders should be treated separately. However, this does not negate the overlap that we see in functional tasks and in cases of dual diagnosis. Another perspective is to take a group with another diagnosed developmental disorder and investigate what percentage might also be diagnosed with DCD. Looking at children with motor difficulties who are also on the autistic spectrum, Green *et al.*[126] found that around 80% had movement difficulties; Hill *et al.*[127] found a 60% prevalence of DCD in a sample of children with specific language impairment; furthermore, in a sample of children with both diagnosed and threshold ADHD, 47% would also have a diagnosis of DCD.[109] A recent literature review searching for studies about children with ADHD and impaired motor skills has revealed that more than half of the children with ADHD have motor skills difficulties.[128]

In the last 5 years there has been a major initiative by Swiss and German colleagues and a world-wide international team of experts to provide a European set of Guidelines for DCD. The first version has been produced[116] and is currently under revision, and will eventually provide a definitive guide to and recommendations for the identification, assessment, diagnosis, and intervention of children with DCD. This new version is currently in press.

Research into most aspects of DCD has increased, but there is a cautionary note that coordination, the core of the disorder, has not been investigated to the same degree as other aspects. For example, many studies examine the cognitive aspects of the condition as exemplified by the studies on executive function and other internal mechanisms, but studies on the actual coordination of body and limbs have been few. With some exceptions, there are limited studies investigating variables like degrees of freedom, coordinative structures, and other aspects of dynamical systems. As Karl Newell[129] declared in a keynote speech at the 2011 conference on DCD, studies of coordination in DCD are notable by their absence.

The topic of learning has also been neglected in children with DCD. There have been intervention studies, which can be classed as a type of learning, but tightly controlled studies of learning are few and far between. It is worth noting here that studying children with DCD and how they control and learn skilled movements will not only aid our understanding of the condition and facilitate better support, but it will also contribute to the understanding of these processes in children who are more typical in their development.

Conclusions

The study of motor development has moved towards self-organizing dynamic systems tuned to both the internal constraints of the child and the external ones embedded in the environment. It is an integral part of the overall development of the child with bi-directional influences on other facilities such as cognition. Thus the study of motor development is not only important for itself, but its transaction with other faculties makes it a crucial player in the holistic development of the child.

An important final point to emphasize is that the underlying theoretical explanations of children's motor development are the same for all children. There are not different explanations for different groups. The setting is a triad:

(i) a child brings a set of resources to

(ii) the context setting, and must interpret

(iii) the manner in which the task is presented. These parameters are the same for all children; it is the metrics within these parameters that are different.

Summary

- Children's motor development involves a description of the changes that take place and an explanation as to how and why these changes occur.
- Early classic studies have given us excellent accounts and descriptions of these changes, and usually use a neuro-maturational explanation.
- During the last 30–40 years explanations from neuro-cognitive approaches have dominated, with empirical studies showing how children improve, with age, on tasks involving information processing variables.
- Although these approaches have taken our understanding further, a more ecological approach to explaining motor development may be better, with roots in the direct perception and dynamical systems camps.
- Explanations of development involve a transaction between the resources the child brings to any movement situation, the environmental context in which it is situated, and the task at hand.
- Motor development becomes a dynamic non-linear process with ever-changing features that are self-organizing and that transact the constituent parts.
- Typical and atypical development is explained in the same way with similar parameters and it is only the metrics that differ.

References

1. Gesell AL. *Infancy and human growth*. New York: Macmillan; 1928.
2. McGraw M. From reflex to muscular control in the assumption of an errect posture and ambulation in the human infant. *Child Dev*. 1932; 3: 291–297.
3. Schmidt R. A schema theory of discrete motor skill learning. *Psychol Rev*. 1975; 82: 225–260.

4. Adams JA. A closed-loop theory of motor learning. *J Mot Behav.* 1971; 3: 111–150.
5. Bernstein N. *The co-ordination and regulation of movement.* Oxford: Pergamon Press; 1967.
6. Gibson EJ, Owsley CJ, Walker A, Megaw-Nyce J. Development of the perception of invariants: substance and shape. *Perception.* 1979; 8: 609–619.
7. Gibson EJ. The concept of affordances in development: The renaissance of functionalism. In: Collins W (ed.) *The concept of development.* Hillsdale, NJ: Erlbaum; 1982. p. 55–81.
8. Turvey MT. Preliminaries to a theory of action with reference to vision. In: Shaw R, Bransford J (eds.) *Perceiving acting and knowing.* Hillsdale, NJ: Erlbaum; 1997. p. 211–265.
9. Turvey M, Shaw R, Mace W. Issues in the theory of action: Degrees of freedom, coordinative structures and coalitions. In: Requin J (ed.) *Attention and Performance VII.* Hillsdale, NJ: Lawrence Erlbaum Associates; 1978. p. 557–595.
10. Lopresti-Goodman SM, Turvey MT, Frank TD. Behavioral dynamics of the affordance 'graspable'. *Atten Percept Psychophys.* 2011; 73: 1948–1965.
11. Lopresti-Goodman SM, Turvey MT, Frank TD. Negative hysteresis in the behavioral dynamics of the affordance 'graspable'. *Atten Percept Psychophys.* 2013; 75: 1075–1091.
12. Adolph KE, Eppler MA, Gibson EJ. Crawling versus walking: infants' perception of affordances for locomotion over sloping surfaces. *Child Dev.* 1993; 64: 1158–1174.
13. Adolph KE, Vereijken B, Denny MA. Learning to crawl. *Child Dev.* 1998; 69: 1299–1312.
14. Adolph KE, Vereijken B, Shrout PE. What changes in infant walking and why. *Child Dev.* 2003; 74: 475–497.
15. Joh AS, Adolph KE, Campbell MR, Eppler MA. Why walkers slip: shine is not a reliable cue for slippery ground. *Percept Psychophys.* 2006; 68: 339–352.
16. Tamis-LeMonda CS, Adolph KE, Lobo SA, Karasik LB, Ishak S, Dimitropoulou KA. When infants take mothers' advice: 18-month-olds integrate perceptual and social information to guide motor action. *Dev Psychol.* 2008; 44: 734–746.
17. Soska KC, Adolph KE. Postural position constrains multimodal object exploration in infants. *Infancy.* 2014; 19: 138–161.
18. Sugden D, Wade M. *Typical and atypical motor development.* London: MacKeith Press; 2013.
19. Staples KL, Reid G. Fundamental movement skills and autism spectrum disorders. *J Autism Dev Disord.* 2010; 40: 209–217.
20. Crawford SG. *Addressing adapted physical activity interventions for children and adults with autism.* Dublin: Dept of Health, Health Action Zone; 2013.
21. Connolly K, Elliott J. The evolution and ontogeny of hand function. In: Jones M (ed.) *Ethological studies of child behavior.* Cambridge: Cambridge University Press; 1972. p. 329–380.
22. Haywood K, Getchell N. *Life span motor development*, 6th ed. Champagne, IL: Human Kinetics; 2014.
23. Gallahue D, Ozmun J. *Understanding motor development: Infants, children, adolescents, adults*, 6th ed. Boston: McGraw-Hill; 2006.
24. Haibach P, Reid G, Collier D. *Motor learning and development.* Champaign, IL: Human Kinetics; 2011.
25. McGraw M. *The neuromuscular maturation of the human infant.* New York: Hafner Publishing Company; 1963.
26. Ulrich B. Dynamic systems theory and skill development in infants and children. In: Connolly K, Forssberg H (eds.) *Neurophysiology and neuropsychology of motor development.* London: MacKeith Press; 1997. p. 319–345.
27. Tulving E. How many memory systems are there? *Am Psychol.* 1985; 40: 385–398.
28. Brown AL. The development of memory: knowing, knowing about knowing, and knowing how to know. *Adv Child Dev Behav.* 1975; 10: 103–152.
29. Zwicker JG, Missiuna C, Harris SR, Boyd LA. Brain activation of children with developmental coordination disorder is different than peers. *Pediatrics.* 2010; 126: e678–686.
30. Zwicker JG, Missiuna C, Harris SR, Boyd LA. Brain activation associated with motor skill practice in children with developmental coordination disorder: an fMRI study. *Int J Dev Neurosci.* 2011; 29: 145–152.
31. Sherwood DE, Lee TD. Schema theory: critical review and implications for the role of cognition in a new theory of motor learning. *Res Q Exerc Sport.* 2003; 74: 376–382.
32. Schmidt RA. Motor schema theory after 27 years: reflections and implications for a new theory. *Res Q Exerc Sport.* 2003; 74: 366–375.
33. Shea CH, Wulf G. Schema theory: a critical appraisal and reevaluation. *J Mot Behav.* 2005; 37: 85–101.
34. Wolpert DM, Ghahramani Z, Flanagan JR. Perspectives and problems in motor learning. *Trends Cogn Sci.* 2001; 5: 487–494.
35. Wolpert DM, Flanagan JR. Motor learning. *Curr Biol.* 2010; 20: R467–472.
36. Karniel A. Open questions in computational motor control. *J Integr Neurosci.* 2011; 10: 385–411.
37. Ruddock SR, Hyde CE, Piek JP, Sugden D, Morris S, Wilson PH. Executive systems constrain the flexibility of online control in children during goal-directed reaching. *Dev Neuropsychol.* 2014; 39: 51–68.
38. Barclay CR, Newell KM. Children's processing of information in motor skill acquisition. *J Exp Child Psychol.* 1980; 30: 98–108.
39. Bruner J. The growth and structure of skill. In: Connolly K (ed.) *Mechanisms of motor skill development.* London: Academic Press; 1970. p. 63–92.
40. Cerella J, Hale S. The rise and fall in information-processing rates over the life span. *Acta Psychol (Amst).* 1994; 86: 109–197.
41. Kail R, Salthouse TA. Processing speed as a mental capacity. *Acta Psychol (Amst).* 1994; 86: 199–225.
42. Elliott J, Connolly K. Hierarchical structure in skill development. In: Connelly K, Bruner J (eds.) *The Development of competence in childhood.* London: Academic Press; 1974. p. 135–168.
43. Newell KM, Carlton LG. Developmental trends in motor response recognition. *Dev Psychol.* 1980; 14: 531–536.
44. Salmoni A, Pascoe C. Fitts' reciprocal tapping task: A developmental study. In: Roberts C, Newell KM (eds.) *Psychology of motor behavior.* Champaign, IL: Human Kinetics; 1978. p. 288–294.
45. Simon H. What is visual imagery? An information processing interpretation. In: Gregg L (ed.) *Cognition in learning and memory.* New York: Wiley; 1972. p. 164–203.
46. Sugden DA. Visual motor short term memory in educationally subnormal boys. *Br J Educ Psychol.* 1978; 48: 330–339.
47. Sugden DA. Developmental strategies in motor and visual motor short-term memory. *Percept Mot Skills.* 1980; 51: 146.
48. Sugden DA. Movement speed in children. *J Mot Behav.* 1980; 12: 125–132.
49. Sugden DA, Gray SM. Capacity and strategies of educationally subnormal boys on serial and discrete tasks involving movement speed. *Br J Educ Psychol.* 1981; 51: 77–82.
50. Wickens C, Benel D. The development of time-sharing skills. In: Kelso JAS (ed.) *Motor development.* New York: John Wiley and Sons; 1982. p. 253–272.
51. Gibson EJ, Walk RD. The 'visual cliff'. *Sci Am.* 1960; 202: 64–71.
52. Newell KM. Constraints on the development of coordination. In: Wade M, Whiting H (eds.) *Motor development in children: Aspects of coordination and control.* Amsterdam: Martinus Nijhoff Publishers; 1986. p. 341–361.
53. Keogh J, Sugden D. *Movement skill development.* New York: Macmillan; 1985.
54. Newell KM, Scully DM, McDonald PV, Baillargeon R. Task constraints and infant grip configurations. *Dev Psychobiol.* 1989; 22: 817–831.
55. Sporns O, Edelman GM. Solving Bernstein's problem: a proposal for the development of coordinated movement by selection. *Child Dev.* 1993; 64: 960–981.
56. Thelen E. Motor development. A new synthesis. *Am Psychol.* 1995; 50: 79–95.

57. Prechtl H. Prenatal and early postnatal development of human motor behavior. In: Kalverboer A, Gramsbergen A (eds.) *Handbook of brain and behavior in human development*. Dordrecht: Kluwer; 2001. p. 415–428.
58. Hadders-Algra M. Development of postural control during the first 18 months of life. *Neural Plast*. 2005; 12: 99–108; discussion 263–272.
59. Thelen E. Rhythmical stereotypies in normal human infants. *Anim Behav*. 1979; 27: 699–715.
60. Thelen E, Bradshaw G, Ward JA. Spontaneous kicking in month-old infants: manifestation of a human central locomotor program. *Behav Neural Biol*. 1981; 32: 45–53.
61. Thelen E, Fisher DM. The organization of spontaneous leg movements in newborn infants. *J Mot Behav*. 1983; 15: 353–377.
62. Goldfield EC, Kay BA, Warren WH. Infant bouncing: the assembly and tuning of action systems. *Child Dev*. 1993; 64: 1128–1142.
63. Thelen E, Smith LB. *A dynamic systems approach to the development of cognition and action*. Cambridge, MA: MIT Press; 1994.
64. Kretch KS, Adolph KE. No bridge too high: infants decide whether to cross based on the probability of falling not the severity of the potential fall. *Dev Sci*. 2013; 16: 336–351.
65. Kretch KS, Adolph KE. Cliff or step? Posture-specific learning at the edge of a drop-off. *Child Dev*. 2013; 84: 226–240.
66. Kretch KS, Franchak JM, Adolph KE. Crawling and walking infants see the world differently. *Child Dev*. 2014; 85: 1503–1518.
67. Stoffregen TA, Schmuckler MA, Gibson EJ. Use of central and peripheral optical flow in stance and locomotion in young walkers. *Perception*. 1987; 16: 113–119.
68. Thelen E. Three-month-old infants can learn task-specific patterns of interlimb coordination. *Psychol Sci*. 1994; 5: 280–285.
69. von Hofsten C. Development of visually directed reaching: the approach phase. *J Hum Mov Stud*. 1979; 5: 160–178.
70. Braddick O, Atkinson J, Wattam-Bell J. Normal and anomalous development of visual motion processing: Motion coherence and 'dorsal-stream vulnerability'. *Neuropsychologia*. 2003; 41: 1769–1784.
71. Braddick O. Binocularity in infancy. *Eye*. 1996; 10: 182–188.
72. Lee DN. The optic flow field: the foundation of vision. *Philos Trans R Soc Lond B Biol Sci*. 1980; 290: 169–179.
73. Lee D, Aronson E. Visual proprioceptive control of standing in human infants. *Percept Psychophys*. 1974; 15: 529–532.
74. Lee D, Lishman R. Visual proprioceptive control of stance. *J Hum Mov Stud*. 1975; 1: 87–95.
75. Butterworth G, Hicks L. Visual proprioception and postural stability in infancy. A developmental study. *Perception*. 1977; 6: 255–262.
76. von Hofsten C. On the development of perception and action. In: Connolly K, Valsiner J (eds.) *Handbook of developmental psychology*. London: Sage; 2003. p. 114–140.
77. Corbetta D, Thurman SL, Wiener RF, Guan Y, Williams JL. Mapping the feel of the arm with the sight of the object: on the embodied origins of infant reaching. *Front Psychol*. 2014; 5: 576.
78. Campos J, Anderson D, Barbu-Roth M, Hubbard E, Hertenstein M, Witherington D. Travel broadens the mind. *Infancy*. 2000; 1: 149–219.
79. Hamilton M. Effect of optokinetic stimulation on gait initiation in children ages four and ten. In: Woollacott M, Horak F (eds.) *Posture and gait: control mechanisms, Volume II*. Portland: University of Oregon Press; 1992. p. 255–258.
80. Hirschfeld H, Forssberg H. Development of anticipatory postural adjustments during locomotion in children. *J Neurophysiol*. 1992; 68: 542–550.
81. Cesari P, Formenti F, Olivato P. A common perceptual parameter for stair climbing for children, young and old adults. *Hum Mov Sci*. 2003; 22: 111–124.
82. Smith T, Wade M. Variability in human motor and sport performance. In: Smith T, Henning R, Wade M, Fisher T (eds.) *Variability in human performance*. Boca Raton, FL: CRC Press, Taylor & Francis Group; 2015. p. 31–50.
83. Kuhtz-Buschbeck JP, Stolze H, Jöhnk K, Boczek-Funcke A, Illert M. Development of prehension movements in children: a kinematic study. *Exp Brain Res*. 1998; 122: 424–432.
84. Lenoir M, Savelsbergh GJ, Musch E, Thiery E, Uyttenhove J, Janssens M. Intercepting moving objects during self-motion: effects of environmental changes. *Res Q Exerc Sport*. 1999; 70: 349–360.
85. Chohan A, Savelsbergh GJP, van Kampen P, Wind M, Verheul MHG. Postural adjustments and bearing angle use in interceptive actions. *Exp Brain Res*. 2006; 171: 47–55.
86. Chohan A, Verheul MHG, Van Kampen PM, Wind M, Savelsbergh GJP. Children's use of the bearing angle in interceptive actions. *J Mot Behav*. 2008; 40: 18–28.
87. Smits-Engelsman BCM, Sugden D, Duysens J. Developmental trends in speed accuracy trade-off in 6–10-year-old children performing rapid reciprocal and discrete aiming movements. *Hum Mov Sci*. 2006; 25: 37–49.
88. Engel AK, Maye A, Kurthen M, König P. Where's the action? The pragmatic turn in cognitive science. *Trends Cogn Sci*. 2013; 17: 202–209.
89. Glenberg AM, Gallese V. Action-based language: A theory of language acquisition, comprehension, and production. *Cortex*. 2012; 48: 905–922.
90. Coey CA, Varlet M, Richardson MJ. Coordination dynamics in a socially situated nervous system. *Front Hum Neurosci*. 2012; 6: 1–12.
91. Oudgenoeg-Paz O, Leseman PPM, Volman M (Chiel) JM. Exploration as a mediator of the relation between the attainment of motor milestones and the development of spatial cognition and spatial language. *Dev Psychol*. 2015; 51: 1241–1253.
92. Piaget J. *The origins of intelligence in children*. New York: International Universities Press; 1952.
93. Smith L, Gasser M. The development of embodied cognition: six lessons from babies. *Artif Life*. 2005; 11: 13–29.
94. Bornstein MH, Hahn C-S, Suwalsky JTD. Physically developed and exploratory young infants contribute to their own long-term academic achievement. *Psychol Sci*. 2013; 24: 1906–1917.
95. Dellatolas G, De Agostini M, Curt F, *et al.* Manual skill, hand skill asymmetry, and cognitive performances in young children. *Laterality*. 2003; 8: 317–338.
96. Noten M, Wilson P, Ruddock S, Steenbergen B. Mild impairments of motor imagery skills in children with DCD. *Res Dev Disabil*. 2014; 35: 1152–1159.
97. Ferguson GD, Wilson PH, Smits-Engelsman BCM. The influence of task paradigm on motor imagery ability in children with Developmental Coordination Disorder. *Hum Mov Sci*. 2015; 44: 81–90.
98. Adams ILJ, Lust JM, Wilson PH, Steenbergen B. Compromised motor control in children with DCD: a deficit in the internal model? A systematic review. *Neurosci Biobehav Rev*. 2014; 47: 225–244.
99. Groen SE, de Blécourt ACE, Postema K, Hadders-Algra M. General movements in early infancy predict neuromotor development at 9 to 12 years of age. *Dev Med Child Neurol*. 2005; 47: 731–738.
100. Hadders-Algra M, Groothuis AM. Quality of general movements in infancy is related to neurological dysfunction, ADHD, and aggressive behaviour. *Dev Med Child Neurol*. 1999; 41: 381–391.
101. Hadders-Algra M. General movements: A window for early identification of children at high risk for developmental disorders. *J Pediatr*. 2004; 145: S12–S18.
102. Magalhães LC, Missiuna C, Wong S. Terminology used in research reports of developmental coordination disorder. *Dev Med Child Neurol*. 2006; 48: 937–941.
103. Henderson SE, Henderson L. Toward an understanding of developmental coordination disorder: terminological and diagnostic issues. *Neural Plast*. 2003; 10: 1–13.
104. American Psychiatric Association. *DSM-III-R Diagnostic and statistical manual of mental disorders*. Washington, DC: American Psychiatric Association; 1987.
105. American Psychiatric Association. *DSM 5 Diagnostic and statistical manual of mental disorders*. Washington, DC: American Psychiatric Association; 2013.
106. Gaines R, Missiuna C, Egan M, McLean J. Interprofessional care in the management of a chronic childhood condition: Developmental Coordination Disorder. *J Interprof Care*. 2008; 22: 552–555.

107. Wright HC, Sugden DA. A two-step procedure for the identification of children with developmental co-ordination disorder in Singapore. *Dev Med Child Neurol.* 1996; 38: 1099–1105.
108. Lingam R, Hunt L, Golding J, Jongmans M, Emond A. Prevalence of developmental coordination disorder using the DSM-IV at 7 years of age: a UK population-based study. *Pediatrics.* 2009; 123: e693–e700.
109. Kadesjö B, Gillberg C. Attention deficits and clumsiness in Swedish 7-year-old children. *Dev Med Child Neurol.* 1998; 40: 796–804.
110. Summers J, Larkin D, Dewey D. Activities of daily living in children with developmental coordination disorder: dressing, personal hygiene, and eating skills. *Hum Mov Sci.* 2008; 27: 215–229.
111. Prunty MM, Barnett AL, Wilmut K, Plumb MS. Handwriting speed in children with Developmental Coordination Disorder: are they really slower? *Res Dev Disabil.* 2013; 34: 2927–2936.
112. Prunty MM, Barnett AL, Wilmut K, Plumb MS. An examination of writing pauses in the handwriting of children with Developmental Coordination Disorder. *Res Dev Disabil.* 2014; 35: 2894–2905.
113. Huau A, Velay JL, Jover M. Graphomotor skills in children with developmental coordination disorder (DCD): Handwriting and learning a new letter. *Hum Mov Sci.* 2015; 42: 318–332.
114. Smyth M, Anderson H. Coping with clumsiness in the school playground: social and physical play in children with coordination impairments. *Br J Dev Psychol.* 2000; 18: 389–413.
115. Cairney J, Hay JA, Veldhuizen S, Missiuna C, Faught BE. Developmental coordination disorder, sex, and activity deficit over time: a longitudinal analysis of participation trajectories in children with and without coordination difficulties. *Dev Med Child Neurol.* 2010; 52: e67–e72.
116. Blank R, Smits-Engelsman B, Polatajko H, Wilson P. European Academy for Childhood Disability (EACD): recommendations on the definition, diagnosis and intervention of developmental coordination disorder (long version). *Dev Med Child Neurol.* 2012; 54: 54–93.
117. de Oliveira RF, Wann JP. Driving skills of young adults with developmental coordination disorder: regulating speed and coping with distraction. *Res Dev Disabil.* 2011; 32: 1301–1308.
118. de Oliveira RF, Wann JP. Driving skills of young adults with developmental coordination disorder: Maintaining control and avoiding hazards. *Hum Mov Sci.* 2012; 31: 721–729.
119. Reynolds JE, Licari MK, Elliott C, Lay BS, Williams J. Motor imagery ability and internal representation of movement in children with probable developmental coordination disorder. *Hum Mov Sci.* 2015; 44: 287–298.
120. Licari MK, Billington J, Reid SL, *et al.* Cortical functioning in children with developmental coordination disorder: a motor overflow study. *Exp Brain Res.* 2015; 233: 1703–1710.
121. McLeod KR, Langevin LM, Goodyear BG, Dewey D. Functional connectivity of neural motor networks is disrupted in children with developmental coordination disorder and attention-deficit/hyperactivity disorder. *Neuro Image Clin.* 2014; 4: 566–575.
122. Hoare D. Subtypes of developmental coordination disorder. *Adapt Phys Act Q.* 1994; 11: 158–169.
123. Wright HC, Sugden DA. The nature of developmental coordination disorder: Inter- and intragroup differences. *Adapt Phys Act Q.* 1996; 13: 357–371.
124. Green D, Baird G. DCD and overlapping conditions. In: Sugden D, Chambers ME (eds.) *Children with developmental coordination disorder.* London: Whurr; 2005. p. 93–118.
125. Goulardins JB, Rigoli D, Licari M, *et al.* Attention deficit hyperactivity disorder and developmental coordination disorder: Two separate disorders or do they share a common etiology. *Behav Brain Res.* 2015; 292: 484–492.
126. Green D, Charmant T, Pickles A, Chandler S, Loucas T, Simonoff E, *et al.* Impairment in movement skills of children with autistic spectrum disorders. *Dev Med Child Neurol.* 2009; 51: 311–316.
127. Hill EL. A dyspraxic deficit in specific language impairment and developmental coordination disorder? Evidence from hand and arm movements. *Dev Med Child Neurol.* 1998; 40: 388–395.
128. Kaiser ML, Schoemaker MM, Albaret JM, Geuze RH. What is the evidence of impaired motor skills and motor control among children with attention deficit hyperactivity disorder (ADHD)? Systematic review of the literature. *Res Dev Disabil.* 2014; 36C: 338–357.
129. Newell KM. *Movement coordination in developmental co-ordination disorder.* Keynote address. 24th June, 2011: Lausanne, IX World DCD Conference.

CHAPTER 5

Exercise and hormones

Alon Eliakim and Dan Nemet

Introduction

Exercise and physical activity (PA) both play an important role in tissue anabolism, growth, and development, but the mechanisms that link patterns of PA with tissue anabolism are not completely understood. Anabolic effects of exercise are not limited to participants in competitive sports, since substantial anabolic stimuli arise even from relatively modest physical activities.[1]

The exercise-associated anabolic effects are age and maturity dependent. Naturally occurring levels of PA are significantly higher during childhood, and during adolescence there is a simultaneous substantial increase in muscle mass and strength. Thus, the combination of rapid growth, high levels of PA, and spontaneous puberty-related increases in anabolic hormones (growth hormone [GH], insulin-like growth factor-I [IGF-I], and sex steroids) suggests the possibility of integrated mechanisms relating exercise with anabolic responses. In contrast, participation of young athletes in intense competitive training, especially if associated with inadequate caloric intake, may be associated with health hazards, and may reduce growth potential.[2]

Training efficiency depends on the exercise intensity, volume, duration, and frequency, as well as on the athlete's ability to tolerate it. An imbalance between the training load and the individual's tolerance may result in under- or overtraining. Therefore, efforts are made to develop objective methods to quantify the fine balance between training load and the athlete's tolerance. The endocrine system, by modulation of anabolic and catabolic processes, seems to play an important role in the physiological adaptation to exercise training[3] (interested readers are referred to Chapter 33 for a discussion of hormones and training). For example, changes in the cortisol/testosterone ratio, as an indicator of the anabolic-catabolic balance, have been used for several years, with limited success, to determine training strain.[4] In recent years changes in circulating components of the GH/IGF-I axis, a system of growth mediators that control somatic and tissue growth,[5] have been used to quantify the effects of training.[6] Interestingly, exercise is also associated with remarkable changes in catabolic hormones and inflammatory cytokines, and the exercise-related response of these markers can be also used to gauge exercise load.[7,8] Anabolic response dominance eventually leads to increased muscle mass and improved fitness, while prolonged dominance of the catabolic response, particularly if combined with inadequate nutrition, may ultimately lead to overtraining. Therefore, it was suggested that the evaluation of changes in these antagonistic circulating mediators may assist in quantifying the effects of different types of single and prolonged exercise training and recovery modalities.

This chapter focuses on the effects of a *single* exercise bout on the endocrine system, and will emphasize the unique relationship between exercise-related anabolic and catabolic responses. Moreover, an important goal of this chapter is to share our experience and introduce to elite competitive athletes, coaches, and their supporting staff, how exercise-induced hormonal changes may be used to evaluate practice load throughout the competitive season.

Exercise and the growth hormone—insulin-like growth factor-I axis

The growth hormone—insulin-like growth factor-I axis

The GH/IGF-I axis is composed of hormones, growth factors, binding proteins (BP), and receptors that regulate essential life processes. The axis starts at the central nervous system where several neurotransmitters (catecholamines, serotonin, cholinergic agents, etc.) stimulate the hypothalamus to synthesize growth hormone-releasing hormone (GHRH) and somatostatin (SMS). Growth hormone releasing hormone stimulates the anterior pituitary to secrete GH, while SMS inhibits GH secretion.

Growth hormone is the major product of the axis. One of GH's most important functions is the stimulation of hepatic IGF-I synthesis. However, some GH effects on metabolism, body composition, and tissue differentiation are IGF-I independent. Tissue GH bioactivity results from interaction between GH and its receptor. The GH receptor is composed of intra- and extracellular transmembrane domains. The extracellular domain is identical in structure to GH binding protein (GHBP),[9] thus, measuring circulating GHBP levels reflect GH receptor number, and activity.

Insulin-like growth factor-I is one of the insulin-related peptides. Some of IGF-I's effects are GH dependent, but the majority of its actions occur due to autocrine or paracrine secretion and regulation, which are only partially GH-dependent. Insulin-like growth factor-I is responsible for most, but not all, the anabolic and growth related effects of GH. It stimulates SMS secretion, and inhibits GH by a negative feedback mechanism.[10]

The bulk of circulating IGF-I is bound to IGFBPs. The most important circulating BP is IGFBP-3, which accounts for 80% of all IGF binding. Some IGFBPs are GH dependent (e.g. IGFBP-3), while others (IGFBP-1 and -2) are insulin dependent (being high when insulin level is low). The interaction between IGF-I and its BPs is even more complicated since some BPs stimulate (e.g. IGFBP-5), while others inhibit (e.g.IGFBP-4) IGF-I anabolic effects.[11]

Some hormones in the GH-IGF-I axis (i.e. GHRH and GH) have a pulsatile secretion pattern, and it has been shown that GH pulsatility is important for growth rate acceleration.[12] In contrast, IGF-I and IGFBPs level are relatively stable throughout the day.

Several components of the axis are age and maturity dependent. Growth hormone, GHBP, IGF-I, and IGFBP-3 reach their peak levels during puberty,[13] and decrease with aging.[14] These changes are partially sex-hormone mediated. Nutritional status influences the GH-IGF-I axis as well. Prolonged fasting and malnutrition increases GH secretion, but despite elevated GH, IGF-I levels remain low due to reduced levels of GH receptors.[15] All these factors must be taken into account when studying the effect of exercise on the GH-IGF-I axis.

The effect of an exercise bout

Growth hormone

The GH response to exercise depends on the duration and intensity of the exercise bout. Additionally, the fitness level of the exercising individual, the timing of blood sampling, refractoriness of pituitary GH secretion and other environmental factors also affect the GH response.[16]

Aerobic exercise

Most of our knowledge on the exercise-associated GH response is related to aerobic-type exercise. Previous reports suggested that *less fit* subjects exhibit a greater GH response to exercise.[17] However, individuals in these early studies performed exercise at the same *absolute,* rather than *relative*, capacity. Since fitness level varied markedly among participants, some subjects exercised below, while others above, their lactate/anaerobic threshold (T_{LAC}). This is important since, although GH secretion is related to exercise intensity in a linear dose-dependent fashion,[18] exercise intensities above the T_{LAC} yielded greater GH rise than milder loads.[19,20] These results demonstrate simply that, as individuals become fitter, the stress associated with exercise at an absolute work rate diminishes. For practical research purposes, this suggests that similar *relative* exercise intensity should be used preferably to study the 'real' GH response. This scientific approach therefore mandates evaluation of the maximal oxygen uptake ($\dot{V}O_2$ max) and/or T_{LAC}, and calculation of the relative exercise intensity. The obvious implication for the young athlete is that as he/she becomes fitter, a more intense exercise should be performed to stimulate GH secretion. This is consistent with the common coaching modality of training cycles with increased intensity within each cycle and throughout the training season.

Aerobic-type exercise duration for the stimulation of GH secretion should be at least 10 min.[21] The exercise-induced GH peak occurs 25–30 min after the start of the exercise, irrespective of the exercise duration,[22,23] and occurs a few minutes earlier in females.[24] Thus, in a brief exercise (e.g. 10 min), GH peak will be reached after the end of exercise, while in a long exercise (e.g. 60 min), this peak will be reached while the individual is still exercising. Growth hormone blood sampling, therefore, should be timed to the exercise-induced GH peak. The important possible implication for athletes is that brief training sessions, especially in female athletes, can be good enough to stimulate GH, and to achieve anabolic 'training effects'.

Analysis of the GH response to exercise must also consider pituitary refractoriness, which is the time in which the normal pituitary gland will not respond sufficiently to exercise stimulation for GH release. It was previously demonstrated[23] that the GH response to exercise was inhibited if a spontaneous, early morning GH pulse had occurred within 1 h prior to exercise. This inhibition most likely resulted from GH auto-inhibition (previously elevated circulating GH attenuated the pituitary's response to exercise). Cappon *et al.*[25] demonstrated at least a 1-h refractory period following exercise-induced GH secretion (i.e. a subsequent GH response to exercise was blunted), and suggested that an exercise-induced increase in free fatty acids or alterations in parasympathetic/sympathetic tone might have been responsible. Ronsen *et al.*[26] showed that if the second high-intensity endurance exercise bout was performed 3 h after the first session, GH peak did occur. Similarly, integrated 1.5-h GH concentrations were found to be significantly greater if the difference between exercise bouts (30 min, 70% $\dot{V}O_2$ max) was 3.5 h.[27] A practical application for young athletes who train several times per day should be that in order to achieve optimal GH secretion, the rest interval between multiple daily training sessions should be long enough (probably more than 3 h) to allow pituitary recovery.

Anaerobic exercise

Major progress was made in recent years in the understanding of the effects of anaerobic exercise on the GH-IGF-I axis. Stokes *et al.*[28] studied the effect of a single supramaximal 30-s sprint on a cycle ergometer against different levels of resistance. They found that the increase in GH levels was significantly greater when resistance was 7% (faster cycling) and not 9% (slower cycling) of body mass. Consistent with that, it was shown that heavier loads were lifted, more total work was performed, and higher IGF-I levels were found using faster, compared to slower, tempo resistance training.[29] The possible implication for athletes is that lower levels of resistance and faster anaerobic efforts may better stimulate the GH-IGF-I axis, and thus should be preferred by coaches and young athletes.

Interval training is one of the most frequent training methods used in anaerobic and aerobic-type sports.[30] The intensity of such training depends on the running distance (sprint versus long distance), running speed (% of maximal speed), the number of repetitions, and the length of the rest interval between runs. In addition, coaches and athletes quite often change the style of the interval training and use constant running distances (e.g. 6 × 200 m), increasing distance interval sessions (e.g. 100–200–300–400 m), decreasing distance interval sessions (e.g. 400–300–200–100 m), or a combination of increasing-decreasing distance interval sessions (e.g. 100–200–300–200–100 m). While these style differences may seem negligible, they may involve different physiological demands, since in the increasing distance protocol, metabolic demands (e.g. lactate levels) increase gradually and are highest toward the end of practice, while in the decreasing distance protocol metabolic demands are high from the beginning of the session.[31]

Recently, we demonstrated a significant increase in GH levels following a typical constant distance (4 × 250 m) interval training session.[31] Consistent with previous findings in aerobic exercise, changes in the GH-IGF-I axis following the brief sprint interval exercise suggested exercise-related anabolic adaptations. More recently, we evaluated the effect of increasing (100–200–300–400 m) and decreasing (40–300–200–100 m) distance sprint interval training protocols, on the balance between anabolic, catabolic and inflammatory mediators.[31] Both sprint interval training types led to a significant increase in lactate and GH and IGF-I. Interestingly, the lactate and GH area under the curve was significantly greater in the decreasing distance session. In contrast, rate of perceived exertion (RPE) was higher in the increasing distance session. Thus, despite similar running distance, running speed, and total resting period in the two interval training sessions, the decreasing distance interval was associated with a greater metabolic (lactate) and anabolic (GH) response. Interestingly, these greater metabolic and anabolic responses were not accompanied by an increase in RPE, which suggests that physiological and psychological responses to interval training do not necessarily correlate. When the athletes were asked to explain why the increasing distance training protocol was perceived as more intense (i.e. higher RPE), they replied that the response was that the longest and hardest run (400 m) was at the end of the session and was very difficult to tolerate. Coaches and athletes should be aware of these differences, and as a consequence, of the need for specific recovery adaptations after different types of interval training sessions. Differences in physiological and psychological responses to competitive sport training, and their influence on the training course and recovery process, should also be addressed (interested readers are referred to Chapter 15 for a discussion of RPE).

Both aerobic and anaerobic-type exercises that stimulated GH secretion involved high metabolic demands. In contrast, we previously demonstrated a smaller but still significant GH response to exercise input that was perceived as difficult by the participants (i.e. 10 min of unilateral wrist flexion; a small relatively unused muscle group), but had no systemic effect on heart rate or circulating lactate levels.[32,33] This suggests that other factors, such as the individual's perceived exertion and associated psychological stress, may also activate the hypothalamic-pituitary axis and GH release, even in exercise involving small muscle groups.

Resistance exercise

Previous studies have demonstrated increases in GH following a session of resistance exercise in adolescent and prepubertal boys. No comparable data are available for girls. Children and adolescents demonstrate a lower GH response to resistance exercise compared with adults, presumably due to higher baseline GH levels. The increases in growth hormone are likely not related to a hypertrophic response and may reflect a general stress response.

As mentioned before, GH is secreted in a pulsatile manner, with highest secretion during deep sleep, especially in children. Interestingly, Nindl *et al.*[34] reported that in men, an afternoon resistance-training session affected the GH secretion pattern during rest. While mean GH secretion did not change, a lower rate of secretion in the first half of sleep and a higher rate of secretion in the second half of sleep was detected. This could be a direct effect of the resistance exercise on GH secretion, or an indirect effect on sleep quality. Considering the importance of nighttime GH secretion during childhood and adolescence, resistance training during different times of day may have different effects on sleep quality, or directly on GH secretion pattern. Likewise, effects on the pulsatile secretion pattern may potentially even affect linear growth. There is a need for further research in this area.

'Real-life' exercise studies

The majority of studies on the effect of exercise on the GH-IGF-I axis are laboratory based. There is no doubt that laboratory-based science is important for understanding the exercise-related endocrine response. However, the translation of this knowledge to everyday use by competitive young athletes is complicated, and there is a severe lack of 'real-life' studies on the endocrine effect of exercise training. One of the main obstacles of executing real-life training studies is exercise standardization. We recently compared previous reports on the effect of real-life typical field individual (i.e. cross country running and wrestling—representing combat versus non-combat sports) and team sports practice (i.e. volleyball and water-polo—representing water and land team sports) on GH levels.[35] We were unable to control for the participants' fitness level or for each practice's intensity. In order to achieve some standardization, participants did not train during the day before the study, the duration of each practice was 60–90 min, and the practice was performed during the initial phases of the training season when athletes are at a relatively lower fitness level. All practice sessions were performed in the morning hours, and each typical practice included warm-up, main part, and cool-down. Blood samples were collected immediately before and at the end of practice, and the effect of the typical practice on hormonal and cytokine levels was calculated as the % change. Despite these limitations, several important observations and conclusions can be drawn about the real-life training-related GH response from this unique comparison. Cross-country running practice and volleyball practice in both males and females were associated with significant increases of GH. The magnitude (% change) of the GH response to the different practices was determined mainly by pre-exercise GH levels. There was no difference in the GH response between individual and team sports practices. Interestingly, the GH response to the typical practices was not influenced by the practice-associated lactate change.

Another important finding is the effect of training on the endocrine response to a single practice. The hormonal response to a typical 60 min volleyball practice was assessed before and after 7 weeks of training during the initial phase of the season in elite national team-level male players.[36] Training resulted in a significantly greater GH increase along with significantly reduced IL-6 response to the same relative intensity volleyball practice. The results suggest that along with the training-associated improvement of power, anaerobic, and aerobic characteristics, part of the adaptation to training is that a single practice becomes more anabolic and less catabolic and inflammatory during initial phases of the training season (Figure 5.1). It is suggested that real-life training hormonal measurement can assist athletes and their coaching staff in assessing the training programme adaptation throughout different stages of the competitive season.

Nutrition

Environmental factors like nutrition may affect the GH response to exercise. For example, intravenous administration of the amino acid arginine is a strong stimulator of GH release and is used as one of the common provocation tests for GH secretion in the assessment of children with short stature. In contrast, the ingestion of a lipid-rich meal 45–60 min prior to an intermittent 30 min cycle ergometer exercise resulted in a significant >40% reduction in the GH secretion in healthy children.[37] The effect of prior high-fat meal ingestion appeared to be selective for GH, as other counter-regulatory responses to exercise, such as glucagon, cortisol, and epinephrine, were not affected. In adults, the high-fat meal related exercise-induced GH secretion inhibition was correlated with circulating somatostatin levels.[38] Interestingly, a high-carbohydrate meal with a similar caloric content was not associated with a significant decrease in GH response to exercise. The effect

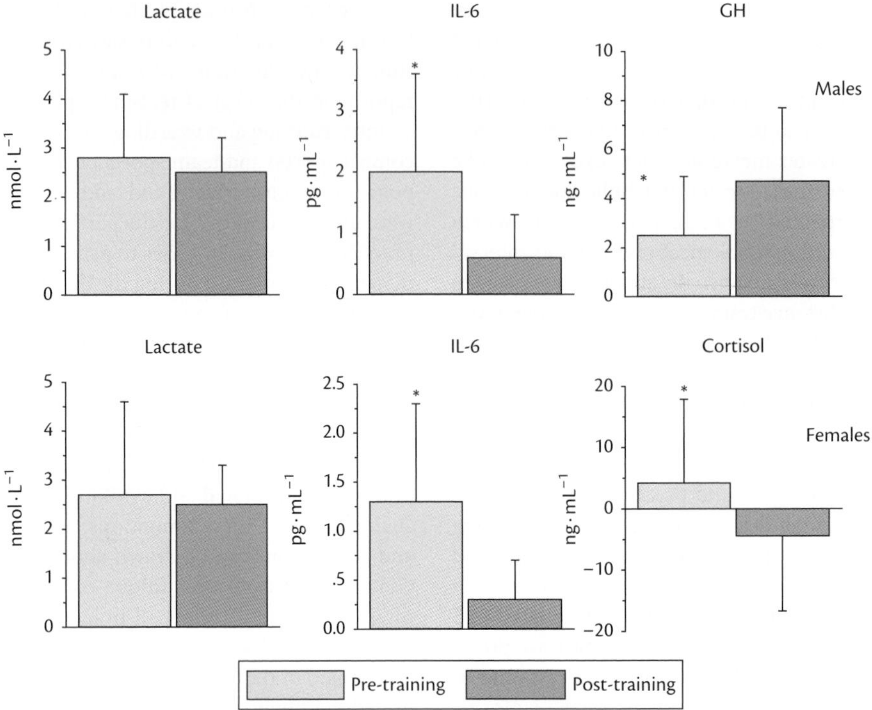

Figure 5.1 The effect of training on the hormonal response to a single volleyball practice in male (upper panel) and female (lower panel) adolescent players.

of a high-protein meal on exercise-induced GH secretion in children was not studied. Since the GH response to exercise plays an important role in the muscle adaptation to exercise, these studies indicate that food consumption prior to practice should be carefully selected, since a consumption of a high-fat meal may limit the beneficial effect of practice. In contrast, longer periods (3 days) of high-fat consumption (61% of total caloric consumption) had no effect on the exercise-induced GH secretion (30 min cycling at 60% of $\dot{V}O_2$ max) in young adults,[39] suggesting that the effect of acute and prolonged fat consumption on the GH response to exercise may differ.

Obesity

Pathological conditions such as childhood obesity may also affect the GH response to exercise. A significantly reduced exercise-associated GH response was reported in otherwise healthy obese children and adolescents.[40] Growth hormone response of obese individuals was also attenuated following other commonly used agents for GH provocation tests.[41] This is important since childhood obesity has now reached epidemic proportions in Westernized societies. It is possible that the blunted GH response may, at least partially, explain the difficulties in achieving body composition changes and in increasing muscle mass via exercise interventions in obese children.

Insulin-like growth factor-I

Several studies demonstrated that acute exercise increases circulating IGF-I levels. Interestingly, exercise-induced IGF-I increase occurred following very short supra-maximal exercise (i.e. 90 s),[42] 10 min following the onset of endurance exercise, and in exercise below and above the T_{LAC}.[43] Exercise led also to an increase in urinary IGF-I.[44]

The mechanism for this exercise-induced transient increase is not clearly understood. It is clear that the classic mechanism of increased hepatic IGF release due to exercise-induced secretion of GH is not the cause for IGF-I release. Growth hormone increases mainly follow high-intensity exercise, while IGF-I increases after both low- and high-intensity aerobic exercise. In addition, circulating IGF-I reaches its peak *before* the GH peak (i.e. 10 min compared to 30 min), while *de novo* hepatic IGF-I synthesis and transport to the circulation occurs several hours *after* administration of exogenous GH.[45] Moreover, exercise resulted in increases in IGF even in subjects with pituitary insufficiency.[46] These studies suggest that the exercise-associated increase in IGF-I must reflect rapid changes in IGF-I distribution in the circulation due to release from marginal pools or changes in IGF-I removal, and that the increase is not GH dependent.

The increase in circulating IGF-I may result from its release from the exercising muscle. To test this, we performed a unilateral repeated wrist flexion against relatively high resistance, and collected blood samples during and post-exercise simultaneously from the basilic vein of the exercising (representing local release) and resting arm (representing systemic response). We found a bilateral, simultaneous increase in IGF-I suggesting that the local exercising muscle was not the source of the IGF-I increase.[33]

Interestingly, Elias *et al.*[47] showed a transient rise in circulating IGF-I immediately after an exercise test to exhaustion, followed by a significant drop to reach nadir level 60–90 min after the exercise, with gradual return to baseline levels. Consistent with this observation, prolonged and intense exercise sessions (1.5 h of intense soccer practice in children,[48] intense Taekwondo fighting day simulation [three fights, 6 min each, 30 min rest between fights][49] or 1.5 h of wrestling practice in adolescents[8]) were associated with decreases in circulating IGF-I levels. Interestingly, these sessions were also associated with increases in pro-inflammatory cytokines, and the authors suggested that the increase in these inflammatory markers mediated the decrease in circulating IGF-I.

The effect of resistance exercise on circulating IGF-I is inconsistent and was studied mainly in adults.[50] An increase in circulating IGF-I and free IGF-I following strength exercise was found by several investigators. Moreover, eccentric exercise was associated with increases in muscle IGF-I mRNA, suggesting that IGF-I may modulate tissue regeneration after mechanical damage.[51] Other studies found no change in circulating IGF-I following heavy-resistance exercise,[52] or even reduced IGF-I levels the morning after a high and moderate intensity resistance workout.[53] These conflicting results probably reflect differences in exercise protocols, timing of blood sampling, individual fitness levels, etc.

Previous studies have found that a higher social rank/status was associated with higher levels of IGF-I in both men and women, independent of the wide range of known confounders like age, ethnicity, body weight, nutrition, and exercise.[54] Recently Bogin *et al.*[55] studied high-level male and female competitive athletes from different university team sports (men: lacrosse, handball, rugby, and volleyball; women: football, rugby, netball, and volleyball) and assumed that what determines the social rank in this unique social network is the level of success (and not economic status). Therefore the athletes were divided to winners and losers. The main finding of the study was that both pre- and post-competition IGF-I levels were about 11% higher among winners. There was no difference in the competition-related changes in IGF-I levels between the groups, suggesting that it is the baseline levels of IGF-I and not the change in IGF-I levels during the competition that may contribute to winning. This is the first study to relate IGF-I levels with winning. It seems that IGF-I integrates the multiple genetic, nutritional, social, and emotional influences to a coherent signal that regulates growth and possibly athletic performance. This suggests a novel cycle: both single practice and prolonged training increase IGF-I levels, which in turn increase the chances of an athlete to win (Figure 5.2). However, future larger studies that analyse other types of team sports, individual sports, and that better control for nutritional, training, and doping status are needed to confirm this very interesting finding.

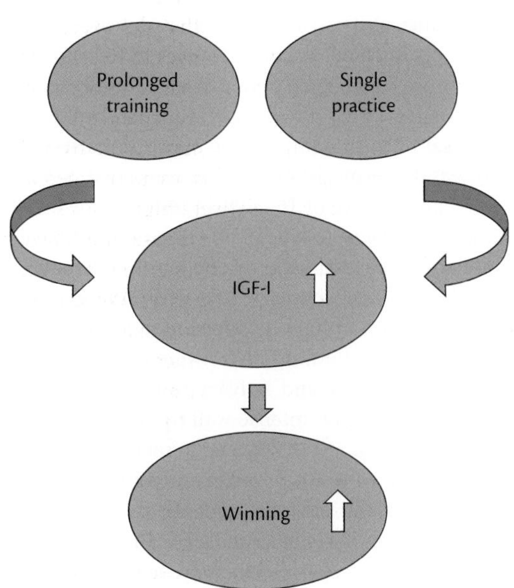

Figure 5.2 The exercise-training-IGF-I cycle.

Both single practice and prolonged training increase IGF-I levels, which in turn increase the chances of an athlete to win.

Recovery modalities and the growth hormone-insulin-like growth factor-1 axis

The use of additional aids in the training process plays a relatively minor role in athletic performance. However, in competitive sports, where one hundredth of a second, or a few millimeters could make a difference between fame and shame in the life of an athlete, the search for legal methods to improve training ability and performance becomes critical.

The development of methods to enhance the recovery of elite athletes from intense training and/or competition has been a major target of athletes and their accompanying staff for many years. Recently, it was shown that bicarbonate supplementation prior to high-intensity interval training attenuated the GH response.[56] The authors suggested that acidosis increases the GH response to interval training, and that these findings might be relevant to selection of active or passive recovery. While active recovery between intervals improves lactate clearance, reduces acidosis, and allows longer training, its effect may attenuate the GH response to training. This information has to be accounted for by athletes and coaches when planning interval training.

Cryotherapy is widely used to treat sports-associated traumatic injuries, and as a recovery modality following training and competition that may cause some level of traumatic muscle injury.[57,58] However, evidence regarding the effectiveness and appropriate guidelines for the use of cryotherapy are limited. We evaluated the effect of cold ice pack application following brief sprint interval training on the balance between anabolic, catabolic, and circulating pro- and anti-inflammatory cytokines in 12 male, elite junior handball players.[59] The interval practice (4 × 250 m) was associated with a significant increase in GH and IL-6 levels. Local cold-pack application was associated with significant decreases in IGF-I, and IGF binding protein-3 during the recovery from exercise (Figure 5.3), which supports some clinical evidence for possible negative effects of cryotherapy on athletic performance. These results, along with previously reported evidence for some negative effects of ice application on athletic performance, and no clear effect on muscle damage or delayed onset muscle soreness (DOMS), may suggest that the use of cold packs should probably be reserved for traumatic injuries or used in combination with active recovery and not

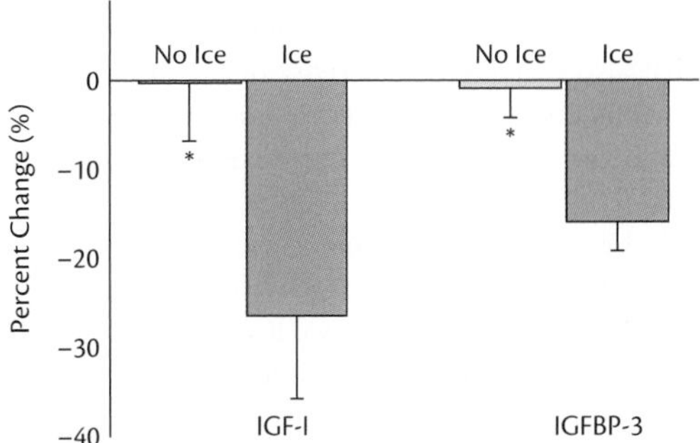

Figure 5.3 The effect of ice-pack application following exercise on anabolic mediators.

Cold-pack application was associated with significant decreases in IGF-I, and IGF binding protein-3 during the recovery from exercise.

with complete rest. However, this is an example of how exercise-induced changes in the GH-IGF-I axis and other catabolic and inflammatory markers may be used to fit in the complete puzzle of optimizing competitive training. Further studies are needed to explore the beneficial use of anabolic, catabolic, and inflammatory markers measurement in many other aspects of the recovery from exercise.

Exercise and sex hormones

The hypothalamic-pituitary-gonadal axis

The hypothalamic-pituitary-ovarian axis regulates the female reproductive system. Pulsatile secretion of gonadotropin-releasing hormone (GnRH) from the hypothalamus stimulates pulsatile secretion of luteinzing hormone (LH) and follicle stimulating hormone (FSH) from the anterior pituitary gland. An optimal frequency of pulsatile secretion and monthly rhythmic stimulation of LH and FSH is necessary for ovarian follicle growth and oestrogen secretion. Eventually one of these follicles becomes dominant. The rising levels of oestrogen impose positive feedback on the pituitary gland that leads to LH surge, which causes the dominant follicle to rupture and release an egg cell in a process called ovulation. The remaining dominant follicle becomes the corpus luteum which secretes progesterone and oestrogen. Oestrogen and progesterone stimulate proliferation and vascularization of the uterine endothelium in an effort to create optimal conditions for successful fertilized egg implantation. If fertilization does not occur, the corpus luteum's ability to secrete progesterone diminishes, the endometrium cells collapse and menstruation occurs. The period from menses to ovulation is called the follicular phase, and the interval from ovulation until the next menses is termed the luteal phase.

The hypothalamic-pituitary-testicular axis regulates the male reproductive system. Similar to females, pulsatile hypothalamic secretion of GnRH stimulates the anterior pituitary to secrete LH and FSH. Pulsatile secretion of FSH stimulates testicular Sertoli cells to promote spermatogenesis while pulsatile secretion of LH stimulates testicular Leidig cells to produce testosterone. Some testosterone can be derived peripherally from adrenal androgens. Adrenal androgens (DHEA, androstenedione) are significantly less potent than testosterone and therefore play a minor role in males. However, due to the low testosterone levels, they may play a greater role in females.[60] Similarly, adrenal androgens may also play an important anabolic role in pre-pubertal children. The anabolic effect of testosterone results from its interaction with androgen receptors. Therefore, a complete understanding of testosterone effects must also consider the activity of the androgen receptors. Due to obvious ethical reasons, such assessment requires muscle biopsies, and therefore has not been carried out in children or adolescents.

The link between testosterone concentration and strength development during growth emerges from the parallel increases in testosterone and strength in boys. Round *et al.*[61] studied these associations longitudinally over a 4-year period in boys and girls 8- to 17-years-old. An increase in strength was demonstrated in girls, with a concomitant increase in oestrogen. But increases in strength among the girls were proportional to body-size changes and not to changes in oestrogen. In contrast, in the boys, strength increases were independently related to increased testosterone levels. Interestingly, the differences in testosterone concentrations explained sex-related differences in quadriceps strength, but could not fully explain the difference in elbow-flexor strength.

Testosterone

The majority of previous studies have concentrated on the effect of resistance exercise on testosterone levels in males. Similar to other hormones, testosterone response to exercise depends on the exercise protocol, the exercising individual's fitness level, blood sampling timing, and other environmental factors. An increase in testosterone concentration was demonstrated following a weightlifting session in trained adolescent boys.[62] Interestingly, the testosterone response was higher in athletes with greater than 2 years experience, compared with less-experienced athletes, although there was no age difference between the two groups.[63] It is not clear whether the bigger response of the experienced athletes related simply to greater motivation and hence higher exercise intensity, or instead to intrinsic changes in testosterone secretion and clearance. Pullinen *et al.*[64] demonstrated a testosterone increase in adolescent boys and young men following a session of resistance exercise. However, both pre- and post-exercise testosterone levels were lower in the boys and the increase in the boys was smaller than in adults. The lower, or even lack, of response in boys and adolescents compared with men may be explained by smaller testicular volume, fewer or less-differentiated Leydig cells, or reduced synchronized regulation of the hypothalamic-pituitary-gonadal axis.[65]

We previously described an increase in testosterone levels following a typical volleyball practice in adolescent males and females.[66] Baseline and post-exercise testosterone levels were significantly higher in the males compared with females. However, training was associated with an increase in testosterone levels in both genders, and the response to training was not significantly different between genders. The testosterone increase may indicate an exercise-associated anabolic adaptation. Results suggest, therefore, that an increase in testosterone levels may play an important role in the anabolic response to exercise in female athletes as well. While the effect of different types of exercise on testosterone levels in males are well studied, few previous studies examined the effect of endurance and resistance exercise on testosterone level in females (e.g. Consitt *et al.*[67]). Circulating levels of testosterone have been shown to increase in response to acute bouts of endurance exercise in females across a wide age range (from young adult to pre-menopausal[67,68]). In contrast, the effect of resistance training on circulating testosterone levels was less consistent. Several studies demonstrated an increase of 16–25% in testosterone levels following resistance exercise in females.[69,70] Other studies have failed to demonstrate an increase in testosterone levels in females at different stages of the menstrual cycle.[71,72] Very few studies examined the effect of team sports training on testosterone levels in female athletes. In contrast to our findings, there were no significant changes in circulating testosterone and salivary testosterone levels in elite female players following an intense water-polo practice and handball match, respectively.[73,74] In contrast to male athletes, the source of the exercise-induced testosterone production in female athletes is the adrenal gland and obviously not the testicles. Accordingly, post-exercise increases in testosterone levels in female athletes were usually accompanied by a parallel increase in cortisol, DHEA, and/or androstenedione levels.[67,70,74]

Finally, we evaluated the effect of fighting simulation (three fights, 6 min each, 30 min rest between fights) on anabolic and catabolic hormones in elite, male and female adolescent (12–17 years)

Taekwondo fighters.[49] The fighting simulation practice led to significant decreases in LH and FSH in both genders. Fighting simulation led to decreases in testosterone and free androgen index in both genders as well; however, these decreases were significant only in male fighters. In addition, the fighting simulation was associated with a significant increase in cortisol in both sexes. These results raise two important points; first, the fighting simulation-induced decrease in testosterone among males resulted from central hypothalamic-pituitary suppression and not from peripheral inhibition. Second, while testosterone usually increased following a single exercise session, the combination of physiological and psychological strain in a competition, and as shown in the present study, also in competition simulation, may lead to central suppression of testosterone level and to a catabolic-type hormonal response (in this case increased cortisol/testosterone ratio).

Amenorrhea and performance

The inhibitory effect of exercise training, particularly when associated with nutritional deprivation, on the pulsatile hypothalamic GnRH and pituitary LH and FSH secretion is well established. This inhibition results in increased risk of athletic amenorrhea, and hypoestrogenism.[75] It was shown that the exercise-associated GH release is attenuated in amenorrheic athletes. The mechanism for the attenuated amenorrhea-associated exercise-induced GH response is not completely understood. However, it was found recently[76] that low oestrogen leads to decreased post-exercise type 1 deiodinase (an enzyme that converts T4 to the more active thyroid hormone T3), reduced T3 levels, and blunted GH response. This is particularly relevant to the adolescent female athlete, since the prevalence of amenorrhea among these athletes is 4–20 times higher than the general population. Athletic amenorrhea appears mainly in younger athletes, in sports types where leanness provide a competitive advantage (e.g. aesthetic-type sports, long distance running, etc.), and in particular, when intense training is accompanied by inadequate nutrition.[75] The reduced exercise-induced GH response in these athletes should be considered since it most likely indicates reduced training effectiveness and performance. Additionally, Vanheest *et al.*[77] showed that reduced energy intake and availability that was associated with ovarian suppression was also accompanied by lower T3 and IGF-I levels and by a 9.8% decline in 400 m swim velocity compared to 8.2% improvement among female swimmers without ovarian suppression at the end of 12 weeks of training (in total, 18% difference!). This occurred despite similar training protocols and while the ovarian suppressed swimmers were still menstruating (although less regularly). This is important because many coaches and young athletes promote energy restrictive practices with the belief that it improves competitive performance. The results of this study emphasize that athletes can maintain chronic energy deficit for varied periods with continued success in sport, although prolonged negative energy balance results in training maladaptation and reduced performance. This may be particularly relevant for athletes during adolescence, a time with greater energy needs for growth and maturation (interested readers are referred to Chapter 47 for further discussion of nutrition and disordered eating).

Exercise and adrenal hormones

The adrenal gland is comprised of two main tissue types: the outer cortex and the medulla. The adrenal medulla is a sympathetic ganglion. Sympathetic ganglion fibers end in secretory vesicles that, following nervous system stimulation, secrete hormones (i.e. epinephrine). Adrenal medullary hormones are produced and secreted in response to stress. The adrenal cortex is essential for life. It secretes glucocorticoids (i.e. cortisol) that regulate carbohydrate and protein metabolism, mineralocorticoids (i.e. aldosterone) responsible for extracellular fluid volume maintenance, and sex hormones.

Cortisol

The stress hormone cortisol is secreted from the adrenal cortex under the central regulation of hypothalamic corticotropine-releasing hormone (CRH) and pituitary adreno-corticotropic hormone (ACTH). Cortisol has both metabolic and anti-inflammatory functions. It stimulates gluconeogenesis and lipolysis, inhibits growth factors secretion and function, up-regulates several interleukins, and also inhibits the production of numerous inflammatory factors. As a consequence, cortisol is considered a catabolic hormone known to increase protein degradation and decrease protein synthesis in skeletal muscles. However, cortisol can also play a role in tissue remodeling since the catabolic effect provides free amino acids, increasing their pool for later protein synthesis and renewal.

The acute exercise-induced cortisol response generally reflects a stress response and is related to the intensity and duration of exercise.[78] A significant increase in cortisol levels in aerobic exercise requires duration of at least 20 min and an intensity of at least 60% of $\dot{V}O_2$ max.[3] Following resistance exercise, most adult studies report increases in cortisol in both genders (see Kraemer *et al.*[60] and Crewther *et al.*[79] for review). Studies in adolescent males have shown a greater cortisol increase in the more experienced males following an intense resistance exercise session.[62] Whether the greater cortisol increase in the more experienced boys reflects greater effort ability is not clear. Moreover, a greater cortisol increase compared with men following a session of resistance exercise showed that the cortisol (along with epinephrine) response to resistance exercise among untrained adolescent boys, was twice as high compared with men who performed exercise at a similar relative intensity to exhaustion.[64,80] The fact that the exercise-associated increases in cortisol were similar to increases in epinephrine reflects possibly a greater anxiety or stress in the adolescent boys.[64] Alternatively, the greater acute cortisol increase may also reflect an exercise-associated catabolic response. Altogether, the higher catabolic (cortisol) along with the lower anabolic (testosterone) responses in boys may explain their lower hypertrophic adaptation to resistance training.

Consistent with that, as mentioned earlier in both male and female adolescents,[49] Taekwondo fighting simulation practice led to a significant increase in the cortisol/testosterone ratio. This ratio is commonly used as an indicator of exercise-induced catabolic state.[3] It should be noted that the significant increase in cortisol levels occurred despite its diurnal circadian rhythm, which is associated with a decrease in cortisol level throughout the day; this suggests that the increase in cortisol level was even higher. Indeed, cortisol levels were found to be increased in fighting sports during competition, and were higher among the winners compared to losers.[81,82] However, a greater practise-associated cortisol response or cortisol/testosterone ratio may reflect a catabolic response to training. While such a response might be important and even necessary, following some practices, for the overall success of the athlete, the training staff should be aware and plan an adequate recovery following such practices, since prolonged catabolic training response may eventually lead to overtraining.

Finally, we studied the hormonal response to a typical 60 min volleyball practice before and after 7 weeks of training during the initial phase of the season in elite national team-level female players.[36] Training resulted in significantly lower cortisol and IL-6 increase to the same relative intensity volleyball practice. The results suggest that along with training-associated improvement of power, anaerobic, and aerobic characteristics, part of the training adaptation is that a single practice becomes less catabolic and inflammatory (Figure 5.1).

Catecholamines

The catecholamine response to exercise is generally examined acutely, rather than chronically, mainly due their relatively short half-life. Catecholamines are stress hormones that affect fuel-substrate mobilization and performance. Some catecholamines are produced in the adrenal medulla (i.e. epinephrine), while others are produced in the sympathetic chain (i.e. norepinephrine) and the central nervous system (i.e. dopamine). Generally, plasma catecholamine concentrations increase following resistance exercise, although that increase is dependent on the exercise intensity and rest intervals. The acute catecholamine (epinephrine and norepinephrine) response to resistance exercise in adolescents compared to adults appears to be inconsistent.[64,65] Moreover, catecholamines may increase even before exercise, in what has been termed 'anticipatory rise.'[83]

One of the most interesting findings is that the catecholamine response to exercise differs between obese and normal-weight children. The effect of intense exercise (ten 2 min bouts of constant work rate cycle ergometry at 50% between the T_{LAC} and $\dot{V}O_2$ max, with a 1 min rest interval between bouts) on both GH and neuroadrenergic hormones was assessed in obese compared with normal-weight children and adolescents.[40] The major finding of the study was that despite equivalent cardiovascular responses to the exercise, both GH and catecholamine (epinephrine, norepinephrine, and particularly dopamine) responses were attenuated in the obese subjects (Figure 5.4). The reduced epinephrine and norepinephrine responses and the absent dopamine response to exercise in obese subjects suggest the possibility of a centrally mediated attenuation of sympathetic adrenal-medullary function. Reduced central dopaminergic tone, due to reduced dopamine-2 receptor (D2) gene expression in obese subjects,[84] could explain the findings of blunted catecholamines and GH in response to exercise in obese subjects. It is possible that the blunted GH and catecholamine response to exercise leads to reduced carbohydrate and fat utilization during exercise in obese children,[85] and as a result to a greater protein utilization. This may, at least partially, explain the difficulties in achieving changes in body composition and in increasing muscle mass via exercise interventions in obese children. Consistent with this, previous studies have demonstrated that elevated body mass index (BMI) was associated with a reduced training effect in children following a prolonged resistance training intervention.[86] Therefore, it is possible that the GH and catecholamine response to exercise might be used prior to participation in weight reduction interventions to predict outcome. A sufficient GH and catecholamine response will suggest success, while insufficient response will indicate a need for a more intense intervention. Further studies are needed to clarify the extent to which these hormonal abnormalities persist after weight loss and/or improved fitness following exercise training programmes in obese children and adolescents.

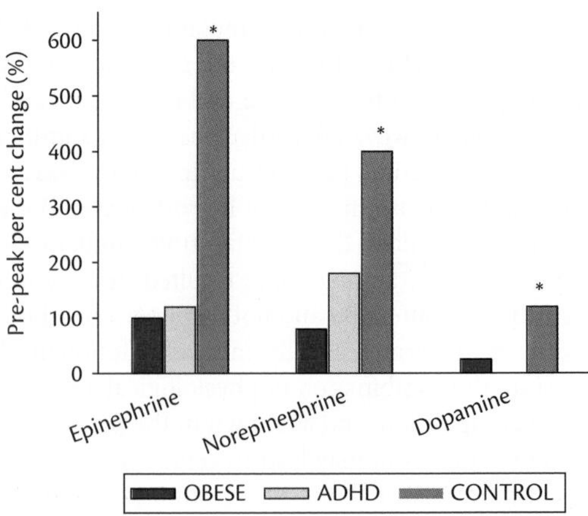

Figure 5.4 The effect of exercise on percent change in epinephrine, norepinephrine, and dopamine.
In both obese and ADHD children, exercise leads to a significant lower response in all three markers.

Moreover, similarly reduced epinephrine and norepinephrine responses and an absent dopamine response to exercise was found in children with attention deficit hyperactive disorder (ADHD).[87] It is possible that the catecholamine response to exercise might be used to predict medication use success (e.g. methylphenidate) in children with ADHD. An insufficient catecholamine response will suggest a need for medication, while sufficient response will allow a trial of lifestyle and behavioral changes prior to the use of medication. Further studies are needed to expand our understanding of the exercise-associated hormonal responses and their possible practical applications in this unique population.

Conclusions

Many efforts have been made to find objective parameters to quantify the balance between training load and the athlete's tolerance, with limited success. The complexity of hormonal responses to different types of exercises, in a diversity of sports disciplines, during different phases of the training season, and following competitions has become increasingly apparent in recent years. This chapter suggests that the evaluation of exercise-induced hormonal changes, particularly in the growing adolescent athlete, may be used as an objective tool to assess the physical strain of training.

Summary

- The endocrine system, by modulation of anabolic and catabolic processes, seems to play an important role in the physiological adaptation to exercise.
- The balance between anabolic and catabolic responses to exercise may be used to gauge exercise load.
- Aerobic, anaerobic, and resistance exercise lead to an increase in growth hormone levels.
- Following training, along with the training-associated improvement of power, anaerobic, and aerobic characteristics, a

single practice becomes more anabolic and less catabolic and inflammatory.

- The growth hormone response to a single exercise bout is influenced by environmental factors such as nutrition, and by pathological states like obesity and amenorrhea.
- The anabolic adaptation to exercise is influenced by recovery modalities (e.g. cryotherapy).
- Exercise leads to an increase in testosterone levels in both genders.
- Amenorrhea-associated decrease in thyroid hormone and growth hormone leads to reduced exercise performance.
- The magnitude of the hormonal response to exercise is influenced by the intensity and type of sports, the participants' fitness level, and the timing along the competitive season.
- The usage of the hormonal response to exercise as a practical tool to monitor training load and response should be individualized.
- Obese and attention-deficit hyperactive disorder children have a blunted catecholamine response to exercise. This response may be used to test treatment modalities.

References

1. Krebs JM, Schneider VS, Evans H, Kuo MC, LeBlanc AD. Energy absorption, lean body mass, and total body fat changes during 5 weeks of continuous bed rest. *Aviat Space Environ Med.* 1990; 61: 314–318.
2. Theintz GE, Howald H, Weiss U, Sizonenko PC. Evidence for a reduction of growth potential in adolescent female gymnasts. *J Pediatr.* 1993; 122: 306–313.
3. Urhausen A, Kindermann W. The endocrine system in overtraining. In: M.P. Warren, N.W. Constantini (eds.) *Sports endocrinology.* New Jersey: Humana Press; 2000. p. 347–370.
4. Hoffman JR, Falk B, Radom-Isaac S, *et al.* The effect of environmental temperature on testosterone and cortisol responses to high intensity, intermittent exercise in humans. *Eur J Appl Physiol Occup Physiol.* 1997; 75: 83–87.
5. LeRoith D, Roberts CT, Jr. Insulin-like growth factors and their receptors in normal physiology and pathological states. *J Pediatr Endocrinol.* 1993; 6: 251–255.
6. Eliakim A, Nemet D, Cooper DM. Exercise, training and the GH—>IGF-I axis. In: Kraemer WJ, Rogol A.D (eds.) *The endocrine system in sports and exercise.* Oxford: Wiley-Blackwell; 2005. p. 165–179.
7. Nemet D, Rose-Gottron CM, Mills PJ, Cooper DM. Effect of water polo practice on cytokines, growth mediators, and leukocytes in girls. *Med Sci Sports Exerc.* 2003; 35: 356–363.
8. Nemet D, Oh Y, Kim HS, Hill M, Cooper DM. Effect of intense exercise on inflammatory cytokines and growth mediators in adolescent boys. *Pediatrics.* 2002; 110: 681–689.
9. Leung DW, Spencer SA, Cachianes G, *et al.* Growth hormone receptor and serum binding protein: purification, cloning and expression. *Nature.* 1987; 330: 537–543.
10. Berelowitz M, Szabo M, Frohman LA, Firestone S, Chu L, Hintz RL. Somatomedin-C mediates growth hormone negative feedback by effects on both the hypothalamus and the pituitary. *Science.* 1981; 212: 1279–1281.
11. Rajaram S, Baylink DJ, Mohan S. Insulin-like growth factor-binding proteins in serum and other biological fluids: regulation and functions. *Endocr Rev.* 1997; 18: 801–831.
12. Clark RG, Jansson JO, Isaksson O, Robinson IC. Intravenous growth hormone: growth responses to patterned infusions in hypophysectomized rats. *J Endocrinol.* 1985; 104: 53–61.
13. Mauras N, Blizzard RM, Link K, Johnson ML, Rogol AD, Veldhuis JD. Augmentation of growth hormone secretion during puberty: evidence for a pulse amplitude-modulated phenomenon. *J Clin Endocrinol Metab.* 1987; 64: 596–601.
14. Corpas E, Harman SM, Blackman MR. Human growth hormone and human aging. *Endocr Rev.* 1993; 14: 20–39.
15. Merimee TJ, Zapf J, Froesch ER. Insulin-like growth factors in the fed and fasted states. *J Clin Endocrinol Metab.* 1982; 55: 999–1002.
16. Eliakim A, Nemet D. Exercise provocation test for growth hormone secretion: methodologic considerations. *Pediatr Exerc Sci.* 2008; 20: 370–378.
17. Buckler JM. Exercise as a screening test for growth hormone release. *Acta Endocrinol.* 1972; 69: 219–229.
18. Pritzlaff-Roy CJ, Widemen L, Weltman JY, *et al.* Gender governs the relationship between exercise intensity and growth hormone release in young adults. *J Appl Physiol.* 2002; 92: 2053–2060.
19. Sutton J, Lazarus L. Growth hormone in exercise: comparison of physiological and pharmacological stimuli. *J Appl Physiol.* 1976; 41: 523–527.
20. Hartley LH, Mason JW, Hogan RP, *et al.* Multiple hormonal responses to graded exercise in relation to physical training. *J Appl Physiol.* 1972; 33: 602–606.
21. Felsing NE, Brasel JA, Cooper DM. Effect of low and high intensity exercise on circulating growth hormone in men. *J Clin Endocrinol Metab* 1992; 75: 157–162.
22. Bar-Or O. Clinical implications of pediatric exercise physiology. *Ann Clin Res.* 1982; 14(suppl 34): 97–106.
23. Eliakim A, Brasel JA, Cooper DM. GH response to exercise: assessment of the pituitary refractory period, and relationship with circulating components of the GH-IGF-I axis in adolescent females. *J Pediatr Endocrinol Metab* 1999; 12: 47–55.
24. Wideman L, Weltman JY, Shah N, Story S, Veldhuis JD, Weltman A. Effects of gender on exercise-induced growth hormone release. *J Appl Physiol.* 1999; 87: 1154–1162.
25. Cappon J, Brasel JA, Mohan S, Cooper DM. Effect of brief exercise on circulating insulin-like growth factor I. *J Appl Physiol.* 1994; 76: 2490–2496.
26. Ronsen O, Haug E, Pedersen BK, Bahr R. Increased neuroendocrine response to a repeated bout of endurance exercise. *Med Sci Sports Exerc.* 2001; 33: 568–575.
27. Kanaley JA, Weatherup-Dentes MM, Alvarado CR, Whitehead G. Substrate oxidation during acute exercise and with exercise training in lean and obese women. *Eur J Appl Physiol.* 2001; 85: 68–73.
28. Stokes KA, Sykes D, Gilbert KL, Chen JW, Frystyk J. Brief, high intensity exercise alters serum ghrelin and growth hormone concentrations but not IGF-I, IGF-II or IGF-I bioactivity. *Growth Horm IGF Res.* 2010; 20: 289–294.
29. Headley SA, Henry K, Nindl BC, Thompson BA, Kraemer WJ, Jones MT. Effects of lifting tempo on one repetition maximum and hormonal responses to a bench press protocol. *J Strength Cond Res.* 2011; 25: 406–413.
30. Kubukeli ZN, Noakes TD, Dennis SC. Training techniques to improve endurance exercise performances. *Sports Med.* 2002; 32: 489–509.
31. Meckel Y, Nemet D, Bar-Sela S, *et al.* Hormonal and inflammatory responses to different types of sprint interval training. *J Strength Cond Res.* 2011; 25: 2161–2169.
32. Nemet D, Hong S, Mills PJ, Ziegler MG, Hill M, Cooper DM. Systemic vs. local cytokine and leukocyte responses to unilateral wrist flexion exercise. *J Appl Physiol.* 2002; 93: 546–554.
33. Eliakim A, Oh Y, Cooper DM. Effect of single wrist exercise on fibroblast growth factor-2, insulin-like growth factor, and growth hormone. *Am J Physiol Regul Integr Comp Physiol.* 2000; 279: R548–R553.
34. Nindl BC, Hymer WC, Deaver DR, Kraemer WJ. Growth hormone pulsatility profile characteristics following acute heavy resistance exercise. *J Appl Physiol.* 2001; 91: 163–172.
35. Eliakim A, Cooper DM, Nemet D. The GH-IGF-I response to typical field sports practices in adolescent athletes: a summary. *Pediatr Exerc Sci.* 2014; 26: 428–433.

36. Nemet D, Portal S, Zadik Z, *et al.* Training increases anabolic response and reduces inflammatory response to a single practice in elite male adolescent volleyball players. *J Pediatr Endocrinol Metab.* 2012; 25: 875–880.
37. Galassetti P, Larson J, Iwanaga K, Salsberg SL, Eliakim A, Pontello A. Effect of a high-fat meal on the growth hormone response to exercise in children. *J Pediatr Endocrinol Metab.* 2006; 19: 777–786.
38. Cappon JP, Ipp E, Brasel JA, Cooper DM. Acute effects of high fat and high glucose meals on the growth hormone response to exercise. *J Clin Endocrinol Metab.* 1993; 76: 1418–1422.
39. Sasaki H, Ishibashi A, Tsuchiya Y, *et al.* A 3-day high-fat/low-carbohydrate diet does not alter exercise-induced growth hormone response in healthy males. *Growth Horm IGF Res.* 2015; 25: 304–311.
40. Eliakim A, Nemet D, Zaldivar F, *et al.* Reduced exercise-associated response of the GH-IGF-I axis and catecholamines in obese children and adolescents. *J Appl Physiol.* 2006; 100: 1630–1637.
41. Patel L, Skinner AM, Price DA, Clayton PE. The influence of body mass index on growth hormone secretion in normal and short statured children. *Growth Regul.* 1994; 4: 29–34.
42. Kraemer WJ, Harman FS, Vos NH, *et al.* Effects of exercise and alkalosis on serum insulin-like growth factor I and IGF-binding protein-3. *Can J Appl Physiol.* 2000; 25: 127–138.
43. Schwarz AJ, Brasel JA, Hintz RL, Mohan S, Cooper DM. Acute effect of brief low- and high-intensity exercise on circulating insulin-like growth factor (IGF) I, II, and IGF-binding protein-3 and its proteolysis in young healthy men. *J Clin Endocrinol Metab.* 1996; 81: 3492–3497.
44. De Palo EF, Gatti R, Lancerin F, *et al.* Effects of acute, heavy-resistance exercise on urinary peptide hormone excretion in humans. *Clin Chem Lab Med.* 2003; 41: 1308–1313.
45. Marcus R, Butterfield G, Holloway L, *et al.* Effects of short-term administration of recombinant human growth hormone to elderly people. *J Clin Endocrinol Metab.* 1990; 70: 519–527.
46. Bang P, Brandt J, Degerblad M, *et al.* Exercise-induced changes in insulin-like growth factors and their low molecular weight binding protein in healthy subjects and patients with growth hormone deficiency. *Eur J Clin Invest.* 1990; 20: 285–292.
47. Elias AN, Pandian MR, Wang L, Suarez E, James N, Wilson AF. Leptin and IGF-I levels in unconditioned male volunteers after short-term exercise. *Psychoneuroendocrinology.* 2000; 25: 453–461.
48. Scheett TP, Mills PJ, Ziegler MG, Stoppani J, Cooper DM. Effect of exercise on cytokines and growth mediators in prepubertal children. *Pediatr Res.* 1999; 46: 429–434.
49. Pilz-Burstein R, Ashkenazi Y, Yaakobovitz Y, *et al.* Hormonal response to Taekwondo fighting simulation in elite adolescent athletes. *Eur J Appl Physiol.* 2010; 110: 1283–1290.
50. Bermon S, Ferrari P, Bernard P, Altare S, Dolisi C. Responses of total and free insulin-like growth factor-I and insulin-like growth factor binding protein-3 after resistance exercise and training in elderly subjects. *Acta Physiol Scand.* 1999; 165: 51–56.
51. Bamman MM, Shipp JR, Jiang J, *et al.* Mechanical load increases muscle IGF-I and androgen receptor mRNA concentrations in humans. *Am J Physiol Endocrinol Metab.* 2001; 280: E383–E390.
52. Nindl BC, Kraemer WJ, Marx JO, *et al.* Overnight responses of the circulating IGF-I system after acute, heavy-resistance exercise. *J Appl Physiol.* 2001; 90: 1319–1326.
53. Raastad T, Bjoro T, Hallen J. Hormonal responses to high- and moderate-intensity strength exercise. *Eur J Appl Physiol.* 2000; 82: 121–128.
54. Kumari M, Tabassum F, Clark C, Strachan D, Stansfeld S, Power C. Social differences in insulin-like growth factor-1: findings from a British birth cohort. *Ann Epidemiol.* 2008; 18: 664–670.
55. Bogin B, Hermanussen M, Blum WF, Assmann C. Sex, sport, IGF-1 and the community effect in height hypothesis. *Int J Environ Res Public Health.* 2015; 12: 4816–4832.
56. Wahl P, Zinner C, Achtzehn S, Bloch W, Mester J. Effect of high- and low-intensity exercise and metabolic acidosis on levels of GH, IGF-I, IGFBP-3 and cortisol. *Growth Horm IGF Res.* 2010; 20: 380–385.
57. Barnett A. Using recovery modalities between training sessions in elite athletes: does it help? *Sports Med.* 2006; 36: 781–796.
58. Wilcock IM, Cronin JB, Hing WA. Physiological response to water immersion: a method for sport recovery? *Sports Med.* 2006; 36: 747–765.
59. Nemet D, Meckel Y, Bar-Sela S, Zaldivar F, Cooper DM, Eliakim A. Effect of local cold-pack application on systemic anabolic and inflammatory response to sprint-interval training: a prospective comparative trial. *Eur J Appl Physiol.* 2009; 107: 411–417.
60. Kraemer WJ, Ratamess NA. Hormonal responses and adaptations to resistance exercise and training. *Sports Med.* 2005; 35: 339–361.
61. Round JM, Jones DA, Honour JW, Nevill AM. Hormonal factors in the development of differences in strength between boys and girls during adolescence: a longitudinal study. *Ann Hum Biol.* 1999; 26: 49–62.
62. Fry AC, Kraemer WJ, Stone MH, *et al.* Endocrine and performance responses to high volume training and amino acid supplementation in elite junior weightlifters. *Int J Sport Nutr.* 1993; 3: 306–322.
63. Kraemer WJ, Fry AC, Warren BJ, Stone MH, Fleck SJ, Kearney JT, *et al.* Acute hormonal responses in elite junior weightlifters. *Int J Sports Med.* 1992; 13: 103–109.
64. Pullinen T, Mero A, MacDonald E, Pakarinen A, Komi PV. Plasma catecholamine and serum testosterone responses to four units of resistance exercise in young and adult male athletes. *Eur J Appl Physiol Occup Physiol.* 1998; 77: 413–420.
65. Pullinen T, Mero A, Huttunen P, Pakarinen A, Komi PV. Resistance exercise-induced hormonal response under the influence of delayed onset muscle soreness in men and boys. *Scand J Med Sci Sport.* 2011; 21: e184–e194.
66. Eliakim A, Portal S, Zadik Z, *et al.* The effect of a volleyball practice on anabolic hormones and inflammatory markers in elite male and female adolescent players. J *Strength Cond Res.* 2009; 23: 1553–1559.
67. Consitt LA, Copeland JL, Tremblay MS. Endogenous anabolic hormone responses to endurance versus resistance exercise and training in women. *Sports Med.* 2002; 32: 1–22.
68. Copeland JL, Consitt LA, Tremblay MS. Hormonal responses to endurance and resistance exercise in females aged 19–69 years. *J Gerontol A Biol Sci Med Sci.* 2002; 57: B158–B165.
69. Nindl BC, Kraemer WJ, Gotshalk LA, *et al.* Testosterone responses after resistance exercise in women: influence of regional fat distribution. *Int J Sport Nutr Exerc Metab.* 2001; 11: 451–465.
70. Cumming DC, Wall SR, Galbraith MA, Belcastro AN. Reproductive hormone responses to resistance exercise. *Med Sci Sports Exerc.* 1987; 19: 234–238.
71. Kraemer WJ, Fleck SJ, Dziados JE, *et al.* Changes in hormonal concentrations after different heavy-resistance exercise protocols in women. *J Appl Physiol.* 1993; 75: 594–604.
72. Kraemer WJ, Patton JF, Gordon SE, *et al.* Compatibility of high-intensity strength and endurance training on hormonal and skeletal muscle adaptations. *J Appl Physiol.* 1995; 78: 976–989.
73. Filaire E, Lac G. Dehydroepiandrosterone (DHEA) rather than testosterone shows saliva androgen responses to exercise in elite female handball players. *Int J Sports Med.* 2000; 21: 17–20.
74. Hale RW, Kosasa T, Krieger J, Pepper S. A marathon: the immediate effect on female runners' luteinizing hormone, follicle-stimulating hormone, prolactin, testosterone, and cortisol levels. *Am J Obstet Gynecol.* 1983; 146: 550–556.
75. Eliakim A, Beyth Y. Exercise training, menstrual irregularities and bone development in children and adolescents. *J Pediatr Adolesc Gynecol.* 2003; 16: 201–206.
76. Ignacio DL, da S Silvestre DH, Cavalcanti-de-Albuquerque JP, Louzada RA, Carvalho DP, Werneck-de-Castro JP. Thyroid hormone and estrogen regulate exercise-induced growth hormone release. *PLOS One.* 2015; 10: e0122556.
77. Vanheest JL, Rodgers CD, Mahoney CE, De Souza MJ. Ovarian suppression impairs sport performance in junior elite female swimmers. *Med Sci Sports Exerc.* 2014; 46: 156–166.
78. Falk B, Eliakim A. Endocrine response to resistance training in children. *Pediatr Exerc Sci.* 2014; 26: 404–422.

79. Crewther B, Keogh J, Cronin J, Cook C. Possible stimuli for strength and power adaptation: acute hormonal responses. *Sports Med.* 2006; 36: 215–238.
80. Pullinen T, Mero A, Huttunen P, Pakarinen A, Komi PV. Resistance exercise-induced hormonal responses in men, women, and pubescent boys. *Med Sci Sports Exerc.* 2002; 34: 806–813.
81. Filaire E, Sagnol M, Ferrand C, Maso F, Lac G. Psychophysiological stress in judo athletes during competitions. *J Sports Med Phys Fit.* 2001; 41: 263–268.
82. Salvadora A, Suay F, Martinez-Sanchis S, Simon VM, Brain PF. Correlating testosterone and fighting in male participants in judo contests. *Physiol Behav.* 1999; 68: 205–209.
83. Kraemer WJ, Fleck SJ, Maresh CM, *et al.* Acute hormonal responses to a single bout of heavy resistance exercise in trained power lifters and untrained men. *Can J Appl Physiol.* 1999; 24: 524–537.
84. Pijl H. Reduced dopaminergic tone in hypothalamic neural circuits: expression of a 'thrifty' genotype underlying the metabolic syndrome? *Eur J Pharmacol.* 2003; 480: 125–131.
85. Lopes IM, Forga L, Martinez JA. Effects of leptin resistance on acute fuel metabolism after a high carbohydrate load in lean and overweight young men. *J Am Coll Nutr.* 2001; 20: 643–648.
86. Falk B, Sadres E, Constantini N, Zigel L, Lidor R, Eliakim A. The association between adiposity and the response to resistance training among pre- and early-pubertal boys. *J Pediatr Endocrinol Metab.* 2002; 15: 597–606.
87. Wigal SB, Nemet D, Swanson JM, *et al.* Catecholamine response to exercise in children with attention deficit hyperactivity disorder. *Pediatr Res.* 2003; 53: 756–761.

CHAPTER 6

Muscle metabolism during exercise

Neil Armstrong, Alan R Barker, and Alison M McManus

Introduction

Skeletal muscle metabolism during exercise in adulthood is well-documented[1] but research into paediatric muscle metabolism has been ethically constrained, with few studies interrogating the exercising muscles. Research with youth has been generally limited to blood and respiratory gas indicators of substrate and energy use, measures of maximal aerobic and anaerobic performance, and models of recovery from maximal or intermittent high-intensity exercise, rather than potentially more informative studies at the level of the myocyte.[2] Metabolic profiles estimated in this manner are useful indicators of muscle exercise metabolism but they require confirmation at muscle cell level and do not provide the quality or specificity of data required to tease out age-, biological maturity-, and sex-related changes in muscle metabolism during exercise of various intensities and durations.

The few muscle biopsy studies that have been performed with healthy youth must be interpreted cautiously. They are generally confounded by large individual variations in muscle fibre profiles, classification of teenagers by chronological age without assessing biological maturity, comparisons with previously published studies of adult data from elsewhere, utilization of resting and post-exercise measures rather than data collected during exercise, and investigation of small numbers of boys with very few studies including girls. However, the emergence of rigorous techniques to measure pulmonary oxygen uptake ($p\dot{V}O_2$) kinetics[3] and non-invasive technologies such as ^{31}P magnetic resonance spectroscopy ($^{31}PMRS$)[4] and stable isotope tracers[5] have enhanced our understanding of muscle exercise metabolism during youth.[6]

This chapter reviews what can be inferred from conventional studies of skeletal muscle metabolism during exercise in relation to chronological age, biological maturity, and sex. It critiques key studies using recently developed techniques and technologies, explores new insights, and synthesizes current views of developmental muscle exercise metabolism. The focus throughout is on healthy young people.

Few studies of muscle metabolism during exercise have reported participants' stage of maturity and for clarity the chapter uses the terms 'prepubertal children' when prepuberty is confirmed in the research cited; 'children' represents those 12 years and younger but without proof of pubertal status; 'adolescents' refers to 13–18 year-olds; and 'youth' or 'young people' describes both children and adolescents. Throughout the chapter use of 'age' refers to chronological age.

Anaerobic and aerobic exercise metabolism

Participation in exercise of different intensities, durations, and frequencies is dependent on interplay between anaerobic and aerobic metabolism. This section provides a brief primer and readily accessible resource for subsequent sections, particularly the sections Muscle energy stores, Muscle enzymes activity, and Substrate utilization. In-depth coverage of the biochemistry of exercise is beyond the scope of the chapter and interested readers are encouraged to access textbooks devoted to the topic[1] for further detail.

High-energy phosphates

Muscle contraction is enabled by the energy released during the hydrolysis of adenosine triphosphate (ATP) via adenosine diphosphate (ADP), adenosine monophosphate (AMP), and inorganic phosphate (Pi) catalysed by myosin ATPase:

$$ATP + H_2O \rightarrow ADP + Pi + H^+ + energy$$

$$ADP + H_2O \rightarrow AMP + Pi + H^+ + energy$$

The intramuscular stores of ATP are sufficient to support maximal exercise for only ~2 s but ATP is rapidly re-synthesized by the breakdown of phosphocreatine (PCr) to creatine (Cr) and phosphate (Pi), which are transferred to ADP to re-form ATP. The reaction is catalysed by creatine kinase (CK):

$$PCr + ADP + H^+ \rightarrow ATP + Cr$$

There is three to four times as much PCr stored in skeletal muscles as there is ATP (see section Muscle energy stores). However, re-synthesis of ATP through the enzymatic breakdown of PCr reaches its peak within ~2 s and PCr is depleted rapidly during exercise. For exercise to be sustained beyond a few seconds ATP supply must be maintained and this is ensured in the short-term by anaerobic glycolysis in the muscles.

Anaerobic metabolism

Carbohydrates (CHOs) are stored in the muscles and liver as glycogen. Muscle glycogen is immediately available to re-synthesize ATP during exercise whereas liver glycogen is broken down and released into the blood as glucose where it is transported to tissues as an energy substrate. This chapter focuses on the exercising muscles where glycogenolysis is the breakdown of muscle glycogen to glucose-1-phosphate, and glycolysis is the sequence of reactions which convert glucose (from the blood) or glucose-1-phosphate

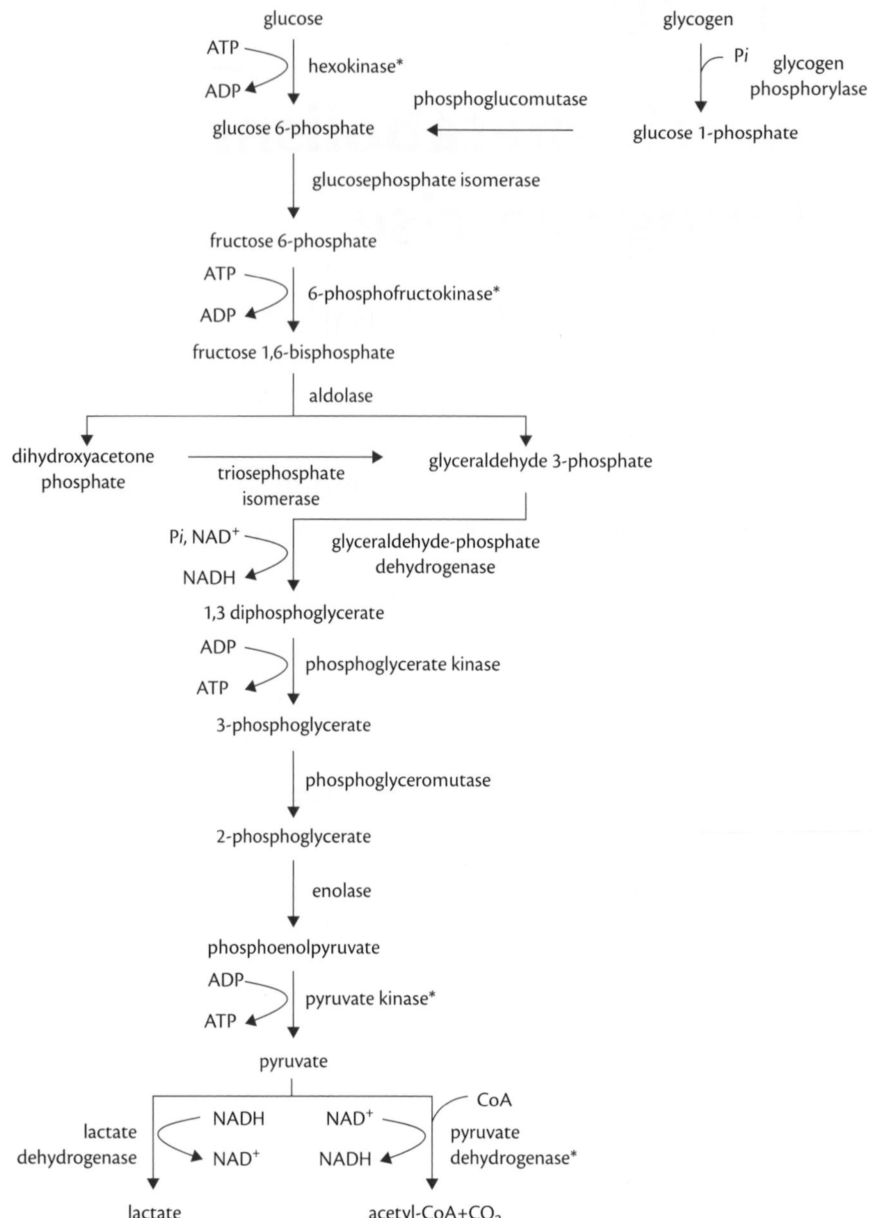

Figure 6.1 The reactions of glycogenolysis and glycolysis.
ATP is adenosine triphosphate; ADP is adenosine diphosphate; CoA is coenzyme A; NAD^+ is nicotinamide adenine dinucleotide; Pi is inorganic phosphate; * irreversible reactions.
Maughan R, Gleeson M, Greenhaff PL. Biochemistry of exercise and training. Oxford: Oxford University Press: 1997.

to pyruvate (Figure 6.1). Despite the number of reactions involved glycolysis responds rapidly to exercise with a time constant (τ) of ~1.5 s. Peak production of ATP is therefore reached within ~5 s and the glycolytic pathway becomes the major provider of ATP within ~10 s of the onset of maximal exercise. At its peak glycolysis re-synthesizes ATP at ~50% of the rate of re-synthesis from PCr.

Pyruvate can be converted into acetyl coenzyme A catalysed by pyruvate dehydrogenase (PDH) or reduced to lactate catalysed by lactate dehydrogenase (LDH). (Other pathways are described in detail elsewhere[1]). When the demand for energy is high lactate accumulates in the muscle and some diffuses into the blood where it is often used as an indicator of glycolytic activity. (See the section Muscle lactate production and blood lactate accumulation and interested readers are referred to Chapter 12 for wider discussion of blood lactate accumulation).

Aerobic metabolism

The initial steps of aerobic (oxidative) carbohydrate (CHO) metabolism are the transport of pyruvate into the mitochondria and its conversion into acetyl coenzyme A, which then enters the tricarboxylic acid cycle (TCA cycle) by condensing with 4-carbon molecule oxaloacetate to form 6-carbon molecule citrate. The reaction is catalysed by citrate synthase (CS). One complete turn of the TCA cycle results in the re-formation of oxaloacetate, and the production of ATP, carbon dioxide (CO_2), and hydrogen atoms (H^+) as shown in Figure 6.2. The H^+ are then oxidized via the electron transport chain with the re-synthesis of ATP from ADP as illustrated in Figure 6.3.

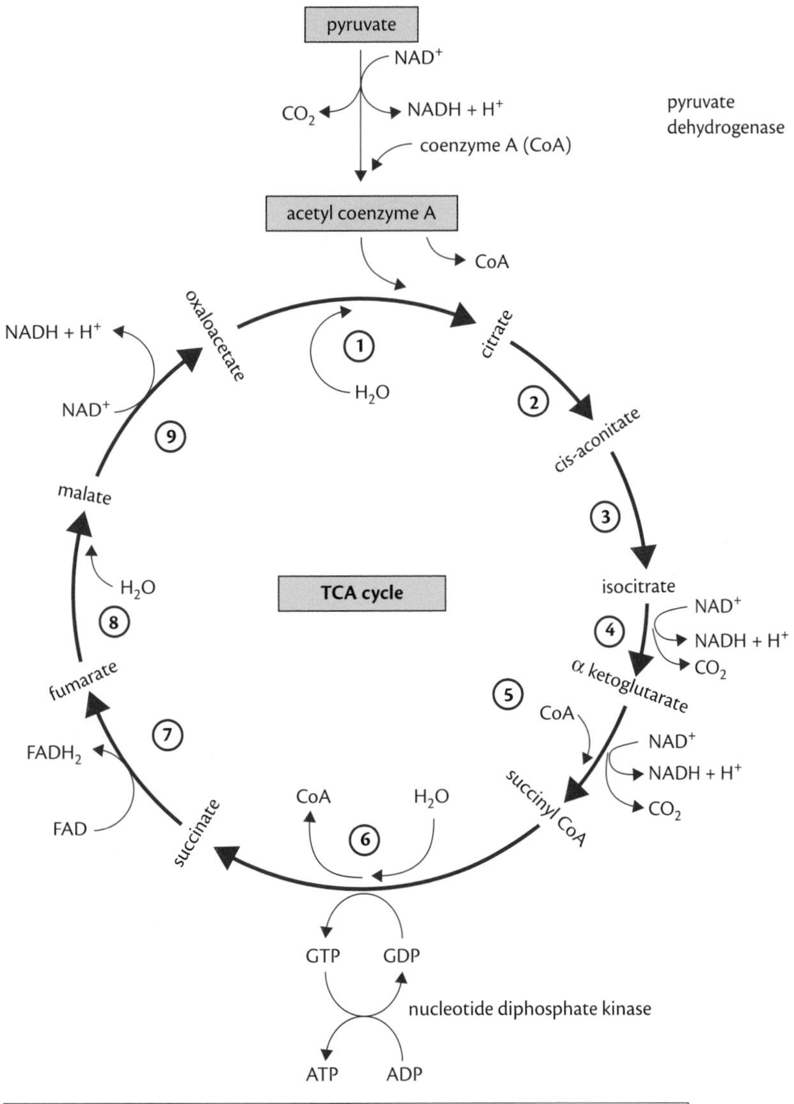

Figure 6.2 Summary of the reactions of the tricarboxylic acid cycle.
The figure shows sites of substrate level phosphorylation and nicotinamide adenine dinucleotide (NAD^+) and flavin adenine dinucleotide (FAD) reduction. ATP is adenosine triphosphate; ADP is adenosine diphosphate; CO_2 is carbon dioxide; GTP is guanosine triphosphate; GDP is guanosine diphosphate.
Maughan R, Gleeson M, Greenhaff PL. Biochemistry of exercise and training. Oxford: Oxford University Press: 1997.

Lipids (or fats), principally stored in adipose tissue but also in muscle as triacylglycerol, provide a much larger reservoir of energy-rich substrate than CHOs. Lipolysis catalysed by lipases breaks down triacylglycerol into free fatty acids (FFAs) and glycerol, which are transported in the blood to the muscles. The uptake of FFAs by skeletal muscle is directly related to the plasma FFA concentration. Free fatty acids from adipose tissue are transported into the muscle cell by facilitated diffusion which occurs if the intracellular FFA concentration is less than that in solution in the extracellular fluid. On entry into the muscle cell the FFAs are converted to acyl coenzyme A through the action of ATP-linked acyl coenzyme A synthetase. The acyl coenzyme A molecules move across the mitochondrial membranes through the action of carnitine acyltransferase (CAT). Once released into the mitochondria acyl coenzyme A undergoes a series of sequential reactions (β oxidation) involving the release of two carbon units in the form of acetyl coenzyme A. Acetyl coenzyme A combines with oxaloacetate to form citrate which is degraded in the TCA cycle to ATP, CO_2, and H^+. The H^+ are then oxidized via the electron transport system generating ATP (see Figure 6.3).

Oxidative metabolism is relatively slow to adapt to the demands of exercise and the τ of children's response to heavy intensity exercise is ~20–25 s. The rate at which ATP can be generated aerobically is much slower than that of anaerobic ATP synthesis, but as oxidative metabolism can use CHOs, FFAs, and even amino acids as substrates it has much greater capacity than anaerobic pathways. Amino acids only make a small contribution to energy provision during exercise, perhaps ~5%. Adequate protein is vital for healthy

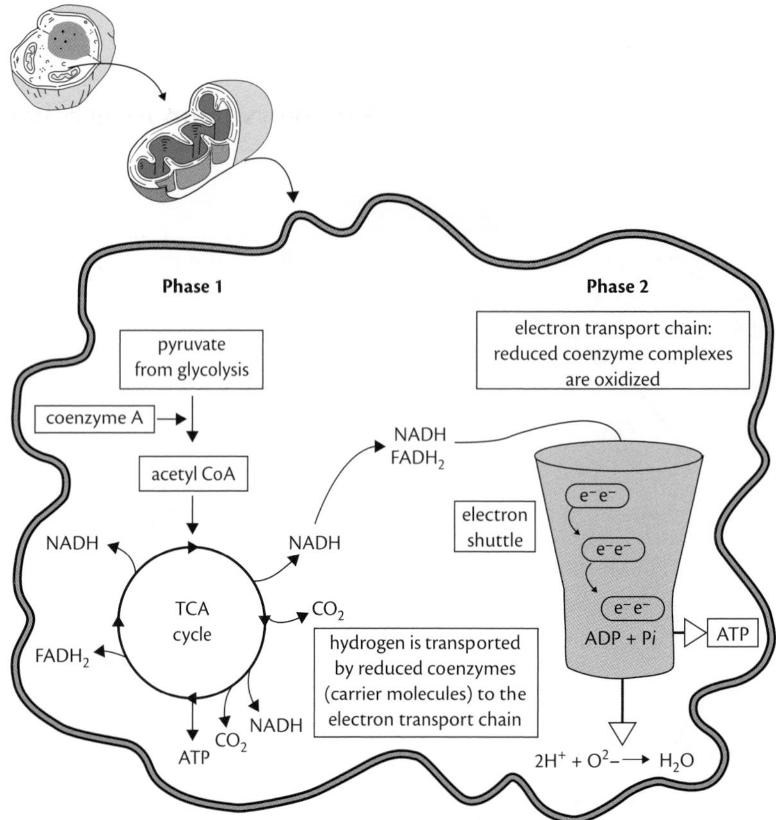

Figure 6.3 Schematic diagram showing the relationship of the tricarboxylic acid cycle to the electron transport chain.
ATP is adenosine triphosphate; ADP is adenosine diphosphate; CO_2 is carbon dioxide; FAD is flavin adenine dinucleotide; H_2O is water; NAD^+ is nicotinamide adenine dinucleotide; Pi is inorganic phosphate; TCA cycle is tricarboxylic acid cycle.
Maughan R, Gleeson M, Greenhaff PL. Biochemistry of exercise and training. Oxford: Oxford University Press: 1997.

growth and biological maturation but as appropriate nutrient intake is discussed in detail in Chapter 47 and the present chapter is focused on energy to support muscular exercise, amino acids will only receive passing references herein.

In comparison with the anaerobic pathways oxidative metabolism plays a minor role in ATP re-synthesis during short-term high-intensity exercise, but the aerobic contribution progressively increases with time and is dominant during exercise longer than ~70–80 s. The overlapping contributions of the aerobic and anaerobic energy systems during high-intensity exercise of different durations in youth can be nicely illustrated by considering performance in various track events. A 100-m sprint (~11–13 s) is primarily supported by the catabolism of PCr and anaerobic glycolysis with ~10% of the energy being provided by aerobic metabolism. A 400-m sprint (~50–60 s) is ~60–70% supported by anaerobic metabolism, predominantly glycolysis, with minor support from aerobic sources. The 1500 m (~250–300 s) is a ~80% aerobic event although increases in pace (e.g. final sprint) have high anaerobic components.

Substrate utilization during submaximal exercise is addressed in the section on Substrate utilization but, in general, CHOs are the principal substrate during the early stages of submaximal exercise with lipids becoming the primary contributor over time. During exercise below the lactate threshold (T_{LAC}) the lipid contribution increases with the intensity of the exercise until Fatmax, the relative exercise intensity that elicits the highest fat oxidation rate is attained. There are wide individual variations in Fatmax but in youth it has been reported to lie between 30–60% of peak $\dot{V}O_2$[7] although it may be relatively higher in prepubertal boys.[8] As the relative intensity of exercise increases above Fatmax the contribution of fat falls and CHOs again become the predominant energy substrate. The relative contribution of fat and CHO to metabolism is crucial during prolonged exercise. The precise balance of energy stores is dependent on diet, but both muscle glycogen stores (see Muscle energy stores section) and blood glucose (from liver glycogen stores) are limited whereas triacylglycerol in adipose tissue and muscles provides a vast reservoir of potential energy-generating substrate. Increased utilization of triacylglycerol can therefore spare CHOs, delay the onset of fatigue, and enhance performance.

The response of the endocrine system to exercise varies with biological maturation and several hormones influence interplay between CHO and FFA availability and utilization during exercise.[8] Detailed analysis of hormonal influences sit outside the scope of this chapter, as Chapter 5 is devoted to this topic, but reference will be made to relevant hormonal actions where appropriate.

Maximal-intensity exercise

Maximal 'anaerobic'[9] and 'aerobic'[10] exercise during childhood and adolescence are independently well-documented without always being well-defined, or the metabolic anaerobic/ aerobic interplay addressed. Maximal anaerobic and aerobic power will only be summarized briefly herein focusing on their comparative development with aging and biological maturation. (Interested readers are referred to Chapter 8 and Chapter 12 where maximal-intensity exercise and maximal aerobic power are comprehensively discussed).

Maximal anaerobic power

In contrast with maximal aerobic power, there is no 'gold standard' laboratory technique for the assessment of maximal anaerobic power. There is a plethora of 'maximal anaerobic tests' which have been critiqued elsewhere[11] but research has primarily focused on the assessment of cycling peak power output (CPP) estimated using variants of the Wingate anaerobic test (WAnT).[12] Cross-sectional data indicate that from ages 7 to 17 years, girls' CPP increases by ~295% compared to a ~375% increase in boys' CPP over the same age range. Sex differences in CPP appear to be minimal until ~12–13 years of age, when boys experience a marked spurt in CPP through to young adulthood; by 17 years the sex difference in CPP is ~50%.[13] Data are, however, confounded by the fact that few studies have simultaneously considered the age and biological maturity of the participants.

Maximal aerobic power

Peak $\dot{V}O_2$ is widely recognized as the best single indicator of young people's maximal aerobic power and its assessment and interpretation are well-documented.[14] Cross-sectional data are consistent and show boys' and girls' peak $\dot{V}O_2$ to increase in a near-linear manner by ~150% and ~80% respectively from age 8 to 16 years. The sex difference increases from ~10% at 8 years to ~35% at 16 years of age.[15] Longitudinal data follow a similar trend with a tendency for girls' values to level-off at ~14 years.[16] Peak $\dot{V}O_2$ is strongly correlated with body mass and when body mass is appropriately controlled for using allometry or multi-level modelling,[17] boys' values progressively increase from childhood into young adulthood, whereas girls' peak $\dot{V}O_2$ increases from childhood into mid-teens, and then remains relatively stable into young adulthood.[18] Longitudinal data demonstrate that in both sexes biological maturity exerts an additional positive effect on peak $\dot{V}O_2$ independent of age and body mass.[19]

Comparison of maximal anaerobic and aerobic power

In the current context it must be noted that i) peak $\dot{V}O_2$ is a function not only of oxygen utilization by the muscle (aerobic metabolism) but also oxygen delivery to the muscle[20] and, ii) age- and biological maturity-related increases in CPP are enhanced by changes in muscle fibre size, % muscle fibre type, and the ability to recruit and more fully use higher threshold motor units, as well as enhanced muscle anaerobic metabolism.[21] Nevertheless, cross-sectional data strongly suggest that CPP and peak $\dot{V}O_2$ increase at different rates during the teen years. This has been confirmed in a longitudinal study of 12- to 17-year-olds where CPP was reported to increase by ~120% in boys and ~65% in girls respectively, with increases in peak $\dot{V}O_2$ somewhat smaller at ~70% for boys and ~25% for girls, respectively.[19,22] Independent of age there is a more marked effect of biological maturity on CPP than peak $\dot{V}O_2$, which was clearly illustrated in a study of 200 (100 boys) 12-year-olds. Children were classified according to the stages of maturation described by Tanner.[23] Girls and boys in maturation stage 4 for pubic hair (PH4) were reported to have respectively, 51% and 66% higher CPP and 25% and 32% higher peak $\dot{V}O_2$ than those in PH1. With body mass controlled for using allometry, the difference between stage 4 and stage 1 in CPP and peak $\dot{V}O_2$ was 20% and 12% respectively, in girls and 31% and 14% respectively, in boys.[24,25]

Recovery from intermittent maximal or high-intensity exercise

Boys have been reported to recover more rapidly than men from intermittent bouts of maximal or high-intensity running[26,27] or cycling,[26,28] and maximal isokinetic contractions.[29,30] Research with females is less extensive but shows a similar trend, at least into the mid-teens.[31,32] It has been persuasively argued that, as children generate lower power output than adults, their faster recovery from high-intensity exercise is not directly comparable because they have less to recover from.[33] However, studies have consistently reported that the ability to recover from repeated bouts of high-intensity exercise progressively declines from childhood to young adulthood in males, whereas in females an adult profile appears to be established by ~14–15 years of age.[32,34,35]

Children's faster recovery from high-intensity exercise has been related to maturational changes in aerobic and anaerobic metabolism and attributed to factors including an enhanced oxidative capacity, more rapid PCr re-synthesis, better acid-base regulation, lower production and/or more efficient removal of metabolic by-products compared to adults.[36–38] (Interested readers are referred to Chapter 9 for further discussion of fatigue and recovery).

Muscle biopsies

The muscle biopsy technique was first introduced in the early 1900s to study muscular dystrophy but it was Bergstrom's re-introduction of the biopsy needle to exercise science in 1962 which stimulated research into muscle biochemistry during exercise.[39] The technique involves local anaesthesia followed by a small incision through the skin, subcutaneous tissue, and fascia. A hollow needle is inserted into the belly of the muscle and, via a plunger in the centre of the needle, a small piece of muscle is excised and the needle containing the muscle withdrawn. The muscle sample is cleaned and quickly frozen for subsequent microscopy or biochemical analysis. Despite problems related to the size of the muscle sample,[40] the depth of the incision in relation to muscle size,[41] and the variability of fibre type distributions within and between human muscles[42,43] muscle biopsies have greatly enhanced our understanding of muscle metabolism. In many laboratories muscle biopsies are used almost routinely in adult investigations but ethical considerations have limited the number of healthy young people subjected to the technique.

Muscle fibre types

Muscle fibres consist of a continuum of biochemical and contractile features, but they are conventionally classified into type I (slow twitch), type IIa (fast twitch, or fatigue resistant), and type IIX (fast twitch, or fatiguable) fibres. It is sometimes possible to detect type IIc fibres but they normally account for less than 1% of the total muscle fibre pool. Type I fibres have a high oxidative capacity and are characterized by a rich capillary blood supply, numerous mitochondria, and high activity of oxidative enzymes. The high lipid content of type I fibres supports fat oxidation during submaximal exercise with a glycogen sparing effect. Type II fibres are better equipped for high-intensity exercise with higher glycolytic enzymes activity and greater glycogen and PCr stores than type I fibres. In type II fibres the rate of pyruvate production by glycolysis is greater than the rate at which it can be oxidized and the excess pyruvate is reduced to lactate to allow regeneration of nicotinamide adenine dinucleotide (NAD) and the continuation of glycolysis (see Figure 6.1). Type I fibres have a low threshold of activity and preferentially respond to low- to moderate-intensity exercise, but type IIa and type IIX fibres are better equipped to support more severe exercise and they are sequentially recruited as exercise intensity increases.[44]

It has been suggested that maturation of skeletal muscle fibre patterns might account for age-related changes in the metabolic response to high-intensity exercise,[45] but published studies of muscle biopsies from children or adolescents are sparse, generally involve few participants, and the interpretation of data has been confounded by large variations in fibre profiles.[46] Nevertheless, some patterns have emerged from the extant literature.

Muscle fibre size appears to increase linearly with age from birth to adolescence[13] and, at least in males, into young adulthood.[40] Some studies have indicated that during adolescence muscle fibre areas for all fibre types are larger in boys than in girls, but girls' values are similar to those of young adult females.[46,47]

In an often-cited early study, Bell *et al.*[48] obtained biopsies from the vastus lateralis of thirteen 6-year-old Swiss children and reported that their fibre type distribution pattern was essentially similar to normal adult tissue. However, it should be noted that the 'normal adult tissue' referred to was extracted from previous studies performed by others elsewhere. Oertel[49] reported data from an autopsy study of 113 subjects, aged from 1 week to 20 years, and revealed that the % of type I fibres in the vastus lateralis muscle of 15- to 20-year-olds tended to be lower than in younger subjects. This trend was subsequently supported in a similar autopsy study of 22 previously healthy males between the ages of 5 to 37 years, where a highly significant negative relationship between % of type I fibres in the vastus lateralis and age was observed. The % of type I fibres decreased from ~65% at age 5 years to ~50% at age 20 years.[40] Further support for an age-related decline in % of type I fibres, at least in males, was provided in what appears to be the only published study involving young people in which data have been collected longitudinally. Biopsies taken from the vastus lateralis of 55 males and 28 females at age 16 years and again at 27 years were analysed for fibre type. The % of type I fibres was reported to significantly decrease with age in males but no significant change in females was observed.[47]

Jansson[41] critically reviewed the extant literature to examine the hypothesis that % of type I fibres in the vastus lateralis is a function of age. She concluded that the % of type I fibres decreases in sedentary to moderately active males, without any known diseases, between the ages of 10 and 35 years. No clear age-related fibre type changes were observed in females, but this might be a methodological artefact as few data on girls and young women are available.

Studies comparing the muscle fibre distribution of boys and girls are particularly sparse. Small participant samples, often including fewer girls than boys, and large inter individual differences confound statistical analyses. Statistically significant sex differences in the % of type I fibres have not been reported but there is a consistent trend with adolescent boys and young men exhibiting, on average, 4–15% more type I fibres in the vastus lateralis than similarly aged females in the same study.[46,47,50,51] No published study has indicated that girls have a higher % of type I fibres than boys.

Methodological concerns demand that paediatric muscle biopsy studies be interpreted cautiously but the extant data are consistent in showing an age-related decline in % of type I fibres from childhood to young adulthood, at least in boys. Similarly, published work indicates a strong trend in which adolescent boys present a higher % of type I fibres than girls. Further research is clearly warranted and the potential of magnetic resonance imaging (MRI) and ^{31}PMRS to provide non-invasive methods of indirectly estimating muscle fibre types might open ethical avenues of resolving intriguing issues concerning age-, biological maturity, and sex-related differences in muscle fibre type.[52–54]

Muscle energy stores

In a series of innovative muscle biopsy studies of 11- to 16-year-old boys, Eriksson and his colleagues[55–60] made a significant contribution to understanding young people's muscle metabolism. They focused on energy stores and the activity of key enzymes in the muscle at rest, following exercise of different intensities, and post-training. Their data, which have often been interpreted uncritically, have influenced the interpretation of paediatric exercise metabolism for almost 50 years.

Eriksson and Saltin[59] took muscle biopsies from the vastus lateralis of boys aged 11.6 years, 12.6 years, 13.5 years, and 15.5 years, with eight or nine participants per year. They analysed the samples for concentrations of ATP, PCr, glycogen, and lactate at rest and immediately after both submaximal exercise and exercise to peak$\dot{V}O_2$ (which they termed 'maximal exercise') on a cycle ergometer. They reported mean resting values but as variances were not recorded the data are difficult to interpret. Resting ATP stores of ~5 mmol·kg^{-1} wet weight of muscle which were invariant with age and similar to values they had earlier observed in adults[61] were reported. The concentration of ATP remained essentially unchanged following 6-min bouts of submaximal exercise but minor reductions were observed following maximal exercise.

The authors concluded that boys' PCr concentration at rest was comparable to that of adults but noted that there was, 'a tendency towards higher values with increasing age'[59(p260)]. The mean PCr concentration of the 11-year-olds was 14.5 mmol·kg^{-1} wet weight of muscle, but 15-year-olds' PCr concentration was ~63% higher at 23.6 mmol·kg^{-1} wet weight of muscle and similar to values recorded in men in their earlier studies.[61] Phosphocreatine concentration gradually declined following exercise sessions of increasing intensity with values of <5 mmol·kg^{-1} wet weight of muscle observed following maximal exercise. Subsequent research using ^{31}PMRS and modelling equations to interrogate the gastrocnemius and soleus confirmed the invariance of ATP with age but no differences in PCr concentrations between 10-year-old boys and adults were observed.[62]

In the 11-year-olds, muscle glycogen concentration at rest averaged 54 mmol·kg^{-1} wet weight of muscle and progressively increased with age, reaching 87 mmol·kg^{-1} wet weight of muscle in the 15-year-olds, which is comparable to muscle glycogen concentrations, but not absolute values, they had previously observed in men.[61] With exercise a gradual decrease in glycogen was reported in all groups but the decrease was three times greater in the oldest compared to the youngest boys, thus suggesting enhanced glycolysis with age.[58]

Muscle lactate production and blood lactate accumulation

Lactate is continuously produced in skeletal muscles, even at rest, but the onset of exercise stimulates glycolysis and lactate production increases as a function of the imbalance between anaerobic and aerobic metabolism of pyruvate. Lactate metabolism is a dynamic process and while some fibres produce lactate, adjacent fibres consume it as an energy source. The net muscle lactate accumulation derived from a single muscle biopsy is therefore not a direct measure of lactate production and, at best, only reflects the glycolytic contribution to the synthesis of ATP during exercise. There are very few data on young people's muscle lactate accumulation either at rest or following exercise.

In the initial report of their muscle biopsy studies, Eriksson *et al.*[55] observed, in 13-year-old boys, a mean resting muscle lactate accumulation of 1.3 $mmol \cdot kg^{-1}$ wet weight of muscle. At low exercise intensities muscle lactate increased very little but at exercise intensities above 60% of peak $\dot{V}O_2$ (presumably above the boys' T_{LAC}) a more rapid increase was observed. When the research was extended to 11- to 16-year-old boys[59] it was noted that muscle lactate accumulation increased with increasing relative exercise and that muscle lactate immediately following submaximal exercise was higher in older boys. An age-related increase in the anaerobic glycolytic contribution to metabolism after maximal exercise was indicated by observations of muscle lactate accumulations of 8.8, 10.7, 11.3, and 15.5 $mmol \cdot kg^{-1}$ wet weight of muscle for boys aged 11.6, 12.6, 13.5, and 15.5 years, respectively.[59]

In his thesis, Eriksson[56] suggested a possible maturation effect on muscle lactate as, at age 13.6 years, those with higher muscle lactate had a greater testicular volume although this relationship was only 'almost significant'. Eriksson *et al.*[55] commented that boys' 'blood lactate concentration reflected their muscle lactate concentration'[55(p156)]. In subsequent paediatric studies blood lactate accumulation has often been used to reflect muscle lactate production, but the relationship is complex and the limits of the assumption are addressed in Chapter 12.

There is evidence which suggests that age-related differences in the kinetics of blood lactate reflect a faster elimination of lactate out of the blood in children rather than differences in muscle lactate,[63] but this interpretation has been criticized on methodological grounds[31] and conflicting data are available.[64]

The interpretation of blood lactate accumulation, as a surrogate of muscle lactate production, in relation to sex, age, and biological maturity is also clouded by methodological issues. There appears to be a positive relationship between age and blood lactate accumulation during both submaximal and maximal exercise, but a direct relationship with biological maturity has proved difficult to establish. Some studies have indicated that girls exhibit a greater accumulation of blood lactate during both submaximal and maximal exercise, but data are equivocal and sex differences remain to be proven.[65–67] (Interested readers are referred to Chapter 12 for further discussion of blood lactate accumulation).

In the present context, the work of Pianosi *et al.*,[68] who monitored the blood lactate and pyruvate concentrations of 28 young people following 6 min of cycling at two-thirds of maximal exercise, is noteworthy. The data were analysed in relation to three age groups; 7- to 10-year-olds, 11- to 14-year-olds, and 15- to 17-year-olds. They reported that following exercise, lactate increased out of proportion to that of pyruvate such that the lactate to pyruvate ratio rose in an age-related manner. These data suggest an enhanced glycolytic function rather than a compromised oxidative capacity with increasing age. On the other hand, using the WAnT as an exercise model, another study concluded that lower post-exercise blood lactate accumulation in children reflects a lower muscle mass combined with a facilitated aerobic metabolism.[69]

Muscle enzymes activity

Eriksson *et al.*'s[58] pioneering research described levels of succinic dehydrogenase (SDH) and phosphofructokinase (PFK) activity in the vastus lateralis of five boys, mean age 11.2 years, before and after a 6-week training programme. They demonstrated a ~29% increase in SDH and a ~83% increase in PFK activity following training. However, it was the pre-training activities of SDH and PFK, which were observed to be ~25% higher and ~67% lower respectively than adult values reported by the same research group,[70] that generated the most interest among paediatric exercise physiologists. Despite the small sample size, the fact that the muscle biopsies were carried out at rest, and Eriksson's[56] revealing comment in his thesis that his results must be interpreted with caution, numerous authors (particularly of textbooks) have uncritically cited these data to unequivocally support the view that children have a low glycolytic and enhanced oxidative capacity during exercise. Subsequent studies of enzyme activity in the vastus lateralis have provided more comprehensive analyses of young people's enzymes activity.

In a series of studies Haralambie[71,72] determined the activity of a number of enzymes from biopsies of the vastus lateralis taken at rest. She acknowledged the limitations of extrapolating in vitro data to in vivo conditions and focused on measuring enzyme activity as near as possible to optimal conditions, including physiological temperature. To maximize insights into the mechanisms controlling the functional characteristics and capacity of muscle, the importance of investigating as many enzyme activities of a specific metabolic pathway as possible was emphasized.

Haralambie[71] compared enzyme activity in twelve 11–14-year-old girls with ten 36-year-old women. She reported significantly higher activity of two TCA enzymes, namely fumarase and isocitrate dehydrogenase (ICDH), in the girls and concluded that this may reflect enhanced oxidation of substrate in the younger participants. She also observed higher LDH activity in the girls, but commented somewhat glibly that this, 'simply suggests a daily physical activity directed towards more intensity than endurance in this group'[71(p265)].

In a more comprehensive investigation, Haralambie[72] determined the activity of 22 enzymes involved in energy metabolism in seven boys and seven girls, aged 13–15 years, and seven women and seven men, aged 22–42 years. The activity of glycolytic enzymes was not significantly different between adults and adolescents. In contrast with her earlier report, Haralambie observed no significant age difference in LDH activity, and her observation of no age-related change in PFK activity is in direct conflict with Eriksson *et al.*'s[58] findings. The activity of enolase was lower in females in both age groups, but no difference due to age was noted; this was the only sex difference in anaerobic enzyme activity recorded. Of the studies by Haramblie[72] all oxidative enzymes, with the exception of CS, were more active in adolescents compared with adults. The activities of ICDH and fumarase were ~44% and ~25% higher respectively in adolescents compared to adults. No significant adult-adolescent differences were noted in activities of three enzymes involved in fatty acid metabolism, but enzymes involved in amino acid metabolism showed a tendency to higher activity in adolescents.

Berg and his associates[73,74] biopsied resting samples from the vastus lateralis and determined the activity of CK, hexose phosphate isomerase, aldolase, pyruvate kinase (PK), LDH, CS, and fumarase in 33 participants categorized into three age groups, i.e. children (four males, four females), mean age 6.4 years; 'juveniles' (five males, seven females) mean age 13.5 years; and, 'young adults' (five males, eight females) mean age 17.1 years. The activity of glycolytic enzymes was positively correlated with age and the activity of TCA cycle enzymes was negatively correlated with age, although no correlations reached statistical significance. Mean activity increases of ~32%, ~85%, ~48%, ~143%, and ~25% were observed in CK, aldolase, PK, LDH, and hexose phosphate isomerise respectively, from 6 to 13 years. However, with wide intra-group standard deviations, changes were only significant for aldolase, PK, and LDH. With the exception of LDH, which decreased in activity from 13–17 years, but remained significantly higher than at 6 years, there were no significant changes from 13–17 years. The activity of TCA cycle enzymes CS and fumarase declined by ~28% and ~40% respectively from 6 to 17 years, with the decrease in fumarase activity being statistically significant.

The work of Haralambie[72] and Berg *et al.*[73,74] provides the opportunity for further insights into muscle metabolism through the exploration of ratios of specific glycolytic to oxidative enzymes activity. A re-calculation of Berg's data indicates PK to fumarase ratios of 3.585, 3.201, and 2.257 for 'young adults', 'juveniles', and children respectively. In other words, the glycolytic to oxidative enzyme activity ratio was ~59% higher in 17-year-olds than in 6-year-old children. Haralambie's[72] data allow a comparison of the activity of potential rate-limiting enzymes of glycolysis and the TCA cycle, namely PFK and ICDH. Unfortunately, data are only available on eight adolescents and eight adults, but the ratio PFK to ICDH was reported to be 93% (and significantly) higher in adults than in adolescents at 1.633 and 0.844 respectively.

Kaczor *et al.*[75] collected samples of the obliquus abdominis muscle from twenty 3- to 11-year-olds and twelve 29- to 54-year-old hernia patients and determined the enzyme activity of adenylate kinase (AK), CK, CAT, LDH, and α-ketoglutarate dehydrogenase (KDH), a rate-limiting enzyme in the TCA cycle. They reported lower activity of the 'anaerobic' enzymes (AK, CK, and LDH) in children and suggested that this difference, particularly the 3.5-fold lower LDH activity, is likely to be a major factor in children's lower anaerobic performance (and muscle/blood lactate concentration) compared to adults. They observed KDH activity to be slightly lower in children and, in accord with Haralambie,[72] CAT activity to be similar for children and adults. The ratio of CAT to LDH was threefold (i.e. significantly) higher in children and the ratio of CAT to KDH also tended to be higher in children (16%) without being statistically significant. The authors commented that their results indicate that children have a greater ability than adults to oxidize lipids during exercise, although the mechanisms are not clear.

Substrate utilization

Indirect calorimetry

Carbohydrates and lipids are the principal energy substrates during submaximal exercise with amino acids playing a minor role which, in adults, has been estimated to be in the range of providing between 1–8% of total energy.[76] The relative contribution of CHO and fat to energy provision during exercise can be computed from indirect calorimetry by calculating the respiratory exchange ratio (R; $\dot{V}CO_2/\dot{V}O_2$) measured at the mouth and computing fat and CHO utilization from conventional conversion equations.

Estimation of substrate utilization through R is conducive for use with children but data must be interpreted cautiously. Indirect calorimetry relies on the assumptions that $\dot{V}CO_2$ and $\dot{V}O_2$ measured at the mouth replicate gas exchange at the level of the tissue, that a physiological steady state has been reached, and that there is a negligible effect of other metabolic processes such as lipogenesis, gluconeogenesis, and ketogenesis on oxygen consumption and carbon dioxide production.[77] Nevertheless, under well-controlled steady-state conditions in the moderate exercise intensity domain, the R reflects the respiratory quotient (RQ; gas exchange at tissue level) and studies with adults suggest that estimates of substrate utilization through R compare well with those from stable isotope techniques, up to ~75% peak $\dot{V}O_2$.[7] During exercise above the T_{LAC}, fat oxidation is likely to be underestimated as R increases in response to the bicarbonate buffering of H^+ production and the increased release of CO_2 in the expired gas. No published studies with youth appear to have taken into account individual T_{LACs} when evaluating R in relation to age, biological maturity, or sex, and data need to be interpreted in this context.

The R is also influenced by prior exercise, state of training, fitness, nutritional intake before and during exercise, type, mode, and duration of exercise.[78] In addition, indirect calorimetry is unable to clarify the various lipid (intramuscular triglyceride vs blood FFAs) and CHO (muscle glycogen vs blood glucose) sources and the validity of the conventional conversion equations based on calculations of the balance of glucose and glycogen oxidation has been questioned.[79]

Age and sex

Despite the limitations of the technique indirect calorimetry has been used extensively to characterize substrate utilization in children, adolescents, and adults. Almost 80 years ago, in the first laboratory-based study of youth oxygen consumption during exercise, Robinson[80] noted that Rs were lower in young boys than in teenage boys and lower in teenage boys than in men. Subsequent studies have consistently reported significantly lower R values (and therefore a higher fat contribution to energy provision) in boys than in men during exercise at the same relative[81–83] or absolute intensity.[84–86] During cycling, at ~70% peak $\dot{V}O_2$, for two 30-min periods separated by a 5-min rest period, pre- and early pubertal 12-year-old boys have been reported to oxidize ~70% more fat and ~23% less CHO compared with young men.[87] Differences in substrate use have also been observed in youth with 12-year-old boys reported to have a twofold higher rate of fat oxidation than 14-year-old boys during submaximal cycling for 60 min at ~70% peak $\dot{V}O_2$.[88]

The vast majority of paediatric muscle exercise metabolism data are from boys; well-designed studies of girls are sparse. Some studies of females have reported significantly lower R values in young girls compared to young women treadmill running at the same relative exercise intensity.[89] In contrast to studies of males, however, others have observed no significant differences in the R of young women compared with premenarcheal girls during cycling[90] or prepubertal girls during treadmill running[91] at the same relative exercise intensity.

The conflicting age-related data from females might be related to the general consensus that adult women rely more than men on fat oxidation during submaximal exercise.[92–94] The mechanisms responsible for sex differences in substrate utilization in adults have been widely debated but remain elusive.[95] Sex differences in fat utilization during submaximal exercise have been generally attributed to the hormonal environment and in particular to oestrogen and progesterone in women and testosterone in men.[95–97] However, data showing a more than twofold higher rate of fat oxidation in 12-year-old girls compared with 14-year-olds during cycling for 60 min at ~70% peak $\dot{V}O_2$, despite the older girls having nearly 50% higher circulating oestradiol levels,[98] suggests that sex hormones might not be wholly responsible for sex differences in fat oxidation in youth.[8]

Biological maturity

Little is known about the independent influence of biological maturity on substrate utilization and to explore the problem evidence from the few relevant investigations will be examined in detail. (Interested readers are referred to Chapter 1 for further discussion of the assessment and interpretation of biological maturation).

Two studies of boys[99,100] and one of girls[98] have provided some insights but all are weakened by not controlling for chronological age.[101] Stephens *et al.*[99] investigated the effect of biological maturation on substrate utilization by observing R responses of 43 males, between the ages of 9 and 27 years during steady state cycling exercise at ~30%, ~40%, ~50%, ~60%, and ~70% peak$\dot{V}O_2$. They reported higher lipid and lower CHO utilization in a mid-pubertal (n = 14; mean age 12 years; PH2–PH3) group compared to late-pubertal (n = 11; mean age 15 years; PH4 or PH5) and young adult (n = 9; mean age 22 years; assumed to be fully mature) groups. However, no significant differences in fuel utilization between prepubertal (n = 9; mean age 10 years; PH1) and mid-pubertal groups at most of the submaximal exercise intensities were observed. It was concluded that the development of an adult fuel-utilization profile occurs sometime in the transition between mid-puberty and late-puberty and is complete on reaching full maturity.[99]

Riddell *et al.*[100] studied five 11- to 12-year-old boys (mean age 12.0 years) classified as prepubertal (self-assessed PH1) and determined their rate of lipid oxidation during 3-min bouts of cycling across a wide range of exercise intensities using indirect calorimetry. The boys were re-tested at mean ages 13.2 years (PH2 or PH3) and 14.7 years (PH4). In addition, nine men (mean age 23.8 years) were tested on a single occasion using the same techniques. They observed that compared with men, prepubertal boys had considerably higher relative rates of fat oxidation and that their peak fat oxidation rate occurred at a significantly higher relative metabolic rate. Furthermore, it was reported that in boys both peak fat oxidation rate and Fatmax decreased with advancing pubertal stage (and chronological age), with the greatest decreases occurring during the final stages of puberty.

A study from the same laboratory recruited twelve 12-year-old and ten 14-year-old girls who cycled for 60 min at ~70% peak $\dot{V}O_2$ with substrate utilization calculated for the final 15 min of exercise. Pubertal status was self-assessed from breast development[23] which ranged from stage B2–B5 in the younger group and from stage B3–B5 in the older group. All of the girls in the older group were experiencing regular menstrual cycles and four of the 12-year-olds had experienced their first menstrual period but none experienced regular cycles. Mean serum oestradiol levels were 88 ± 15 and 157 ± 29 $pg \cdot mL^{-1}$ respectively for the 12- and 14-year-olds. As specifically noted in the study, the younger group presented a more than twofold higher rate of fat oxidation than the older, more mature group, but the difference in ages preclude this being solely attributed to biological maturity.[98]

A study which controlled for chronological age and reported eighty seven 12-year-old boys' responses to steady state treadmill running at ~70% peak $\dot{V}O_2$ provided a conflicting snapshot of R in relation to biological maturation. The boys were classified into PH stages 1–4 and it was noted that there was no significant difference in the R (R = 0.89–0.90) across the four stages of pubic hair development.[102]

These findings were confirmed in a study which divided twenty 12-year-old boys into prepubertal (PH1), early pubertal (PH2), and mid-to-late- pubertal (PH3–PH5) groups on the basis of self-assessed PH. The boys cycled, at ~70% peak $\dot{V}O_2$, for two 30-min periods interspersed with a 5- to 7-min rest with R being determined during the final 15 min of the second exercise session. The R varied from 0.89–0.93 across the three groups, but no significant differences in fat oxidation were reported. Again, as noted specifically in the study, 14-year-old boys in the same study had a much lower rate of fat oxidation than the 12-year-olds.[88]

It must therefore be concluded that although indirect calorimetry studies have demonstrated that substrate utilization during submaximal exercise varies with age, an independent effect of biological maturity remains to be proven.

Stable isotope tracers

An isotope is an atom of a given element that has a different number of neutrons than protons and is classified as unstable or stable. Stable isotopes are more balanced than unstable isotopes with respect to the relative number of protons and neutrons, and consequently do not decay or emit radiation. In exercise metabolism studies stable isotopes can be chemically attached to metabolically similar compounds and act as tracers to monitor their subsequent utilization. The stable isotope tracer can be administered orally in the form of a labelled beverage and with R data the utilization of the major nutrients used during exercise can be safely investigated.[5]

A series of innovative studies using ^{13}C-glucose ingested as 6% or 8% CHO-enriched drinks to investigate young people's metabolism during prolonged exercise has recently emerged from McMaster University in Canada.[87,88,98,103–105] The detailed assumptions and calculations necessary to estimate metabolism from stable isotope tracer studies are available elsewhere[106] and the experimental techniques and methodologies underpinning the McMaster studies have been concisely described in a recent review.[5] Herein the focus is on exploring the data on 9- to 17-year-olds' utilization of exogenous CHO (CHOexo) in relation to age, biological maturity, and sex.

In their initial studies of healthy children, the effect of ingestion of ^{13}C-glucose labelled enriched CHO drinks (CHOexo) before and during prolonged submaximal exercise on 10- to 17-year-old males was investigated.[103,104] In the first study[103] eight 13–17-year-olds performed four 30 min exercise bouts at ~60% peak $\dot{V}O_2$, interspersed with 5 min rest periods, on two occasions. In one trial (control trial; CT) the participants ingested water intermittently and in the other (glucose trial; GT) they intermittently ingested a ^{13}C-glucose labelled 8% CHO-enriched drink. It was observed that, compared to the CT, ingestion of CHOexo elevated blood glucose concentration and increased total CHO utilization but decreased endogenous CHO (CHOendo) utilization by ~16% and fat utilization by ~45%. The boys' rating of perceived exertion was also lowered, a finding which was not confirmed in 9- and 10-year-old boys in a subsequent study.[105]

In a follow-up investigation twelve 11- to 14-year-old boys cycled, at ~55% of peak $\dot{V}O_2$, for three 30 min periods which were separated by 5 min of rest, over three trials. In the CT the boys ingested flavoured water and in the other trials they intermittently ingested either 6% glucose-enriched (GT) or 3% fructose plus 3% glucose-enriched (FGT) drinks. Both CHO-enriched labelled beverages similarly spared CHOendo and fat by ~14% and ~17% respectively. Following a 10 min rest after each trial the boys were required to cycle to exhaustion at 90% of their predetermined peak power. Compared with flavoured water, it was reported that exhaustion was delayed following the FGT by ~40% and following the GT by a non-statistically significant ~25%.[104]

Having established that young people's consumption of CHOexo is associated with improved endurance performance, subsequent studies in the series used ^{13}C-glucose labelled 6% enriched CHO drinks and 60-min cycling protocols at ~70% peak $\dot{V}O_2$ to investigate the influence of age and biological maturity on substrate utilization.[87,88,98] Participant details in these studies are available in the previous section on Indirect calorimetry.

In a comparison of the oxidation rate of CHOexo between young men and 9-year-old boys, it was reported that relative to body mass the boys' oxidation rate of CHOexo was ~37% higher and contributed proportionally more to the total energy expended.[87] As the % contribution of CHOexo to total energy expenditure in the pre- or early-pubertal 9-year-olds was higher than that calculated in the laboratory's earlier studies of older boys,[103,104] the authors speculated that, 'the relative utilization of CHOexo to meet energy demands during exercise depends on age and/or pubertal status'.[87(p283)]

To test their hypothesis that CHOexo depends on age and/or pubertal status, they recruited twenty 12-year-old boys and classified them as prepubertal, early-pubertal, and mid- to late-pubertal on the basis of self-reported PH. They noted that the contribution of CHOexo to the total energy expenditure was ~27% higher in the pre- and early-pubertal boys than in the mid- to late-pubertal boys of the same age. The CHOexo oxidation rates of mid- to late-pubertal boys were very similar to nine 14-year-old boys (PH5) who followed the same protocols. The oxidation rate of CHOexo as a % of energy expenditure was inversely and significantly related to testosterone levels ($r = -0.51$). They therefore concluded that in boys CHOexo oxidation rates are sensitive to pubertal status independent of chronological age. The authors commented that age-related differences in reliance on muscle glycogen during exercise might be due to lower resting muscle glycogen levels rather than a reduced capacity to utilize glycogen. Boys may therefore compensate for reduced muscle glycogenolysis by increasing their use of extra-muscle sources of energy such as adipose-derived FFAs, liver gluconeogenesis, or CHOexo when available. It was concluded that the data do not support the view that less mature boys have a reduced capacity for glycolytic flux in the muscles, but do indicate that they might have a lower rate of liver glycogenolysis and delivery of blood glucose to the exercising muscles.[88]

Intriguingly, a similar study with 12- and 14-year-old girls found no significant difference in the contribution of CHOexo to total energy expenditure or the balance between CHOexo and CHOendo utilization during exercise.[98] On the face of it these data suggest sex differences in substrate utilization during exercise in youth, but the overlap in stage of maturation between the two groups of girls B2–B5 vs B3–B5 might have clouded the issue. Further research with girls in more discreet stages of maturity and with chronological age controlled is required.

Magnetic resonance spectroscopy

Magnetic resonance spectroscopy (MRS) has the potential to revolutionize understanding of exercise metabolism in youth as it offers in real time a window through which muscle can be interrogated during exercise. The safety of MRS for research with humans is well-documented,[107] and as the technique is non-invasive and does not involve ionizing radiation, it can be ethically applied to examine aspects of developmental muscle metabolism during exercise.[4,108]

To date, few studies have used MRS techniques to examine age-, biological maturity- or sex-related effects on muscle metabolism during exercise. Intriguing insights have been generated but the extant data must be interpreted in the light of methodological concerns regarding mixed age and/or sex participant groups, generally little consideration of biological maturity, inadequate habituation to exercising in a MR scanner, inter-study differences in body position (e.g. prone or supine), varying exercise protocols (e.g. incremental exercise, constant intensity exercise, intermittent exercise, isometric exercise), interrogation of different muscle groups (e.g. quadriceps, calf, forearm), and, in some studies, use of inappropriate data normalization techniques. Moreover, the technique is expensive and participant groups are generally small.

This section briefly describes the methodological challenges of using MRS with children, and outlines the basic theory underpinning MRS. It critiques relevant studies, and analyses the current contribution of MRS to understanding developmental muscle metabolism. To allow detailed consideration of key studies the discussion will be focused on the metabolic responses of leg muscles to exercise.

Methodological issues and theoretical concepts

The theoretical concepts underpinning MRS and the methodological challenges of MRS research with children have been addressed elsewhere.[4,109] Interested readers are referred to these sources for further information as herein only the main issues will be reviewed.

Methodological issues

Magnetic resonance spectroscopy studies of leg exercise are constrained by exercising within a small bore tube and the requirement to synchronize the acquisition of data with the rate of muscle contractions. This can be challenging for young participants and the construction of a to-scale replica scanner which allows children to overcome any fears of exercising within a tube is a useful tool in studies of this type. Lying prone the children can practise matching the movement of their leg(s) to moving vertical bars thrown on to a visual display without using expensive magnet time. When they are comfortable exercising in the enclosed space of the replica scanner, fully habituated to the exercise regimen, and capable of maintaining the required knee cadence they can transfer to the MR scanner with confidence. In our laboratory this usually requires three 20-min sessions with young children.[4,109]

Some early ^{31}PMRS studies of developmental muscle metabolism might have clouded interpretation of metabolic responses through examination of the calf muscles.[35,110,111] The calf is composed of two muscle groups with very different muscle fibre populations.

The gastrocnemius is composed of ~50% type I and ~50% type II fibres whereas the soleus consists of ~80–90% type I fibres.[112] Given the heterogeneity in calf muscle size between prepubertal children, adolescents, and adults, the use of an unlocalized ^{31}PMRS signal is likely to result in disproportionate sampling of the soleus and gastrocnemius muscles between groups, such that the soleus will represent a greater portion of the total ^{31}PMRS signal in the smaller participants (i.e. the children).[4] More recent investigations have generally monitored developmental leg muscle energetics by more judicious examination of the quadriceps muscles which do not display the muscle fibre type expression heterogeneity of the calf muscles.[113–115] Analysis of the quadriceps also facilitates comparisons with muscle biopsy data which were generally obtained from the vastus lateralis or rectus femoris.

Theoretical concepts

With the child comfortable in the scanner the magnetic field is activated and following a period of rest, the exercise protocol is initiated and carefully monitored. In a typical MR scanner experiment, the software driving the rhythmic movement incorporates signals from a non-magnetic ergometer to record changes in, for example, leg stroke frequency, stroke amplitude, work done, and power output.

Once the magnet is activated the nuclei of atoms align with the magnetic field, a second oscillating magnetic field is applied and the subsequent nuclear transitions allow spectral analysis of the interrogated muscles. Molecules produce their own individual spectra and once the molecules have been identified changes in the spectral lines can be interpreted. The principal nucleus used in metabolic studies is the naturally occurring phosphorus nucleus ^{31}P which enables the monitoring of ATP, PCr, and Pi, which play a central role in exercise metabolism. Typical ^{31}PMRS spectra obtained during rest, incremental exercise, and recovery are shown in Figure 6.4 where, from left to right, the spectral peaks represent Pi, the single phosphorus nucleus of PCr, and the three phosphate nuclei of ATP. During incremental exercise Pi increases with a corresponding decline in PCr. Spectral areas are quantified and exercise-induced changes in PCr and Pi are expressed as the % change from baseline

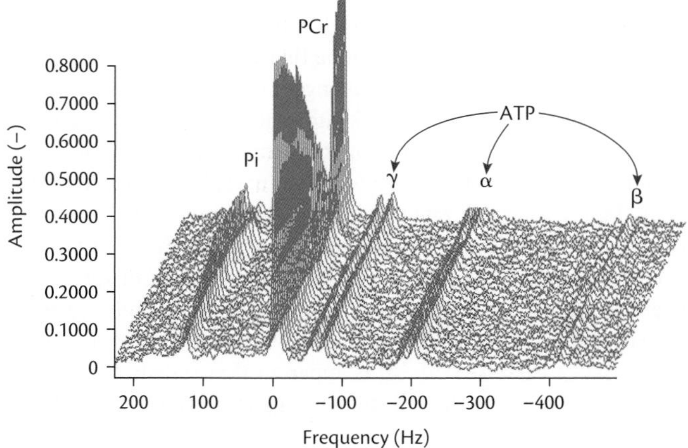

Figure 6.4 ^{31}P-magnetic resonance spectra obtained from a 9-year-old boy during rest, exercise, and recovery.
From left to right the peaks represent inorganic phosphate (Pi), phosphocreatine (PCr), and the three phosphorus nuclei of adenosine triphosphate.

using the PCr and Pi spectral areas obtained during the preceding rest period. Furthermore, skeletal muscle oxidative capacity can be assessed from the rate of PCr re-synthesis during recovery.

The chemical shift of the Pi spectral peak relative to the PCr peak reflects the acidification of the muscle and intracellular pH can be determined using the relationship:

$$pH = 6.75 + \log(\sigma - 3.27)/(5.96 - \sigma)$$

where σ represents the chemical shift in parts per million between the Pi and the PCr resonance peaks. The change in pH during exercise provides an indication of muscle glycolytic activity, but it is not a direct measure of glycolysis.[4]

Intracellular thresholds

An incremental exercise test to exhaustion results in non-linear changes in the ratios Pi to PCr plotted against power output and in pH plotted against power output. As power output increases, an initial shallow slope is followed by a second steeper slope and the transition point is known as the intracellular threshold ($IT_{Pi/PCr}$ and IT_{pH}). Muscle intracellular thresholds are similar to whole body metabolic thresholds (e.g. T_{LAC} or ventilatory threshold [T_{VENT}]) determined during incremental cycle ergometer exercise and are recognized as an estimation of the oxidative capacity of the muscle and therefore mitochondrial function.[4] Intracellular thresholds have been demonstrated to have good test-retest reliability even with prepubertal children.[109]

Incremental exercise to exhaustion

The first ^{31}PMRS study of exercise metabolism to include healthy child participants involved two girls and eight boys, aged 7–10 years, and three women and five men, aged 20–40 years, who carried out supine, incremental, treadle plantar-flexion exercise to voluntary exhaustion. Intracellular thresholds (ITs)were detected in 50% of the children and 75% of the adults. The characteristics of the initial linear slopes to $IT_{Pi/PCr}$ and IT_{pH} were similar regardless of age, but following the ITs the incline in the Pi to PCr ratio and decline in pH in relation to power output were both steeper in adults than in children. The change in pH from rest to end-exercise was significantly greater in adults than in children, whose end-exercise Pi to PCr ratio was, on average, only ~27% of adult values. These findings were interpreted as being indicative of a comparable capacity for oxidative metabolism (mitochondrial function) in children and adults during low- to moderate-intensity exercise, but to reflect children's lower reliance on substrate level phosphorylation (i.e. PCr and anaerobic glycolysis) during exercise above ITs.[110]

This pioneering research[110] characterized the interpretation of ^{31}PMRS studies of children's exercise metabolism for ~15 years despite several methodological concerns.[6] The exercise protocol with large increments in power output only elicited a $IT_{Pi/PCr}$ in 50% of children and 75% of adults, whereas other researchers have observed an $IT_{Pi/PCr}$ in 100% of both children and adults.[115] As the children's end-exercise Pi to PCr ratio was only 0.54 and ratios in excess of 2.0 have been reported by others[109] it is likely that they did not achieve true maximal values. Furthermore, interrogation of the calf muscle might have biased the lower accumulation of Pi, breakdown of PCr, and fall in pH in child compared to adult muscle.[4]

Nevertheless, Zanconato *et al's*[110] observations were subsequently supported by a study of 14 trained and 23 untrained 12–15-year-old boys and six adults with an average age of 25 years.[113] Magnetic resonance spectra were collected from the quadriceps during supine, incremental exercise to exhaustion and higher values of intracellular pH and the ratio PCr to (PCr + Pi) were noted in boys at exhaustion.

A study of ageing effects on skeletal muscle compared ^{31}PMRS spectra at rest, during incremental calf muscle exercise to exhaustion and recovery from exercise of fifteen 6- to 12-year-olds with twenty 20- to 29-year-olds. Both groups consisted of unspecified numbers of males and females. The children presented a higher pH during exercise, indicating a lower anaerobic glycolytic contribution to metabolism, and a faster re-synthesis of PCr during recovery than adults. As PCr recovery kinetics has been shown to reflect muscle oxidative capacity,[116] the authors concluded that the oxidative capacity of skeletal muscle is highest in childhood.[35] In contrast, a study of recovery from maximal quadriceps exercise observed no differences between boys and adults in the PCr τ and concluded that the invariant PCr kinetics were indicative of a comparable mitochondrial oxidative capacity between child and adult muscle.[113] However, the experimental conditions (i.e. cellular acidosis) under which PCr recovery dynamics were determined in these studies raise methodological concerns which preclude any firm conclusions being drawn.

The first ^{31}PMRS study to investigate the effects of biological maturity on exercise metabolism evaluated the responses of nine 10-year-old, 'prepubertal' (both PH and B in maturity stage 1 or 2) and nine 15-year-old 'pubertal' (both PH and B in at least maturity stage 3) trained female swimmers to 2 min of light calf exercise (40% of predetermined maximal work capacity) followed by 2 min of 'supramaximal' calf exercise (140% of maximal work capacity) using a plantar flexion ergometer. At the end of the exercise, intracellular pH was lower (6.66 vs 6.76) and the Pi to PCr ratio was higher (2.18 vs 1.31) in the 15-year-olds, but the differences were not statistically significant. The authors concluded that glycolytic metabolism in physically active children is not maturity dependent. This conclusion, however, should be interpreted with caution as scrutiny of the magnitude of the difference between the two groups in the Pi to PCr ratio (66%) suggests that the observed differences might be of biological significance.[111]

A more comprehensive study[115] monitored 15 boys and 18 girls, aged 9–12 years, and eight men and eight women, aged 22–26 years, during a single-legged quadriceps incremental test to exhaustion. Quadriceps muscle mass was determined using MR imaging and log-linear allometric regression models used to determine power function ratios to normalize absolute power output measurements for quadriceps muscle mass. The participants were well-habituated to exercising within a magnet and an $IT_{Pi/PCr}$ was detected in 100% of cases in both children and adults. Using the derived power function ratio to normalize power output for muscle mass, no age- or sex-related differences in power output were identified between children and adults below the $IT_{Pi/PCr}$. The increase in the Pi to PCr ratio at the $IT_{Pi/PCr}$ was comparable between boys and men, girls and women, boys and girls, and men and women. However, above the ITs age- and sex-related differences in muscle phosphate and pH responses were readily apparent, indicating that for a given increase in power output during exercise above $IT_{Pi/PCr}$, adults require a greater breakdown of PCr and accumulation of Pi compared to children (i.e. a greater anaerobic energy contribution). This was also observed to be the case when girls were compared to boys. Similarly, above the IT_{pH} pH changes were significantly less in boys compared to men and girls, indicating lower anaerobic glycolytic flux during high intensity exercise. In girls, a number of significant relationships between ^{31}PMRS derived indices of anaerobic metabolism and biological maturity, which was estimated from the offset score from the age at peak height velocity,[117] were observed. In conflict with the conclusions of Petersen *et al.*,[111] the authors suggested that the higher anaerobic energy contribution of the girls during exercise above the $IT_{Pi/PCr}$ might be attributable to their more advanced level of biological maturity than the boys who were largely pre- and early-pubertal. The age- and sex-related responses to exercise observed are strikingly similar to those in adult studies comparing muscle phosphate and pH responses during exercise in muscles with different fibre type profiles.[118,119]

Constant intensity exercise

An investigation of potential age- and sex-related differences in the kinetics of muscle PCr breakdown included eighteen 9-year-olds (ten girls) and sixteen 23- to 25-year-olds (eight women). Following an incremental quadriceps exercise test to exhaustion to determine their $IT_{Pi/PCr,}$ the participants carried out a series of constant exercise intensity transitions corresponding to 80% of the power output at the $IT_{Pi/PCr}$ (i.e. moderate intensity exercise). No significant age- or sex-related differences were found in the PCr kinetics τ, either at the onset or offset of exercise. It appears, on the basis of these findings (which are consistent with the authors' earlier study of incremental exercise), that the kinetics of muscle PCr are unrelated to age and sex during the transition to and recovery from moderate intensity exercise.[114]

A subsequent investigation from the same laboratory examined the response of eleven 13-year-olds (5 girls) and eleven 24-year-olds (five women) to heavy intensity exercise. The methodology was similar to the earlier study except that the constant intensity exercise was set at 20% of the difference (20%Δ) between the power output at the participants' $IT_{Pi/PCr}$ and their maximal power output, as determined in an incremental test to exhaustion. In accord with the investigation into constant moderate intensity exercise, no statistically significant age or sex differences in the PCr τ at the onset of heavy intensity exercise were noted.[120]

Collectively the results of the two studies are consistent with the view that in both moderate- and heavy-intensity exercise, the phosphate-linked regulation of muscle oxygen utilization is fully mature in children. The authors suggested that this might be attributable to a comparable capacity for mitochondrial oxidative phosphorylation in child and adult muscle. However, two points are worthy of note. First, it might be that the predetermined 20%Δ is not high enough to clearly distinguish between moderate- and heavy-intensity exercise. Second, although differences in the PCr τ between boys and men were not statistically significant, the men's PCr τ at the onset of exercise was 24% and 42% longer than the boys' PCr τ for moderate- and heavy-intensity exercise, respectively. The notion that this scale of difference might be of biological significance is supported by ^{31}PMRS studies of finger flexion exercise which have reported prepubertal boys to rely more on oxidative metabolism and less on PCr than men at both the onset and offset of exercise.[121,122] It is apparent that statistically higher-powered research with well-defined age and biological maturity groups is required.

Intermittent exercise

Some intriguing results emerged from an elegant study of sixteen 9-year-olds (eight girls) and sixteen 26-year-olds (eight women) designed to explore why children have been consistently reported to recover faster than adults from bouts of intermittent high-intensity exercise. The exercise protocol consisted of supine calf exercise consisting of ten bouts of 30 s exercise interspersed with 20 s rest periods. In each exercise period participants lifted a load of 25% of their individually estimated one-repetition maximum 24 times. Following the last exercise bout participants rested for 10 min while recovery data were collected. The data revealed that PCr breakdown was significantly greater in adults compared to children only during the first exercise interval. In subsequent exercise the PCr breakdown and recovery was similar in children and adults. The overall PCr concentration therefore oscillated between exercise and recovery intervals at a higher level in children than in adults. Taken together with their recorded higher intracellular pH, this suggests that children are more able to support muscle contraction by oxidative metabolism than adults who rely more on anaerobic energy sources (i.e. PCr and anaerobic glycolysis). No metabolic differences between boys and girls, or men and women, were observed.[123]

Muscle phosphocreatine kinetics and pulmonary oxygen uptake kinetics

Magnetic resonance spectroscopy is currently too expensive and too labour intensive to be used routinely in most paediatric exercise science laboratories. However, the measurement of muscle (m) $\dot{V}O_2$ using the Fick technique has been shown, in adults, to agree with $p\dot{V}O_2$ within ~10%.[124] This relationship has been confirmed by simultaneously determining both intramuscular PCr kinetics (as a surrogate of $m\dot{V}O_2$) and $p\dot{V}O_2$ kinetics at the onset and offset of knee extensor exercise within a MR scanner.[125] The coherence between PCr and $p\dot{V}O_2$ kinetics during the off-transient is consistent with the correlation of PCr recovery kinetics and muscle oxidative capacity.[126] Children present a much lower $p\dot{V}O_2$ signal amplitude than adults, which makes analysis of $p\dot{V}O_2$ kinetics at the onset and offset of knee flexor exercise infeasible. Simultaneous measurement of PCr and $p\dot{V}O_2$ kinetics in a MR scanner has therefore not been replicated with children. However, a close relationship between children's intramuscular PCr kinetics during prone quadriceps exercise in a MR scanner and $p\dot{V}O_2$ kinetics during upright cycling at both the onset and offset of exercise has been demonstrated.[127] These studies indicate that $p\dot{V}O_2$ kinetics has the potential to provide a readily accessible window into developmental muscle metabolism during exercise.

Pulmonary oxygen uptake kinetics

Young people's $p\dot{V}O_2$ kinetics has been reviewed elsewhere[128–130] and the theoretical concepts, the methodological challenges, and the age-, sex-, and biological maturity-related responses of $p\dot{V}O_2$ kinetics at the onset and offset of exercise in different domains are extensively examined in Chapter 13. Herein, for context, a brief reference is made to methodological issues but the emphasis is on reviewing the contribution of $p\dot{V}O_2$ kinetics studies to the elucidation of paediatric exercise metabolism. (Interested readers are referred to Chapter 13 for individual study details and critiques).

Methodological issues

Children's inherently erratic breathing pattern, low signal to noise ratio, and large inter-breath fluctuations reduce confidence in resolving parameters of the $p\dot{V}O_2$ kinetics response, particularly the primary τ.[131] As children have a lower peak $\dot{V}O_2$ than adults the scope of the metabolic transitions to exercise possible within each exercise domain is therefore reduced.[132] Interpretation of data is further confounded by several studies using suboptimal numbers of repeat transitions and not reporting confidence intervals, not accurately defining exercise domains, and applying an array of analytical models with limited physiological rationales.[133–135] Nevertheless, despite concerns over the rigour of several investigations, a consensus on $p\dot{V}O_2$ kinetics responses in youth is emerging, at least for exercise in the moderate and heavy intensity domains.

Moderate-intensity exercise

The moderate intensity exercise domain encompasses all exercise intensities below T_{LAC} and is characterized by three phases (see Figure 12.3). Phase I is independent of $m\dot{V}O_2$ and is predominantly a reflection of an increase in pulmonary blood flow with exercise. Phase II (the primary phase) is a rapid exponential increase in $p\dot{V}O_2$ that develops as a result of an additional effect of an increased oxygen extraction in the blood perfusing the exercising muscles. The speed of the $p\dot{V}O_2$ kinetics is described by the τ. During phases I and II the need for ATP re-synthesis is not fully satisfied by $p\dot{V}O_2$ and the oxygen deficit is primarily met by ATP re-synthesis from the breakdown of PCr, with minor contributions from muscle oxygen stores and anaerobic glycolysis. Phase III is the subsequent steady state in $p\dot{V}O_2$ that occurs within ~2 min.[128]

The weight of evidence supports the view that compared with adults, children's $p\dot{V}O_2$ kinetics response at the onset of exercise is faster and the oxygen cost of the exercise (gain) during phase II is greater.[126,136,137] There are no sex differences in children's $p\dot{V}O_2$ kinetic responses to moderate intensity exercise.[138] Children's shorter τ and greater gain indicates a higher aerobic contribution to ATP re-synthesis and therefore an enhanced oxidative capacity, which might be due to superior oxygen delivery or better oxygen utilization by the muscle during childhood, or both. There is no compelling evidence to show that delivery of oxygen to the mitochondria is enhanced in children compared to adults, or that increased delivery of oxygen to the muscle increases the rate of $p\dot{V}O_2$ kinetics during moderate intensity exercise. It is therefore likely that children's shorter phase II τ and greater gain reflects an enhanced capacity for oxygen utilization by the mitochondria.[3,126,129]

Heavy-intensity exercise

The heavy-intensity exercise domain lies between T_{LAC} and the maximal lactate steady state. During phase II anaerobic glycolysis makes a larger contribution to the oxygen deficit, but over time blood lactate accumulation is stable. When expressed as $p\dot{V}O_2$ ($mL \cdot min^{-1} \cdot W^{-1}$) above that during unloaded pedalling the phase II gain is similar to that observed in the moderate exercise domain. However, within ~2–3 min of the beginning of exercise a slow component of $p\dot{V}O_2$ kinetics is superimposed upon the primary $p\dot{V}O_2$ response and the achievement of a steady state is delayed by ~10 min (see Figure 12.3). The mechanisms underlying the $p\dot{V}O_2$ slow component are speculative, but compelling arguments support the view that, at least in adults, ~85% of the additional $p\dot{V}O_2$ originates from the exercising muscle.[136] Muscle fibre type recruitment patterns (e.g. less efficient type II fibres) and/or fatigue processes within select fibre populations are thought to underlie the emergence of the $p\dot{V}O_2$ slow component.[126]

Children have a significantly shorter phase II τ, smaller oxygen deficit, and higher oxygen cost of exercise during phase II than adults. Even prepubertal children exhibit a slow component of $p\dot{V}O_2$, but it is smaller than that of adults and increases with age through adolescence. In contrast to exercise in the moderate domain, boys have a shorter phase II τ than girls during exercise above T_{LAC} and the $p\dot{V}O_2$ slow component contribution to the total change in $p\dot{V}O_2$ amplitude during exercise is greater in girls.[140,141]

The higher oxygen cost of exercise and shorter τ during the primary component support an enhanced oxidative function during childhood. This might be indicative of a higher % of type I fibres in children as, in adults, the ratio of type I to type II muscle fibres has been demonstrated to be positively related to the oxygen cost of exercise, and negatively correlated with the speed of $p\dot{V}O_2$ kinetics. Preferential recruitment of type I fibres by children would also help to explain the increase in amplitude of the $p\dot{V}O_2$ slow component with age. Why there are sex differences in the primary τ during moderate- but not heavy-intensity exercise is not readily apparent. At exercise intensities above T_{LAC} oxygen delivery might play a more prominent role in limiting $p\dot{V}O_2$ kinetics and boys might have a faster cardiac output response than girls at the onset of exercise. However, if boys have a greater % of type I fibres than girls, this would be consistent with their $p\dot{V}O_2$ kinetics responses[3] (see section on Muscle fibre types).

Synthesis of data across methodologies

Cycling peak power and peak $\dot{V}O_2$ increase in an asynchronous manner with biological maturation and with aging (at least from 8 to 18 years). The data strongly infer that maximal anaerobic energy generation is less well-developed in youth than maximal aerobic energy generation. Prepubertal children are particularly disadvantaged compared to those in late puberty who are, in turn, disadvantaged compared to young adults during short-duration, maximal or high-intensity exercise supported predominantly by anaerobic metabolism.

Children recover more rapidly than adults from intermittent bouts of high-intensity exercise. Although conventional exercise models cannot refute the view that adults' slower recovery is simply a direct consequence of their ability to generate more power, there are persuasive hypotheses to support young people's superior resistance to muscle fatigue. Potential explanatory metabolic mechanisms of age-related differences include children's enhanced oxidative capacity, faster recovery kinetics of cardiopulmonary variables, differential motor unit recruitment and usage, better acid-base regulation, and lower production and/or more efficient removal of metabolic by-products than adults. The hypothesis of children's faster PCr re-synthesis than adults between exercise bouts has been recently developed further by ^{31}PMRS support of a model, where PCr breakdown is only greater in adults during the first exercise interval and PCr concentration subsequently oscillates between exercise and recovery intervals at a higher level in children.

Despite methodological limitations and some equivocal data, muscle biopsy studies have provided valuable insights into paediatric exercise metabolism although studies have focused on changes with chronological age and generally have not considered biological maturity. The higher % of type I fibres in young people is consistent with enhanced aerobic function in youth. Lactate is an inhibitor of FFA mobilization and uptake by the muscles and both muscle and blood lactate accumulations are negatively related to age. The ratios of various glycolytic and oxidative enzyme activities are of particular interest. The balance of evidence suggests that young children have lower glycolytic enzymes activity than adolescents but, although the data are equivocal, adolescents' glycolytic enzymes activity appears to be similar to that of adults. However, the reported activity of oxidative enzymes indicates that children are able to oxidize pyruvate and FFAs at a higher rate than adolescents, and adolescents have an enhanced oxidative capacity compared to adults. A consistent finding is that the ratio of glycolytic to oxidative enzymes activity is higher in adults than in adolescents or children. Muscle biopsy studies strongly suggest that children have a well-developed capacity for oxidative metabolism during exercise, but might be disadvantaged in activities supported by anaerobic metabolism when compared to adults.

Evidence from indirect calorimetry that boys rely relatively more on fat oxidation during submaximal exercise than men is unequivocal. Data on females are less clear but, on balance, it appears that the contribution of fat oxidation to total energy expenditure during moderate intensity exercise is negatively related to age in both sexes, at least from ~10 years until young adulthood. Sex differences in adults' substrate utilization during exercise are extensively documented, although the underlying mechanisms are still being debated. Well-designed comparative studies of sex differences in substrate utilization in youth are not available, but age-matched cross-study comparisons infer differences which might be related to the timing and tempo of maturation. A relationship between endogenous substrate utilization during exercise and biological maturity independent of chronological age remains to be proven. However, research with stable isotope tracers suggests that boys' CHOexo oxidation rates are sensitive to pubertal status independent of chronological age. This relationship remains to be demonstrated in girls.

The oxidation rate of CHOexo during exercise is higher in boys than in men. These data have raised the question of whether boys have a reduced capacity for glycolytic flux or whether their lower rate of endogenous muscle glycogen utilization is a glycogen sparing issue related to lower muscle glycogen stores and/or inferior delivery of blood glucose following liver glycogenolysis.

There is a paucity of ^{31}PMRS studies of healthy young people during exercise and the extant data are clouded by methodological flaws in study design and execution. On balance the data support the view that age- and sex-related differences in muscle metabolism are dependent on the intensity of the imposed exercise. In contrast to data from $p\dot{V}O_2$ kinetics studies, during moderate-intensity exercise no age-related differences in metabolism have been observed. But, during incremental exercise above the $IT_{Pi/PCr}$ the anaerobic energy contribution for a given increase in normalized power has been demonstrated to be lower in children than adults, and in boys compared to girls. In females the increased glycolytic activity has been related to biological maturity. A statistically significant age-related PCr kinetics response at the onset of heavy exercise remains to be verified. Recovery data following both maximal and intermittent high-intensity exercise have demonstrated children's ability to re-synthesize PCr at a higher rate than adults and support the view that children have an enhanced oxidative capacity compared to adults. Sex differences in recovery data from high-intensity intermittent exercise have not been reported.

There are few well-designed and rigorously executed studies of children's and adolescents' $p\dot{V}O_2$ kinetics responses at the onset of exercise but the extant data are quite consistent. In both the moderate and heavy exercise domains the phase II τ becomes progressively longer and the oxygen cost of the exercise decreases with age. During exercise above the T_{LAC} the size of the $p\dot{V}O_2$ slow component increases during the transition from prepuberty to adulthood. To date no studies have rigorously explored $p\dot{V}O_2$ kinetics in relation to biological maturity. Collectively $p\dot{V}O_2$ kinetics responses are consistent with the notion that children have an enhanced oxidative but attenuated anaerobic energy transfer during exercise, compared with adults. The mechanisms supporting child-adult differences in $p\dot{V}O_2$ kinetics are poorly understood, but are likely to reside in age-related changes in oxidative phosphorylation, oxygen delivery, and muscle fibre recruitment strategies. (Interested readers are referred to Chapter 13 where the mechanisms underpinning age- and sex-related differences in $p\dot{V}O_2$ kinetics are analysed in detail).

Scrutiny of data relating to developmental muscle metabolism during exercise illustrates the myriad potential confounding factors, methodological considerations, and analytical issues which need to be considered. Collectively, evidence from a range of invasive and non-invasive methodologies supports the view that during exercise there is interplay of anaerobic and aerobic energy metabolism in which children present a relatively higher oxidative capacity than adolescents or adults. There is a progressive increase in anaerobic glycolytic flux with age at least into adolescence and possibly young adulthood. Independent effects of biological maturation on muscle metabolism during exercise remain to be empirically proven.

An amalgam of findings (e.g. muscle fibre profile, muscle enzymes activity, muscle energy stores, substrate utilization, rate of PCr re-synthesis, $p\dot{V}O_2$ and mPCr kinetics) contribute to a plausible model of an age- and sex-specific developing metabolic profile, but the precise mechanisms underpinning anaerobic and aerobic interaction during exercise require further clarification.

There is a persuasive argument that muscle fibre recruitment patterns are a fundamental component of age- (and perhaps sex-) related differences. An intriguing recent hypothesis even suggests that children's different metabolic profile might not be the underlying cause of their lower anaerobic power and capacity, but rather the result of their under-recruitment of type II muscle fibres. It is argued that under-use of type II muscle fibres would attenuate development of their glycolytic capacity and relative size. Similarly, over-use of type I muscle fibres would enhance oxidative capacity and possibly relative hypertrophy.[142]

A plethora of unanswered questions remain, but experimental techniques and non-invasive technologies pioneered with adults have been successfully developed and modified for use with children. New avenues of research into developmental muscle metabolism during exercise have been unlocked and now need to be pursued with rigour and vigour.

Conclusions

Research in paediatric muscle exercise metabolism has been limited by ethical considerations and the lack, until recently, of accessible non-invasive techniques of interrogating exercising muscles. Much remains to be revealed, but the weight of evidence from a wide range of techniques indicates that during exercise there is interplay of anaerobic and aerobic metabolism in which young people respond to an exercise challenge with relatively higher fat oxidation than adults. Anaerobic glycolytic flux progressively increases with age at least into adolescence and possibly into young adulthood. An independent relationship between biological maturity and substrate utilization remains to be proven. Several studies across methodologies have suggested the presence of intriguing sex differences in exercise metabolism in youth, but the influence of biological maturity is still obscure. Further research is required to tease out and explain underlying mechanisms, but there is compelling evidence that age-related differences in muscle fibre recruitment patterns play a central role.

The rigorous application of non-invasive technologies such as stable isotope tracers, ^{31}PMRS, and breath-by-breath determination of $p\dot{V}O_2$ kinetics has the potential to enhance understanding of developmental exercise metabolism. In particular, ^{31}PMRS studies have opened up new research potential with insights into the exercising muscle in real time. However, the high cost of obtaining MR spectra, the time-consuming habituation of children to an exercise protocol confined within a tube, and the restricted availability of MR scanners for research with healthy children has limited the development and application of the technique with the exercising child. More research using ^{31}PMRS is urgently required, but in the absence of ^{31}PMRS data, the close relationship between mPCr and $p\dot{V}O_2$ kinetics encourages the use of more child-friendly and less expensive $p\dot{V}O_2$ kinetics as an additional non-invasive window into developmental muscle metabolism during exercise.

Summary

- Independent of chronological age and body size, biological maturity has a positive and independent effect on maximal performance, with young people experiencing a more marked increase in maximal anaerobic power than maximal aerobic power during adolescence.
- Children recover from repeated bouts of high-intensity exercise faster than adults. This has been attributed to factors such as children's more rapid initial phosphocreatine (PCr) re-synthesis and subsequent maintenance of higher concentration of PCr through enhanced oxidative metabolism.
- Muscle biopsy studies indicate an age-related decline in the % of type I fibres from childhood to young adulthood and a consistent trend showing adolescent boys and young adult males to exhibit a higher % of type I fibres than similarly aged females.
- Resting ATP stores are invariant with age and glycogen stores progressively increase from childhood into young adulthood. Age-related data are equivocal but PCr stores appear to increase with age, at least in the quadriceps muscles.
- Children have higher oxidative enzymes activity and lower glycolytic enzymes activity than adolescents and adults. Adolescents have an enhanced oxidative capacity compared to adults but the evidence indicating differences in glycolytic enzymes activity of adolescents and adults is equivocal.
- Substrate utilization studies of prolonged submaximal exercise consistently report fat oxidation to be negatively related to age.
- Indirect calorimetry studies have been unable to clearly demonstrate a relationship between biological maturity and substrate utilization which is independent of chronological age.

- Studies using stable isotope tracers and enriched carbohydrate drinks have showed oxidation rates of exogenous carbohydrate to be sensitive in boys to pubertal status independent of chronological age. This relationship remains to be demonstrated in girls.
- The ingestion of carbohydrate can spare muscle glycogen and potentially enhance the endurance performance of children and adolescents.
- ^{31}P-magnetic resonance studies indicate that during incremental exercise to exhaustion children and adults have a similar rate of mitochondrial oxidative metabolism below the intracellular threshold ($IT_{Pi/PCr}$) but adults exhibit higher glycolytic activity during exercise above the $IT_{Pi/PCr}$.
- No statistically significant sex- or age-related differences in the kinetics of PCr breakdown during quadriceps exercise have been reported.
- Children's shorter primary time constant and greater oxygen cost at the onset of both moderate- and heavy-intensity exercise and smaller pulmonary oxygen uptake ($p\dot{V}O_2$) slow component during exercise above the lactate threshold support the presence of an enhanced oxidative function.
- The sex difference in children's $p\dot{V}O_2$ kinetics responses to heavy- but not moderate-intensity exercise is consistent with boys having a higher % of type I fibres than girls.
- Taken together, evidence from a range of techniques suggest that i) during submaximal exercise there is interplay of anaerobic and aerobic metabolism in which young people exhibit higher oxidative activity than adults, ii) there is a progressive increase in glycolytic activity with age, at least into adolescence and possibly into young adulthood, iii) sex differences have been identified in some studies and require further exploration, iv) an independent influence of biological maturity on muscle metabolism during exercise remains to be proven but represents an intriguing avenue for future research, and v) age-related differences in muscle fibre recruitment patterns might play a central role in developmental muscle metabolism during exercise.

References

1. Maughan R, Gleeson M, Greenhaff PL. *Biochemistry of exercise and training*. Oxford: Oxford University Press: 1997.
2. Armstrong N, Barker AR, McManus AM. Muscle metabolism changes with age and maturation: How do they relate to youth sport performance? *Br J Sport Med*. 2015; 49: 860–864.
3. Armstrong N, Barker AR. Oxygen uptake kinetics in children and adolescents. A review. *Pediatr Exerc Sci*. 2009; 21: 130–147.
4. Barker AR, Armstrong N. Insights into developmental muscle metabolism through the use of ^{31}P-magnetic resonance spectroscopy. A review. *Pediatr Exerc Sci*. 2010; 22: 350–368.
5. Mahon AD, Timmons BW. Application of stable isotope tracers in the study of exercise metabolism in children: A primer. *Pediatr Exerc Sci*. 2014; 26: 3–10.
6. Armstrong N, Barker AR. New insights in paediatric exercise metabolism. *J Sport Health Sci*. 2012; 1: 18–26.
7. Zakrzewski J, Tolfrey K. Fatmax in children and adolescents. A review. *Eur J Sport Sci*. 2011; 11: 1–18.
8. Riddell MC. The endocrine response and substrate utilization during exercise in children and adolescents. *J Appl Physiol*. 2008; 105: 725–733.
9. Van Praagh E. *Pediatric anaerobic performance*. Champaign, IL: Human Kinetics; 1998.
10. Armstrong N, Tomkinson GR, Ekelund U. Aerobic fitness and its relationship to sport, exercise training and habitual physical activity during youth. *Br J Sports Med*. 2011; 45: 849–858.
11. Van Praagh E. Testing anaerobic performance. In: Hebestreit H, Bar-Or O (eds.) *The young athlete*. Oxford: Blackwell; 2008. p. 469–485.
12. Inbar O, Bar-Or O, Skinner JS. *The Wingate anaerobic test*. Champaign, IL: Human Kinetics; 1996.
13. Van Praagh E, Dore E. Short-term muscle power during growth and maturation. *Sports Med*. 2002; 32: 701–728.
14. Armstrong N, Fawkner SG. Aerobic fitness. In: Armstrong N (ed.) *Paediatric exercise physiology*. Edinburgh: Elsevier; 2007. p. 161–188.
15. Armstrong N, Welsman JR. Assessment and interpretation of aerobic fitness in children and adolescents. *Exerc Sport Sci Rev*. 1994; 22: 435–476.
16. Kemper HCG, Twisk JWR, Van Mechelen W. Changes in aerobic fitness in boys and girls over a period of 25 years: Data from the Amsterdam Growth and Health Longitudinal Study revisited and extended. *Pediatr Exerc Sci*. 2013; 25: 534–535.
17. Welsman JR, Armstrong N. Scaling for size: Relevance to understanding effects of growth on performance. In: Hebestreit H, Bar-Or O, eds. *The young athlete*. Oxford: Blackwell; 2008. p. 50–62.
18. Welsman JR, Armstrong N, Kirby BJ, Nevill AM, Winter EM. Scaling peak $\dot{V}O_2$ for differences in body size. *Med Sci Sports Exerc*. 1996; 28: 259–265.
19. Armstrong N, Welsman JR. Peak oxygen uptake in relation to growth and maturation in 11–17-year-old humans. *Eur J Appl Physiol*. 2001; 85: 546–551.
20. Armstrong N, Welsman JR. Aerobic fitness. What are we measuring? *Med Sport Sci*. 2007; 50: 5–25.
21. Inbar O, Chia M. Development of maximal anaerobic performance: An old issue revisited. In: Hebestreit H, Bar-Or O (eds.) *The young athlete*. Oxford: Blackwell; 2008. p. 27–38.
22. Armstrong N, Welsman JR, Chia MYA. Short-term power output in relation to growth and maturation. *Br J Sports Med*. 2001; 35: 118–124.
23. Tanner JM. *Growth at adolescence*, 2nd ed. Oxford: Blackwell; 1962.
24. Armstrong N, Welsman JR, Kirby BJ. Performance on the Wingate anaerobic test and maturation. *Pediatr Exerc Sci*. 1997; 9: 253–261.
25. Armstrong N, Welsman JR, Kirby BJ. Peak oxygen uptake and maturation in 12-year-olds. *Med Sci Sports Exerc*. 1998; 30: 165–169.
26. Ratel S, Williams CA, Oliver J, Armstrong N. Effects of age and mode of exercise on power output profiles during repeated sprints. *Eur J Appl Physiol*. 2004; 92: 204–210.
27. Ratel S, Williams CA, Oliver J, Armstrong N. Effects of age and recovery duration on performance during multiple treadmill sprints. *Int J Sports Med*. 2005; 26: 1–8.
28. Hebestreit H, Meyer F, Htay H, Heigenhauser GJ, Bar-Or O. Recovery of muscle power after short-term exercise: Comparing boys and men. *J Appl Physiol*. 1993; 74: 2875–2880.
29. Zafeiridis A, Dalamitros A, Dipla K, *et al*. Recovery during high-intensity intermittent anaerobic exercise in boys, teens and men. *Med Sci Sports Exerc*. 2005; 37: 505–512.
30. Paraschos I, Hassani A, Bassa E, *et al*. Fatigue differences between adults and prepubertal males. *Int J Sports Med*. 2007; 28: 958–963.
31. Chia M. Power recovery in the Wingate anaerobic test in girls and women following prior sprints of short duration. *Biol Sport*. 2001; 18: 45–53.
32. Dipla K, Tsirini T, Zafeiridis A, *et al*. Fatigue resistance during high-intensity intermittent exercise from childhood to adulthood in males and females. *Eur J Appl Physiol*. 2009; 106: 645–653.
33. Falk B, Dotan R. Child-adult differences in the recovery from high-intensity exercise. *Exerc Sport Sci Rev*. 2006; 34: 107–112.
34. Ratel S, Duche P, Williams CA. Muscle fatigue during high-intensity exercise in children. *Sports Med*. 2006; 36: 1031–1065.
35. Ratel S, Kluka V, Vicencio SG, *et al*. Insights into the mechanisms of neuromuscular fatigue in boys and men. *Med Sci Sports Exerc*. 2015; 47: 2319–2328.

36. Taylor DJ, Bore PJ, Styles P, Gadian DG, Radda GK. Bioenergetics of intact human muscle. A ^{31}P nuclear magnetic resonance study. *Mol Biol Med.* 1983; 1: 77–94.
37. Ratel S, Martin V. Is there a progressive withdrawal of physiological protections against high-intensity induced fatigue during puberty? *Sports.* 2015; 3: 346–357.
38. Ratel S, Lazaar N, Williams CA, Bedu M, Duche P. Age differences in human skeletal muscle fatigue during high-intensity intermittent exercise. *Acta Paediatr.* 2003; 92: 1248–1254.
39. Bergstrom J. Muscle electrolytes in man determined by neutron activation analysis on needle biopsy specimens. *Scand J Clin Lab Invest.* 1962; 14(suppl 68): 1–110.
40. Lexell J, Sjostrom M, Nordlund AS, Taylor CC. Growth and development of human muscle: A quantitative morphological study of whole vastus lateralis from childhood to adult age. *Muscle Nerve.* 1992; 15: 404–409.
41. Jansson, E. Age-related fiber type changes in human skeletal muscle. In: Maughan RJ, Shirreffs SM (eds.) *Biochemistry of exercise IX.* Champaign, IL: Human Kinetics; 1996. p. 297–307.
42. Elder GCB, Bradbury K, Roberts R. Variability of fiber type distributions within human muscles. *J Appl Physiol.* 1982; 53: 1473–1481.
43. Lexell J, Taylor C, Sjostrom M. Analysis of sampling errors in biopsy techniques using data from whole muscle cross sections. *J Appl Physiol.* 1985; 59: 1228–1235.
44. Armstrong N, Welsman JR. Exercise metabolism. In: Armstrong N (ed.) *Paediatric exercise physiology.* Edinburgh: Elsevier; 2007. p. 71–98.
45. Boisseau N, Delmarche P. Metabolic and hormonal responses to exercise in children and adolescents. *Sports Med.* 2000; 30: 405–422.
46. Jansson E, Hedberg G. Skeletal muscle fibre types in teenagers: relationship to physical performance and activity. *Scand J Med Sci Sports.* 1991; 1: 31–44.
47. Glenmark BC, Hedberg G, Jansson E. Changes in muscle fibre type from adolescence to adulthood in women and men. *Acta Physiol Scand.* 1992; 146: 251–259.
48. Bell RD, MacDougall JD, Billeter R, Howald H. Muscle fibre types and morphometric analysis of skeletal muscles in six-year-old children. *Med Sci Sports Exerc.* 1980; 12: 28–31.
49. Oertel, G. Morphometric analysis of normal skeletal muscles in infancy, childhood and adolescence. *J Neurol Sci.* 1988; 88: 303–313.
50. Komi PV, Karlsson J. Skeletal muscle fibre types, enzyme activities and physical performance in young males and females. *Acta Physiol Scand.* 1978; 103: 210–218.
51. du Plessis MP, Smit PJ, du Plessis LAS, Geyer HJ, Mathews G. The composition of muscle fibers in a group of adolescents. In: Binkhorst RA, Kemper HCG, Saris WHM (eds.) *Children and exercise XI.* Baltimore: University Park Press; 1985. p. 323–324.
52. Houmard JA, Smith R, Jendrasiak GL. Relationship between MRI relaxation time and muscle fibre composition. *J Appl Physiol.* 1995; 78: 807–809.
53. Kuno S, Katsuta S, Inouye T, Anno I, Matsumoto K, Akisada M. Relationship between MR relaxation time and muscle fiber composition. *Radiology.* 1988; 169: 567–568.
54. Meyer RA, Brown TR, Kushmerick MJ. Phosphorus nuclear magnetic resonance of fast- and slow-twitch muscle. *Am J Physiol.* 1985; 248: C279–C287.
55. Eriksson BO, Karlsson J, Saltin B. Muscle metabolites during exercise in pubertal boys. *Acta Paediatr Scand.* 1971; 217:154–157.
56. Eriksson BO. Physical training, oxygen supply and muscle metabolism in 11–13-year-old boys. *Acta Physiol Scand.* 1972; 384(suppl): 1–48.
57. Eriksson BO, Gollnick PD, Saltin B. Muscle metabolism and enzyme activities after training in boys 11–13 years old. *Acta Physiol Scand.* 1973; 87: 485–499.
58. Eriksson BO, Gollnick PD, Saltin B. The effect of physical training on muscle enzyme activities and fiber composition in 11-year-old boys. *Acta Paediatr Belg.* 1974; 28: 245–252.
59. Eriksson BO, Saltin B. Muscle metabolism during exercise in boys aged 11 to 16 years compared to adults. *Acta Paediatr Belg.* 1974; 28: 257–265.
60. Eriksson BO. Muscle metabolism in children—a review. *Acta Physiol Scand.* 1980; 283: 20–28.
61. Karlsson J, Diamant B, Saltin B. Muscle metabolites during submaximal and maximal exercise in man. *Scand J Clin Invest.* 1970; 26: 385–394.
62. Garoid L, Binzoni T, Ferretti G, *et al.* Standardisation of ^{31}phosphorus-nuclear magnetic resonance spectroscopy determinations of high energy phosphates in humans. *Eur J Applied Physiol.* 1994; 68: 107–110.
63. Beneke R, Hutler M, Jung M, Leithauser RM. Modeling the blood lactate kinetics at maximal short-term exercise conditions in children, adolescents and adults. *J Appl Physiol.* 2005; 99: 499–504.
64. Dotan R, Ohana S, Bediz C, Falk B. Blood lactate disappearance dynamics in boys and men following exercise of similar and dissimilar peak-lactate concentrations. *J Pediatr Endocrinol Metab.* 2003; 16: 419–429.
65. Pfitzinger P, Freedson P. Blood lactate responses to exercise in children: Part 1. Peak lactate concentration. *Pediatr Exerc Sci.* 1997; 9: 210–222.
66. Pfitzinger P, Freedson P. Blood lactate responses to exercise in children: Part 2. Lactate threshold. *Pediatr Exerc Sci.* 1997; 9: 299–307.
67. Welsman J, Armstrong N. Assessing postexercise blood lactates in children and adolescents. In: Van Praagh E (ed.) *Pediatric anaerobic performance.* Champaign, IL: Human Kinetics; 1998. p. 137–153.
68. Pianosi P, Seargeant L, Haworth JC. Blood lactate and pyruvate concentrations, and their ratio during exercise in healthy children: developmental perspective. *Eur J Appl Physiol.* 1995; 71: 518–522.
69. Beneke R, Hutler M, Leithauser RM. Anaerobic performance and metabolism in boys and male adolescents. *Eur J Appl Physiol.* 2007; 101: 671–677.
70. Gollnick PD, Armstrong RB, Saubert CW, *et al.* Enzyme activity and fiber composition in skeletal muscle of trained and untrained men. *J Appl Physiol.* 1972; 33: 312–319.
71. Haralambie G. Skeletal muscle enzyme activities in female subjects of various ages. *Bull Eur Physiopath Resp.* 1979; 15: 259–267.
72. Haralambie G. Enzyme activities in skeletal muscle of 13–15 year old adolescents. *Bull Eur Physiopath Resp.* 1982; 18: 65–74.
73. Berg A Keul J. Biochemical changes during exercise in children. In: Malina RM (ed.) *Young athletes.* Champaign, IL: Human Kinetics; 1988. p. 61–78.
74. Berg A, Kim SS, Keul J. Skeletal muscle enzyme activities in healthy young subjects. *Int J Sports Med.* 1986; 7: 236–239.
75. Kaczor JL, Ziolkowski W, Popinigis J, Tarnopolsky MA. Anaerobic and aerobic enzyme activities in human skeletal muscle from children and adults. *Pediatr Res.* 2005; 57: 331–335.
76. Poortmans JR. Protein metabolism. *Med Sport Sci.* 2004; 46: 227–228.
77. Frayn KF. Calculation of substrate oxidation rates in vivo from gaseous exchange. *J Appl Physiol.* 1983; 55: 628–634.
78. Aucouturier J, Baker JS, Duche P. Fat and carbohydrate metabolism during submaximal exercise in children. *Sports Med.* 2008; 38: 213–238.
79. Jeukendrup AE, Wallis GA. Measurement of substrate oxidation during exercise by means of gas exchange measurements. *Int J Sports Med.* 2004; 26: 28–37.
80. Robinson S. Experimental studies of physical fitness in relation to age. *Arbeitsphysiologie.* 1938; 10: 251–323.
81. Foricher JM, Ville N, Gratas-Delamarche A, Delamarche P. Effects of submaximal intensity cycle ergometry for one hour on substrate utilization in trained prepubertal boys versus trained adults. *J Sports Med Phys Fit.* 2003; 43: 36–43.
82. Asano K, Hirakoba K. Respiratory and circulatory adaptation during prolonged exercise in 10–12-year-old children and in adults. In: Imarinen J, Valimaki I (eds.) *Children and sport.* Berlin: Springer-Verlag; 1984. p. 119–128.

83. Eynde BV, Van Gerven D, Vienne D, *et al.* Endurance fitness and peak height velocity in Belgian boys. In: Osseid S, Carlsen (eds.) *Children and exercise XIII.* Champaign, IL: Human Kinetics; 1989. p. 19–27.
84. Morse M, Schlutz FW, Cassels DE. Relation of age to physiological responses of the older boy to exercise. *J Appl Physiol.* 1949; 1: 683–709.
85. Montoye HJ. Age and oxygen utilization during submaximal treadmill exercise in males. *J Gerontol.* 1982; 37: 396–402.
86. Rowland TW, Auchinachie JA, Keenan TJ, Green GM. Physiologic responses to treadmill running in adult and prepubertal males. *Int J Sports Med.* 1987; 8: 292–297.
87. Timmons BW, Bar-Or O, Riddell MC. Oxidation rate of exogenous carbohydrate during exercise is higher in boys than in men. *J Appl Physiol.* 2003; 94: 278–284.
88. Timmons BW, Bar-Or O, Riddell MC. Influence of age and pubertal status on substrate utilization during exercise with and without carbohydrate intake in healthy boys. *Appl Physiol Nutr Metab.* 2007; 32: 416–425.
89. Martinez LR, Haymes EM. Substrate utilization during treadmill running in prepubertal girls and women. *Med Sci Sports Exerc.* 1992; 24: 975–983.
90. Rowland TW, Rimany TA. Physiological responses to prolonged exercise in premenarchael and adult females. *Int J Sports Med.* 1995; 7: 183–191.
91. Armstrong N, Kirby BJ, Welsman JR, McManus AM. Submaximal exercise in prepubertal children. In: Armstrong N, Kirby BJ, Welsman JR (eds.) *Children and exercise X1X.* London: Spon; 1997. p. 221–227.
92. Horton TJ, Pagliassotti MJ, Hobbs K, Hill JO. Fuel metabolism in men and women during and after long-duration exercise. *J Appl Physiol.* 1998; 85: 1823–1832.
93. Tarnopolsky LJ, MacDougall JD, Atkinson SA, Tarnopolsky MA, Sutton JR. Gender differences in substrate for endurance exercise. *J Appl Physiol.* 1990; 68: 302–308.
94. Tarnopolsky MA. Gender differences in substrate metabolism during endurance exercise. *Can J Appl Physiol.* 2000; 25: 312–327.
95. Braun B, Horton T. Endocrine regulation of exercise substrate utilization in women compared to men. *Exerc Sport Sci Rev.* 2001; 29: 149–154.
96. Friedlander AL, Casazza GA, Hornig MA, *et al.* Training-induced alterations of carbohydrate metabolism in women: Women respond differently from men. *J Appl Physiol.* 1998; 85: 1175–1186.
97. D'Eon TM, Sharoff C, Chipkin SR, Grow D, Ruby BC, Braun B. Regulation of exercise carbohydrate metabolism by estrogen and progesterone in women. *Am J Physiol Endocrinol Metab.* 2002; 283: 1046–1055.
98. Timmons BW, Bar-Or O, Riddell MC. Energy substrate utilization during prolonged exercise with and without carbohydrate intake in preadolescent and adolescent girls. *J Appl Physiol.* 2007; 103: 995–1000.
99. Stephens BR, Cole AS, Mahon AD. The influence of biological maturation on fat and carbohydrate metabolism during exercise in males. *Int J Sport Nutr Exerc Metab.* 2006; 16: 166–179.
100. Riddell MC, Jamnik VK, Iscoe KE, Timmons BW, Gledhill N. Fat oxidation rate and the exercise intensity that elicits maximal fat oxidation decreases with pubertal status in young male subjects. *J Appl Physiol.* 2008; 105: 742–748.
101. Malina RM, Bouchard C, Bar-Or O. *Growth, maturation and physical activity*, 2nd ed. Champaign, IL: Human Kinetics; 2004.
102. Armstrong N, Welsman JR, Kirby BJ. Submaximal exercise and maturation in 12-year-olds. *J Sports Sci.* 1999; 17: 107–114.
103. Riddell MC, Bar-Or O, Schwarcz P. Substrate utilization in boys during exercise with [^{13}C]-glucose ingestion. *Eur J Appl Physiol.* 2000; 83: 441–448.
104. Riddell MC, Bar-Or O, Wilk B, Parolin ML, Heigenhauser GJF. Substrate utilization during exercise with glucose plus fructose ingestion in boys ages 10–14 yr. *J Appl Physiol.* 2001; 90: 903–911.
105. Timmons BW, Bar-Or O. RPE during prolonged cycling with and without carbohydrate ingestion in boys and men. *Med Sci Sports Exerc.* 2003; 35: 1901–1907.
106. Wolfe RR, Chinkes DL. *Isotope tracers in metabolic research.* Hoboken NJ: John Wiley & Sons; 2005.
107. Kent-Braun JA, Miller RG, Weiner MW. Human skeletal muscle metabolism in health and disease: Utility of magnetic resonance spectroscopy. *Exerc Sports Sci Rev.* 1995; 23: 305–347.
108. Cooper DM, Barstow TJ. Magnetic resonance imaging and spectroscopy in studying exercise in children. *Exerc Sport Sci Rev.* 1996; 24: 475–499.
109. Barker AR, Welsman JR, Welford D, Fulford J, Williams C, Armstrong N. Reliability of ^{31}P-magnetic resonance spectroscopy during an exhaustive incremental exercise test in children. *Eur J Appl Physiol.* 2006; 98: 556–565.
110. Zanconato S, Buchthal S, Barstow TJ, Cooper DM. ^{31}P-magnetic resonance spectroscopy of leg muscle metabolism during exercise in children and adults. *J Appl Physiol.* 1993; 74: 2214–2218.
111. Peterson SR, Gaul CA, Stanton MM, Hanstock CC. Skeletal muscle metabolism during short-term high-intensity exercise in prepubertal and pubertal girls. *J Appl Physiol.* 1999; 87: 2151–2156.
112. Johnson MA, Polgar J, Weightman D, Appleton D. Data on the distribution of fibre types in thirty six human muscles, an autopsy study. *J Neurol Sci.* 1973; 18: 111–129.
113. Kuno S, Takahashi H, Fujimoto K, *et al.* Muscle metabolism during exercise using phosphorus-31 nuclear magnetic resonance spectroscopy in adolescents. *Eur J Appl Physiol.* 1995; 70: 301–304.
114. Barker AR, Welsman JR, Fulford J, Welford D, Williams CA, Armstrong N. Muscle phosphocreatine kinetics in children and adults at the onset and offset of moderate intensity exercise. *J Appl Physiol.* 2008; 105: 446–456.
115. Barker AR, Welsman JR, Fulford J, Welford D, Armstrong N. Quadriceps muscle energetics during incremental exercise in children and adults. *Med Sci Sports Exerc.* 2010; 42: 1303–1313.
116. McCully KK, Fielding RA, Evans WJ, Leigh ESJr, Posner JD. Relationships between in vitro and in vivo measurements of metabolism in young and old human calf muscles. *J Appl Physiol.* 1993; 75: 813–819.
117. Mirwald RL, Baxter-Jones AD, Bailey DA, Beunen GP. An assessment of maturity from anthropometric measurements. *Med Sci Sports Exerc.* 2002; 34: 689–694.
118. Kushmerick MJ, Meyer RA, Brown TR. Regulation of oxygen consumption in fast- and slow-twitch muscle. *Am J Physiol Cell Physiol.* 1992; 263: C598–C606.
119. Minzo M, Secher NH, Quistorff B. ^{31}P-NMR spectroscopy, EMG and histochemical fiber types of human wrist flexor muscles. *J Appl Physiol.* 1994; 76: 531–538.
120. Willcocks RJ, Williams CA, Barker AR, Fulford J, Armstrong N. Age-and sex-related differences in muscle phosphocreatine and oxygenation kinetics during high-intensity exercise in adolescents and adults. *NMR Biomed.* 2010; 23: 569–577.
121. Ratel S, Tonson A, Le Fur Y, Cozzone P, Bendahan D. Comparative analysis of skeletal muscle oxidative capacity in children and adults: a ^{31}P-MRS study. *Appl Physiol Nutr Metab.* 2008; 33: 720–727.
122. Tonson A, Ratel S, Le Fur Y, Vilmen C, Cozzone P, Bendahan D. Muscle energetics changes throughout maturation: a quantitative ^{31}P-MRS analysis. *J Appl Physiol.* 2010; 109: 1769–1778.
123. Kappenstein J, Ferrauti A, Runkel B, Fernandez-Frenadez J, Zange J. Changes in phosphocreatine concentration of skeletal muscle during high-intensity intermittent exercise in children and adults. *Eur J Appl Physiol.* 2013; 113: 2769–2779.
124. Grassi B, Poole DC, Richardson RS, Knight Dr, Erickson BK, Wagner PD. Muscle $\dot{V}O_2$ kinetics in humans: implications for metabolic control. *J Appl Physiol.* 1996; 80: 988–998.
125. Rossiter HB. Exercise; Kinetic considerations for gas exchange. *Compr Physiol.* 2011; 1: 203–244.
126. Poole DC, Jones AM. Oxygen uptake kinetics. *Compr Physiol.* 2012; 2: 933–996.

127. Barker AR, Welsman JR, Fulford J, Welford D, Williams CA, Armstrong N. Muscle phosphocreatine and pulmonary oxygen uptake kinetics in children at the onset and offset of moderate intensity exercise. *Eur J Appl Physiol.* 2008; 102: 727–738.
128. Fawkner SG, Armstrong N. Oxygen uptake kinetic response to exercise in children. *Sports Med.* 2003; 33: 651–659.
129. Barstow TJ, Scheuermann BW. Effects of maturation and aging on $\dot{V}O_2$ kinetics. In: Jones AM, Poole DC (eds.) *Oxygen uptake kinetics in sport, exercise and medicine.* Routledge: London; 2006. p. 332–352.
130. Fawkner SG, Armstrong N. Oxygen uptake kinetics. In: Armstrong N (ed.) *Paediatric exercise physiology.* Edinburgh: Elsevier; 2007. p. 189–211.
131. Potter CR, Childs DJ, Houghton W, Armstrong N. Breath-to-breath noise in the ventilatory gas exchange responses of children to exercise. *Eur J Appl Physiol.* 1999; 80: 118–124.
132. Fawkner SG, Armstrong N. The slow component response of $\dot{V}O_2$ to heavy intensity exercise in children. In: Reilly T, Marfell-Jones M (eds.) *Kinanthropometry viii.* Routledge: London; 2003. p. 105–113.
133. Fawkner SG, Armstrong N. Modelling the kinetic response to moderate-intensity exercise in children. *Acta Kinesiol Univ Tartuensis.* 2002; 7: 80–84.
134. Fawkner SG, Armstrong N. Modelling the $\dot{V}O_2$ kinetic response to heavy-intensity exercise in children. *Ergonomics.* 2004; 47: 1517–1527.
135. Fawkner SG, Armstrong N. Can we confidently study $\dot{V}O_2$ kinetics in young people? *J Sport Sci Med.* 2007; 6: 277–285.
136. Fawkner SG, Armstrong N, Potter CR, Welsman JR. Oxygen uptake kinetics in children and adults after the onset of moderate-intensity exercise. *J Sports Sci.* 2002; 20: 319–326.
137. Armon Y, Cooper DM, Flores R, Zanconato S, Barstow TJ. Oxygen uptake dynamics during high-intensity exercise in children and adults. *J Appl Physiol.* 1991; 70: 841–848.
138. Fawkner SG, Armstrong N. Sex differences in the oxygen uptake kinetic response to heavy-intensity exercise in prepubertal children. *Eur J Appl Physiol.* 2004; 93: 210–216.
139. Gaesser GA, Poole DC. The slow component of oxygen uptake kinetics in humans. *Exerc Sport Sci Rev.* 1994; 24: 35–71.
140. Fawkner SG, Armstrong N. Longitudinal changes in the kinetic response to heavy-intensity exercise in children. *J Appl Physiol.* 2004; 97: 460–466.
141. Breese BC, Williams CA, Barker AR, *et al.* Longitudinal changes in the oxygen uptake response to heavy intensity exercise in 14–16-year old boys. *Pediatr Exerc Sci.* 2010; 22: 314–325.
142. Dotan R, Mitchell C, Cohen R, Klentrou P, Gabriel D, Falk B. Child-adult differences in muscle activation—a review. *Pediatr Exerc Sci.* 2012; 24: 2–21.

CHAPTER 7

Muscle strength

Mark BA De Ste Croix

Introduction

The development of equipment, technology, and an increased understanding of growth and maturation issues have provided new insights into paediatric strength development in the last decade. Since writing the chapter for the second edition of this book, there has been an increase in the number of studies that have examined strength and neuromuscular function in children. In fact, published studies utilizing isokinetic dynamometry to measure dynamic strength in children have doubled in the last 5 years alone. Despite this increase, the total volume of work that has explored age- and sex-associated changes in strength is relatively small. The majority of data that have emerged in recent years has focused on strength performance in elite youth populations, especially in professional soccer, and may in part be due to the development of the strength and conditioning profession. The lack of recent descriptive studies exploring changes in strength with age is probably due to the perception that this change is already well described and understood and that those studies available on age- and sex-associated changes in dynamic strength are relatively consistent. To some extent this is true, as generally strength appears to increase in both boys and girls until about the age of 14 years, when it begins to plateau in girls and a spurt is evident in boys. By 18 years, there are few overlaps in strength between boys and girls with force production generally greater in males. The exact age at which sex differences become apparent is unclear and the extent of any sex differences is both muscle group and muscle action specific.[1,2] For example, the male-female difference in strength is much greater in the trunk and upper extremity than in the lower extremity.[1,2]

Recent studies have focused on trying to integrate strength data with other forms of data to explore the complex changing mechanisms that are involved in the development of dynamic strength with age. For example, the integration of isokinetic strength data with electromyography (EMG) has allowed the exploration of co-contraction, rate of torque development, torque kinetics, and electromechanical delay (EMD) for both sports performance and injury prevention. Integration with magnetic resonance imaging (MRI) and ultrasound have also allowed observation of the influence of muscle cross-sectional area (mCSA), (including determining physiological cross-sectional area [PCSA]), muscle moment arms, and pennation angles on strength changes with age. The understanding of the complex interactions of both morphological and neuromuscular factors that explain differences in strength during childhood and adolescence is continuing to be developed.[1] However, there are few well-controlled longitudinal studies of muscle strength that have concurrently examined the influence of known explanatory variables using appropriate statistical techniques.[3–5]

In longitudinal studies employing such analyses, stature and limb length consistently appear to be key factors in strength development alongside muscle size, body mass, and neuromuscular control. The importance of stature and limb length may be attributed to changes in mechanical advantage, including muscle moment arm lengths and the stimulation of muscle growth as a consequence of long bone growth. Evidence suggests that although these variables have a significant role to play when examined individually, when they are analysed concurrently with other known variables, the contribution of some factors becomes non-significant. For example, most studies have shown that maturation does not exert a significant independent effect when stature and body mass are accounted for.[6] Current data indicate the importance of muscle size as an independent predictor in the development of strength with age,[7] but when examined alongside other known explanatory variables it appears that mCSA cannot fully account for age and sex differences in strength during childhood.[6,8] O'Brien *et al.*[9] suggested that changes in PCSA alongside changes in muscle moment arms and voluntary activation levels could account for maturation-related changes in strength.

Understanding the age- and sex-associated changes in strength also requires measurement of muscle agonist/antagonist activation, muscle size, muscle architecture, and muscle tendon moment arms/mechanical advantage. This presents many challenges to researchers, especially in the paediatric population due to the individual timing and tempo of growth and maturation. One of the biggest issues for readers wanting to understand age- and sex-associated changes in strength is that there are very few longitudinal studies which have tracked changes in strength throughout childhood. Thus although there is a growing consensus regarding the change in strength with growth and maturation, and the potential mechanisms associated with this change, caution must be taken as the evidence base is not comprehensive. Table 7.1 provides details of the available longitudinal studies exploring age- and sex-associated changes in strength.

Defining muscle strength

There are various definitions of muscle strength probably attributable to the numerous factors that interact to form the expression of strength. However, during dynamic movements we know that both concentric and eccentric muscle actions occur. Given the significance of these muscle actions in everyday life, investigations of age- and sex-associated strength development should consider concurrently the ability of the individual to perform both types of action. Underpinning the choice of muscle action to examine must be the activity or sport-specific component under investigation.

Table 7.1 Longitudinal studies examining age- and sex-associated changes in muscle strength.

Citation	Sample size	Age (y)	Sex	Duration	Dependent Variable	Independent Factors
De Ste Croix *et al.*[5]	41	10–14y	M=20 F=21	4 years (8 test occasions)	Isokinetic concentric knee extension and flexion	Stature, body mass, skinfolds, maturation
Kanehisa *et al.*[31]	12	11–13y	M=6 F=6	2 years (3 test occasions)	Isokinetic concentric knee extension	Stature, body mass, bone age, muscle CSA
Round *et al.*[15]	100	8–17y	M=50 F=50	3 years (3 test occasions)	Isometric elbow flexors and knee extensors	Stature, body mass, testosterone, peak height velocity
Holm *et al.*[32]	12	10–21y	M	11 years (6 test occasions)	Isokinetic concentric knee extension and flexion	Stature, mass, bone age
Kanehisa *et al.*[33]	10	13–15y	M	2 years (3 test occasions)	Isokinetic elbow flexors and knee extensors	Stature, mass, muscle thickness
Wood *et al.*[3]	37	13–16y	M=18 F=19	3 years (3 test occasions)	Isokinetic concentric and isometric elbow extension and flexion	Stature, mass, arm length, muscle CSA
Peltonen *et al.*[34]	66	13–17y	F	3 years (3 test occasions)	Trunk isometric extension and flexion	Stature, mass, muscle CSA
Seger and Thoreston[99]	16	11–16y	M=9 F=7	5 years (2 test occasions)	Isokinetic concentric and eccentric knee extension	Stature, body mass, BMI, femur and tibia length, thigh and calf circumference, muscle activation
Newcomer *et al.*[35]	96	10–19y	M=53 F=43	4 years (2 test occasions)	Trunk isometric extension and flexion	Back pain questionnaire
Quatman *et al.*[99]	33	14–15y	M=17 F=16	2 years (2 test occasions)	Take off force, vertical jump height	Loading rate, maturation
Quatman-Yates *et al.*[86]	39	11–13y	F	3 years (3 test occasions)	Knee extension and flexion, hip abduction	Stature, maturation
Pitcher *et al.*[7]	20	5–11y	M=9 F=11	6 months (2 test occasions)	Isometric and isokinetic concentric knee extension and flexion	Stature, mass, Tanner stage, muscle volume

For example, in sports where maximal strength is an important component it may be wise to assess children's strength at very slow velocities, based on the force-velocity relationship. However, during activities where fast velocity movements are common it may be prudent to assess functional strength at faster velocities rather than maximal strength.

Definitions of force and torque

Up to this point, the term 'strength' rather than force or torque (moment of force) has been used. Force represents the tension generated during voluntary/involuntary muscle activation and is appropriate to use when strength is measured *in vivo* at the point of load application.[10,11] This includes direct measurement within muscle-tendons[12] as well as forces measured using strain gauge transducers mounted in line with the applied force.[13–15] If load is applied distal to the joint axis/centre of rotation and measurement is made at the axis of rotation (for example, in isokinetic dynamometry), the term torque is appropriate. Torque can be defined as the product of the force and the perpendicular distance from the line of action of the force to the axis/centre of rotation. It represents the tendency of a force to cause body segment rotation about an axis/centre of rotation.[16] In most instances, more than one force may be acting about the axis of rotation; therefore the measured torque represents the net torque (sum of all of the forces acting and their moment arms). The joint torque will vary depending on joint angle and velocity of movement.

When using an isokinetic dynamometer, isometric torques or gravity corrected joint torques may be recorded. Assuming sufficient body stabilization and joint isolation, these can be defined as the net torque resulting from both agonist and antagonist activation. Therefore when measuring concentric isokinetic knee extension torque, greater activation of the hamstrings would reduce the net knee extension torque.[17] An estimation of maximal knee extensor muscle torque must therefore take into account muscle co-activation. This can be achieved by deriving the torque/EMG relationship for the antagonist muscles (hamstrings) and adding the estimated antagonist torque to the net knee extension torque.[9,18–20] Failure to consider antagonist co-activation would lead to an underestimation of knee extensor torque and consequently causes inaccuracies in any subsequent calculations and comparisons of strength development. The torque (adjusted for any contribution from the antagonists) represents the resultant torque from all of the agonist muscles. This assumes that the angular acceleration is zero (the measurement of joint torque occurs within the isokinetic window). For knee extension the adjusted knee extension torque acting via the patella tendon can be considered to be a resultant torque generated by the individual quadriceps muscles. For the purpose of this chapter the terms force and torque will be used where appropriate, but readers should be cautious of making comparisons between paediatric studies that have measured and interpreted 'strength' in differing ways.

Assessment of muscle strength

Determining strength in paediatric populations

It is beyond the scope of this chapter to discuss fully the implications and limitations of the numerous assessment tools used to determine force and torque in children, and interested readers are directed to earlier reviews.[1,2,6] However, it is important for readers to understand that differing methods of assessment of strength should not always be considered valid and reliable strength measures in children. Often indirect or surrogate measures of strength are used and these should be viewed with a degree of caution. Numerous authors have discussed changes in children's neuromuscular function based on field tests (in particular counter movement jumps), without any direct measurement of neuromuscular capability.

Laboratory-based versus field-based tests

Generally within the sport and exercise literature there has been a drive towards more ecological validity of strength, in particular determining strength and neuromuscular performance during applied sporting movements. In some ways this makes sense as the limb never moves through a range of movement at a fixed angular velocity, as is performed during isokinetic testing. For example, there are a growing number of paediatric studies measuring neuromuscular capability utilising EMG and ground reaction forces using force plates. The development in portable force plates and wireless EMG technology permits the paediatric researcher to undertake more ecologically relevant work. Likewise it is almost impossible to measure the closed-open-closed kinetic chain of jumping and landing using a dynamometer. The importance of not applying adult procedures to paediatric testing will be reinforced throughout this chapter, especially where equipment and protocols have been designed for adults. Most manufacturers now supply paediatric attachments/consumables for their equipment (e.g. paediatric attachments are available for the Biodex isokinetic dynamometer; see Figure 7.1) and where this is not readily available paediatric researchers should adapt their equipment in-house to improve the trustworthiness of the data they produce.

Most important, irrespective of the method used to determine changes in strength, is the sensitivity of the measurement to ascertain changes due to growth and maturation. In order for any strength measurement to be used as an objective and accurate measure of maximum strength it must be documented to be a reliable measurement tool. Poor reliability may lead to erroneous conclusions about the strength parameter being measured. Experimental error can be minimized effectively by standardization of test protocols that will provide greater sensitivity to detect biological sources of variation in a child's ability to exert maximum muscular effort.

A habituation period is critical for paediatric strength testing as this essential period of learning facilitates a phase in which the specific movements, neuromuscular patterns, and demands of the test become familiar to the individual. It is difficult to compare results across studies as different statistical methods, many of which are questionable, have been used to assess reliability that is also protocol, measured parameter, and dynamometer specific. Previous studies have reported good reliability in repeated isokinetic actions of the knee (extension $r = 0.95$; flexion $r = 0.85$), the elbow (extension $r = 0.97$; flexion $r = 0.87$), and isometric hand grip data ($r = 0.92$). Others have reported limits of agreement showing no systematic difference in knee and elbow peak torque measured on two

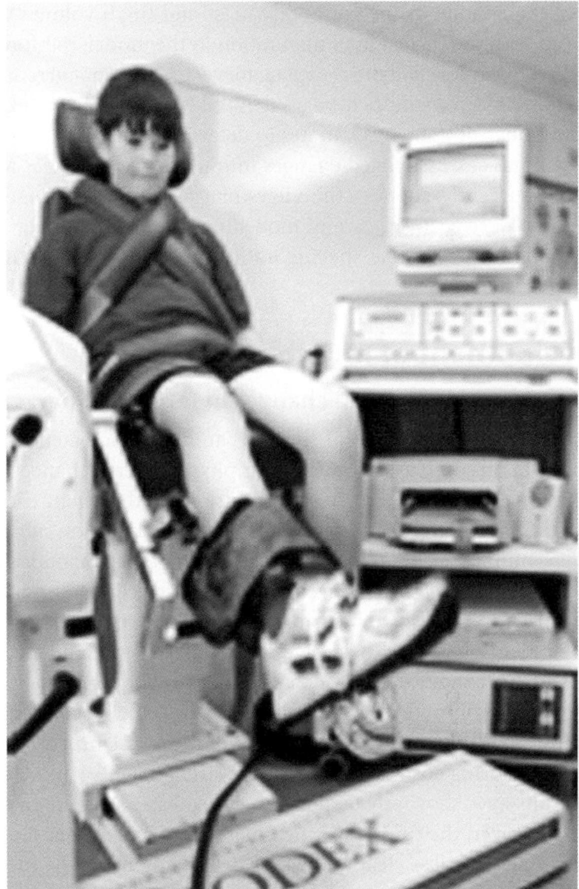

Figure 7.1 Boy on Biodex isokinetic dynamometer using paediatric attachments.
Photograph courtesy of the Children's Health and Exercise Research Centre, with participant permission.

separate occasions.[21] A study of prepubertal soccer players reported systematic bias in concentric and eccentric knee torque, although these improvements, 3–7%, were relatively small.[22] The available literature also suggests that extension movements are more reliable than flexion movements and that concentric actions are more reliable than eccentric actions. It would appear that strength testing in children, irrespective of muscle action or muscle joint assessed, has a test-retest variation of 5–10%.

Interpretation of paediatric strength data—issue of scaling

In the following discussion of the age- and sex-associated changes in force/torque it is important to be aware of the subtleties of how changes due to growth and maturation are accounted for by paediatric researchers. It has become common in the literature to express strength in absolute terms, with isometric data expressed in Newtons (N) and isokinetic data expressed in Newton metres (Nm). In the study of muscle strength in relation to growth and maturation, comparisons are made between individuals of different sizes and therefore it is important that a size-free strength variable is used for comparative purposes.

The most commonly used technique to partition out differences in size is the ratio standard, with body mass as the most widely used denominator. However, stature and fat-free mass (FFM) have also featured as covariates.[15,23] This was highlighted in a recent study using allometric scaling techniques, which demonstrated that the size of the exponents for both body mass and thigh volume were reduced with the inclusion of maturation in the model, reinforcing the need to explore potential explanatory variables concurrently.[24] Three longitudinal studies have used multilevel modelling to examine a number of known covariates to determine their influence on the age- and sex-associated changes in muscle strength.[3,5,15] Most authors currently support the view that suitable scaling factors should be derived from careful modelling of individual data sets, and therefore be sample specific, rather than adopting assumed scaling indices.

Development of muscle strength

Age- and sex-associated changes in force/torque

Most early understanding of the age- and sex-associated development in strength was restricted to physical performance tests that frequently measured muscle endurance rather than muscle strength. Studies that have used pull-ups as the criterion measure for determining sex differences in muscle strength have clouded our understanding of strength development during growth and maturation. It is important to bear in mind that understanding of the development of strength with age is influenced by the nuances of the testing procedures used, such as subject positioning, degree of practice, level of motivation, lateral dominance, and level of understanding about the purpose and nature of the test. Unsurprisingly, studies exploring absolute differences in strength between children and adults have shown that adults generate greater forces than children. However, the timing of when males and females reach adult strength levels is less clear and varies depending upon the muscle joint and action that is assessed.

Body mass-related strength increases with age in boys but there is no age-related increase in girls. This may be due to the increase in body fat as a percentage of total body mass as girls move through the pubertal period. These data support a recent study examining changes in concentric and eccentric torque profiles of male youth professional footballers (11–18 years old).[25] Peak torque per body mass increased with age until 15 years, where it appeared to plateau as there were no significant age related increases between 15–18 years.[25] Polynominal regression analysis has shown that isokinetic strength increases with age (11–18 years old) even when torque is co-varied for body mass, stature, and fat free weight.[26] Interestingly the cross-sectional data are relatively consistent and support the work of Camic *et al.*,[26] but longitudinal studies reveal conflicting data.[5] This demonstrates the difficulties in describing the age-related changes in strength and discrepancies between studies might be due to differences in study design, age range, or training status of participants. Additionally, the statistical methods for accounting for covariates within cross-sectional compared to longitudinal studies may provide differing insights.

When examining data relating to changes in strength due to growth and maturation it is important to remember that a large amount of data have been derived from isometric testing.[14,15,27–29] Children may not produce maximal force during isometric actions, and this has been attributed to inhibitory mechanisms that preclude children from giving a maximal effort. Therefore, the whole motor pool may not be activated due to a reduction in the neural drive under high tension loading conditions.[30] No studies appear to have described the torque or force deficit in children during growth and maturation. This requires some measure of force-generating capacity (using electrical stimulation) and removal of force-generating capability. Recent years have seen an increase in the number of longitudinal studies, which have focused predominantly on knee function,[5,15,31–33] but there are also studies on elbow strength[3,15] and back strength[34,35] (see Table 7.1). Even though there are a few longitudinal studies, most have not taken repeated measurements throughout the maturational period, and are either follow-up studies restricted to a 2–3-year period and/or have small sample sizes. Indeed, when critically reviewing the evidence base the total number of participants from longitudinal studies is ~410 with only 157 female participants and one study exploring eccentric torque. Few studies have examined strength of the trunk muscles, but a comprehensive study by Mueller *et al.*[36] reported significant age-related changes (twofold increase) in concentric trunk extensor and flexor strength in 11- to 15-year-olds.

Data from isometric and isokinetic muscle actions indicate that in both boys and girls strength increases in a fairly linear fashion from early childhood up until the onset of puberty in boys, and until about the end of the pubertal period in girls. The marked difference seen between boys and girls is a strength spurt in boys throughout the pubertal period, which is not evident in girls. Girls' strength appears to increase during puberty at a similar rate to that seen during the prepubertal phase and then appears to plateau post puberty. However, data from elite youth athletes suggests that, at least in boys, strength might plateau by around 15 years.[25] There is some disagreement about the age at which sex differences become evident and although conflicting evidence is available, it is generally agreed that before the male adolescent growth spurt there are considerable overlaps in strength between boys and girls. By the age of 16–17 years of age, very few girls out-perform boys in strength tests, with boys demonstrating 54% more strength on average than girls (see Figures 7.2 and 7.3).

Throughout childhood and puberty, particularly in males, isometric elbow flexor and knee extensor strength are highly correlated with chronological age.[10] In line with isometric data, most cross-sectional and longitudinal studies of changes in dynamic strength have demonstrated a significant increase with age.[5,21,25,26,31–33,37–39] For example, increases in children's absolute knee extensor (range 143–314%) and flexor (range 131–285%) strength have been noted from the ages of 9 to 21 years.[32,39] A recent study of 9- to 22-year-old males and females has suggested that whole lower limb strength (including knee, ankle, and hip strength) is a more appropriate composite measure for exploring age- and sex-associated differences in strength.[40] Despite this, age-related differences in composite lower limb strength were still observed, although the age-related effects were minimized when stature and body mass were accounted for.

Some studies have suggested that age exerts an independent effect on strength development over and above maturation and stature.[41] Others have indicated that even when mCSA is accounted for using a multilevel modelling procedure age explains a significant amount of the additional variance for isometric elbow extensors.[3] It was suggested that this positive age term may be explained by the shared variance with maturation, as maturation was not included in the model. However, another longitudinal data set, using multilevel modelling, suggested that age is a non-significant explanatory variable of isokinetic knee torque once stature and mass are accounted for.[5] This is probably attributable to differing rates of anatomical growth and maturation, which vary independently and thus their effects on strength do not correlate simply with chronological age. It would appear that although there is a strong correlation between strength and age, a large portion of this association is probably

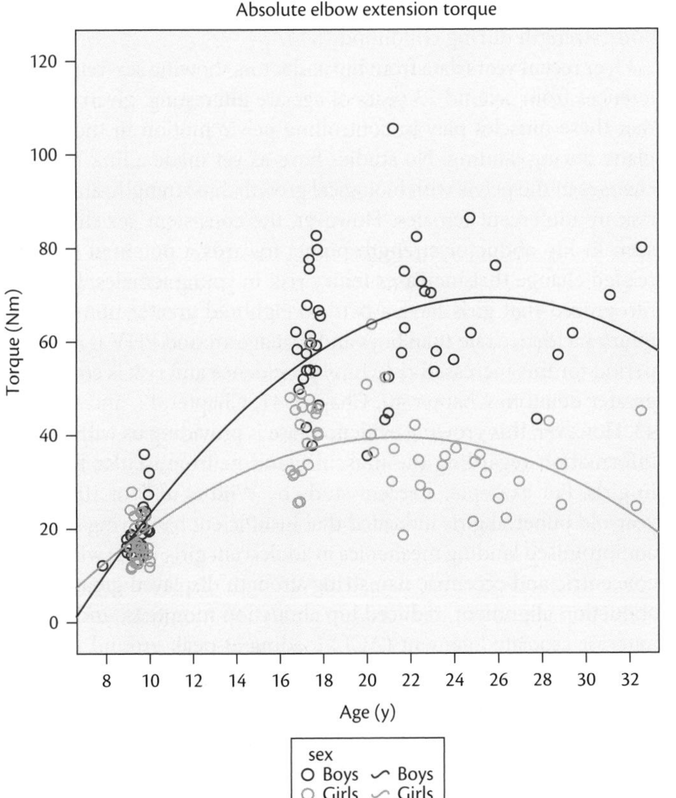

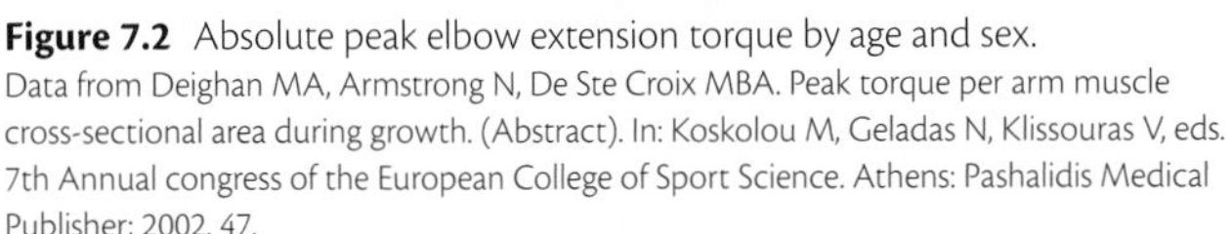

Figure 7.2 Absolute peak elbow extension torque by age and sex.
Data from Deighan MA, Armstrong N, De Ste Croix MBA. Peak torque per arm muscle cross-sectional area during growth. (Abstract). In: Koskolou M, Geladas N, Klissouras V, eds. 7th Annual congress of the European College of Sport Science. Athens: Pashalidis Medical Publisher; 2002. 47.

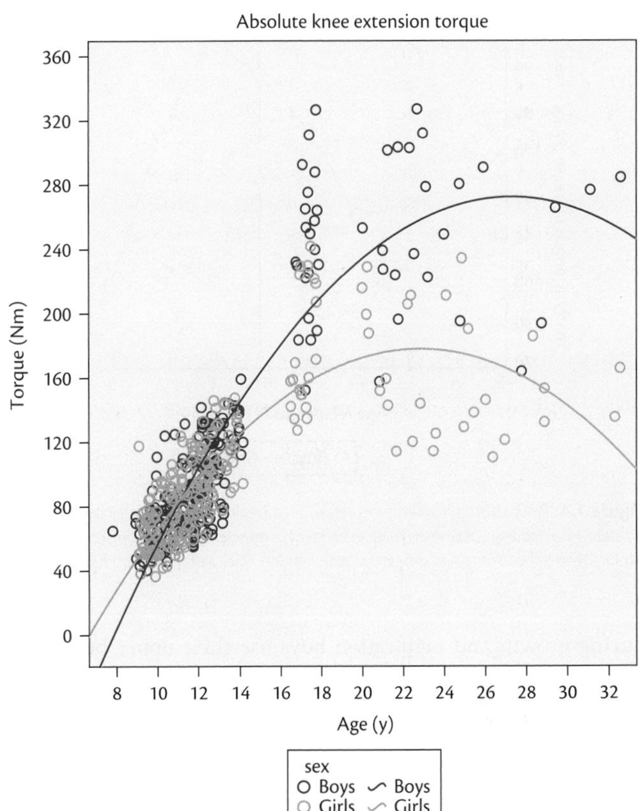

Figure 7.3 Absolute peak knee extension torque by age and sex.
Data from Deighan MA, Armstrong N, De Ste Croix MBA. Peak torque per arm muscle cross-sectional area during growth. (Abstract). In: Koskolou M, Geladas N, Klissouras V, eds. 7th Annual congress of the European College of Sport Science. Athens: Pashalidis Medical Publisher; 2002. 47.

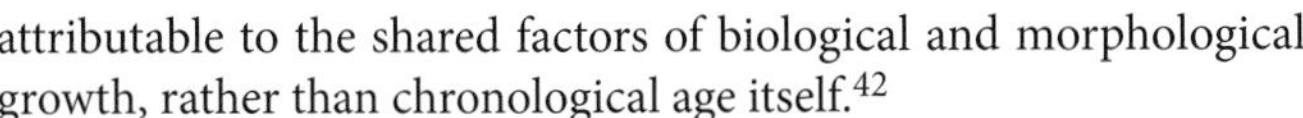

attributable to the shared factors of biological and morphological growth, rather than chronological age itself.[42]

There is little consensus about when sex differences in muscle strength become apparent. Some authors have suggested that sex differences in muscle strength are evident from as early as 3 years, or at least by 9–10 years.[31,43] A recent study exploring sex differences in back strength demonstrated significant sex differences in all age groups (11–15 years) even when body mass was controlled for.[36] Other studies have shown clear sex differences by 11–14 years.[10,27,44] A large cross-sectional study of 1140 boys and girls aged 9–17 years demonstrated that sex differences in absolute dynamic knee strength occur at 14 years.[38] This study suggests that girls' quadriceps torque peaks at 13 years but that hamstring strength peaks as young as 11 years, compared to 14 years in boys.[38] Recent studies focusing on sex difference in hip torque[29,45,46] have also demonstrated significant sex differences in absolute eccentric hip torque in adolescents (14–18 years), which remained even when torque was normalized to body mass.[45] Bittencourt *et al.*[46] found no significant sex difference in isometric hip abductor torque in 10- to 14-year-olds but sex differences were evident in 15- to 19-year-olds. These hip data are supported by a well-controlled longitudinal study, which indicated that there are no sex differences in dynamic strength up until the age of 14 years.[5] After 14 years boys out-perform girls in muscle strength irrespective of the muscle action examined, even with body size accounted for. It is important at this point to remind ourselves that factors relating to biological growth and maturation probably play a key role in the factors behind the timing of sex differences in strength development. For example, some authors have attributed the non-significant sex difference observed at 13–14 years to earlier biological maturation in girls, and the associated neural maturation that accompanies biological maturation.[5,15] However, as little is known about neural maturation, it is probably more likely that the well-recognized relationship between peak strength velocity (PSV) and peak height velocity (PHV) play a key role in sex differences. As seen in Figure 7.4, PSV occurs about a year after PHV at ~11.4–12.2 years in girls and ~13.4–14.4 years in boys.

Therefore 13- to 14-year-old girls are more likely to have benefited from peak strength gains while boys are still in the PHV phase and will have not experienced a strength spurt. In addition, there is evidence that PSV, in boys at least, lags behind peak gains in muscle mass velocity by 0.4 years and thus boys do not gain an advantage in strength, based on the growth in muscle size, until about 15 years.[47] Data from a study using allometric scaling techniques suggest that in boys the PSV occurs 2 years after PHV.[24]

Isometric data suggest that sex differences in strength are relatively greater in muscles of the upper compared to the lower body in children. Gilliam *et al.*[43] reported no significant sex difference in 15–17-year-olds' knee extension peak torque, but sex differences were apparent for the elbow extensors. This has been attributed to the weight-bearing role of the leg muscle. It has been suggested that

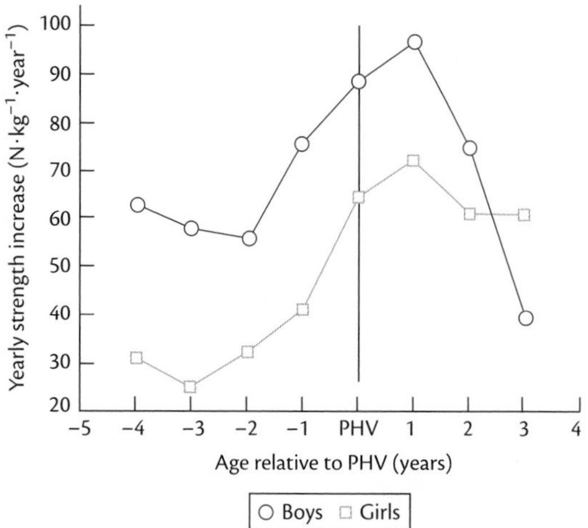

Figure 7.4 Peak strength velocity in relation to peak height velocity by sex.
Adapted from Froberg K, Lammert O. Development of muscle strength during childhood. In: Bar-Or O (ed.) The child and adolescent athlete. London: Blackwell Scientific; 1996: 25–41.

during growth and maturation boys use their upper body more than girls through habitual physical activities (such as climbing). This sociocultural explanation has recently been challenged as there is no overlap in strength between sexes as would be expected with physically active girls and sedentary boys if this contention was true.[15] A recent longitudinal study also demonstrated that sex differences are apparent in elbow flexion and extension from 13–15 years, even when stature and arm length are accounted for. However, when mCSA was accounted for, sex differences disappeared, leading the authors to conclude that the use of linear dimensions to account for sex differences in upper body strength has clouded our understanding. Thus caution must be exercised when describing sex-associated differences in upper and lower body strength during childhood.

Over recent years data from hip abductors showing sex-related differences from around 13 years of age are interesting, given the role that these muscles play in controlling pelvic motion in the frontal plane during landing. No studies have as yet made a link between changes in the pelvis with biological growth, hip strength, and injury risk in adolescent females. However, the consistent sex difference seen in hip abductor strength points towards a potential growth-related change that increases injury risk in young females. It is well recognized that girls have a two- to eightfold greater non-contact injury incidence rate than boys and that age around PHV is a critical period for this increased risk. Injury incidence and risk is covered in greater detail in Chapter 40, Chapter 41, Chapter 42, and Chapter 43. However, this growing evidence base is providing us with greater information regarding the muscular and neuromuscular function in girls. For example, a recent study by Wild *et al.*[48] of 10- to 13-year-old pubertal girls indicated that insufficient hamstring strength compromised landing mechanics in adolescent girls. Girls with lower concentric and eccentric hamstring strength displayed greater knee abduction alignment, reduced hip abduction moments, and greater anterior cruciate ligament (ACL) loading at peak ground reaction force. It is beyond the scope of this chapter to explore the biomechanical and hormonal differences between boys and girls in relation to knee mechanics, but a number of comprehensive studies have demonstrated sex differences across all stages of maturation.[49]

Determinants of strength development

The mechanisms associated with the age- and sex-associated development in strength are complex and multifaceted. Kellis *et al.*[50] recently presented a schematic (Figure 7.5) providing a summary of the proposed factors behind the child-adult differences in strength.

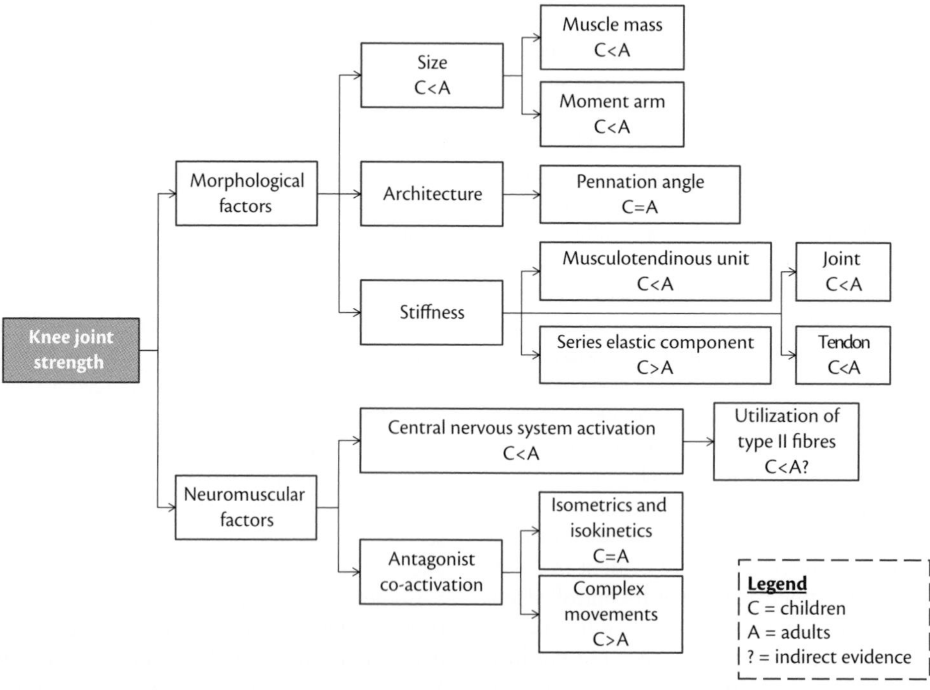

Figure 7.5 Schematic summary of comparisons between children (C) and adults (A) regarding factors influencing knee joint strength.
Kellis E, Mademli L, Patikas D, Kofotolis N. Neuromuscular interactions around the knee in children, adults and elderly. World J Ortho. 2014; 5: 469–485.

As discussed, most growth-related factors are independent predictors of the age and sex-associated changes in strength, although when explanatory variables are investigated concurrently certain parameters become non-significant. Kellis *et al.*[50] suggest that although hormonal changes that promote muscle mass augmentation and limb size increases (which influence the muscle moment arm) probably play a significant role in the development of strength, they do not fully explain these growth- and maturation-related changes. A growing body of evidence indicates that neural adaptations probably account for some of the strength gains observed during developmental ages, as well as changes in muscle tendon unit (MTU) architecture and stiffness.

Stature, mass, and strength development

The influence of gross body size on strength development has been examined in many studies. Stature and mass are traditionally the size variables of choice because they can be quickly and easily measured. Early longitudinal studies demonstrated that isometric strength per body mass varied only slightly during childhood and through puberty in girls.[51,52] In contrast, around the time of boys' PHV, i.e. age ~14 years, an increase in strength per body mass in boys which was still increasing by age 18 years has been demonstrated.[52]

Body mass has been found to be correlated with isometric strength of elbow flexors and knee extensors.[10] However, age-specific correlation coefficients between strength and body mass for males are generally low to moderate during the mid-childhood years, increase, then peak during puberty, and abate in the late teens.[14] Figure 7.6 demonstrates the strong positive correlation between isokinetic knee and elbow extension torque and body mass in 7- to 32-year-old males and females.

In a well-designed, allometrically scaled study, isokinetic strength was found to be mostly mediated by corresponding changes in overall body mass in adolescent males.[24] Data on this relationship are sparse for females but moderate positive coefficients between strength and body mass for females during the prepubertal years and at the onset of puberty and low correlations at the end of puberty and during puberty have been reported.[14,52] Others have found the relationship between female strength and body mass to be high during the teen years and to decline during young adulthood.[39] When related to shorter periods of growth (in which the range of the anthropometric variable in question is small), correlations become weaker. It is worth noting here that when isokinetic knee extension and flexion torque are adjusted for body mass using the ratio standard, the rate of change in strength might be underestimated compared to mass-adjusted data using allometric techniques.[39]

Three longitudinal studies have used multilevel modelling to examine the influence of stature and body mass on strength development. Round *et al.*[15] reported that isometric knee extensor strength in girls increased in proportion to the increase in stature and mass in 8- to 13-year-olds. De Ste Croix *et al.*[5] also demonstrated that stature and mass are significant explanatory variables of isokinetic knee extension and flexion torque in 10- to 14-year-olds. This was further reinforced by Wood *et al.*,[3] who demonstrated a significant influence of stature on the development of isometric and

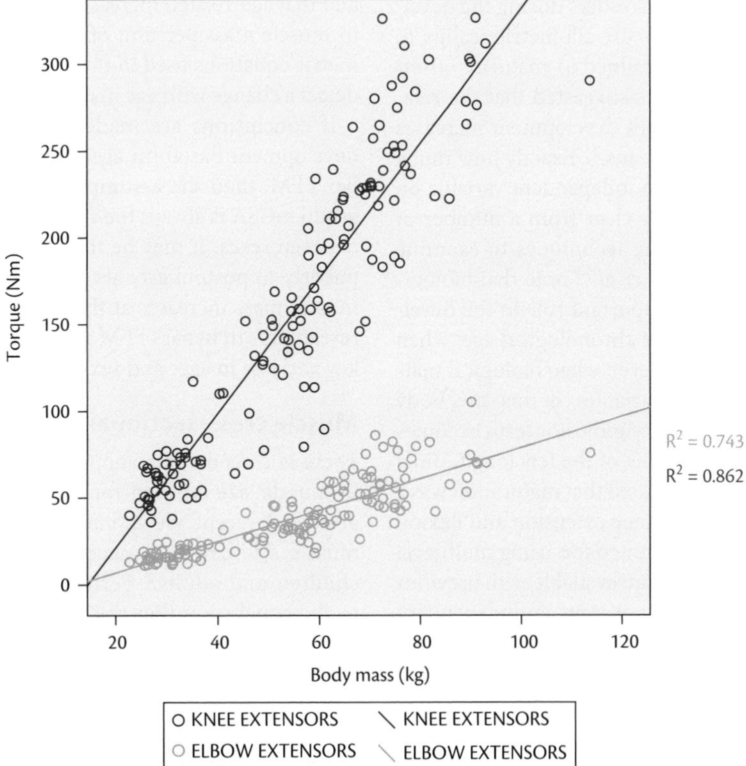

Figure 7.6 Relationship between knee and elbow extension torque and body mass.

Data from Deighan MA, Armstrong N, De Ste Croix MBA. Peak torque per arm muscle cross-sectional area during growth. (Abstract). In: Koskolou M, Geladas N, Klissouras V, eds. 7th Annual congress of the European College of Sport Science. Athens: Pashalidis Medical Publisher; 2002. 47.

isokinetic elbow flexion and extension strength in 13- to 15-year-olds. Conflicting data are available and the study of Round *et al.*[15] suggested that in boys the strength of the knee extensors was disproportionate to the increase in body size. This difference was explained once testosterone was added to the multilevel model.

Although both stature and mass appear to be important explanatory variables of the age- and sex-associated development in strength, it is important to consider that it may be the simultaneous development of other biological factors that are contributing to this increase. For example, it has been postulated that the linear increase in bone with age produces a stimulus for muscle growth and therefore increases in stature with age are associated with increases in muscle size. Changes in stature are also associated with changes in the muscle moment arm. Likewise the changes in proportions of body fat and lean tissue, as a percentage of total body mass, are important factors in the expression of strength with age. Therefore, although simple body dimensions appear to be important in the development of strength with age, only between 40–70% of the variance in strength of 5- to 17-year-olds could be accounted for by age, sex, stature, and body mass, which leaves a large portion of the variance unexplained.[10] This is supported by recent data from Camic *et al.*,[26] who suggested that the age-related changes in isokinetic strength could not be fully accounted for by changes in stature, body mass, or fat-free weight

Maturation and hormonal influences on strength development

A number of studies have shown that strength increases with biological maturation, mapping a similar trend to chronological age.[25,52,53] Gerodimos *et al.*[53] reported a significant maturation-related increase in handgrip strength in wrestlers during the developmental years. One of the few studies to use allometric scaling to account for maturational changes (determined as maturity offset) in muscle size in 14- to 16-year-old boys suggested that the relationship between maturation and strength development increases up until 2 years after PHV, and then plateaus.[24] Exactly how much influence biological maturation has as an independent variable on the development of strength is relatively clear from a number of studies that have used allometric scaling techniques to examine known variables concurrently. Carvalho *et al.*[24] note that biological maturation probably plays a more important role in the development of strength with age than simple chronological age, when examined as an independent factor. However, when biological maturation is explored alongside body size variables (in this case, body mass and thigh volume), then the maturity indicator term becomes non-significant.[24] This is reinforced by one of the few longitudinal studies in 10- to 14-year-olds which indicated that maturation was a non-significant explanatory variable in knee extension and flexion torque, once stature and mass were accounted for, using multilevel modelling procedures.[5] Supporting data are available with previous studies indicating that maturation does not exert an independent effect upon isometric strength development in 10- to 18-year-old athletes[41] and 12- to 14-year-old football players[54] once age and body size have been controlled for. Interestingly, Carvalho *et al.*[24] reported that the maturity indicator term remained significant in their allometric model when only thigh volume was included and only in late adolescence. The authors suggest that this may reflect some form of neuromuscular development during the later stages of maturation.

Well-controlled longitudinal studies that concurrently examine testosterone and maturation, alongside other known variables, are still needed before firm conclusions about the independent influence of maturation on strength development can be established. There is a growing body of literature looking at the influence of biological maturation on adaptations to strength training[55] and this is explored in Chapter 36.

Fat-free mass and strength development

Typically, during childhood and puberty, strength increases coincide with changes in FFM.[10] Moderate to strong correlations have been found between knee extension and flexion torque and FFM in 8- to 13-year-old wrestlers.[56] However, other studies have reported age-related increases in torque per FFM for knee extensors and elbow extensors and flexors that could not be accounted for by changes in FFM.[26,57,58] The age effect for increases in strength, independent of FFM, may be attributable to an increase in muscle mass per unit of FFM or neural maturation which allows for a greater expression of strength. The proportion of FFM which is skeletal muscle has been suggested to increase with age. In addition, the proportion of muscle mass that is distributed at various sites is thought to vary and at birth ~40% of total muscle mass is located in the lower extremities, increasing to ~55% at sexual maturity in both boys and girls.

Studies that have used anthropometric estimations of total body muscle mass have reported that estimated total body muscle mass cannot account for the age-related increase in strength and that non-significant correlations exist between age and estimated muscle mass co-varied for FFM.[56] This suggests that there are nearly proportional increases in total body muscle mass and FFM with age and that age-related increases in strength are not due to an increase in muscle mass per unit of FFM. It is possible that the anthropometric equations used in these studies were not sensitive enough to detect a change with age in the contribution of muscle mass to FFM.

If conclusions are made about the factors affecting strength development based on age- or sex-related differences in strength per FFM, then the assumption must be that a muscle or muscle group mCSA is always the same proportion of FFM across ages and between sexes. It may be that regional mCSA increases from prepuberty to postpuberty at the same rate as FFM and not that total muscle mass increases at the same rate as FFM. This has led most researchers to bypass FFM and investigate changes in mCSA as the key variable in age- and sex-associated development in strength.

Muscle cross-sectional area and strength development

There is considerable support for the contention that differences in muscle size account for differences in muscle strength during growth. A recent 'viewpoint' statement asked the question whether muscle size can fully account for strength differences between children and adults.[8] Perhaps unsurprisingly, the authors came to the conclusion that this remains an open question due to the lack of studies concurrently exploring muscle activation, pennation angles and length, muscle moment arms, and tendon stiffness during childhood. One of the earliest studies of strength and mCSA indicated that strength 'is fairly proportional' to elbow flexor mCSA regardless of age or training status,[59] but the relationship was weaker for girls than boys. Others have reported a strong correlation between muscle size and isometric knee strength (r = 0.87), isokinetic knee strength (r = 0.73), isokinetic elbow strength

($r = 0.82$), and isokinetic triceps surae strength ($r = 0.91$).[10,11,51,76] A recent study has indicated that quadriceps femoris muscle volume accounts largely for the increase in strength that occurs with maturation in boys and girls, not only in kinematically constrained knee extensions but also in multijoint tasks.[9] Numerous longitudinal studies have shown that as an independent covariate mCSA is a significant explanatory variable in the age-associated development of strength.[3,5] However, it would appear that when additional variables are examined concurrently alongside mCSA its influence lessens or disappears.

Age differences in strength per muscle cross-sectional area

There is still some debate about whether strength per mCSA increases with age. Early studies demonstrated increasing strength per mCSA from 7 to 13 years, with greater isokinetic strength per mCSA observed in older (18 years) than younger (7 years) age groups.[60] It is hypothesized that children in the early stages of puberty may not develop strength in proportion to their muscle (plus bone) anthropometric cross-sectional area (ACSA). It is likely that the deficiency of strength per mCSA in the younger age groups might be related to a lack of the ability to mobilize the muscle voluntarily. Kanehisa *et al.*[33] also found that isometric strength of the ankle dorsi flexors and plantar flexors per mCSA was significantly greater only for plantar flexion in 16- to 18-year-old boys compared to the younger age groups. Others have reported a significant increase in isokinetic knee and elbow torque per MRI-determined mCSA from 9 to 16 years, but no significant difference from 16–24 years.[21,61] Further investigation is required to establish whether these differences in torque per mCSA are due to biomechanical or neuromuscular factors. What these data do suggest is that torque per mCSA of the elbow and knee extensors and flexors are at adult levels by around 16 years. Conflicting data are available indicating that, despite smaller MRI determined triceps surae mCSA, early pubertal boys' torque scaled to muscle size is not different from adult males.[62] These conflicting data emphasize the need to measure the strength per mCSA ratio in a variety of muscles as the strength development characteristics of one muscle or group of muscles may not be the same as another, even within the same joint.

Sex differences in strength per muscle cross-sectional area

Whether sex differences exist in strength per mCSA is also debatable. Early work reported that absolute isometric strength differences between sexes disappeared when data were normalized to ACSA in 9- to 12-year-olds. Sunnegardh *et al.*[27] showed that boys had significantly greater torque per ACSA than girls at 13 years. Deighan *et al.*[61] recently reported significant sex differences in isokinetic elbow flexion per mCSA in 9- to 10-year-olds and 16- to 17-year-olds. These studies are in contrast to others that have demonstrated similar strength to mCSA ratios between sexes.[3,57] Deighan *et al.*[21,61] reported no significant sex differences in isokinetic torque per mCSA of the knee extensors and flexors and elbow flexors in 9- to 10-year-olds, 16- to 17-year-olds, and adults. Using multilevel modelling procedures on longitudinal data, Wood *et al.*[3] also reported that sex effects for isokinetic elbow extensors and flexors became non-significant once mCSA was controlled for. The majority of recent studies would lead us therefore to the conclusion that there is no significant sex difference in strength per mCSA irrespective of the muscle joint or action examined. It would appear that factors in addition to mCSA may account for the age- and sex-associated development in strength. For example, the peak gain in muscle strength in boys occurs more often after peak stature and mCSA velocity but there is no such trend for girls. Consequently, this would seem to suggest either a biomechanical effect or a qualitative change in muscle tissue as puberty progresses and perhaps a neuromuscular maturation affecting the volitional demonstration of strength.

Biomechanical factors and strength development

The mechanical advantage of the musculoskeletal system is variable across different muscle groups and is considered unfavourable because the measured force or torque is somewhat smaller than the corresponding tension developed in the muscle tendon. Another unfavourable biomechanical influence on the measured force lies in the internal muscle architecture, i.e. the greater the angle of pennation to the long axis of the muscle the smaller proportion of force in the muscle fibres that is transmitted to the muscle tendon. The age-associated relationships between these factors have not yet been extensively investigated in children.

It is difficult to account for biomechanical factors but some authors have divided strength by the product of mCSA and stature ($Nm \cdot cm^{-3}$), i.e. the product of mCSA and moment arm length which they assume to be proportional to stature.[21,61,63] There are few published data on the relationship between strength per mCSA and mechanical advantage covering age, sex, and different muscle groups but it seems sensible to correct strength for differences in mechanical advantage, especially if comparing children of different sizes.[11] One of the major assumptions with using this method is that muscle moment arm and limb length are proportional to one another.

Kanehisa *et al.*[63] found that isokinetic torque was significantly correlated to mCSA*thigh length ($r = 0.72–0.83$). When 'local' body size measures (limb segment length, ACSA, limb circumferences, and skinfolds) have been used to scale strength data significant age effects persist. Blimkie[10] reported that age effects were the same whether dividing torque by the product of mCSA and stature or just mCSA. Young adults have been found to have significantly higher ratios of isokinetic knee extension torque per unit of mCSA*thigh length than children, with the difference becoming greater with increasing velocity of movement. Kanehisa *et al.*[64] normalized isometric force of the ankle dorsiflexors and plantarflexors to ACSA multiplied by lower leg length to approximate muscle volume and possibly PCSA in 7- to 18-year-old boys and girls. The ratio of plantar flexion force to ACSA*leg length (LL) was significantly higher in the 16- to 18-year-old boys compared to other age groups. Similar age effects between children and adults when isokinetic knee extensor torque was normalized to ACSA*thigh length have been observed.[60,63] Grip force normalized to ACSA*forearm length has also been shown to increase with age in 6- to 23-year-olds.[65] Longitudinal data from isometric and concentric elbow flexion and extension has suggested that age effects are both action and muscle group specific.[3,21,61] Deighan *et al.*[21,61] reported non-significant age effects for the elbow extensors and flexors but a significant difference between 9- to 10-year-olds and 16- to 17-year-olds in knee extension and flexion torque per mCSA*LL. The elbow data findings are supported by the work of Falk *et al.*,[66] who demonstrated no significant difference between prepubertal girls and women in isometric elbow flexion torque normalized to ACSA. Knee data have suggested that mCSA*LL alone cannot account for the age differences in strength.[21,61] It is difficult to attribute physiological reasons to the muscle group differences but it is possible that the differing function of the arms and legs play a part.

No significant sex differences were observed in isometric plantar flexor or dorsi flexor force in boys and girls aged 7–18 years,[64] or in grip force normalized to ACSA*forearm length in 6- to 23-year-olds.[65] Similarly, no significant sex differences were reported in isokinetic knee and elbow extensors and flexors torque per mCSA*LL in 9- to 25-year-olds;[21,61] in prepubertal children when isometric elbow flexion torque was scaled using ACSA;[4] or in isometric/concentric elbow flexion and extension torques per ACSA*arm length in adolescent children over the course of a 3-year longitudinal study.[3] All these data would therefore suggest that sex differences in strength cannot be accounted for by the product of mCSA and limb length.

Muscle strength and tendon/limb stiffness

There has recently been a greater focus on both tendon and limb stiffness in children as they play important roles both in physical performance and injury prevention. Leg stiffness incorporating muscle, tendon, and joint stiffness, is an example of a neuromuscular feed-forward mechanism, acting as protective mechanisms to counteract the external forces placed on the tibiofemoral joint, particularly during dynamic movements.[67,68] Greater levels of leg stiffness increase the ability of the dynamic mechanisms to generate rebound movements during the stretch shortening cycle,[69,70] and strong associations between leg stiffness and sprinting performance have been reported in children.[71,72] Therefore, determining leg stiffness in children may be a useful monitor of neuromuscular function for coaches and clinicians.

Leg stiffness data from paediatric populations are growing and providing us with some compelling information regarding neuromuscular feed-forward mechanisms in children, especially in relation to fatigue.[73,74] Therefore, there is an increasing demand for coaches and clinicians to accurately measure muscle/limb/tendon stiffness in athletes. It is beyond the scope of this chapter to describe fully changes in tendon stiffness with age and interested readers are directed to Blazevich *et al.*[75] The comparability of previous studies can be difficult due to the adoption of different methods to calculate leg stiffness and small sample sizes.[76] Additionally, it is essential for paediatric researchers to normalize stiffness data to body mass and stature/limb length.

Oliver and Smith[72] found significantly higher leg stiffness in adult males compared to prepubescent boys during submaximal hopping at high hopping frequencies. Subsequently others have reported age and maturation-related increases in relative leg stiffness and reactive strength index (RSI).[77–79] Lloyd *et al.*[79] found prepubescent boys (9–12 years) to have lower leg stiffness compared to adolescent boys aged 15 years. This suggests a potential tendency for prepubescent males to rely on feedback mechanisms, with a shift towards feed-forward mechanisms as age increases. This is further highlighted by the greater ground contact times, and shorter flight times demonstrated in prepubescent children.[79] The efficiency of neural control has been reported to increase with age[78] as a child's musculoskeletal system develops.[80] Therefore, the underdeveloped neural control demonstrated in prepubescent children could contribute to the notably lower stiffness levels.[72] Data on leg stiffness in females are sparse, but De Ste Croix[73] found no significant age differences in relative leg stiffness in 12- to 17-year-old girls. Although not statistically significant, lower stiffness was noticeable in 16- to 17-year-olds compared to younger age groups. This contradicts previous studies on males noting increases in leg stiffness with age[72,77–79] but this may be due to the limited maturational range in studies on boys. Whether there are no age-related increases in stiffness in girls remains to be determined.

Torque/force kinetics

As discussed, biological changes in growth and maturation cannot fully account for the age-related development in muscle strength, as children demonstrate lower maximal voluntary force even after age and maturation have been accounted for. This has led authors to propose that children have a lower level of maximal voluntary muscle activation than adults, termed the *activation deficit*.[81] This has led to a number of studies exploring force or torque kinetics during dynamic muscle actions and proposing that slower kinetics can indirectly support the view that there is reduced type II motor unit utilization in children compared to adults. This is compelling given the difficulty in directly determining activation of different fibre types. The determination of torque or force kinetics rather than absolute maximal force/torque also has some ecological validity, as a high rate of force development is often more important than maximal force in most sporting activities. Despite this, few studies have explored rate of force development or force kinetics in children. Those that are available have examined adult/child differences rather than explore changes throughout childhood due to growth and maturation. Dotan *et al.*[81,82] have described the adult/child-related differences in torque kinetics showing significantly faster and greater torque kinetics in adults compared to 8- to 11-year-old boys (see Figure 7.7). All torque kinetic parameters were significantly lower in young boys compared to adults and were greater for the elbow flexors than knee extensors. Time to both 30% and 80% of maximal voluntary contraction (MVC) was 24% and 48% longer, respectively, in the boys. This kinetic disparity in part probably explains young children's disadvantage in tasks requiring speed or explosive force compared to adults.

Dotan *et al.*[81,82] proposed that these child/adult differences cannot be explained by muscle composition and/or musculo-tendinous-stiffness and must reflect children's lower utilization of type II motor units. There appear to be no studies that have explored torque kinetics in young girls and only one study that has examined time to peak torque in young females. This study demonstrated that there were no significant sex differences in the knee and elbow extensor and flexor muscles' isokinetic time to reach peak torque.[83] This may suggest that child-adult differences might also be evident for females, although only direct measurement will determine if child-adult differences in torque kinetics are as pronounced in females as they are in males. Interestingly, when a highly trained young group were added into the analysis their torque kinetics were similar to adults, indicating potential strength training effects in developing torque kinetics in children.[82] If changes in torque kinetics support the data demonstrating lower motor unit activation in children compared with adults,[9,84] then it may be a simple indirect method to examine age-related changes in neuromuscular function.

Time to peak twitch torque and twitch relaxation indices can be used as a measure of rate of energy turnover and fibre type

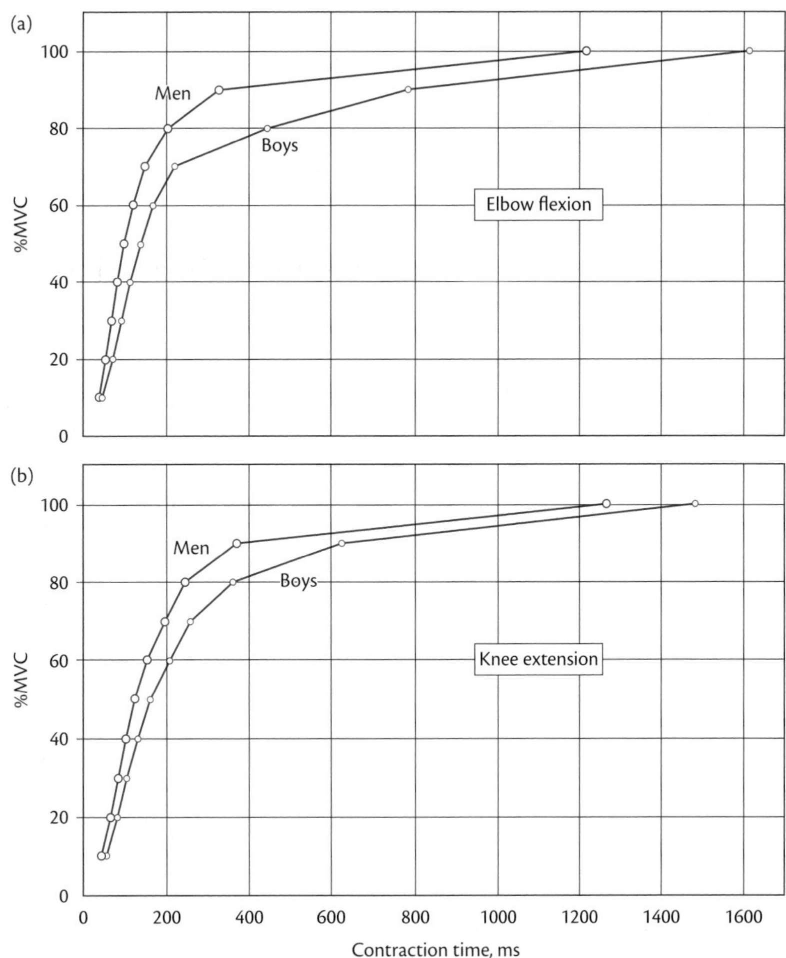

Figure 7.7 Child and adult differences in torque kinetics during elbow flexion (a) and knee extension (b).
Dotan R, Mitchell C, Cohen R, Gabriel D, Klentrou P, Falk B. Child–adult differences in the kinetics of torque development. J Sports Sci. 2013; 31: 945–953.

composition. Twitch relaxation times have been shown to be similar in boys and girls and are not influenced by age. Also, it has been found that time to peak twitch force and relaxation times are the same regardless of age during childhood.[85] Likewise, similar time to peak twitch tension was demonstrated in 3-year-olds as in 25-year-olds. These data suggest that muscle fibre composition and muscle activation speed are similar between these age groups and that there is no difference in the fibre type distribution from the age of approximately 7 years. Previous authors have suggested that the neuromuscular system is still maturing with respect to the myelination of the nerves in younger children.[85] Also muscle fibre conduction velocity has been seen to increase with age in children. The influence that neuromuscular factors have on the development of muscle strength, concurrently with other known variables, remains to be established.

Neuromuscular function

Methodological issues in measuring neuromuscular function

One of the key issues with understanding neuromuscular development with age and maturation is the difficulty in determining neuromuscular function. Many studies that profess to determine neuromuscular capability in children are often based on indirect measures of neuromuscular function. The preferred method to explore neuromuscular capability is to measure muscle activation using surface EMG. It is beyond the scope of this chapter to describe all of the associated potential sources of error in using surface EMG, although the potential to provide some indication of different elements that make up neuromuscular performance means that surface EMG is still seen as the method of choice. Relatively few studies have used EMG with children, although the data that are available have allowed us to explore if child-adult differences may be associated with a neuromuscular deficit, similarly to that of the described force deficit. Unfortunately, the majority of paediatric data purporting to determine neuromuscular function have either used indirect measures of neuromuscular capability or not looked at the sub-components of neuromuscular function that are important for differing performance and injury related reasons. For example Quatman *et al.*[86] conducted a 2-year longitudinal study examining sex differences in landing force and jump performance in adolescent athletes, suggesting that a neuromuscular spurt during puberty is evident in boys but not in girls. These data must be viewed with some caution as the neuromuscular measurement was vertical jump height and landing force. A recent comprehensive review of neuromuscular function around the knee states that the effects of growth and maturation on neuromuscular function during childhood are poorly understood and have not been thoroughly investigated.[50] However, available data would appear to suggest that children display different neuromuscular profiles compared with adults, which may vary depending upon both muscle action and/or movement velocity. What is relatively well known is that age-related changes in force generation are generally accompanied to some degree by changes in neuromuscular activation patterns. Age-related changes in torque kinetics reinforce the likelihood that neuromuscular factors probably play a significant role in the adult/child related differences in muscle strength (e.g. the observed force deficit).

There are a number of well designed studies that show that children have a reduced ability to recruit their motor unit pool compared to adults.[81,82,87,88] The study of O'Brien *et al.*[9] suggests that adults have the ability to activate a greater percentage of their MU pool compared with boys (87% vs 75%) and girls (87% vs 68%). We would assume that at some stage this ability to activate a greater percentage of motor units develops with age and maturation. However, no studies have longitudinally explored changes in % motor unit activation so how/when this occurs during growth and maturation remains to be elucidated. It is surprising that this is still unknown, given the performance and injury risk implications of reduced % motor unit recruitment.

Neuromuscular feedforward and feedback mechanisms

There are few studies that have examined the age- and sex-associated changes in knee muscle activation during landing or pivoting tasks, but studies have shown reduced pre-activation of hamstring muscles prior to landing in children compared with adults.[89,90] These data suggest that neuromuscular feed-forward mechanisms are more mature in adults compared with children, which provides an interesting insight into neuromuscular feed-forward mechanisms.

Electromechanical delay during growth and maturation

Electrochemical delay has been implicated as a risk factor for knee injury in children[91] and EMD varies between 30–50 ms up to as much as a few hundred milliseconds depending on the muscle examined and movement velocity.[92] Very few studies have examined EMD during childhood and there appears to be only one longitudinal study.[66,93–95]

The work of Gosset *et al.*[95] focused on ankle stiffness and EMD of the triceps surae and reported a longer EMD in children suffering with Legg-Calve-Perthes disease (a hip disorder) compared to healthy controls, albeit only in six children. Cohen *et al.*[93] also found significantly longer EMD in young children (9–12 years) compared to adults (65 vs 57 ms, respectively) for knee and elbow extension and flexion during isometric actions. However, they did not show any significant difference between the endurance trained and untrained children, suggesting that level of training status did not have an effect on EMD. Falk *et al.*[66] and Zhou *et al.*[94] both reported a significantly longer EMD in prepubertal boys compared with adult males and in 8- to 12-year-olds compared with 13- to 16-year-olds and adults respectively. Recently, Dotan *et al.*[82] showed significantly slower EMD in 8- to 12-year-old boys compared with adult males. Interestingly, in young trained gymnasts EMD was identical to untrained males indicating the potential effects of reducing EMD in children through training. A recent study exploring changes in EMD after simulated soccer match play in 12- to 17-year-old girls indicated that EMD increases when fatigue is present in all age groups, compromising neuromuscular feedback mechanisms.[96]

This longer EMD in children may be as a result of differences in muscle composition. However, limited evidence suggests that differences in muscle composition are not sufficient to account for the child-adult differences. Therefore differences in muscle activation, such as excitation-contraction coupling and muscle fibre conduction velocity, have been implicated in this longer EMD. Therefore, this lower rate of force development may reduce muscle-tendinous stiffness and increase the potential for injury in children. However, Grosset *et al.*[84] reported greater electrically stimulated EMD for the triceps surae in 7-year-olds compared with 11-year-old prepubertal children. This indicates a potential increase in muscle-tendinous stiffness with age independent of maturation. However, this hypothesis requires further investigation employing longitudinal studies throughout childhood and including female participants.

Only one study appears to have explored sex differences in EMD of the knee extensors during childhood, and no sex differences were reported in either the 8- to 12-year-old or 13- to 16-year-old age groups.[94] Whether EMD accounts for the greater relative risk of non-contact ACL injury in girls is unclear as there are no studies that have examined sex differences in EMD in children during eccentric muscle actions. It is surprising that there is only one study on the EMD of young girls, given that they are the most at risk group for non-contact ACL injury. It remains to be identified how EMD may change during childhood, particularly for the knee flexors and eccentric actions. Further study is needed to explore the age- and sex-related changes in EMD, linked to performance and the relative risk of injury.

Conclusions

Despite a growing literature base exploring differing strength-related factors in paediatric populations there is still a distinct lack of well-controlled longitudinal investigations into the static and dynamic development of muscle strength. As the current evidence base reveals muscle group- and muscle action-specific differences in the age- and sex-associated development in strength, then caution is advised when describing strength changes during childhood. Although there is disagreement about when sex differences occur it is recognized that few girls outperform boys by 15 years. Importantly, many of the factors discussed in this chapter play a role in strength development when examined as independent variables. However, the picture changes when known variables are examined concurrently. It would appear that for dynamic muscle actions in particular, mechanical and neuromuscular factors may play a large role in the development of strength with age. The greatest challenge still, is to elucidate the factors that contribute to the age- and sex-associated development in strength, concurrently with other known explanatory variables. Researchers are turning to new technologies to advance the understanding of the mechanisms that contribute to the development of force (e.g. determining muscle pennation angle to calculate PCSA and muscle tendon stiffness).[97]

Summary

- There are distinct differences in static and dynamic strength characteristics in children which must be acknowledged when examining age- and sex-associated changes in strength.

- Age- and sex-associated changes in muscle strength, combined with the factors that contribute to this development, appear to be muscle group and muscle action specific.
- The age-associated development in strength is attributable to the shared variance in growth and maturation. Sex differences appear at around 14 years of age and very few girls outperform boys in strength tests at 18 years.
- Stature and mass appear to be important explanatory variables in the development of muscle strength but may be reflective of changes in biomechanical factors, such as the muscle moment arm. Peak height velocity is a particularly important time for maximal gains in strength during childhood.
- Biological maturation does not appear to exert an influence on strength development but circulating hormones, such as testosterone, appear to stimulate the development in muscle size.
- Neuromuscular maturation is poorly understood and may contribute to the improvement in motor unit activation with age.
- More understanding is needed to elucidate the age- and sex-associated changes in torque/force kinetics and potential utilization of type II motor units.
- Studies should attempt to directly determine the neuromuscular deficit during childhood to help explain the role that neuromuscular capability plays in the age- and sex-associated changes in strength.
- Investigation of muscle tendon force and stiffness is needed that encompasses the maturational period.

References

1. De Ste Croix MBA. Isokinetic assessment and interpretation in paediatric populations: Why do we know relatively little? *Iso Exerc Sci.* 2012; 20: 275–291.
2. De Ste Croix MBA. Advances in paediatric strength testing: changing our perspective on age and sex associated differences in muscle strength. *J Sports Sci Med.* 2007; 6: 292–304.
3. Wood LE, Dixon S, Grant C, Armstrong N. Elbow flexion and extension strength relative to body size or muscle size in children. *Med Sci Sports Exerc.* 2004; 36: 1977–1984.
4. Wood LE, Dixon S, Grant C, Armstrong N. Elbow flexor strength, muscle size, and moment arms in prepubertal boys and girls. *Pediatr Exerc Sci.* 2006; 18: 457–469.
5. De Ste Croix MBA, Armstrong N, Welsman JR, Sharpe P. Longitudinal changes in isokinetic leg strength in 10–14 year olds. *Ann Hum Biol.* 2002; 29: 50–62.
6. De Ste Croix MBA, Deighan MA, Armstrong N. Assessment and interpretation of isokinetic strength during growth and maturation. *Sports Med.* 2003; 33: 727–743.
7. Pitcher CA, Elliott CM, Williams SA, *et al.* Childhood muscle morphology and strength: alterations over six months of growth. *Muscle and Nerve.* 2012; 46: 360–366.
8. Bouchant A, Martin V, Maffiuletti NA, Ratel S. Can muscle size fully account for strength differences between children and adults? *J Appl Physiol.* 2011; 110: 1748–1749.
9. O'Brien TD, Reeves ND, Baltzopoulos V, Jones DA, Maganaris CN. In vivo measurements of muscle specific tension in adults and children. *Exper Physiol.* 2010; 95: 202–210.
10. Blimkie CJR Age and sex-associated variation in strength during childhood: Anthropometric, morphologic, neurologic, biomechanical, endocrinologic, genetic and physical activity correlates. In: Gisolf CV, Lamb DR (eds.) *Perspectives in exercise science and sports medicine: Youth, exercise and sport Vol. 2.* Indianapolis: Benchmark Press; 1989. p. 99–163.
11. Blimkie CJR, Macauley D Muscle strength. In: Armstrong N, Van-Mechelen W (eds.) *Paediatric exercise science and medicine.* Oxford: Oxford University Press; 2000. p. 23–36.
12. Ravary B, Pourcelot P, Bortolussi C, Konieczka S, Crevier-Denoix N. Strain and force transducers used in human and veterinary tendon and ligament biomechanical studies. *Clin Biomech.* 2004; 19: 433–447.
13. Nevill AM, Holder RL, Baxter-Jones A, Round JM, Jones DA. Modeling developmental changes in strength and aerobic power in children. *J Appl Physiol.* 1998; 84: 963–970.
14. Parker DF, Round JM, Sacco P, Jones DA. A cross-sectional survey of upper and lower limb strength in boys and girls during childhood and adolescence. *Ann Hum Biol.* 1990; 17: 199–211.
15. Round JM, Jones DA, Honour JW, Nevill AM. Hormonal factors in the development of differences in strength between boys and girls during adolescence: a longitudinal study. *Ann Hum Biol.* 1999; 26: 49–62.
16. Pandy MG. Moment arm of a muscle force. *Exerc Sport Sci Rev.* 1999; 27: 79–118.
17. Baltzopoulos B, King M, Gleeson N, De Ste Croix M. The BASES expert statement on measurement of muscle strength with isokinetic dynamometry. *Sport and Exerc Sci.* 2012; 31: 12–13.
18. Aagaard P, Simonsen EB, Trolle M, Bangsbo J. Klausen K. Isokinetic hamstring/quadriceps strength ratio: influence from joint angular velocity, gravity correction and contraction mode. *Acta Physiol Scand.* 1995; 154: 421–427.
19. Kellis E. Antagonist moment of force during maximal knee extension in pubertal boys: effects of quadriceps fatigue. *Eur J Appl Physiol.* 2003; 89: 271–280.
20. Kellis E, Baltzopoulos V. The effects of antagonist moment on the resultant knee joint moment during isokinetic testing of the knee extensors. *Eur J Appl Physiol Occ Physiol.* 1997; 76: 253–259.
21. Deighan MA, Armstrong N, De Ste Croix MBA. Peak torque per MRI-determined cross-sectional area of knee extensors and flexors in children, teenagers and adults. (Abstract). *J Sports Sci.* 2003; 21: 236.
22. Iga J, George K, Lees A, Reilly T. Cross-sectional investigation of indices of isokinetic leg strength in youth soccer players and untrained individuals. *Scand J Med Sci Sports.* 2009; 19: 714–720.
23. Weir JP, Housh TJ, Johnson GO, Housh DJ, Ebersole KT. Allometric scaling of isokinetic peak torque: The Nebraska wrestling study. *Eur J Appl Physiol.* 1999; 80: 240–248.
24. Carvalho HM, Coelho-e-Silva M, Valente-dos-Santos J, Gonçalves RS, Philippaerts R, Malina R. Scaling lower-limb isokinetic strength for biological maturation and body size in adolescent basketball players. *Eur J Appl Physiol.* 2012; 112: 2881–2889.
25. Forbes H, Bullers A, Lovell A, McNaughton LR, Polman RC, Siegler JC. Relative torque profiles of elite male youth footballers: effects of age and pubertal development. *Int J Sports Med.* 2009; 30: 592–597
26. Camic CL, Housh TJ, Weir JP, *et al.* Influences of body-size variables on age-related increases in isokinetic peak torque in young wrestlers. *J Strength Cond Res.* 2010; 24: 2358–2365.
27. Sunnegardh J, Bratteby LE, Nordesjo LO, Nordgren B. Isometric and isokinetic muscle strength, anthropometry and physical activity in 8- and 13-year-old Swedish children. *Eur J Appl Physiol.* 1988; 58: 291–297.
28. Carron AV, Bailey DA. Strength development in boys from 10 through 16 years. *Monogr Soc Res Child Dev.* 1974; 39: 1–37.
29. Eek MN, Kroksmark AK, Beckung E. Isometric muscle torque in children 5 to 15 years of age: Normative data. *Arch Phys Med Rehab.* 2006; 87: 1091–1099.
30. Backman E, Henriksson KG. Skeletal muscle characteristics in children 9–15 years old: force, relaxation rate and contraction time. *Clin Physiol.* 1988; 8: 521–527.
31. Kanehisa H, Kuno S, Katsuta S, Fukunaga T. A 2-year follow-up study on muscle size and dynamic strength in teenage tennis players. *Scand J Med Sci Sports.* 2006; 16: 93–99.

32. Holm I, Steen H, Olstad M. Isokinetic muscle performance in growing boys from pre-teen to maturity. An eleven-year longitudinal study. *Iso Exerc Sci*. 2005; 13: 153–156.
33. Kanehisa H, Abe T, Fukunaga T. Growth trends of dynamic strength in adolescent boys. A 2-year follow-up survey. *J Sports Med Phys Fit*. 2003; 43: 459–464.
34. Peltonen JE, Taimela S, Erkintalo M, Salminen JJ, Oksanen A, Kujala UM. Back extensor and psoas muscle cross-sectional area, prior physical training, and trunk muscle strength—a longitudinal study in adolescent girls. *Eur J Appl Physiol*. 1998; 77: 66–71.
35. Newcomer K, Sinaki M, Wollan P. Physical activity and four year development of back strength in children. *Am J Phys Med Rehab*. 1997; 76: 52–58.
36. Mueller J, Mueller S, Stoll J, Baur H, Mayer F. Trunk Extensor and Flexor Strength Capacity in Healthy Young Elite Athletes Aged 11–15 Years. *J Strength Cond Res*. 2014; 28: 1328–1334.
37. Deighan, MA, De Ste Croix MBA, Armstrong N. Measurement of maximal muscle cross-sectional area of knee and elbow extensors and flexors in children, teenagers and adults *J Sports Sci*. 2006; 24: 543–546.
38. Barber-Westin SD, Noyes FR, Galloway M. Jump-land characteristics and muscle strength development in young athletes. A gender comparison of 1140 athletes 9 to 17 years of age. *Am J Sports Med*. 2006; 34: 375–384.
39. De Ste Croix MBA, Armstrong N, Welsman JR Concentric isokinetic leg strength in pre-teen, teenage and adult males and females. *Biol Sport*. 1999; 16: 75–86.
40. Buchanan PA, Vardaxis VG. Lower-extremity strength profiles and gender-based classification of basketball players ages 9–22 years. *J Strength Cond Res*. 2009; 23: 406–419.
41. Maffulli N, King JB, Helms P. Training in elite youth athletes: Injuries, flexibility and isometric strength. *Br J Sports Med*. 1994; 28: 123–136.
42. Davies CTM. Strength and mechanical properties of muscle in children and young adults. *Scand J Sport Sci*. 1985; 7: 11–15.
43. Gilliam TB, Villanacci JF, Freedson PS, Sady SP. Isokinetic torque in boys and girls ages 7 to 13: Effect of age, height and weight. *Res Q*. 1979; 50: 599–609.
44. Falk B, Tenenbaum G. The effectiveness of resistance training in children: a meta-analysis. *Sports Med*. 1996; 22: 176–186.
45. Silva RS, Serrão FV. Sex differences in trunk, pelvis, hip and knee kinematics and eccentric hip torque in adolescents. *Clin Biomech*. 2014; 29: 1063–1069.
46. Bittencourt NF, Santos TR, Gonçalves GG, *et al*. Reference values of hip abductor torque among youth athletes: Influence of age, sex and sports. *Phys Ther Sport*. 2016. doi: 10.1016/j.ptsp.2015.12.005
47. Rasmussen B, Kalusen K, Jespersen B, Jensen K. A longitudinal study of development in growth and maturation of 10- to 15-year old girls and boys. In: Oseid S, Carlsen HK (eds.) *Children and exercise XIII*. Champaign, IL: Human Kinetics; 1990. p. 103–111.
48. Wild CY, Steele JR, Munro BJ. Insufficient hamstring strength compromises landing technique in adolescent girls. *Med Sci Sports Exerc*. 2013; 45: 497–505.
49. Sigward SM, Pollard CD, Havens KL, Powers CM. The influence of sex and maturation on knee mechanics during side-step cutting. *Med Sci Sports Exerc*. 2012; 44: 1497–1503.
50. Kellis E, Mademli L, Patikas D, Kofotolis N. Neuromuscular interactions around the knee in children, adults and elderly. *World J Ortho*. 2014; 5: 469–485.
51. National children and youth fitness study. *J Phys Ed Rec Dance*. 1985; 56: 45–50.
52. Faust MS. Somatic development of adolescent girls. *Soc Res Child Dev*. 1977; 42: 1–90.
53. Gerodimos V, Karatrantou K, Dipla K, Zafeiridis A, Tsiakaras N, Sotiriadis S. Age-related differences in peak handgrip strength between wrestlers and nonathletes during the developmental years. *J Strength Cond Res*. 2013; 27: 616–623.
54. Forbes H, Sutcliffe S, Lovell A, McNaughton LR, Siegler JC. Isokinetic thigh muscle ratios in youth football: effect of age and dominance. *Int J Sports Med*. 2009; 30: 602–606.
55. Meylan C, Malatesta D. Effects of in-season plyometric training within soccer practice on explosive actions of young players. *J Strength Cond Res*. 2009; 23: 2605–2613.
56. Housh TJ, Johnson GO, Housh DJ, Stout JR, Weir JP, Weir LL. Isokinetic peak torque in young wrestlers. *Pediatr Exerc Sci*. 1996; 8: 143–155.
57. Housh TJ, Stout JR, Housh DJ, Johnston GO. The covariate influence of muscle mass on isokinetic peak torque in high school wrestlers. *Pediatr Exerc Sci*. 1995; 7: 176–182.
58. Housh TJ, Stout JR, Weir JP, Weir LL, Housh DJ, Johnson GO. Relationships of age and muscle mass to peak torque in high school wrestlers. *Res Q Exerc Sport*. 1995; 66: 256–261.
59. Ikai M, Fukunaga T. Calculation of muscle strength per unit cross-sectional area of human muscle by means of ultrasonic measurement. *Int Z Angew Physiol Einschl Arbeitsphysiol*. 1968; 26: 26–32.
60. Kanehisa H, Ikegawa S, Tsunoda N, Fukunaga T. Strength and cross-sectional areas of reciprocal muscle groups in the upper arm and thigh during adolescence. *Int J Sports Med*. 1995; 16: 54–60.
61. Deighan MA, Armstrong N, De Ste Croix MBA. Peak torque per arm muscle cross-sectional area during growth. (Abstract). In: Koskolou M, Geladas N, Klissouras V (eds.) *7th Annual congress of the European College of Sport Science*. Athens: Pashalidis Medical Publisher; 2002. p. 47.
62. Morse CI, Tolfrey K, Thom JM, Vassilopoulos V, Maganaris CN, Narici MV. Gastrocnemius muscle specific force in boys and men. *J Appl Physiol*. 2008; 104: 469–474.
63. Kanehisa H, Ikegawa S, Tsunoda N, Fukanaga T. Strength and cross-sectional area of knee extensor muscles in children. *Eur J Appl Physiol*. 1994; 68: 402–405.
64. Kanehisa H, Ikegawa S, Fukunaga T. Comparison of muscle cross-sectional area and strength between untrained women and men. *Eur J Appl Physiol*. 1994; 68: 148–154.
65. Neu CM, Rauch F, Rittweger J, Manz F, Schoenau E. Influence of puberty on muscle development at the forearm. *Am J Physiol Endoc Metab*. 2002; 283: 103–107.
66. Falk B, Usselman C, Dotan R, *et al*. Child-adult differences in muscle strength and activation pattern during isometric elbow flexion and extension. *Appl Physiol Nutr Metabol*. 2009; 34: 609–615.
67. Riemannn BL, Lephart SM. The Sensorimotor System, Part I: The physiologic basis of functional joint stability. *J Athl Train*. 2002; 37: 71–79.
68. Hughes G, Watkins J. A risk-factor model for anterior cruciate ligament injury. *Sports Med*. 2006; 36: 411–426.
69. Granata KP, Padua DA, Wilson SE. Gender differences in active musculoskeletal stiffness. Part II. Quantification of leg stiffness during functional hopping tasks. *J Electro Kinesiol*. 2002; 12: 127–135.
70. Padua DA, Carcia CR, Arnold BL, Granata KP. Gender differences in leg stiffness and stiffness recruitment strategy during two-legged hopping. *J Motor Behav*. 2005; 37: 111–125.
71. Chelly SM, Dennis C. Leg power and hopping stiffness: relationship with sprint running performance. *Med Sci Sports Exerc*. 2001; 33: 326–333.
72. Oliver JL, Smith PM. Neural control of leg stiffness during hopping in boys and men. *J Electro Kinesiol*. 2010; 20: 973–979.
73. De Ste Croix MBA. The effect of football specific fatigue on dynamic knee stability in female youth players: *UEFA Research Grant Programme Final Report*. Unpublished Report. 2012.
74. De Ste Croix MBA. Neuromuscular readiness to reperform in female youth footballers *FIFA Research Grant Programme Final Report*. Unpublished Report. 2014.
75. Blazevich AJ, Waugh CM, Korff T. Development of musculo-skeletal stiffness. In: De Ste Croix MBA, Korff T (eds.) *Paediatric biomechanics and motor control: Theory and application*. Oxford: Routledge; 2011. p. 96–118.
76. Serpell BG, Ball NB, Scarvell JM, Smith PN. A review of models of vertical, leg, and knee stiffness in adults for running, jumping or hopping tasks, *J Sports Sci*. 2012; 30: 1347–1363.

77. Lambertz D, Mora I, Grosset JF, Perot C. Evaluation of musculotendinous stiffness in prepubertal children and adults, taking into account muscle activity. *J Appl Physiol.* 2003; 95: 64–72.
78. Lloyd RS, Oliver JL, Hughes MG, Williams CA. Specificity of test selection for the appropriate assessment of different measures of stretch-shortening cycle function in children. *J Sports Med Phys Fit.* 2011; 51: 595–602.
79. Lloyd RS, Oliver JL, Hughes MG, Williams CA. The influence of chronological age on periods of accelerated adaptation of stretch-shortening cycle performance in pre- and post-pubescent boys. *J Strength Cond Res.* 2011; 25: 1889–1897.
80. De Ste Croix MBA, Deighan MA. Development of joint stability during childhood. In: De Ste Croix MBA and Korff T (eds.) *Paediatric biomechanical and motor control: Theory and application.* Oxford: Routledge; 2011. p. 233–258.
81. Dotan R, Mitchell C, Cohen R, Gabriel D, Klentrou P, Falk B. Child–adult differences in the kinetics of torque development. *J Sports Sci.* 2013; 31: 945–953.
82. Dotan R, Mitchell C, Cohen R, Klentrou P, Gabriel D, Falk B. Child–adult differences in muscle activation—a review. *Pediatr Exerc Sci.* 2012; 24: 2–21.
83. De Ste Croix MBA, Deighan MA, Armstrong N. Time to peak torque for knee and elbow extensors and flexors in children, teenagers and adults. *Iso Exerc Sci.* 2004; 12: 143–148.
84. Grosset JF, Lapole T, Mora I, Verhaeghe M, Doutrellot PL, Perot C. Follow-up of ankle stiffness and electromechanical delay in immobilized children: three case studies. *J Electro Kines.* 2010; 20: 642–647.
85. Houmard JA, Smith R, Jendrasiak GL. Relationship between MRI relaxation time and muscle fibre composition. *J Appl Physiol.* 1995; 78: 807–809.
86. Quatman-Yates CC, Myer GD, Ford KR, Hewett TE. A longitudinal evaluation of maturational effects on lower extremity strength in female adolescent athletes. *Pediatr Phys Ther.* 2013; 25: 271–276.
87. Blimkie CJR, Ebbesen B, MacDougall D, Bar-Or O, Sale D. Voluntary and electrically evoked strength characteristics of obese and non-obese preadolescent boys. *Hum Biol.* 1989; 61: 515–532.
88. Fox EJ, Moon H, Kwon M, Chen YT, Christou EA. Neuromuscular control of goal-directed ankle movements differs for healthy children and adults. *Eur J Appl Physiol.* 2014; 114: 1889–1899.
89. Russell PJ, Croce RV, Swartz EE, Decoster LC. Knee-muscle activation during landings: Developmental and gender comparisons. *Med Sci Sports Exerc.* 2007; 39: 159–169.
90. Lazaridis S, Bassa E, Patikas D, Giakas G, Gollhofer A, Kotzamanidis C. Neuromuscular differences between prepubescents boys and adult men during drop jump. *Eur J Appl Physiol.* 2010; 110: 67–75.
91. Troy BJ, Bell D, Norcross M, Hudson J, Engstrom L. Comparison of hamstring neuromechanical properties between healthy males and females and the influence of musculotendinous stiffness. *J Electro Kines.* 2009; 19: e362–369.
92. Shultz S, Perrin D. Using surface electromyography to assess sex differences in neuromuscular response characteristics. *J Athl Train.* 1999; 34: 165–176.
93. Cohen R, Mitchell C, Dotan R, Gabriel D, Klentrou P, Falk B. Do neuromuscular adaptations occur in endurance-trained boys and men? *Appl Physiol Nutrit Metabol.* 2010; 35: 471–479.
94. Zhou S, Lawson DL, Morrison WE, Fairweather I. Electromechanical delay of knee extensors: the normal range and the effects of age and gender. *J Hum Move Stud.* 1995; 28: 127–146.
95. Grosset J F, Mora I, Lambertz D, Perot C. Changes in stretch reflexes and muscle stiffness with age in prepubescent children. *J Appl Physiol.* 2007; 102: 2352–2360.
96. De Ste Croix MB, Priestley AM, Lloyd RS, Oliver JL. ACL injury risk in elite female youth soccer: Changes in neuromuscular control of the knee following soccer-specific fatigue. *Scand J Med Sci Sports.* 2015; 25: 531–538.
97. Maganaris CN, Baltzopoulos V, Ball D, Sargeant AJ. In vivo specific tension of human skeletal muscle. *J Appl Physiol.* 2001; 90: 865–872.
98. Froberg K, Lammert O. Development of muscle strength during childhood. In: Bar-Or O (ed.) *The child and adolescent athlete.* London: Blackwell Scientific; 1996. p. 25–41.
99. Quatman CE, Ford KR, Myer GD, Hewett TE. Maturation leads to gender differences in landing force and vertical jump performance A longitudinal study. *Am J Sports Med.* 2006; 34: 806–813.

CHAPTER 8

Maximal-intensity exercise

Craig A Williams and Sébastien Ratel

Introduction

Most studies of paediatric maximal intensity exercise have used the Wingate Anaerobic Test (WAnT) devised by Cumming *et al.*[1] and popularized by Ayalon *et al.*,[2] Bar-Or,[3] and Inbar *et al.*[4] from the Wingate Institute in Israel. This test measures several indices of external mechanical power production; peak power (PP) usually over 1 or 5 s, mean power (MP) over 30 s, and the Fatigue Index (FI). Although other protocols such as the Force-Velocity (F-V) test or isokinetic cycle sprint tests have been developed, the contribution from the Wingate Institute should not be underestimated.

Despite advances in methodological techniques that have enabled informative inferences to be drawn about young people's maximal intensity exercise, it is still poorly understood. This observation is interesting for a number of reasons. Firstly, during the prepubertal years, children's physical activity patterns generally consist of short duration but intermittent maximal intensity bouts of effort that are difficult to characterize.[5] Secondly, despite new technology, investigators are still limited to the assessment of external, but indirect, mechanical indices of maximal intensity exercise upon which to infer changes in metabolism. Thirdly, there are few data on females. Finally, due to the importance of maximal intensity efforts during sports and the increasing emphasis on organized youth sport programmes, the differentiation between growth and maturation and training adaptations of maximal intensity still need to be addressed. Consequently, important reliability and validity issues need to be resolved prior to paediatric exercise scientists determining which key factors influence maximal intensity exercise during childhood and adolescence. This chapter focuses on the variables that are most commonly measured and reviews the determinants of young people's maximal intensity exercise and the consequential effects of growth and maturation.

Definition of maximal-intensity of exercise

In both the adult and paediatric exercise science literature there has been a plethora of terms (short-term muscle power, supramaximal, and maximal intensity) used to describe exercise that is 'all-out'. This descriptor could conveniently be applied to peak or maximal oxygen uptake ($\dot{V}O_2$), but in the absolute sense of 'all-out' exercise, the mechanical power production during a peak $\dot{V}O_2$ determination only represents 25–33% of the possible maximal power output. For example, a child who reaches the criteria for peak $\dot{V}O_2$ and produces a maximal power output of 185 W on a cycle ergometer can produce two or three times as much power in a 30-s sprint cycle ride. The power output during short maximal-intensity sprints and peak $\dot{V}O_2$ have been examined between boys and men, and between adolescent boys and girls.[6,7] As predicted, both found significantly higher PP during a 90 s maximal sprint compared to maximal minute power obtained during the peak $\dot{V}O_2$ test. More interestingly however, the adolescent boys and girls were able to attain $\dot{V}O_2$ values that were closer to their peak $\dot{V}O_2$ (~93%) than adults. These results demonstrate that the limits to the maximum sustainable ATP turnover rate in the muscle are dependent on the maximum flux capacity for ATP production, in tandem with the duration of the required sprint. For short-duration sprints, all three metabolic pathways will contribute to the sustainable rate. However, the important principle is the balance of the maximum flux capacities relative to each other and their differing elasticizes to calcium and net ATP hydrolysis.[8] The synchronous effect of the three pathways is represented by the power output profile in Figure 8.1 where at the end of the 90 s test, the maximum sustainable rate of exercise is becoming more dependent upon oxidative phosphorylation than the glycolytic and high-energy phosphates. The misconception of the synchrony between the three flux capacities has often led to an assertion that the aerobic system responds slowly to the energy demands of maximum-intensity exercise, thereby playing little part in short-duration exercise.[9]

Accounting for the discrepancy between power output produced in peak $\dot{V}O_2$ tests compared to shorter-duration sprint exercise tests, the descriptor 'supramaximal' has often been used to describe this intensity of all-out exercise. However, this descriptor is contradictory because it implies that a subject's maximal effort can be exceeded. Therefore, the appropriate term should not focus on the measurement variable per se (i.e. power output, distance, speed, and impulse) but that the metabolism that supports the exercise demonstrates a higher anaerobic ATP yield than oxidative phosphorylation.[10]

Assessment of maximal-intensity exercise

The two main components of maximal-intensity exercise assessment are peak power output and mean power output. Peak power output (PP) is the maximum rate at which energy is transferred to the external system and mean power output (MP) is the total work done during the performance test divided by the time taken.[11] Young people's PP has been assessed using jumping, cycling, running, and isokinetic dynamometry, but the validity of these tests is difficult to assess. For a test to be valid it must also be reliable, and because of the widespread and inappropriate use of the correlation coefficient as a measure of test–retest reliability[12,13] there is little information on the variation in repeated measurements by the same participant on the same performance test. Even if performance tests have acceptable reliability it is difficult to confirm their validity, as there is no 'gold standard' test against which to compare.

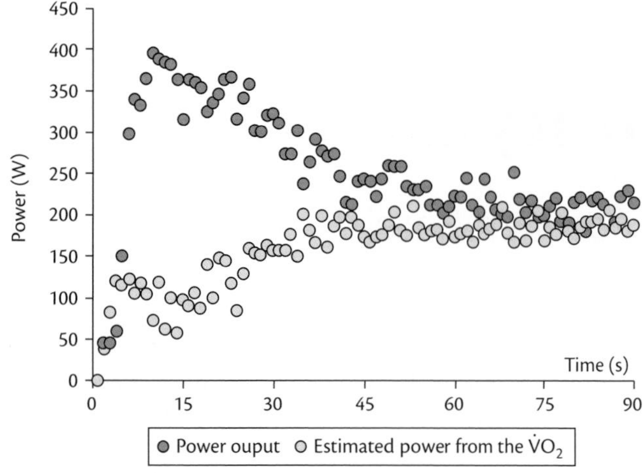

Figure 8.1 Power output profile of a 90 s maximal isokinetic cycling sprint and estimated power from a peak oxygen uptake test for one adolescent boy.
Courtesy of the Children's Health and Exercise Research Centre, University of Exeter.

Furthermore, as maximal-intensity power output is predominantly dependent on energy supply intrinsic to the active muscles, performance test data are specific to the movement pattern used.[14] Therefore, it cannot be assumed that power output in running tests will be similar to power output generated during cycling, as the contribution of the muscles involved may vary markedly between the two activities.[14]

Jump tests

Sargent[15] popularized the vertical jump (VJ) as a measure of muscular power and a range of protocols have evolved from his original test. But it was work first conducted by Marey[16] that initiated the investigation of leg muscle power. Typically in a VJ protocol, participants perform a counter-movement (e.g. momentary crouch, forward arm swing) to aid their performance,[17] but other protocols prevent the use of a counter-movement.[18]

Vertical jump performance is highly dependent on protocol and the general lack of standardization across studies confounds inter-study comparisons.[19] The VJ as described by Sargent[15] has the dimension of work, not power, and several formulae have been proposed to add velocity to the body mass and vertical height components;[20,21] the validity of these formulae is questionable.[19] Jumping is more related to impulse, with the height jumped being a function of the product of force and time and not the product of force and velocity. The VJ has been strongly criticized as a measure of power output[22] and although a popular field test, it is not considered a valid laboratory measure of young people's maximal intensity performance.

Monoarticular force-velocity tests

Using isokinetic dynamometers, torque during movement across a single joint can be measured[23] and because the angular velocity is pre-set, power output is calculated. This approach enables the characteristics of single muscle groups to be measured under controlled conditions. There are several potential problems associated with the use of commercially available isokinetic dynamometers, not least being the necessity to modify equipment that was designed for adults. Isokinetic dynamometer readings are rarely generated under true constant angular velocity[24] and the difficulty of voluntarily accelerating a limb to optimal velocity for PP output has been noted.[14] Torque results are often difficult to interpret because of the range of angular velocities reported. Van Praagh[25] reported that the F-V relationship is highly specific and the torque–velocity relationship cannot be simply evaluated by an isolated movement at a markedly different velocity.

Monoarticular F-V data from children are sparse and focus on peak torque rather than power output.[26–31] Research in our Centre (De Ste Croix and Armstrong, unpublished data), with 23 10-year-old boys tested 1 week apart, found repeatability coefficients varied from 12.4 to 21.8 N·m (mean torque values, 42.7–66.3 N·m) for extension and from 12.6 to 21.0 N·m (mean torque values, 33.7–48.2 N·m) for flexion, across velocities from 0.52 to 3.14 $rad \cdot s^{-1}$. At slower velocities, repeatability was more variable. For isokinetic reliability data on girls interested readers are directed to De Ste Croix *et al.*[32]

Cycle tests

The Wingate anaerobic test

The WAnT involves pedalling a cycle ergometer against a constant braking force, with maximal intensity for 30 s; the majority of data on young people's performance have been generated using this test. An advantage of this test is that it can be easily modified for upper body assessment and several studies of children's and adolescents' maximal power output during arm cranking have been published.[33–36] The WAnT has been demonstrated to be highly related to young people's performance in a range of predominantly anaerobic tasks.[37] McGawley[38] and colleagues in a novel application of the WAnT assessed a 90 s maximal-intensity cycle test, in order to fully deplete the anaerobic energy reserves, and compared responses to data from the WAnT. Mean power, FI, total work done, and anaerobic work capacity were not significantly different between the WAnT and after 30 s of the 90 s test. However, the 95% limits of agreement exhibited large variations between the two tests when comparing all anaerobic parameters. The authors concluded that the validity of the 90-s isokinetic maximal test to assess anaerobic performance remains unconfirmed. The WAnT has also been found to be both feasible and informative when used with children with a neuromuscular disability.[39] High test–retest correlation coefficients have been reported,[37] but to date the only study to investigate the repeatability and validity of the WAnT is by Sutton *et al.*[40]

The WAnT requires both a cycle ergometer in which the braking force can be kept constant as well as a means of monitoring and recording pedal or flywheel revolutions. Various commercial software packages are now available. Important protocol considerations include the use of toe clips, which has been demonstrated to improve power output by 5–12% in adults.[41] With small children, the cycle crank length may be problematic and the muscle length–tension relationship may adversely affect power output.[42]

Several laboratories have modified the original Wingate protocol and the lack of standardization across studies has resulted in confounding interpretation of data. Other protocol considerations include the use of a pre-test warm-up,[43] the use of a rolling start, and the inertia-corrected method of calculation applied to PP.[44] The Wingate team initially recommended calculating PP over a 5 s time interval and assumed that this was a reflection of alactic anaerobic performance. However, subsequent research in adults demonstrated a dramatic surge in muscle lactate concentration during the first few seconds of the test,[45] and the convention was adopted that PP represented the highest mechanical power generated during a cycling or arm-cranking motion without reference to the energy pathways supporting the activity.[39] Experimenters have reported PP over 1 s, 3 s, or 5 s time segments, and it has been recommended that, with the relative ease of computer-driven data collection systems, PP over several time periods should be reported to facilitate cross-study comparisons.[44] The total work done over 30 s was originally referred to as 'anaerobic capacity'[3] but as protocols longer than 30 s have yielded more anaerobic work than the WAnT,[46] the term MP has been adopted to describe the power output over the 30 s period. The 30 s WAnT can result in a significant contribution from the aerobic energy pathway, which in children may be as high as 40%;[44] investigators should beware that MP is not an exclusively anaerobic variable. Some studies have indicated that during the WAnT children and adolescents attain about 70% of their peak $\dot{V}O_2$.[47] As power is the product of force and velocity and each combination of braking force and pedal revolutions may produce a different power output, optimal performance on the WAnT is therefore dependent on the selection of an appropriate braking force for each subject. The prototype of the WAnT[1] used the same braking force for all participants, but subsequent versions of the test have related the braking force to body mass. Bar-Or[37] published tables of optimal braking forces for both boys and girls according to body mass, but there is evidence, that, at least with 6- to 12-year-olds, PP is independent of braking force on the Monark cycle ergometer, in the range 0.64–0.78 $N \cdot kg^{-1}$.[48] A braking force of 0.74 $N \cdot kg^{-1}$ is commonly used with older children and adolescents.[49,50]

However, as the WAnT progresses, fatigue causes a decrease in pedalling rate, affecting the power/velocity ratio and consequently a further fall in power output. In practice, the braking force will not be optimal for both MP and PP. This problem has been addressed with the development of isokinetic cycle ergometers, which maintain constant velocity throughout the test.[51–54] Identification of an appropriate braking force is difficult during growth and maturation due to the complex changes in body composition.[55] The limitations of setting a braking force in relation to body mass when performance is better related to muscle mass are readily apparent.[14,56,57] Most data on young people's anaerobic performance are from the WAnT using body mass-related braking forces, the calculated PP may not have been optimal. Therefore, these factors may have clouded understanding of sex, growth, and maturational differences and changes in PP and MP.

The Force-Velocity test

The F-V test focuses on optimized peak power (OPP) and overcomes the WAnT methodological problem of selecting the appropriate braking force to elicit PP. The test consists of a series (typically four to eight) of maximal 5 s to 8 s sprints, performed against a range of constant braking forces. In contrast to the characteristic curvilinear relationship between force and velocity in the contracting muscle, quasi-linear braking force–velocity and parabolic braking force–power relationships have been observed during cycling at pedal rates between 50 and 150 rev · min^{-1}.[18,19] These relationships enable the optimal velocity (V_0) and braking force (F_0) for OPP to be identified for each participant. According to Vandewalle *et al.*,[19] the force (F) and velocity (V), which elicit OPP, are about 50% of F_0 and V_0 respectively, where F_0 corresponds to the extrapolation of F for zero braking force and V_0 corresponds to the extrapolation of V for zero velocity. Optimized peak power is therefore equal to 25% of the product of F_0 and V_0. Winter[58,59] has provided details of the calculation of OPP from the relationship between pedalling rate and braking force and a simple computer programme facilitates the process. Dore *et al.*[60–62] have utilized the protocol of 'all-out' sprint cycling to determine cycling PP (maximal power value averaged per half revolution), optimal velocity, force which corresponds to the velocity, force at cycling PP, and the time to reach cycling PP. Dore *et al.*[62] determined anthropometric characteristics of 520 males, aged 8 to 20 years, and found PP increased with growth but slowed after 15–16 years of age. The highest correlations were found between cycling PP, fat-free mass, and lean leg volume. The authors argued that although it might make sense to standardize cycling measurements to lean muscle volume, age and fat-free mass can provide as consistent a prediction of cycling PP during growth. From a practical approach, fat-free mass estimations are easier to determine than leg volumes, but other age-related qualitative characteristics should not be ignored. Santos *et al.*[63] used the F–V test to examine OPP in 12- to 14-year-old boys and girls over four occasions at 6-month intervals. The longitudinal design of the study, although relatively short, was strengthened by a multilevel modelling procedure. In contrast to the findings of Dore *et al.*,[62] who proposed a single braking force across a wide range of ages for boys (8–20 years) to determine cycling PP, this study found that the braking force increased with age and that a single braking force did not adequately estimate changes in power due to growth during adolescence. In addition, sex differences in OPP were not significant in contrast to previous WAnT investigations.[64] This is most likely to be explained by the effects of a fixed braking force protocol in the WAnT compared to the optimized protocol of the F–V test. The F–V test has been used in studies of young people,[63,65–70] but the number of sprints employed, the rest period between sprints, the use of a rolling or standing start, the randomization and increments of braking forces applied, and the standardization of warm-ups all still need to be standardized to enhance interpretation across studies. The principal disadvantage of the F–V test is the total time required for completion in relation to other anaerobic tests and there is a possibility of lactate stacking over the series of sprints.[66] Some investigators have advocated the use of the F–V test to identify the optimal braking force for the WAnT,[39,66] but this is contentious as the optimal braking force for a sprint of about 5 s is unlikely to also be optimal for a 30-s sprint. The F–V test provides a promising model in its own right and not just as a pre-requisite for another test.

Isokinetic cycle ergometers

In the early 1980s researchers began to develop isokinetic cycle ergometers by maintaining a constant cadence and measuring force at the pedal cranks.[51,71] These early ergometers have been constantly refined, resulting in commercially available but expensive cycle ergometers (e.g. SRM, Lode, and Biodex). To overcome the financial cost of commercial ergometers, Williams and Keen[72] developed an innovative cycle mounted to a large treadmill. This purpose-built ergometer resolved two of the major disadvantages of a traditional friction-braked flywheel ergometer. First, the dynamometry allowed control of the cadence and therefore application of the fundamental muscle force–velocity characteristics. Second, as the ergometer measured force at the cranks and cadence was controlled to within ±1 rev·min^{-1}, issues related to problems of inertial load of the flywheel and variation in velocity due to acceleration and deceleration were resolved. Several studies using this device have measured maximal intensity exercise in both boys and girls.[54] Data generated using this ergometer have been found to be reliable.[53,73] In the only published study of comparisons between different cycle ergometers, a commercially available isokinetic ergometer (SRM performance Ergo, Julich, Germany), a modified friction-braked Monark, and a modified friction-braked Ergomeca cycle ergometer were compared.[53] Maximal sprint cycling (modified 20-second WAnT) on all three ergometers over 3 consecutive days were performed by 14 boys (8.9 ± 0.3 y). Common indices of PP and MP produced similar mean values. Typical error for PP varied from 27–34 W between the three ergometers. The typical error for the MP ranged from a low of 23 W to a high of 29 W. Intra-class correlations were higher for PP indices (r = 0.60–0.77) than MP (r = 0.45–0.66). Despite contrasting instrumentation and measurement of power output, it was concluded that the typical errors were similar for all ergometers.

In summary, if PP is to be measured during cycling then the external force should be optimally matched with the ability of the muscle groups exercised to operate at their optimal velocity. The F–V test is therefore the method of choice as it provides information on the force and velocity components of power output. Data on young people, however, are sparse and the reliability of the test with this population requires further investigation. For a more sustained test of power output (i.e. >10 s), the WAnT retains its current popularity despite the well-documented problems associated with an appropriate braking force to determine PP and MP. Isokinetic cycle ergometers have a role but remain costly.

Running tests

Margaria step test

In the original Margaria step test (MST) protocol, after a 2 min run participants sprinted up a flight of stairs, two steps of 17.5 cm each at a time. The recorded time up an even number of stairs was measured with an electronic clock and two photoelectric cells. The choice of an even number of steps was to have the participant break the beam of light while in the same position and in the same phase of movement. Margaria *et al.*[74] reported that maximal speed was attained in 1.5–2 s and then maintained constant for at least 4 s to 5 s. It was assumed that all the external work was done in raising the centre of mass of the body and that this rise was the same as the level difference between the steps.

Margaria *et al.*[74] reported data on 131 subjects of both sexes, aged from 10 to 70 years. The authors claimed the data to be 'very reproducible', with repeat tests in the same session giving values that never exceeded ± 4% of the average. Disadvantages of the test are its requirement for good motor coordination, which is essential for optimal performance, and the likelihood of a considerable learning effect, especially with young children. These factors have resulted in its popularity waning. But it should not be forgotten that Margaria provided the first data to indicate that children's anaerobic performance may be inferior to adults.[74]

Non-motorized treadmill test

A 30 s maximal sprint on an non-motorized treadmill (NMT) was first proposed by Lakomy and his associates[75,76] as a way of investigating responses to brief periods of high-intensity exercise. Van Praagh and colleagues used the test with trained and untrained 8- to 13-year-olds, but only for periods of less than 10 s. Although reported in abstract form, a correlation of r = 0.94 between PP on the NMT and PP during an F–V test was found.[77,78] Peak power during the F–V test was significantly higher than 'running power' on the NMT and Van Praagh and Franca[79] reported that, whereas no learning effects were observed during the F–V test, a significant learning effect was observed (test–retest) during running on the NMT. No further details on reliability were reported and, despite stressing the potential of NMT tests for the measurement of an individual's running power, this group do not appear to have published further research on this topic.

Falk *et al.*[80,81] tested 11–17-year-old athletes on an NMT and reported PP over 2.5 s. The young athletes were instructed to sprint 'all-out' for 30 s but as most participants found this duration of exercise too difficult to complete, MP was reported over a 20 s period. The PP and MP scores were compared to WAnT performances of untrained young people of a similar age. Non-motorized treadmill scores were generally higher but as the WAnT PP and MP were calculated over 5 s and 30 s periods, this was not unexpected. The participants appear to have only experienced the test once and no habituation period was described. Test–retest reliability was determined with 29 males and females aged 10–31 years who performed the test twice. Nineteen of these participants performed the test three times. Test–retest coefficients of 0.80 and 0.81 for PP and MP, respectively, were found between the second and third tests but the relationship between the first and second tests was found to be less consistent.[81] Falk and Van Praagh emphasized the importance of a habituation period prior to the NMT.

Sutton *et al.*[40] refined Lakomy's model and developed a permanent anaerobic test station for children as illustrated in Figure 8.2. Power output is calculated from the product of the restraining force and the treadmill belt velocity, which is monitored online with an electronic sensor. Sutton *et al.*[40] reported a study on 19 well-habituated 10-year-olds who completed two NMTs and two WAnTs counterbalanced over 2 days. Correlations between PP and MP on the NMT and WAnT were 0.82 and 0.88 ($p < 0.01$), respectively. The NMT demonstrated PP and MP repeatability coefficients of 26.6 W and 15.3 W respectively. The corresponding WAnT values were 44.5 W for PP and 42.1 W for MP. The same authors[40] demonstrated that following habituation the NMT was appropriate for 8-year-olds where repeatability coefficients were 28.4 W and 14.1 W for PP and MP, respectively.

Oliver *et al.*[82] tested 12 adolescent boys (15.3 ± 0.3 years) for the reliability of laboratory tests of repeated sprint ability (7 × 5 s sprints) using the NMT. In a well-controlled study, mean coefficients of variation (CVs) calculated across all the trials were <2.9% for velocity and <8.4% for power output. This study also analysed the FI (mean results over the first two and last two sprints) to represent the drop-off, but recommended that the resulting CV which was >46% did not support its use in future studies. These authors appear to be the first to differentiate the reliability of the resulting power output. The measurement of power output during the test was found to be less reliable than velocity. A recalculation of Sutton *et al's.*[40] reported coefficients of repeatability data found CV values of 6.3% and 5.1%, respectively. The variability of Sutton *et al.*'s MP is similar to the data of Oliver *et al.*,[82] with the larger variability in PP a likely function of the subject starting each sprint from a rolling start and hence slightly different velocities each time.

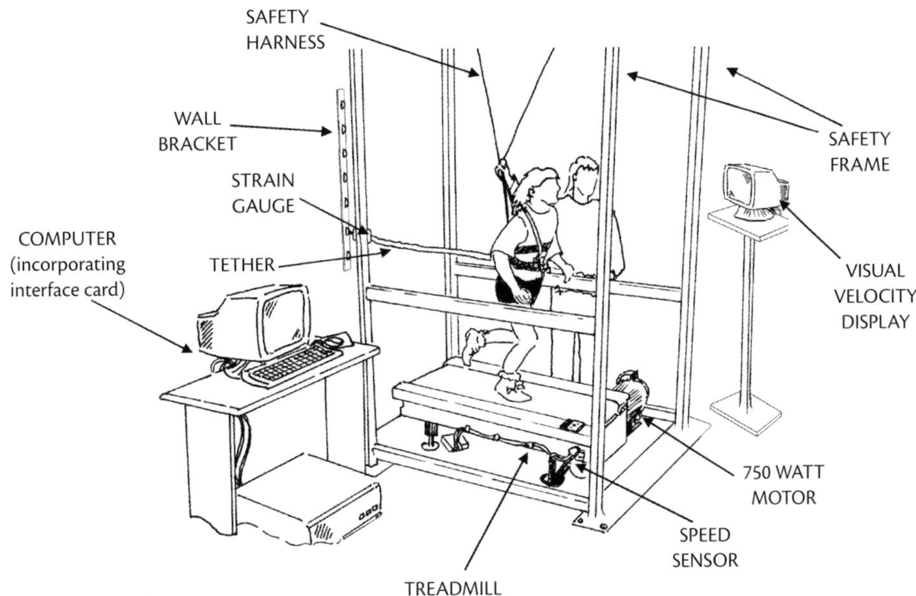

Figure 8.2 The non-motorized treadmill test.
Courtesy of the Children's Health and Exercise Research Centre, University of Exeter.

However, when data are averaged to represent MP, the effect of this variation in the rolling start is reduced. These small reliability changes in the PP and MP are subtle but important because the more reliable the measure, the greater the confidence to detect observed differences. To the best of our knowledge, these are the only studies that have reported the test–retest repeatability of an NMT test in young people.

In summary, the NMT test offers a promising laboratory model for research into young people's maximal power output during running, but more research is required before its potential can be evaluated fully. The use of both cycling and running tests with the same children may provide further insights into maximal-intensity exercise during growth and maturation.

Determinants of maximal-intensity exercise

A major methodological obstacle in assessing maximal-intensity exercise, via the production of mechanically measured power output on ergometers, is the multitude of variables that comprise the resultant muscle performance (see Figure 8.3). These variables include the length-force relationship, the force-velocity and power-velocity relationships, muscle fibre composition, muscle size, muscle geometry, muscle force, and muscle dimension. Given the complexities of muscle geometry (i.e. pennation angles, the unknown degrees of activation and contribution of different muscles acting around a joint, the length of the lever arm, fibres and their tension, the intrinsic speed of active muscle fibres, and how mechanical output is modulated during growth), it is unsurprising that without further improvements in technology, major advancements in our understanding are unlikely. In-vitro experiments have allowed some of these factors to be investigated using a controlled and standardized animal model,[83] but the examination of whole-body performance to examine differences in force between children and adults is too blunt an experimental tool to definitively establish differences.

Cadence and neuromuscular inferences

Force-velocity tests to infer relationships between power, velocity, and neuromuscular performance have found similar optimal cadences for maximal power production between boys and girls and between children and adults. Optimal cadences range from 114 and 109 rev · min^{-1} for 12.8-year-old boys and girls[84], 116 and 118 rev · min^{-1} for 15-year-old girls and 21-year-old women, 110 rev · min^{-1} [85] and 119.5 rev · min^{-1} [86] for female adults, 122 and 126 rev · min^{-1} for 14-year-old boys and 29-year-old men.[52] Even though there are some subtle differences between studies, which all used either isokinetic or friction-braked ergometers, there does not appear to be any significant difference for optimal cadence (optimal velocity) for maximal power production.

These findings could explain similar evidence from the electrically evoked twitch and titanic tension method. Although results from electrically stimulated methods must be interpreted carefully because the implication that failure to initiate muscle action under electrically stimulated isometric action translates directly to dynamic muscle actions is not supported. Using the electrical stimulation technique, Davies *et al.*[87] found no differences in relaxation time, specific muscle force per cross-sectional area, fatiguability, or contraction velocity between pubescent boys and girls. It is also reported that corticospinal tract maturity in conduction velocity increases to approximately 15 years of age, thus reaching maturity in the second decade of life.[10] Maximal intensity power differences between adolescents and adults do not appear to be related to the influence of the contractile properties.

However, there may appear to be an age or maturation effect. Prepubertal boys have been reported as possessing significantly higher ratios of twitch peak force to maximal voluntary force of the plantar flexor muscles compared to pubertal boys and men.[88] The inference from these findings is that the increase in isometric voluntary muscle strength during and after puberty is correlated with an increase in motor unit activation. The earlier findings of Blimkie

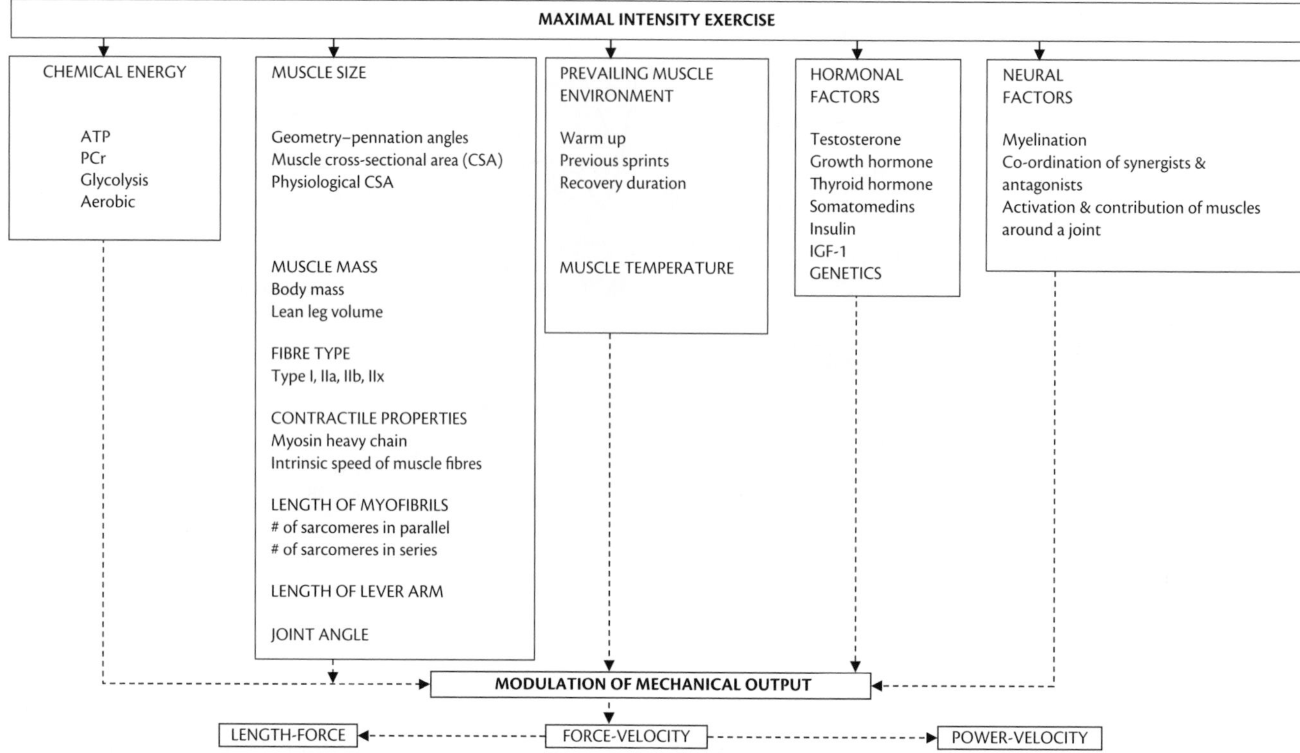

Figure 8.3 Determinants of maximal-intensity exercise.

et al.[89] found that 16-year-old boys could voluntarily activate a greater available percentage of knee extensor motor units during a maximal voluntary contraction (MVC) trial compared to 11-year-olds. In the same year, Belanger and McComas[90] also confirmed the difficulty of some prepubertal 11-year-old boys compared to pubertal 16.5-year-old boys, in being able to fully and optimally activate the motor neuron pool of the plantar flexor muscles during an isometric trial. However, there was no significant age difference for the percentage motor unit activation. Although the area of neuromuscular activation has been ignored as a possible contributor to child and adult differences, care is warranted when transferring the inferences from isometric contractions to dynamic protocols. However, if there is a lower ability in prepubertal children this would result in a low voluntary activation of muscle groups as well as in a lower muscle force and power production. This line of investigation has shown encouraging findings including lower voluntary activation level in children for different muscle groups compared to adults.[90–94]

Although it is difficult to conclude that there are differences in intrinsic force and power production capabilities between children and adults using whole body exercise, animal models may help. In one study to determine isometric force and power in rat muscle, muscle mass, physiological cross-sectional area (PCSA), and fibre CSA were carefully standardized.[83] In young rats whose fibre differentiation was complete, but whose muscle fibre length was still lengthening, the specific force was ~30% less than young mature rats, whose muscle fibre length had ceased changing. It is still unclear why these differences exist but de Haan and colleagues[83] suggest possible factors as the increased density of myofibrillar packing, connective tissue changes in the muscle, more effective cross bridge kinetics, or a compromise of the force transmission related to growth processes.

Power and muscle size related inferences

During skeletal muscle growth from childhood to adulthood there are important changes in muscle mass and increases in protein content. It is known that between the 14th week of gestation and adulthood there is a fourfold increase in myofibrillar fraction, accompanied by a twofold increase in sarcoplasmic protein.[95] These changes in myofibrillar proteins, particularly during maturation, have often been proposed to explain the maximal intensity differences between children and adults. However, even taking into account these muscle growth changes and appropriate normalization for power output, differences still remain between children and adults. This is despite a fivefold increase in muscle mass (7.5 kg to ~37 kg) in 5-year-old to 18-year-old males or a threefold increase (7 kg to ~24 kg) for similarly aged females.

In the 1980s Saltin and Gollnick demonstrated that growth in muscle circumference is associated with increases in fibre CSA and that there is a positive correlation between age and fibre area.[96] The moderate to strong correlation (~ $r = 0.85$) between age and fibre area has been long associated with the relationship between CSA and force production. Correlations in children between CSA and MVCs are moderate to strong across a variety of muscle groups and in both sexes, despite a variety of methods to assess muscle CSA. This line of investigation is partially supported by findings related to lower relative muscle mass (as reflected by lower levels of blood lactate concentration) combined with a facilitated aerobic metabolism[97] in boys compared to adolescents. It is not until mid-puberty that muscle size differences between the sexes begin to emerge.

These differences are more marked in the upper limbs compared to the lower, where adolescent females have only 50% of the upper limb size but 70% of the lower limb size compared to similarly aged males. However, if absolute force is normalized by CSA, age and sex differences disappear, highlighting the importance of CSA, rather than age and sex as a factor influencing force production during growth.[98]

One way to isolate quantitative factors is to compare the same chronologically aged children with similar body mass and volume values. This experimental design was utilized by Martin *et al.*[99] when they compared similarly aged boys (n = 132, aged 9.5–16.5 years) who possessed similar lean leg volume (LLV), % body fat (%BF), and leg length (LL) to highlight the qualitative determinants of maximal power (P_{max}). By completing a modified F-V test[100], P_{max}, optimal force (F_{opt}), and pedalling velocity (V_{opt}) values were obtained. As expected the P_{max} increased with age and was statistically significant at the time of the adolescent growth spurt (around 14 years in this study). The V_{opt} in this study increased significantly in boys classified as prepubertal (n = 37), a finding explained by the possible development of motor coordination providing a basis for skill improvement. There were no significant differences for V_{opt} found between the older boys, as confirmed by other V_{opt} studies that found no differences in adolescent boys or girls compared to adults.[52,53] Therefore, V_{opt} changes in cycling sprint performance appear during the period of prepubescence. Optimal force, however, showed significant increases after the prepubertal period, a factor explained by the increase in ability to activate the motor units of the muscles. The increasing P_{max} with age demonstrated by the boys was the result of differing components of the power equation. Similar groups for LLV, %BF, and LL increased PP by 17.2%, 19.8%, and 14.2% between the ages 10–12, 12–14, and 14–16 years, respectively. When grouped according to maturation, prior to puberty the increase in P_{max} was associated with an increase in V_{opt} of 9.3%, whereas the pubertal and post-pubertal boys increased their P_{max} with a F_{opt} increase of 12.2% and 13.2% respectively. Therefore, further investigations exploring qualitative factors that influence F_{opt} and V_{opt} are needed.

Power and muscle fibre type inferences

In adult studies, the optimal velocity for maximal power production has been related to muscle fibre type composition. Hautier and colleagues[101] determined force, velocity, and power averaged over each down pedal stroke in ten participants (eight men and two women). Muscle fibre composition was determined from the vastus lateralis muscle. The relative proportion of fast twitch fibres (CSA) correlated to optimal velocity was found to be high (r = 0.88, P < 0.001) as was squat jump performance (r = 0.78, P < 0.01), but was not significantly correlated to maximal anaerobic power relative to body mass (r = 0.60, P > 0.06). The authors suggested that the strong correlation between optimal velocity and fibre composition supported the proposition that optimal velocity in maximal sprint cycling is related to muscle fibre composition. It is difficult to equate high optimal velocity with high maximal-intensity scores, thereby implying a high proportion of fast twitch fibres in children. However, the interpretation of these inferences is sound. A participant having a large proportion of fast twitch fibres should produce more power and greater force at high shortening velocities than a participant with a greater proportion of slow twitch fibres. This inference should equally apply to the participant who possesses more fast twitch fibres being able to accelerate their body mass during sprint running to a greater extent than another participant. Currently, no biopsy work coupled with force-velocity testing has established this association in children, but the use of magnetic resonance imaging (MRI) to measure fibre type could be a possibility.[102]

Limited data from muscle biopsies in children show that children have a higher proportion of type I fibres than adults.[103–106] Both Lexell *et al.*[105] and Oertel *et al.*[106] have shown that the proportion of type I fibres decreases with age from childhood to adulthood. Declines of between 54–65% of type I fibres at age 5–6 years to between 42–50% at age 20 years were reported. A review by Jansson[104] reported the percentage of type I fibres to demonstrate an inverted U shaped curve with males from birth to 9 years and a decrease, which was significantly lower at 19 years compared to 9-year-olds. However, this relationship was not found for females. The majority of studies have in fact reported a higher percentage of type II fibres in adolescent females than in males.[107–109] Bell *et al.*[103] found that by age 6 years, histochemical analyses compared to adults were similar. In agreement with the higher proportion of type I fibres were the findings from Colling-Saltin *et al.*,[110] Fournier *et al.*,[111] and Hedberg *et al.*,[112] who reported lower proportions of type II fibres in early childhood compared to adults. It is not clear if there is a greater prevalence of type IIa versus type IIb fibres during childhood and adolescence compared to adulthood as studies have found both for[107] and against this proposition.[103]

Other biopsy studies by Eriksson,[113,114] Haralambie,[115] Fournier *et al.*,[111] and Berg *et al.*[116] have all examined biochemical changes following strenuous cycling exercise but not necessarily after maximal-intensity exercise. Therefore, inferences from biopsy studies must be examined carefully because of the differing exercise protocols, the sample of muscle examined, and the training status of the participants.

The pioneering work of Eriksson *et al.*[113,114] in the 1970s examining muscle metabolism and children's exercise performance led to the suggestion that glycolytic activity is lower in children than in adults and was dependent on maturational status. The frequent citing of this work in the literature has led to these results appearing to be established as an accepted tenet. However, the acceptance of this principle is despite the fact that Eriksson's studies were not designed to test the effects of maturation and employed very small sample sizes.[117]

Eriksson *et al.*[117] found phosphofructokinase (PFK) levels to be threefold lower in 11- to 13-year-old boys compared to men. Although this finding was supported by another study,[116] other groups have found similar glycolytic enzymatic activity in children aged 13–15 years and adults.[115] Allied to the lower glycolytic enzymatic capacity and lower maximal intensity exercise of children is the reported lower blood lactate accumulation after maximal exercise. Kaczor *et al.*,[118] examined the effects of age on creatine kinase (CK), adenylate kinase (AK), lactate dehydrogenase (LDH), carnitine palmitoyl-transferase (CPT), and 2-oxoglutarate dehydrogenase (OGDH) in 20 children (3–11 years) and 12 adults (29–54 years). All measurements were collected at rest and from participants who had been admitted to hospital for hernia surgery. Muscle samples were taken of the obliquus internus abdominis muscle. Significant lower values for CK, AK, and LDH enzymes activity were found for children compared to adults. The enzyme LDH remained significantly lower, even when the concentration was expressed relative to total protein in milligrams. The authors proposed 'the significantly lower LDH is likely to be a major factor of decreased anaerobic performance'.[118(p334)] This assertion is despite the fact that these measures were taken at rest and no indication is given of the maturity of the children's group or any activity status. The authors, however, concluded at the end of the paper that 'mechanisms behind the enzymatic differences reported here in children and adults are not clear'.[118(p334)]

Power and hormonal related inferences

Maximal-intensity exercise differences between children and adults that are due to hormonal changes during puberty have been suggested.[119] It is known that during puberty there are substantial increases in growth hormone, testosterone in males, and oestradiol in females.[120] It is also speculated that the anabolic effect of physical activity is somehow mediated by increases in insulin-like growth factor-1 (IGF-1), which is independent of growth hormone.[121] Levels of IGF-1 certainly appear to increase both in the lead up to and after peak height velocity (PHV) and tend to occur in advance of significant increases in sex hormones.[122] In the longitudinal study of Round *et al.*[122] who investigated muscle strength and power related to circulating IGF-1 and testosterone, for girls, quadriceps muscle strength was proportional to height and total body mass. In boys, the additional factor of testosterone was found to explain the quadriceps strength. Testosterone in the boys was found to increase 1 year prior to PHV, then continue to increase and attain adult values 3 years post PHV.

Maximal-intensity exercise and age

There is unequivocal evidence that male and female maximal-intensity exercise increases with age. This observation has been confirmed mainly by cross-sectional (see Table 8.1), but also by a few longitudinal, studies. Less information is available beyond the age of 40 years, probably because maximal-intensity exercise is mainly regarded as a measure of performance rather than a health indicator. Van Praagh and Franca[79] showed that the growth curves of sprinting events, which are indicative of maximal-intensity performance, improved with age from childhood to adolescence to adulthood. The maximal intensity typically plateaus for men in the third decade of life and for women in the second decade.

Athletic performance data also support data from laboratory testing.[39,123,124] In males, absolute PP increases from childhood to adolescence to adulthood with a typical surge in power output from the teenage years to adulthood. For females, PP also increases through childhood and adolescence, although there appears to be more of a plateau in power output during the latter adolescent years into adulthood. However, some caution is warranted for two reasons. Firstly, the lack of standardized protocols, e.g. duration of warm-up, differences in load, rolling or a static start, and inertia, uncorrected or corrected data have meant considerable variation during measurement. Secondly, there are considerably fewer data from females available.

Peak power output from F-V sprint protocols lasting less than 10 s were obtained across an age range of 7–21 years.[124] In total 1200 participants were tested and Figures 8.4 and 8.5 show a significant increase in power with age. Interestingly, if the figures are examined carefully a number of observations can be made. Firstly, there is less variance in the male data compared to the female data throughout the age range. Hence, the degree of heteroscedasticity, that is, the spread of the scores widening with age, is less for males than females. Secondly, there is a smaller linear increase for boys up to the age of 12–13 years before what appears to be a second and steeper linear increase is observed. For females the increase appears to be more consistently linear throughout the age range.

From the F-V test and the WAnT, the average PP and MP scores for 10- to 12-year-old boys are ~ 43% and 47% compared to that of 25- to 35-year-old men. For similarly aged girls, the scores are slightly higher for PP and MP, at 44% and 55% compared to females aged between 18- to 25 years. Maximal intensity scores obtained from arm cranking, although fewer in number than data obtained from cycling, show that the upper limbs generate ~60–70% of the power compared to the legs.

Despite these concerns, unlike peak aerobic power, no matter how it is standardized, children always have a significantly lower score than adolescents, who are in turn significantly lower than adults. These findings have been interpreted as size dependent (quantitative) factors which become less important with age, whereas the size independent (qualitative) factors, i.e. neuromuscular, genetics, and hormonal factors, become more important in explaining age differences. However, there is considerably less information on qualitative factors and this imbalance needs redressing.

Dore *et al.*[60] investigated the influence of age on PP in 506 males aged between 7.5–18 years using three maximal cycle sprints of <10 s duration to calculate the force, velocity, and power curves. Using allometric modelling, a multiple stepwise regression equation predicted PP from age and fat-free mass. It was found that age (2.3%) contributed to a negligible part of the explanatory variable to PP and that other anthropometric variables were more predictive, e.g. free-fat mass and lean leg volume. Interestingly, although the contribution of age to the optimal velocity at PP was as low as 1.3% it did provide a significant contribution to the prediction model. This small contribution of age might be a surrogate for other changes, which are occurring at the level of motor unit activation, or fibre type distribution, or hormonal influences, or a combination of all three factors. These three factors have mostly been ignored by paediatric researchers and more research is required to elucidate the influence of neuromuscular and hormonal factors.

In a study designed to examine the applicability of a regression model for PP and total mechanical work (TMW) for children, adolescents, and adults at the extremes of stature, mass, and hence body mass index (BMI), 454 participants between 6 to 20 years were studied.[125] All participants completed two unilateral WAnTs, one with each leg. The braking force was determined according to body mass equations and some modification based on practice tests. Peak power output and TMW were averaged for the right and left leg of each participant. In total, 267 participants within the normal anthropometric range (defined as between 10th and 90th percentile for mass and stature) were used to establish the log-transformed regression equation. The major finding was that for children, adolescents, and adults who were heavier than the reference group (n = 267) predictions for PP and TMW were overestimated compared to reference group values on the WAnT. This observation also held true for those individuals who were taller than the reference group. However, the regression prediction equation worked adequately for those participants at the lower distribution of mass and stature.

Table 8.1 Indicative data for maximal intensity exercise.

Study	Participants	Sample	Gender	Age (y)	Test	Peak power (PP)/torque/ force	Mean power (MP)	PP in ratio with body mass	MP in ratio with body mass
De Ste Croix *et al.*[27]	School age children (SAC)	15	M	10.2 ± 0.3	Wingate anaerobic test (WAnT; W)	267 ± 49.7	193 ± 36.8		
		19	F	9.9 ± 0.2		225 ± 62.4	173 ± 43.3		
		15	M	11.9 ± 0.3		486 ± 77.1	303 ± 67.5		
		18	F	11.6 ± 0.2		431 ± 143	261 ± 86.9		
De Ste Croix *et al.*[32]	SAC				Isokinetic knee extension and flexion torque (Nm)	MaxExT			
		16	M	12.2 ± 0.3		85.6 ± 24.3			
		14	F	12.2 ± 0.3		88.0 ± 26.0			
						MaxFlexT			
		16	M	12.2 ± 0.3		47.6 ± 13.1			
		14	F	12.2 ± 0.3		48.1 ± 12.8			
Santos *et al.*[63]	SAC	17	M	12.4 ± 0.3	Force—Velocity Test (W)	306.7 ± 58.1			
		18	F	12.2 ± 0.2		299.5 ± 53.8			
		22	M	12.8 ± 0.3		368.3 ± 71.9			
		18	F	12.6 ± 0.2		360.2 ± 74.3			
		20	M	13.3 ± 0.3		414.3 ± 76.7			
		15	F	13.2 ± 0.3		395.2 ± 75.2			
		20	M	13.8 ± 0.3		453.1 ± 90.6			
		16	F	13.6 ± 0.2		417.1 ± 67.8			
Armstrong *et al.*[64]	SAC	97	M	12.2 ± 0.4	WAnT (W)	321 ± 83	269 ± 64		
		100	F	12.2 ± 0.4		333 ± 88	275 ± 65		
		95	M	13.2 ± 0.4		468 ± 121	356 ± 85		
		80	F	13.2 ± 0.4		454 ± 108	325 ± 58		
		28	M	17.0 ± 0.3		707 ± 114	573 ± 89		
		17	F	17.0 ± 0.3		553 ± 122	439 ± 100		
Beneke *et al.*[97]	SAC	10	M	11.8 ± 0.5	WAnT (W·kg^{-1})			10.8 ± 0.7	6.1 ± 0.7
		10		16.3 ± 0.7				11.5 ± 0.6	6.9 ± 0.9
Pääsuke *et al.*[133]	Prepubertal school age children (PC)	18	M	9.5 ± 0.1	Maximal voluntary contraction force (N)	395 ± 24.2			
		14	F	9.6 ± 0.1		339 ± 36.2			
Hebestreit *et al.*[134]	PC	8	M	10.3 ± 1.4	WAnT T (W; W·kg^{-1})	289 ± 84 (mean of 3 trials)		8.5 ± 0.7	
								8.0 ± 0.5	
								8.4 ± 0.6	
	Adults	8	M	21.6 ± 1.6		1005 ± 111 (mean of 3 trials)		13.7 ± 0.4	
								13.3 ± 0.3	
								13.3 ± 0.4	
Chia[135]	SAC	19	F	13.6 ± 1.0	WAnT (W; W·kg^{-1})	471 ± 61	422 ± 58	9.0 ± 0.7	
	Adults	21	F	25.1 ± 2.7		584 ± 145	439 ± 65	10.1 ± 2.0	

These results demonstrate the difficulties in adequately expressing mass to body fat and muscle ratios in extremely heavy participants. In particular, there is a potential to overestimate muscle mass in these participants. Armstrong and colleagues[123] corroborated these findings, reporting a significant negative correlation between skinfold thickness and log-transformed PP and TMW. Regional distributions of fat, bone, and muscle are likely to be different in very heavy individuals and are likely to change with age. The observation of the 'wobble-gait' in overweight individuals when walking or running, mean it is likely that body mass to

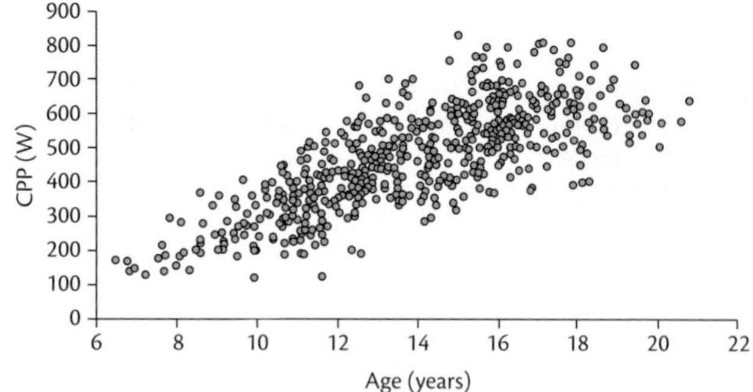

Figure 8.4 Relationship between cycling peak power and age in females.
Van Praagh E. Development of anaerobic function during childhood and adolescence. Pediatr Exerc Sci. 2000; 21: 150–173.

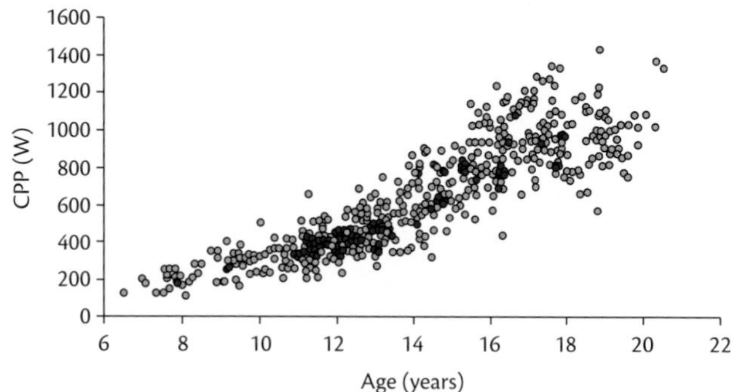

Figure 8.5 Relationship between cycling peak power and age in males.
Van Praagh E. Development of anaerobic function during childhood and adolescence. Pediatr Exerc Sci. 2000; 21: 150–173.

bone-muscle-adiposity imbalances result in increased strain on tendons and joints, and therefore limit cycling performance. The authors also postulated that hypoactivity and muscle fibre recruitment might differ in overweight children, resulting in a reduced anaerobic capacity. Although this inactivity recruitment paradigm might exist in the overweight individuals it does not explain those individuals with greater stature. We cannot conclude that the capacity of the anaerobic system is deficient in these individuals, as the WAnT cannot measure capacity of the anaerobic metabolism, and it is more likely that Unnithan *et al.*[125] meant mechanical power performance.

Maximal-intensity exercise and sex

More cross-sectional and longitudinal data are available on males than females, but it is often confined to a narrow age range, typically 11–16 years of age. Comparisons between boys and girls using the WAnT have reported no sex differences for PP and MP,[40,123] higher PP and MP for girls, and a higher MP in boys.[126] In fact, a careful examination of most data up to the age of 13 years shows there are no discernible absolute differences between boys and girls. Hence, it is possible that for differences for PP and MP, girls could have higher performances in these later childhood years. In one of the first studies to examine sex differences in anaerobic PP and MP in relation to body composition, it was found that absolute PP and MP were similar in both sexes.[84] Interestingly, when PP and MP scores were related to lean thigh volume (LTV), PP and MP were significantly higher in boys than girls. The girls had a higher LTV than boys, 6.0 ± 1.4 and 5.1 ± 1.7 L respectively, but the difference was not statistically significant. Van Praagh and colleagues explained part of these sex differences as due to qualitative factors, which might favour the higher relative power output in boys. Firstly, the lack of a significant difference in the LTV negated differences due to a quantitative factor. Secondly, it was noted that the boys developed more power than girls at the beginning of the exercise. Thirdly, isometric evidence was presented to suggest a longer time rise of isometric force in adolescent girls than boys, and thus a lower neuromotor efficiency and power output. However, each of these three explanations is not without repudiation. Firstly, it has been established that the Jones and Pearson method of estimating LTV significantly underestimates volumes.[127] Winsley and colleagues[128] found that in 16 boys (mean age 9.9 years), the anthropometric technique underestimated the total, lean, and fat thigh volume by 36%, 31%, and 52%, compared to MRI. The size of this underestimation of LTV ranged from 0.4–1.3 L. In the original Jones and Pearson[127] method, validation was against water displacement and X-ray techniques, a process unlikely to account for differing quantities and distribution of fat and fat-free mass of growing children. In the Van Praagh *et al.*[84] study, although this under-prediction is likely to be similar for both sexes, expressing the thigh volume as wholly indicative of muscle ignores intramuscular fat and other constituent tissues.

Secondly, if the development of TMW across time figure in the work of Van Praagh *et al.*[84] is studied, although the maximum work achieved is higher in boys than girls, it is not significantly different in its rate of development. In most instances across the abscissa, work in Joules and the standard deviation lines appear to cross both sexes. Finally, the justification of isometric muscle actions for a concentric cycling action is not valid. Although Van Praagh *et al.*[84] supports this observation by citing the significantly higher optimal braking force in boys compared to girls (F_{opt}, 0.085 ± 0.02 and 0.068 ± 0.01 kp·kg^{-1} body mass respectively, $P < 0.01$), they ignored the lack of significant differences in predicted unloaded and maximal cycling (V_o, 228 ± 18 and 218 ± 21 rev·min^{-1} respectively) and optimal velocity (V_{opt}, 114 ± 9 and 109 ± 11 rev·min^{-1} respectively). These latter two variables would be more indicative of neuromuscular factors than either the optimal force variables or isometric muscle actions.

Armstrong and colleagues[49] found that for absolute PP and MP derived from the WAnT with 100 boys and 100 girls aged 12 years, the girls had significantly higher PP and MP than boys. This observation is contrary to peak $\dot{V}O_2$ values where sex differences, in favour of the boys, have already significantly developed. This significant sex difference in maximal intensity exercise is likely due to the advanced biological maturation of girls who, despite being at the same chronological age, are on average 2 years ahead of the boys.[55] These findings re-iterate the importance of the assessment of biological maturation alongside chronological age.

Potential sex differences in absolute PP and MP also highlight the difficulty of adequately controlling for body size differences between girls and boys. It is common to report maximal-intensity power standardized to body mass (W·kg^{-1}). However, this statistical technique fails to appropriately account for body size.[129] Dore[126] examined PP relative to body mass (W·kg^{-1}) of 535 males and 510 females between the ages of 7 and 21 years, and found sex-related differences from as early an age as 10 to 11 years, and that it continued through to age 21 years. Although cross-sectional in design (and the statistical analyses can be criticized for not appropriately controlling for body size differences) inferences from the study for PP were later confirmed by a study appropriately accounting for body size. Armstrong and colleagues[123] appropriately controlled for body size using a log-linear model, and found that boys' PP and MP were significantly higher than those of the girls. This finding was despite the fact that their earlier analyses comparing absolute power output in W had found girls to be significantly higher in PP and MP than boys.[49] The analyses for PP showed significant explanatory variables of mass and stature, but not maturity.[123] The age by sex interaction was non-significant but the age parameter was positive and similar for both boys and girls. The negative parameter for sex reflected girls' lower PP. The significant negative covariance between the level two random age/constant parameters indicated a smaller rate of increase in PP for higher starting values of PP. A second model showed when skinfolds were entered as an additional variable it rendered stature non-significant. For MP mass, stature, and age were once again significant explanatory variables. Similar to PP, girls' MP was significantly lower compared to boys, but a significant and negative age by sex interaction was found. This result represents the smaller increase for MP in girls compared to boys. An additional parameter maturity effect (last two stages of the indices described by Tanner) was also found to explain MP. However, like PP, the addition of the skinfolds parameter removed both stature and maturity from the model. The two key findings from this study were firstly that age, mass, and stature, as significant explanatory variables, revealed an incremental effect for early maturity on MP, but not PP. Secondly, that stature, which previously was associated with a significant prediction of aerobic and strength performance, was rendered non-significant by the skinfolds parameter.

Santos and colleagues[65] investigated both age- and sex related differences during the F-V test for optimal peak power (PP_{opt}) in 41 participants aged 9–10 years (21 males and 20 females), 45 participants aged 14–15 years (23 males and 22 females) and 41 participants aged 21–22 years (20 males and 21 females). As expected, absolute PP_{opt} was found to significantly increase with age in both boys and girls, while significant sex differences were only found between teenagers and adults, but not pre-teens. For mass-related PP_{opt} sex differences were non-significant between pre-teens, but males obtained significantly higher scores than females in both teen and adult groups. In this study females were not disadvantaged by cycling against a fixed braking force. Fixed braking forces penalize females as the braking force cannot account for differences in body composition or muscularity between the sexes. Additionally, the power output produced during a WAnT is usually lower than that achieved during a F-V test. Most importantly, despite the observation of a mass-related PP_{opt} across the age ranges for males and an increase for females in the teenage years followed by a subsequent plateau into adulthood, allometric scaling revealed a different pattern for females. Using analysis of covariance (ANCOVA) on log-transformed data, it was reported that PP_{opt} was found to significantly increase across all age groups for the females, not just the males. Therefore, when body mass differences were appropriately adjusted, the age-related increases remained for both sexes, even though this effect was masked in females when conventional ratio scaling ($W \cdot kg^{-1}$) was utilized.

The results of Santos *et al.*[65] were confirmed in a later study by Martin and colleagues[130], who used the F-V test with two randomized braking loads, where individual power-velocity relationships determined maximal power, defined as the apex of the power-velocity relationship. Using multilevel modelling procedures, including allometric approaches to describe the developmental changes in PP, mass, lean leg volume, and age proved to be significant explanatory variables. Martin *et al.*[130] found a 273% increase for girls in maximal power from age 7 to 16 years with a plateau between 16 and 17 years. Boys increased by 375% from 7 to 17 years. More interestingly the difference between the sexes did not emerge until after 14 years of age, an observation supported by the negative age by sex interaction reflecting a smaller increase of maximal power with age in girls. Although all three independent variables, age, sex, and LLV, were significant explanatory variables, for girls LLV was the best predictor (68%, $P < 0.05$) as was age for boys (57%, $P < 0.05$). Both leg length (83%, $P < 0.05$) and LLV (48%, $P < 0.05$) were significant explanatory variables for V_{opt} and F_{opt} respectively for boys and girls combined as one group. For the V_{opt} data, it was shown that for the same LL, boys had a significantly higher V_{opt}. Hautier *et al.*[101] had previously shown a strong relationship between muscle fibre typing and V_{opt}. Therefore, Martin *et al.*[130] concluded that sex differences in V_{opt} might be due to differences in glycolytic ability, proportion and recruitment of type II muscle fibres, and/or motor co-ordination differences. They also concluded that children should develop neuromuscular determinants of contraction velocity rather than LLV, but did not suggest how or what the training effect is on such systems.

Maximal-intensity exercise and maturation

It is recognized that age and sex differences are important differentiators of maximal intensity exercise alongside that of maturation. The most appropriate research design to investigate maturation in explaining PP and MP differences is through longitudinal studies. However, these are limited in number. Currently, there have only been five paediatric longitudinal studies (defined as re-testing on three or more occasions) investigating maximal intensity exercise, with three from the same research group (see Table 8.2).

The first study by Duche *et al.*[67] investigated the bioenergetic profiles of boys aged from 9 to 14 years. In total, 13 prepubertal boys were studied for 3 years at ages 9, 10.5, and 11.5 years, with 11 more boys being studied at ages 12 (prepubertal stage) and 14 years (pubertal stage). Significant increases in PP and MP over 30 s were observed between nine and 10.5, and 12 and 14 years. The authors commented that the most important increases related to anaerobic performance appeared to occur at the time of puberty. Although the relatively small sample numbers and simplistic statistical analyses restricted more detailed explanations of the data, this study highlighted the importance of accounting for growth via a longitudinal design to examine the evolution of anaerobic performance.

The second study by Falk and Bar-Or[50] which reported PP and MP of 27 boys over an 18-month period found that mass-related PP appeared to increase at each stage of maturity. Indeed, 2 years later these findings were confirmed by Williams,[131] who similarly found mass-related increases at increasing stages of maturational development. However, both of these studies were restricted in their interpretations of the results as both statistical analyses were confined to ratio standard and ANCOVA methods.

The first of three longitudinal studies from the Exeter Children's Health and Exercise Research Centre investigated maximal intensity exercise in relation to age, sex, and maturation.[64] This study is

Table 8.2 Summary of published longitudinal data for maximal intensity exercise.

Study	Sample size	Age	Sex	Duration	Dependent measures analyses	Statistical
Duche *et al.*[67]	13	9 y	M	Once a year for 3 years	Max power by F-V test & mean 30 s WAnT power	Conventional power-to-body mass ratios
		10.5 y	M			
		11.5 y	M			
Falk and Bar-Or[50]	11 (prepubertal)	10.9 y	M	Four times at 6-month intervals for 18 months	Peak power over 3 s & mean 30 s WAnT power	MANOVA with repeated measures
	11 (midpubertal)	13.2 y	M			
	5 (pubertal)	16.2 y	M			
Armstrong *et al.*[64]	97	12.2 y	M	Once a year for 2 years then once 4 years later	Peak power over 1 s & mean 30 s WAnT power	Multi-level modelling
	95	13.2 y	M			
	28	17 y	M			
	100	12.2 y	F			
	80	13.2 y	F			
	17	17 y	F			
De Ste Croix *et al.*[130]	20	10.1 y	M	Eight times over 4 years	Peak extension & flexion torque	Multi-level modelling
	20	10.9 y	M			
	20	11.4 y	M			
	20	11.9 y	M			
	16	12.3 y	M			
	20	12.7 y	M			
	17	13.2 y	M			
	19	13.7 y	M			
	21	9.9 y	F			
	20	10.6 y	F			
	21	11.1 y	F			
	21	11.6 y	F			
	17	12.2 y	F			
	17	12.7 y	F			
	13	13.3 y	F			
	13	13.7 y	F			
Santos *et al.*[63]	17	12.4 y	M	Four times at approx. 6-monthly intervals	Optimized peak power, force, and velocity	Multi-level modelling
	22	12.8 y	M			
	20	13.3 y	M			
	20	13.8 y	M			
	18	12.2 y	F			
	18	12.6 y	F			
	15	13.2 y	F			
	16	13.6 y	F			

probably the most comprehensive. Using a large sample size, inertia-corrected measurements of the WAnT, and appropriate multi-level modelling analyses, participants were measured at 12, 13, and 17 years. It was found that males' absolute PP and MP increased by 121% and 113% respectively. Females, however, only increased by 66% and 60% for PP and MP respectively. Multilevel regression models on log-transformed data demonstrated that boys generated higher PP and MP than girls, even when body mass and fatness were appropriately and concurrently controlled. Age showed a positive but non-linear effect on PP and MP. The negative age by sex interaction for MP illustrated a smaller increase in MP with age for the girls over the 5-year time span. However, unlike the earlier studies of Duche *et al.*[67] and Bar-Or and Falk[50], once age, body size, and body composition were controlled, sexual maturity (as indicated by the indices of pubic hair development described by Tanner) did not exert an independent effect on PP and MP.

De Ste Croix *et al.*[132] studied younger children commencing at 10 years of age, changes in PP and MP over a 21.6 month period. Like the Armstrong *et al.*[64] paper, multilevel modelling was utilized and found, albeit in a narrower age range, that neither sex nor maturity exhibited a significant explanatory variable, although an age effect was reported for MP. Measures of thigh muscle volume (TMV) as determined from MRI scans exhibited a significant and independent effect on both PP and MP.

Santos and colleagues[63] conducted a study over a 2-year period with four test occasions which investigated the F-V test derived PP_{opt} in boys and girls aged 12–14 years. As with previous studies, PP_{opt} increased with age but was not significantly different between the sexes. Like the study of De Ste Croix *et al.*,[132] even with body size controlled for, TMV was shown to be a significant and independent explanatory variable for PP_{opt}.

Conclusions

Systematic data on the development of maximal-intensity exercise performance in children and adolescents have increased over the decade. Although many of the data are cross-sectional rather than longitudinal, and are more focused on quantitative determinants in contrast to qualitative ones, they have enabled researchers to further interpret findings in respect of changes in growth and maturation and by sex.

Researchers in this area are faced with two main challenges. Firstly, continued investigations of the determinants of maximal intensity by sex, growth, maturation, and by mode, and different durations of exercise are still required. More research is required in muscle dimension and geometry that precede neuromuscular changes and dynamic movement. The second and more applied challenge is to utilize maximal-intensity exercise as a protocol to examine potential mechanisms. These types of experiments should include manipulating different muscle actions during exercise bouts, e.g. isometric versus dynamic, affecting the end exercise pH values, or influencing different fatigue profiles to investigate recovery patterns. By using maximal-intensity exercise as a method to examine underlying anaerobic physiological change, researchers will advance current knowledge as opposed to describing it. This second challenge will require a certain amount of creativity from the researcher in terms of experimental design and methodologies.

Summary

- Definitions of maximal-intensity exercise for children and adolescents, as in the adult literature, are numerous. Although it is easier to focus on a measurement variable (i.e. power or speed), it is better to opt for the particular metabolism supplying the exercise (i.e. a higher anaerobic ATP yield than oxidative metabolism) to determine the definition.
- Assessments of maximal-intensity exercise have relied on mechanical power to infer anaerobic metabolism. These tests have been shown to be reliable, although validity is more difficult to confirm because of a lack of a comparative direct gold standard test.
- During childhood maximal-intensity exercise scores between the sexes are minimal but become significantly different during the teenage years.
- Conventional usage of peak power (PP) and mean power (MP) in ratio with body mass results in the masking of a 'true' age-related increase for females in PP_{opt}, an effect revealed when allometric scaling is performed to show age-related increases for both males and females from 10 to 21 years.
- A fixed braking force, as commonly used in the Wingate Anaerobic test, can reduce the magnitude of age and sex differences in maximal power output.
- Unlike cross-sectional studies, which have reported a significant effect of biological maturation in explaining maximal-intensity exercise, longitudinal studies have shown that once the effects of age, body size, and body composition have been accounted for, maturation is not a significant independent explanatory variable.
- The determinants for quantitative factors have been more systematically studied than qualitative ones. Muscle mass, muscle volume, and lean leg volume are important determinants of power production, but the relative importance can only be evaluated when such factors as geometric influences, length of lever arms, and interaction of tendon-bone-muscle have been investigated.
- The determinants of the qualitative factors need to be investigated more thoroughly. As velocity of movement forms one half of the power production equation, more studies in this area would make a significant contribution. Current information has found that prepubertal children have a lower ability to voluntarily activate muscle groups. This evidence has been used to explain lower power scores and a greater resistance to fatigue. However, these studies need to be replicated.
- New instruments which can investigate maximal intensity exercise *in vivo* and which are ethically acceptable for use with children will undoubtedly advance knowledge of this area.

References

1. Cumming GR. Correlation of athlete performance and aerobic power in 12- to 17-year-old children with bone age, calf muscle, total body potassium, heart volume, and two indices of anaerobic power. In Bar-Or O (ed.) *Pediatric work physiology*. Natanya: Wingate Institute; 1973. p. 109–134.
2. Ayalon A, Inbar O, Bar-Or O. Relationships between measurements of explosive strength and anaerobic power. In: Nelson RC, Morehouse CA (eds.) *International series on sports sciences: Vol 1, Biomechanics IV*. Baltimore: University Park Press; 1974. p. 527–532.
3. Bar-Or O. *Pediatric sports medicine for the practitioner*. New York: Springer; 1983.
4. Inbar O, Bar-Or O, Skinner JS. *The Wingate anaerobic test*. Champaign, IL: Human Kinetics; 1996.
5. Bailey RC, Olson J, Pepper SL, *et al.* The level and tempo of children's physical activities: an observational study. *Med Sci Sports Exerc.* 1995; 27: 1033–1041.
6. Carter H, Dekerle J, Brickley G, Williams CA. Physiological responses to 90 s all out isokinetic sprint cycling in boys and men. *J Sports Sci Med.* 2005; 4: 437–445.
7. Williams CA, Ratel S, Armstrong N. The achievement of peak $\dot{V}O_2$ during a 90 s maximal intensity cycle sprint in adolescent children. *Can J Appl Physiol.* 2005; 30: 157–171.
8. Meyer RA, Wiseman RW. The metabolic systems: Control of ATP synthesis in skeletal muscle. In Tipton CM, Sawka MN,

Tate CA, Terjung RL (eds.) *ACM's advanced exercise physiology*. Philadelphia: Lippincott Williams and Wilkins; 2006. p. 370–384.

9. Gastin PB. Energy system interaction and relative contribution during maximal exercise. *Sports Med.* 2001; 31: 725–741.
10. Sargeant AJ. Anaerobic performance. In: Armstrong N and Van Mechelen W (eds.) *Pediatric exercise science and medicine*. Oxford: Oxford University Press; 2000. p. 143–151.
11. Lakomy HKA. Assessment of anaerobic power. In: Harries M, Williams C, Stanish WD, Micheli LJ (eds.) *Oxford textbook of sports medicine*. Oxford: Oxford University Press; 1994. p. 180–187.
12. Hopkins WG. Measures of reliability in sports medicine and science. *Sports Med.* 2000; 30: 1–15.
13. Atkins G, Nevill AM. Statistical methods for assessing measurement error (reliability) in variables relevant to sports medicine. *Sports Med.* 1998; 26: 217–238.
14. Sargeant A. Short-term muscle power in children and adolescents. In Bar-Or O (ed.) *Advances in paediatric sports sciences*. Champaign, IL: Human Kinetics; 1989. p. 41–63.
15. Sargent LW. The physical test of a man. *Am Phys Educ Rev.* 1921; 26: 188–194.
16. Marey EJ, Demeny G. Locomotion humaine: méchanisme du saut (Human locomotion: the jump mechanism). *Compte Rendu Séances Acad Sci.* 1885; 489–494.
17. Kirby RF. *Kirby's guide for fitness and motor performance tests*. Cape Girardeau: Ben Oak; 1991.
18. Ferretti G, Gussoni M, di Prampero PE, Ceretelli P. Effects of exercise on maximal instantaneous muscular power of humans. *J Appl Physiol.* 1987; 62: 2288–2294.
19. Vandewalle H, Pérès G, Monad H. Standard anaerobic exercise tests. *Sports Med.* 1987; 4: 268–289.
20. Gray RK, Start KB, Glencross DJ. A test of leg power. *Res Quart.* 1962; 33: 44–50.
21. Fox EL, Bowers R, Foss M. *The physiological basis for exercise and sport*. Madison: Brown and Benchmark; 1993.
22. Adamson GT, Whitney RJ. Critical appraisal of jumping as a measure of human power. *Med Sport.* 1971; 6: 208–211.
23. Baltzopoulos V, Kellis E. Isokinetic strength during childhood and adolescence. In: Van Praagh E (ed.) *Pediatric anaerobic performance*. Champaign, IL: Human Kinetics; 1998. p. 225–240.
24. Murray DA, Harrison E. Constant velocity dynamometer: an appraisal using mechanical loading. *Med Sci Sports Exerc.* 1986; 6: 612–624.
25. Van Praagh E. Testing of anaerobic performance. In: Bar-Or O (ed.) *The child and adolescent athlete*. London: Blackwell Scientific; 1996: 602–616.
26. Faro A, Silva J, Santos A, Iglesias P, Ning Z. A study of knee isokinetic strength in preadolescence. In: Armstrong N, Kirby BJ, Welsman JR (eds.) *Children and exercise XIX*. London: E and FN Spon; 1997. p. 313–318.
27. De Ste Croix MBA, Armstrong N, Welsman JR, Winsley RJ, Parsons G, Sharpe P. Relationship of muscle strength with muscle volume in young children. In: Armstrong N, Kirby BJ, Welsman JR (eds.) *Children and exercise XIX*. London: E and FN Spon; 1997. p. 319–324.
28. Weltman A, Tippett S, Janney C *et al.* Measurement of isokinetic strength in prepubertal males. *J Orthop Sports Phys Ther.* 1988; 9: 345–351.
29. Gilliam TB, Villanacci JF, Freedson PS. Isokinetic torque in boys and girls ages 7 to 13: effect of age, height and weight. *Res Quart.* 1979; 50: 599–609.
30. Burnie J, Brodie DA. Isokinetic measurement in preadolescent males. *Int J Sports Med.* 1986; 7: 205–209.
31. Kanecisa H, Ikagawa S, Tsunoda N, Fukunaga T. Strength and cross-sectional areas of knee extensor muscles in children. *Eur J Appl Physiol.* 1994; 65: 402–405.
32. De Ste Croix MBA, Armstrong N, Welsman JR. The reliability of an isokinetic knee muscle endurance test in young children. Pediatr *Exerc Sci.* 2003; 15: 313–323.
33. Blimkie CJR, Roache P, Hay JT, Bar-Or O. Anaerobic power of arms in teenage boys and girls: relationship to lean tissue. *Eur J Appl Physiol.* 1988; 57: 677–683.
34. Nindle BC, Mahar MT, Harman EA, Patton JF. Lower and upper body anaerobic performance in male and female adolescent athletes. *Med Sci Sports Exerc.* 1995; 27: 235–241.
35. McNarry MA, Welsman JR, Jones AM. Influence of training and maturity status on the cardiopulmonary responses to ramp incremental cycle and upper body exercise in girls. *J Appl Physiol.* 2011; 110: 375–381.
36. McNarry MA, Welsman JR, Jones AM. The influence of training and maturity status on girls' responses to short-term, high-intensity upper- and lower-body exercise. *Appl Physiol Nutr Metab.* 2011; 36: 344–352.
37. Bar-Or O. Noncardiopulmonary pediatric exercise tests. In: Rowland TW (ed.) *Pediatric laboratory exercise testing*. Champaign, IL: Human Kinetics; 1993. p. 165–185.
38. McGawley K, Leclair E, Dekerle J, Carter H, Williams CA. A test to assess aerobic and anaerobic parameters during maximal exercise in young girls. *Pediatr Exerc Sci.* 2012; 24: 262–274.
39. Bar-Or O. Anaerobic performance. In: Docherty D (ed.) *Measurement in pediatric exercise science*. Champaign, IL: Human Kinetics; 1996. p. 161–182.
40. Sutton NC, Childs DJ, Bar-Or O, Armstrong N. A nonmotorized treadmill test to assess children's short-term power output. *Pediatr Exerc Sci.* 2000; 12: 91–100.
41. Lavoie N, Dallaier J, Brayne S, Barrett D. Anaerobic testing using the Wingate and the Evans-Quinney protocols with and without toe stirrups. *Can J Appl Sport Sci.* 1984; 9: 1–5.
42. Sargeant AJ. The determinants of anaerobic muscle function during growth. In: Van Praagh E (ed.) *Pediatric anaerobic performance*. Champaign, IL: Human Kinetics; 1998. p. 97–117.
43. Inbar O, Bar-Or O. The effects of intermittent warm-up on 7- to 9-year-old boys. *Eur J Appl Physiol.* 1975; 34: 81–89.
44. Chia M, Armstrong N, Childs D. The assessment of children's anaerobic performance using modifications of the Wingate anaerobic test. *Ped Exerc Sci.* 1997; 9: 80–89.
45. Jacobs I, Tesch PA, Bar-Or O, Karlsson J, Dotan R. Lactate in human skeletal muscle after 10 and 30 s of supramaximal exercise. *J Appl Physiol.* 1983; 55: 365–367.
46. Katch V, Weltman A, Martin R, Gray L. Optimal test characteristics for maximal anaerobic work on the bicycle ergometer. *Res Quart.* 1977; 48: 319–327.
47. Van Praagh E, Bedu M, Falgairette G, Fellmann N, Coudert J. In: Frenkl R, Szmodis I (eds.) *Children and exercise: pediatric work physiology XV*. Budapest: National Institute for Health Promotion; 1991. p. 281–287.
48. Carlson J, Naughton G. Performance characteristics of children using various braking resistances on the Wingate anaerobic test. *J Sports Med Phys Fit.* 1994; 34: 362–369.
49. Armstrong N, Welsman JR, Kirby BJ. Performance on the Wingate anaerobic test and maturation. *Pediatr Exerc Sci.* 1997; 9: 253–261.
50. Falk B, Bar-Or O. Longitudinal changes in peak aerobic and anaerobic mechanical power of circumpubertal boys. *Pediatr Exerc Sci.* 1993; 5: 318–331.
51. Sargeant AJ, Hoinville E, Young A. Maximum leg force and power output during short-term dynamic exercise. *J Appl Physiol.* 1981; 51: 1175–1182.
52. Williams CA, Keen P. Isokinetic measurement of maximal muscle power during leg cycling—A comparison of adolescent boys and adult men. *Ped Exerc Sci.* 2001; 13: 154–166.
53. Williams CA, Dore E, Albaan J, Van Praagh E. Short term power output in 9-year-old children: Typical error between ergometers and protocols. *Pediatr Exerc Sci.* 2003; 15: 302–312.
54. Williams CA, Hammond A, Doust JH. Short-term power output of females during isokinetic cycling. *Isokin Exerc Sci.* 2003; 11: 123–131.
55. Malina RM, Bouchard C. *Growth, maturation and physical activity*. Champaign, IL: Human Kinetics; 1991.
56. Sargeant AJ. Problems in, and approaches to, the measurement of short term power output in children and adolescents. In: Coudert J, Van Praagh E (eds.) *Children and exercise XVI, Pediatric work physiology*. Paris: Masson; 1992. p. 11–17.
57. Welsman JR, Armstrong N, Kirby BJ, Winsley RJ, Parson G, Sharp P. Exercise performance and magnetic resonance imaging

determined thigh muscle volume in children. *Eur J Appl Physiol.* 1997; 76: 92–97.
58. Winter EM. Cycle ergometry and maximal exercise. *Sports Med.* 1991; 11: 351–357.
59. Winter EM, Brown D, Roberts NKA, Brookes FBC, Swaine IL. Optimized and corrected peak power output during friction-braked cycle ergometry. *J Sports Sci.* 1996: 14: 513–521.
60. Dore E, Diallo O, Franca NM, Bedu M, Van Praagh E. Dimensional changes cannot account for all differences in short-term cycling power during growth. *Int J Sports Med.* 2000; 21: 360–365.
61. Dore E, Bedu M, Franca NM, Van Praagh E. Anaerobic cycling performance characteristics in prepubescent, adolescent and young adult females. *Eur J Appl Physiol.* 2001; 84: 476–481.
62. Dore E, Bedu M, Franca NM, Diallo O, Duche P, Van Praagh E. Testing peak cycling performance: effects of braking force during growth. *Med Sci Sports Exerc.* 2000: 32: 493–498.
63. Santos AMC, Armstrong N, De Ste Croix, Sharpe P, Welsman JR. Optimal peak power in relation to age, body size, gender, and thigh muscle volume. *Pediatr Exerc Sci.* 2003; 15: 406–418.
64. Armstrong N, Welsman JR, Chia MYH. Short-term power output in relation to growth and maturation. *Br J Sports Med.* 2001; 35: 118–124.
65. Santos AM, Welsman JR, De Ste Croix MB, Armstrong N. Age-and sex-related differences in optimal peak power. *Pediatr Exerc Sci.* 2002; 14: 202–212.
66. Williams C, Armstrong N. Optimized peak power output of adolescent children during maximal sprint pedalling. In: Ring FJ (ed.) *Children in sport.* Bath: University Press; 1995. p. 40–44.
67. Duché P, Falgairette G, Bedu M, *et al.* Longitudinal approach of bio-energetic profile in boys before and during puberty. In: Coudert J, Van Praagh E (eds.) *Pediatric work physiology.* Paris: Masson; 1992. p. 43–55.
68. Falgairette G, Bedu M, Fellmann N, Van Praagh E, Coudert J. Bioenergetic profile in 144 boys aged from 6 to 15 years with special reference to sexual maturation. *Eur J Appl Physiol.* 1991; 62: 151–156.
69. Mercier B, Mercier J, Ganier P, La Gallais D, Préfaut C. Maximal anaerobic power: relationship to anthropometric characteristics during growth. *Int J Sports Med.* 1992; 13: 21–26.
70. Dore E, Duche P, Rouffer D, Ratel S, Bedu M, Van Praagh E. Measurement error in short-term power testing in young people. *J Sports Sci.* 2003; 21: 135–142.
71. McCartney N, Heigenauser GJF, Sargeant AJ, Jones NL. A constant-velocity cycle ergometer for the study of dynamic muscle function. *J Appl Physiol.* 1983; 55: 212–217.
72. Williams CA, Keen P. Test-retest reproducibility of a new isokinetic cycle ergometer. In: Armstrong N, Kirby B, Welsman JR (eds.) *Children and exercise XIX.* London: E & FN Spon; 1997. p. 300–305.
73. Jones SM, Passfield L. The dynamic calibration of bicycle power measuring cranks. In: SJ Haake (ed.) *The engineering of sport.* Oxford: Blackwell Science; 1998. p. 265–274.
74. Margaria R, Aghemo P, Rovelli E. Measurement of muscular power (anaerobic) in man. *J Appl Physiol.* 1966; 21: 1662–1664.
75. Lakomy HKA. The use of a non-motorized treadmill for analysing sprint performance. *Ergonomics.* 1987; 30: 627–637.
76. Cheetham MF, Williams C, Lakomy HKA. A laboratory running test: metabolic responses of sprint and endurance trained athletes. *Br J Sports Med.* 1985; 19: 81–84.
77. Fargeas MA, Van Praagh E, Léger L, Fellmann N, Coudert J. Comparison of cycling and running power outputs in trained children. (Abstract). *Pediatr Exerc Sci.* 1993; 5: 415.
78. Van Praagh E, Fargeas MA, Léger L, Fellmann N, Coudert J. Short-term power output in children measured on a computerized treadmill ergometer.(Abstract). *Pediatr Exerc Sci.* 1993; 5: 482.
79. Van Praagh E, Franca NM. Measuring maximal short-term power output during growth. In: Van Praagh E (ed.) *Pediatric anaerobic performance.* Champaign, IL: Human Kinetics; 1998. p. 155–189.
80. Falk B, Weinstein Y, Epstein S, Karni Y, Yarom Y. Measurement of anaerobic power among young athletes using a new treadmill test. (Abstract). *Pediatr Exerc Sci.* 1993; 5: 414.
81. Falk B, Weinstein Y, Dotan R, Abramson DA, Mann-Segal D, Hoffman JR. A treadmill test of sprint running. *Scand J Med Sci Sports.* 1996; 6: 259–264.
82. Oliver JL, Williams CA, Armstrong N. Reliability of a field and laboratory test of repeated sprint ability. *Pediatr Exerc Sci.* 2006; 18: 339–350.
83. de Haan A, de Rutier CJ, Lind A, Sargeant AJ. Growth-related change in specific force but not in specific power of fast rat skeletal muscle. *Exp Physiol.* 1992; **77**: 505–508.
84. Van Praagh E, Fellmann N, Bedu M, Falgairette G, Coudert J. Gender difference in the relationship of anaerobic power output to body composition in children. *Pediatr Exerc Sci.* 1990; 2: 336–348.
85. Sargeant AJ, Dolan P and Thorne A. Isokinetic measurement of leg force and anaerobic power output in children. In: Ilmarinen J, Valimaki I (eds.) *Children and sport.* Berlin: Springer-Verlag; 1984. p. 93–98.
86. Sargeant AJ, Dolan P. Optimal velocity of muscle contraction for short-term (anaerobic) power output in children and adults. In: Rutenfranz J, Mocellin R, Klimt F (eds.) *Children and exercise XII.* Champaign, IL: Human Kinetics; 1986. p. 39–42.
87. Davies CTM, White MJ, Young K. Muscle function in children. *Eur J Appl Physiol.* 1983; 52: 111–114.
88. Paasuke M, Ereline J, Gapeyeva H. Twitch contraction properties of plantar flexor muscles in pre- and post-pubertal boys and men. *Eur J Appl Physiol.* 2000; 82: 459–464.
89. Blimkie CJR. Age- and sex-associated variation in strength during childhood: anthropometric, morphologic, neurologic, biomechanic, endocrinologic, genetic and physical activity correlates. In: Gisolfi CV, Lamb DR (eds.) *Perspectives in exercise science and sport medicine: Youth, exercise and sport,* Vol. 2. Indianapolis: Benchmark Press; 1989. p. 99–163.
90. Belanger AY, McComas AJ. Contractile properties of human skeletal muscle in childhood and adolescence. *Eur J Appl Physiol.* 1989; 58: 563–567.
91. Martin V, Kluka V, Vicencio SG, Maso F, Ratel S. Children have a reduced maximal voluntary activation level of the adductor pollicis muscle compared to adults. *Eur J Appl Physiol.* 2015; 19: 1–7.
92. Kluka V, Martin V, Vicencio SG, *et al.* Effect of muscle length on voluntary activation level in children and adults. *Med Sci Sports Exerc.* 2015; 47: 718–724.
93. O'Brien TD, Reeves ND, Baltzopoulos V, Jones DA, Maganaris CN. The effects of agonist and antagonist muscle activation on the knee extension moment–angle relationship in adults and children. *Eur J Appl Physiol.* 2009; 106: 849–856.
94. O'Brien TD, Reeves ND, Baltzopoulos V, Jones DA, Maganaris CN. In vivo measurements of muscle specific tension in adults and children. *Exper Physiol.* 2010; 95: 202–210.
95. Dickerson JWT, Widdowson EM. Chemical changes in skeletal muscle during development. *J Biochem.* 1960: 74; 247.
96. Saltin B, Gollnick PD. Skeletal muscle adaptability: significance for metabolism and performance. In: Peachy LD (ed.) *Handbook of physiology.* Bethesda: American Physiological Society; 1983. p. 555–631.
97. Beneke R, Hütler M, Leithäuser RM. Anaerobic performance and metabolism in boys and male adolescents. *Eur J Appl Physiol.* 2007; 101: 671–677.
98. Blimkie JR, Sale DG. Strength development and trainability during childhood. In: Van Praagh E (ed.) *Pediatric anaerobic performance.* Champaign, IL: Human Kinetics; 1998. p. 193–224.
99. Martin RJF, Dore E, Hautier CA, Van Praagh E, Bedu M. Short-term peak power changes in adolescents of similar anthropometric characteristics. *Med Sci Sports Exerc.* 2003; 35: 1436–1440.
100. Arsac LM, Belli A, Lacour JR. Muscle function during brief maximal exercise: accurate measurements ion a friction-loaded cycle ergometer. *Eur J Appl Physiol.* 1996; 74: 100–106.
101. Hautier CA, Linnossier MT, Belli A, Lacour JR, Arsac LM. Optimal velocity for maximal power production in non-isokinetic cycling is

related to muscle fibre type composition. *Eur J Appl Physiol.* 1996; 74: 114–118.
102. Ratel S, Williams CA. Children's musculoskeletal system: New research perspectives. In: Beaulieu NP (ed.) *Physical activity and children: New research.* Hauppauge: Nova Science; 2008. p. 117–135.
103. Bell RD, MacDougall JD, Billeter R, *et al.* Muscle fibre types and morphometric analysis of skeletal muscle in six-year old children. *Med Sci Sports Exerc.* 1980; 12: 28–31.
104. Jansson E. Age-related fiber type changes in human skeletal muscle. In: Maughan RJ, Shireffs SM (eds.) *Biochemistry of exercise IX.* Champaign, IL: Human Kinetics; 1996. p. 297–307.
105. Lexell J, Sjostrom M, Nordlund AS, *et al.* Growth and development of human muscle: a quantitative morphological study of whole vastus lateralis from childhood to adult age. *Muscle Nerve.* 1992; 15: 404–409.
106. Oertel G. Morphometric analysis of normal skeletal muscles in infancy, childhood, and adolescence. An autopsy study. *J Neurol Sci.* 1988; 88: 303–313.
107. Jannson E, Hedberg G. Skeletal muscle fibre types in teenagers: relationship to physical pereformance and activity. *Scand J Med Sci Sports.* 1991; 1: 31–44.
108. du Plessis MP, Smit PJ, du Plessis LAS, *et al.* The composition of muscle fibers in a group of adolescents. In: Binkhorst RA, Kemper HCG, Saris WHM (eds.) *Children and exercise XI.* Champaign, IL: Human Kinetics; 1985. p. 323–328.
109. Glenmark B, Hedberg G, Kaijser L, *et al.* Muscle strength from adolescence to adulthood-relationship to muscle fibre types. *Eur J Appl Physiol.* 1994; 68: 9–19.
110. Colling-Saltin AS. Skeletal muscle development in human fetus and during childhood. In: Berg K, Eriksson BO (eds.) *Children and exercise IX.* Baltimore, MD: University Park Press; 1980. p. 193–207.
111. Fournier M, Ricca J, Taylor AW, *et al.* Skeletal muscle adaptation in adolescent boys: sprint and endurance training and detraining. *Med Sci Sports Exerc.* 1982; 14: 453–456.
112. Hedberg G, Jansson E. Skeletal muscle fibre distribution, capacity and interesting different physical activities among students in high school. *Pedag Rapp* (English abstract). 1976; 54.
113. Eriksson BO, Karlsson J, Saltin B. Muscle metabolites during exercise in pubertal boys. *Acta Paed Scand.* 1971; 217: 154–157.
114. Eriksson BO, Gollnick PD, Saltin B. Muscle metabolism and enzyme activities after training in boys 11–13 years old. *Acta Physiol Scand.* 1973; 87: 485–497.
115. Haralambie G. Enzyme activities in skeletal muscle of 13–15 years old adolescents. *Bull Eur Physiopathol Resp.* 1982; 18: 65–74.
116. Berg A, Kim SS, Keul J. Skeletal muscle enzyme activities in healthy young subjects. *Inter J Sports Med.* 1986; 7: 236–239.
117. Eriksson BO. Muscle metabolism in children-a review. *Acta Paediatr Scand.* 1980; 283: 20–27.
118. Kaczor JJ, Ziolkowski W, Popinigis J, *et al.* Anaerobic and aerobic enzyme activities in human skeletal muscle from children and adults. *Pediatr Res.* 2005; 57: 331–335.
119. Ferretti G, Narici MV, Binzoni T, *et al.* Determinants of peak muscle power: effects of age and physical conditioning. *Eur J Appl Physiol.* 1994; 68: 111–115.
120. Costin G, Kaufman FR, Brasel J. Growth hormone secretory dynamics in subjects with normal stature. *J Pediatr.* 1989; 115: 537–544.
121. Cooper DM. New horizons in pediatric exercise research. In: Blimkie CJR, Bar-Or O (eds.) *New horizons in pediatric exercise science.* Champaign, IL: Human Kinetics; 1995. p. 1–24.
122. Round JM, Jones DA, Honor JW, Nevill AM. Hormonal factors in the development of differences in strength between boys and girls during adolescence: a longitudinal study. *Ann Hum Biol.* 1999; 26: 49–62.
123. Armstrong N, Welsman JR, Williams CA, Kirby BJ. Longitudinal changes in young people's short-term power output. *Med Sci Sport Exerc.* 2000; 32: 1140–1145.
124. Van Praagh E. Development of anaerobic function during childhood and adolescence. *Pediatr Exerc Sci.* 2000; 21: 150–173.
125. Unnithan VB, Nevill A, Lange G, Eppel J, Fischer M, Hebestreit H. Applicability of an allometric power equation to children, adolescents and young adults of extreme body size. *J Sports Med Phys Fit.* 2006; 46: 202–208.
126. Dore E. *Evolution de la puissance maximale anaérobie dans une population non-selectionnée de filles et de garçons agés de 7 à 21 ans.* Unpublished PhD Thesis, Blaise Pascal University, Clermont-Ferrand II, France, 1999.
127. Jones PRM, Pearson J. Anthropometric determination of leg fat and muscle plus bone volumes in young male and female adults. *J Physiol.* 1969; 204: 63P–66P.
128. Winsley R, Armstrong N, Welsman J. The validity of the Jones and Pearson anthropometric method to determine thigh volumes in young boys: A comparison with magnetic resonance imaging. *Port J Sport Sci.* 2003; 3: 94–95.
129. Armstrong N, Welsman JR. *Young people and physical activity.* Oxford: Oxford University Press; 1997.
130. Martin RJF, Dore E, Twisk J, Van Praagh E, Hautier CA, Bedu E. Longitudinal changes of maximal short-term peak power in girls and boys during growth. *Med Sci Sports Exerc.* 2004; 36: 498–503.
131. Williams CA. *Anaerobic performance of prepubescent and adolescent children.* Unpublished doctoral dissertation. University of Exeter: United Kingdom, 1995.
132. De Ste Croix MBA, Armstrong N, Welsman JR, *et al.* Longitudinal changes in isokinetic leg strength in 10–14-year-olds. *Ann Hum Biol.* 2002; 29: 50–62.
133. Paasuke M, Ereline J, Gapeyeva H, Toots M, Toots L. Comparison of twitch contractile properties of plantar flexor muscles in 9–10-year-old girls and boys. *Pediatr Exerc Sci.* 2003; 15: 324–332.
134. Hebestreit H, Minura K-I, Bar-Or O. Recovery of muscle power after high intensity short-term exercise comparing boys to me. *J Appl Physiol.* 1993; 74: 2875–2880.
135. Chia M. Power recovery in the Wingate anaerobic test in girls and women following prior sprints of a short duration. *Biol Sport.* 2001; 18: 45–53.

CHAPTER 9

Neuromuscular fatigue

Sébastien Ratel and Craig A Williams

Introduction

Over the last two decades, exercise-induced neuromuscular fatigue in children has received much more attention. One reason for this growing interest is the increasing involvement of children and adolescents in high-level sports. Today's prepubertal children are often exposed to training regimens that are considered highly demanding, even compared to adult standards. In some sports, such as female gymnastics, children and adolescents excel and reach world-class standards. In other sports, such as athletics or swimming, most children do not reach their peak performance levels before the second decade of life, but their specialized training might start as early as the first decade. Knowledge of muscle performance and physiological demand under fatigue conditions in children is therefore of fundamental importance for coaches and practitioners in paediatric research. This chapter principally provides the reader with an overview of the effects of age on the development and aetiology of neuromuscular fatigue during exercise. The chapter focuses on the investigation of neuromuscular fatigue in children during maximal-intensity exercise.

The conceptual framework of fatigue

Definition

Fatigue, as a concept, has initiated many debates over the last century. Often, fatigue has been conceptualized as a 'negative' feature of the neuromuscular system.[1] However, fatigue should be considered as a protective phenomenon, which prevents a metabolic crisis and preserves the integrity of the muscle fibre. In other words, fatigue should be considered as the result of the manifestation of one or several 'fail-safe' mechanisms in the organism that call for temperance before damage occurs. Aside from conceptualizing what fatigue represents, the investigation of this topic has been limited by a lack of agreement on a common definition of fatigue. This disagreement about a suitable definition is not surprising given the numerous paradigms to study it, for example, in vivo and in vitro methods and the task dependency nature of fatigue. In this chapter, the term 'fatigue' is defined as 'any exercise-induced reduction in the maximal capacity to generate force or power output',[2] because this definition is an observable functional definition that applies to dynamic or isometric, voluntary, or evoked muscle contractions or whole-body dynamic activities. Maximal-intensity exercise will be defined as any exercise that exceeds the adenosine triphosphate (ATP) turnover rate of the maximal power of the oxidative metabolism, such as maximal voluntary contraction (MVC) or 'all-out' sprints.[3] Finally, the terms 'prepubertal' and 'child' will refer to girls and boys prior to the development of secondary sex characteristics, approximately defined as up to the age of 11 years for girls and up to age 13 years for boys. The terms 'pubertal' and 'adolescent' will be applied to girls aged 12–18 years and boys aged 14–18 years.

Aetiology

Historically, potential factors involved in neuromuscular fatigue were classified into two categories: i) central factors involving the central nervous system and neural pathways, and ii) peripheral factors occurring within the muscle, beyond the neuromuscular junction.[4] It has been shown in adults that peripheral factors account for a larger part of fatigue after repeated MVC compared to prolonged exercise, where central fatigue is prominent.[5,6] Typically, central fatigue translates into a progressive reduction of voluntary activation of muscles during exercise (activation failure) that could be due to supraspinal and/or spinal mechanisms.[7] In contrast, peripheral fatigue is produced by changes at, or distal to, the neuromuscular junction, and could include transmission and/or contractile failure (excitation–contraction coupling failure). To date, the relative contribution of central and peripheral mechanisms to neuromuscular fatigue has been poorly investigated in children as compared to adults. However, the available data on this topic will be discussed in the section Interplay between peripheral and central factors.

Fatigue protocols used with children

Whole-body dynamic activities

Maximal, but intermittent, intensity exercise either using treadmill or cycle ergometry has been used consistently to investigate the rate of fatigue, the effect of prior bouts of exercise, and performance on subsequent bouts in children. Invariably, these protocols have employed a series of sprints, often as many as 10 of 6 to 30 s in duration.[8,9] Recovery duration during each successive sprint has also varied from 30–300 s. A variety of physiological measures has been associated to the changes in peak and mean power outputs during repeated cycling or running events. These measurements have included arterialized blood lactate, H^+ ions, bicarbonate concentrations, and the partial pressure of carbon dioxide. They have showed, for instance, that the regulation of blood acid-base balance during repeated cycling sprints was more efficient in prepubertal boys as compared with men.[9] However, whole-body dynamic activities are limited to investigating the central and peripheral mechanisms of neuromuscular fatigue because numerous skeletal muscle groups are involved during the task. In addition, whole-body fatigue is not only attributed to neuromuscular mechanisms, but also could be associated with the capacity of the respiratory and cardiovascular systems to deliver adequate supplies of oxygen and glucose to working muscles and the removal of products of metabolism. Therefore, other modalities of exercise on isokinetic dynamometers, including more specific muscle groups (i.e. knee extensors, plantar flexors, elbow flexors) and different forms of muscle contractions (isometric vs. isokinetic, stimulated vs. voluntary, sustained vs. intermittent), have been used in children compared to adults.[10–12]

Maximal voluntary contraction

The most common approach with children to investigate the mechanisms of neuromuscular fatigue consists of performing a series of MVCs, with concomitant electromyography (EMG) and force recordings.[13,14] In the these studies, fatigue was investigated from the measurements of torque and EMG signals of agonist and antagonist muscles during repeated MVCs in children compared to adults either over a fixed number of contractions[14] or until the MVC torque reached a given percentage of its initial value.[13] Therefore, fatigue was evaluated from the reduction of MVC torque, the number of repetitions, and/or the reduction of EMG activity.

To gain more insight into the mechanisms of neuromuscular fatigue, other studies have used non-invasive electrical or magnetic stimuli applied at the level of superficial peripheral nerves or over the muscle, and analysed evoked EMG and force recording.[11,12,15] In these studies, central fatigue was measured from the reduction of voluntary activation of agonist muscles during exercise using the twitch interpolation technique,[16] by applying either trains of electrical stimuli over the muscle[17] or single electrical/magnetic stimuli at the level of superficial peripheral nerves.[11,12] Furthermore, peripheral fatigue was determined from the time course of evoked torque and the analysis of the compound muscle action potential (or M-wave) recorded by surface EMG in children compared to adults.[11,12,15] However, these studies are scarce and notably reported conflicting results on central fatigue in children. These results will be discussed in the section Factors underpinning age differences.

Age-related differences in fatigue

Until now, it has been widely demonstrated that prepubertal children fatigue less than adults when performing whole-body dynamic activities, such as maximal cycling,[9,18,19] short running bouts,[19,20] maximal isometric,[11–13,21] or isokinetic contractions.[10,14,22,23] Studies that investigated fatigue during whole-body dynamic actions and MVC in children, adolescents, and adults are summarized in the Tables 9.1 and 9.2, respectively.

Whole-body dynamic activities

Running

Under laboratory conditions, Ratel *et al.*[20] compared the effects of ten consecutive 10 s sprints on a non-motorized treadmill separated by 15 s and 180 s passive recovery between 12 boys (mean age 11.7 years) and 13 men (mean age 22.1 years). Results showed that boys decreased their performance much less than men during the ten repeated sprints with 15 s recovery intervals. The lower decrease in running velocity of the boys was related to a lower decline in their relative step rate because the shortening in their relative step length was similar to the men. With 180 s recovery, boys were able to maintain running performance over the 10 s sprints. However, the men decreased their power and force outputs significantly, although they were able to maintain running speed by increasing the relative step length to counteract the decline of the

Table 9.1 Summary of studies that investigated fatigue during whole-body activities in children, adolescents, and adults.

Study	Age (y)	Sex	Ergometer/ equipment	Protocol	Measurements	Fatigability
Running						
Ratel *et al.*[20]	C: 11.7 (0.5) Adu: 22.1 (2.9)	M M	Non-motorized treadmill	10 × 10 s sprints, r = 15 s 10 × 10 s sprints, r = 3 min	Run distance Total work	E < Adu E < Adu
Lazaar *et al.*[25]	C: 11.0 (0.6) Adu: 21.3 (2.0)	M M	Field track	10 × 10 s sprints, r = 30 s, 1- or 5-min	Run distance	E < Adu
Dupont *et al.*[24]	C: 11.6 (1.0) Adu: 18.4 (2.4)	M M	Field track	6 × 20 s sprints, r = 1 min	Run distance	E < Adu
Cycling						
Ratel *et al.*[19]	C: 11.7 (0.5) Adu: 22.1 (2.9)	M M	Cycle ergometer	10 × 10 s sprints, r = 15 s	Maximal power Total work	E < Adu
Ratel *et al.*[18]	C: 9.6 (0.7) Ado: 15.0 (0.7) Adu: 20.4 (0.8)	M M M	Cycle ergometer	10 × 10 s sprints, r = 30 s or 1 min 10 × 10 s sprints, r = 5 min	Maximal power	E < A; Ado < Adu E = Ado = Adu
Chia[77]	Ado: 13.6 (1.0) Adu: 25.1 (2.7)	F F	Cycle ergometer	3 × 15 s sprints, r = 45 s	Maximal power	Ado < Adu
Hebestreit *et al.*[8]	C: 10.3 (1.4) Adu: 21.6 (1.6)	M M	Cycle ergometer	2 × 30 s sprints, r = 1- or 2 –min	Maximal power Total work	E < Adu

Mean (standard deviation), C = children, Ado = adolescents, Adu = adults, F = female, M = male, r = recovery duration, 1-RM: one repetition maximum.

Table 9.2 Summary of studies that investigated neuromuscular fatigue during maximal voluntary contraction (isokinetic vs. isometric conditions) in children, adolescents, and adults.

Study	Age (y)	Sex	Ergometer	Protocol	Measurements	Fatigability
Isokinetic conditions						
Chen *et al.*[27]	C: 9.4 (0.5) Ado: 14.3 (0.4) Adu: 22.6 (2.0)	M M M	Isokinetic dynamometer	5 × 6 maximal eccentric contractions of the elbow flexors at $90°\cdot s^{-1}$, r = 120 s	Concentric maximal torque of the elbow flexors	C < Ado < Adu
Murphy *et al.*[15]	C: 9.7 (0.9) Adu: 25.7 (2.4)	M M	Isokinetic dynamometer	3 × high-repetition maximum or low-repetition maximum dynamic knee extensions (tempo of 1-s concentric and 1-s eccentric contraction), r = 60 s	Number of repetitions	C < Adu
Bottaro *et al.*[78]	C: 11.1 (0.5) Ado: 15.8 (0.5)	M M	Isokinetic dynamometer	3 × 10 concentric knee extensions at $60°\cdot s^{-1}$ or $180°\cdot s^{-1}$, r = 60 s or 120 s	Maximal torque of the knee extensors	C < Ado
De Ste Croix *et al.*[10]	C: 12.2 (0.3) C: 12.2 (0.3) Adu: 29.9 (5.8) Adu: 29.5 (5.9)	M F M F	Isokinetic dynamometer	50 repeated concentric knee flexions and extensions at $180°\cdot s^{-1}$	Maximal torque of the knee flexors and extensors	C < Adu M = F for C and Adu
Dipla *et al.*[22]	C: 11.3 (0.5) C: 10.9 (0.6) Ado: 14.7 (0.3) Ado: 14.4 (0.7) Adu: 24.0 (2.1) Adu: 25.2 (1.4)	M F M F M F	Isokinetic dynamometer	4 × 18 concentric knee flexions and extensions at $120°\cdot s^{-1}$, r = 1 min	Maximal torque of the knee flexors and extensors	C < Adu; Ado < Adu for M; Ado = Adu for F M = F for C, Ado and Adu
Paraschos *et al.*[14]	C: 10.5 (0.6) Adu: 24.3 (2.5)	M M	Isokinetic dynamometer	25 repeated concentric knee extensions at $60°\cdot s^{-1}$	Maximal torque of the knee extensors	C < Adu
Zafeiridis *et al.*[23]	C: 11.4 (0.5) Ado: 14.7 (0.4) Adu: 24.1 (2.0)	M M M	Isokinetic dynamometer	4 × 18 concentric knee flexions and extensions at $120°\cdot s^{-1}$, r = 1 min 2 × 34 concentric knee flexions and extensions at $120°\cdot s^{-1}$, r = 2 min	Maximal torque of the knee flexors and extensors	C < Ado < Adu
Kanehisa *et al.*[79]	Ado: 14.0 Adu: 18–25	M M	Isokinetic dynamometer	50 repeated concentric knee extensions at $180°\cdot s^{-1}$	Maximal torque of the knee extensors	Ado < Adu
Isometric conditions						
Ratel *et al.*[12]	C: 9.9 (1.2) Adu: 23.9 (3.5)	M M	Isokinetic dynamometer	Repeated 5-s maximal voluntary contractions separated by 5-s recovery intervals until the torque reached 60% of its initial value	Number of repetitions	C < Adu
Hatzikotoulas *et al.*[11]	C: 10.7 (0.2) Adu: 26.4 (0.7)	M M	Isokinetic dynamometer	Sustained maximal voluntary contraction of the plantar flexors until the torque reached 50% of its initial value	Endurance time	C < Adu
Armatas *et al.*[13]	C: 10.0 (0.8) Adu: 26.1 (4.2)	M M	Isokinetic dynamometer	Repeated 5-s maximal voluntary contractions separated by 5-s recovery intervals until the torque reached 50% of its initial value	Number of repetitions	C < Adu
Streckis *et al.*[17]	C: 13.9 (0.3) C: 13.6 (0.2) Adu: 22.2 (0.9) Adu: 20.8 (0.5)	M F M F	Isokinetic dynamometer	Sustained 2-min maximal voluntary contraction of the knee extensors	Maximal torque of the knee extensors Tetanic torque 100 Hz of the knee extensors	C = Adu C < Adu M = F for C and Adu
Halin *et al.*[21]	C: 10.5 (0.9) Adu: 21.5 (4.5)	M M	Constructed device	30-s isometric maximal voluntary contraction of the biceps brachii	Peak torque of the biceps brachii	C < Adu

Mean (standard deviation), C = children, Ado = adolescents, Adu = adults, F = female, M = male, r = recovery duration.

relative step rate. Under field conditions, the results were consistent with those found in laboratory conditions, where repeated sprint ability was found to be significantly higher in prepubertal children compared to adults.[24,25] For instance, Lazaar *et al.*[25] have indicated that after ten 10 s track sprints separated by 30 s recovery intervals, the decline in maximal run distance was less evident in young boys than in men (−12% vs. −20%, respectively). The same finding was obtained after six 20 s track sprints separated by 1 min recovery periods in prepubertal boys compared to young men.[24]

Cycling

Repeated sprint ability protocols have also been applied to sprint cycling and children. Hebestreit *et al.*,[8] using a Wingate anaerobic test protocol on three different occasions, had subjects complete two consecutive 30 s maximal-intensity cycle sprints separated by 1, 2, and 10 min recoveries. Eight prepubertal boys (9–12 years) and eight young men (19–23 years) completed the protocol, which was devised to determine the difference in ability to recover from the sprint cycling bouts. It was found that boys' mean power reached 89.9 ± 3.6% of the first sprint value after 1 min recovery, 96.4 ± 2.3% after 2 min recovery, and 103.5 ± 1.3% after 10 min recovery. For the men, the values were 71.2 ± 2.6%, 77.1 ± 2.4%, and 94.0 ± 1.3%, respectively. It was concluded by the authors that boys recovered faster than men from the sprint cycling exercise. Similar conclusions were drawn by other researchers when investigating the effects of age and recovery duration on cycling peak power during repeated sprints.[18] Eleven prepubescent (9.6 ± 0.7 years) and nine pubescent boys (15.0 ± 0.7 years) and ten men (20.4 ± 0.8 years) completed ten 10 s cycling sprints separated by 30 s, 1 min, or 5 min of passive recovery. For the prepubescent boys, whatever recovery duration was chosen, peak power remained unchanged during the 10 s sprints. In the pubescent boys, peak power decreased significantly by 20% during the 30 s recovery, by 15% during the 1 min recovery, and was unchanged by the 5 min recovery. For the men, peak power significantly decreased by 29%, 11%, and slightly but non-significantly during the 30 s, 1 min, and 5 min recovery periods, respectively (Figure 9.1).

Running vs. cycling

Ratel *et al.*[19] also utilized both sprint cycling and running to examine any possible difference in fatigue due to the mode of exercise for both boys and men. As hypothesized, the extent of the fatigue was greater in mean power output during sprint running for both boys and adult men compared to cycling. This observation is in contrast to the decline in peak power output for all participants, which was not dependent on the mode of exercise. The authors concluded that as peak power was obtained within similar time periods for cycling and running that the maximal utilization of phosphocreatine stores was similar. The greater fall in mean power for both boys and men in running indicated a more stressful situation indicated by the higher perceived exertion and blood lactate concentrations (Figure 9.2). In addition, the higher recruitment of body balance and weight-bearing muscles during running will likely have an impact on contractile force production. Further work is required to investigate children's recovery from sprints, particularly applied to the sporting context.

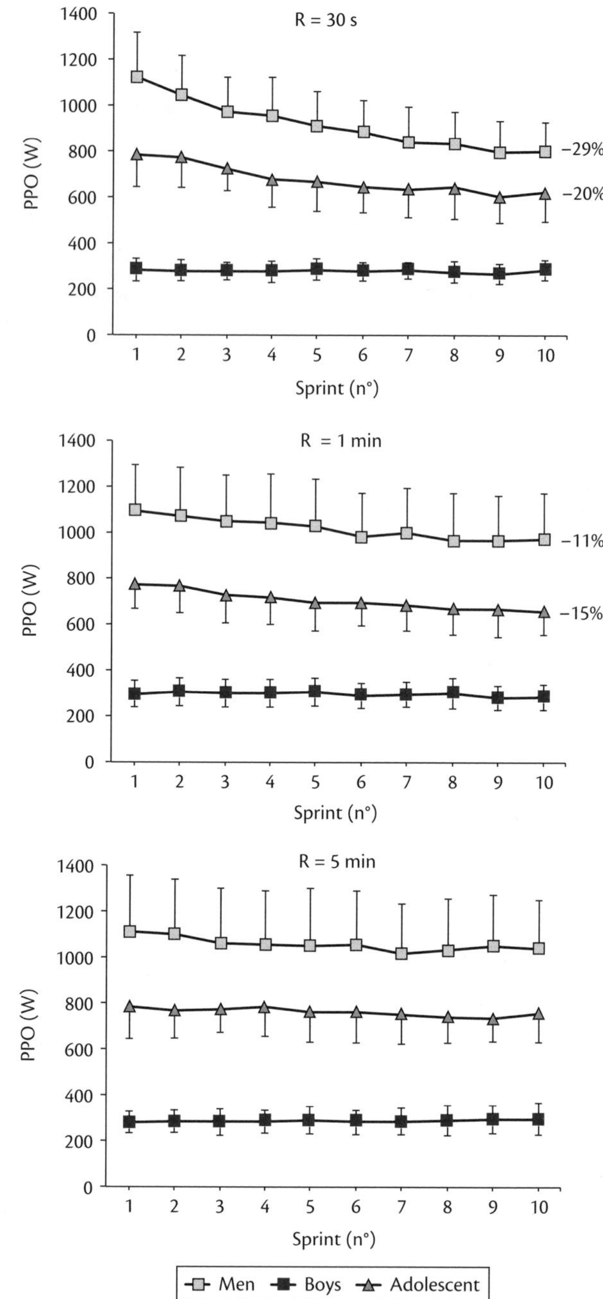

Figure 9.1 Time course of peak power output (PPO) during ten repeated 10 s cycling sprints separated by 30 s, 1 min or 5 min recovery periods in boys, male adolescents, and men.

Data from Ratel S, Bedu M, Hennegrave A, Dore E, Duche P. Effects of age and recovery duration on peak power output during repeated cycling sprints. Int J Sports Med. 2002; 23: 397–402.

Maximal voluntary contraction

The lower fatigability in children has been confirmed during sustained or repeated MVCs whatever the nature of contraction and the muscle group investigated. Some authors have reported a lower reduction of peak torque and total work during repeated maximal knee extensions and flexions on an isokinetic dynamometer in prepubertal children compared to adults.[10,22,23] Similar results were obtained during repeated MVCs of the knee extensors under concentric[14] and isometric contraction conditions,[12] with prepubertal children compared to adults. For instance, during a fatigue protocol consisting of the repetition of 5 s isometric MVCs of the knee extensors, separated by 5 s passive recovery periods until the torque reached 60% of its initial value, Ratel *et al.*[12] showed that the number

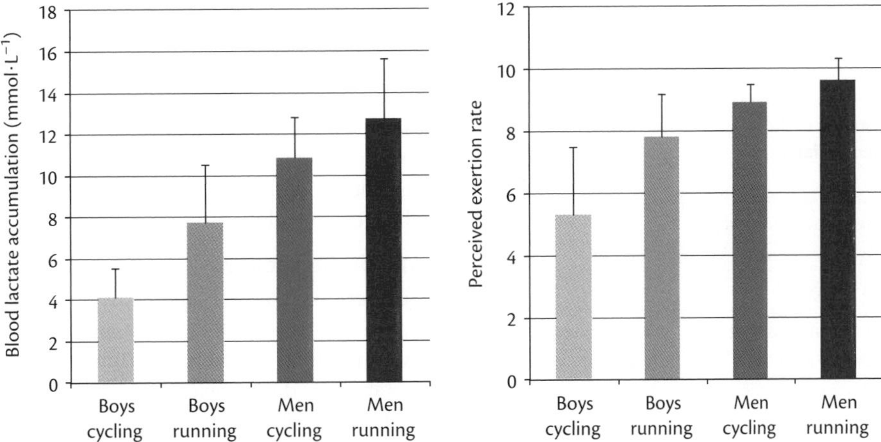

Figure 9.2 Blood lactate accumulation and perceived exertion rate obtained after ten repeated 10 s sprints separated by 15 s recovery periods on cycle ergometer or non-motorized treadmill in boys and men.
Data from Ratel S, Williams CA, Oliver J, Armstrong N. Effects of age and mode of exercise on power output profiles during repeated sprints. Eur J Appl Physiol. 2004; 92: 204–210.

of repetitions was significantly lower in men compared to prepubertal boys (34.0 ± 19.6 vs 49.5 ± 16.8 repetitions, respectively), suggesting a lower fatigability in children. Also, when muscle contractions included repeated eccentric phases (i.e. repeated stretch phases of the active muscle), the decline of concentric peak torque of the elbow flexors was found to be lower in prepubertal children compared to adolescents and lower in adolescents compared to adults.[27] Moreover, the magnitude of symptoms appearing during the days after repeated eccentric contractions (i.e. stiffness, oedema, decreased range of motion) was lower in prepubertal children compared to adolescents and lower in adolescents compared to adults.[27]

In summary, whatever the nature of the task performed (whole-body dynamic activities or MVCs) and the muscle group investigated, high-intensity exercise-induced fatigue differs according to age. Indeed, adults fatigue faster than prepubertal children. Also, the fatigability may be maturity-dependent in childhood given that adolescents fatigue faster than children but slower than adults.[12,22,23,27] This lower muscle fatigability in prepubertal children could be explained by peripheral (i.e. muscular) and central (i.e. nervous) changes that occur during adolescence and these factors underpinning age differences have been investigated.

Factors underpinning age differences

Peripheral factors

Some studies have shown a lower twitch torque decrement after sustained or repeated MVCs in children or adolescents compared to adults.[11,12,15,17] Furthermore, following repetitive stretch shortening cycles, Gorianovas *et al.*[28] reported a lower low-frequency fatigue, as evaluated by the low-to-high frequency tetanic force ratio, in children compared to adults, suggesting a lower alteration of the excitation-contraction coupling. However, the contribution of sarcolemmal excitability changes to peripheral fatigue in children still remains to be elucidated. Indeed, while some authors reported a similar decrement[11] or no change of the M-wave[12] in response to exercise in prepubertal children compared to adults, others showed an increase in children and a significant decrease in adults.[15] These discrepancies could result from a different balance of potentiation and fatigue on the M-wave during exercise between children and adults. However, further studies are required to confirm this assumption, since the M-wave changes have been poorly described during the course of fatigue protocols in children. Therefore, although the underlying factors are not all fully acknowledged, there is a consensus that prepubertal children develop lower peripheral fatigue compared to adults (Table 9.3).

This lower peripheral fatigue in children could be attributed to different factors such as absolute force, muscle phenotype, muscle metabolism, and musculo-tendinous stiffness.

Absolute force

The higher peripheral fatigue in adults during high-intensity exercise could be associated with their larger active muscle mass involved during exercise and their superior maximal force-generating capacity. This assumption is supported by the recent work published by Ratel *et al.*,[12] which shows a significant positive relationship between the first MVC and the twitch torque decrement during repeated maximal contractions of the knee extensors in children and adults. Furthermore, when the initial MVCs torque was used as a covariate, no significant difference in the course of the twitch torque was observed between groups, suggesting the importance of MVC torque in the development of fatigue. This finding is consistent with other studies that showed the fatigability of the knee extensors during repeated MVCs was no longer different between obese and non-obese adolescent girls when the initial MVC torque was used as covariate in statistical analyses.[29] Furthermore, other studies reported that the greater fatigue observed in men vs. women was eliminated when subjects were matched for absolute force.[30] This greater muscle mass involved during exercise in adults could be the cause of the greater metabolic disturbances that are usually observed during high-intensity exercise in adults compared to children.[31] An alternative hypothesis, often proposed when comparing the fatigability between groups that produce different levels of force (women vs. men; elderly vs. young adults; obese vs. non-obese) is that individuals with higher force levels have greater vascular occlusion during exercise. The resulting decrease in blood flow could contribute to the increased accumulation of muscle by-products (i.e. lactate, H^+ ions, inorganic phosphate) and to the reduced supply of nutrients and oxygen. However, this suggestion

Table 9.3 Factors potentially involved in the development of neuromuscular fatigue during high-intensity exercise in children and adults

Category (central vs. peripheral)	Factors involved in the development of fatigue	Child-adult comparison
Central factors (nervous)	Motor cortex activation deficit	?
	Neural drive alteration (cortex ◊ spinal cord)	?
	Motor unit activation deficit (voluntary activation loss)	Child = adult Hatzikotoulas *et al.*[11] Child > adult Streckis *et al.*[12] Child < adult Gorianovas *et al.*[28]
Peripheral factors (muscular)	Sarcolemmal excitability alteration (M-wave alteration)	Child = adult Hatzikotoulas *et al.*[11] Child < adult Murphy *et al.*[15] No alteration in both groups Ratel *et al.*[12]
	Excitation-contraction coupling alteration (low-frequency fatigue)	Child < adult Gorianovas *et al.*[28]
	Energy substrates depletion (glycogen, phosphocreatine)	Child < adult Kappenstein *et al.*[31]
	Metabolites accumulation	Child < adult Kappenstein *et al.*[31]
	Contractile properties alteration (twitch torque alteration)	Child < adult Streckis *et al.*[11] Murphy *et al.*[12]
	Blood flow alteration	?

is purely speculative because this has never been demonstrated in adults compared to children. However, the removal rate of some muscle by-products (i.e. H^+ ions) and the re-synthesis rate of some energy substrates such as phosphocreatine were found to be lower in adults compared to children,[31–34] suggesting that the vascular occlusion could be increased in adults because of their higher absolute force. Finally, some studies have suggested that the extent of muscle damage could be dependent on the absolute force produced during eccentric contractions.[35,36] Therefore, the gradual increase in the maximal force-generating capacity during growth may explain the increased post-exercise muscle damage with advancing age. However, this statement has recently been questioned[27] and remains to be verified.

Muscle phenotype

Muscle phenotype could also account for the differences in peripheral fatigue between children and adults. It has been previously shown that individuals with predominantly fast-twitch fibres develop greater peripheral fatigue compared to subjects with a higher proportion of slow-twitch fibres.[37] Furthermore, it has been reported that adults have a lower percentage of fatigue-resistant slow-twitch fibres than children.[38–41] The decrease in the % of slow-twitch fibres from childhood to adolescence could be explained by the transformation of slow-twitch fibres into fast-twitch fibres.[41] However, the influence of muscle typology on fatigability in children remains to be established, since another study showed no significant difference in muscle fibre type composition between children and adults.[42]

Muscle metabolism

Furthermore, several studies using ^{31}phosphorus-magnetic resonance spectroscopy (^{31}PRMS) and muscle biopsies have provided evidence that children rely more on oxidative than anaerobic metabolism during exercise.[33,34,43] With the exception of citrate synthase, the enzymes of the tricarboxylic acid cycle (e.g. fumarase, nicotinamide-adenine dinucleotide phosphate (NADP), isocitrate dehydrogenase (ICDH), malate dehydrogenase, and succinate dehydrogenase) were found to show higher activities in children and adolescents compared to young adults.[44–46] Furthermore, it has been shown that the ratio of PFK (phosphofructokinase)/ICDH activity was 1.633 in adults and 0.844 in 13- to 15-year-old adolescents[46] and the muscle enzyme activity ratio fumarase to PFK was higher in children compared to adolescents and young adults.[43] These observations have been used to propose that the tricarboxylic acid cycle, as compared with glycolysis, functions at a higher rate in children than in adults. In addition, recent studies using ^{31}PRMS showed that post-exercise phosphocreatine re-synthesis rates were higher in children compared to adults, suggesting a higher muscle oxidative activity during exercise in children.[32–34,47] This specific metabolic profile in children could lead to a lower accumulation of muscle by-products (i.e. H^+ ions and inorganic phosphate) and a lower phosphocreatine depletion during high-intensity intermittent exercise in children compared to adults.[31] As these muscle by-products promote peripheral fatigue through an alteration of the contractile processes[48] and the excitation-contraction coupling,[48] a lower accumulation of metabolites could translate into a reduced peripheral fatigue, which is usually observed in prepubertal children.[11,12,15,17]

Musculo-tendinous stiffness

Finally, recent reports show that compliant tendinous tissues may act as a 'mechanical buffer' that may protect the muscle from extensive damage and fatigue.[49,50] As the musculo-tendinous stiffness has been reported to be lower in children,[51] part of the constraints imposed on the muscle-tendon unit could be better absorption by the tendon itself in children and explain their lower peripheral fatigue during repeated maximal contractions. Nevertheless, these results were obtained from adult and animal models during dynamic contractions,[49,50] and need to be confirmed in children during isometric and dynamic contractions. Alternatively, it can be argued that a greater compliance puts the muscle in a less-productive force condition. This effect results in a rightward shift of the force-length relationship.[52] Therefore, greater tendon compliance would result in a greater shortening of the muscle fibres, even at the optimal muscle-tendon length. The consequence would be that the children, who have a greater musculo-tendinous compliance,[51] would exercise at a shorter relative muscle fibre length than adults. Such conditions could reduce the peripheral fatigue[53] and increase the central fatigue.[54] This is consistent with the results of Streckis *et al.*[17] and Ratel *et al.*,[12] who showed lower peripheral fatigue and greater central fatigue in children compared to adults (Figure 9.3). However, further studies are required to confirm this issue.

Central factors

Beyond the peripheral factors, central factors (i.e. the nervous system) may also be responsible for the lower fatigability of children. These factors could include the capacity to maximally activate the motor units of agonist muscles (i.e. agonist activation) and the co-activation level of antagonist muscles (i.e. antagonist activation). However, contrary to peripheral fatigue, there is still no consensus regarding the implication of central factors in the development of fatigue in children and adults.[11,12,17,28]

Agonist activation

In adults, some studies have emphasized the importance of maximal voluntary activation (VA) of agonist muscles on the development of peripheral fatigue.[55] For instance, Nordlund *et al.*[55] showed during repeated maximal voluntary isometric plantar flexions that adults who had a poor ability to maximally activate their motor units before fatigue ensued, developed less peripheral fatigue but similar central fatigue, compared to their counterparts with a high VA. This lower peripheral fatigue during incomplete activation could be brought about via redistributing muscle activation within or between agonist muscles.[55] Furthermore, according to the 'size principle',[56] individuals with a low VA could recruit a greater relative proportion of slow-twitch motor units, which are known to be more resistant to the metabolic disturbances and muscle damage. As a result, individuals with a low VA could be characterized by a delayed peripheral fatigue via a lower accumulation of metabolites that are likely to impair the muscle contractile properties.

Contrary to adolescents and adults, prepubertal children could be considered as a low-VA group. Indeed, some studies have reported lower VA of the knee extensor muscles in prepubertal (10 years) compared with that in postpubertal boys (16 years)[57] and between prepubertal children (8–12 years) and adults.[58,59] A lower maximal VA level was also reported on the adductor pollicis muscle in prepubertal boys (11 years) compared with men.[60] Furthermore, the maximal VA level of the plantar flexor muscles was found to increase between 7 and 10–11 years of age, when maximal activation level was no longer different from adult values.[61] Therefore, prepubertal children may have a lower impairment in muscle activation during fatiguing exercise than older subjects. As stated by Halin *et al.*,[21] less fatigable fast-twitch motor units may be involved in prepubertal children resulting in fewer metabolic by-products being accumulated during fatigue.[31] This lower impairment in children's muscle metabolic and ionic state could be responsible for a lower reflex-induced decrease of motor units firing rates in prepubertal children compared with adults. However, although the VA level is likely to affect the amount of peripheral fatigue, its relationship with central fatigue (i.e. VA reduction) still remains to be demonstrated in children and adults.

Antagonist co-activation

Co-activation, also known as co-contraction, has an important link to the central theories of fatigue because the decline in force can be related to an increased activation of antagonist muscles during repeated or sustained MVC.[62] Indeed, numerous studies have confirmed that antagonist activation produces forces in the opposite direction to agonist muscles during isometric and dynamic MVCs.[62] For instance, when running or cycling the knee extensors are producing force and any increase in knee flexors force because of co-activation will delimit knee extensors force. Several studies have postulated that if co-activity was shown to increase during acute exercise, it could add to the loss of the force-generating capacity associated with fatigue. Conversely, a decrease in co-activity could help extend the limit of endurance and delay fatigue.

Studies that have investigated the antagonist co-activation during acute exercise in children are few and reported inconsistent results. Some studies found no significant difference in antagonist co-activation of the vastus lateralis and biceps femoris muscles between prepubertal children and adults,[63] or between pubertal children and adults,[64] during isokinetic concentric and eccentric knee extension and flexion tasks. Similar conclusions were reported between prepubertal children and adults on the co-activation level of the biceps femoris during isometric MVCs of the knee extensors.[12,58] However, some authors observed higher co-activation

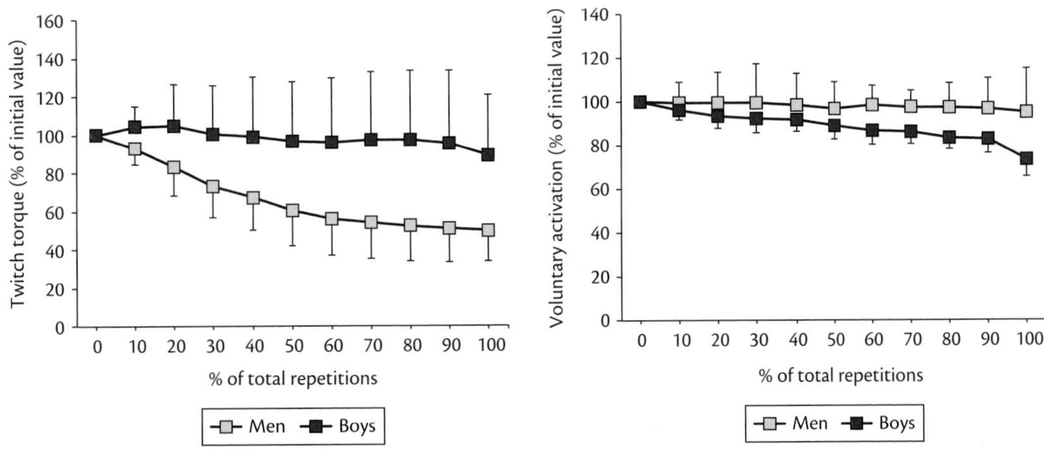

Figure 9.3 Time course of the twitch torque (left panel) and maximal voluntary activation level (right panel) of the knee extensors during a series of repeated isometric maximal voluntary contraction (MVC) until the MVC torque reached 60% of its initial value in boys and men.
Data from Ratel S, Kluka V, Vicencio SG, *et al.* Insights into the mechanisms of neuromuscular fatigue in boys and men. Med Sci Sports Exerc. 2015; 47: 2319–2328.

levels of the tibialis anterior muscle during submaximal isometric plantar flexions in prepubertal children compared to adults,[61] with a level of antagonist co-activation, which tended to decline from 7 to 11 years. Conversely, O'Brien *et al.*[59] reported higher co-activation levels of the biceps femoris muscle in adults compared to prepubertal children during isometric MVC of the knee extensor muscles. Finally, higher co-activation levels were found in children during polyarticular movements such as walking[65] and drop jumps.[66] Therefore, the nature of the task could be a factor accounting for the agonist and antagonist activity in children compared to adults. Whether the antagonist co-activation is different between children and adults and whether it significantly accounts for the differences in peripheral fatigue between both age groups remains to be determined. Further studies are required to clarify this issue as a function of the nature of the task performed.

Interplay between peripheral and central factors

Noakes[67] proposed the 'central governor' theory, which suggests that physiological responses are essentially determined and limited by the central nervous system. Indeed, the central nervous system could limit the recruitment of motor units to prevent any extensive homeostasis disturbance, muscle damage, and biological harm.[67] As such, Amann and Dempsey[68] proposed the existence of a 'critical threshold' of peripheral fatigue and demonstrated that when the inhibitory feedback from group III/IV afferents was reduced by pharmacological blockade, the exercising adult subjects 'tolerated' the development of peripheral muscle fatigue substantially beyond their critical threshold.[69] It is currently unknown if this critical threshold is different between children and adults, but the lower peripheral and the higher central fatigue reported by Streckis *et al.*[17] and Ratel *et al.*[12] suggest the critical threshold could be centrally set at a higher level in children (Figure 9.3). Interestingly, Hatzikotoulas *et al.*[11] recently reported a comparable amount of central fatigue in children and adults, but lower peripheral fatigue in children. The authors suggested that at similar peripheral fatigue, children could have developed more central fatigue. This finding also supports the assumption that the central nervous system could not tolerate the development of an extensive peripheral fatigue in children, contrary to adults. Whether a higher limitation is set at a supraspinal level[70] and/or whether the sensitivity of the III-IV afferent fibres differ between children and adults remains to be determined. However, the specificity of physiological responses during exercise in prepubertal children leads us to believe that the activity of type III and IV afferents could be different between children and adults. Indeed, if these afferents are involved in the mechano- and metabo-sensitivity, they are also involved in nociception (i.e. the sensation or perception of pain) and regulation of cardiovascular and ventilatory responses. Given that the prepubertal children have a greater sensitivity to pain[71] and exacerbated cardiorespiratory responses to exercise (relative to their body dimensions)[72] that promotes aerobic metabolism,[73] they could therefore be characterized by a greater sensitivity of type III and IV afferents. However, this hypothesis remains to be verified. Furthermore, as the nature of the regulation (i.e. inhibitory or facilitatory) of the neural drive by the group III-IV afferents may vary across muscles,[74] other muscles should be investigated before generalization of these findings. Finally, we cannot exclude the additional contribution of other regulatory mechanisms, acting extrinsically or intrinsically on the motoneuron pool,[7] to account for the difference of central fatigue between children and adults. Thus, other nervous adjustments could also account for the lower fatigability in children, but these remain to be identified.

Beyond the influence of this potential central regulation of force output during a fatiguing task, the exercise duration could promote the development of central fatigue in children.[12,13] Indeed, the lower fatigability of prepubertal children translates into a longer exercise duration when repeating MVC until the same level of exhaustion, i.e. a predetermined percentage of initial MVC.[12,13] This assumption is supported by recent work[12] showing a positive relationship between the decrement in VA and the number of repeated isometric maximal contractions of the knee extensor muscles until the same level of exhaustion in prepubertal children and adults.

Regarding the central regulation of the antagonist co-activation under fatigue conditions, studies have reported different patterns between children and adults. Ratel *et al.*[12] showed that antagonist activity of the biceps femoris remained constant in adults whereas it significantly decreased in prepubertal children during repeated maximal voluntary isometric knee extensions. This observed decrease in antagonist co-activation in children may contribute to limit the loss of force, and therefore to delay peripheral fatigue.[12] Also, in this same study, the decrement of co-activation in children was positively correlated with the decrement of VA, which is consistent with the theory of 'common drive'.[62] Such a phenomenon could serve to maintain the balance between agonist and antagonist force in children, to preserve their joint integrity.[62] However, these results should be confirmed since other studies have reported contradictory results. Indeed, it has been shown during repeated isokinetic knee extensions that antagonist activity of the biceps femoris remained constant in adults and increased in prepubertal children because of a potential discomfort.[14,15] Furthermore, Armatas *et al.*[13] showed during repeated maximal voluntary isometric knee extensions that antagonist activity of the biceps femoris did not change in prepubertal children and adults and this could not explain the differences of fatigability between children and adults. Therefore, this issue requires further research.

Conclusions

The majority of the available scientific evidence supports the notion that prepubertal children fatigue less than adults when performing whole-body dynamic actions such as maximal cycling and short running bouts, or maximal voluntary isometric and isokinetic muscle contractions. Although the mechanisms underpinning differences in neuromuscular fatigue between children and adults are not fully understood, there is however a consensus that children experience less peripheral fatigue (i.e. muscular fatigue) than their older counterparts. This translates typically into a reduced twitch torque decrement and a lower low-frequency fatigue in children, which links to a lower alteration of excitation-contraction coupling and/or muscle contractile properties. Factors such as a lower maximal force-generating capacity, a more oxidative metabolic profile, and a higher percentage of fatigue-resistant slow-twitch fibres in children could account for these differences. Central factors may be also responsible for the lower fatigability in children. Some studies have reported a higher VA decrement during fatiguing exercise in children compared to adults. This observation could reflect a strategy of the central nervous system aimed at limiting the recruitment of motor units, in order to prevent any extensive peripheral fatigue. However, further studies examining the interplay of central vs peripheral factors on the development of neuromuscular fatigue in children compared to adults are required to clarify this assumption.

Summary

- Prepubertal children fatigue less than adults when performing maximal isometric or isokinetic muscle contractions, or whole-body dynamic activities, such as maximal cycling and short running bouts.
- The fatigability may be maturity-dependent during childhood given that adolescents fatigue more than children but less than adults during high-intensity intermittent exercise.
- Although the underlying factors are not fully identified, based on current evidence, there is a consensus that children develop lower peripheral fatigue compared to adults. This lower peripheral fatigue in children translates into a reduced twitch torque decrement and a lower low-frequency fatigue, suggesting a lower alteration of the excitation-contraction coupling and/or muscle contractile properties. However, the contribution of sarcolemmal excitability changes (i.e. M-wave changes) to peripheral fatigue in children remains contested.
- Children's metabolic profile, which is better reflective of oxidative than anaerobic metabolism during high-intensity exercise could explain their lower peripheral fatigue, through a lower depletion of phosphocreatine and a lower accumulation of H^+ ions and inorganic phosphate, which is known to impair muscle contractile properties. Other contributing factors such as a lower maximal force generating capacity and a higher % of fatigue resistant slow-twitch fibres in children are likely to account for these differences.
- Central factors may also be responsible for the lower fatigability in prepubertal children. Although the relative supraspinal and spinal contributions to the development of central fatigue remains to be determined in children compared to adults, the loss of voluntary activation of motor units was found to be higher in prepubertal children. This greater central fatigue observed in children could reflect a strategy of the central nervous system aimed at limiting the recruitment of motor units in order to prevent any extensive peripheral fatigue. However, further studies are required to clarify this issue.
- A practical implication from neuromuscular studies is that during maximal-intensity intermittent training, young children may cope better with shorter rest periods than are commonly used by adults. As a consequence, the combination between the various training parameters (number of sets, duration/intensity of exercise, and duration of recovery) should be chosen not only as a function of the aims of the training but also according to age and maturation level of individuals.[75,76]

References

1. Williams CA, Ratel S. Definitions of muscle fatigue. In: Williams CA, Ratel S (eds.) *Human muscle fatigue*. London: Routledge; 2009. p. 3–16.
2. Vollestad NK. Measurement of human muscle fatigue. *J Neurosci Methods*. 1997; 74: 219–227.
3. Sargeant AJ. Anaerobic performance. In: Armstrong N, Van Mechelen W (eds.) *Pediatric exercise science and medicine*. Oxford: Oxford University Press; 2000. p. 143–151.
4. Enoka RM, Stuart DG. Neurobiology of muscle fatigue. *J Appl Physiol*. 1992; 72: 1631–1648.
5. Kent-Braun JA. Central and peripheral contributions to muscle fatigue in humans during sustained maximal effort. *Eur J Appl Physiol Occup Physiol*. 1999; 80: 57–63.
6. Martin V, Kerherve H, Messonnier LA, *et al*. Central and peripheral contributions to neuromuscular fatigue induced by a 24-h treadmill run. *J Appl Physiol*. 2010; 108: 1224–1233.
7. Gandevia SC. Spinal and supraspinal factors in human muscle fatigue. *Physiol Rev*. 2001; 81: 1725–1789.
8. Hebestreit H, Mimura K, Bar-Or O. Recovery of muscle power after high-intensity short-term exercise: comparing boys and men. *J Appl Physiol*. 1993; 74: 2875–2880.
9. Ratel S, Duche P, Hennegrave A, Van Praagh E, Bedu M. Acid-base balance during repeated cycling sprints in boys and men. *J Appl Physiol*. 2002; 92: 479–485.
10. De Ste Croix MB, Deighan MA, Ratel S, Armstrong N. Age- and sex-associated differences in isokinetic knee muscle endurance between young children and adults. *Appl Physiol Nutr Metab*. 2009; 34: 725–731.
11. Hatzikotoulas K, Patikas D, Ratel S, Bass E, Kotzamanidis C. Central and peripheral fatigability in boys and men during maximal contraction. *Med Sci Sports Exerc*. 2014; 46: 1326–1333.
12. Ratel S, Kluka V, Vicencio SG, *et al*. Insights into the mechanisms of neuromuscular fatigue in boys and men. *Med Sci Sports Exerc*. 2015; 47: 2319–2328.
13. Armatas V, Bassa E, Patikas D, Kitsas I, Zangelidis G, Kotzamanidis C. Neuromuscular differences between men and prepubescent boys during a peak isometric knee extension intermittent fatigue test. *Pediatr Exerc Sci*. 2010; 22: 205–217.
14. Paraschos I, Hassani A, Bassa E, Hatzikotoulas K, Patikas D, Kotzamanidis C. Fatigue differences between adults and prepubertal males. *Int J Sports Med*. 2007; 28: 958–963.
15. Murphy JR, Button DC, Chaouachi A, Behm DG. Prepubescent males are less susceptible to neuromuscular fatigue following resistance exercise. *Eur J Appl Physiol*. 2014; 114: 825–835.
16. Merton PA. Voluntary strength and fatigue. *J Physiol*. 1954; 123: 553–564.
17. Streckis V, Skurvydas A, Ratkevicius A. Children are more susceptible to central fatigue than adults. *Muscle Nerve*. 2007; 36: 357–363.
18. Ratel S, Bedu M, Hennegrave A, Dore E, Duche P. Effects of age and recovery duration on peak power output during repeated cycling sprints. *Int J Sports Med*. 2002; 23: 397–402.
19. Ratel S, Williams CA, Oliver J, Armstrong N. Effects of age and mode of exercise on power output profiles during repeated sprints. *Eur J Appl Physiol*. 2004; 92: 204–210.
20. Ratel S, Williams CA, Oliver J, Armstrong N. Effects of age and recovery duration on performance during multiple treadmill sprints. *Int J Sports Med*. 2006; 27: 1–8.
21. Halin R, Germain P, Bercier S, Kapitaniak B, Buttelli O. Neuromuscular response of young boys versus men during sustained maximal contraction. *Med Sci Sports Exerc*. 2003; 35: 1042–1048.
22. Dipla K, Tsirini T, Zafeiridis A, *et al*. Fatigue resistance during high-intensity intermittent exercise from childhood to adulthood in males and females. *Eur J Appl Physiol*. 2009; 106: 645–653.
23. Zafeiridis A, Dalamitros A, Dipla K, Manou V, Galanis N, Kellis S. Recovery during high-intensity intermittent anaerobic exercise in boys, teens, and men. *Med Sci Sports Exerc*. 2005; 37: 505–512.
24. Dupont G, Berthoin S, Gerbeaux M. Performances lors d'un exercice intermittent anaérobie: comparaison entre enfants et sujets matures. *Sci. Sports*. 2000; 15: 147–153.
25. Lazaar N, Ratel S, Rudolf P, Bedu M, Duché P. Etude de la performance au cours d'un exercice intermittent en course à pied: influence de l'âge et de la durée de récupération. *Biométrie Humaine et Anthropologie*. 2002; 20: 29–34.

26. Williams JG, Eston R, Furlong B. CERT: a perceived exertion scale for young children. *Percept Mot Skills*. 1994; 79: 1451–1458.
27. Chen TC, Chen HL, Liu YC, Nosaka K. Eccentric exercise-induced muscle damage of pre-adolescent and adolescent boys in comparison to young men. *Eur J Appl Physiol*. 2014; 114: 1183–1195.
28. Gorianovas G, Skurvydas A, Streckis V, Brazaitis M, Kamandulis S, McHugh MP. Repeated bout effect was more expressed in young adult males than in elderly males and boys. *Biomed Res Int*. 2013; doi: 10.1155/2013/218970.
29. Garcia-Vicencio S, Martin V, Kluka V, *et al*. Obesity-related differences in neuromuscular fatigue in adolescent girls. *Eur J Appl Physiol*. 2015; 115: 2421–2432.
30. Hunter SK, Critchlow A, Shin IS, Enoka RM. Fatigability of the elbow flexor muscles for a sustained submaximal contraction is similar in men and women matched for strength. *J Appl Physiol*. 2004; 96: 195–202.
31. Kappenstein J, Ferrauti A, Runkel B, Fernandez-Fernandez J, Muller K, Zange J. Changes in phosphocreatine concentration of skeletal muscle during high-intensity intermittent exercise in children and adults. *Eur J Appl Physiol*. 2013; 113: 2769–2779.
32. Fleischman A, Makimura H, Stanley TL, *et al*. Skeletal muscle phosphocreatine recovery after submaximal exercise in children and young and middle-aged adults. *J Clin Endocrinol Metab*. 2010; 95: E69–E74.
33. Ratel S, Tonson A, Le Fur Y, Cozzone P, Bendahan D. Comparative analysis of skeletal muscle oxidative capacity in children and adults: a 31P-MRS study. *Appl Physiol Nutr Metab*. 2008; 33: 720–727.
34. Tonson A, Ratel S, Le Fur Y, Vilmen C, Cozzone PJ, Bendahan D. Muscle energetics changes throughout maturation: a quantitative 31P-MRS analysis. *J Appl Physiol*. 2010; 109: 1769–1778.
35. McCully KK, Faulkner JA. Characteristics of lengthening contractions associated with injury to skeletal muscle fibers. *J Appl Physiol*. 1986; 61: 293–299.
36. Warren GL, Hayes DA, Lowe DA, Armstrong RB. Mechanical factors in the initiation of eccentric contraction-induced injury in rat soleus muscle. *J Physiol*. 1993; 464: 457–475.
37. Hamada T, Sale DG, MacDougall JD, Tarnopolsky MA. Interaction of fibre type, potentiation and fatigue in human knee extensor muscles. *Acta Physiol Scand*. 2003; 178: 165–173.
38. Du Plessis MP, Smit PJ, Du Plessis LAS, Geyer HJ, Mathews G, Louw HNJ. The composition of muscle fibers in a group of adolescents. In: Binkhorst RA, Kemper HCG, Saris WHM (eds.) *Children and exercise XI*. Champaign, IL: Human Kinetics; 1985. p. 323–328.
39. Fournier M, Ricci J, Taylor AW, Ferguson RJ, Montpetit RR, Chaitman BR. Skeletal muscle adaptation in adolescent boys: sprint and endurance training and detraining. *Med Sci Sports Exerc*. 1982; 14: 453–456.
40. Glenmark B, Hedberg G, Kaijser L, Jansson E. Muscle strength from adolescence to adulthood—relationship to muscle fibre types. *Eur J Appl Physiol Occup Physiol*. 1994; 68: 9–19.
41. Lexell J, Sjostrom M, Nordlund AS, Taylor CC. Growth and development of human muscle: a quantitative morphological study of whole vastus lateralis from childhood to adult age. *Muscle Nerve*. 1992; 15: 404–409.
42. Bell RD, MacDougall JD, Billeter R, Howald H. Muscle fiber types and morphometric analysis of skeletal msucle in six-year-old children. *Med Sci Sports Exerc*. 1980; 12: 28–31.
43. Berg A, Keul J. Biochemical changes during exercise in children. In: Malina R (ed.) *Young athletes/biological, psychological and educational perspectives*. Champaign, IL: Human Kinetics; 1988. p. 61–77.
44. Berg A, Kim SS, Keul J. Skeletal muscle enzyme activities in healthy young subjects. *Int J Sports Med*. 1986; 7: 236–239.
45. Eriksson BO, Gollnick PD, Saltin B. Muscle metabolism and enzyme activities after training in boys 11–13 years old. *Acta Physiol Scand*. 1973; 87: 485–497.
46. Haralambie G. Enzyme activities in skeletal muscle of 13–15 years old adolescents. *Bull Eur Physiopathol Respir*. 1982; 18: 65–74.
47. Taylor DJ, Kemp GJ, Thompson CH, Radda GK. Ageing: effects on oxidative function of skeletal muscle in vivo. *Mol Cell Biochem*. 1997; 174: 321–324.
48. Allen DG, Lamb GD, Westerblad H. Skeletal muscle fatigue: cellular mechanisms. *Physiol Rev*. 2008; 88: 287–332.
49. Hicks KM, Onambele-Pearson GL, Winwood K, Morse CI. Gender differences in fascicular lengthening during eccentric contractions: the role of the patella tendon stiffness. *Acta Physiol (Oxf)*. 2013; 209: 235–244.
50. Lichtwark GA, Barclay CJ. A compliant tendon increases fatigue resistance and net efficiency during fatiguing cyclic contractions of mouse soleus muscle. *Acta Physiol (Oxf)*. 2012; 204: 533–543.
51. Waugh CM, Korff T, Fath F, Blazevich AJ. Rapid force production in children and adults: mechanical and neural contributions. *Med Sci Sports Exerc*. 2013; 45: 762–771.
52. Marginson V, Eston R. The relationship between torque and joint angle during knee extension in boys and men. *J Sports Sci*. 2001; 19: 875–880.
53. Fitch S, McComas A. Influence of human muscle length on fatigue. *J Physiol*. 1985; 362: 205–213.
54. Desbrosses K, Babault N, Scaglioni G, Meyer JP, Pousson M. Neural activation after maximal isometric contractions at different muscle lengths. *Med Sci Sports Exerc*. 2006; 38: 937–944.
55. Nordlund MM, Thorstensson A, Cresswell AG. Central and peripheral contributions to fatigue in relation to level of activation during repeated maximal voluntary isometric plantar flexions. *J Appl Physiol*. 2004; 96: 218–225.
56. Henneman E, Somjen G, Carpenter DO. Excitability and inhibitability of motoneurons of different sizes. *J Neurophysiol*. 1965; 28: 599–620.
57. Blimkie CJ. Age- and sex-associated variations in strength during childhood: Anthopometric, morphologic, neurologic, biomechanic, endocrinologic, genetic and physcial activity correlates. In: Gisolfi C, Lamb D (eds.) *Perspectives in exercise science and sport medicine: youth, exercise and sport*. Indianapolis: Benchmark Press; 1989. p. 99–163.
58. Kluka V, Martin V, Vicencio SG, *et al*. Effect of muscle length on voluntary activation level in children and adults. *Med Sci Sports Exerc*. 2015; 47: 718–724.
59. O'Brien TD, Reeves ND, Baltzopoulos V, Jones DA, Maganaris CN. In vivo measurements of muscle specific tension in adults and children. *Exp Physiol*. 2010; 95: 202–210.
60. Martin V, Kluka V, Garcia Vicencio S, Maso F, Ratel S. Children have a reduced maximal voluntary activation level of the adductor pollicis muscle compared to adults. *Eur J Appl Physiol*. 2015; 115: 1485–1491.
61. Grosset JF, Mora I, Lambertz D, Perot C. Voluntary activation of the triceps surae in prepubertal children. *J Electromyogr Kinesiol*. 2008; 18: 455–465.
62. Psek JA, Cafarelli E. Behavior of coactive muscles during fatigue. *J Appl Physiol*. 1993; 74: 170–175.
63. Bassa E, Patikas D, Kotzamanidis C. Activation of antagonist knee muscles during isokinetic efforts in prepubertal and adult males. *Pediatr Exerc Sci*. 2005; 17: 171–181.
64. Kellis E, Unnithan VB. Co-activation of vastus lateralis and biceps femoris muscles in pubertal children and adults. *Eur J Appl Physiol Occup Physiol*. 1999; 79: 504–511.
65. Frost G, Dowling J, Dyson K, Bar-Or O. Cocontraction in three age groups of children during treadmill locomotion. *J Electromyogr Kinesiol*. 1997; 7: 179–186.
66. Lazaridis SN, Bassa EI, Patikas D, Hatzikotoulas K, Lazaridis FK, Kotzamanidis CM. Biomechanical comparison in different jumping tasks between untrained boys and men. *Pediatr Exerc Sci*. 2013; 25: 101–113.
67. Noakes TD, St Clair Gibson A, Lambert EV. From catastrophe to complexity: a novel model of integrative central neural regulation of effort and fatigue during exercise in humans: summary and conclusions. *Br J Sports Med*. 2005; 39: 120–124.
68. Amann M, Dempsey JA. The concept of peripheral locomotor muscle fatigue as a regulated variable. *J Physiol*. 2008; 586: 2029–2030.
69. Amann M, Blain GM, Proctor LT, Sebranek JJ, Pegelow DF, Dempsey JA. Implications of group III and IV muscle afferents for high-intensity endurance exercise performance in humans. *J Physiol*. 2011; 589: 5299–5309.

70. Millet GY. Can neuromuscular fatigue explain running strategies and performance in ultra-marathons?: the flush model. *Sports Med.* 2011; 41: 489–506.
71. Sandrini G, Alfonsi E, Ruiz L, Livieri C, Verri AP, Nappi G. Age-related changes in excitability of nociceptive flexion reflex. An electrophysiological study in school-age children and young adults. *Funct Neurol.* 1989; 4: 53–58.
72. Rowland TW, Cunningham LN. Development of ventilatory responses to exercise in normal white children. A longitudinal study. *Chest.* 1997; 111: 327–332.
73. Ratel S, Duche P, Hennegrave A, Van Praagh E, Bedu M. Acid-base balance during repeated cycling sprints in boys and men. *J Appl Physiol.* 2002; 92: 479–485.
74. Martin PG, Smith JL, Butler JE, Gandevia SC, Taylor JL. Fatigue-sensitive afferents inhibit extensor but not flexor motoneurons in humans. *J Neurosci.* 2006; 26: 4796–4802.
75. Ratel S, Duche P, Williams CA. Muscle fatigue during high-intensity exercise in children. *Sports Med.* 2006; 36: 1031–1065.
76. Ratel S, Lazaar N, Dore E, *et al.* High-intensity intermittent activities at school: controversies and facts. *J Sports Med Phys Fitness.* 2004; 44: 272–280.
77. Chia M. Power recovery in the Wingate anaerobic test in girls and women following prior sprints of a short duration. *Biol Sport.* 2001; 18: 45–53.
78. Bottaro M, Brown LE, Celes R, Martorelli S, Carregaro R, de Brito Vidal JC. Effect of rest interval on neuromuscular and metabolic responses between children and adolescents. *Pediatr Exerc Sci.* 2011; 23: 311–321.
79. Kanehisa H, Okuyama H, Ikegawa S, Fukunaga T. Fatigability during repetitive maximal knee extensions in 14-year-old boys. *Eur J Appl Physiol Occup Physiol.* 1995; 72: 170–174.

CHAPTER 10

Pulmonary function

Alison M McManus and Neil Armstrong

Introduction

Episodic breathing movements begin in utero, with an intrinsic rhythmicity already established so that from birth the continuous movement of air into and out of the lungs, ventilation, is possible.[1] Ventilation is a remarkably adaptive process, modifying with structural changes as the lungs and respiratory muscles grow and mature, and adjusting to alterations in environmental conditions such as exercise or hypoxia. Pulmonary gas exchange depends on ventilation as the primary step in the oxygen transport pathway, allowing oxygen uptake ($\dot{V}O_2$) and carbon dioxide removal ($\dot{V}CO_2$) to be tightly regulated. Even when metabolic demands change, such as the onset of moderate intensity exercise, ventilation maintains the partial pressures of arterial oxygen (PaO_2) and carbon dioxide ($PaCO_2$) and pH close to resting levels. As exercise becomes increasingly more intense, additional demands are placed on $\dot{V}O_2$ and $\dot{V}CO_2$, yet the exquisite control of ventilation enables adequate gas exchange.

The principles of pulmonary ventilation are the same for children and adults, but the child's pulmonary system is immature and it is well established that the pulmonary responses to exercise are not the same for the child as the adult. The lungs may be ready to function from birth, but are not structurally mature until adulthood, with lung weight increasing three-fold and lung surface area increasing tenfold from birth to 18 years of age.[2,3] Changes in body size impact both the structure and function of the lung, with, for example, alterations in mechanical properties of the lung as the child grows, resulting in decreases in airway resistance and increases in compliance.[4] Similar to adults, ventilation adjusts to alterations in metabolic demand during moderate intensity exercise in the child, but for a given exercise intensity there is a greater ventilation when expressed relative to body mass, and a higher energetic cost of breathing in the child compared to the adult.[5,6]

The reasons for the child-adult differences in pulmonary responses to exercise remain unclear, and our understanding is limited by a paucity of research in the child. The control of breathing during exercise in adults has been a topic of intense debate for over a century and remains one of the most challenging physiological questions under scrutiny.[7–9] Various control mechanisms for exercise hyperpnoea have been proposed. Two theories dominate. The first is a feed-forward system, whereby neural signals from higher brain centres are responsible for the locomotor and cardiorespiratory responses to exercise. Alternatively, a feedback system relays signals from a variety of afferents, such as the muscle contraction itself, blood-borne metabolites, or respiratory muscle action, to the central controller to effect changes in breathing.[8] As exercise increases in intensity toward maximum, ventilation increases out of proportion to metabolic need and the response again changes, with the ensuing hyperventilation thought to be driven by both peripheral and central signals, including limb fatigue and chemoreceptors.[7] Limited evidence suggests the differing pulmonary response to exercise of the child may be a result of immature chemoreception,[10,11] a greater drive to breathe,[12] and/or differences in airway dimensions and the mechanical work of breathing.[5] Understanding the ontogenetic changes in pulmonary function during exercise is therefore important to both the paediatric exercise scientist and the clinician.

Resting pulmonary function

Lung volumes

To appreciate exercise ventilation, an understanding of resting lung volumes is important. These volumes refer to various gas-containing spaces in the lungs, as shown in Figure 10.1. The volume of each breath during normal breathing is the tidal volume (V_T). Absolute V_T increases with age, but when body mass and body surface area are taken into consideration values decrease with age.[13] The frequency of breaths taken per minute (f_R) declines from ~24–25 breaths·min^{-1} during early childhood, to ~13–15 breaths·min^{-1} by 16 years of age.[14]

Using a spirometer, when a child takes a maximal inspiration, the volume of air inhaled above the V_T is the inspiratory reserve volume (IRV). If the child now exhales maximally, the volume of air expired beyond the V_T is the expiratory reserve volume (ERV). Any air left in the lungs after a maximal expiration is the residual volume (RV). The IRV, ERV, and V_T comprise the vital capacity (VC). Using the same manoeuver, if the child is asked to exhale as hard and completely as possible, the total volume exhaled is the forced vital capacity (FVC). The gas that remains in the lung after a normal expiration is the functional residual capacity (FRC). As can be seen from Figure 10.1, the total lung capacity (TLC) is the sum of IRV, V_T, ERV, and RV.

Lung volumes are related to body size, with increases in TLC with age in the child primarily reflecting growth of the chest wall in both boys and girls.[15] Lung growth appears to lag behind growth in stature and the relationship between lung volume and stature alters between childhood and adolescence.[16,17] Sitting height is a preferred reference variable for growth spurts in the lung because of the close association with trunk development and thus thoracic size.[15] Sex differences in lung volumes are apparent even when stature has been accounted for, and this is likely an outcome of differences in thoracic size.[15] With increasing age, the ratio of chest width to sitting height becomes greater in boys, but remains constant in girls, contributing to the increasing sex differences in lung

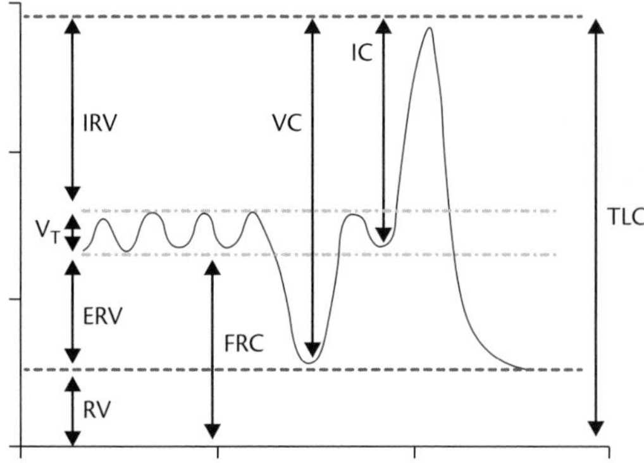

Figure 10.1 Lung volumes as they appear on a spirographic tracing.
Note that the total lung capacity, functional residual capacity, and residual volume cannot be measured with the spirometer.
V_T = tidal volume, IRV = inspiratory reserve volume, ERV = expiratory reserve volume, RV = residual volume, FRC = functional residual capacity, VC = vital capacity, IC = inspiratory capacity, TLC = total lung capacity.

volumes.[15] This also possibly reflects sex divergence in the mechanical properties of the lung.[18] As with many physiological variables, because of the heteroscedastic scatter of the residuals around the regression of lung volumes on either body mass or stature, log-linear transformations are the preferred model for understanding the variance in resting lung volumes with size in the growing child, but have seldom been used.[19]

Assessing the FRC and RV requires more complex measurement than simple spirometry. Available techniques include gas dilution (such as helium [He] dilution or nitrogen [N_2] washout measurements), whole body plethysmography using various methodologies (based on Boyle's law, which assumes that in a closed container changes in lung volume can be calculated from changes in pressure under constant temperature), and radiographic imaging methods using standard posterior-anterior and lateral chest radiographs or computerized tomography (CT).[20]

The multi-breath He dilution technique is a commonly used approach with the younger child; however, when comparing FRC values obtained from plethysmography and He gas-dilution, derived FRC values have been found to be between 130–320 mL lower using the He gas-dilution method for children of varying stature.[21] In contrast, Kraemer and colleagues[22] found no significant differences in FRC values derived from plethysmography, N_2 washout, and He dilution in children aged 7–17 years of age. Repeated measures of FRC are recommended to keep the coefficient of variation below 5%; however this is less feasible with gas-dilution or washout techniques because of the interval necessary between repeated tests. In comparison repeated measures are simple and quick with plethysmography. Usually three to five repeated manoeuvers provide a coefficient of variation within 5% for plethysmographic FRC values in the child.[18] As such, plethysmographic measures of FRC and RV are now more commonly used with healthy children than gas dilution or washout techniques.[23]

Flow rates

The combined assessment of forced expiratory volume (FEV) and flow rates provide dynamic measures of lung function and a marker of airway patency.[24] This is most commonly achieved using the flow-volume loop. The flow-volume loop combines forced expiratory flow rates with timed FEVs. A timed FEV is defined as the volume of air exhaled in a given time during a FVC measurement, such as in 1 s (FEV_1). Forced expiratory volume in 1 s is normally ~85–86% of the FVC in children,[25] with the FEV_1/FVC_1 ratio decreasing with increasing age and stature.[26] This suggests a physiological narrowing of small and large airways relative to lung size with growth. The flow-volume loop of a healthy child is shown in Figure 10.2a. When the child inspires to total lung capacity, then exhales as hard as possible to RV the flow-volume loop can be recorded. As can be seen in Figure 10.2a, flow rises rapidly during inspiration then declines through expiration. The peak expiratory flow rate falls early in the expiratory manoeuver in the healthy child, the FEV_1 is usually recorded at ~85–86% of FVC.[26] Forced expiratory volume in 1 s provides an indicator of large airway patency, while the FEV flow rate between 25% and 75% of FVC (FEV_{25-75}) provides a marker of small airway patency. These measures are useful for identifying restrictive and obstructive limitations. An obstructive limitation, such as in asthma, would be characterized by an expiratory flow that ends prematurely (see Figure 10.2b). In the case of asthma this would be because of early airway closure reducing the FEV_1.[27] A restrictive limitation, as seen in scoliosis,[28] would be noted by normal flow but limited inspiration and hence a reduced FVC (see Figure 10.2c). This may be because of the reduced compliance of the lung and /or weakness of the inspiratory muscles.

Dead space

For each tidal breath some of the inhaled air remains in the conducting airways where no gas exchange takes place. This air is the anatomic dead space, which can be estimated non-invasively using a variety of methods, including single breath analyses of expired CO_2. Kerr[29] found anatomic dead space in children increases from ~38 mL at 110 cm in stature, to ~60 mL at a stature of 140 cm and ~80 mL at 160 cm. This is estimated to be approximately 18% of V_T in 5- to 16-year-olds.[29] The first part of each breath effectively flushes the anatomic dead space. The volume of inspired air that does enter the alveoli and is available for gas exchange is the alveolar ventilation ($\dot{V}_A$); however, a portion of this air does not participate in gas exchange and is known as the physiologic dead space (V_D). In healthy adults it is assumed that the physiologic and anatomic dead spaces are almost the same. Anatomic and physiologic dead spaces are smaller in children than in adults and a difference between anatomic and physiologic dead spaces of ~44.5 mL has been shown to exist between the ages of 5 and 16 years.[29] Measurement of physiologic dead space requires invasive measurement of the $PaCO_2$; however, this is not always feasible or desirable in the healthy child. Instead, physiologic dead space is usually estimated using the Bohr equation,[30] estimating $PaCO_2$ from end-tidal CO_2 ($P_{ET}CO_2$; the CO_2 recorded at the end of the breath). Using this non-invasive approach, estimates of physiologic dead space of approximately 70 mL were reported for children of 1.10 m in stature, 110 mL for those at 1.40 m, and 140 mL at 1.60 m.[29] These represent ~33 ± 4.6% of V_T, from 5 to 16 years of age, similar to findings in adults from directly assessed physiologic dead space.[31]

The use of $P_{ET}CO_2$ as a surrogate for $PaCO_2$ is commonplace, however, there are a number of important assumptions that should be considered. The difference between $PaCO_2$ and $P_{ET}CO_2$ is a result of the relationship between ventilation, airflow to the alveoli and perfusion, reflecting ventilation-perfusion matching. Calculation of the arterial to end-tidal CO_2 difference requires

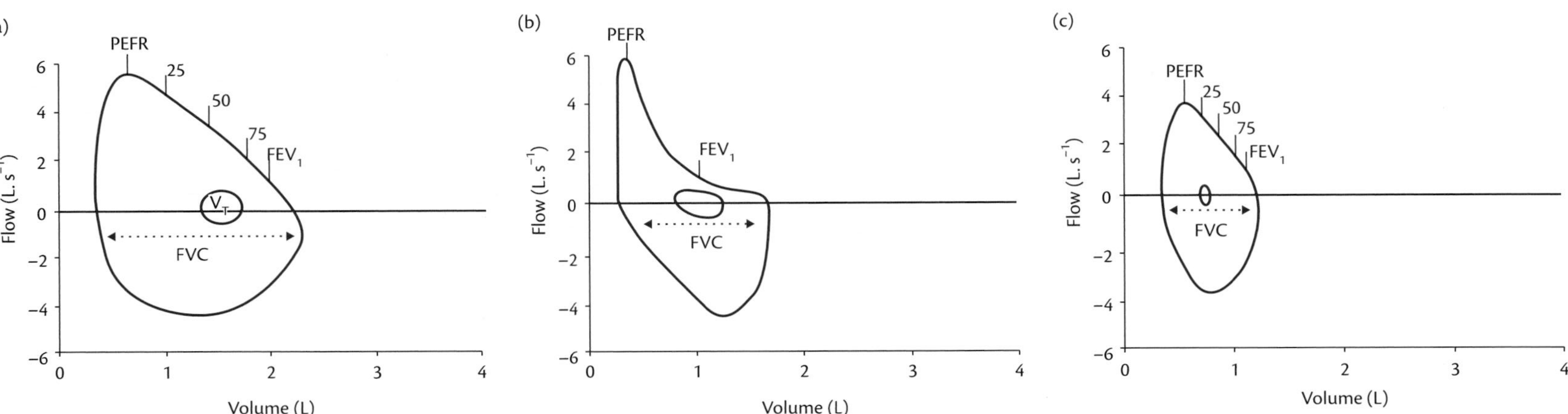

Figure 10.2 Flow-volume loops.

Flow-volume loops obtained by recording expiratory flow rates and timed forced expiratory volumes. The figure illustrates flow-volume loops for (a) a healthy child, (b) a child with an obstructive lung limitation and (c) a child with a restrictive lung limitation. Tidal volume loop (V_T), peak expiratory flow rate (PEFR), forced expiratory volume in 1 s (FEV_1) and forced expiratory volume at 25%, 50%, and 75% of forced vital capacity (FVC) are labelled.

simultaneous assessment of arterial blood gases and an end-tidal measurement. In healthy adults there is a good match between alveolar ventilation and perfusion to the pulmonary capillaries at rest and despite $P_{ET}CO_2$ underestimating resting $PaCO_2$, $P_{ET}CO_2$ is a widely accepted surrogate for $PaCO_2$ and used to estimate the dead space to tidal volume ratio (V_D/V_T).

Using $P_{ET}CO_2$ as a noninvasive index for $PaCO_2$ during exercise violates the assumption that there is a constant relationship between $P_{ET}CO_2$ and $PaCO_2$.[32] Exercise increases pulmonary capillary recruitment, intrapulmonary shunting, and mixed venous PCO_2, widening the gradient between $P_{ET}CO_2$ and $PaCO_2$. This results in an over-prediction of $PaCO_2$. Although correction factors have been developed, the most common of these being the Jones equation[33] ($PaCO_2 = 5.5 + 0.9\,P_{ET}CO_2 — 0.0021\,V_T$), prediction of V_D/V_T during exercise from $P_{ET}CO_2$ is tenuous. Evidence in children is limited largely to the critically ill, but similar to adults, alterations in $PaCO_2$ at rest are closely followed by alterations in $P_{ET}CO_2$, with $P_{ET}CO_2$ generally lower than $PaCO_2$.[34] Ohuchi and colleagues[35] explored the relationship between $P_{ET}CO_2$ and $PaCO_2$ during exercise in a small group of children and adolescents, establishing that the prediction of $PaCO_2$ could be improved by including age, $\dot{V}_E/\dot{V}CO_2$, respiratory exchange ratio (R), and $P_{ET}CO_2$ within the regression equation:

$$PaCO_2 = 12.0 + 0.54\,P_{ET}CO_2 + 0.15\,\dot{V}_E/\dot{V}CO_2 - 3.6\,R + 0.22\,\text{age}$$

Using the above equation predicted $PaCO_2$ was only fractionally less (–0.1 mmHg) than the actual $PaCO_2$ in the younger child and provided a good fit (slope = 1.0, r = 0.86). In comparison, the Jones equation[33] resulted in a shallower slope (slope = 0.59; r = 0.72) and a significant inverse correlation between the measured and predicted values and the mean of the two $PaCO_2$ values.[35] The improved prediction of $PaCO_2$ most likely relates to the developmental differences in the response of CO_2 and $\dot{V}_E$ (pulmonary ventilation) during exercise in children.[5,6] It should be noted however, that the control children in Ohuchi *et al.*'s study[35] had Kawasaki's disease and it is possible that this could affect the lung vasculature, perhaps leading to differences in lung dead space, and hence an altered $P_{ET}CO_2$—$PaCO_2$ relationship. Despite the improved prediction of $PaCO_2$, V_D/V_T estimated using $P_{ET}CO_2$ resulted in a wide limit of agreement (± 5%), highlighting the limitations of this noninvasive index in children.[35]

Perhaps it is timely to re-visit approaches which would allow more detailed investigations of $PaCO_2$ and thus adequacy of ventilation during exercise in children. Arterialized capillary blood can be used as a surrogate for arterial blood, with arterial $PaCO_2$, PaO_2, and pH values closely mirrored by arterialized capillary blood values. There are limitations however if multiple samples during continuous steady-state exercise are required. Alternatively PCO_2 and pH can be obtained with a high degree of precision from arterialized venous blood (usually drawn from the superficial dorsal hand veins).[36] This technique is particularly advantageous in exercise pulmonary studies where there is the need for repeated samples during steady-state exercise without disruption to the exercise and therefore without disruption to ventilation. The disadvantage for children is the insertion of a thin-wall vein needle and the need for hand warming; however, in adults the procedure is accomplished with little or no discomfort,[36] and with carefully designed habituation this may be feasible with young people.

Methodological considerations

Whether at rest or during exercise, the assessment of pulmonary function can be technically challenging in the child.[37] To detect volume and flow measurement requires either a mouthpiece and nose-clip or facemask. The choice of equipment and its dead space influences the assessment of pulmonary function, as does the child's cooperation, ability, and/or willingness to perform respiratory manoeuvers properly.

The child's ability to perform a respiratory manoeuver with acceptable reliability can be challenging if the manoeuver requires effort, such as the assessment of forced expiratory volumes and flow. Children need a calm, relaxed environment, and if taught well the manoeuvers can be performed properly and with sufficient reliability, even in younger children. The importance of experienced and well-trained staff, combined with lots of patience, as well as appropriate participant training and habituation cannot be overstated in achieving reliable pulmonary measures in children.

Changes in the pattern of ventilation have been associated with the equipment used to measure it.[38,39] The switch from nasal to oral breathing has resulted in a 60 mL increase in V_T in adults, which corresponds with the volume of the buccal cavity.[38] Mouthpieces, if too large, may impose uncomfortable constraints on the child, which might be expected to affect the pattern of breathing. Mouthpieces have been found to cause an increase in electromyographic activity in the diaphragm, the scalene, and sternocleidomastoid muscles.[40] A drop in f_R can also occur with mouthpiece use, which may be explained by the inhibition of respiration by stimulation of the trigeminal receptors. Maxwell and colleagues[39] found that noseclips also appear to slow breathing, again probably due to stimulation of trigeminal receptors. Increases have been noted in T_V, most likely because of the change from nasal to oral breathing, likely offset the drop in f_R noted above. Although mouthpiece use may affect breathing patterns, the alternative, the facemask is often poorly fitting and the resultant leakage is a more persistent problem.

Masks, mouthpieces, and valves must have an appropriate dead space, so that gas analysis reflects the dead space ventilation of the child and not that of the equipment.[41] Equipment dead space may significantly confound the measurement and interpretation of $\dot{V}_E$ in children.[42] For example, a higher ventilatory equivalent for oxygen ($\dot{V}_E/\dot{V}O_2$) or carbon dioxide ($\dot{V}_E/\dot{V}CO_2$) is often used as a marker of ventilatory inefficiency in the child. This may however, reflect equipment dead space that is overly large. Using a modeling approach, the effects of apparatus dead space on $PaCO_2$ and f_R was explored in infants and children of hypothetical body mass from 2–17 kg.[43] Findings demonstrated that the lighter the mass the greater the impact of increasing apparatus dead space on increases in $PaCO_2$. The rise in $PaCO_2$ also led to an exponential increase in f_R in an effort to maintain normocapnia. It has been recommended that apparatus dead space should not exceed 59 mL in children with a body surface area over 1.0 m^2 and 39 mL in smaller children.[42]

Pulmonary responses to exercise

Ventilation adapts to exercise in an intensity specific manner through increases in both f_R and T_V. At lower intensities $\dot{V}_E$ matches metabolic demand closely mirroring changes in $\dot{V}O_2$ and $\dot{V}CO_2$. As intensity reaches and exceeds the ventilatory threshold (T_{VENT}), a non-invasive marker of the lactate threshold (T_{LAC}), the slope of increase in $\dot{V}_E$ steepens, as bicarbonate buffering of lactic acid increases, limiting the fall of pH_a. As exercise intensity approaches maximum, $\dot{V}_E$ breaks away from $\dot{V}CO_2$ and CO_2 is washed out of body stores, resulting in hyperventilation and a fall in $PaCO_2$. It is clear that, like adults, the response of $\dot{V}_E$ to exercise more closely matches the need for CO_2 clearance rather than the need for increased PaO_2. This has been elegantly described in adults using the integrated influence of $\dot{V}CO_2$and $PaCO_2$ on $\dot{V}_E$ for a given exercise intensity, taking into consideration the influence of dead space ventilation.[44] The ventilatory requirement for a particular exercise intensity has therefore been expressed using the following equation:

$$\dot{V}_E(BTPS) = \frac{863 \times \dot{V}CO_2(STPD)}{PaCO_2\left(1 - \frac{V_D}{V_T}\right)}$$

Changes to the components $PaCO_2$, $\dot{V}CO_2$, or V_D/V_T are readily seen in adjustments to $\dot{V}_E$. For example, as $PaCO_2$ falls with hyperventilation at maximal exercise, a greater $\dot{V}_E$ is required to support the increase in $\dot{V}CO_2$. A rise in V_D/V_T in the same individual (such as in the less-compliant lung) would further increase the $\dot{V}_E$ response.[44] These principles are the same for children, except the input components respond in an age- and maturity-dependent manner resulting in exercise $\dot{V}_E$ responses that are both quantitatively and qualitatively different in the child compared to the adult.

Breathing patterns during exercise

Breathing patterns are diverse and variable both within and between children.[45] Breathing pattern is determined primarily by alterations in T_V, f_R, inspiratory (T_I), and expiratory durations (T_E). End-inspiratory and end-expiratory lung volumes (EILV and EELV respectively) and the drive to breathe are also believed to be important in determining the pattern of breathing.

During moderate intensity exercise both f_R and V_T increase to achieve the necessary $\dot{V}_E$ response. As exercise intensity increases beyond moderate intensity, a higher reliance on f_R has been shown in children than adults,[46] accompanied by an increased f_R/V_T ratio.[47] This rise in f_R at higher intensities is believed to result from decreases in both T_I and T_E and is often referred to as a 'tachypneic' breathing pattern. In adults, a plateau in V_T is apparent in higher intensity exercise at ~50–60% of FVC.[48] Limiting the increase in V_T is important because there is a concomitant reduction in EELV below resting levels, which minimizes the elastic work of breathing and maximizes the mechanical efficiency of breathing.[48] Increasing V_T further is thought to result in a greater metabolic cost than simply increasing the f_R. In the child, there is evidence that f_R plateaus at ~65–70% of maximal exercise.[49,50] Further increases in $\dot{V}_E$ are achieved through increases in V_T, with a corresponding fall in the f_R/V_T ratio, suggesting a lower ventilatory efficiency and higher metabolic cost of breathing in the child.[49,50]

The drive and timing of components of $\dot{V}_E$ provide physiologically relevant markers of the breathing pattern. Inspiratory drive can be calculated from V_T divided by the T_I. When normalized for body mass, inspiratory drive decreases with age, with a drop of ~31% from age 8 to 18 years.[12,51] It is unclear what aspect of drive, V_T or T_I, is responsible for this decrease, but a greater increase in T_I with age (~42%) is apparent compared to a small decrease in V_T per kg body mass (~11%), suggesting T_I is more influential.[51] The timing of inspiration over a respiratory cycle (T_I/T_{TOT}) also decreases with age.

Both inspiratory drive and timing increase with exercise intensity and this increase is believed to relate to changes in $PaCO_2$ with increasing intensity of exercise. Estimating $PaCO_2$ from $P_{ET}CO_2$, Ondrak and Murray[51] investigated the relationship between $PaCO_2$, respiratory drive and timing at rest and during exercise in 8- to 18-year-olds. The relationship between inspiratory drive and $P_{ET}CO_2$ was strongest at rest and weakest at high intensity exercise in 8- to 18-year-olds, suggesting that $P_{ET}CO_2$ plays only a limited role in inspiratory timing and drive at higher exercise intensities during childhood.

Responses to acute moderate-intensity exercise

As a child ages $\dot{V}_E$ relative to body size declines for the same submaximal exercise intensity.[52] The decline in size-relative $\dot{V}_E$ is thought to relate largely to the decline in f_R, but may also relate to changes in ventilatory control mechanisms with age. Absolute V_T in contrast increases with age, but when scaled to body mass is stable with age during submaximal exercise.[47]

At absolute submaximal exercise intensities there is a wide range of sex differences in the ventilatory response. Girls demonstrate higher f_R, adjusted $\dot{V}_E$, f_R/V_T, $\dot{V}_E/\dot{V}O_2$, and $\dot{V}_E/\dot{V}CO_2$ in comparison to boys.[47] Accounting for the higher peak $\dot{V}O_2$ in boys, Armstrong and colleagues[47] also compared ventilatory responses at 70–75% and 80–85% of peak $\dot{V}O_2$. Sex differences in f_R, $\dot{V}_E/\dot{V}O_2$, $\dot{V}_E/\dot{V}CO_2$, and V_T/FVC were no longer apparent at these relative submaximal exercise intensities.[47] Mass adjusted $\dot{V}_E$ and V_T remained higher in boys, suggesting that at the same relative intensity boys support their higher $\dot{V}O_2$ with a higher $\dot{V}_E$.

Normalizing exercise intensity using a percentage of maximal oxygen uptake ($\dot{V}O_2$ max) is problematic because of the smaller absolute $\dot{V}O_2$ max of the child, which severely compresses the range of intensities within a given exercise intensity domain.[53] Anchoring intensity to the T_{VENT} provides greater methodological rigour. The T_{VENT} reflects the highest exercise intensity that can be performed at the expense of oxidative energy production, therefore reflecting the oxidative potential of the working muscle. Exercise at intensities below the T_{VENT} does not result in sustained metabolic acidosis and is considered moderate in intensity.[54] The T_{VENT} is commonly determined using the relationship between the ventilatory equivalents, where there is an abrupt increase in the $\dot{V}_E/\dot{V}O_2$, without an accompanying increase in the $\dot{V}_E/\dot{V}CO_2$. Figure 10.3 provides an illustration of the T_{VENT} determined by the ventilatory equivalents method.

Since ventilation can be erratic and lag behind $\dot{V}O_2$ in certain conditions e.g. in obese patients or those with airway obstruction, an alternative procedure avoiding the use of ventilation in the calculation is the V-slope method.[55] This involves regressing CO_2 production against $\dot{V}O_2$. The V-slope method is based upon the intersection of the two regression lines explaining $\dot{V}CO_2$ as a function of $\dot{V}O_2$ and is illustrated in Figure 10.4. The T_{VENT} is chosen from the point at which the residual sum of squares is minimized. Plotting ventilatory variables against $\dot{V}O_2$ rather than time improves detection rates and therefore the V-slope method is the preferred mode of determination.

The ventilatory response to moderate intensity exercise has been used to assess efficiency or ventilation/perfusion mismatch. As noted earlier a non-invasive marker of ventilation/perfusion

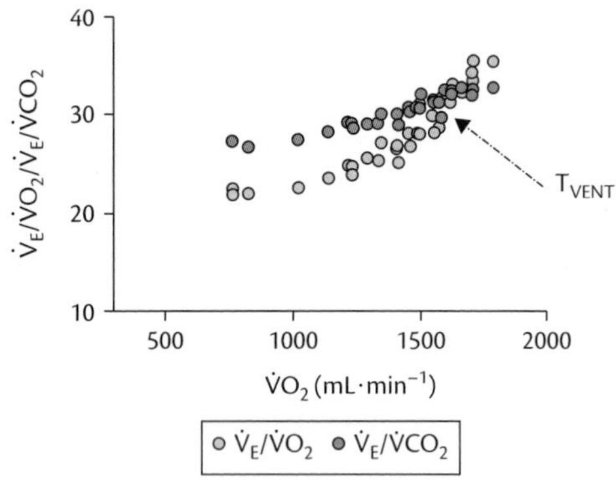

Figure 10.3 Ventilatory threshold determined using the ventilatory equivalents method.

The ventilatory threshold is noted by the arrow and is the point at which the $\dot{V}_E/\dot{V}O_2$ begins to increase without an accompanying increase in $\dot{V}_E/\dot{V}CO_2$.

mismatch is V_D/V_T calculated from $P_{ET}CO_2$. Data indicate that resting and exercise V_D/V_T remain constant with age through childhood.[29,56] Resting V_D/V_T remains stable at ~0.33 from 5 to 16 years of age[29]. Exercise V_D/V_T declines with increasing intensity, with values of 0.21, 0.18, and 0.14 reported for cycle ergometer exercise at 400, 600, and 800 kpm·min^{-1} (i.e. 65.4, 98.0, and 130.7 W) respectively, but these values were again similar from 9 to 15 years of age in boys.[56]

As discussed, exercise V_D/V_T estimated from $P_{ET}CO_2$ is unconvincing as a measure and an alternative noninvasive marker for ventilatory/perfusion mismatch is the use of the $\Delta\dot{V}_E/\Delta\dot{V}CO_2$. Data from contrast radionuclide lung perfusion scans demonstrate good correlations between the degree of pulmonary blood flow maldistribution and the slope elevation of $\Delta\dot{V}_E/\Delta\dot{V}CO_2$, providing evidence that the $\Delta\dot{V}_E/\Delta\dot{V}CO_2$ is an acceptable marker of ventilatory/perfusion matching or ventilatory efficiency in children.[57] A high $\Delta\dot{V}_E/\Delta\dot{V}CO_2$ slope may also indicate impaired breathing control or deconditioning. At maximum exercise, a greater change in $\dot{V}_E$ for a given change in $\dot{V}CO_2$ has been shown in younger compared to older children[58] and in girls compared to boys.[59] Differences in the $\Delta\dot{V}_E/\Delta\dot{V}CO_2$ may therefore simply reflect the higher relative percentage of maximum that younger children and girls are working at in comparison to older children and boys respectively, and may not denote true inefficiency.[60] If ventilatory equivalents are compared

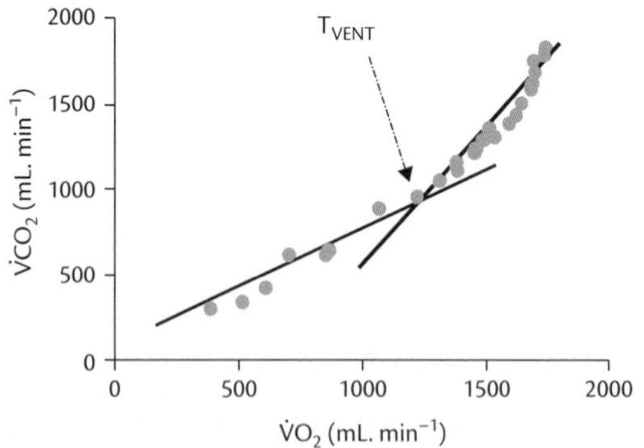

Figure 10.4 Ventilatory threshold determined using the V-slope method.

The ventilatory threshold is noted by the arrow and is the point at which two regression lines explaining $\dot{V}CO_2$ as a function of $\dot{V}O_2$ intersect, and is expressed as the $\dot{V}O_2$ where the residual sum of squares is minimized.

at the same relative exercise intensities, values are remarkably similar between the sexes.[47]

Ventilatory kinetic response to moderate-intensity exercise

The ventilatory kinetic response provides important information on the dynamic response to exercise, as well as insight into ventilatory control mechanisms. How $\dot{V}_E$ adjusts to abrupt changes in metabolic need provides a more ecologically valid reflection of the day-to-day stresses on the metabolic system, in comparison to either the steady state or maximal $\dot{V}_E$ response described earlier. The ventilatory kinetic response to moderate-intensity exercise has been eloquently described in adults,[61] but there is scant information from children.

In adults, in response to a step change in exercise below the T_{VENT}, $\dot{V}_E$ follows a similar time course to $\dot{V}O_2$, characterized by three distinct phases. (Readers interested in pulmonary $\dot{V}O_2$ kinetics are referred to Chapter 13). The first is an immediate, rapid increase in $\dot{V}_E$, which is followed by phase II, a slower gradual increase in $\dot{V}_E$ to a plateau, defined as phase III. The initial phase I response is believed to be too rapid to be the outcome of blood gases and is more likely mediated by cardiodynamic control, with $\dot{V}_E$ being driven by the increase in cardiac output at the onset of exercise.[61] Alternatively phase I may reflect a common neurogenic drive, or be a result of changes in intramuscular vascular pressure at the skeletal muscle site.[62] Characterizing the phase I response in children is confounded by the large noise to signal ratio in breath-by-breath data in the child compared to the adult. This greater noise in breath-by-breath data in children is thought to relate to the greater variability in the breathing pattern.[63] Potter *et al.*[63] noted that the variability in both V_T and f_R was large, with a range in V_T of 0.15–2.29 L for a mean V_T of 1.15 L. As a consequence the child's $\dot{V}_E$ phase I kinetics are not well understood. Limited evidence does show that in comparison to 25-year-old men, phase I changes in both inspiratory $\dot{V}_E$ and V_T are blunted in 11-year-old boys.[64] In contrast, f_R was higher, albeit non significantly, in the boys compared to the men.

The rate at which $\dot{V}_E$ rises in phase II has been described by a first-order exponential in adults.[65] The resultant phase II $\dot{V}_E$ time constant tau (τ) in adults is only slightly slower than $\dot{V}CO_2$, with values for $\dot{V}_E$ τ of 55–65 s, closely following $\dot{V}CO_2$ (τ = ~50–60 s), but is considerably slower than $\dot{V}O_2$ (τ = ~30–40 s).[44] There is ample evidence that the rate at which CO_2 is cleared from skeletal muscle tissue and exchanged at the lung drives the phase II $\dot{V}_E$ kinetic response and results in the close coupling of $\dot{V}CO_2$ and $\dot{V}_E$. For example, voluntary hyperventilation induced hypocapnia results in a slower $\dot{V}CO_2$ τ and corresponding slowing of $\dot{V}_E$ τ.[61] Evidence in children has also shown a close coupling of $\dot{V}CO_2$ and $\dot{V}_E$ during exercise in the moderate exercise intensity domain and this is illustrated in Figure 10.5.

Cooper and coleagues[6] demonstrated that in 8- to 10-year-olds exercising at 75% of the T_{VENT}, $\dot{V}_E$ τ (41.3 s) was marginally slower than $\dot{V}CO_2$ τ (39.9 s), but considerably slower than $\dot{V}O_2$ τ (26.4 s). Haouzi *et al.*[66] provide evidence of a faster phase II $\dot{V}_E$ τ in the younger child. Likewise, Cooper *et al.* [6] report a mean $\dot{V}_E$ τ value of 41.3 s in 8- to 10-year-olds compared to 52.5 s in 16–18 year-olds. Similarly, Welsman *et al.*[67] showed that $\dot{V}_E$ τ in 12-year-old boys (37.9 s) and girls (41.9 s) was faster than in 19–27-year-old men (60.1 s) and women (52.8 s), illustrating a developmental pattern in the pulmonary kinetic response to exercise. What is unknown is the mechanistic basis for these developmental

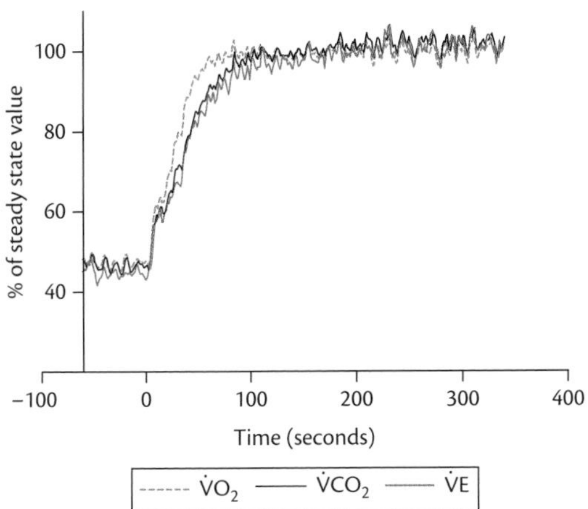

Figure 10.5 Mean oxygen uptake, and expired carbon dioxide and ventilation response to the onset of moderate intensity exercise.

Ventilatory responses of 24 children (11–12 years of age) from baseline pedaling to 80% of T_{VENT}, imposed as a square wave forcing function at $t = 0$ s. Each child completed at least four transitions, which were time aligned and averaged. The average response was normalized to give a percentage of the moderate intensity steady state before time aligning and averaging the group data.

Armstrong N, Fawkner SG, Welsman JR, unpublished data. Figure reprinted from Fawkner SG,[69] with permission.

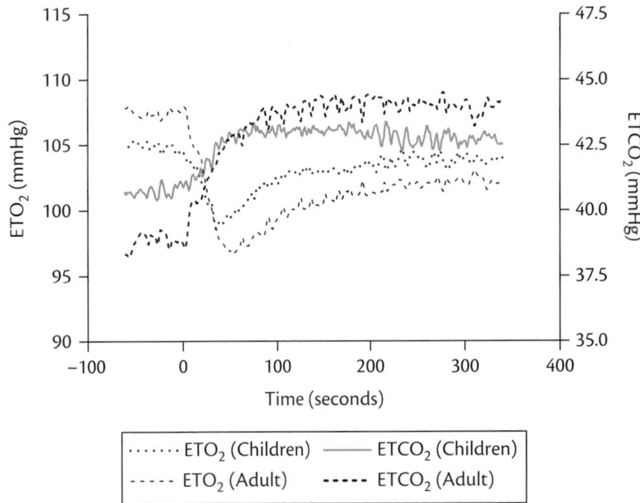

Figure 10.6 Mean end-tidal oxygen and carbon dioxide responses in children and adults from baseline pedaling to 80% of ventilatory threshold.

Mean end-tidal oxygen and carbon dioxide response of 24 children (11–12 years of age) and 22 adults (19–26 years of age) from baseline pedaling to 80% of T_{VENT}, imposed as a square wave forcing function at $t = 0$ s. ETO_2 = end-tidal O_2, $ETCO_2$ = end-tidal CO_2.

Armstrong N, Fawkner SG, Welsman JR, unpublished data. Figure reprinted from Fawkner SG,[69] with permission.

adjustments in the dynamic response of ventilation to moderate intensity exercise. The extant evidence suggests this may be an outcome of a smaller storage capacity for CO_2 in the child.[68] The time constant for $\dot{V}_E$ only lags behind $\dot{V}CO_2$ by a few seconds (Figure 10.5) and thus it is unlikely that an increased sensitivity to $\dot{V}CO_2$ in children compared to adults accounts for the age-related differences in the phase II $\dot{V}_E$ response. It is more likely that the smaller storage capacity for CO_2 in haemoglobin and body tissues in the child means metabolically produced CO_2 is detected earlier, with a proportional effect on the rate of the rise in $\dot{V}_E$. This may explain the greater input from peripheral chemoreceptors in the control of $\dot{V}_E$ in children (discussed further in the Control of breathing section), enabling changes in metabolically produced CO_2 to be rapidly dealt with. This results in a closer coupling of $\dot{V}_E$ to $\dot{V}O_2$ in children at the onset of exercise, a smaller disruption to $P_{ET}O_2$ during phase II compared to adults and a smaller rise in $P_{ET}CO_2$ as exercise progresses to steady-state in the child (Figure 10.6).

The plateau in $\dot{V}_E$ in phase III is in linear proportion to $\dot{V}CO_2$ and enables $PaCO_2$ and pHa to be maintained close to resting values. This steady state condition remains stable for about 20 min, at which point $\dot{V}_E$ begins to drift upwards. In adults this drift is believed to result from a rise in core temperature, causing an increase in f_R and a slight decrease in V_T.[69] There is also evidence of ventilatory drift in girls who cycled for 40 min at 63% of peak $\dot{V}O_2$. An increase of 7.1% in $\dot{V}_E$ was noted in the girls with an accompanying increase in f_R of 15%, while V_T declined by 6%.[70]

Heavy, very heavy, severe, and maximal exercise

When exercise intensity increases above the T_{VENT} it can be classified as heavy, very heavy, or severe. Heavy-intensity exercise is above T_{VENT}, but below critical power (CPo) and is normally set as 40% of the difference (40%Δ) between the $\dot{V}O_2$ at the T_{VENT} and peak $\dot{V}O_2$.[54] At this exercise intensity a steady state is elicited, albeit delayed. Very heavy-exercise intensity is defined as above CPo but below peak $\dot{V}O_2$ and is normally set as 60% of the difference (60%Δ) between the $\dot{V}O_2$ at the T_{VENT} and peak $\dot{V}O_2$. Severe exercise is exercise exceeding the exercise intensity attained at peak $\dot{V}O_2$ [54] (see Figure 12.3).

Ventilation at heavy-, very heavy-, and severe-exercise intensities is not a well-defined variable, because of the dependence of $\dot{V}_E$ on the protocol. As noted earlier $\dot{V}_E$ is to a large extent driven by changes in $PaCO_2$ and protocols that involve large incremental increases in exercise intensity raise the blood lactate accumulation and the subsequent release of CO_2 artificially drives the ventilation. Maximal $\dot{V}_E$ values of 49–95 $L \cdot min^{-1}$ have been recorded for girls between the ages of 9 and 16 years and a consistent sex difference has been observed with values somewhat higher in boys (58–105 $L \cdot min^{-1}$) over the same age span.[52,71] Maximum ventilation remains higher in boys, whether controlled for body size using a ratio standard or allometric adjustment with either stature and/or body mass.[47,52] (Interested readers are referred to Chapter 12 for a discussion of scaling physiological variables to body size).

Ventilatory reserve (the ratio of maximal ventilation during incremental exercise to voluntary exhaustion to maximal voluntary ventilation (MVV) at rest) offers an assessment of the pulmonary contribution to exercise limitation. A limitation is thought to be present when the $\dot{V}_E$ at maximum is similar to or exceeds the MVV.[41] In healthy children, a substantial ventilatory reserve exists at maximal exercise (60–70% of MVV), which suggests that the lungs do not limit exercise. One of the limitations of resting MVV as a marker is the inability of younger children to satisfactorily perform the resting MVV test. This may result in $\dot{V}_E$ equaling or exceeding the determined MVV, reflecting test effort as opposed to a true ventilatory limitation. Additionally, respiratory muscle recruitment patterns, operating lung volumes, and breathing patterns during exercise are quite different to those during a brief burst of voluntary hyperpnoea.[72] As such the use of MVV should therefore be treated with caution with children. Alternatively, better insight into exercise ventilatory limitation during exercise may be gained from the assessment of operational lung volumes and tidal flow-volume loops during exercise. This is discussed in the section on Breathing mechanics.

Long-term pulmonary adaptations to exercise

There are conflicting data regarding the impact exercise training may have on pulmonary function. Training studies in children are inherently challenging and much of the extant evidence is from ex post facto study designs. It is therefore extremely difficult to discern between a training-induced effect on ventilatory parameters or morphological optimization for sports where enhanced pulmonary responses are advantageous, such as swimming. Elevated lung volumes and enhanced diffusion capacity have been noted in trained swimmers, either suggesting that large lungs may be a characteristic of those selected for swim teams, or that swim training may induce pulmonary training adaptations.[73–75] Data from young athletes from land-based sports has not found evidence of a pulmonary advantage in the trained child. Comparing trained prepubertal and pubertal ice-hockey players and untrained matched controls, Hamilton and Andrew[76] found no differences in pulmonary capillary blood flow or pulmonary diffusing capacity. Similarly, no differences were found in either dynamic or static lung function in trained and untrained female track athletes (10 to 14 years old).[77] Comparison of trained swimmers and youngsters in other sports has shown superior functional residual volume in the swimmers.[78] This may signify pulmonary conditioning in young swimmers, which may be an outcome of the stimulus of breathing under water and breath-holding procedures used during swim training. Alternatively the authors conclude that this may simply reflect the genetic predisposition to optimized pulmonary morphology in children who are training in swimming, rather than the training per se.[78] Longitudinal evidence from the Training of Young Athletes (TOYA) study supports this contention.[79] Baxter-Jones and Helms[79] demonstrated that the young swimmers who entered the TOYA study did indeed have higher FVC and FEV_1, although these parameters did not change with subsequent training, suggesting exercise training has no discernable impact on lung volumes or flow.

Breathing mechanics

Insight into the mechanics of breathing during exercise in the child can be gained through the use of inspiratory capacity (IC) manoeuvers, and the interpretation of tidal flow-volume in relation to maximal expiratory flow-volume (MEFV; the flow-volume relationships during a maximal expiration). The calculated operational lung volumes provide information on where tidal breathing occurs relative to TLC and RV, offering insight into the breathing strategy during exercise and the degree of expiratory or inspiratory flow constraints. For example, if the child breathes close to their RV this will result in a reduced maximal airflow and reduced chest wall compliance. In the reverse, if the child breathes near to their TLC, they will increase the inspiratory elastic load and the work of breathing.

The IC manoeuver is usually performed in the final 20 s of each stage of graded exercise tests and at maxiumum.[48] The inspiratory manoeuver entails a five- to ten-breath cycle of normal breathing to ensure the breathing cycle is stable and then at the end of a normal breath children are asked, 'to take a deep breath in until you feel you are full'. End-expiratory lung volume is calculated from TLC minus IC and because TLC remains constant during exercise, changes in IC reflect an inverse change in EELV. End-inspiratory lung volume can be calculated from EELV and V_T.

An exercise pulmonary mechanical limitation has been noted in both healthy-weight and overweight children during exercise,[80,81] characterized by a shorter total time for each breath and shorter inspiratory time. Reductions in ERV and FRC may force overweight youngsters to breathe closer to RV. McMurray and Ondrak[80] noted an increased f_R in overweight children, which was possibly an attempt to reduce the elastic and resistive components of the work of breathing that are a consequence of breathing close to RV. The greater effort needed to achieve the same ventilation as the healthy-weight child would likely result in unpleasant sensations of breathing or dyspnoea, although no measurement of perceived breathlessness was reported. Breathing a helium-oxygen (He-O_2) inspiratory gas mix during exercise has been shown to reduce the sensations of breathlessness, primarily because of decreases in f_R and $\dot{V}_E$.[82] This in turn reduces the work of breathing and the respiratory drive to breathe. Using He-O_2 in obese 16-year-olds, a decrease in the mean inspiratory flow rate and the perception of dyspnoea was reported, suggesting a reduction in inspiratory muscle work. Although there was no direct measure of exercise tolerance, the amplitude of the $\dot{V}O_2$ slow component was reduced, in other words the onset of fatigue was delayed when breathing He-O_2 during vigorous intensity exercise.[82] Dead space loading also provides an elegant way to non-invasively probe pulmonary mechanics, since dead space loading reduces the ability to expand V_T, resulting in an inability to increase end inspiratory lung volume and $\dot{V}_E$.[83] This technique needs to be explored with the healthy child.

Expiratory flow limitation

Although the pulmonary system is not thought to limit exercise performance, an expiratory flow limitation has been noted in adult women, resulting in a greater oxygen cost of breathing and the onset of arterial desaturation, which may limit exercise tolerance.[84] An expiratory flow limitation can be assessed by superimposing exercise tidal flow-volume loops on the MEFV. Using the IC manoeuver the tidal flow-volume loops can be accurately placed within the MEFV and an expiratory flow limitation is usually defined as an exercise tidal flow volume curve intersecting the MEFV by ≥5% (see Figure 10.7).[48] The determinants of the higher prevalence of EFL in women include a reduced diffusion capacity relative to stature[85] and smaller airways relative to lung volume or dysanapsis.[84,86]

Similar to women, children have smaller airways relative to lung size and a high prevalence of expiratory flow limitation has been confirmed in both trained and untrained prepubertal children.[87,88] In a study of untrained prepubescent girls and boys, 93% of the children presented with expiratory flow limitation during exercise to maximum, but without declines in arterial saturation.[88] Of note, there was no evidence of sex differences in expiratory flow limitation prior to puberty, with prevalence rates almost identical for boys and girls. Further work from this group indicated that although the prevalence of expiratory flow limitation declines with increasing age, there is a greater prevalence of expiratory flow limitation in pubertal boys compared to girls.[89] This higher prevalence of expiratory flow limitation in pubertal boys compared to girls is in contrast

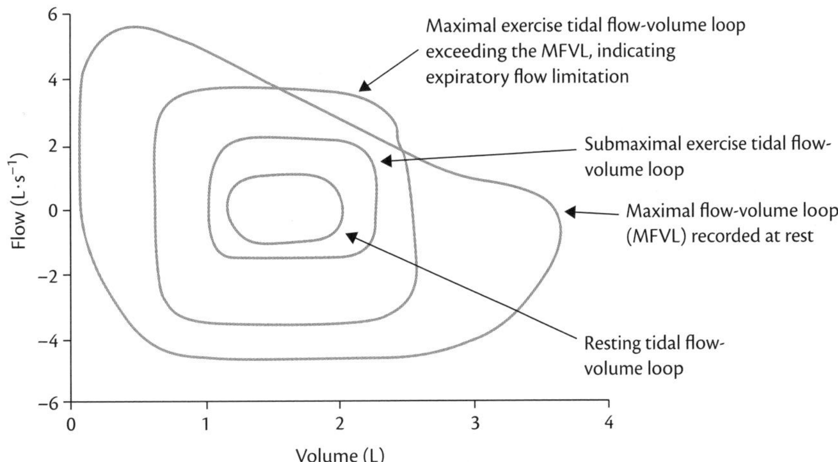

Figure 10.7 Exercise tidal flow-volume loops.
Exercise tidal flow-volume loops superimposed on the resting forced maximal flow-volume loop, illustrating how the end expiratory lung volume can encroach upon the maximal flow volume loop, indicating an expiratory flow limitation.

to adult data, which indicate that women have a higher prevalence of expiratory flow limitation compared to men.[90] The authors suggest that maturation timing and tempo differences between girls and boys might explain these findings. Indeed the girls in this study at 14.1 years would have likely reached peak height velocity, while the boys aged 15.3 years may not. Given lung maturation is in lag with stature,[16,17] this is a plausible hypothesis. Determining when the sex divergence in the prevalence of expiratory flow-limitation occurs would provide important information relating to changes in pulmonary function with growth and development.

A strong relationship between the degree of expiratory flow limitation and an increased ERV relative to FVC (i.e. an increased EELV) has been noted. At maximum exercise the flow-limited children have been shown to breathe at high lung volumes, which would likely increase the work of breathing. Nourry *et al.*[87] also demonstrated expiratory flow limitation during exercise in children, with over 50% of prepubescent children tested presenting with an expiratory flow limitation. There was evidence of arterial desaturation at maximum exercise in seven of the ten children who were expiratory flow-limited. This is in contrast with Swain *et al.*'s[88] findings of no exercise-induced arterial hypoxaemia in those with expiratory flow limitation. The differing findings may relate to the physical conditioning of the participants given the children in Nourry *et al.*'s[87] study were highly trained, and arterial desaturation is more common in highly trained athletes than non-athletes. Interestingly, those who did not present with an expiratory flow limitation breathed at a higher lung volume at peak exercise; although it should be noted that peak $\dot{V}O_2$ was higher in the non-flow-limited group.

From the extant data, it would appear that the ventilatory demands of exercise can exceed the capacity of some children's pulmonary system; however, in all these studies $\dot{V}_E$ was sufficient to supply the demands of maximal exercise, and generally did not result in arterial desaturation. The ventilatory constraint apparent in some children may not severely limit exercise tolerance, but may result in a higher work of breathing. An interesting continuation of this work would be to use a He-O_2 inspiratory gas mix during exercise in expiratory flow-limited youngsters to see whether the work of breathing decreases and exercise capacity increases.

Control of breathing

Breathing is largely an involuntary act and requires very careful control. To this end, the control of breathing requires three basic elements: a central controller, sensors, and an effector. The central controller for breathing is located in the pons and medulla of the brainstem, and this is where signals are integrated so the rhythm, pattern, and timing can be coordinated. An extensive system of sensors is available, and this comprises chemoreceptors, metabolic, stretch, irritant receptors and other receptors in the upper airways, muscle, aortic, and carotid baroreceptors, as well as temperature and pain sensors. Precise integration of the input signals and the central controller with the effector, the respiratory musculature, creates the necessary adjustments in ventilation.[91] The level of sensitivity in this control system is extraordinary, with $PaCO_2$ held close to resting values (~38 ± 4 mmHg in children[92]) throughout normal daily activities via minute adjustments in $\dot{V}_E$.

There is still lively debate over the precise details of the regulatory pathway controlling exercise ventilation. There are multiple potential regulators. Theories include feed-forward stimuli from higher brain centres, feedback stimuli from blood borne metabolites, and more recently, evidence of adaptive control strategies.[7–9,93] Far less attention has been given to the developmental pattern of $\dot{V}_E$ control from childhood through adolescence. Uncovering developmental changes is challenging because of methodological limitations when working with children, and the focus of attention in children has largely been on the chemoreceptor mediated $\dot{V}_E$ response of the child,[5,6] probably because the manipulation of inspired gases is relatively straightforward and well tolerated in the child.

Both central and peripheral chemoreceptors play a role in the maintenance of PaO_2 and $PaCO_2$ homeostasis. Central chemoreceptors are located near the ventral surface of the medulla and respond to changes in hydrogen ion (H^+) concentration, and thus the pH of the medullary extracellular fluid that surrounds them.

The cerebrospinal fluid (CSF) is separated from the blood by the blood-brain barrier, which is fairly impermeable to H^+ and HCO_3^-, but molecular CO_2 can diffuse into the CSF from the cerebral blood vessels, liberating H^+ ions that stimulate the central chemoreceptors. An important distinction here is that it is actually central PCO_2 as opposed to $PaCO_2$ that is responsible for shifts in the central chemoreflex mediated $\dot{V}_E$ response.[91] The central chemoreflex response is slower than peripheral chemoreceptor feedback because of the delay between a change in $PaCO_2$ and the sensing of changes in central PCO_2. The peripheral chemoreceptors are primarily located in the carotid bodies at the bifurcation of the carotid artery and are stimulated by changes in PaO_2, $PaCO_2$, and H^+.

A great deal of attention has been given to comparing the relative contribution of the peripheral and central chemoreceptors to the ventilatory response.[94] In adults, it has been estimated that less than 20% of the ventilatory response can be attributed to the peripheral chemoreceptors.[91] It is thought that this is because of the higher sensitivity of the peripheral chemoreceptors to alterations in PaO_2. Evidence for this hypothesis is provided by the maintenance of the $\dot{V}_E$ response to changes in CO_2 during hyperoxic gas administration, which is believed to blunt the peripheral chemoreceptor response.[95] Although the evidence is limited, a striking developmental difference in the chemoreceptive relationship with $\dot{V}_E$ has been demonstrated.[96,97] In comparison to adults peripheral chemoreceptor responsiveness to $PaCO_2$ appears to be heightened in children, suggesting the peripheral chemoreceptor contribution to the ventilatory response is more prominent during childhood and attenuates with increasing age and maturation.[97] Using a step protocol comprising a single breath of 15% CO_2 in 85% O_2, Gozal and colleagues[97] showed that when corrected for FVC, the slope in the ventilatory response to step hypercapnic stimuli ($\dot{V}_E$ vs $P_{ET}CO_2$) was greater in children than in adults (0.507 vs 0.183 respectively). Springer and colleagues[96] also demonstrated a greater role of the peripheral chemoreceptors during exercise (75% of T_{VENT} under hypoxic [15% O_2] conditions). Using a switching technique, alternating room air or hypoxia with hyperoxic breaths (80% O_2), they established that in comparison to adults, the peripheral chemoreceptor feedback was significantly greater in children following a hyperoxic switch during exercise under hypoxic conditions. A rapid and marked decline in $\dot{V}_E$ of 57.6% was noted in the children, compared to a smaller reduction of only 38.9% in $\dot{V}_E$ in adults. There was a 7.1 mmHg increase in $P_{ET}CO_2$ in the children compared to 4.3 mmHg in the adults in response to the hyperoxic stimuli.[96] The increase in $P_{ET}CO_2$ means it was unlikely that changes in VD/V_T would account for the decrease in $\dot{V}_E$ and these findings suggest that when hyperoxia is used to inhibit the carotid chemoreceptors, the greater decrease in $\dot{V}_E$ noted in the child compared to the adult supports the evidence that peripheral chemoreceptor sensitivity is enhanced during childhood.

Possible mechanisms for this greater reliance on the peripheral chemoreceptors during childhood may be greater exposure to hypoxia because of the longer time period the child spends sleeping compared to the adult and a smaller CO_2 storage capacity in the child. Evidence from animal work suggests that a segregated view of peripheral and central chemoreceptor CO_2 sensitivity is inappropriate and instead a synergistic relationship exists, whereby the sensitivity of the central chemoreceptor mediated $\dot{V}_E$ response is dependent on peripheral chemoreceptor inputs. As this interaction changes with age and maturation, the magnitude of the interaction between peripheral and central chemoreceptor stimuli would be anticipated to change. It seems reasonable to suggest that the increased sensitivity in the peripheral chemoreflex in childhood reflects a developmentally dependent interaction between the peripheral and central chemoreceptors[98] whereby the greater magnitude of the ventilatory response to a step change in $PaCO_2$ (or $P_{ET}CO_2$) that has been noted in the child,[5,6,10,11] is defined by the strength of this interaction, and the greater chemoreceptor sensitivity to CO_2. This remains to be established, but is certainly deserving of future research attention.

Future avenues of research

The study of the pulmonary responses to exercise in the child is by no means complete. There are a number of questions that remain unanswered regarding exercise pulmonary responses during youth. To address some of these non-invasive experimental approaches such as manipulation of inspired gases, skeletal muscle blood flow occlusion, pedal frequency stimulation, or alterations in the mechanics of breathing will be needed. Some of these techniques are discussed to illustrate how, with a little creative experimentation, fascinating insight into the mechanisms responsible for the exercise hyperpnoea in children is possible.

Development of chemoreceptor sensitivity can be probed using chemoreceptor inhibition and stimulation strategies by altering inspiratory gases during exercise, an approach that has been used with children.[5,10,99] It is also possible to use voluntary hyperventilation to blunt the drive to breathe because of reductions in $PaCO_2$. Additionally, chemoreceptor manipulations can be combined with the assessment of cerebral blood flow regulation to provide an integrative understanding of the sensitivity of the central and peripheral chemoreceptors. Cerebral blood flow (CBF) can be assessed from the Transcranial Doppler ultrasound measure of cerebral blood flow velocity, an approach that is well-tolerated by children.[100,101] Cerebral blood flow alters in response to CO_2, with hypercapnia causing vasodilation of the cerebral vasculature and an increase in CBF in order to washout CO_2 from the brain tissue. Hypocapnia on the other hand causes vasoconstriction and a decrease in CBF.[102] The role central and peripheral chemoreceptors play in the control of $\dot{V}_E$ can be elegantly expressed using the integrated responses of both CBF and $PaCO_2$ (or the surrogate $P_{ET}CO_2$).[102] Although the integrated ventilatory and CBF response during exercise has been extensively studied in adults,[103–105] there are, to date, no data documenting the exercise CBF responses of the child.[106] It would be reasonable to expect that a heightened peripheral ventilatory response during exercise in childhood would limit an increase in brain tissue PCO_2 and therefore blunt changes in CBF in comparison to adults; but this remains to be determined.

Increasing the work of breathing by asking participants to breathe through a narrow tube will reduce the ventilatory response to CO_2. This occurs even though the neural output from the brainstem control centres is maintained, but the increased airway resistance results in a smaller ventilatory response. Similarly, assessing the drive to breath from inspiratory pressure during temporary airway occlusion provides a measure of respiratory centre output. This has been used to show how inspiratory flow and mouth occlusion pressure decline with age[12].

As noted, the rapid phase I kinetic response of $\dot{V}_E$ to the onset of moderate intensity exercise is thought to be too quick to be controlled by a blood-borne metabolic signal. Instead it may originate from mechanoreceptor[107] or metaboreceptor[108] signals. The role skeletal muscle afferents play in the regulation of $\dot{V}_E$ can be probed using a variety of approaches including venous occlusion and limb movement. Using sub-systolic venous occlusion of the bilateral proximal quadriceps, Keller-Ross and colleagues[109] quantified the influence of venous distention on ventilation and breathing patterns. The sub-systolic pressures used were 20, 40, 60, 80, and 100 mmHg, and an increase in $\dot{V}_E$ was found at each of these pressures, with the greatest increase occurring at 100 mmHg. No changes were noted in V_T, but f_R increased from 24.8 breaths · min^{-1} in the control condition to 30.9 breaths · min^{-1} at 100 mmHg. Inspiratory flow also increased significantly at each occlusion pressure compared to the unoccluded control condition. Sub-systolic cuff inflations of only 2 min in duration would be easily tolerated in children given supra-systolic pressures for 5 min in duration have been successfully employed for the assessment of endothelial flow-mediated dilation of the lower limb in children.[110] This approach has the potential to establish whether venous distension increases ventilation in children, and would provide insight into the role of mechanoreceptors and metaboreceptors in determining exercise hyperpnoea in the child.

The coupling of limb movement frequency to $\dot{V}_E$ is not a new hypothesis and it is thought that the alterations in $\dot{V}_E$ to increased limb movement frequency originate from peripheral feedback from the exercising muscles to the central medullary command. Caterini and colleagues[111] used sinusoidal speed and load adjustments in adults to demonstrate that ventilation was modulated by limb movement frequency. Sinusoidal changes in pedaling speed resulted in larger and more rapid increases in ventilation compared to sinusoidal changes in pedal loading. Interestingly the role limb movement frequency plays in determining the initial exercise drive to breathe was attenuated with exercise training. This may account for changes noted with exercise training and illustrates that the control of $\dot{V}_E$ is indeed an adaptive process. Pedal speed manipulations have been used to alter the $\dot{V}O_2$ kinetic response,[112] and this presents a feasible experimental approach to probe exercise ventilatory control mechanisms in children.

Conclusions

The lungs play an essential role in maintaining metabolic homeostasis, but despite this fundamental biological function our understanding of exercise pulmonary responses in the child and the underlying mechanisms of these remains basic.

As the lungs, thorax, and airways develop in the child lung volumes change, mechanical properties of the lungs alter, and alongside a maturing chemosensitivity to $PaCO_2$, developmentally divergent breathing patterns are apparent. Children show a high prevalence of expiratory flow limitation in comparison to adults, which are likely an outcome of smaller airways relative to lung volume. Whether this actually constitutes a ventilatory constraint that limits exercise tolerance has yet to be established.

Critical questions remain unanswered with regard to exercise hyperpnoea in the child. The child exhibits a different breathing strategy to exercise compared to the adult, which suggests the control of breathing is dependent on age and maturation. Is the control of ventilation during mild or moderate exercise in the child primarily driven by feed-forward stimuli? Or is the tight regulation of ventilation achieved by sensory feedback? How do these adaptive control strategies alter in response to other environmental challenges such as altitude in the child? How does the control strategy alter with increasing age and maturation? Considerable research will be necessary before we have a full appreciation of pulmonary function during exercise in the child.

Summary

- There are discrepant patterns of lung growth and smaller lungs and narrower airways may predispose the child to mechanical limitations during exercise. The timing and tempo of changes in stature, body mass, chest dimensions, lung volumes, and dynamic lung function are not well understood, and there may be a period where girls' lung function is superior to boys. At all other times boys outperform girls in measures of pulmonary function.
- Children ventilate more for a given metabolic demand compared to adults. The underlying reason for this is poorly understood, but likely relates to immature chemoreception, neural drive, and changing mechanical properties of the lung.
- There are few studies investigating the dynamic ventilatory response to moderate intensity exercise and none to heavy or very heavy intensity exercise in the child. Yet the kinetic response of ventilation provides intriguing insight into both the ventilatory strategy during exercise and the underlying control mechanisms. There is certainly the need for more research attention to be dedicated to children's pulmonary dynamic responses to exercise.
- The extant literature is small, and there is sparse evidence that exercise training has any discernable impact on the pulmonary system. Differences in static lung volumes and flow have been documented between swimmers and non-swimmers, but it is more likely this reflects a genetic predisposition to optimized pulmonary morphology in children who enter swim training.
- A number of questions remain unanswered regarding the control of exercise hyperpnoea in the child. There are a number of techniques which could be employed to investigate exercise hyperpnoea *in vivo* and which are ethically acceptable for use with children. Creative physiological experiments using an integrative approach are desperately needed to develop knowledge around the child's regulation of breathing.

References

1. Carroll JL, Agarwal A. Development of ventilatory control in infants. *Paediatr Respir Rev*. 2010; 11: 199–207.
2. Thurlbeck WM. Postnatal human lung growth. *Thorax*. 1982; 37: 564–571.
3. Davies G, Reid L. Growth of the alveoli and pulmonary arteries in childhood. *Thorax*. 1970; 25: 669–681.
4. Lanteri CJ, Sly PD. Changes in respiratory mechanics with age. *J Appl Physiol*. 1993; 74: 369–378.
5. Gratas-Delamarche A, Mercier J, Ramonatxo M, Dassonville J, Prefaut C. Ventilatory response of prepubertal boys and adults to carbon dioxide at rest and during exercise. *Eur J Appl Physiol*. 1993; 66: 25–30.
6. Cooper DM, Kaplan MR, Baumgarten L,Weiler-Ravell D, Whipp BJ, Wasserman K. Coupling of ventilation and CO_2 production during exercise in children. *Pediatr Res*. 1987; 21: 568–572.

7. Dempsey JA. Challenges for future research in exercise physiology as applied to the respiratory system. *Exerc Sport Sci Rev.* 2006; 34: 92–98.
8. Forster HV, Haouzi P, Dempsey JA. Control of breathing during exercise. *Compr Physiol.* 2012; 2: 743–777.
9. Casaburi R. The mechanism of the exercise hyperpnea. The ultrasecret revisited. *Am J Respir Crit Care Med.* 2012; 186: 578–579.
10. Nagano Y, Baba R, Kuraishi K, *et al.* Ventilatory control during exercise in normal children. *Pediatr Res.* 1998; 43: 703–707.
11. Ohuchi H, Kato Y, Tasato H, Arakaki Y, Kamiya T. Ventilatory response and arterial blood gases during exercise in children. *Pediatr Res.* 1999; 45: 389–396.
12. Gaultier V, Perret L, Boule M, Buvry A, Girard F. Occlusion pressure and breathing pattern in healthy children. *Respir Physiol.* 1981; 46: 71–80.
13. Cassels DE, Morse M. *Cardiopulmonary data for children and young adults.* Springfield, IL: Charles C Thomas; 1962.
14. Fleming S, Thompson M, Stevens R, *et al.* Normal ranges of heart rate and respiratory rate in children from birth to 18 years of age: a systematic review of observational studies. *Lancet.* 2011; 377: 1011–1018.
15. Kivastik J, Kingisepp P. Differences in lung function and chest dimensions in school-age girls and boys. *Clin Physiol.* 1997; 17: 149–157.
16. Degroodt EG, Quanjer PH, Wise ME, Van Zomeren BC. Changing relationships between stature and lung volumes during puberty. *Respir Physiol.* 1986; 65: 139–153.
17. Wang X, Dockery DW, Wypij D, *et al.* Pulmonary function growth velocity in children 6 to 18 years of age. *Am Rev Respir Dis.* 1993; 148: 1502–1508.
18. Taussig LM, Cota K, Kaltenborn W. Different mechanical properties of the lung in girls and boys. *Am Rev Respir Dis.* 1981; 123: 640–643.
19. Stocks J, Quanjer PH. Reference values for residual volume, functional residual capacity and total lung capacity. *Eur Respir J.* 1996; 8: 492–506.
20. Wanger J, Clausen JL, Coates A, *et al.* Standardisation of the measurement of lung volumes. *Eur Respir J.* 2005; 26: 511–522.
21. Cogswell JJ, Hull D, Milner AD, Norman AP, Taylor B. Lung function in childhood. 2. Thoracic gas volumes and helium functional residual capacity measurements in healthy children. *Br J Dis Chest.* 1975; 69: 118–124.
22. Kraemer R, Zehnder M, Meister B. Intrapulmonary gas distribution in healthy children. *Respir Physiol.* 1986; 65: 127–137.
23. Halvorsen T, Skadberg BT, Eide GE, Roksund OD, Bakke P, Thorsen E. Assessment of lung volumes in children and adolescents: comparison of two plethysmographic techniques. *Clin Physiol Funct Imaging.* 2005; 25: 62–68.
24. Miller MR, Hankinson J, Brusasco V, *et al.* Standardisation of spirometry. *Eur Respir J.* 2005; 26: 319–338.
25. Zapletal A. Lung function in children and adolescents. *Prog Respir Res.* 1987; 22: 1–20.
26. Zapletal A, Hladíková M, Chalupová J, Svobodová T, and Vávrová V. Area under the maximum expiratory flow-volume curve—a sensitive parameter in the evaluation of airway patency. *Respiration.* 2008; 75: 40–47.
27. in't Veen JC, Beekman AJ, Bel EH, Sterk PJ. recurrent exacerbations in severe asthma are associated with enhanced airway closure during stable episodes. *Am J Respir Critical Care Med.* 2000; 161: 1902–1906.
28. Tsiligiannis T, Grivas T. Pulmonary function in children with idiopathic scoliosis. *Scoliosis.* 2012; 7: 7.
29. Kerr AA. Dead space ventilation in normal children and children with obstructive airways disease. *Thorax.* 1976; 31: 63–69.
30. Comroe JH, Forster R E, DuBois AB, Briscoe WA, Carlsen E. *The lung: clinical physiology and pulmonary function tests,* 2nd ed. Chicago, IL: Year Book Medical Publishers: 1962.
31. Nunn JF, Hill WD. Respiratory dead space and arterial to end-tidal CO_2 tension difference in anesthetized man. *J Appl Physiol.* 1960; 15: 383–389.
32. Whipp BJ, Ward SA. The respiratory system. In: Tipton C (ed.) *History of exercise physiology.* Champaign, IL: Human Kinetics; 2014. p. 211–245.
33. Jones NL, Robertson DG, Kane JW. Difference between end-tidal and arterial PCO_2 in exercise. *J Appl Physiol.* 1979; 47: 954–960.
34. McDonald MJ, Montgomery VL, Cerrito PB, Parrish CJ, Boland KA, Sullivan JE. Comparison of end-tidal CO_2 and $PaCO_2$ in children receiving mechanical ventilation. *Pediatr Crit Care Med.* 2002; 3: 244–249.
35. Ohuchi H, Hayashi T, Yamada O, Echigo S. Estimation of $PaCO_2$ during exercise in children and postoperative pediatric patients with congenital heart disease. *Chest.* 2005; 128: 3576–3584.
36. Forster HV, Dempsey JA, Thomson J, Vidruk E, doPico GA. Estimation of arterial PO_2, PCO_2, pH and lactate from arterialized venous blood. *J Appl Physiol.* 1972; 32: 134–137.
37. Vogt B, Falkenberg C, Weiler N, Frerichs I. Pulmonary function testing in children and infants. *Physiol Meas.* 2014; 35: R59–R90.
38. Bloch KE, Barandun J, Sackner MA. Effect of mouthpiece breathing on cardiorespiratory response to intense exercise. *Am J Respir Critical Care Med.* 1995; 151: 1087–1092.
39. Maxwell DL, Cover D, Hughes JMB. Effect of respiratory apparatus on timing and depth of breathing in man. *Respir Physiol.* 1985; 61: 255–264.
40. Druz WS, Sharp JT. Activity of respiratory muscles in upright and recumbent humans. *J Appl Physiol.* 1981; 51: 1552–1561.
41. Orenstein DM. Assessment of exercise pulmonary function. In: Rowland TW (ed.) *Pediatric laboratory exercise testing.* Champaign, IL: Human Kinetics; 1993. p. 141–164.
42. Staats BA, Grinton SF, Mottram CD, Driscoll DJ, Beck KC. Quality control in exercise testing. *Prog Pediatr Cardiol.* 1993; 2: 11–17.
43. Pearsall MF, Feldman JM. When does apparatus dead space matter for the pediatric patient? *Anesth Analg.* 2014; 118: 776–780.
44. Ward SA. Ventilatory control in humans: constraints and limitations. *Exp Physiol.* 2007; 92: 357–366.
45. Benchetrit G. Breathing pattern in humans: diversity and individuality. *Respir Physiol.* 2000; 122: 123–129.
46. McMurray RG, Baggett C, Pennell M, Bangdiwala S, Harrell J. Gender differences in ventilatory responses of youth are related to exercise intensity. *Port J Sport Sci.* 2003; 3: 101–102.
47. Armstrong N, Kirby BJ, McManus AM, Welsman JR. Prepubescents' ventilatory responses to exercise with reference to sex and body size. *Chest.* 1997; 112: 554–1560.
48. Guenette JA, Chin RC, Cory JM, Webb KA, O'Donnell DE. Inspiratory capacity during exercise: measurement, analysis, and interpretation. *Pulm Med.* 2013; 2013: 956081.
49. Boule M, Gaultier C, Girard F. Breathing pattern during exercise in untrained children. *Respir Physiol.* 1989; 75: 115–234.
50. Rowland TW, Green GM. The influence of biological maturation and aerobic fitness on ventilator responses to treadmill exercise. In: Dotson CO, Humphrey JH (eds.) *Exercise physiology: current selected research.* New York: AMS Press; 1990. p. 51–59.
51. Ondrak KS, McMurray RG. Exercise-induced breathing patterns in youth are related to age and intensity. *Eur J Appl Physiol.* 2006; 98: 88–96.
52. Rowland TW, Cunningham LN. Development of ventilatory responses to exercise in normal white children. A longitudinal study. *Chest.* 1997; 111: 327–332.
53. Armstrong N, Barker AR. Oxygen uptake kinetics in children and adolescents: a review. *Pediatr Exerc Sci.* 2009; 21: 130–147.
54. Fawkner SG, Armstrong N. Can we confidently study VO_2 kinetics in young people? *J Sports Sci Med.* 2007; 6: 277–285.
55. Beaver WL, Wasserman K, Whipp BJ. A new method for detecting anaerobic threshold by gas exchange. *J Appl Physiol.* 1986; 60: 2020–2027.
56. Gadhoke S, Jones NL. The responses to exercise in boys aged 9–15 years. *Clin Sci.* 1969; 37: 789–801.
57. Rhodes J, Dave A, Pulling MC, *et al.* Effect of pulmonary artery stenoses on the cardiopulmonary response to exercise following repair of tetralogy of Fallot. *Am J Cardiol.* 1998; 81: 1217–1219.

58. Pianosi P, Wolstein R. Carbon dioxide chemosensitivity and exercise ventilation in healthy children and in children with cystic fibrosis. *Pediatr Res*. 1996; 40: 508–513.
59. Lintu N, Viitasalo A, Tompuri T, *et al.* Cardiorespiratory fitness, respiratory function and hemodynamic responses to maximal cycle ergometer exercise test in girls and boys aged 9–11 years: the PANIC Study. *Eur J Appl Physiol*. 2015; 115: 235–243.
60. Parazzi PL, Marson FA, Ribeiro MA, Schivinski CI, Ribeiro JD. Ventilatory efficiency in children and adolescents: a systematic review. *Dis Markers*. 2015; 2015: 546891.
61. Ward SA. *Control of breathing during exercise*. New Jersey: Morgan & Claypool Life Sciences; 2014.
62. Haouzi P, Hill JM, Lewis BK, Kaufman MP. Responses of group III and IV afferents to distension of the peripheral vascular bed. *J Appl Physiol*. 1999; 87: 545–553.
63. Potter CR, Childs DJ, Houghton W, Armstrong N. Breath-by-breath 'noise' in the ventilatory and gas exchange responses of children to exercise. *Eur J Appl Physiol*. 1999; 80: 118–124.
64. Sato Y, Katayama K, Ishida K, Miyamura. Ventilatory and circulatory responses at the onset of voluntary exercise and passive movement in children. *Eur J Appl Physiol*. 2000; 83: 516–523.
65. Ward SA. Control of the exercise hyperpnoea in humans: a modeling perspective. *Respir Physiol*. 2000; 122: 149–166.
66. Haouzi P, Fukuba Y, Peslin R, Chalon B, Marchal F, Crance JP. Ventilatory dynamics in children and adults during sinosuidal exercise. *Eur J Appl Physiol*. 1992; 64: 410–418.
67. Welsman JR, Fawkner SG, Armstrong N. Respiratory response to non-steady state exercise in children and adults (abstract). *Pediatr Exerc Sci*. 2001; 45: 263–264.
68. Zanconato S, Cooper DM, Barstow TJ, Landaw E. $^{13}CO_2$ washout dynamics during intermittent exercise in children and adults. *J Appl Physiol*. 1992; 73: 2476–2482.
69. Fawkner SG. Pulmonary function. In: Armstrong N, van Mechelen W (eds.) *Paediatric exercise science and medicine*, 2nd ed. Oxford: Oxford University Press; 2008. p. 243–254.
70. Rowland TW, Rimmey TA. Physiological responses to prolonged exercise in premenarchal girls and adult females. *Pediatr Exerc Sci*. 1995; 7: 183–191.
71. Godfrey S. *Exercise testing in children*. London: WB Saunders; 1974.
72. Klas JV, Dempsey JA. Voluntary versus reflex regulation of maximal exercise flow volume loops. *Am Rev Respir Disease*. 1989; 139: 150–156.
73. Astrand PO, Eriksson BO, Nylander I, *et al.* Girl swimmers. With special reference to respiratory and circulatory adaptation and gynecological and psychiatric aspects. *Acta Paediatr*. 1963; 147(Suppl): 1–75.
74. Andrew GM, Becklake MR, Guleria JS, Bates DV. Heart and lung function in swimmers and nonathletes during growth. *J Appl Physiol*. 1972; 32: 245–251.
75. Zinman R, Gaultier C. Maximal static pressures and lung volumes in young swimmers. *Respir Physiol*. 1986; 64: 229–239.
76. Hamilton P, Andrew GM. Influence of growth and athletic training on heart and lung functions. *Eur J Appl Physiol Occup Physiol*. 1976: 36: 27–38.
77. Vaccaro P, Poffenbarger A. Resting and exercise respiratory function in young female child runners. *J Sports Med Phys Fitness*. 1982; 22: 102–107.
78. Doherty M, Dimitriou L. Comparison of lung volumes in Greek swimmers, land-based athletes and sedentary controls using allometric scaling. *Br J Sports Med*. 1996; 31: 337–341.
79. Baxter-Jones ADG, Helms PJ. Effects of training at a young age: a review of The Training of Young Athletes (TOYA) Study. *Pediatr Exerc Sci*. 1996: 8: 310–327.
80. McMurray RG, Ondrak KS. Effects of being overweight on ventilatory dynamics of youth at rest and during exercise. *Eur J Appl Physiol*. 2011; 111: 285–292.
81. Swain KE, Rosenkranz SK, Beckman B, *et al.* Expiratory flow limitation during exercise in prepubescent boys and girls: prevalence and implications. *J Appl Physiol*. 2010; 108: 1267–1274.
82. Salvadego D, Sartorio A, Agosti F. Acute respiratory muscle unloading by normoxic helium–O_2 breathing reduces the O_2 cost of cycling and perceived exertion in obese adolescents. *Eur J Appl Physiol*. 2015; 115: 99–109.
83. Jensen D, O'Donnell DE, Li R, *et al.* Effects of dead space loading on neuro-muscular and neuro-ventilatory coupling of the respiratory system during exercise in healthy adults: Implications for dyspnea and exercise tolerance. *Resp Physiol Neurobiol*. 2011; 179: 219–226.
84. Sheel AW, Dominelli PB, Molgat-Seon Y. Revisiting dysanapsis: sex-based differences in airways and the mechanics of breathing during exercise. *Exp Physiol*. 2016; 101: 213–218.
85. Mead J. Dysanapsis in normal lungs assessed by the relationship between maximal flow, static recoil, and vital capacity. *Am Rev Respir Dis*. 1980; 121: 339–342.
86. Smith JR, Rosenkranz SK, Harms CA. Dysanapsis ratio as a predictor for expiratory flow limitation. *Respir Physiol Neurobiol*. 2014; 198: 25–31.
87. Nourry C, Deruelle F, Fabre C, *et al.* Evidence of ventilatory constraints in healthy exercising prepubescent children. *Pediatr Pulmonol*. 2006; 41: 133–140.
88. Swain KE, Rosenkranz SK, Beckman B, Harms CA. Expiratory flow limitation during exercise in prepubescent boys and girls: prevalence and implications. *J Appl Physiol*. 2010; 108: 1267–1274.
89. Emerson SR, Kurt SP, Rosenkranz SK, Smith JR, Harms CA. Decreased prevalence of exercise expiratory flow limitation from pre- to postpuberty. *Med Sci Sports Exerc*. 2015: 47: 1503–1511.
90. Guenette JA, Witt JD, McKenzie DC, Road JD, Sheel AW. Respiratory mechanics during exercise in endurance-trained men and women. *J Physiol*. 2007; 581: 1309–1322.
91. West JB. *Respiratory physiology. The essentials*, 8th ed. Philadelphia: Lippincott Williams & Wilkins: 2008.
92. Marcus CL, Glomb WB, Basinksi DJ, Davidson Ward SL, Keens TG. Developmental pattern of hypercapnic and hypoxic ventilatory responses from childhood to adulthood. *J Appl Physiol*. 1994; 76: 314–320.
93. Mitchell GS, Babbs TG. Layers of exercise hyperpnea: modulation and plasticity. *Respir Physiol Neurobiol*. 2006; 151: 251–266.
94. Dempsey JA, Forster HV. Mediation of ventilatory adaptations. *Physiol Rev*. 1982; 62: 262–346.
95. Ward SA, Blesovsky L, Russack S, Ashjian A, Whipp B. Chemoreflex modulation of ventilatory dynamics during exercise in man. *J Appl Physiol*. 1987; 63, 2001–2007.
96. Springer C, Cooper DM, Wasserman K. Evidence that maturation of the peripheral chemoreceptors is not complete in childhood. *Respir Physiol*. 1988; 74: 55–64.
97. Gozal D, Arens R, Omlin KJ, Marcus CL, Keens TG. Maturational differences in step vs. ramp hypoxic and hypercapnic ventilator responses. *J Appl Physiol*. 1994; 76: 1968–1975.
98. Blain GM, Smith CA, Henderson KS, Dempsey JA. Peripheral chemoreceptors determine the respiratory sensitivity of central chemoreceptors to CO_2. *J Physiol*. 2010; 588: 2455–2471.
99. Pianosi R, Wolstein R. Carbon dioxide chemosensitivity and exercise ventilation in healthy children and in children with cystic fibrosis. *Pediatr Res*. 1996; 40: 508–513.
100. Schoning M, Staab M, Walter J, *et al.* Transcranial color duplex sonography in childhood and adolescence. Age dependence of flow velocities and waveform parameters. *Stroke*. 1993; 24: 1305–1309.
101. Tontisirin N, Muangman SL, Suz P, *et al.* Early childhood gender differences in anterior and posterior cerebral blood flow velocity and autoregulation. *Pediatrics*. 2007; 119: e610.
102. Ainslie PN, Duffin J. Integration of cerebrovascular CO_2 reactivity and chemoreflex control of breathing: mechanisms of regulation, measurement and interpretation. *Am J Physiol Regul Integr Comp Physiol*. 2009; 296: R1473–R1495.
103. Fan JL, Burgess KR, Basnyat R, *et al.* Influence of high altitude on cerebrovascular and ventilator responsiveness to CO_2. *J Physiol*. 2010; 588: 539–549.

104. Peebles K, Celi L, McGrattan K, Murrell C, Thomas K, Ainslie PN. Human cerebrovascular and ventilator CO_2 reactivity to end-tidal, arterial and internal jugular vein PCO_2. *Hum J Physiol.* 2007; 584: 347–357.
105. Ainslie PN, Smith KJ. Integrated human physiology: breathing, blood pressure and blood flow to the brain. *J Physiol.* 2011; 589: 2917.
106. Ainslie PN, McManus AM. Big brain, small body: towards a better understanding of cerebrovascular physiology in children. *J Physiol.* 2016; 594:2563.
107. Amann M, Runnels S, Morgan DE, *et al.* On the contribution of group III and IV muscle afferents to the circulatory response to rhythmic exercise in humans. *J Physiol.* 2011; 589: 3855–3866.
108. Haouzi P. Theories on the nature of the coupling between ventilation and gas exchange during exercise. *Respir Physiol Neurobiol.* 2006; 151: 267–279.
109. Keller-Ross ML, Sarkinen AL, Cross T, Johnson BD, Olson TP. Ventilation increases with lower extremity venous occlusion in young adults. *Med Sci Sports Exerc.* 2016; 48: 377–383.
110. McManus AM, Ainslie PN, Green DJ, Simair RG, Smith K, Lewis N. Impact of prolonged sitting on vascular function in young girls. *Exp Physiol.* 2015; 100: 1379–1387.
111. Caterini JE, Duffin J, Wells GD. Limb movement frequency is a significant modulator of the ventilatory response during submaximal cycling exercise in humans. *Respir Physiol Neurobiol.* 2016; 220: 10–16.
112. Breese BC, Armstrong N, Barker AR, Williams CA. The effect of pedal rate on pulmonary O_2 uptake kinetics during very heavy intensity exercise in trained and untrained teenage boys. *Respir Physiol Neurobiol.* 2011; 177: 149–54.

CHAPTER 11

Cardiovascular function

Thomas W Rowland

Introduction

Appropriate increases in circulatory blood flow are critical for the performance of endurance exercise. The rise in metabolic demand of exercising muscle must be met with parallel and closely matched increases in oxygen supply provided by circulating blood flow, while control of body temperature, provision of energy substrate, elimination of metabolic waste products, and hormonal responses are also all highly dependent on augmentation of cardiovascular function.

Understandably, then, considerable research attention by exercise physiologists has focused on understanding the nature and limitations of circulatory responses to acute bouts of exercise. These investigations have revealed an intricate system orchestrated by the interplay of the functions and dimensions of the cardiac pump in concert with alterations in systemic vascular resistance and regional blood flow. The magnitude of these adaptations is highly controlled such that together, with remarkable precision, the volume of circulatory flow to contracting muscle conforms to the metabolic demands of endurance exercise.

These tenets of circulatory responses to endurance exercise are no different in growing children than in their adult counterparts. Historically, however, two concerns have been raised suggesting that the heart of the immature child might be less effective in responses to exercise than that of mature individuals. The first, which dates back to the late 1800s, held that during the childhood years there existed a discrepancy between the increases in heart volume (which grows in respect to body mass) and the circumference of the aorta and pulmonary artery (which increase linearly with body height).[1] This 'natural disharmony' was considered to place undue strain on the heart that would 'diminish the child's vigour at this period', leading to recommendations that children might be best limited from intensive exercise.[1]

A second, more recent observation, indicated that when all research studies are considered, children typically exhibit a lower average cardiac output ($\dot{Q}$) for any given level of oxygen uptake ($\dot{V}O_2$) during exercise compared to adults.[2] For example, at an $\dot{V}O_2$ of 1.4 $L \cdot min^{-1}$ an exercising adult is expected to demonstrate a $\dot{Q}$ of approximately 14 $L \cdot min^{-1}$, while that observed in a child is about 11 $L \cdot min^{-1}$. This discrepancy has been interpreted as a hypokinetic response of the heart to exercise in children, one which might limit performance in high-intensity exercise, particularly in the heat[3] (interested readers are referred to Chapter 14 for further discussion).

Both of these concerns have been subsequently dispelled. In the former, Karpovich[1] pointed out that it is the area of the great vessels, not the circumference, which needs to accept blood volume, and with this geometric error corrected, growth in cardiac stroke volume (delivered as area over time) of the child is now recognized to be appropriately matched to that of dimensions of the aorta and pulmonary artery. The second issue is best interpreted as biologically irrelevant, since children and adults do not exercise at the same absolute $\dot{V}O_2$. In fact, a child has a lower stroke volume (SV) at a given absolute $\dot{V}O_2$ than an adult because of his or her smaller heart size, and when this SV is expressed appropriately to body size, as this chapter explores, values are similar to those of mature individuals.

Compared to adults, children do exhibit certain quantitative differences in exercise variables (heart rate (HR), blood pressure (BP), SV, and $\dot{Q}$). Still, current research information indicates that i) these child/adult differences are accounted for by changes in body dimensions, and that ii) myocardial function, pattern of SV response, relative ventricular dimensional changes, systolic and diastolic filling periods, and exercise factor (ratio of increase in $\dot{Q}$ to that of $\dot{V}O_2$) are similar during endurance exercise in children and adults.

This chapter reviews this information in light of current insights into the normal cardiovascular responses within the model of an acute bout of progressive exercise in euthermic conditions. It should be noted that the discussion will be limited to such responses in lean, healthy youth, with a focus on the prepubertal period. Readers are referred to other sources for information regarding cardiovascular responses to exercise in obese youth,[4] in the heat,[5] and during isometric (resistance) and sustained steady-rate exercise.[6] Small sex differences in certain cardiac variables, particularly SV, are largely accounted for by differences in body composition between boys and girls. Some studies have suggested, however, that other unexplained factors could be responsible; this issue is addressed in Chapter 12.

Measurement of cardiac output

The importance of accurate measurement of cardiac responses notwithstanding, the assessment of cardiovascular changes during exercise, particularly at high intensities, has proven highly challenging. In fact, the availability of a safe, accurate, feasible, and inexpensive means of determining $\dot{Q}$ with exercise remains elusive. Consequently, the exercise scientist is currently handicapped in possessing no single gold standard for the measurement of $\dot{Q}$. This lack of a reference standard has proven to be a particular difficulty when researchers attempt to evaluate the accuracy of newer methodologies, since the various means of assessing $\dot{Q}$ with exercise can only be compared with each other.

A full discussion of the different techniques for estimating $\dot{Q}$ during exercise in children is beyond the purview of this chapter and will only be briefly summarized here. The reader is referred to other sources for a detailed review (e.g. Warburton *et al.*[7]).

Measurement of $\dot{Q}$ in children at rest began as an invasive procedure during heart catheterization of youth with cardiac disease. Most particularly, this involved the direct Fick method, by which $\dot{Q}$ was calculated as $\dot{V}O_2$ divided by the difference between the oxygen content of arterial and mixed venous blood (a-vO_2 diff) according to the Fick equation. While accurate values of $\dot{Q}$ are obtained at rest or even during steady state submaximal exercise, this approach is unsuitable for estimation of $\dot{Q}$ with exercise in paediatric studies due to the need for vascular and cardiac catheter placement and the inability to record valid data at non-steady state or maximal exercise. Other invasive, catheter-based techniques, such as dye dilution and thermodilution suffer identical weaknesses.

Given the inappropriate nature of these invasive methodologies during exercise testing of healthy paediatric subjects, a number of safe, noninvasive techniques for estimating $\dot{Q}$ or SV during exercise have been developed over the past several decades. At present, establishing the value of each of these approaches awaits a broader experience in paediatric subjects.

Carbon dioxide rebreathing

The carbon dioxide rebreathing technique utilizes the Fick equation for estimating $\dot{Q}$ but substitutes measures of carbon dioxide (CO_2) for O_2, which are obtained non-invasively. Carbon dioxide output ($\dot{V}CO_2$), is measured from expired gas, which is then divided by the difference of arterial and venous CO_2 content to provide $\dot{Q}$. Estimate of arterial CO_2 content is calculated from end tidal CO_2, while that of mixed venous CO_2 content can be obtained by two different indirect methodologies (the Collier and the Defares methods), both which require inhalation of CO_2 gas mixtures during exercise.

Although safe and noninvasive, this methodology suffers a number of weaknesses in estimating $\dot{Q}$ with exercise: a) the multiple assumptions and equations involved reduce its accuracy, b) estimates of $\dot{Q}$ with exercise are limited to steady-state (i.e. submaximal) states, and c) children may feel discomfort in inhaling CO_2 at high work intensities.

Acetylene rebreathing

In this technique, pulmonary blood flow (assumed to be equivalent to $\dot{Q}$) is estimated by the rate at which inhaled acetylene enters and leaves the blood in the lungs. The recent development of rapid, low-cost gas analysers has increased the feasibility of this method and permitted assessment of $\dot{Q}$ at maximal exercise with spontaneous breathing.

Doppler echocardiography

Cardiac SV can be estimated as the product of the velocity of blood flow leaving the heart and the cross-sectional area through which it passes. Doppler echocardiography permits estimation of the former during exercise, while two-dimensional ultrasound measures the latter. Cardiac output is then calculated by multiplying SV by HR. This technique bears the advantages of being safe and non-obtrusive to the subject, while providing beat-to-beat SV values to maximal exercise. The weakness of this technique is that it necessitates highly trained personnel and expensive ultrasound equipment.

Bioimpedance cardiography

Bioimpedance cardiography estimates SV during exercise by its calculated relationship to alterations in electrical compliance of the chest. These changes in electrical resistance are recorded by electrodes applied to the chest. The ease of this method and its ability to estimate SV at peak exercise are appealing. However, controversy surrounds its accuracy, and its theoretical construct has been questioned.

Expressing cardiac output with exercise to body size

Paediatric exercise scientists and clinicians face the challenge of identifying appropriate means of adjusting exercise physiological variables for differences in body size. During the growing years a number of circulatory variables, such as HR and a-vO_2 diff, are largely independent of body dimensions. On the other hand, SV (and, consequently, $\dot{Q}$) are direct reflections of left ventricular chamber size. These variables are therefore expected to increase in the process of normal growth as children age. Between the years of 8 and 15, for instance, heart volume of the healthy child more than doubles.[8]

Size-related variables therefore need to be expressed relative to some marker of body size in order to i) establish normative values, ii) permit comparisons between different individuals or groups, and iii) allow assessment of intra-individual change serially over time. A number of such normalizing factors have been utilized in paediatric exercise science, including body mass, height, body surface area (BSA), and lean mass, sometimes expressed in exponential or allometric form (interested readers are referred to Chapter 12 for further discussion). Current research has divulged the advantages and weaknesses surrounding many of these anthropomoetric markers and has indicated the importance of utilizing an accurate and appropriate means of expressing exercise physiologic variables to avoid spurious conclusions.

Appropriate anthropometric variables for adjusting $\dot{Q}$ and SV to body size are best derived through the process of allometric scaling. In this approach, any given physiological variable Y (in this case $\dot{Q}$ or SV) is scaled to the adjusted anthropometric factor X (i.e. BSA, height, weight, lean body mass) according to the equation:

$$Y = aX^b$$

where a is the proportionality constant and b is the scaling factor which describes the influence of that anthropometric variable on $\dot{Q}$ and SV. Solving this equation after logarithmic transformation provides the value of X^b, which then serves as an appropriate size-normalizing denominator for the physiological variable in question in the particular subjects being considered.

If the value of b is equal or close to 1.0, the absolute value of the anthropometric variable is a proper size-adjusting factor. The greater the discrepancy from 1.0, the greater the error that can be expected from using the absolute factor and, in that case, the anthropometric factor raised to the empirically derived exponent (X^b) should be employed to adjust the physiological variables to body size. The validity of the derived scaled anthropometric variable to serve in such adjustment can be confirmed by the failure of demonstrating any significant statistical relationship between Y/X^b and X.

Cardiac output and SV have traditionally been adjusted for differences in body size by the BSA in square metres as the cardiac index and stroke index, respectively. This convention developed from its use in normalizing values of basal and resting metabolic rate which are linked to metabolic heat lost through the body surface (which is directly related to $\dot{V}O_2$ and $\dot{V}CO_2$). This approach is convenient, requiring only consultation of tables relating body height and weight to BSA based on empirically derived equations, and size-related values can be compared to others previously described by the same manner in the scientific literature. Additionally, the use of BSA is supported by dimensionality theory, which holds that volume flow rates (such as $\dot{Q}$ in $L \cdot min^{-1}$) should be related to length cubed divided by length (considered equivalent to time), or length (or body height) squared. And, again mathematically, BSA, expressed in metres squared, is expected to similarly relate to the square of body height (e.g. length).

Nonetheless, the use of BSA as a means of adjusting SV and $\dot{Q}$ has often been criticized.[9] It has been claimed that the formulae on which BSA is estimated from height and weight are inaccurate (and not relevant to children), and that BSA does not take into consideration differences in body composition, particularly fat content which does not contribute to metabolic expenditure.

These arguments notwithstanding, a number of empirical observations have supported the use of BSA to adjust $\dot{Q}$ and SV for body size during exercise in children, at least in non-obese populations. Rowland[10] found allometric exponents of 1.08 and 1.05 for BSA in measures of maximal $\dot{Q}$ and SV, respectively, in 24 girls (age 12.2 ± 0.5 years). No significant relationship was observed between $\dot{Q}$/BSA and BSA (r = 0.04). In a similar study in boys the allometric exponent for BSA related to maximal SV was 1.03.[11] Armstrong and Welsman[12] found that changes in $\dot{Q}$ during submaximal exercise increased over 2 years in direct proportion to BSA. However, Turley and Wilmore[13] found that $\dot{Q}$/BSA and SV/BSA were not independent of body size in children, with correlations to BSA of r = −0.82 and r = 0.29, respectively.

Conceptually, measures of $\dot{Q}$ and SV as functions closely matched to metabolic demand should be expected to relate most closely to the volume of metabolically active tissue. During exercise, this means the actively contracting muscle mass, and this volume should be expected to serve as the ideal denominator by which to normalize $\dot{Q}$ and SV to body size. As this is practically impossible to quantify, the value of lean (fat-free) body mass has often been used as a surrogate marker. This is an improvement over the use of body mass (which includes metabolically inert body fat), but still encompasses tissues not involved in the exercise performed (e.g. bone mass, organ protein, non-contracting muscle). In a group of prepubertal children, Vinet *et al.*[14] found that maximal SV and $\dot{Q}$ related to lean body mass by exponents of 0.79 and 0.76, respectively.

From this information, it can be recommended that the optimal means of expressing $\dot{Q}$ or SV during exercise is by expressing values in respect to fat-free mass raised to an empirically derived allometric scaling exponent calculated from the subjects involved.[15] This approach, of course, requires an accurate measurement of body composition to provide reliable values of lean body mass. Using body height adjusted allometrically provides an alternative approach.

If BSA is used to adjust maximal $\dot{Q}$ or SV (as maximal stroke index and cardiac index), the relationship of $\dot{Q}$ max/BSA or SV max/BSA to BSA in the study group should be examined to assure that the calculated scaling exponent for BSA is approximately 1.0 (i.e. allometric analysis should ensure that the 95% confidence limits of the scaling exponent should include the value 1.0). If not, BSA raised to the calculated scaling exponent b should be used to adjust values of $\dot{Q}$ and SV. Based on the degree of variability that has been observed in scaling exponents for anthropometric variables published in the research literature, 'off-the-shelf', i.e. assumed, exponents should not be used with a high level of confidence.

Dynamics of cardiovascular responses to progressive exercise

The onset of a bout of progressive exercise triggers a complex interplay of cardiac SV, HR, and vascular reactivity which eventuates in augmentation of circulatory blood flow. A full understanding of this response does not yet exist, and controversy and debate continue to surround a number of the details. Still, it should be expected that any construct of such circulatory dynamics as exercise intensity rises should conform to certain empirically derived observations:

Total systemic vascular resistance: observed progressive decline

Autonomic action on vascular smooth muscle effects regionally specific alterations in peripheral vascular resistance during exercise. Arterioles which feed exercising muscle undergo vasodilatation, while those supplying non-exercising tissues (such as renal and mesenchymal) vasoconstrict. As a result of this redistribution of circulatory flow with exercise, approximately 80% of total $\dot{Q}$ is shunted to the skeletal muscle, compared to 20% at rest. In sum, the balance of these alterations produces a progressive fall in total systemic vascular resistance, calculated by the simplified Poiseuille Law as mean arterial pressure divided by $\dot{Q}$. A review of eight reports describing the response of calculated systemic vascular resistance to maximal exercise in youth revealed an average of 18.8 ± 2.0 units at rest, declining to 7.1 ± 1.8 units at peak exercise, an overall reduction of 62% at the point of maximal exercise.[16]

A number of locally generated vasodilatory agents contribute to the fall in resistance within the exercising muscle. This response may explain the tight quantitative link between augmentation of circulatory flow and the rise in metabolic demand of the contracting muscle. Such biochemical actions on peripheral vascular tone with exercise have not been studied in paediatric subjects. Still, that these effects are quantitatively and qualitatively similar in children and adults is indicated by identical, age-independent alterations in systemic vascular resistance with progressive exercise. For example, during such exercise, Nottin *et al.*[17] described a decline in average systemic vascular resistance from 15 units at rest to seven units at peak exercise in boys (mean age 11.7 years) and from 15 units to 6 units in young men (mean age 21.2 years).

Stroke Volume change in various levels of exercise intensity

At the onset of running, walking, or upright cycle exercise, SV typically increases by approximately 25% above resting values. However, at intensities above that equivalent to 50% $\dot{V}O_2$ max remains essentially stable (± 5%) to the point of maximal exertion. This pattern is one of the most consistently observed responses in cardiac exercise physiology, having been documented by each of the various assessment methodologies and evident in both child and adult males and females, fit and unfit youth in the general population, and highly trained child athletes.[18]

The small rise in SV at the onset of upright exercise has been explained as follows. Gravity profoundly affects the cardiovascular system, causing substantial amounts of venous pooling of blood in the dependent lower extremities (estimated to be 500–1000 mL in adults) when assuming the upright position. As a result SV and $\dot{Q}$ normally decline by 20–40%, reflecting diminution of central blood volume (i.e. that flowing through the heart). At the onset of exercise, this dependent blood is mobilized through the joint effects of arteriolar dilatation and the pumping action of leg muscles.[19] Consequently, central blood volume is restored, and SV rises by approximately 25% to its original supine value. By these observations, then, the initial increase in SV can reasonably be explained as a re-filling phenomenon, the result of mobilization of blood sequestered in the lower extremity at the onset of exercise.

A number of early studies supported this conclusion. Stegall[20] reported that pressures in the superficial and deep veins at the ankle fell from 90 mmHg at rest to less than 10 mmHg with running. Pollack and Wood[21] found that with the onset of walking exercise venous pressure at the ankle fell from 100 mmHg to approximately 40 mmHg. Similarly, Stick *et al.*[22] observed that venous pressures of 24–30 mmHg at the ankle during treadmill walking and running compared to 84 mmHg with quiet standing.

More recently, Rowland *et al.*[23] documented this scenario by measuring alterations in SV in ten healthy adolescent males (mean age 15.3 ± 0.5 years) using Doppler echocardiography. As indicated in Figure 11.1, SV fell by 25% when these boys moved from the supine position to sitting upright on a cycle ergometer. At the onset of exercise, values rose to approximate those observed supine, then subsequently remained stable to the point of maximal exercise.

This explanation for the early rise of SV during exercise is further supported by observations that no such initial increase is evident in situations in which gravity does not influence cardiovascular dynamics. A study comparing SV responses to progressive cycle exercise performed in the supine and upright positions in the same circumpubertal boys (mean age 12.5 ± 1.4 years) revealed that at rest, mean values for SV were 16.4% lower in the upright posture compared to supine.[24] With increasing work intensities, SV remained stable when supine, but in the upright position rose by 29% initially to become statistically similar to those supine.

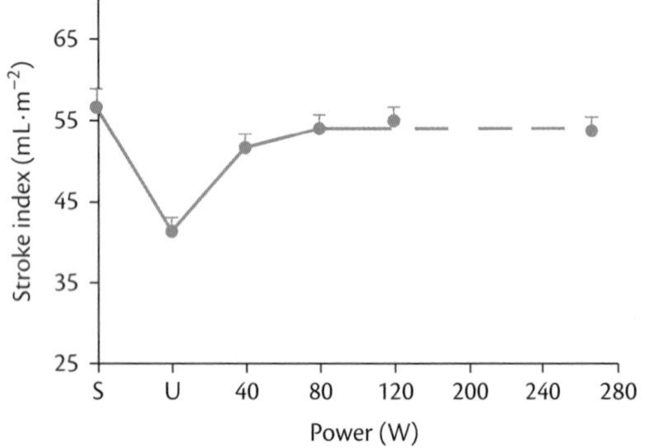

Figure 11.1 Stroke index at rest supine, then when assuming the upright position, followed by progressive exercise to exhaustion in a study of 17-year-old males.
S = supine; U = upright.
Rowland T, Unnithan V. Stroke dynamics during progressive exercise in healthy adolescents. Pediatr Exerc Sci. 2013: 25: 173–185.

This failure to demonstrate an initial rise in SV during supine exercise is consistent with the findings in a number of studies performed in adults.[25–28] Some investigations in adults have demonstrated a rise in SV during supine exercise, but of lower magnitude than when subjects were exercising upright.[29,30] For example, Thadani and Parker[29] reported increases in SV during exercise of 22% and 71% with subjects supine and upright, respectively.

Similarly, a 'flat' SV response to increasing work intensities has typically been observed in other conditions not expected to be affected by gravity. These include prone simulated swimming,[31] astronauts in zero gravity,[32] arm exercise,[33] and upright exercise in a swimming pool.[34]

In summary, this information indicates that the initial rise in SV during upright exercise does not represent an inherent response for augmenting the circulatory response to the metabolic demands of exercise. Moreover, other than a refilling of the central circulation at the onset of upright exercise, SV does not contribute to the rise in $\dot{Q}$ and circulatory flow during a bout of progressive exercise.

Left ventricular end-diastolic dimension

There exists a popular conception that the heart, being engaged in a volume overload (increased $\dot{Q}$), enlarges in size during a bout of endurance exercise. In fact, the end-diastolic volume, as indicated by early radiographic studies and more recently by echocardiography[17,24,35–37] and radionuclide ventriculography[38,39], changes little from rest to the point of maximal exercise. Often a minor rise (~2 mm) in dimension is observed at the onset of upright exercise, consistent with the transient increase in cardiac filling from blood mobilized from the legs. This is typically followed by a gradual decline, with change in values from rest to maximal exercise escaping any statistically significant difference.

This stability of left ventricular end-diastolic dimension through the course of a bout of progressive exercise has been documented by echocardiography in children[17,24,35,36] as well as adults[17,37] and is evident when exercise is performed in the supine as well as the upright position.[24]

Nottin *et al.*[17] performed a direct comparison of left ventricular end-diastolic dimensions during exercise by echocardiography in 10- to 12-year-old and 19- to 24-year-old males. Rest-to-maximal declines were from 44.4 ± 3.8 to 41.0 ± 5.1 mm and from 51.9 ± 3.6 to 49.7 ± 3.8 mm in the two groups, respectively.

This constancy of left ventricular end-diastolic size is assumed to reflect a stability of ventricular filling pressure with increasing work intensities. Two observations further support this conclusion.

First, during exercise the ratio of the peak early transmitral filling velocity (measured echocardiographically as the E wave) and the diastolic relaxation velocity of the ventricular myocardium (the E′ wave by tissue Doppler imaging) is considered to reflect left ventricular filling pressure.[40] While values of both E and E′ normally rise during progressive exercise with augmentation of myocardial diastolic function, the ratio E/E′ has repeatedly been demonstrated to remain unchanged or gradually decline, in a manner similar to that of measures of left ventricular end diastolic dimension.[16]

These observations imply that, with the exception of brief increases at the onset of upright exercise, ventricular preload is not influenced by increasing work intensities. Despite threefold to fivefold increases in total ventricular output, left ventricular end-diastolic volume remains essentially stable during a bout of progressive exercise.

Myocardial systolic and diastolic function

As work intensity rises, all markers of myocardial contractility (inotropy) rise. By necessity—since what goes in must come out—diastolic function (ventricular filling) improves in a parallel fashion.

Myocardial systolic function

Myocardial contractility is here defined in a global sense as the velocity and force of heart muscle contraction. This broad description is utilized, since, by this definition, myocardial contractility during progressive exercise is influenced by a multitude of factors—ventricular preload, afterload, HR, sympatho-adrenal stimulation—the individual contributions of which are impossible to decipher, particularly in the intact exercising human.[41]

In the past, assessment of changes in myocardial contractility with exercise was limited to investigations utilizing radionuclide angiography.[42,43] These studies revealed an improvement of left ventricular ejection fraction (volume of blood expelled per beat expressed as a percentage of end-diastolic volume) during a progressive exercise test in a healthy adult from approximately 60% at rest to 70–90% at peak exercise (i.e. an expected rise in myocardial contractility of about 15%). In children, using gated equilibrium nuclear angiograms, DeSouza *et al.*[44] found a rise in average ejection fraction from 63% at rest to 81% with supine exercise (an 18% increase) in subjects ages 8–18 years with familial hypercholesterolaemia (but no overt evidence of cardiac disease).

As this methodology requires the use of radioactive material, information in healthy children awaited the advent of cardiac ultrasound techniques. Studies utilizing two-dimensional and M-mode echocardiography have provided measures of the ventricular shortening fraction (the difference of end-diastolic dimension and end-systolic dimension divided by the end-diastolic dimension, expressed as a percentage), the one-dimensional analogue of the ejection fraction. The mean rise in these reports has been from 34 ± 6% at rest to 46 ± 6% at maximal exercise, an average increase of 32%.[41] This rise in shortening fraction is explained by the observation that, although end-diastolic dimension remains stable, end-systolic dimension progressively falls with augmented contractility as exercise intensity increases. A similar magnitude of augmentation of left ventricular shortening fraction values has been observed in studies involving paediatric and adult subjects.[41]

The advent of Doppler echocardiography to measure vascular and tissue velocities provided a means of assessing myocardial contractility non-invasively at rest and during exercise. As noted previously, per-beat SV is estimated by this technique by multiplying the integrated aortic flow velocity (the velocity-time integral, VTI, obtained either from the suprasternal notch or inferiorly from an apical five-chamber view) by the cross-sectional area of the aortic outflow tract. The VTI also offers a means of determining systolic ejection time. The ventricular systolic ejection rate, or SV over time, then provides a marker of rate of generation of myocardial force and velocity.[45] In comparisons between groups or individuals, the ejection rate needs to be adjusted for ventricular mass.

Eight studies of changes in systolic ejection rate with progressive exercise in children have indicated an average increase of 70–80% above pre-exercise values.[41] Similarly, the peak velocity of aortic flow, an indicator of generation of ventricular pressure, can be estimated by the same approach. Values typically rise from 110 $cm \cdot s^{-1}$ at rest to 181 $cm \cdot s^{-1}$ at peak exercise (+70%).[41]

The technique of tissue Doppler imaging (TDI) permits estimation of the velocity of the left ventricular myocardium during systolic contraction in the longitudinal (i.e. vertical) plane. Several studies have indicated that this velocity (TDI-S) approximately doubles in the course of a bout of progressive exercise in both children and adults.[41]

The latest generation of advances in Doppler echocardiographic technology has provided new tools for assessing ventricular contractility with exercise. Speckle tracking, which measures both regional myocardial displacement (strain) and rate of displacement (strain rate), permits estimation of ventricular myocardial velocities in all planes of orientation. The most realistic means of measuring ventricular contractility is Doppler assessment of the extent of the 'twist' of the heart during systole. The myocardium normally contracts in a spiral fashion, creating a 'wringing out' effect on the ventricular chamber to expel blood. Quantifying the magnitude and velocity of the opposite rotations of the cardiac base (clockwise) and apex (counterclockwise) by Doppler techniques thereby provides a true reflection of the contractility of the heart in three-dimensional space.

The use of these newer methodologies during exercise has been currently tempered by the inability to assess contractility at high-exercise intensities. Consequently, studies at present have generally been limited to supine and submaximal exercise. However, responses of markers of myocardial contractility to exercise in these studies have been predictable. In a group of 17-year-old males, Unnithan *et al.*[46] demonstrated increases in longitudinal, radial, and circumferential strain from rest to upright cycle exercise to a work load of 80 watts. Doucende *et al.*[47] reported approximate doubling of measures of ventricular twist when young men cycled in the semisupine position to a work rate equivalent to 40% $\dot{V}O_2$ max (HR 121 ± 12 $beats \cdot min^{-1}$).

Myocardial diastolic function

Similar echocardiographic techniques have been used to assess diastolic function (ventricular relaxation and filling properties) during exercise. Not surprisingly, research findings indicate that such changes mirror those of increases in systolic function as workload intensifies.

Filling of the left ventricle during diastole is contingent upon the pressure gradient across the mitral valve created between 'upstream' left atrial pressure and 'downstream' of factors such as rate of ventricular relaxation and suction effect. This gradient can be estimated at rest and during exercise by measuring the E-wave velocity across the valve in early diastole (corresponding to the rapid filling phase) by Doppler echocardiography and converting this velocity (v) to pressure gradient (g) by the Bernoulli equation $g = 4v^2$.

Mitral E velocity in healthy children normally rises twofold from rest to peak exercise.[48–50] Data from a study of 10- to 14-year-old boys indicated, consequently, that the pressure gradient driving blood across the mitral valve in diastole increases by a factor of four in the course of a progressive upright cycle exercise test.[48] The A wave during late diastole, reflecting atrial systole, has not been considered in exercise studies, since E and A waves fuse beyond a HR of approximately 110 beats·min^{-1}. Based on pacing studies, it has generally been considered that atrial systole does not contribute meaningfully to left ventricular filling during exercise.[51]

The rate of relaxation of the left ventricular myocardium in the longitudinal plane (a component of the 'downstream' influence on mitral valve pressure gradient) can be estimated by tissue Doppler imaging. Paralleling findings of augmented systolic function, this TDI-E′ velocity normally doubles during the course of progressive exercise to exhaustion.[41]

A synthesis

The empirically derived observations described in the previous section are consistent with a model in which circulatory responses to a bout of progressive exercise are facilitated and controlled by changes in peripheral vascular resistance. Additionally, since each of these individual findings is evident in studies of both adults and children, it can be assumed that this construct of how the cardiovascular system works with exercise holds true for both groups.

The cardiovascular response to progressive exercise appears to be dictated by Poiseuille's Law, which, simplified, indicates that $\dot{Q} \sim P/R$, where $\dot{Q}$ is level of systemic blood flow, P is the pressure head, and R is the systemic vascular resistance. During exercise, it is the fall in R which increases $\dot{Q}$, while the cardiac pump is required to maintain P. That the level of vasodilatation of the arterioles feeding exercising muscle is the controlling factor to blood flow conveniently explains how local vasodilatory factors, produced in response to metabolic need, match so tightly such demand to circulatory supply.

This model, supported by contemporary research data, is consistent with conclusions drawn from early studies of humans and instrumented dogs in the 1950s. These findings indicated that,

> The heart serves as a force-feed pump designed to discharge whatever volume it receives by increasing its rate or stroke volume. Unless there is dilatation of resistance vessels in some systemic vascular bed, mediated by local humoral or nervous mechanisms, an increased rate will not result in an increase in cardiac output.[52(p180)]

Or, as Guyton put it, 'the heart has little effect on the normal regulation of cardiac output'.[53]

Essentially, therefore, as noted by Braunwald and Ross,[54] the circulatory system during exercise mimics that of a large arterial-venous fistula (a connection between the two that bypasses the high resistance arteriolar vessels), which lowers total systemic vascular resistance and increases $\dot{Q}$ (sometimes to the point of causing congestive heart failure). In fact, Binak *et al.*[55] demonstrated experimentally that the rise in $\dot{Q}$ with exercise replicated that seen in patients with such a pathologic fistula.

In this model, the rise in systemic venous return to the heart with exercise must be met precisely with a concomitant increase in HR to account for the observed stability of left ventricular end-diastolic size. Indeed, it appears that the rise in HR serves to defend left ventricular size as exercise intensity increases, since a failure to do so would result in a progressive enlargement of left ventricular end-diastolic dimension that would unfavourably augment left ventricular wall stress.[55] Only by invoking a means which cardiac venous return and HR are closely linked can the stability of left ventricular filling size and a fourfold rise in volume of blood return to the right atrium during progressive exercise be explained.

The mechanism for this matching of sinus node discharge rate with increases in atrial volume is uncertain. The Bainbridge reflex, by which increases in right atrial pressure stimulate reflex sympathetic stimulation of the sinus node, is a reasonable explanation. While the existence of this reflex has always been surrounded by controversy,[56] its function has been demonstrated in both humans and subhuman primates.[57] Others have proposed that the afferent limb of such a reflex involves receptors within the skeletal muscle, while, as another possibility, brain centres might in parallel activate both sympathetic signals to accelerate sinus node discharge and trigger skeletal muscle activation (so called central command).[58]

In examining these empirically-derived observations, one is faced with the need to explain how SV can remain essentially unchanged with increasing exercise intensities while myocardial contractility increases. The answer must be that the increase in contractile force serves to eject the same volume of blood (i.e. a stable SV) in a progressively shortening ejection time. As illustrated in one report, a 20% increase in shortening fraction in such a test was observed with a concomitant 24% fall in ejection time while SV remained unchanged.[59] That is, the observed augmented systolic function acts to maintain rather than increase SV during a bout of progressive exercise. Predictably, then, a failure of such a myocardial response, as is observed in patients with myocardial dysfunction, is manifest by a decline in SV during progressive exercise.[60]

The same action must occur in diastole as well. Following the initial phase of incremental upright exercise, SV exhibits little change, and left ventricular end-diastolic dimension (reflecting ventricular preload) is stable. By necessity, then, the volume of blood crossing the mitral valve to enter the left ventricle per beat during diastole must remain unchanged as work intensity increases. Yet all evidence indicates a progressively increasing LA-LV pressure gradient with augmentation of transmitral flow velocity. These observations can only be reconciled if the rise in diastolic function serves to deliver the same volume of blood to the ventricle per beat in diastole in a shorter time period (i.e. the decline in typical duration of diastole at rest of 0.49–0.15 s at peak exercise.)

Normative values

As indicated in the preceding section, children do not differ from adults in the means by which the cardiovascular system responds to the metabolic demands of progressive exercise. The following now examines potential age- and size-dependent quantitative differences in the elements of that response that might distinguish the two groups.

Heart rate

The frequency of electrical discharge of the sinus node, which triggers sequential atrial-ventricular contraction, is governed by the rate of its spontaneous depolarization/repolarization. Superimposed on this intrinsic function are the additional effects of parasympathetic (deceleration) and sympathetic (acceleration) neural influences, as well as, to a lesser extent, the stimulating action of circulating catecholamines. Pharmacologic autonomic blocking studies have generally indicated that a) the resting HR reflects a suppressant effect of parasympathetic action on the intrinsic node firing rate, which is approximately 40–50 beats higher in both children and adults,[61] and b), at least in adults, parasympathetic withdrawal, replaced by augmented sympathetic stimulation, is largely responsible for the rise in HR with exercise.

Normal values for resting HR for children were initially established almost 100 years ago in studies that were examining basal metabolic rate in young subjects.[62] These values describe HR in standardized basal conditions (lying quietly in the post-absorptive state). Average basal HRs decline gradually during the paediatric years, from about 91 beats $\cdot$ min^{-1} at age 5 to 74 beats $\cdot$ min^{-1} at age 15 years in males. Corresponding values in females are approximately 6 beats $\cdot$ min^{-1} faster. It should be remembered that 'resting' HRs as described in most contemporary exercise studies of children are expected to be higher, being influenced by pre-test anxiety.

The cause of this developmental decline in resting HR during the course of childhood is not entirely clear. The fall in HR with age parallels that of size-related basal metabolic rate. Basal metabolic rate (related to BSA) declines by approximately 23% in females from age 6 to 16 years, while the basal HR falls over the same time span by 20%.[63] Considering that the magnitude of rise of resting HR after parasympathetic blockade is similar in children and adults, it seems likely that the rise in resting HR during childhood reflects progressive alterations in the intrinsic firing rate (such as rate of ion flux) of the sinoatrial node rather than developmental changes in autonomic influence.

During progressive exercise, HR rises linearly with increasing work load, but beyond moderate intensities HR is often observed to taper as work load rises. In a group of 12-year-old children, all 13 subjects demonstrated such a taper when exercise intensity exceeded 60% $\dot{V}O_2$ max on treadmill testing, and approximately one third showed a plateau in HR (defined as less than a three-beat increase in the final stage).[64] The aetiology of this pattern is uncertain. A number of explanations have been offered, including increases in lactate production and alterations in autonomic balance.

The HR at a given work load during an exercise test falls as children age. As muscle energy efficiency is independent of age or body size, absolute values of $\dot{V}O_2$ and $\dot{Q}$ at a specific exercise intensity will be similar in children and adults. But as children age, the absolute values of SV will increase with growth of the cardiac chambers. Consequently, HR, as the dividend of $\dot{Q}$/SV, will progressively fall at that workload with age and increasing body size.

This rate of decline in submaximal HR has been documented in both cycle and treadmill protocols. Cassels and Morse[65] demonstrated that the average HRs while walking at 3.5 miles $\cdot$ h^{-1} on an 8.6% grade in 10- and 16-year-old subjects were 167 and 147 beats $\cdot$ min^{-1} respectively. While pedaling at a workload of 30 W, Bouchard *et al.*[8] found 8-year-old children to have a mean heart rate of 138 beats $\cdot$ min^{-1}, while that of 18-year-olds was 100 beats $\cdot$ min^{-1}.

Measures of HR in children during a specific exercise challenge are highly reliable. Amorim *et al.*[66] found no significant differences in submaximal HRs in 14 children (mean age 10.1 ± 1.4 years) during three sessions of treadmill walking at four different speeds.

Maximal HR achieved by children during a truly exhaustive effort on a progressive test depends on testing modality (e.g. treadmill or cycle ergometer) as well as form of exercise (e.g. running or walking), but not age or sex. In most reports involving studies of treadmill running, subjects achieve an average maximal HR of about 200 beats $\cdot$ min^{-1}.[67,68] With treadmill walking protocols, peak values are typically 5–10 beats $\cdot$ min^{-1} lower.[68,69] Average maximal HRs in children while cycling are usually 185–195 beats $\cdot$ min^{-1}.[68] In these studies boys and girls generally show similar values.

Both cross-sectional and longitudinal studies have indicated that while resting HR falls with age, peak values remain stable, at least to the mid-teen years. Bailey *et al.*[70] used a treadmill running protocol to test 51 boys serially over a period of 8 years, beginning at age 8. During this time the mean maximal HR was 196 beats $\cdot$ min^{-1}. With the exception of the first year of testing (when peak HR was 193 beats $\cdot$ min^{-1}), average maximal rates did not vary by more than 3 beats $\cdot$ min^{-1}. In an unpublished study, Rowland and Cunningham showed no systematic changes in maximal HR during treadmill walking in either boys or girls (±2 beats $\cdot$ min^{-1} and ±4 beats $\cdot$ min^{-1}, respectively) in a 5-year longitudinal study starting at age 9 years.

Beginning in the late teen years, maximal HR declines steadily over the lifetime. The peak HR during progressive exercise in a 60-year-old man, for instance, is expected to be approximately 160 beats $\cdot$ min^{-1}.[71]

Two observations here are particularly important. First, since maximal HR during exercise testing remains stable across the paediatric years, formulae for estimating maximal HR used in adults (such as 220-age) are not appropriate for use in children. Second, although the normative figures for peak HRs in children have been used as target rates for maximal testing, it should be recognized that a significant inter-individual variability exists in these values. Most studies of children indicate a standard deviation of 5–10 beats $\cdot$ min^{-1}, a variability that presumably is not explained by differences in peak effort, since elite athletes demonstrate a similar range. The difficulty posed by this variability is well-illustrated in the report of Sheehan *et al.*[72] The subjects in this study had an average maximal HR of 202 beats $\cdot$ min^{-1} during treadmill running with a standard deviation of 9 beats $\cdot$ min^{-1}. In these subjects, then, 17% would be expected to demonstrate a peak HR less than 193 beats $\cdot$ min^{-1}, while an equal number would have a maximal value over 211 beats $\cdot$ min^{-1}. If a criterion of >200 beats $\cdot$ min^{-1} were selected to identify a peak effort, a significant number of the children would have been inappropriately excluded, while others might have fallen short of an exhaustive effort (interested readers are referred to Chapter 12 for further discussion).

While maximal HR remains stable during the growing years, the rate of fall in HR after exhaustive exercise progressively declines. For example, following maximal cycle testing, 1 min recovery HRs for boys grouped by BSA as <1.0 m^2, 1.0–1.19 m^2, and >1.2 m^2 were 133, 138, and 148 beats $\cdot$ min^{-1}, respectively, in the study by Washington *et al.*[73] This trend during childhood growth and development has been attributed to possible changes in catecholamine levels and/or lactate production and clearance.

Stroke volume and cardiac output

Normal growth in cardiac ventricular dimensions is uniquely responsible for the increases in resting SV and $\dot{Q}$ during the course of the childhood years. In early cross-sectional studies, resting absolute values for SV and $\dot{Q}$ during cardiac catheterization were found to correlate closely with both BSA and body mass across the paediatric age span.[74,75] Blimkie *et al.*[76] described a significant association between left ventricular end-diastolic diameter, mass and SV in boys 10–14 years old. At the same time, evidence indicates that myocardial systolic function at rest is independent of age and therefore does not contribute to developmental increases in SV (and, consequently, of $\dot{Q}$). Colan *et al.*[77] demonstrated that resting values of left ventricular shortening fraction show little change between the ages of 1 week and 19 years. Progressively increasing values of TDI-S and TDI-E′ (reflecting systolic and diastolic function, respectively) described by Eidem *et al.*[78] for children between the ages of 1 and 18 years were explained by the rise in left ventricular end-diastolic dimension. In that study left ventricular shortening fraction was also stable over the same age span.

Similar trends are evident for SV and $\dot{Q}$ at maximal exercise. A number of important clues indicate that at peak exercise, as at rest, values a) reflect ventricular volume, independent of myocardial systolic and diastolic functional responses, and b) when expressed relative to body size, are not influenced by age.

As noted previously, values of maximal SV and $\dot{Q}$ have been closely linked to measures of BSA.[10–12] A study of maximal prone swim bench exercise in 11-year-olds revealed a strong correlation between resting left ventricular end-diastolic dimension and maximal SV ($r = 0.78$).[31] Similarly, Obert *et al.*[79] demonstrated a close relationship between left ventricular size and maximal SV in 10- to 11-year-old boys and girls during incremental cycle exercise.

The magnitude of augmentation of myocardial systolic and diastolic function during a maximal progressive exercise is independent of values of maximal SV. This was demonstrated by Rowland *et al.*[23] in a study of 12 male adolescent soccer players and 10 untrained boys. Maximal values of stroke index were 59 ± 8 and 46 ± 10 $mL \cdot m^{-2}$ in the two groups, respectively, while no differences were observed in increases or peak values of systolic ejection rate, peak aortic velocity, TDI-E, and mitral E velocity. Similar findings were observed in a follow-up study in adolescent females.[80]

Information regarding longitudinal changes in maximal values of SV and $\dot{Q}$ during the growing years is limited. McNarry *et al.*[81] estimated maximal cardiovascular variables by thoracic bioimpedance with cycle testing in 15 untrained boys and girls annually for 3 years beginning at age ten. Mean values for maximal cardiac index were 10.78, 9.84, and 10.38 $L \cdot min^{-1} \cdot m^{-2}$, while those for stroke index were 56, 52, and 55 $mL \cdot m^{-2}$. In a cross-sectional study of 10 prepubertal, 16 pubertal, and 10 postpubertal girls, McNarry *et al.*[82] found no significant differences in maximal stroke index and cardiac index by the thoracic bioimpedance technique during an incremental ramp cycle test.

These findings suggest that in the paediatric age group neither age nor sexual maturation influences size-adjusted values, which is consistent with previous reports indicating similar maximal stroke index and cardiac index in direct comparisons of prepubertal boys and girls compared to their young adult counterparts.[8,17,83] In a comparison of 24 premenarcheal girls (mean age 11.7 years) and 17 young adult women (mean age 27.4 years), allometric analysis revealed no group differences in average maximal $\dot{Q}$ (10.50 and 10.07 $L \cdot min^{-1} \cdot BSA^{-1.11}$, respectively) nor maximal SV (53 and 56 $mL \cdot BSA^{-1.13}$, respectively).[83] In a similar study by the same research group, maximal stroke index values for 11-year-old boys and 31-year-old men during upright cycle exercise were not significantly different (59 ± 11 vs. 61 ± 14 $mL \cdot m^{-2}$, respectively).[84]

Nottin *et al.*[17] found no significant difference in maximal cardiac index or stroke index between 12-year-old boys and young men during maximal upright cycle exercise. Others have demonstrated similar maximal stroke index and/or cardiac index values in comparisons of 10- and 18-year-old subjects,[85] 12- and 32-year-old men,[86] and 9- to 20-year-old males.[87]

Additional evidence of comparable cardiac performance between children and adults comes from a consideration of the exercise factor, the ratio of change in $\dot{Q}$ to that of $\dot{V}O_2$ as work intensifies. Considered a marker of myocardial performance during exercise, the expected value among healthy adults is approximately 6.0, while reduced values are observed in patients with myocardial dysfunction. Among six exercise studies in children the average exercise factor was 6.1 (see Rowland[88] for review).

Representative values for maximal stroke index and cardiac index in studies of children and adolescents are outlined in Table 11.1. Typical values for males of stroke index at peak exercise are 50–60 $mL \cdot m^{-2}$ and cardiac index 9–11 $L \cdot min^{-1} \cdot m^{-2}$. The slightly lower values in female subjects have been attributed to sex differences in lean body mass. As discussed in Chapter 12, some investigations have indicated small residual differences between boys and girls in maximal SV even with body composition considered.

Blood pressure

Systolic/diastolic BP taken at rest rises during the course of childhood from approximately 70/55 mmHg in a newborn baby to 115/65 mmHg at age 15 years. With dynamic exercise, systolic pressure rises, while diastolic pressure remains stable or declines slightly. The value of maximal systolic pressure is directly related to that at rest. As a consequence of these influences, maximal systolic BP steadily rises as a child ages.[89]

Maximal systolic pressure is typically about 40 mmHg above that measured at rest, although the magnitude of rise may be greater in larger subjects.[69] Values are influenced by body size, sex, athleticism, and ethnicity. Riopel *et al.*[69] provided normative data for maximal systolic pressure during maximal treadmill walking. Subjects with the smallest BSA (0.7–1.09 m^2) had average peak values of 142–147 mmHg, while the largest children (BSA 1.90–2.31 m^2) reached a maximal BP of 200–206 mmHg. Males had greater values than females only among the larger subjects, where values in males were about 15–20 mmHg higher.

Normative data for cycle testing have been published by Alpert *et al.*[90] in 405 children ages 6–15 years. Again, maximal systolic pressure was directly related to body size, with an approximate 30 mmHg greater values in youth with BSA of 2.0 m^2 compared to those with a BSA of 1.0 m^2. Similar findings have been described by Washington *et al.*[73] and James *et al.*[91] In both the reports of Alpert *et al.*[90] and Riopel *et al.*,[69] black children exhibited greater values of maximal BP with exercise. Dlin[92] found that the BP response to exercise was higher in adolescent athletes than non-athletes.

The 'meaning' of cardiovascular fitness

Cardiovascular fitness in children has attracted the attention not only of paediatric exercise scientists but the popular media as well. Level of cardiovascular fitness has been linked to salutary health outcomes, and research into links between the development of endurance performance and aerobic fitness has been a central issue in characterizing unique aspects of child endurance athletes. The

Table 11.1 Representative studies estimating values of stroke index and cardiac index at maximal exercise during progressive upright cycling in children

Study	N	Age	Sex	Method	Cardiac index ($L \cdot min^{-1} \cdot m^{-2}$)	Stroke index ($mL \cdot m^{-2}$)
Rowland *et al.*[80]	9	15	F	Dopp	7.80	41
Rowland *et al.*[23]	10	15	M	Dopp	9.02	46
Rowland *et al.*[86]	8	12	M	Dopp	11.14	62
Rowland *et al.*[35]	10	11	M	Dopp	11.79	62
Rowland *et al.*[49]	14	10	M	Dopp	11.42	58
Rowland *et al.*[83]	24	12	F	Dopp	10.90	55
Nottin *et al.*[17]	17	10–13	M	Dopp	11.3	59
McNarry *et al.*[82]	10	12	F	Bioimp	11.1	57
	16	14	F	Bioimp	11.1	58
	10	17	F	Bioimp	10.1	58
Welsman *et al.*[106]	11	11	F	Bioimp	9.6	49
	9	11	M	Bioimp	9.5	49
Yamaji & Miyashita[85]	8	10–12	M	CO_2	10.4	
Cyran *et al.*[107]	17	8–15	M, F	Acetyl	10.8	62

Acetyl = acetylene rebreathing; CO_2 = carbon dioxide rebreathing; Dopp = Doppler ultrasound; Bioimp = thoracic bioimpedance.

efficacy of cardiac rehabilitation programmes for youth with heart disease has often hinged on responses of cardiovascular fitness to such interventions.

It should be recognized that cardiovascular fitness has been interpreted by a number of differing definitions. It is important that one be aware of such distinctions when assessing values in respect to health or performance outcomes.

Cardiovascular fitness has often been interpreted by finish times on field endurance tests (e.g. 1 mile run, 20 m shuttle run), given the recognized link between such forms of performance and certain physiologic measures (e.g. $\dot{V}O_2$ max, $\dot{Q}$ max). However, it is critical to recognize that cardiovascular functional capacity contributes only a portion to such performance and that other factors, particularly body fat content, are equally important. Fat is an inert load that the body must carry around during weight-bearing tasks, and body fat content is inversely correlated with performance on such exercise tests. For example, in a study of thirty six 12-year-old boys with a wide range of physical fitness, 1 mile run time velocity was closely linked to $\dot{V}O_2$ max per kg body mass measured in a laboratory ($r = 0.77$), yet run performance was also associated with maximal cardiac index ($r = 0.41$) and body fat content ($r = -0.56$).[93] In that study, body fat and $\dot{V}O_2$ max per kg (adjusted for body fat) accounted for 31% and 28% of the variance in run velocity, respectively.

In the exercise testing laboratory, the same problem arises. Physiologic cardiovascular fitness is typically expressed as $\dot{V}O_2$ max per kg body mass. But the denominator, again, includes body fat, which artefactually deflates the value, irrespective of the functional capacity of the cardiovascular system. This is particularly a problem when studies attempt to relate $\dot{V}O_2$ max per kg to health outcome measures, since body fat itself is a strong mediator of such risks factors (hypertension, dyslipidaemia, glucose intolerance).

The most precise definition of true cardiovascular fitness is the ability of the heart to generate $\dot{Q}$ (absolute $\dot{Q}$ max), and, in an ideal world, such fitness would be expressed relative to the volume of body tissue which generates metabolic demand during exercise. As noted, given the impossibility to define such an ideal size-normalizing factor, lean body mass expressed by an empirically-derived allometric exponent for the specific study group is a reasonable surrogate.

The potential confusion arising from misuse of the term cardiovascular fitness, particularly as it relates to differences in body composition, can be illustrated by the changes that would be expected to occur if a lean youngster were to become progressively obese. With increasing body fat content, cardiovascular fitness expressed as his performance on a 1 mile run time will progressively decline, irrespective of his cardiac functional capacity. At the same time, in the exercise testing laboratory, his cardiovascular fitness expressed as $\dot{V}O_2$ max per kg body mass will also fall. Because of the concomitant increase in volume of muscle tissue (which occurs with obesity), his true cardiovascular fitness (absolute $\dot{Q}$ max and SV max) will increase as he becomes more obese, yet these variables expressed relative to lean body mass should be expected to remain stable. Meanwhile, $\dot{Q}$ max and SV max relative to total body mass will decline. Thus, in this scenario, this child's cardiovascular fitness will increase, decrease, or remain the same as he becomes increasingly obese, depending on its definition and means of size-normalization.

We must then ask what it means, physiologically, when one child is said to be 'in good physical shape' and another is not. Insights into this question are gained by a consideration of the Fick equation: $\dot{V}O_2$ max = HR max × SV max × a-vO_2 diff max. Heart rate and peripheral oxygen extraction at peak exercise in children are independent of $\dot{V}O_2$ max.[94,95] That is, a poorly fit and a highly fit child will (if satisfactorily motivated) exhibit similar values of HR and a-vO_2 diff during exercise testing. Consequently, the physiological factor which serves to differentiate individuals with different levels of aerobic fitness is the ability to generate maximal SV.

Research efforts in adult subjects to explain this observation have indicated that end-diastolic volume of the ventricle is responsible for this inter-individual variability in maximal SV.[96] The determinants of ventricle dimensions, which include plasma volume and resting HR, may be dictated by genetic as well as environmental (i.e. physical activity) factors. Studies in children tend to support this conclusion, although findings have been less clear. For instance, Rowland *et al.*[94] described mean resting left ventricular diameters (measured supine) of 3.60 ± 0.17 and 3.46 ± 0.21 cm · $BSA^{0.61}$ in high and low fit boys, respectively, but the difference was not statistically significant. Such studies are hampered by the necessity of comparing $\dot{V}O_2$ max during upright cycling with left ventricular diastolic dimension determined at rest in the supine position instead of—as would be more appropriate—upright at peak exercise.

Limited information suggests that myocardial functional responses to exercise are independent of aerobic fitness. In studies of early adolescent males and females echocardiographic markers of both systolic and diastolic function have been reported to respond equally to progressive exercise in those with high and average values of $\dot{V}O_2$ max.[23,80] That is, the contractile health of the myocardium appears to be equal in children with high and low levels of aerobic fitness.

Myocardial damage

The ventricular myocardium is challenged during exercise to augment contractile force at an increased frequency. The work involved in sustained periods of exercise might be expected, as observed in skeletal muscle, to eventuate in myocardial fatigue. In fact, in adult studies, biochemical and echocardiographic evidence of transient myocardial damage have been observed following sustained exercise such as triathlons and marathon races.[97,98] Such myocardial insult is transient, with findings resolving usually within 24 h post-event, but its implications remain of concern.

Reductions in echocardiographic markers of systolic function (ejection fraction, shortening fraction) as well diastolic properties (mitral flow velocities) have been described post-exercise in adult studies. Investigations of children and adolescents have provided conflicting findings. Hauser *et al.*[99] performed echocardiography in 27 children (mean age 12.6 years) before and after an age-adapted triathlon circuit. No changes in ventricular ejection fraction were observed following the race, but the subjects demonstrated a reduction in longitudinal and circumferential strain. Nie *et al.*[100] found a reduction of ejection fraction and early-to-late atrial peak filling velocities (E/A ratio) in 14-year-old adolescent athletes following two 45 min submaximal runs.

On the other hand, Rowland *et al.*[101] observed no adverse echocardiographic changes from a competitive 4 km road race in male child distance runners (ages 9–14 years). Unnithan *et al.*[102] found no significant echocardiographic effects on systolic or diastolic function in 15-year-old boys following a simulated 5 km cross-country race.

In the same types of ultra-endurance exercise, studies in adults indicate that approximately half of athletes will demonstrate transient, mild increases in serum levels of cardiac troponins, which are indicators of myocardial damage.[103] However, while elevated, these levels do not approach those observed with overt clinical myocardial ischemia (i.e. in patients with myocardial infarction). The mechanisms and clinical significance of this postexercise rise in troponins remain in doubt.

Two studies have examined troponin levels following exercise in adolescent athletes. Tian *et al.*[104] studied 10 trained males (mean age 16.2 ± 0.6 years) who performed a 21 km run and graded treadmill exercise on two separate days. Four hours post-exercise showed mild elevations of troponin levels in 60% of subjects, which returned toward pre-exercise levels by 24 h afterwards. Fu *et al.*[105] found similar results in 14-year-old runners who performed two 45 min and two 90 min constant treadmill runs. Elevations in serum troponin levels were most closely related to exercise intensity than duration. This limited information suggests that serum troponin response to endurance exercise is similar in young and older athletes.

Conclusions

The current body of research literature indicates that, when adjusted appropriately for body size, the dynamics of the cardiovascular response to an acute bout of endurance exercise are neither qualitatively nor quantitatively different in children and young adults. As in adults, inter-individual variations in physiological aerobic fitness among children are mediated by the ability to generate maximal SV, which, in turn, is governed by dimensional differences in the cardiovascular system. How such cardiovascular fitness is defined is contingent on its context and size-normalization. While certain information suggests that myocardial fatigue and perhaps transient damage can occur following sustained periods of high $\dot{Q}$ in adults, little information is available regarding possible myocardial fatigue (and its implications) in young athletes.

Summary

The current body of research literature regarding the cardiovascular responses to an acute bout of endurance exercise in youth is consistent with the following:

- The magnitude of increased circulatory flow in response to the metabolic and thermoregulatory demands of an acute bout of endurance exercise is regulated primarily by changes in peripheral vascular resistance. This response involves the finely tuned interplay between changes in autonomic, sinus node, and myocardial function.
- When adjusted for body size, the dynamics of this cardiovascular response are neither qualitatively nor quantitatively different in children and young adults.
- Defining cardiovascular fitness is contingent on its context and means of size-normalization.
- Variations in physiological aerobic fitness among children are mediated by the ability to generate maximal stroke volume, which, in turn, is governed by dimensional differences in the cardiovascular system.
- Little information is available regarding possible myocardial fatigue (and its implications) in young athletes.

References

1. Karpovich V. Textbook fallacies regarding the development of the child's heart. (Originally published in *Research Quarterly*. 1937; 8). Reprinted in *Pediatr Exerc Sci*. 1991; 3: 278–282.
2. Bar-Or O. *Pediatric sports medicine for the practitioner*. New York: Springer Verlag, 1983.
3. Falk B. Dotan R. Temperature regulation. In: Armstrong N, van Mechelen W (eds.) *Paediatric exercise science and medicine*, 2nd ed. Oxford: Oxford University Press, 2008. p. 309–324.
4. Rowland TW. Effect of obesity on cardiac function in children and adolescents: a review. *Clin J Sports Sci Med*. 2007; 6: 319–326.
5. Rowland TW. Thermoregulation during exercise in the heat in children: old concepts revisited. *J Appl Physiol*. 2008; 105: 718–724.
6. Rowland TW. Cardiovascular function. In: Armstrong N, van Mechelen W (eds.) *Paediatric exercise science and medicine*, 2nd ed. Oxford: Oxford University Press, 2008. p. 255–267.
7. Warburton DER, Nettlefold L, McGuire KA, Bredin SSD. Cardiovascular function. In: Armstrong N, van Mechelen W (eds.) *Paediatric exercise science and medicine*, 2nd ed. Oxford: Oxford University Press; 2008. p. 77–95.
8. Bouchard C, Malina RM, Hollman W, Leblanc C. Submaximal working capacity, heart size, and body size in boys 8–18 years. *Eur J Appl Physiol*. 1977; 36: 115–126.
9. Burch GE, Giles TD. A critique of the cardiac index. *Am Heart J*. 1971; 32: 425–426.
10. Rowland T, Goff D, Martel L, Ferrone L, Kline G. Normalization of maximal cardiovascular variables for body size in premenarcheal girls. *Pediatr Cardiol*. 2000; 21: 429–432.
11. Rowland T, Goff D, Martel L, Ferrone L. Influence of cardiac functional capacity on gender differences in maximal oxygen uptake in children. *Chest*. 2000; 117: 629–635.
12. Armstrong N, Welsman JR. Cardiovascular response to submaximal treadmill running in 11- to 13-year olds. *Acta Paediatr*. 2002; 91: 125–131.
13. Turley KR, Wilmore JH. Ratio scaling of submaximal data: is it appropriate [abstract]. *Med Sci Sports Exerc*. 1998; 30 (Suppl): S242.
14. Vinet A, Mandigout S, Nottin S, *et al*. Influence of body composition, hemoglobin concentration, cardiac size, and function on gender differences in maximal oxygen uptake in prepubertal children. *Chest*. 2003; 124: 1494–1499.
15. Batterham AM, George KP, Whyte G, Sharma S, McKenna W. Scaling cardiac structural data by body dimensions: a review of theory, practice and problems. *Int J Sports Med*. 1999; 20: 495–502.
16. Rowland T. Echocardiography and circulatory responses to progressive exercise. *Sports Med*. 2008; 38: 541–551.
17. Nottin S, Agnes V, Stecken N, *et al*. Central and peripheral cardiovascular adaptations during maximal cycle exercise in boys and men. *Med Sci Sports Exerc*. 2002; 34: 456–463.
18. Rowland T, Unnithan V. Stroke dynamics during progressive exercise in healthy adolescents. *Pediatr Exerc Sci*. 2013: 25: 173–185.
19. Tschakovsky ME, Shoemaker JK, Hughson RL. Vasodilation and muscle pump contribution to immediate exercise hyperemia. *Am J Physiol*. 1996; 271: H1697–H1701.
20. Stegall HF. Muscle pumping in the dependent leg. *Circ Res*. 1966; 19: 180–190.
21. Pollack A, Wood EH. Venous pressure in the saphenous vein at the ankle in man during exercise and changes in posture. *J Appl Physiol*. 1949; 1: 649–662.
22. Stick C, Jaeger H, Witzleb E. Measurements of volume changes and venous pressures in the human lower leg during walking and running. *J Appl Physiol*. 1992; 72: 2063–2068.
23. Rowland T, Garrard M, Marwood S, Guerra M, Roche D, Unnithan V. Myocardial performance during progressive exercise in athletic adolescent males. *Med Sci Sports Exerc*. 2009; 41: 1721–1728.
24. Rowland T, Garrison A, Deulio A. Circulatory responses to progressive exercise: insights from positional differences. *Int J Sports Med*. 2003; 24: 512–517.
25. Bevegard S, Holmgren A, Johnsson B. The effect of body position on the circulation at rest and during exercise, with special reference to the influence on the stroke volume. *Acta Physiol Scand*. 1960; 49: 279–298.
26. Leyk D, Essfield D, Hoffman U, Wunderlich HE, Baum K, Stegeman J. Postural effect on cardiac output, oxygen uptake, and lactate during cycle exercise of varying intensity. *Eur J Appl Physiol*. 1994; 68: 30–35.
27. Stenberg J, Astrand P-O, Ekblom B, Royce B, Saltin B. Hemodynamic response to work in different muscle groups, sitting and supine. *J Appl Physiol*. 1967: 22: 61–70.
28. Loeppky JA, Greene ER, Hoekenga DE. Beat-by-beat stroke volume assessment by pulsed Doppler in upright and supine exercise. *J Appl Physiol*. 1981; 50: 1173–1182.
29. Thadani U, Parker JO. Hemodynamics at rest and during supine and sitting bicycle exercise in normal subjects. *Am J Cardiol*. 1978; 41: 52–59.
30. Poliner LR, Dehmer GJ, Lewis SE, Parkey RW, Blomqvist CG, Willerson JT. Left ventricular performance in normal subjects: a comparison of the responses to exercise in the upright and supine positions. *Circulation*. 1980; 62: 528–534.
31. Rowland T, Bougault V, Walter G, Nottin S, Vinet A, Obert P. Cardiac responses to swim bench exercise in age-group swimmers and non-athletic children. *J Sci Med Sport*. 2009; 12: 266–272.
32. Atkov OY, Bednenko VS, Formina GA. Ultrasound techniques in space medicine. *Aviat Environ Med*. 1987; 58(Suppl): A69–A73.
33. Magel JR, McArdle WD, Toner M, Delio DJ. Metabolic and cardiovascular adjustment to arm training. *J Appl Physiol*. 1978; 45: 75–79.
34. Christie JL, Sheldahl LMN, Tristahi FE. Cardiovascular regulation during head-out water immersion. *J Appl Physiol*. 1990; 69: 657–664.
35. Rowland T, Blume JW. Cardiac dynamics during upright cycle exercise in boys. *Am J Hum Biol*. 2000; 12: 749–757.
36. Kimball TR, Mays WA, Khoury PR, Mallie R, Claytor RP. Echocardiographic determination of left ventricular preload, afterload, and contractility during and after exercise. *J. Pediatr*. 1993; 122: S89–S94.
37. Pokan R, Von Duvillard SP, Hofman P, Smekal G, Fruhwald FM, Gasser R. Change in left atrial and ventricular dimensions during and immediately after exercise. *Med Sci Sports Exerc*. 2000; 32: 1713–1718.
38. Higginbotham M, Morris KG, Williams RS, McHale PA, Coleman RE, Cobb FR. Regulation of stroke volume during submaximal and maximal upright exercise in normal man. *Circ Res*. 1986; 58: 281–291.
39. Parrish MD, Boucek RJ, Burger J, Artman MF, Partain C, Graham TP. Exercise radionuclide ventriculography in children: normal values for exercise variables and right and left ventricular function. *Br Heart J*. 1985; 54: 509–516.
40. Talreja DR, Nishimura RA, Oh JK. Estimation of left ventricular filling pressure with exercise by Doppler echocardiography in patients with normal systolic function: a simultaneous echocardiographic-cardiac catherization study. *J Am Soc Echocardiogr*. 2007: 20: 477–479.
41. Rowland T, Unnithan V. Myocardial inotropic response to progressive exercise in healthy subjects: a review. *Curr Sports Med Rep*. 2013; 12: 93–100.
42. Borer JS, Kent KM, Bacharach SL. Sensitivity, specificity, and predictive accuracy of radionuclide cineangiography during exercise in patients with coronary artery disease. *Circulation*. 1979; 60: 572–579.
43. Rerych SK, Scholz PM, Sabiston DC, Jones RH. Effects of exercise training on left ventricular function in normal subjects: a longitudinal study by radionuclide angiography. *Am J Cardiol*. 1980; 45: 244–251.
44. DeSouza M, Schaffer MS, Gilday DL, Rose V. Exercise radionuclide angiography in hyperlipidemic children with apparently normal hearts. *Nucl Med Comm*. 1984; 5: 13–17.
45. Braunwald E, Sarnoff JJ, Stainsby WN. Determinants of duration and mean rate of ventricular ejection. *Circ Res*. 1958; 6: 319–325.
46. Unnithan V, Rowland T, Lindley MR, Roche D, Garrard M, Barker P. Cardiac strain during upright cycle ergometry in adolescent males. *Echocardiography*. 2015; 32: 638–643.

47. Duocende G, Schuster I, Rupp T. Kinetics of left ventricular strain and torsion during incremental exercise in healthy subjects. *Circ Cardiovasc Imaging*. 2010; 3: 133–148.
48. Rowland T, Mannie E, Gawle I. Dynamics of left ventricular filling during exercise. *Chest*. 2001; 120: 145–150.
49. Rowland T, Heffernan K, Jae SY, Fernhall B. Tissue Doppler assessment of ventricular function during cycling in 7–12-year-old boys. *Med Sci Sports Exerc*. 2006; 38: 1216–1222.
50. Chang RC, Qi N, Rose-Gottron C. Comparison of upright and semi-supine postures for exercise echocardiography in healthy children. *Am J Cardiol*. 2005; 95: 918–921.
51. Linde-Edelstam CM, Juhlin-D, Annfelt A, Nordlander R. The hemodynamic importance of atrial systole: a function of the kinetic energy of blood flow? *PACE*. 1992; 15: 1740–1749.
52. Bevegard BS, Shepherd JT. Regulation of the circulation during exercise in man. *Physiol Rev*. 1967; 47: 178–213.
53. Guyton AC. Regulation of cardiac output. *N Engl J Med*. 1967; 277: 805–812.
54. Braunwald E, Ross J. Control of cardiac performance. In: Berne RM (ed.) *Handbook of physiology: the cardiovascular system*. Bethesda, MD: American Physiological Society, 1979. p. 553–579.
55. Binak K, Regan TJ, Christensen RC. Arteriovenous fistula: hemodynamic effects of occlusion and exercise. *Am Heart J*. 1960; 60: 495–502.
56. Hakumaki MOK. Seventy years of the Bainbridge reflex. *Acta Physiol Scand*. 1987: 130: 177–185.
57. Boettcher DH, Zimpfer M, Vatner SF. Phylogenesis of the Bainbridge reflex. *Am J Physiol*. 1982: 242: R244–R246.
58. Mitchell JH. Neural circulatory control during exercise: early insights. *Exp Physiol*. 2013; 98: 867–878.
59. Rowland T, Potts J, Potts T. Cardiac responses to progressive exercise in normal children: a synthesis. *Med Sci Sports Exerc*. 2000; 32: 253–259.
60. Rowland T, Potts J, Potts T, Son-Hing J, Harbison G, Sandor G. Cardiovascular responses to exercise in children and adolescents with myocardial dysfunction. *Am Heart J*. 1999; 137: 126–133.
61. Marcus B, Gillette PC, Garson A. Intrinsic heart rate in children and young adults: an index of sinus node function isolated from autonomic control. *Am Heart J*. 1990; 112: 911–916.
62. Sutcliffe WD, Holt E. The age curve of pulse rate under basal conditions. *Arch Int Med*. 1925; 35: 224–241.
63. Knoebel LK. Energy metabolism. In, Selkurt EE (ed.) *Physiology*. Boston: Little, Brown; 1963. p. 564–579.
64. Rowland TW, Cunningham LN. Heart rate deceleration during treadmill exercise in children [abstract]. *Pediatr Exerc Sci*. 1993; 5: 463.
65. Cassels DE, Morse M. *Cardiopulmonary data for children and young adults*. Springfield, IL: Charles C. Thomas; 1962.
66. Amorim PR, Byrne NM, Hills AP. Within- and between-day repeatability and variability in children's physiological responses during submaximal treadmill exercise. *Res Q Exerc Sport*. 2009; 80: 575–582.
67. Cumming GR, Everatt D, Hastman L. Bruce treadmill test in children: normal values in a clinic population. *Am J Cardiol*. 1978; 41: 69–75.
68. Cumming GR, Langford S. Comparison of nine exercise tests used in pediatric cardiology. In: Binkhorst RA, Kemper HCG, Saris WHM (eds.) *Children and exercise XI*. Champaign, IL: Human Kinetics; 1985. p. 58–68.
69. Riopel DA, Taylor AB, Hohn HR. Blood pressure, heat rate, pressure-rate product, and electrocardiographic changes in healthy children during treadmill exercise. *Am J Cardiol*. 1979; 44: 697–704.
70. Bailey DA, Ross WD, Mirwald RL, Weese C. Size dissociation of maximal aerobic power during growth in boys. *Med Sport*. 1978; 11: 140–151.
71. Robinson S. Experimental studies of physical fitness in relation to age. *Arbeitsphysiol*. 1938; 10: 251–323.
72. Sheehan JM, Rowland TW, Burke EJ. A comparison of four treadmill protocols for determination of maximal oxygen uptake in 10- to 12-year old boys. *Int J Sports Med*. 1987; 8: 31–34.
73. Washington RL, van Gundy JC, Cohen C, Sondhemier HM, Wolfe RR. Normal aerobic and anaerobic exercise data for North American school-age children. *J Pediatr*. 1988; 112: 223–233.
74. Krovetz LJ, McLoughlin TG, Mitchell MB, Schiebler GL. Hemodynamic findings in normal children. *Pediatr Res*. 1967; 1: 122–130.
75. Sproul A, Simpson E. Stroke volume and related hemodynamic data in normal children. *Pediatrics*. 1964; 33: 912–918.
76. Blimkie CJR, Cunningham DA, Nichol PM. Gas transport capacity and echocardiographically determined cardiac size in children. *J Appl Physiol*. 1980; 49: 994–999.
77. Colan SD, Parness IA, Spevak PJ, Sanders SP. Developmental modulation of myocardial mechanics: age and growth-related alterations in afterload and contractility. *J Am Coll Cardiol*. 1992; 19: 619–629.
78. Eidem BW, McMahon CJ, Cohen RR. Impact of cardiac growth on Doppler imaging velocities: a study of healthy children. *J Am Soc Echocardiogr*. 2004; 17: 22–31.
79. Obert P, Mandigout S, Vinet A. Relationships between left ventricular morphology, diastolic function, and oxygen carrying caacity and maximal oxygen uptake in children. *Int J Sports Med*. 2005; 26: 122–127.
80. Rowland T, Unnithan V, Roche D, Garrard M, Holloway K, Marwood S. Myocardial function and aerobic fitness in adolescent females. *Eur J Appl Physiol*. 2011; 111: 1991–1997.
81. McNarry MA, Mackintosh KA, Stoedefalke K. Longitudinal investigation of training status and cardiopulmonary responses in pre- and early-pubertal children. *Eur J Appl Physiol*. 2014; 114: 1573–1580.
82. McNarry MA, Welsman JR, Jones AM. Influence of training and maturity status on the cardiopulmonary responses to ramp incremental cycle and upper body exercise in girls. *J Appl Physiol*. 2011; 110: 375–381.
83. Rowland T, Miller K, Vanderburgh P, Goff D, Martel L, Ferrone L. Cardiovascular fitness in premenarcheal girls and young women. *Int J Sports Med*. 1999; 20: 117–121.
84. Rowland T, Popowski B, Ferrone L. Cardiac responses to maximal upright cycle exercise in healthy boys and men. *Med Sci Sports Exerc*. 1997; 29: 1146–1151.
85. Yamaji K, Miyashita M. Oxygen transport system during exhaustive exercise in Japanese boys. *Eur J Appl Physiol*. 1977; 36: 93–99.
86. Rowland T, Hagenbuch S, Pober D, Garrison A. Exercise tolerance and thermoregulatory responses during cycling in boys and men. *Med Sci Sports Exerc*. 2008; 40: 282–287.
87. Miyamura M, Honda Y. Maximum cardiac output related to sex and age. *Jpn J Physiol*. 1973; 23: 645–656.
88. Rowland TW. *Developmental exercise physiology*. Champaign, IL: Human Kinetics; 1996.
89. Malina RM, Roche AF. *Manual of physical status and performance in childhood. Volume 2. Physical performance*. New York: Plenum Press; 1983.
90. Alpert BS, Flood NL, Strong WB, *et al*. Response to ergometer exercise in a healthy biracial population of children. *J. Pediatr*. 1982; 101: 538–545.
91. James FW, Kaplan S, Glueck CJ, Tsay JY, Knight MJS, Sarwar CJ. Responses of normal children and young adults to controlled bicycle exercise. *Circulation*. 1980; 61: 902–912.
92. Dlin R. Blood pressure response to dynamic exercise in healthy and hypertensive youth. *Pediatrician*. 1986; 13: 34–43.
93. Rowland T, Kline G, Goff D, Martel L, Ferrone L. One-mile run performance and cardiovascular fitness in children. *Arch Pediatr Adolesc Med*. 1999; 153: 845–849.
94. Rowland T, Kline G, Goff D, Martel L, Ferrone L. Physiological determinants of maximal aerobic power in healthy 12-year-old boys. *Pediatr Exerc Sci*. 1999; 11: 317–326.
95. Thoren CAR, Asano K. Functional capacity and cardiac function in 10-year-old boys and girls with high and low running performance. In: Ilmarinen J, Valimaki I (eds.) *Children and Sport*. Bedin, Italy: Springer Verlag; 1984. p. 182–188.

96. Osborne G, Wolfe LA, Burggraf GW, Norman R. Relationships between cardiac dimensions, anthropometric characteristics, and maximal aerobic power ($\dot{V}O_2$ max) in young men. *Int J Sports Med.* 1992; 13: 219–224.
97. Shave R, George K, Whyte G, Hart E, Middleton N. Post-exercise changes in left ventricular function: the evidence so far. *Med Sci Sports Exerc.* 2008; 40: 1393–1399.
98. Oxborough D, Birch K, Shave R, George K. 'Exercise-induced fatigue'—a review of the echocardiographic literature. *Echocardiography.* 2010; 27: 1130–1140.
99. Hauser M, Petzuch K, Kuhn A. The Munich triathlon heart study: ventricular function, myocardial velocities, and two-dimensional strain in healthy children before and after endurance stress. *Pediatr Cardiol.* 2013; 34: 576–582.
100. Nie J, George KP, Tong TK. Effects of repeated endurance runs on cardiac biomarkers and function in adolescents. *Med Sci Sports Exerc.* 2011; 43: 2081–2088.
101. Rowland T, Goff D, DeLuca P, Popowski B. Cardiac effects of a competitive road race in trained child runners. *Pediatrics.* 1997; 100: E2.
102. Unnithan VB, Rowland T, George K, Lindley MR, Roche DM. Regional and global left ventricular function following a simulated 5 km race in sports-trained adolescents. *Pediatr Cardiol.* 2015; 36: 322–328.
103. Shave R, George KP, Atkinson G, *et al.* Exercise-induced cardiac troponin T release: a meta-analysis. *Med Sci Sports Exerc.* 2007; 39: 2099–2106.
104. Tian Y, Nie J, Tong TK, *et al.* Changes in serum cardiac troponins following a 21 km run in junior male runners. *J Sports Med Phys Fitness.* 2006; 46: 481–488.
105. Fu F, Nie J, Tong TK. Serum cardiac troponin in adolescent runners: effects of exercise intensity and duration. *Int J Sports Med.* 2009; 30: 168–172.
106. Welsman J, Bywater K, Farr C, Welford D, Armstrong N. Reliability of peak VO_2 and maximal cardiac output using thoracic bioimpedance in children. *Eur J Appl Physiol.* 2005; 94: 228–234.
107. Cyran SE, James FW, Daniels S, Mays W, Shukala R, Kaplan S. Comparison of the cardiac output and stroke volume response to upright exercise in children with valvular and subvalvular aortic stenosis. *J Am Coll Cardiol.* 1988; 11: 651–658.

CHAPTER 12

Aerobic fitness

Neil Armstrong and Alison M McManus

Introduction

Aerobic fitness may be defined as the ability to deliver oxygen to the muscles and to utilize it to generate energy to support muscle activity during exercise. Aerobic fitness therefore depends upon the pulmonary, cardiovascular, and haematological components of oxygen delivery and the oxidative mechanisms of exercising muscles.

Maximal oxygen uptake ($\dot{V}O_2$ max), the highest rate at which oxygen can be consumed by the muscles during an exercise test to exhaustion, is widely recognized as the best single measure of aerobic fitness. However, only a minority of children satisfy the classical $\dot{V}O_2$ plateau criterion for achieving $\dot{V}O_2$ max in a single exercise test, and it has become conventional to use the term peak $\dot{V}O_2$ when discussing young people's aerobic fitness. The distinction between $\dot{V}O_2$ max and peak $\dot{V}O_2$ will be clarified in the Methodological issues section and thereafter the term peak $\dot{V}O_2$ will be adopted when referring to children or adolescents. In the meantime, the conventional term $\dot{V}O_2$ max will be used unless the research cited specifically refers to peak $\dot{V}O_2$.

Maximal $\dot{V}O_2$ limits the capacity to perform aerobic exercise but it does not define all aspects of aerobic fitness. The ability to sustain submaximal exercise is aptly represented by blood lactate accumulation, which also provides a sensitive means of evaluating improvements in muscle oxidative capacity with exercise training, often in the absence of changes in $\dot{V}O_2$ max. However, in everyday life young people's spontaneous play and participation in sport are more concerned with short duration, intermittent exercise, and rapid changes in exercise intensity. Under these conditions $\dot{V}O_2$ max and blood lactate accumulation might be considered variables of investigative convenience rather than factors underpinning exercise behaviour, and it is the kinetics of pulmonary $\dot{V}O_2$ (p$\dot{V}O_2$) which best describe this aspect of aerobic fitness.

To provide an appropriate framework for subsequent discussion of aerobic fitness initially the concepts of $\dot{V}O_2$ max, blood lactate accumulation, and p$\dot{V}O_2$ kinetics will be introduced. Thereafter the focus will be on aerobic fitness in relation to chronological age, body size, biological maturity, and sexual dimorphism. It is recognized that aerobic fitness has a genetic component, with the heritability of $\dot{V}O_2$ max estimated to be ~50%,[1] but genetics are outside the scope of this chapter and the topic is addressed in Chapter 20 and Chapter 31.

The following terms are used throughout the chapter: 'prepubertal children' when prepuberty is confirmed in the research cited; 'children' to represent those 12 years and younger but without proof of pubertal status; 'adolescents' to refer to 13- to 18-year-olds; and 'youth' or 'young people' to describe both children and adolescents.

Measures of aerobic fitness

Maximal oxygen uptake

The seminal work of Hill and Lupton[2] in the 1920s gave rise to the concept of $\dot{V}O_2$ max in humans. They were, of course, constrained by the available technology and for context their experimental protocol is worth describing in their own words,

> In determining the rate of oxygen intake during running at various speeds, the subject ran with a constant measured velocity around a grass track carrying a Douglas bag, and breathing through mouthpiece and valves, the tap being turned to allow the expired air to escape into the atmosphere. After continuing this for a time known to be sufficient for the oxygen intake to attain a steady value, the tap was turned for a measured interval (usually about 1 min) to allow a sample of expired air to be collected in the bag, the running being continued at the same speed. After the interval, the running ceased, and the measurement and analysis of the expired air were carried out in the usual manner. Experiments were made at a variety of speeds and on several subjects (which amply confirm one another).[2(p156)]

Their observations revealed a near-linear relationship and eventual plateau between p$\dot{V}O_2$ and running speed during discontinuous, incremental exercise (but see the section on Methodological issues). Hill and Lupton's findings evolved into the development of a range of laboratory protocols designed to investigate the p$\dot{V}O_2$ response to incremental exercise, based on the concept of $\dot{V}O_2$ max being achieved when a levelling-off or plateau in p$\dot{V}O_2$ emerged (see Figure 12.1). By the late 1930s boys were participating in laboratory determinations of $\dot{V}O_2$ max.

The first laboratory-based investigations of boys' $\dot{V}O_2$ max were carried out by Robinson[3] and Morse *et al.*[4] in the US, on either side of the Second World War. They determined 6- to 18-year-old boys' $\dot{V}O_2$ max using a treadmill protocol involving a 15 min walk at 3.5 miles$\cdot$h^{-1} up an 8.6% gradient, followed by a 10 min rest, and a run to exhaustion at a speed of 6 or 7 miles$\cdot$h^{-1} up an 8.6% gradient. Åstrand's[5] doctoral thesis, published in Scandinavia in 1952, was the first study to report the $\dot{V}O_2$ max of both girls and boys, aged 4–18 years. The three studies reported $\dot{V}O_2$ max in ratio with body mass (mL$\cdot$kg$^{-1}\cdot$min^{-1}) but Åstrand insightfully expressed reservations about whether this approach was appropriate with children (see the section on Peak oxygen uptake and body size).

Åstrand[5] criticized the Robinson[3] and Morse *et al.*[4] methodology as 'certainly practical from the investigator's point of view but hardly so from that of the subject, especially if he is 6–10 years old'.[5] He commented that on the basis of the exercise protocol and the post-exercise blood lactate accumulation, 'the work in several cases must have been submaximal',[5(p110)], a point conceded

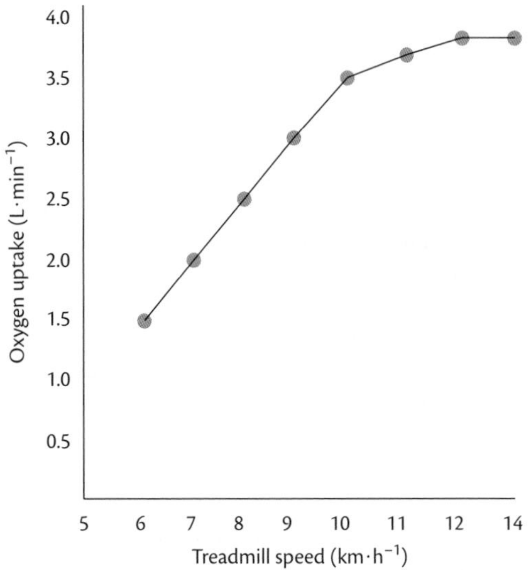

Figure 12.1 Pulmonary oxygen uptake and treadmill speed.
The classical pulmonary oxygen uptake response to incremental treadmill exercise illustrating a near-linear relationship and levelling-off (plateauing) as maximal oxygen uptake approaches.

by Morse *et al.*,[4] who observed that, 'undoubtedly all of the boys did not push themselves to the same state of exhaustion, and some had not reached the limit of their capacity in 5 min of running at 7 m.p.h.'[4(p699)] (see Methodological issues section). In his studies Åstrand used a discontinuous, incremental protocol in which the first session was carried out on a horizontal treadmill running at 7–8 $km \cdot h^{-1}$. He described subsequent sessions as follows: 'after a couple of days the experiment was repeated with a higher speed of 1–2 $km \cdot h^{-1}$ etc. until the intensity was reached which exhausted the subject in 4–6 min. The determinations for each subject were spread over a period of 3 weeks or more'.[5(p19)] The vast majority of subsequent investigations of young people's $\dot{V}O_2$ max followed Åstrand's lead and adopted either a discontinuous or (more recently) a continuous, incremental exercise protocol to voluntary exhaustion.

Oxygen uptake response to incremental exercise

Incremental exercise to $\dot{V}O_2$ max requires the cardiopulmonary oxygen delivery and muscle oxygen utilization mechanisms to accommodate the rising metabolic demands. Interested readers are invited to peruse Chapter 10 for a comprehensive review of pulmonary function during exercise and Chapter 11 for an insightful analysis of cardiovascular function during exercise, but the main points can be summarized as follows.

Pulmonary ventilation ($\dot{V}_E$) increases in accord with exercise intensity, but it is primarily driven by carbon dioxide (CO_2) production and the need to minimize metabolic acidosis. Pulmonary ventilation is therefore only matched with exercise intensity and $p\dot{V}O_2$ until the ventilatory threshold (T_{VENT}) is reached. The T_{VENT} is defined as the point during incremental exercise at which $\dot{V}_E$ begins to increase out of proportion to the increase in $p\dot{V}O_2$. Beyond the T_{VENT} the bicarbonate buffering of hydrogen ions accompanying lactic acid dissociation to lactate causes CO_2 and therefore $\dot{V}_E$ to rise faster than $p\dot{V}O_2$. As $\dot{V}O_2$ max is approached, a further reduction in blood pH causes $\dot{V}_E$ to compensate (ventilatory compensation point) by increasing at a disproportionately higher rate than carbon dioxide expired ($\dot{V}CO_2$).

The general pattern of the $\dot{V}_E$ response to progressive exercise is similar in children and adults, but there are clear age and maturity differences in the quantitative and relative responses of $\dot{V}_E$. Data on sex differences in the pulmonary response to exercise are equivocal.

Children have a higher ratio of respiratory frequency (f_R) to tidal volume than adults and during maximal exercise a $f_R > 60$ $breaths \cdot min^{-1}$ is not uncommon compared with ~40 $breaths \cdot min^{-1}$ in adults. Children display a higher $\dot{V}_E$ and therefore a less efficient response to a given metabolic demand than adults, which suggests that there is some maturation of the ventilation control mechanisms during childhood and adolescence. However, gas exchange in the alveoli is determined by alveolar, rather than pulmonary, ventilation and young people's alveolar ventilation is more than adequate to optimize gas exchange. Although at $\dot{V}O_2$ max the ventilatory equivalent ($\dot{V}_E/\dot{V}O_2$) is generally lower in adults than in children, $\dot{V}_E$ at $\dot{V}O_2$ max seldom exceeds ~70% of maximal voluntary ventilation. With healthy children and adolescents, $\dot{V}_E$ does not normally limit $\dot{V}O_2$ max and will therefore not be considered further in this chapter.[6,7]

Oxygen delivery in the blood and subsequent uptake by the muscles is conventionally described by the Fick equation, where $p\dot{V}O_2$ is the product of cardiac output ($\dot{Q}$) and arteriovenous oxygen difference (a-vO_2 diff), where $\dot{Q}$ is the product of heart rate (HR) and stroke volume (SV). Ethical and methodological issues related to the determination of $\dot{Q}$, SV, and a-vO_2 diff during exercise have clouded the interpretation of cardiovascular data, but the introduction of technologies such as Doppler echocardiography, thoracic bioimpedance, and near-infra red spectroscopy (NIRS) has clarified responses to incremental exercise.

Heart rate rises in a near-linear manner before tapering prior to reaching HR max. Maximal HR is independent of age during youth and typical mean values at $\dot{V}O_2$ max on a treadmill and a cycle ergometer are ~200 and ~195 $beats \cdot min^{-1}$, respectively.[8] In the upright position untrained young people's SV rises progressively with incremental exercise to values ~30–40% higher than resting but at ~50% of $\dot{V}O_2$ max SV plateaus and remains stable to the end of the test.[9] In contrast, trained young people's SV has been reported to increase progressively to exhaustion.[10] (Interested readers are referred to Chapter 34 for more detailed discussion). Stroke volume and $\dot{Q}$ are normally expressed in relation to body surface area, as the stroke or cardiac index respectively. Prepubertal boys' peak cardiac index has been reported to be ~10% higher than that of prepubertal girls, but in both sexes values appear to remain stable from ~10 years of age into young adulthood.[11]

Investigations of a-vO_2 diff during youth are sparse but a-vO_2 diff has been observed to increase with incremental exercise before plateauing at near-maximal exercise in both children and adults, with adults having a greater maximum a-vO_2 diff than children.[12] Data are equivocal, but at least one study has reported prepubertal boys to have a significantly higher maximum a-vO_2 diff than prepubertal girls.[13]

Blood lactate accumulation

At rest, lactate is continuously produced in skeletal muscles, but with the onset of exercise there is an increased production and accumulation of lactate in the muscles. Muscle lactate accumulation is a dynamic process where active muscle fibres produce lactate and adjacent fibres simultaneously consume it as an energy source.

Some of the lactate diffuses into the blood where it can be sampled and assayed to provide an estimate of the anaerobic contribution to exercise and therefore an indication of submaximal aerobic fitness. Lactate is, however, continuously removed from the blood by oxidation in the heart or skeletal muscles or through conversion to glucose in the liver or kidneys. Blood lactate accumulation must therefore be interpreted cautiously as lactate sampled in the blood cannot be assumed to reflect a consistent or direct relationship with muscle lactate production.

Hill and Lupton[2] described the production of lactate in humans in relation to the 'limit of muscular exertion', but much of the subsequent research concerned the interpretation of blood lactate accumulation during submaximal exercise and was initially published in the post-Second World War German literature. The hypothesis of an 'anaerobic threshold' to describe blood lactate accumulation during progressive exercise was popularized in the 1970s, but more recent research has both challenged and defended the threshold hypothesis.[14] Current thought on lactate thresholds in adults can be found in the work of Wassermann and his colleagues.[15]

Blood lactate accumulation during incremental exercise

During an incremental exercise test to exhaustion blood lactate accumulation typically increases, as illustrated in Figure 12.2. The onset of the test stimulates minimal change in blood lactate accumulation, which often does not significantly rise above resting values. It is not unusual for blood lactate accumulation to initially increase and then fall back to near resting values due to the interplay between type I and type II muscle fibre recruitment. However, as the exercise progresses blood lactate accumulation gradually increases until an inflection point is reached where lactate begins to accumulate rapidly. The blood lactate accumulation inflection point is defined as the lactate threshold (T_{LAC}), which serves as a useful estimate of submaximal aerobic fitness.[16]

The highest exercise intensity which can be sustained without incurring a progressive increase in blood lactate accumulation is termed the maximal lactate steady state (MLSS). It corresponds to the highest point at which the diffusion of lactate into the blood and removal from the blood are in equilibrium. Exercise can be sustained for prolonged periods at or below the MLSS, and it therefore has the potential to provide an indicator of aerobic fitness, but for methodological reasons secure data from children and adolescents are not currently available.[17]

To avoid taking multiple blood samples from young people, non-invasive alternatives to blood lactate reference values have become the preferred option in many paediatric exercise science laboratories. Robust methods have been developed to determine and evaluate the T_{VENT}[18] (or V-slope[19]) and the critical power (CPo)[20] of children. The V-slope, which is often the preferred method of estimating a threshold, is determined using linear regression to detect the point at which $\dot{V}CO_2$ begins to rise at a more rapid rate than $p\dot{V}O_2$, and is independent of the $\dot{V}_E$ response. Critical power is defined as the power asymptote of the theoretical hyperbolic relationship between muscle power output and the time to exhaustion. The T_{VENT} (or V-slope) and CPo are often used to replace T_{LAC} and MLSS respectively, for example, in defining exercise domains[21] and monitoring training programmes.[22]

Peak blood lactate accumulation following an exercise test to exhaustion has been used routinely to estimate whether a young person has given a maximal effort.[23] Some authors have advocated the use of specific values of post-exercise blood lactate accumulation (e.g. 6 to 9 mmol · L^{-1}) to confirm maximal efforts during tests to determine peak $\dot{V}O_2$.[24] There is, however, considerable variability in young people's blood lactate accumulation. Post-exercise values of blood lactate accumulation at peak $\dot{V}O_2$ of untrained 11- to 13-year-olds have been observed to range from 4 to 13 mmol · L^{-1}, using the same exercise protocol, blood sampling, and assay techniques.[25] Post-exercise blood lactate accumulation is dependent on mode of exercise, protocol employed (see variations of blood lactate accumulation with different exercise test protocols in Table 12.1), and timing of the post-exercise blood sample relative to the cessation of the exercise.[26] The recommendation of a specific minimum post-exercise blood lactate accumulation to validate peak $\dot{V}O_2$ as a maximal effort during youth is therefore untenable.

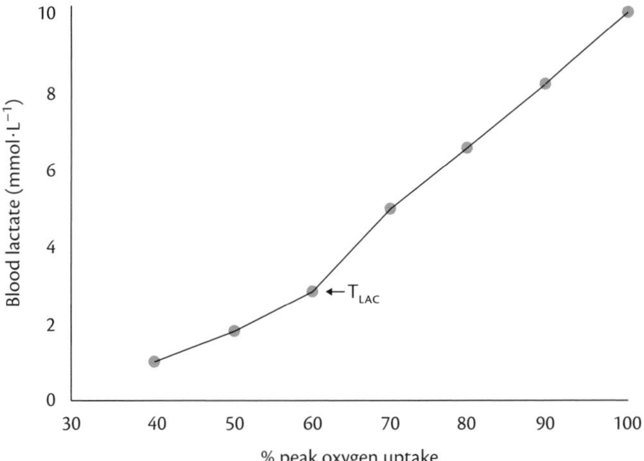

Figure 12.2 Blood lactate accumulation and % peak oxygen uptake.
Blood lactate accumulation in relation to % peak oxygen uptake during incremental exercise. The lactate threshold (T_{LAC}) is illustrated as the point where blood lactate begins to accumulate more rapidly (the inflection point).

Table 12.1 Peak physiological data of 9-year-olds across three maximal exercise tests

Boys	**Test 1**	**Test 2**	**Test 3**
Oxygen uptake (L · min^{-1})	1.93 (0.23)	1.95 (0.24)	1.98 (0.17)
Heart rate (beats · min^{-1})	203 (8)	196 (10)*	196 (7)*
Respiratory exchange ratio	0.99 (0.05)	1.15 (0.07)*	1.18 (0.09)*
Blood lactate (mmol · L^{-1})	5.7 (1.7)	8.4 (2.2)*	9.3 (1.9)*
Girls	**Test 1**	**Test 2**	**Test 3**
Oxygen uptake (L · min^{-1})	1.85 (0.28)	1.90 (0.26)	1.91 (0.35)
Heart rate (beats · min^{-1})	211 (9)	205 (9)*	206 (10)*
Respiratory exchange ratio	1.00 (0.04)	1.13 (0.06)*	1.13 (0.06)*
Blood lactate (mmol · L^{-1})	6.4 (1.3)	8.3 (1.3)*	8.3 (2.1)*

Values are mean (standard deviation).

* Mean significantly different ($p < 0.05$) from test 1.

Source data from Armstrong N, Welsman JR, Winsley RJ, Is peak $\dot{V}O_2$ a maximal index of children's aerobic fitness? Int J Sports Med. 1996; 17: 356–359.

Pulmonary oxygen uptake kinetics

A high $\dot{V}O_2$ max and/or the ability to sustain submaximal exercise are prerequisites of elite performance in some sports, but exercise of the intensity and duration required to elicit $\dot{V}O_2$ max or to sustain performance at the T_{LAC} or MLSS is rarely experienced by most young people.[27] The outcome is that there is no meaningful relationship between daily (or habitual) physical activity during youth and either $\dot{V}O_2$ max[28] or blood lactate indices of aerobic fitness.[29] The vast majority of young people's daily physical activity is intermittent and consists of periods of rest interspersed with physical activity of short duration. Furthermore, in many sports the ability to engage in rapid changes in exercise intensity is at least as important as $\dot{V}O_2$ max or T_{LAC}. Under these circumstances, it is the kinetics of $p\dot{V}O_2$ which best reflect the effective integrated response of the pulmonary, circulatory, and muscular systems.

The introduction of breath-by-breath respiratory gas exchange technology in the late 1960s enabled innovative scientists, including Margaria, Wasserman, and Whipp, to map out the kinetic response of $p\dot{V}O_2$ following the onset of exercise. Critical reviews of the assessment and interpretation of the respiratory gas kinetics of both adults[30] and youth[31] are available elsewhere. The following paragraphs summarize current understanding of the phenomenon; a more detailed analysis is presented in Chapter 13.

Kinetics of the pulmonary oxygen uptake response at exercise onset

The $p\dot{V}O_2$ response to a step change from rest (experimentally usually from unloaded pedalling on a cycle ergometer) to moderate-intensity exercise (i.e. exercise intensity below the T_{LAC} or T_{VENT}) is characterized by three phases as illustrated in Figure 12.3. Phase I (the cardiodynamic phase), which lasts ~15–20 s in young people, is associated with an increase in $\dot{Q}$ which occurs prior to the arrival at the lungs of venous blood from the exercising muscles and is therefore independent of muscle $\dot{V}O_2$ ($m\dot{V}O_2$). Phase I is followed by an exponential increase in $p\dot{V}O_2$ (phase II) that drives $p\dot{V}O_2$ to a steady state (phase III) within ~2 min. Phase II (the primary component) is described by its time constant (τ), which is the time taken to achieve 63% of the change in $p\dot{V}O_2$. The shorter the primary component τ, the smaller the oxygen deficit and the anaerobic contribution to the energy required for the change in exercise intensity.

In contrast to the $p\dot{V}O_2$ response at the onset of moderate-intensity exercise, a step change from rest to heavy-intensity exercise (i.e. exercise intensity above the T_{LAC} or T_{VENT}, but below CPo or the MLSS) elicits a phase III, where the oxygen cost increases over time as a slow component of $p\dot{V}O_2$ is superimposed and the achievement of a steady state is delayed by ~10 min in children[32] and 10–15 min in adults.[30]

Although largely ignored in the physiology literature for over 60 years, initial indications of the presence of a $p\dot{V}O_2$ slow component lie in the 1913 data of Krogh and Lindhard.[33] Ten years later, Hill and Lupton[2] observed what was probably a $p\dot{V}O_2$ slow component in a subject running at constant speed, but reported that, 'The gradual rise in oxygen consumption is probably to be attributed to a painful blister on the foot causing inefficient movement'.[2(p155)] It required the advent of data from more sophisticated breath-by-breath technology before Gaesser and Poole[34] were able to provide an insightful clarification of the sources of the $p\dot{V}O_2$ slow component. The mechanisms still remain speculative, but compelling arguments suggest that ~85% of the $p\dot{V}O_2$ slow component originates from the exercising muscles, perhaps largely

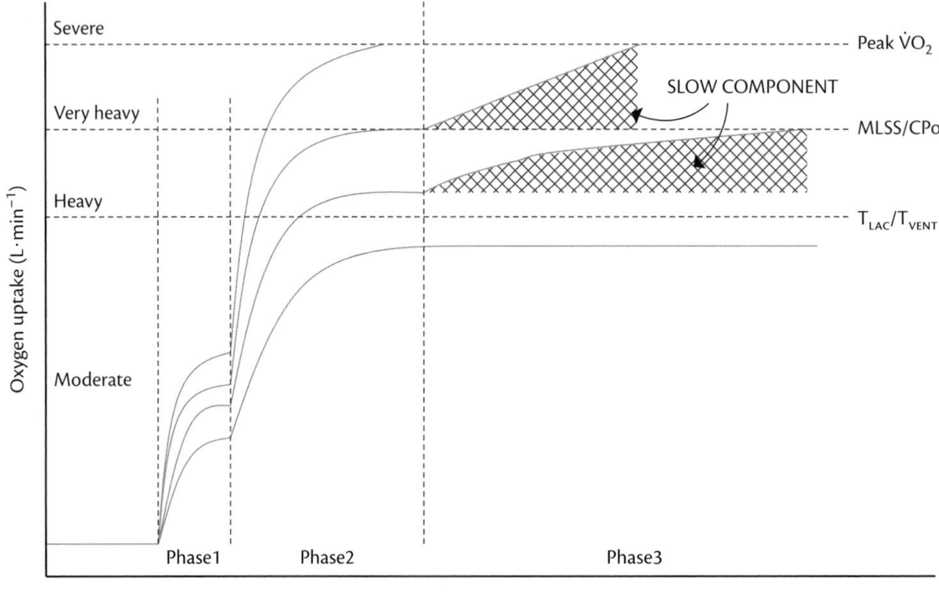

Figure 12.3 Pulmonary oxygen uptake in response to step changes in exercise intensity.

The pulmonary oxygen uptake response at the onset of constant exercise in different exercise intensity domains. The horizontal lines represent the boundaries of the domains where peak $\dot{V}O_2$, MLSS, CPo, T_{LAC}, and T_{VENT} denote peak oxygen uptake, maximal lactate steady state, critical power, lactate threshold, and ventilatory threshold, respectively. The slow component of pulmonary oxygen uptake is represented by the hatched areas.

due to a change in muscle fibre recruitment as exercise progresses. In prepubertal children[32] and adolescents[35] neither the primary component τ nor the p$\dot{V}O_2$ slow component are significantly related to peak $\dot{V}O_2$.

The very heavy-intensity exercise domain encompasses exercise intensities lying between the MLSS (or CPo) and $\dot{V}O_2$ max. In this domain a p$\dot{V}O_2$ steady state is not achieved and in adults the p$\dot{V}O_2$ slow component rises with time and projects to $\dot{V}O_2$ max. The higher the work rate is above CPo the faster the projection of the p$\dot{V}O_2$ slow component to $\dot{V}O_2$ max. This phenomenon has not to date been reported in children where it has been observed that p$\dot{V}O_2$ projects progressively towards peak $\dot{V}O_2$ but stabilizes at ~85–90% of peak $\dot{V}O_2$.[36]

The severe-intensity exercise domain describes step changes in exercise intensity in which the primary component of p$\dot{V}O_2$ is predicted to project to or above $\dot{V}O_2$ max and the maximal rate of p$\dot{V}O_2$ is achieved within 2–3 min of exercise onset. In the severe-intensity exercise domain a p$\dot{V}O_2$ slow component is not discernible from the primary component, but it is unclear whether this is due to the prominence of the primary component of p$\dot{V}O_2$ or insufficient time for a p$\dot{V}O_2$ slow component to be expressed. It has been suggested that as there is a large slow phase in recovery from exercise in this domain it is likely that a p$\dot{V}O_2$ slow component also exists during the onset of exercise.[30]

An alternative classification scheme of p$\dot{V}O_2$ kinetics defines all exercise intensities that achieve $\dot{V}O_2$ max to reside within the severe domain irrespective of whether p$\dot{V}O_2$ projects to $\dot{V}O_2$ max through the primary component or via the p$\dot{V}O_2$ slow component. In this schema there exists a domain termed extreme intensity in which the exercise intensity is so great that fatigue intervenes before $\dot{V}O_2$ max can be attained.[30] As the majority of the paediatric exercise science literature has adopted the terminology illustrated in Figure 12.3 this classification will be adhered to throughout this chapter.

Peak oxygen uptake

Maximal (and later peak) $\dot{V}O_2$ has been the criterion measure of young people's aerobic fitness since the pioneering studies of Robinson,[3] Morse *et al.*,[4] and Åstrand[5], yet the assessment and interpretation of $\dot{V}O_2$ max or (peak $\dot{V}O_2$) during growth and maturation remain shrouded in controversy.[37] This section identifies pertinent methodological issues in the determination of peak $\dot{V}O_2$, clarifies the distinction between $\dot{V}O_2$ max and peak $\dot{V}O_2$, discusses the increase in peak $\dot{V}O_2$ with chronological age, challenges the conventional interpretation of peak $\dot{V}O_2$ in relation to body size; demonstrates the independent contribution of biological maturity to peak $\dot{V}O_2$; and addresses sexual dimorphism in peak $\dot{V}O_2$.

Methodological issues

Maximal or peak oxygen uptake?

Classically, $\dot{V}O_2$ max was determined in a laboratory using a discontinuous, incremental exercise test to exhaustion on a treadmill or cycle ergometer. Typically, the participant exercised at a predetermined, submaximal intensity for about 3–5 min to obtain a steady state p$\dot{V}O_2$ and then rested for ~60 s (in some cases submaximal stages were carried out on different days) before completing a more intense exercise stage. This protocol continued until a stage beyond which a p$\dot{V}O_2$ plateau was reached. The additional energy required to exercise above the point where the p$\dot{V}O_2$ plateau occurred was assumed to be provided exclusively by anaerobic metabolism, resulting in an intracellular accumulation of lactate, acidosis, and eventual termination of exercise. In practice a genuine plateau in p$\dot{V}O_2$ with increasing exercise intensity seldom occurred and less stringent criteria for establishing the existence of a plateau were developed. In order to increase confidence that a true $\dot{V}O_2$ max had been achieved, subsidiary criteria related to HR, respiratory exchange ratio (i.e. $\dot{V}CO_2$/p$\dot{V}O_2$; R), and blood lactate accumulation at the termination of the $\dot{V}O_2$ max test were introduced.[38]

The $\dot{V}O_2$ plateau concept has retained primacy in the literature as the principal criterion for establishing $\dot{V}O_2$ max, but the validity of the classical model has been a topic of lively debate for several years.[39,40] The practice of reporting submaximal p$\dot{V}O_2$ steady states or describing exercise intensities as % $\dot{V}O_2$ max in the heavy- and very heavy-exercise intensity domains has fallen into disrepute with evidence of a p$\dot{V}O_2$ slow component emerging at exercise intensities above the T_{LAC} in adults,[30] adolescents,[35] and prepubertal children.[32]

Åstrand's[5] studies revealed that a p$\dot{V}O_2$ plateau was found in '70 of 140 running experiments with school children'.[5(p23)] It was subsequently argued by some authors that the failure of some children to elicit a p$\dot{V}O_2$ plateau was related to low motivation or low anaerobic capacity.[41] But others demonstrated that with both prepubertal children[42] and adolescents[43] those who exhibited a p$\dot{V}O_2$ plateau at the termination of an incremental exercise test to voluntary exhaustion were indistinguishable in terms of HR, R, or blood lactate accumulation at test termination from those who did not. This raised the question of whether a p$\dot{V}O_2$ plateau was required to indicate a maximal index of aerobic fitness during youth.

The problem was addressed experimentally by determining the peak $\dot{V}O_2$ of 20 boys and 20 girls, mean age 9.9 years, on three occasions, 1 week apart. On the first occasion, the children completed a discontinuous, incremental protocol on a treadmill with the belt speed held at 1.94 $m \cdot s^{-1}$ but with the gradient increasing every 3 min. The children exercised until voluntary exhaustion. Using a <2 $mL \cdot kg^{-1} \cdot min^{-1}$ increase in p$\dot{V}O_2$ as the criterion, six boys and seven girls exhibited a p$\dot{V}O_2$ plateau. No significant differences in either anthropometrical or peak physiological data were revealed between those who did and did not exhibit p$\dot{V}O_2$ plateaus. The second and third tests were performed at the same belt speed as test one (i.e. 1.94 $m \cdot s^{-1}$) but, following a 3 min warm-up running at 1.67 $m \cdot s^{-1}$, the children ran up gradients which were 2.5% and 5% greater, respectively, than the highest gradient achieved on the first test. The children were strongly motivated and the data were accepted if the child ran for at least 2 min up the higher gradient. Eighteen girls and 17 boys completed all tests and although they exhibited significantly higher post-exercise blood lactate accumulation, peak $\dot{V}_E$, and peak R in tests two and three than in the initial test, as illustrated in Table 12.1, there were no significant differences in peak $\dot{V}O_2$ across the three tests.[44]

These data and those from a similar study[45] imply that with well-motivated children 'true' $\dot{V}O_2$ max values can be achieved in a single, incremental test to exhaustion despite the majority of participants not demonstrating a p$\dot{V}O_2$ plateau. There is, however, no easy solution to the problem of whether an individual child has delivered a maximal effort in an incremental test to exhaustion. Habituation to the laboratory environment, subjective criteria of intense effort (e.g. facial flushing, sweating, hyperpnoea, unsteady gait), and the paediatric exercise testing experience of the experimenters are vital ingredients in making this decision. Various other physiological indicators of a maximal effort such as HR and R at peak $\dot{V}O_2$ and peak post-exercise blood lactate accumulation have been proposed as subsidiary criteria,[46] but, as illustrated by the data described in Table 12.1, they are all protocol dependent. Furthermore, there is no 'one size fits all' criterion of a maximal effort. For example, at the termination of an incremental treadmill exercise test HR at peak $\dot{V}O_2$ has a mean ± standard deviation of ~200±7 beats·min^{-1}, in the age range 8–16 years.[8] As ~95% of young people's HRs at peak $\dot{V}O_2$ would therefore be expected to fall in the range 186–214 beats·min^{-1} it is futile to interpret a spot HR of, for example, 195 or 200 beats·min^{-1} as is commonly advocated, as reflecting maximal effort. (Interested readers are referred to Chapter 11 for further detail of the cardiovascular response to exercise).

As the term $\dot{V}O_2$ max conventionally requires a p$\dot{V}O_2$ plateau to be exhibited, it has become common practise in paediatric exercise science to define the highest p$\dot{V}O_2$ observed during a progressive exercise test to exhaustion as peak $\dot{V}O_2$ rather than $\dot{V}O_2$ max.

Respiratory gas analysis

The determination of peak $\dot{V}O_2$ depends upon the accurate measurement of inspired and/or expired air per unit of time and the fraction of oxygen and carbon dioxide therein. Automated respiratory gas analysis systems and sophisticated metabolic carts with appropriate calibration facilities are commercially available and commonplace in research laboratories. Paediatric physiologists must, however, be cautious of measuring children's respiratory responses to exercise using apparatus primarily designed for use with adults.

Most respiratory gas analysis systems measure volume using a breathing valve (normally a lightweight turbine or pneumotachograph) connected to the participant via a mouthpiece and nose clip or facemask. With children it is imperative that the mouthpiece and nose clip or facemask is comfortable and appropriately sized to prevent leakage. To prevent the significant inspiration of previously expired air the combined dead space of the mouthpiece/facemask and breathing valve should be minimized, although this must be balanced against the resulting increase in resistance to flow.

To periodically sample respiratory gases metabolic carts normally use either a mixing chamber, which stores expiratory gases over a given interval, or a breath-by-breath system. Large mixing chambers may cause substantial measurement errors as children have smaller exercise tidal volumes than adults. Breath-by-breath systems with rapid gas analysers allow continuous measurement of volume and respiratory gas content and overcome the potential size limitations of mixing chambers. However, breath-by-breath systems are challenged by the large inter-breath variations of exercising children in relation to their p$\dot{V}O_2$ response amplitude (i.e. high noise-to-signal ratio).[47]

In addition, the breath-by-breath gas sampling interval can have a significant impact on the reported p$\dot{V}O_2$. Short sampling intervals increase the variability in measuring p$\dot{V}O_2$ and with their smaller peak $\dot{V}O_2$ this is more marked in children than in adults. However, large sample intervals may 'over-smooth' the data and artificially reduce the 'true' $\dot{V}O_2$ response. A sampling interval of ~15–30 s is optimum for children and adolescents, but whatever the chosen interval it should be recorded and reported to allow cross-study comparisons.[48]

Ergometry

Young people's peak $\dot{V}O_2$ has been determined using a wide range of ergometers, and although it is important to simulate competitive performance when testing and monitoring young athletes, cycles and treadmills remain the ergometers of choice in most paediatric exercise science laboratories.

Cycle ergometry provides a portable, relatively cheap, and more quantifiable mode of exercise than treadmill running and it tends to induce less anxiety in young children. Cycle ergometer crank lengths may need to be modified for young children who sometimes experience difficulty with the need to maintain a fixed pedal rate when cycling on mechanically braked ergometers. Electronically braked cycle ergometers which adjust resistance to pedalling frequency alleviate this difficulty to some extent, but the increase in resistance required to maintain exercise intensity following a reduction in pedal rate may in itself cause problems with young children.

Limited upper body movement during cycle ergometry facilitates the measurement of ancillary variables such as HR, blood pressure, and blood lactate accumulation. However, a disadvantage of cycle ergometry with young children is that a high proportion of the total power output is developed by the quadriceps muscles[49] and the effort required to push the pedals during the later stages of an incremental test may be high in relation to children's muscle strength.[50] This leads to blood flow through the quadriceps being restricted and results in increased anaerobic metabolism and consequent termination of the test through peripheral muscle fatigue.[51]

Treadmill running engages a larger muscle mass than cycling. The increased venous return and reduced peripheral resistance during running enhances $\dot{Q}$, and peak $\dot{V}O_2$ is more likely to be limited by central than peripheral factors. Peak $\dot{V}O_2$ is typically about 8–10% higher during treadmill running than cycle ergometry, although some adolescents have been reported to achieve higher peak $\dot{V}O_2$ on a cycle ergometer. Pearson product-moment correlations between peak $\dot{V}O_2$ rigorously determined on a treadmill and a cycle ergometer are ~0.90.[52]

Exercise protocols

Peak $\dot{V}O_2$ during youth is a robust variable which, on a specific ergometer, is normally independent of exercise protocol[53] with a coefficient of variation in repeated tests of ~5% on both treadmill and cycle ergometer.[52]

Incremental, continuous, or discontinuous protocols on a treadmill have traditionally been the exercise tests of choice in paediatric exercise research laboratories.[54] However, with clear experimental evidence that children[55] and adolescents[35] exhibit a p$\dot{V}O_2$ slow component during exercise above the T_{LAC}, the availability of commercial breath-by-breath metabolic carts, and the development of electromagnetically braked cycle ergometers, ramp protocols have become popular. In many paediatric exercise science laboratories ramp cycle tests, where power output is increased linearly with time, have replaced classical, discontinuous, 'steady state', incremental protocols. Ramp protocols have the advantages of flexibility of rate and magnitude of power output, short test duration (~10 min), and the ability to determine other parameters of cardiopulmonary function (e.g. V-slope) during a single test.

In a single ramp test to exhaustion a p$\dot{V}O_2$ plateau is an infrequent occurrence. However, a study of 10- and 11-year-old children, across three ramp tests each 1 week apart, reported a typical error in peak $\dot{V}O_2$ of ~4%, which compares favourably with the reliability of adults' $\dot{V}O_2$ max, regardless of protocol.[56] A short duration ramp test coupled with children's ability to recover quickly from exhaustive exercise[57] allows the use of a follow-up supramaximal test to verify whether a maximal effort was elicited in the initial test.

The following protocol has been found to be appropriate for children: After a 3 min period of cycling at 10 W, participants undertake a ramp incremental test to exhaustion with power output increasing by 10 W · min^{-1}. Cycling cadence is maintained at 75 revs · min^{-1} throughout the test and exhaustion is defined as a drop in pedal cadence below 60 revs · min^{-1} for 5 consecutive seconds. Immediately after exhaustion, power output is reduced to 10 W and the child cycles at this intensity for 10 min followed by 5 min of rest. The participant then performs a supramaximal test consisting of 2 min pedalling at 10 W, followed by a step transition to 105% of the peak power achieved during the ramp test. The pedalling cadence is maintained at 75 revs · min^{-1} with the same criterion as in the initial test to define exhaustion. The power output is then returned to 10 W until the HR has recovered to ~120 beats · min^{-1}. With prepubertal children the time to exhaustion in the supramaximal test is ~90 s. On the rare occasions (<5%) that the peak $\dot{V}O_2$ is higher than in the ramp test, the supramaximal test can be repeated at 110% of peak power following full recovery.[58]

Peak oxygen uptake and chronological age

The peak $\dot{V}O_2$ of children and adolescents has been extensively documented with data available from children as young as 3 years of age. The validity of peak $\dot{V}O_2$ determinations in children younger than 8 years has been questioned since the original studies of Robinson.[3] He noted that, 'the youngest boys were unwilling to continue work after it ceased to be fun, whereas all of the boys of 8 years and older could be encouraged to carry on for some time after the first signs of fatigue'.[3(p281)] As very young children typically have short attention spans, poor motivation, and lack sufficient understanding of experimental procedures it is difficult to elicit genuine maximal efforts.[59] Equipment and protocols designed for adults make exercise testing with young children problematic, and the smaller the child, the greater the potential problem. Reports of peak $\dot{V}O_2$ in very young children are often difficult to interpret. Small sample sizes are common and several studies have pooled data from boys and girls. Whether the children exhibited maximal values is unclear in some reports, and there is a strong tendency to report only mass-related data (mL · kg^{-1} · min^{-1}).[46]

One study suggested that it is possible with rigorous techniques to estimate the peak $\dot{V}O_2$ of most young children and reported achieving 'maximal' values in ~84% of 706 6- to 7-year-olds. Boys were noted to have peak $\dot{V}O_2$ values (L · min^{-1}) ~11% higher than girls, confirming the importance of not pooling boys' and girls' values and reporting data in relation to sex, even at a young age.[60] There are, however, few secure data from children aged less than 8 years in the literature and the focus herein will therefore be on the age group 8–18 years.

A comprehensive review of the extant literature generated graphs representing ~10 000 peak $\dot{V}O_2$ determinations of untrained eight- to 16-year-olds. Because of the ergometer dependence of peak $\dot{V}O_2$ data from treadmill and cycle ergometry were graphed separately and the treadmill-determined peak $\dot{V}O_2$ values (n = 4937) are illustrated in Figure 12.4. The data must be interpreted cautiously, as means from a range of studies with varying sample sizes are included. No information is available on randomly selected groups of young people, and since participants are generally volunteers selection bias cannot be ruled out. This type of analysis tends to smooth data, but Figure 12.4 clearly illustrates a near-linear increase in peak $\dot{V}O_2$ in relation to age. Linear regression equations indicate that peak $\dot{V}O_2$ increases by ~80% from 8 to 16 years in girls and by ~150% in boys over the same time period.[46]

Longitudinal studies provide a more granular analysis of peak $\dot{V}O_2$ in relation to age, but few longitudinal studies have reported data from a broad age range and coupled rigorous determination of peak $\dot{V}O_2$ with substantial sample sizes. Data from rigorous longitudinal studies of treadmill-determined peak $\dot{V}O_2$ are illustrated in Figure 12.5 but between studies comparisons should be interpreted with caution.

Longitudinal data from boys are consistent, with a similar trend to that shown in Figure 12.4. The pooled data show an increase in peak $\dot{V}O_2$ of ~150%, from 8 to 18 years, with the largest annual increases occurring between 13–15 years. It has been suggested that the greatest increase in boys' peak $\dot{V}O_2$ accompanies the attainment of peak height velocity (PHV),[66] but others[67] have noted a stable increase in peak $\dot{V}O_2$ from 3 years before to 1 year after PHV. Longitudinal data from girls are sparse and when pooled they indicate an increase in peak $\dot{V}O_2$ of ~98%, from 8 to 17 years. One study observed a growth spurt in peak $\dot{V}O_2$ aligned with PHV,[66] but when data across studies are compared they suggest, on balance, that girls' peak $\dot{V}O_2$ rises progressively from 8 to 13 years and then begins to level off from ~14 years. A trend also noted in some cross-sectional studies.[46]

The most comprehensive longitudinal study reported is the Amsterdam Growth and Health Longitudinal Study (AGHLS) which followed 12- to 14-year-old boys and girls for a period of 25 years.[68] Boys demonstrated a linear increase in peak $\dot{V}O_2$ of

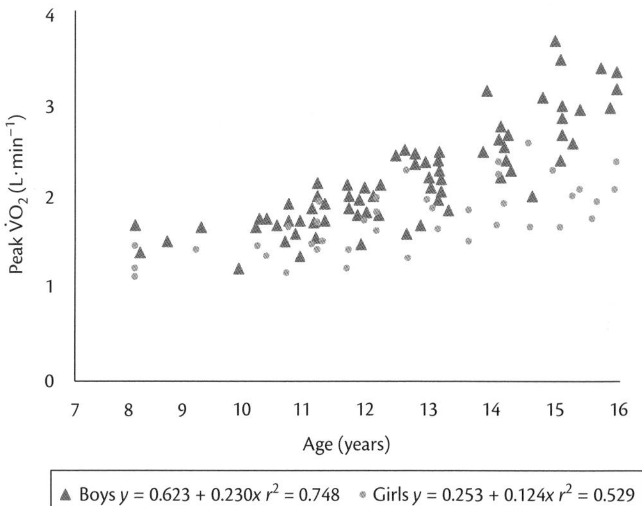

Figure 12.4 Peak oxygen uptake by chronological age and sex.

Treadmill-determined peak oxygen uptake in relation to chronological age and sex in 8- to 16-year-olds. Figure describes peak oxygen uptake data on 3703 boys and 1234 girls.

Source data from Armstrong N, Welsman JR. Assessment and interpretation of aerobic fitness in children and adolescents. Exerc Sport Sci Rev. 1994; 22: 435–476.

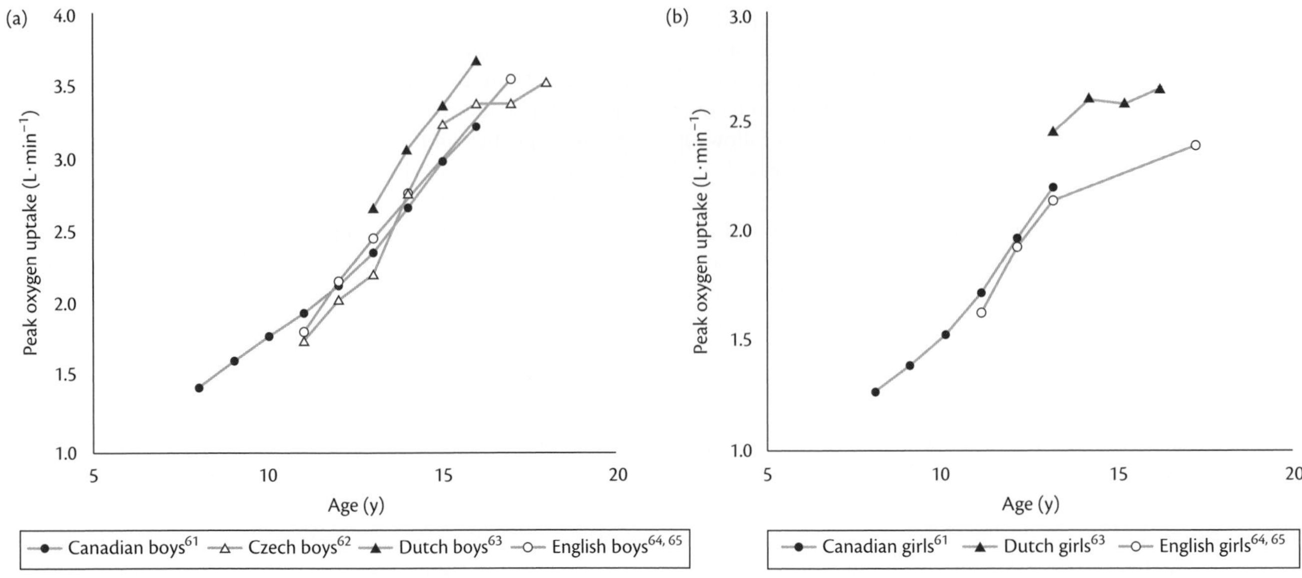

Figure 12.5 (a) Longitudinal studies of boys' peak oxygen uptake and chronological age. (b) Longitudinal studies of girls' peak oxygen uptake and chronological age. Treadmill-determined peak oxygen uptake in relation to age in 8- to 18-year-olds. Figure 12.5a drawn from data in four longitudinal studies[61–65] with 1818 determinations of boys' peak oxygen uptake. Figure 12.5b drawn from data in three longitudinal studies[61,63–65] with 707 determinations of girls' peak oxygen uptake.

~57%, from age 12–17 years. Girls' values increased by ~11% over the same time period, with a marked levelling-off from 14–17 years (~2% change).[69] The Dutch data[63] contrast with a mixed longitudinal study from England, which reported increases in peak $\dot{V}O_2$, from 12–17 years, of ~70% and ~24% for boys and girls respectively.[65] As Dutch values at age 12 years were ~12% and ~22% higher than English values, for boys and girls respectively, the conflicting data may be at least partially explained by the initial high level of aerobic fitness of Dutch youth compared with English youth.

Peak oxygen uptake and body mass

Peak $\dot{V}O2$ is strongly correlated with body mass and, in particular, with lean body mass (LBM). Much of the age-related increase in peak $\dot{V}O_2$ illustrated in Figure 12.4 reflects the increase in muscle mass during the transition from childhood into young adulthood. Because of the problems in assessing LBM, researchers have conventionally focused on controlling for body mass differences by dividing peak $\dot{V}O_2$ by total body mass and expressing it as the simple ratio $mL \cdot kg^{-1} \cdot min^{-1}$ (ratio scaling).[46]

When peak $\dot{V}O_2$ is expressed in this manner a different picture emerges from that apparent when absolute values ($L \cdot min^{-1}$) are used. Cross-sectional data indicate that boys' mass-related peak $\dot{V}O2$ decreases slightly or remains unchanged at ~48 $mL \cdot kg^{-1} \cdot min^{-1}$, from 8 to 18 years, while in girls a progressive decline, from ~45–35 $mL \cdot kg^{-1} \cdot min^{-1}$, is apparent. Boys consistently demonstrate higher mass-related peak $\dot{V}O_2$ than girls throughout childhood and adolescence, with the sex difference being reinforced by the greater accumulation of body fat by girls in puberty.[46] The AGHLS data are intriguing in this context as, in conflict with the extant literature, they indicate that from 12–17 years boys' peak $\dot{V}O_2$ decreases from ~59–52 $mL \cdot kg^{-1} \cdot min^{-1}$ and girls' values fall from ~57–45 $mL \cdot kg^{-1} \cdot min^{-1}$.[69]

Although informative in relation to the performance of, for example, track athletes who carry their body mass,[70] the conventional use of ratio values has clouded the physiological understanding of peak $\dot{V}O_2$ during growth. Rather than removing the influence of body mass, ratio scaling 'over scales' and favours light individuals and penalizes heavy individuals. Tanner[71] described the fallacy of ratio scaling in 1949 and Åstrand[5] noted its limitations in relation to expressing children's peak $\dot{V}O_2$ in 1952, but its use has persisted in the paediatric literature. The interpretation of exercise performance data in relation to body size has been critically reviewed elsewhere,[72] but the inadequacy of ratio scaling can be explained simply.

To create a size-free variable in this context requires a product-moment correlation coefficient between peak $\dot{V}O_2$, expressed in $mL \cdot kg^{-1} \cdot min^{-1}$, and body mass in kg, which is not significantly different from zero. Significant negative correlations between ratio scaled peak $\dot{V}O_2$ and body mass have been reported on numerous occasions,[72] but data drawn from the first year of a longitudinal study[64] of 11- to 13-year-olds and summarized in Figure 12.6 clearly illustrate the phenomenon. Figure 12.6a shows significant positive correlations between peak $\dot{V}O_2$ ($L \cdot min^{-1}$) and body mass (kg). Figure 12.6b describes the presence of significant negative correlations between ratio scaled peak $\dot{V}O_2$ ($mL \cdot kg^{-1} \cdot min^{-1}$) and body mass (kg), and confirms the inability of the simple ratio to remove the influence of body mass from peak $\dot{V}O_2$. Figure 12.6c, however, presents the same data and shows that correlations between allometrically scaled peak $\dot{V}O_2$ ($mL \cdot kg^{-0.68} \cdot min^{-1}$) and body mass (kg) are not significantly different from zero. Body mass has therefore been appropriately controlled for using allometric scaling with, in this case, a common mass exponent of 0.68.

Several studies have generated data illustrating how inappropriate ratio scaling has led to misplaced interpretation of physiological variables, whereas studies in which the use of more appropriate means of controlling for body size have provided new insights into peak $\dot{V}O_2$ during growth.[72] For instance, an early exploration of scaling children's peak $\dot{V}O_2$ used a simple linear regression model to investigate changes in peak $\dot{V}O_2$ with chronological age in two groups of boys aged 10 and 15 years. The mean values for peak $\dot{V}O_2$ were 1.73 and 3.12 $L \cdot min^{-1}$ respectively, but when ratio scaled, the two groups had identical mean values of 49 $mL \cdot kg^{-1} \cdot min^{-1}$. However, the regression lines for the relationship between peak $\dot{V}O_2$ and body mass described two clearly different populations (see Figure 12.7). Intuitively this appears

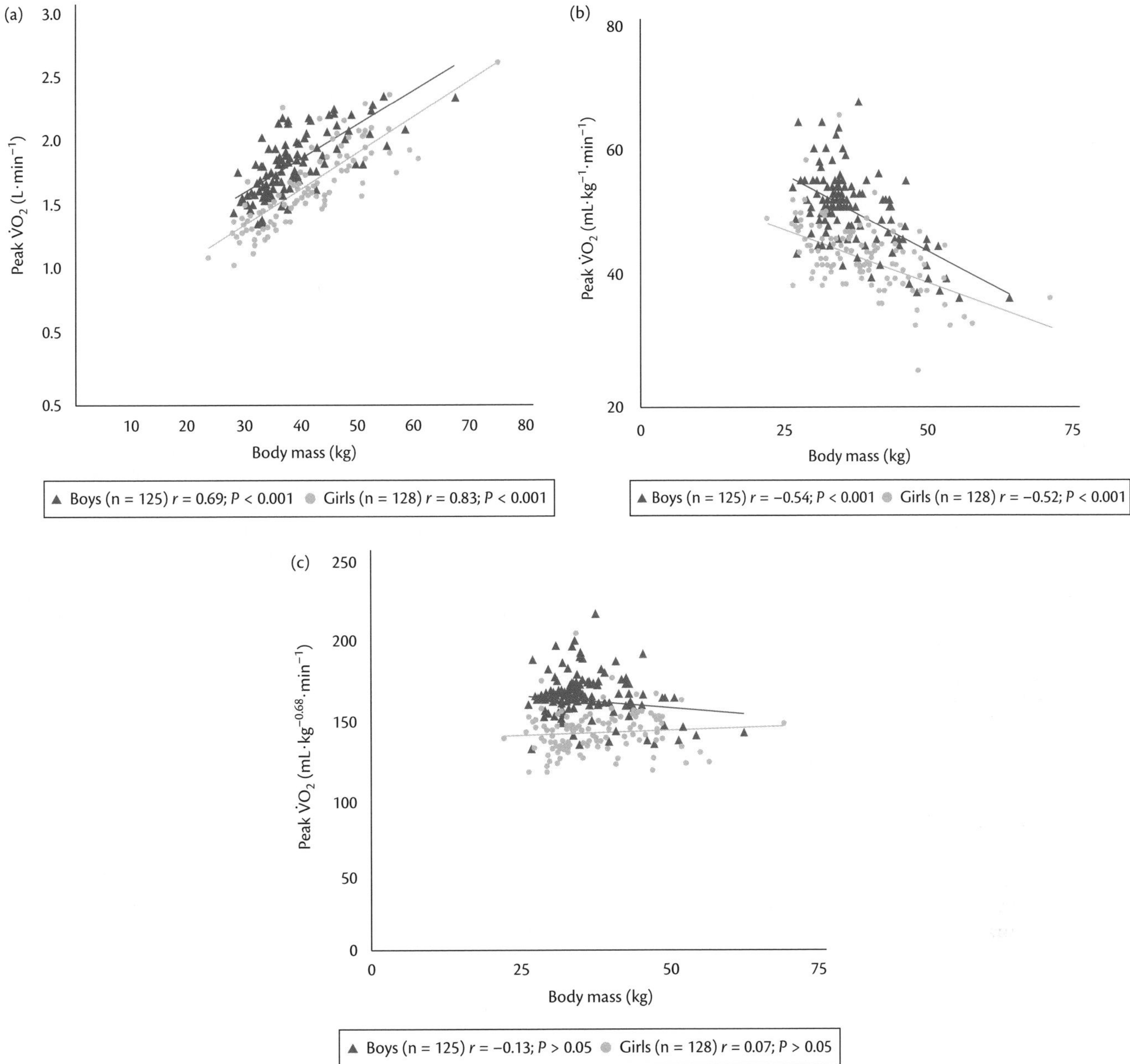

Figure 12.6 (a) Peak oxygen uptake and body mass in 11-year-olds:
This shows significant positive relationships between peak oxygen uptake and body mass in both boys (r = 0.69) and girls (r = 0.83).
(b) Ratio scaled peak oxygen uptake and body mass in 11-year-olds:
This shows significant negative relationships between ratio scaled peak oxygen uptake and body mass in both boys (r = −0.54) and girls (r = −0.52) and illustrates the failure of ratio scaling to deliver a body mass free variable.
(c) Allometrically scaled peak oxygen uptake and body mass in 11-year-olds:
This shows relationships between allometrically scaled peak oxygen uptake and body mass in both boys (r = −0.13) and girls (r = 0.07) are not significantly different from zero and illustrates that body mass has been appropriately controlled for using allometric scaling, with a common mass exponent of 0.68.
Source data from Armstrong N, Welsman JR, Nevill AM, Kirby BJ. Modeling growth and maturation changes in peak oxygen uptake in 11–13 yr olds. J Appl Physiol. 1999; 87: 2230–2236.

appropriate and is in accord with the observed differences in 10- and 15-year-olds' performance in athletic events primarily dependent on aerobic fitness.[73]

A more sophisticated analysis[74] avoiding the limitations of linear regression scaling[75] used both ratio and allometric (log-linear analysis of covariance) scaling to partition size effects from peak $\dot{V}O_2$ data in groups of males and females spanning the age range 11–23 years (see Table 12.2). The results of the ratio analyses conformed to the conventional interpretation with mass-related peak $\dot{V}O_2$ consistent across the three male groups (11, 14, and 23 years). In the females mass-related peak $\dot{V}O_2$ did not change from 11–13 years, but there was a significant decrease in peak $\dot{V}O_2$ from 13–22 years. In direct contrast, allometric scaling revealed significant, progressive increases in peak $\dot{V}O_2$ across male groups demonstrating that, with body size appropriately controlled for, peak $\dot{V}O_2$ is, in fact, increasing during growth rather than remaining static. In females, peak $\dot{V}O_2$ increased significantly from 11–13 years, subsequently remaining constant with no decline into adulthood evident.[74]

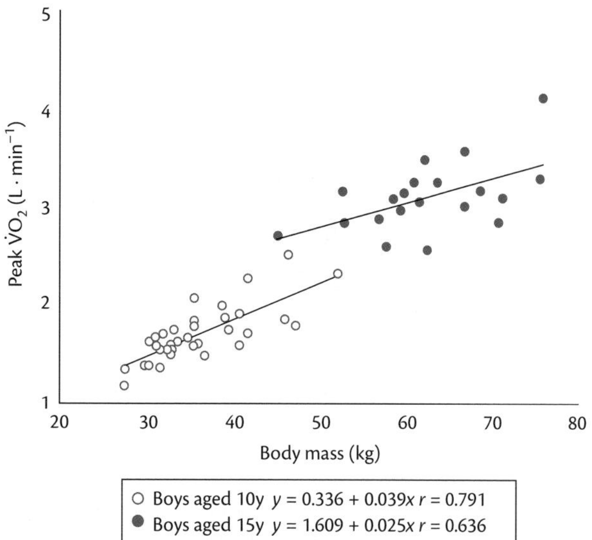

Figure 12.7 Peak oxygen uptake and body mass in 10- and 15-year-old boys. Mean values for peak $\dot{V}O_2$ 1.73 and 3.12 L·min^{-1} for 10- and 15-year-olds respectively. Ratio scaled identical values of 49 mL·kg^{-1}·min^{-1} were revealed; however, the regression lines for the relationship between peak $\dot{V}O_2$ and body mass describe two clearly different populations. Data from Williams JR, Armstrong N, Winter EM, Crichton N. Changes in peak oxygen uptake with age and sexual maturation in boys: Physiological fact or statistical anomaly? In: Coudert J, Van Praagh E, eds. Pediatric work physiology. Paris: Masson; 1992: 35–37.

The application of allometry to longitudinal data is complex, but its use is increasing and evidence to support the cross-sectional analyses is accumulating. Multilevel modelling techniques represent a sensitive and flexible approach to the interpretation of longitudinal exercise data which enable body size, chronological age, and sex effects to be partitioned concurrently within an allometric framework. The interested reader is referred to Welsman and Armstrong,[75] where the theoretical principles of allometry and multilevel modelling are explained and applied to paediatric data sets.

The independent effect of age on peak $\dot{V}O_2$ was clearly demonstrated in a longitudinal study which used multilevel regression modelling to interpret peak $\dot{V}O_2$ in 11–13-year-old boys and girls. The analysis was founded on 590 peak $\dot{V}O_2$ determinations over three annual occasions.[64] A multiplicative, allometric model was adopted based on the model:

$$\text{Peak } \dot{V}O_2(Y) = \text{mass}^{k1} \cdot \text{stature}^{k2} \cdot \exp(\alpha_j + b_j \cdot \text{age} + c \cdot \text{age}^2)\, \varepsilon_{ij}$$

In this model all parameters are fixed, with the exception of the constant (α, intercept term) and age parameters, which are allowed to vary randomly at level two (between individuals), and the multiplicative error ratio ε that varies randomly at level one, describing the error variance between occasions. The subscripts i and j denote this random variation at levels one and two respectively. The variable age is centred on the group mean age of 12.0 years.

In order to allow the unknown parameters to be solved using multilevel regression, the model was linearized by logarithmic transformation and multilevel regression analysis on $\log_e y$ used to solve for the unknown parameters. Once transformed, the initial equation became:

$$\text{Log}_e \text{ peak } \dot{V}O_2(\log_e y) = k_1 \cdot \log_e \text{mass} + k_2 \cdot \log_e \text{stature} + \alpha_j + b_j \cdot \text{age} + c \cdot \text{age}^2 + \log_e(\varepsilon_{ij})$$

From this baseline model the additional explanatory variable sex was incorporated as an indicator variable (i.e. sex, boys = 0; sex,

Table 12.2 Peak oxygen uptake in relation to stage of maturation

Females	Prepubertal girls (Maturation stage 1) (n = 33)	Circumpubertal girls (Maturation stage 3/4) (n = 34)	Adult women (n = 16)
Age (years)	10.7 (0.2)*	13.0 (0.2)**	21.7 (2.8)
Body mass (kg)	32.7 (4.6)*	46.5 (9.6)**	60.5 (6.3)
Peak $\dot{V}O_2$(L·min^{-1})	1.48 (0.2)*	2.14 (0.32)**	2.58 (0.26)
Ratio scaled peak $\dot{V}O_2$ (mL·kg^{-1}·min^{-1})	45 (3)	47 (4)***	43 (3)
Allometrically adjusted peak $\dot{V}O_2$ (L·min^{-1})	1.99*	2.19****	2.13
Males	**Prepubertal boys (Maturation stage 1) (n = 29)**	**Circumpubertal boys (Maturation stage 3/4) (n = 26)**	**Adult men (n = 18)**
Age (years)	10.7 (0.2)*	14.1 (0.3)**	22.8 (2.9)
Body mass (kg)	34.9 (5.4)*	49.5 (8.9)**	78.6 (8.7)
Peak $\dot{V}O_2$(L·min^{-1})	1.76 (0.28)*	2.60 (0.47)**	4.18 (0.47)
Ratio scaled peak $\dot{V}O_2$ (mL·kg^{-1}·min^{-1})	50 (4)	53 (4)	53 (3)
Allometrically adjusted peak $\dot{V}O_2$ (L·min^{-1})	2.25*	2.50**	2.80

Data from Welsman JR, Armstrong N, Kirby BJ, Nevill AM, Winter EM. Scaling peak $\dot{V}O_2$ for differences in body size. Med Sci Sports Exerc. 1996; 28: 259–265.

Values are mean (standard deviation).

level of significance $p < 0.05$.

* Significantly different from circumpubertals and adults.

** Significantly different from prepubertal children and adults.

*** Significantly different from adults.

**** Significantly different from prepubertal children.

Table 12.3 Multilevel regression model for peak oxygen uptake in 11–13-year-olds

Parameters	Estimate (SE)
Fixed	
Constant	−1.3903 (0.0970)
Log_e mass	0.5011 (0.0322)
Log_e stature	0.9479 (0.1162)
Age	0.0585 (0.0111)
Sex	−0.1378 (0.0093)
Age·sex	−0.0134 (0.0068)
Random	
Level 2	
Constant	0.0042 (0.0005)
Age	0.0007 (0.0003)
Covariance	NS
Level 1	
Constant	0.0030 (0.0004

N = 590 NS, not significant.

Data from Welsman JR, Armstrong N, Kirby BJ, Nevill AM, Winter EM Scaling peak VO2 for differences in body size. Med Sci Sports Exerc. 1996; 28: 259–265

girls = 1), which sets the boys' constant as the baseline from which the girls' parameter may deviate. The interaction term age by sex was constructed to investigate whether age effects on peak $\dot{V}O_2$ differed for boys and girls. Age was allowed to vary randomly at level one to investigate within individual variation around the individual growth trajectory. The need to allow each individual their own mass exponent was examined by letting body mass vary at level two. The model is presented in Table 12.3.

The multilevel regression model reveals stature and body mass as significant covariates with an additional significant positive effect for age, which is larger for boys than girls as reflected by the significant age by sex interaction term, which is deducted from the age term for girls. With age, stature, and body mass accounted for, the negative term for sex shows girls' peak $\dot{V}O_2$ to be significantly lower than that of boys. The fixed estimates in the model describe the population mean response, while the random parameters show the variance which remains unaccounted for by the fixed part of the model. Table 12.3 illustrates significant random variation at level two for age, reflecting differential individual growth rates in peak $\dot{V}O_2$. Allowing each individual their own mass exponent proved unnecessary, as there was no random variation between individuals around the fixed (mean) parameter.

Taken together, the cross-sectional and longitudinal data clearly challenge the conventional interpretation of peak $\dot{V}O_2$ during growth in both boys and girls, and demonstrate that there is a progressive increase in peak $\dot{V}O_2$ with chronological age in both sexes, independent of the influence of body size.

Peak oxygen uptake and biological maturation

As young people grow they also mature, and the physiological responses of adolescents must be considered in relation to biological maturity as well as chronological age. Some studies indicate an adolescent growth spurt in peak $\dot{V}O_2$ in boys, with the spurt reaching a maximum gain near the time of PHV, but secure data are insufficient to offer any generalization for girls. With stage of maturity classified using secondary sexual characteristics, more mature young people have been reported to have a higher peak $\dot{V}O_2$ in $L \cdot min^{-1}$ than those less mature, but ratio scaled peak $\dot{V}O_2$ ($mL \cdot kg^{-1} \cdot min^{-1}$) has been reported to be unrelated to state of maturity, indicating no additional effect of biological maturity on peak $\dot{V}O_2$ above that due to growth.[76]

Armstrong *et al.*[77] argued that the true relationship between peak $\dot{V}O_2$ and biological maturity may have been obscured through an inappropriate means of controlling for body mass. They determined the peak $\dot{V}O_2$ of 176 12-year-olds and classified them according to the stages of pubic hair development described by Tanner[78]. In accord with the extant literature, mass-related peak $\dot{V}O_2$ ($mL \cdot kg^{-1} \cdot min^{-1}$) was not significantly different across stages of pubic hair development in either boys or girls. However, when body mass was controlled using allometry (log-linear analysis of covariance with mass as the covariate) peak $\dot{V}O_2$ was demonstrated to significantly increase with biological maturity in both sexes. None of the children were classified as in stage 5 for pubic hair development (PH5), but, with body mass controlled for, boys in PH4 exhibited peak $\dot{V}O_2$ values 14% higher than similarly aged boys in PH1. The corresponding difference in girls was 12%, thus demonstrating that in both boys and girls there is a significant independent effect of biological maturity on peak $\dot{V}O_2$ above that attributed to chronological age and body mass.

Armstrong and Welsman[65] introduced the same criterion of biological maturity into their multilevel regression model of 11–17-year-olds and confirmed their earlier findings on 11–13-year-olds[64] by showing incremental effects of stage of maturity on peak $\dot{V}O_2$ independent of chronological age and body mass (see Table 12.4). The positive effect of biological maturity on aerobic fitness was consistent for both boys and girls. When skinfold thicknesses were introduced into the model, the stage of pubic hair development remained a significant covariate in all but stage PH5, but the magnitudes of the effect were reduced, indicating the relationship between stage of biological maturity and body composition. With body mass, skinfold thicknesses, and pubic hair development accounted for, peak $\dot{V}O_2$ was shown to increase throughout the age range studied in both sexes. The girls' data are noteworthy as earlier longitudinal studies using conventional analyses to control for body mass suggested a decline in females' peak $\dot{V}O_2$ from age ~14 years. The authors concluded that LBM was the predominant influence in the increase in peak $\dot{V}O_2$ through adolescence, but that both chronological age and stage of biological maturity were additional explanatory variables, independent of body size and fatness.[65]

Peak oxygen uptake and sex

Boys' peak $\dot{V}O_2$ values are consistently higher than those of girls by late childhood[60] and the sex difference becomes more pronounced as young people progress through adolescence.[46] The data presented in Figure 12.4 indicate that peak $\dot{V}O_2$ is ~12% higher in boys than in girls at age 10 years, increasing to ~25% higher at 12, ~30% higher at 14, and ~35% higher at 16 years of age. Longitudinal data support this trend, although with small sample sizes there is some variation in the magnitude of sex differences, particularly within the age range 12–14 years, which is likely to be due to individual variations in the speed of biological clocks. These sex differences in peak $\dot{V}O_2$ during adolescence have been attributed to a combination of

Table 12.4 Multilevel regression model for peak oxygen uptake in 11–17-year-olds

Fixed	Estimate (SE)
Constant	−1.9005 (0.1400)
Log_e mass	0.8752 (0.0432)
Log_e stature	NS
Log_e skinfolds	−0.1656 (0.0174)
Age	0.0470 (0.0094)
Sex	−0.1372 (0.0121)
Age·sex	−0.0214 (0.0053)
Maturity 2	0.0341 (0.0094)
Maturity 3	0.0361 (0.0102)
Maturity 4	0.0537 (0.0116)
Maturity 5	NS
Random	0.0030 (0.0004)
Level 2	
Constant	0.0030 (0.0005)
Age	0.0004 (0.0001)
Level 1	
Constant	0.0032 (0.0004)

N = 388 NS, not significant.

Data from Welsman JR, Armstrong N, Kirby BJ, Nevill AM, Winter EM Scaling peak $\dot{V}O2$ for differences in body size. Med Sci Sports Exerc. 1996; 28: 259–265

factors including differences in daily physical activity, body composition, and blood haemoglobin concentration ([Hb]).

Boys are generally more physically active than girls,[27] but reviews of current physical activity patterns demonstrate that both sexes rarely experience the intensity, frequency, and duration of physical activity associated with increases in peak $\dot{V}O_2$.[79] Data are remarkably consistent and demonstrate no meaningful relationship between objectively measured daily physical activity and directly determined peak $\dot{V}O_2$ (see Armstrong *et al.*[80] for a table of relevant studies to date). There is therefore no compelling evidence to suggest that current levels of physical activity are likely to contribute to sexual dimorphism in peak $\dot{V}O_2$.

Muscle mass increases through childhood and adolescence, but although boys generally have more muscle mass than girls, marked sex differences do not become apparent until the adolescent growth spurt. Girls experience a growth spurt in muscle mass but it is less dramatic than that of boys. Between 5 and 16 years of age, boys' relative muscle mass increases from ~42–54% of body mass, whereas in girls muscle mass increases from ~40–45% of body mass between 5 and 13 years of age, and then, in relative terms, it declines due to an increase in fat accumulation during adolescence. Girls have slightly more body fat than boys during childhood, but during the growth spurt, girls' body fat increases to ~25% of body mass while boys decline to ~12–14% of body fat.[59] These dramatic changes in body composition in adolescence contribute to the progressive increase in sex differences in peak $\dot{V}O_2$ over this period. Boys' greater muscle mass not only facilitates the use of oxygen during exercise, but also supplements the venous return to the heart, and therefore augments SV through the peripheral muscle pump.

In adolescence there is a marked increase in [Hb] and hence oxygen-carrying capacity in boys, whereas girls' values plateau in their mid-teens. As [Hb] is significantly correlated with peak $\dot{V}O_2$ during adolescence it would be expected that differences in [Hb] between boys and girls, which are ~11% at 16 years, would be a contributory factor to the observed sex difference in peak $\dot{V}O_2$ during the late teens.[8] However, when [Hb] was investigated longitudinally as an additional explanatory variable to body mass, stature, skinfold thicknesses, age, and pubic hair development (as an indicator of stage of maturity), in a multilevel regression model of peak $\dot{V}O_2$ a non-significant parameter estimate was obtained with 11–17-year-olds.[65]

Prior to the onset of puberty there are only small sex differences in muscle mass and [Hb], but even with body size controlled for, prepubertal boys have consistently been demonstrated to have higher peak $\dot{V}O_2$ than prepubertal girls. For example, in a sample of 164 (53 girls) 11-year-old prepubertal children, boys' peak $\dot{V}O_2$ was observed to be ~22% higher than that of girls. With the removal of the influence of body mass using a log-linear adjustment model, boys' peak $\dot{V}O_2$ remained significantly higher (~16%) than girls' values despite there being no sex difference in either skinfold thickness or [Hb].[42]

Why prepubertal boys have significantly higher values of peak $\dot{V}O_2$ than prepubertal girls is not readily apparent, but the explanation might lie in the Fick equation. (Interested readers are referred to Chapter 11 for further discussion). There is no evidence to indicate sex differences in HR max, but boys have generally been observed to have higher SV max,[81] and therefore higher $\dot{Q}$ max, than girls, although there are conflicting data.[13] The trend for boys to have higher SV max during exercise has been attributed to their greater heart mass (or size) in relation to body mass (or size),[82] but conflicting data indicating no sex differences in relative heart size are available.[83] Exercise SV is, however, not just a function of ventricular size and it is difficult to distinguish between the complex and inter-related effects of ventricular preload, myocardial contractility, and ventricular afterload.

Vinet *et al.*[84] compared the cardiovascular responses of prepubertal boys and prepubertal girls using Doppler echocardiography during maximal cycle exercise. They reported no significant sex differences in a-vO_2 diff or HR at peak $\dot{V}O_2$, but the boys demonstrated significantly higher peak $\dot{V}O_2$ and SV max. They therefore concluded that the only component of peak $\dot{V}O_2$ that distinguished girls from boys was their lower SV max. The data indicated no significant sexual dimorphism in diastolic function indices or shortening or ejection fractions. Vinet and her colleagues[84] concluded that it is unlikely that overall cardiac contractility, relaxation, and compliance properties or loading conditions contribute to the sex difference in SV max, which is therefore due to differences in cardiac size rather than function.

In a similar study, Rowland *et al.*[85] compared prepubertal boys and premenarcheal girls and demonstrated that SV max was the sole cardiac variable responsible for sexual dimorphism in peak $\dot{V}O_2$ These authors noted that a characteristic that distinguished girls from boys was a lower rise in SV at the onset of exercise in girls. They suggested that cardiac functional factors (skeletal muscle pump function, systemic vascular resistance, and adrenergic responses) rather than intrinsic left ventricular size are responsible for the sex differences in SV max during childhood.

There are few secure data on young children's a-vO_2 diff at peak $\dot{V}O_2$, but a study which used thoracic bioelectrical impedance to determine the $\dot{Q}$ at peak $\dot{V}O_2$, of 31 (13 girls) 10-year-olds provided some interesting insights into prepubertal differences in peak $\dot{V}O_2$. The boys had a significantly higher mean peak $\dot{V}O_2$ than the girls (~19%) but no significant sex differences in stature, body mass, LBM, % body fat, body mass index, body surface area, [Hb], HR at peak $\dot{V}O_2$, R at peak $\dot{V}O_2$, SV at peak $\dot{V}O_2$, or $\dot{Q}$ at peak $\dot{V}O_2$ were observed. Furthermore, heart size variables determined at rest using magnetic resonance imaging (MRI) revealed no significant sex differences in left ventricular muscle mass, left ventricular muscle volume, posterior wall thickness, septal wall thickness, left ventricular end-diastolic chamber volume, or left ventricular end-systolic chamber volume. The only significant sex difference was in a-vO_2 diff at peak $\dot{V}O_2$ where boys' values were ~17% higher than those of girls.[13]

The emergence of non-invasive technology has opened up new avenues of research with, for example, NIRS allowing the non-invasive measurement of microcirculatory changes in deoxygenated haemoglobin and myoglobin ([HHb]). An initial study demonstrated a more rapid rate of change in [HHb] during ramp exercise to peak $\dot{V}O_2$ in prepubertal girls than in prepubertal boys. These intriguing data indicate that a poorer matching of muscle oxygen delivery to muscle oxygen utilization in prepubertal girls might contribute to their lower peak $\dot{V}O_2$, but they require confirmatory evidence from different exercise models.[86]

Blood lactate accumulation

PO Åstrand's[5] experimental studies of physical working capacity popularized the use of blood lactate accumulation as an objective measure of young people's effort, and blood sampling for lactate is a common procedure in many paediatric exercise physiology laboratories. The extant literature is, however, confounded by methodological issues which have contributed to the controversy surrounding the interpretation of young people's blood lactate responses to exercise. This section outlines methodological issues, comments on blood lactate thresholds and reference values of performance during youth, and reviews the data on blood lactate responses to exercise in relation to chronological age, biological maturity, and sexual dimorphism.

Methodological issues

Research with children should not employ blood sampling as a routine procedure and for ethical reasons a strong case should always be made to justify it in relation to the research question. Strict practices must be followed at all times in the sampling and handling of blood with the health and safety of both the child and the investigator paramount. Detailed health and safety issues in haematology are beyond the scope of this chapter, and readers are referred to Maughan *et al.*[87] for further guidance. Similarly, a detailed review of blood lactate assessment techniques during youth appears elsewhere,[26] and only key issues are outlined here.

Muscle lactate produced during leg exercise diffuses into the femoral veins, and then rapidly appears in the arterial circulation. It has been demonstrated that blood sampled from the arm arteries provides a close reflection of the extent of lactate diffusion into the systemic circulation.[88] The ethical, technical, and medical hazards associated with arterial blood sampling preclude its use with healthy young people, but it has been shown that arterial lactate levels are closely reflected by capillary lactate levels during treadmill exercise if a good blood flow is maintained at the sampling site.[89] Most paediatric laboratories therefore sample lactate from the capillaries in the fingertip or earlobe. To facilitate blood flow the site can be warmed and to reduce children's anxiety an anaesthetic cream or spray can be applied.

Once sampled, 'whole blood' can be immediately assayed in an automatic analyser and results reported as blood lactate accumulation. Before making cross-study comparisons of blood lactate accumulation during or following exercise, researchers must, however, confirm the comparability of the lactate assay used and the automatic analyser. Prior to the ready availability of automatic analysers, lactate was routinely assayed in preparations such as lysed blood, protein-free blood, plasma, or serum, and often reported as 'blood lactate'. The significant variation in reporting children's blood lactate accumulation from different assays was clearly illustrated in a study which reported lactate values from the same blood sample as 4 $mmol \cdot L^{-1}$ when assayed as whole blood, 4.4 $mmol \cdot L^{-1}$ when the blood was lysed, and 5.5 $mmol \cdot L^{-1}$ from a plasma preparation.[89]

Young people's blood lactate responses to exercise are influenced by mode of exercise, exercise protocol, and time of sampling. Blood lactate reference values are heavily dependent on definition and measurement technique. As discussed in the Ergometry section, when cycling during part of the pedal revolution there is a potential for restriction in children's blood flow through the quadriceps, which will promote anaerobic metabolism. Children's blood lactate accumulation in relation to $p\dot{V}O_2$ is therefore not directly comparable during cycling and treadmill running. Regardless of ergometer, during an incremental exercise test, increments should be small and each exercise stage must be sustained for at least 3 min to allow adequate diffusion of lactate from muscle to blood. If sampled too soon the blood lactate accumulation will not reflect the intensity of the exercise and will profoundly influence the blood lactate reference value.[25]

Numerous fixed blood lactate values (e.g. 4 $mmol \cdot L^{-1}$) have been recommended as submaximal reference measures of adult performance. However, several of these reference values were originally determined using serum or plasma samples and all are problematic when applied to children. A study of 11–13-year-olds, for example, reported that 34% of boys and 12% of girls did not achieve a whole blood lactate value of 4 $mmol \cdot L^{-1}$ at peak $\dot{V}O_2$. The authors suggested that a criterion reference of 2.5 $mmol \cdot L^{-1}$ from a whole blood assay might be more appropriate for children,[17] but any fixed blood lactate value is likely to be inappropriate throughout childhood and adolescence as studies suggest an age-dependent trend in blood lactate responses to exercise.[90]

The T_{LAC}, which represents the individual's response to increasing exercise-induced metabolic demands, has become recognized as an appropriate blood lactate indicator of young people's submaximal aerobic fitness. The T_{LAC} is defined as the first observable increase in blood lactate accumulation above resting levels. It can be determined from visual inspection of the inflection in blood lactate accumulation, but a clear inflection point is not always discernible and some investigators have used mathematical interpolation or defined the point of inflection as a 1 $mmol \cdot L^{-1}$ increase over baseline.[16]

The MLSS represents the upper point at which the processes of blood lactate accumulation and elimination are in equilibrium and theoretically provides a sensitive measure of submaximal aerobic fitness. However, because of the requirement for multiple blood samples over several ~20 min stages at the border of heavy and very heavy-intensity exercise, it is difficult to motivate children to participate in this type of test. Furthermore, there is no consensus over the optimum test time or magnitude of acceptable variation in blood lactate accumulation to represent MLSS.[17] Young people's MLSS data should therefore be interpreted cautiously. Exercise just below CPo has been shown to correspond reasonably well with MLSS in adolescents, and this non-invasive variable may be more appropriate for use during youth.[36]

Chronological age, biological maturity, and sex

Data describing the relationship between chronological age and blood lactate responses to submaximal exercise are equivocal primarily as a result of variation in exercise protocols, threshold and reference value definitions, blood sampling and assay techniques, and the predominance of underpowered and single-sex studies. Data from girls are sparse but there is no compelling evidence of sexual dimorphism in blood lactate responses to submaximal exercise during youth.[90]

Investigations have consistently observed an age-related trend of the T_{LAC} occurring at a higher % of peak $\dot{V}O_2$ in children than in adults.[90] These data have been supported by studies reporting an age-related trend in the T_{VENT} in relation to % of peak $\dot{V}O_2$ during youth.[18] In contrast there is no evidence to support a relationship between blood lactate accumulation at MLSS and age, or between MLSS as a % of peak $\dot{V}O_2$ and age.[17] In general support of differentiating between T_{LAC} and MLSS, a study of 149 11–16-year-olds found no significant relationship between age and % peak $\dot{V}O_2$ at a blood lactate of 4 $mmol \cdot L^{-1}$, but a significant correlation was observed between age and % peak $\dot{V}O_2$ at a reference value postulated to be near T_{LAC} (i.e. 2.5 $mmol \cdot L^{-1}$) in the same 11–16-year-olds studied.[91]

In his seminal thesis Eriksson[92] hypothesized a maturation effect on muscle lactate production, as he observed it to be 'almost significantly' correlated with testicular volume. He proposed that boys' blood lactate accumulation would reflect their muscle lactate production. On the basis of proportion of type I muscle fibres, $p\dot{V}O_2$ kinetics, exercise metabolism, exercise endocrinology, and substrate use during exercise, a compelling theoretical case can be made for a maturational effect on the production of muscle lactate and its accumulation in blood.[93] Empirical studies have, however, been consistent in failing to detect an independent effect of maturity on blood lactate accumulation during exercise. For example, an investigation using multiple regression analyses to examine the effect of salivary testosterone upon the blood lactate responses to exercise of 50 12–16-year-old boys observed no significant, independent effect of testosterone on blood lactate accumulation.[94] Similarly, an analysis of 119 11–16-year-old boys and girls classified into the maturity stages described by Tanner[78] observed no effect of stage of maturity on blood lactate accumulation at peak $\dot{V}O_2$.[91]

Pulmonary oxygen uptake kinetics

During a step change in exercise intensity, once the cardiodynamic phase has been deleted, the exponential rise in $p\dot{V}O_2$ has been demonstrated to reflect in adults the kinetics of $m\dot{V}O_2$ and to therefore provide a non-invasive window into metabolic activity in muscle.[95] The work has not been replicated with children, but a close relationship between children's intramuscular phosphocreatine (PCr) kinetics during prone quadriceps exercise in a MR scanner and $p\dot{V}O_2$ kinetics during upright cycling at both the onset and offset of exercise has been demonstrated.[96] This relationship has opened up new avenues of research in developmental exercise metabolism.[97] The kinetics of $p\dot{V}O_2$ and intramusclular PCr (as a surrogate of $m\dot{V}O_2$) at the onset of exercise are complex, and are comprehensively analysed in Chapter 13 and Chapter 6 where the theoretical principles are explained, the underlying mechanisms explored, and the rigorous methodology required to characterize the kinetic responses critiqued. Discussion here is restricted to identifying methodological issues in the determination of young people's $p\dot{V}O_2$ kinetics responses which might influence their interpretation. The focus is on exploring the $p\dot{V}O_2$ kinetics responses to a step change in exercise intensity in relation to exercise domain, chronological age, and sexual dimorphism. The independent influence (if any) of biological maturity on $p\dot{V}O_2$ kinetics remains to be rigorously investigated.

Methodological issues

The clarification of the $p\dot{V}O_2$ kinetics response at the onset of exercise depends upon the ability to rigorously evaluate the speed and the magnitude of the respiratory gas exchange response to a given metabolic demand. This can be achieved by imposing a predetermined square wave exercise stress and then using non-linear regression and iterative fitting procedures with the response data to fit a specified model to return the rate of the exponential rise and the amplitude of the response. Unfortunately, a wide array of models with various degrees of rigour have been employed to evaluate $p\dot{V}O_2$ kinetics, and interested readers are referred to Fawkner and Armstrong,[98] who have critiqued and tabulated chronological models used with children and adolescents. The confounding effect of different modelling techniques on the interpretation of young people's response parameters has been shown empirically by applying several different models to the same dataset in both the moderate[99] and heavy-intensity exercise domains.[100] The use of different models, several with limited physiological rationales, has made understanding the extant paediatric literature problematic.[31]

Even with an appropriate modelling procedure, the rigorous resolution of the $p\dot{V}O_2$ kinetics of children and adolescents is challenging. Children's inherently erratic breathing pattern reduces the signal-to-noise ratio of their pulmonary gas exchange kinetics.[47] Large inter-breath fluctuations reduce the confidence with which $p\dot{V}O_2$ kinetic responses can be estimated, and confidence intervals are likely to be beyond acceptable limits unless sufficient identical transitions are time aligned and averaged to improve the signal to noise ratio.[101] The number of transitions that are required to achieve suitable confidence is directly proportional to the amount of data being fit, the variability of the data, and the magnitude of the signal, and will thus vary from one person to another. With children, as many as ten transitions may be required in the moderate-intensity exercise domain to establish an acceptable confidence interval for the primary component τ.[102] Fewer transitions are required in heavier-intensity exercise domains because the magnitude of the signal is greater.

Young people's lower peak $\dot{V}O_2$, and therefore smaller range of metabolic rates achievable, may compromise the integrity of working within specific exercise domains. Children's T_{VENT} occurs at ~60–70% of peak $\dot{V}O_2$[19] and to ensure that the prescribed exercise is clearly within the moderate domain, the upper border of exercise intensity is normally set at ~80% of T_{VENT}. With children, the $p\dot{V}O_2$ kinetics responses to exercise intensities above T_{VENT} have rarely been investigated within carefully defined parameters. This is most likely because the assessment of CPo, the upper boundary of heavy-intensity exercise, and the threshold of very heavy-intensity exercise is demanding in terms of both subject effort and testing time.[20] Investigators in adult studies normally use 40–50% of the difference between T_{VENT} and peak $\dot{V}O_2$ (e.g. 40% Δ) as describing exercise within the heavy-intensity domain[30]. It has been demonstrated that CPo occurs at ~70–80% of peak $\dot{V}O_2$ in children, similar to relative values reported for adults, and that exercise at an intensity of 40% Δ is below CPo and falls within the heavy-intensity exercise domain.[103] However, the absolute range of $p\dot{V}O_2$ between T_{VENT} and CPo is small in children and there is considerable individual variation in the relative position of both T_{VENT} and CPo in relation to peak $\dot{V}O_2$. The 40% Δ concept is therefore less secure on an individual basis with children than with adults.

Exercise phases, exercise domains, chronological age, and sex

Macek and Vavra[104] were the first to investigate the half-time of children's transient responses to the onset of exercise, but the initial application of breath-by-breath technology to children's $p\dot{V}O_2$ kinetics was carried out by Dan Cooper and his colleagues.[105] Data from early studies are inconsistent, but recent research using more rigorous methodology, sophisticated mathematical modelling techniques, and emerging technologies has begun to map out young people's transient responses to the onset of a step change in exercise intensity.[31]

Cardiodynamic phase

Following the onset of exercise, $p\dot{V}O_2$ measured at the mouth is dissociated temporarily from $\dot{V}O_2$ at the muscle by the muscle-lung transit delay. The speed of the response is due to the almost instantaneous increase in $\dot{Q}$ which is initiated by vagal withdrawal and the mechanical pumping action of the contracting muscles. The rise in $\dot{V}O_2$ that is evidenced at the mouth during this translational phase is therefore independent from absolute changes in mixed partial pressures arising from the working muscles. If the muscle-lung transit delay is a function of growth, the shorter distance between exercising muscles and the lung in children might suggest an age-related increase in the length of phase I. However, data on phase I in various exercise domains are ambiguous and often confounded by methodological issues. Studies which have attempted to determine the end of phase I visually from response profiles of end-tidal partial pressures of oxygen and carbon dioxide and R must be interpreted cautiously. For the purposes of modelling the primary component the duration of phase I is normally not measured but is assumed to be constant at ~15–20 s.[21,106]

Rigorously determined age- and sex-related data from phase I are sparse. Men have been reported to have a longer duration of phase I than boys in response to the onset of a transition to 50% of peak $\dot{V}O_2$.[107] Longitudinal data show the duration of phase I following the onset of heavy intensity exercise to increase from age 10 to 13 years in both boys (16.7–19.5 s) and girls (20.7–24.3 s).[32] In contrast to adults it has been noted that the duration of phase I in boys is not reduced at higher metabolic rates.[107] Sexual dimorphism has been reported in prepubertal children, with boys noted to have a shorter phase I duration than girls (17.0 vs 19.3 s).[55] This might be indicative of a more rapid increase in SV in boys than in girls, an observation previously noted using Doppler echocardiography.[85] Evidently little is known about age and sex differences and their mechanisms in the duration of phase I. Independent effects of biological maturity on the cardiodynamic phase have not been investigated.

Moderate-intensity exercise

Data from studies of young people's phase II response to the onset of moderate-intensity exercise are equivocal, but several studies are methodologically flawed on the basis of their failure to employ well-defined participant groups, to apply appropriate analytical modelling techniques, to address the low signal-to-noise ratio through adequate exercise transitions, and to report the 95% confidence intervals.[21] These studies and their modelling techniques have been tabulated elsewhere (see Table 13.1), and although often failing to reach statistical significance the strong trend among the studies which used breath-by-breath respiratory gas analysis is for a shorter τ in children and adolescents than in adults.[31]

A carefully designed and modelled study, in which up to ten repeat exercise transitions were completed to ensure the 95% confidence intervals spanning the primary component τ were no more than ± 5 s, addressed the lack of consensus in the extant literature[102]. It was demonstrated unequivocally that the primary component τ was significantly shorter in boys than men (19 vs 28 s) and in girls than women (21 vs 26 s). No sexual dimorphism was observed in the primary component τ despite significant sex differences in peak $\dot{V}O_2$. Peak $\dot{V}O_2$ was not related to the phase II τ, a finding in contrast to earlier data from adults,[22] but later confirmed in a comparison of trained and untrained prepubertal children.[108]

It is not only the speed of the $p\dot{V}O_2$ kinetics responses, but also the magnitude of the response (gain of the primary component or oxygen cost of the response) that provides information on the efficiency of the integrated pulmonary, cardiovascular, and muscle metabolic systems. A substantially higher primary gain in children than in adults has been reported during both treadmill running[109] and cycling.[110] However, in the treadmill running study the gain was expressed in ratio with body mass ($mL \cdot kg^{-1} \cdot km^{-1}$) and, as argued throughout this chapter, in most circumstances this is an inappropriate way to normalize comparative data.[72] Although the balance of evidence supports a higher gain in children,[30] further examination with more rigorous study designs is required to tease out definitive age-related differences in the oxygen cost of the response to moderate intensity exercise.

Children's shorter τ, and therefore greater aerobic contribution to ATP re-synthesis at the onset of exercise, indicates that compared to adults they have an enhanced oxidative capacity, which might be due to greater oxygen delivery or better oxygen utilization in the muscles. Peak $\dot{V}O_2$, which is thought to be primarily dependent on oxygen delivery, is not related to the primary component τ and there is no compelling theoretical hypothesis to indicate that increased delivery of oxygen would speed the rate of healthy young people's $p\dot{V}O_2$ kinetics during moderate-intensity exercise.[30] However, a study utilizing NIRS, HR kinetics, and breath-by-breath technology noted that, compared with men, prepubertal boys presented a shorter primary component τ supported by both a quicker adjustment in [HHb] kinetics and faster local blood flow. It was concluded that faster oxygen extraction and oxygen delivery might both have a role to play in children's faster $p\dot{V}O_2$ kinetics.[111] More research is required to tease out the mechanisms underpinning age-related differences in τ.

Heavy-intensity exercise

Young people's $p\dot{V}O_2$ kinetics responses to the onset of exercise above T_{VENT} are masked in several studies which employ inadequate mathematical models and poor definitions of the heavy- and very heavy-intensity exercise domains, sometimes by simply using % peak $\dot{V}O_2$ to characterize the exercise domain.[98] Nevertheless, despite often-flawed methodology, the literature is consistent in demonstrating that at the onset of heavy-intensity exercise, children have a faster primary component τ than adults.[110]

Two longitudinal studies determined acceptable confidence intervals for the τ and amplitude of the primary component at the onset of heavy-intensity exercise. The first study demonstrated a faster primary component τ in both prepubertal girls and boys than the same children presented 2 years later (boys, 17 vs 21 s; girls, 22 vs 26 s).[32] In the second study 14-year-old boys presented a shorter phase II τ than they did 2 years later (26 vs 30 s).[35] In children, but not adolescent boys, the primary gain decreased over a 2-year period (12.4 vs 12.0 $mL \cdot min^{-1} \cdot W^{-1}$), thus supporting the age-related effect shown in wider age comparisons of children and adults (11.6 vs 9.9 $mL \cdot min^{-1} \cdot W^{-1}$).[110] The same research group demonstrated that, in contrast with their findings at the onset of moderate-intensity exercise, prepubertal boys presented a faster primary component τ than prepubertal girls (18 vs 22 s). No significant sex difference in the primary gain was observed.[55] In accord with exercise in the moderate-intensity domain, but in conflict with adult data, studies consistently show that peak $\dot{V}O_2$ is not related to the phase II τ in prepubertal children[32] or adolescents[35] during exercise in the heavy-intensity domain.

During exercise above T_{VENT} but below CPo adults' phase III is characterized by the oxygen cost increasing over time as a $p\dot{V}O_2$ slow component is superimposed and the achievement of a steady state is delayed[30] (see Figure 12.3). Initial comparisons of children and adults concluded that during heavy-intensity exercise, children demonstrate a negligible $p\dot{V}O_2$ slow component and their responses could be modelled as a mono-exponential process.[109,110] Contrary to these reports, in a series of studies Fawkner and Armstrong[100] demonstrated empirically that a slow component does exist in children and the data should not be modelled mono-exponentially. They showed that with appropriate modelling prepubertal children exhibit a $p\dot{V}O_2$ slow component, which contributes ~10% of the end-exercise $p\dot{V}O_2$ after 9 min of exercise and increases in magnitude with age.[32] It was noted that, despite an increase in the magnitude of the $p\dot{V}O_2$ slow component, the overall oxygen cost at the end of exercise was equal on test occasions 2 years apart. This suggests that the phosphate turnover required to sustain exercise is independent of age and that younger children achieve a larger proportion of their end-exercise $p\dot{V}O_2$ during phase II. A subsequent study identified significant sexual dimorphism in prepubertal children with the $p\dot{V}O_2$ slow component of boys and girls accounting for ~9% and ~12% respectively of the end-exercise $p\dot{V}O_2$.[55] The same research group also demonstrated the presence of a $p\dot{V}O_2$ slow component, which increased in magnitude with age in adolescent boys.[35] Subsequent research has unequivocally established the presence of a $p\dot{V}O_2$ slow component during heavy-intensity exercise in both prepubertal children[112] and adolescents.[113]

There is symmetry between the rate of PCr breakdown and the $p\dot{V}O_2$ primary component τ at the onset of exercise above T_{VENT},[30] which suggests that the shorter phase II τ in young people might be due to an age-dependent effect on mitochondrial oxidative phosphorylation. There is a paucity of data, but this postulate is supported by children's enhanced aerobic enzymes activities and/or lower glycolytic enzymes activities compared to adults.[57] As ~85% of the $p\dot{V}O_2$ slow component originates from the exercising muscles, the increase in the magnitude of the $p\dot{V}O_2$ slow component with age is likely due to progressive changes in muscle fibre recruitment patterns. The enhanced glycogen depletion of type I fibres and the greater recruitment of type II fibres by adults will promote an increased $p\dot{V}O_2$ slow component. The data are in accord with children having a higher % of type I muscle fibres than adults, and the reported sexual dimorphism in the phase II τ and $p\dot{V}O_2$ slow component are consistent with girls having a lower % of type I fibres than similarly aged boys.[57]

Very heavy-intensity exercise

In the very heavy-exercise intensity domain boys have a shorter phase II τ (21 vs 34 s), a greater primary gain (10.8 vs 8.2 $mL \cdot min^{-1} \cdot W^{-1}$), and a smaller relative $p\dot{V}O_2$ slow component (11 vs 16%) than men.[114,115] As demonstrated in other exercise domains, peak $\dot{V}O_2$ is not related to the phase II τ.[114] The presence of a $p\dot{V}O_2$ slow component in prepubertal children[116] and teenage boys[117] during very heavy exercise is not disputed, but sexual dimorphism has not been addressed in this exercise domain. Exploratory investigations of the contribution of oxygen delivery and oxygen utilization to boys' $p\dot{V}O_2$ kinetics have used priming exercise to elevate $\dot{Q}$ and muscle oxygenation prior to and throughout subsequent very heavy-intensity exercise. Phase II $p\dot{V}O_2$ kinetics (i.e. τ) were reported to be unaltered but the $p\dot{V}O_2$ slow component amplitude was reduced, suggesting that phase II $p\dot{V}O_2$ kinetics are principally limited by intrinsic muscle metabolic factors, and that the $p\dot{V}O_2$ slow component is sensitive to oxygen delivery.[118,119]

In conflict with adult data[30] (see Figure 12.3), young people's $p\dot{V}O_2$ slow component when exercising above CPo has not been demonstrated to project to peak $\dot{V}O_2$ over time but to stabilize at ~85–90% of peak $\dot{V}O_2$.[36,] It has been suggested that this may be due to an early termination of exercise by young people through exhaustion.[120]

Severe-intensity exercise

The resolution of the $p\dot{V}O_2$ kinetics response to a system-limited value (i.e. peak $\dot{V}O_2$) is complex and it is problematic to compare investigations using different data collection and modelling techniques. Few studies have been dedicated to unravelling the $p\dot{V}O_2$ kinetics response to severe exercise during youth and available data must be interpreted with caution.[21]

Early studies, which collected $\dot{V}_E$ in gasometers or Douglas bags over 30 s periods, reported boys to achieve a higher percentage of their peak $\dot{V}O_2$ than men during the first 30 s of exercise, requiring at least 100% peak $\dot{V}O_2$.[3,104] However, the lack of temporal resolution of the respiratory gas exchange measurements and the failure to consider phase I compromises the data, and two more recent studies using breath-by-breath technology have failed to confirm these findings.

Hebestreit *et al.*[107] investigated the p$\dot{V}O_2$ kinetics of 9- to 12-year-old boys and of men at the onset of cycling exercise to 100% and 130% of peak $\dot{V}O_2$. On both occasions, once phase I had been excluded, p$\dot{V}O_2$ kinetics could be described by a mono-exponential function (i.e. no p$\dot{V}O_2$ slow component detected) in which no age-related differences were observed for the primary component τ. This study confirmed earlier work which had shown that, when compared to adults, children have higher end-exercise oxygen cost during severe exercise.[121]

Recovery kinetics

Further insights into the development of aerobic fitness undoubtedly lie in the p$\dot{V}O_2$ kinetics of recovery from exercise in different domains, but the only study to specifically investigate the influence of age on p$\dot{V}O_2$ kinetics at the offset of exercise appears to be that of Zanconato *et al.*[121] They analysed the recovery p$\dot{V}O_2$ kinetics of mixed sex groups of children (7–11 years) and adults (26–42 years) following a single 1 min bout of exercise at 80% T_{VENT}, 50% Δ, 100% peak $\dot{V}O_2$, and 125% peak $\dot{V}O_2$. The only significant child-adult difference reported was children's faster recovery from 125% peak $\dot{V}O_2$.

Rigorously determined breath-by-breath data on p$\dot{V}O_2$ kinetics at the offset of exercise during youth are sparse. Lai *et al.*[120] observed similar time courses for recovery p$\dot{V}O_2$ kinetics of male adolescents (14–17-year-olds) when compared with previously published data on adults. They reported that adolescents' recovery p$\dot{V}O_2$ kinetics from both moderate- and heavy-intensity exercise can be described with a single exponential, but that recovery from very heavy-intensity exercise is characterized by two components, one fast and one slow. Lai *et al.*[120] noted that steady states for the p$\dot{V}O_2$ kinetics off-response were attained in ~5 min for moderate- and heavy-intensity exercise and within ~10 min for very heavy-intensity exercise. In contrast, with adults the recovery p$\dot{V}O_2$ slow component from very heavy exercise has been reported to take >20 min to dissipate.[30]

Comparisons of trained and untrained young athletes have confirmed that the p$\dot{V}O_2$ offset kinetics of both moderate- and heavy-intensity exercise can be described with a single exponential. Intriguingly, although the trained athletes displayed faster p$\dot{V}O_2$ kinetics at the onset of both moderate- and heavy-intensity exercise than their untrained peers, only the recovery p$\dot{V}O_2$ kinetics from heavy-intensity exercise were faster in the trained athletes.[122,123] (Interested readers are invited to read Chapter 34 for more detailed discussion).

Conclusions

The laboratory assessment of young people's peak (or max) $\dot{V}O_2$ dates back to 1938 and it is the most researched variable in paediatric exercise science. Yet, debate over the determination and terminology of peak and/or maximal values of $\dot{V}O_2$ persists. The fallacy of expressing peak $\dot{V}O_2$ in ratio with body mass has been documented for over 65 years, but ratios are still reported. Decisive action and insistence on contextual reporting of peak $\dot{V}O_2$ by academic journal editors is required to disseminate the appropriate interpretation of aerobic fitness during growth and maturation. Nevertheless, analysis of data using sophisticated modelling techniques has enhanced understanding of sexual dimorphism and the independent effects of chronological age, body size, and biological maturity on peak $\dot{V}O_2$. The mechanisms underlying sex differences in peak $\dot{V}O_2$ prior to puberty remain to be elucidated, but the introduction of recent non-invasive technology such as NIRS provides promising avenues for future research.

Despite its ubiquity in the literature, the use of fixed post-exercise values of blood lactate accumulation to verify a maximal effort during an exercise test to elicit peak $\dot{V}O_2$ is untenable. The monitoring of blood lactate accumulation and the determination of blood lactate accumulation thresholds (e.g. T_{LAC}) during exercise provides an indicator of the ability to sustain submaximal exercise and a sensitive means of evaluating improvements in muscle oxidative capacity with exercise training. The relationship between blood lactate accumulation and chronological age is well-documented, but sex differences in blood lactate accumulation during youth remain to be proven. A persuasive theoretical argument can be presented for an independent effect of maturity on blood lactate accumulation, although there is no compelling empirical evidence to support the case and more research with appropriate methodology and power to adequately address the problem is required.

Young people's physical activity patterns and participation in most organized sports are reliant on intermittent exercise and rapid changes in exercise intensity. Under these conditions peak $\dot{V}O_2$ and blood lactate accumulation thresholds are variables of investigative convenience rather than factors underpinning exercise behaviour, and it is the kinetics of p$\dot{V}O_2$ which best describe aerobic fitness. Rigorously determined and appropriately analysed studies of young people's p$\dot{V}O_2$ kinetic responses to step changes in exercise intensity are sparse. The extant data describe intriguing chronological age- and sex-related differences across exercise domains, although independent effects of biological maturity are yet to be revealed. Unique insights into aerobic fitness during youth rest in the transient response to and recovery from a forcing exercise regimen. The challenge is to identify and explain the underlying mechanisms and how they evolve during childhood and adolescence.

No single measure describes fully aerobic fitness and this chapter has focused on arguably the three most important variables in relation to chronological age, body mass, biological maturity, and sex. We conclude that although aerobic fitness is the most researched trait in paediatric exercise physiology, much remains to be learned.[124]

Summary

- Aerobic fitness can be defined as the ability to deliver oxygen to the exercising muscles and to utilize it to generate energy during exercise. No single variable describes fully aerobic fitness.
- Boys' peak $\dot{V}O_2$ expressed in $L \cdot min^{-1}$ increases in a near-linear manner with chronological age. Girls' data demonstrate a similar but less consistent trend with several cross-sectional and longitudinal studies indicating a tendency for peak $\dot{V}O_2$ to plateau from ~14 years of age.
- With body mass appropriately controlled for using allometry, boys' peak $\dot{V}O_2$ increases from childhood through adolescence and into young adulthood. Girls' values increase from prepuberty until mid-teens, then level-off as they approach young adulthood.
- Biological maturation exerts a significant and positive effect on the peak $\dot{V}O_2$ of both sexes independent of that due to chronological aging, body composition, and body mass.

- Prepubertal boys have higher peak $\dot{V}O_2$ values than prepubertal girls.
- There is a progressive divergence in sex differences in peak $\dot{V}O_2$ in puberty largely due to sex-related growth in muscle mass.
- Interpretation of blood lactate accumulation during exercise is clouded by methodological issues related to mode of exercise, exercise protocol, timing of blood sample, site of sampling, and assay technique
- The lactate threshold normally occurs at a higher % of peak $\dot{V}O_2$ in children than in adults, and there is no compelling evidence to suggest sexual dimorphism.
- Empirical studies have consistently failed to detect an independent effect of biological maturation on blood lactate accumulation during exercise.
- The confident estimation of the primary component time constant and appropriate modelling of the amplitude of the slow component is challenging and rigorous studies of $p\dot{V}O_2$ kinetics during youth are sparse.
- The primary component time constant is negatively related to chronological age in both sexes across the moderate, heavy, and very heavy exercise domains.
- During exercise above the ventilatory threshold, boys' primary component time constant is shorter than that of girls, whereas the amplitude of the $p\dot{V}O_2$ slow component is greater in girls. Little is known about $p\dot{V}O_2$ kinetic responses to severe exercise.
- The relative contribution of oxygen delivery and oxygen utilization to the speed of the primary component time constant in different exercise domains remains to be elucidated.
- In contrast to adults, the primary component time constant is not related to peak $\dot{V}O_2$ during youth.
- The amplitude of the $p\dot{V}O_2$ slow component of oxygen uptake is positively related to chronological age during exercise above the ventilatory threshold.
- Data on the $p\dot{V}O_2$ kinetics recovery from exercise in different domains are sparse.
- Whether there is an independent effect of biological maturation on the $p\dot{V}O_2$ kinetics response at the onset and offset of exercise is unknown.

References

1. Bouchard C, Daw EW, Rice T, *et al.* Familial resemblance for $\dot{V}O_2$ max in the sedentary state: The HERITAGE family study. *Med Sci Sports Exerc.* 1998; 30: 252–258.
2. Hill AV, Lupton H. Muscular exercise, lactic acid and the supply and utilization of oxygen. *Q J Med.*1923; 16: 135–171.
3. Robinson S. Experimental studies of physical fitness in relation to age. *Arbeitsphysiologie.* 1938; 10: 251–323.
4. Morse M, Schlutz FW, Cassels DE. Relation of age to physiological responses of the older boy to exercise. *J Appl Physiol.* 1949; 1: 683–709.
5. Åstrand PO. *Experimental studies of physical working capacity in relation to sex and age.* Copenhagen: Munksgaard; 1952.
6. Rowland TW, Cunningham LN. Development of ventilatory responses to exercise in normal caucasian children: A longitudinal study. *Chest.* 1997; 111: 327–332.
7. Armstrong N, Kirby BJ, McManus AM, Welsman JR. Prepubescents' ventilatory responses to exercise with reference to sex and body size. *Chest.* 1997; 112: 1554–1560.
8. Armstrong N, Balding J, Gentle P, Williams J, Kirby B. Peak oxygen uptake of British children with reference to age, sex and sexual maturity. *Eur J Appl Physiol.* 1990; 62: 369–375.
9. Nottin S, Agnes V, Stecken N, *et al.* Central and peripheral cardiovascular adaptations during maximal cycle exercise in boys and men. *Med Sci Sports Exerc.* 2002; 33: 456–463.
10. McNarry MA, Jones AM. The influence of training status on the aerobic and anaerobic responses to exercise in children. A review. *Eur J Sport Sci.* 2014; 14(Suppl): 557–568.
11. Vinet A, Nottin S, Lecoq AM, Obert P. Cardiovascular responses to progressive cycle exercise in healthy children and adults. *Int J Sports Med.* 2002; 23: 242–246.
12. Rowland TW, Popowski B, Ferrone L. Cardiac responses to maximal upright cycle exercise in healthy boys and men. *Med Sci Sports Exerc.* 1997; 29: 1146–1151.
13. Winsley RJ, Fulford J, Roberts AC, Welsman JR, Armstrong N. Sex difference in peak oxygen uptake in prepubertal children. *J Sci Med Sport.* 2009; 12: 647–651.
14. Weltman A. *The blood lactate response to exercise*, Champaign, IL: Human Kinetics; 1995.
15. Wasserman K, Hansen JE, Sue DY, *et al. Principles of exercise testing and interpretation. Including pathophysiology and clinical applications*, 5th ed. Philadelphia: Lippincott, Williams and Wilkins; 2012.
16. Pfitzinger P, Freedson P. Blood lactate responses to exercise in children: Part 2. Lactate threshold. *Pediatr Exerc Sci.* 1997; 9: 299–307.
17. Benecke R, Heck H, Schwarz V, Leithauser R. Maximal lactate steady state during the second decade of life. *Med Sci Sports Exerc.* 1996; 28: 1474–1478.
18. Mahon AD, Cheatham CR. Ventilatory threshold in children. A review. *Pediatr Exerc Sci.* 2002; 14: 16–29.
19. Fawkner SG, Armstrong N, Childs DJ, Welsman JR. Reliability of the visually identified ventilatory threshold and V-slope in children. *Pediatr Exerc Sci.* 2002; 14: 189–193.
20. Fawkner SG, Armstrong N. Assessment of critical power with children. *Pediatr Exerc Sci.* 2002; 14: 259–268.
21. Fawkner SG, Armstrong N. Oxygen uptake kinetic response to exercise in children. *Sports Med.* 2003; 33: 651–669.
22. Barker AR, Armstrong, N. Exercise testing elite young athletes. *Med Sport Sci.* 2011; 56: 106–125.
23. Pfitzinger P, Freedson P. Blood lactate responses to exercise in children: Part 1. Peak lactate concentration. *Pediatr Exerc Sci.* 1997; 9: 210–222.
24. Cumming GR, Hastman L, McCort J, McCullough S, High serum lactates do occur in children after maximal work. *Int J Sports Med.* 1980; 1: 66–69.
25. Williams JR, Armstrong N, Kirby BJ. The 4mM blood lactate level as an index of exercise performance in 11–13-year-old children. *J Sports Sci.* 1990; 8: 139–147.
26. Welsman JR, Armstrong N. Assessing postexercise lactates in children and adolescents. In: Van Praagh E (ed.) *Pediatric anaerobic performance.* Champaign, IL: Human Kinetics; 1998. p. 137–153.
27. Ekelund U, Tomkinson GR, Armstrong N. What proportion of youth are physically active? Measurement issues, levels and recent time trends. *Br J Sports Med.* 2011; 45: 859–866.
28. Armstrong N. Young people are fit and active—fact or fiction? *J Sport Health Sci.* 2012; 1: 131–140.
29. Welsman JR, Armstrong N. Daily physical activity and blood lactate indices of aerobic fitness. *Br J Sports Med.* 1992; 26: 228–232.
30. Poole DC, Jones AM. Oxygen uptake kinetics. *Compr Physiol.* 2012; 2: 933–996.
31. Armstrong N, Barker AR. Oxygen uptake kinetics in children and adolescents. A review. *Pediatr Exerc Sci.* 2009; 21: 130–147.
32. Fawkner SG, Armstrong N. Longitudinal changes in the kinetic response to heavy-intensity exercise in children. *J Appl Physiol.* 2004; 97: 460–466.

33. Krogh A, Lindhard J. The regulation of respiration and circulation during the initial stages of muscular work. *J Physiol.* 1913; 47: 112–136.
34. Gaesser GA, Poole DC. The slow component of oxygen uptake kinetics in humans. *Exerc Sport Sci Rev.* 1994; 24: 35–71.
35. Breese BC, Williams CA, Welsman JR, Barker AR, Fawkner SG, Armstrong N. Longitudinal changes in the oxygen uptake kinetic response to heavy intensity exercise in 14–16-year-old boys. *Pediatr Exerc Sci.* 2010; 22: 314–325.
36. Barker AR, Bond B, Toman C, Williams CA, Armstrong N. Critical power in adolescents: physiological bases and assessment using all-out exercise. *Eur J Appl Physiol.* 2012; 112: 1359–1370.
37. Armstrong N, Welsman JR. Development of aerobic fitness during childhood and adolescence. *Pediatr Exerc Sci.* 2000; 12: 128–149.
38. Howley ET, Bassett DR, Welch HG. Criteria for maximal oxygen uptake. Review and commentary. *Med Sci Sports Exerc.* 1995; 29: 1292–1301.
39. Bassett DR, Howley ET. Maximal oxygen uptake: 'classical' versus 'contemporary' viewpoints. *Med Sci Sports Exerc.* 1997; 29: 591–603.
40. Noakes TD. Maximal oxygen uptake: 'classical' versus 'contemporary' viewpoints: a rebuttal. *Med Sci Sports Exerc.* 1998; 30: 1381–1398.
41. Krahenbuhl GS, Skinner JS, Kohrt WM. Developmental aspects of maximal aerobic power in children. *Exerc Sports Sci Rev.* 1985; 13: 503–538.
42. Armstrong N, Kirby BJ, McManus AM, Welsman JR. Aerobic fitness of pre-pubescent children. *Ann Hum Biol.* 1995; 22: 427–441.
43. Armstrong N, Welsman JR. The assessment and interpretation of aerobic fitness in children and adolescents: An update. In: Froberg K, Lammert O, St. Hansen H, Blimkie CJR (eds.) *Exercise and fitness—benefits and limitations.* Odense: University Press; 1997. p. 173–180.
44. Armstrong N, Welsman J, Winsley R. Is peak $\dot{V}O_2$ a maximal index of children's aerobic fitness? *Int J Sports Med.* 1996; 17: 356–359.
45. Rowland TW. Does peak $\dot{V}O_2$ reflect $\dot{V}O_2$ max in children? Evidence from supramaximal testing. *Med Sci Sports Exerc.* 1993; 25: 689–693.
46. Armstrong N, Welsman JR. Assessment and interpretation of aerobic fitness in children and adolescents. *Exerc Sport Sci Rev.* 1994; 22: 435–476.
47. Potter CR, Childs DJ, Houghton W, Armstrong N. Breath-to-breath noise in the ventilatory and gas exchange responses of children to exercise. *Eur J Appl Physiol.* 1998; 80: 118–124.
48. Myers JN. *Essentials of cardiopulmonary exercise testing.* Champaign, IL: Human Kinetics; 1996.
49. Kay C, Shephard RJ. On muscle strength and the threshold of anaerobic work. *Arbeitsphysiol.* 1969; 27: 311–328.
50. Hoes M, Binkhorst RA, Smeekes-Kuyl A, Vissurs AC. Measurement of forces exerted on a pedal crank during work on the bicycle ergometer at different loads. *Arbeitsphysiol.* 1968; 26: 33–42.
51. Wirth A, Trager E, Scheele K, Mayer D, Diehm K, Reisch K. Cardiopulmonary adjustment and metabolic response to maximal and submaximal physical exercise of boys and girls at different stages of maturity. *Eur J Appl Physiol.* 1978; 39: 229–240.
52. Boileau RA, Bonen A, Heyward VH, Massey BH. Maximal aerobic capacity on the treadmill and bicycle ergometer of boys 11–14 years of age. *J Sports Med Phys Fit.* 1977; 17: 153–162.
53. Sheehan JM, Rowland TW, Burke EJ. A comparison of four treadmill protocols for determination of maximal oxygen uptake in 10- to 12-year-old boys. *Int J Sports Med.* 1987; 8: 31–34.
54. McManus AM, Armstrong N. Maximal oxygen uptake. In: Rowland TW (ed.) *Cardiopulmonary exercise testing in children and adolescents.* Champaign, IL: Human Kinetics: 2017. In press.
55. Fawkner SG, Armstrong N. Sex differences in the oxygen uptake kinetic response to heavy-intensity exercise in prepubertal children. *Eur J Appl Physiol.* 2004; 93: 210–216.
56. Welsman JR, Bywater K, Farr C, Welford D, Armstrong N. Reliability of peak $\dot{V}O_2$ and maximal cardiac output assessed using thoracic bioimpedance in children. *Eur J Appl Physiol.* 2005; 94: 228–234.
57. Armstrong N, Barker AR, McManus AM. Muscle metabolism changes with age and maturation with reference to youth sport performance. *Br J Sports Med.* 2015; 49: 860–864.
58. Barker AR, Williams CA, Jones AM, Armstrong N. Establishing maximal oxygen uptake in young people during a ramp test to exhaustion. *Br J Sports Med.* 2011; 45: 498–503.
59. Malina RM, Bouchard C, Bar-Or O. *Growth, maturation and physical activity*, 2nd ed. Champaign, IL: Human Kinetics; 2004.
60. Eiberg S, Hasselstrom H, Gronfeldt V, Froberg K, Svensson J, Andersen LB. Maximum oxygen uptake and objectively measured physical activity in Danish children 6–7 years of age: The Copenhagen school child intervention study. *Br J Sports Med.* 2005; 39: 725–730.
61. Mirwald RL, Bailey DA. *Maximal aerobic power.* London, Ontario: Sports Dynamics: 1986.
62. Sprynarova S, Parizkova J, Bunc S. Relationships between body dimensions and resting and working oxygen consumption in boys aged 11 to 18 years. *Eur J Appl Physiol.* 1987; 56: 725–736.
63. Armstrong N. Van Mechelen W. Are young children fit and active? In: Biddle S, Sallis J, Cavill N (eds.) *Young and active.* London: Health Education Authority; 1998. p. 69–97.
64. Armstrong N, Welsman JR, Nevill AM, Kirby BJ. Modeling growth and maturation changes in peak oxygen uptake in 11-13 yr olds. *J Appl Physiol.* 1999; 87: 2230–2236.
65. Armstrong N, Welsman JR. Peak oxygen uptake in relation to growth and maturation in 11–17-year-old humans. *Eur J Appl Physiol.* 2001; 85: 546–551.
66. Geithner CA, Thomis MA, Vanden Eynde B, *et al.* Growth in peak aerobic power during adolescence. *Med Sci Sports Exerc.* 2004; 36: 1616–1624.
67. Cunningham DA, Paterson DH, Blimkie CJR, Donner AP. Development of the cardiorespiratory system in circumpubertal boys: A longitudinal study. *J Appl Physiol.* 1984; 56: 302–307.
68. Kemper HCG. Amsterdam growth and health longitudinal study. *Med Sport Sci.* 2004; 47: 1–198.
69. Kemper HCG, Twisk JWR, Van Mechelen W. Changes in aerobic fitness in boys and girls over a period of 25 years: Data from the Amsterdam Growth and Health Longitudinal Study revisited and extended. *Pediatr Exerc Sci.* 2013; 25: 534–535.
70. Nevill A, Rowland TW, Goff D, Martell L, Ferrone L. Scaling or normalizing maximum oxygen uptake to predict 1-mile run time in boys. *Eur J Appl Physiol.* 2004; 92: 285–288.
71. Tanner JM. Fallacy of per-weight and per-surface area standards and their relation to spurious correlation. *J Appl Physiol.* 1949; 2: 1–15.
72. Welsman JR, Armstrong N. Interpreting exercise performance data in relation to body size. In: Armstrong N, van Mechelen W (eds.) *Paediatric exercise science and medicine*, 2nd ed. Oxford: Oxford University Press; 2008. p. 13–22.
73. Williams JR, Armstrong N, Winter EM, Crichton N. Changes in peak oxygen uptake with age and sexual maturation in boys: Physiological fact or statistical anomaly? In: Coudert J, Van Praagh E (eds.) *Pediatric work physiology.* Paris: Masson; 1992. p. 35–37.
74. Welsman JR, Armstrong N, Kirby BJ, Nevill AM, Winter EM. Scaling peak $\dot{V}O_2$ for differences in body size. *Med Sci Sports Exerc.* 1996; 28: 259–265.
75. Welsman JR, Armstrong N. Scaling for size: Relevance to understanding effects of growth on performance. In: Hebestreit H, Bar-Or O (eds.) *The young athlete.* Oxford: Blackwell; 2008. p. 50–62.
76. Fahey TD, Del Valle-Zuris A, Oehlsen G, Trieb M, Seymour J. Pubertal stage differences in hormonal and hematological responses to maximal exercise in males. *J Appl Physiol.* 1979; 46: 823–827.
77. Armstrong N, Welsman JR, Kirby BJ. Peak oxygen uptake and maturation in 12-year-olds. *Med Sci Sports Exerc.* 1998; 30: 165–169.
78. Tanner JM. *Growth at adolescence*, 2nd ed. Oxford: Blackwell; 1962.
79. Armstrong N, Welsman JR. The physical activity patterns of European youth with reference to methods of assessment. *Sports Med.* 2006; 36: 1067–1086.
80. Armstrong N, Tomkinson GR, Ekelund U. Aerobic fitness and its relationship to sport, exercise training and habitual physical activity during youth. *Br J Sport Med.* 2011; 45: 849–858.
81. Turley KR. Cardiovascular responses to exercise in children. *Sports Med.* 1997; 24: 241–257.

82. Nagasawa H, Arakaki Y, Yamada O, Nakajima T, Kamiya T. Longitudinal observations of left ventricular end-diastolic dimension in children using echocardiography. *Pediatr Cardiol.* 1996; 97: 169–174.
83. Nidorf SM, Picard MH, Triulzi MO, *et al.* New perspectives in the assessment of cardiac chamber dimensions during development and adulthood. *J Am Coll Cardiol.* 1992; 19: 938–988.
84. Vinet A, Mandigout S, Nottin S, *et al.* Influence of body composition, hemoglobin concentration, and cardiac size and function on gender differences in maximal oxygen uptake in prepubertal children. *Chest.* 2003; 124: 1494–1499.
85. Rowland T, Goff D, Martel L, Ferrone L. Influence of cardiac functional capacity on gender differences in maximal oxygen uptake in children. *Chest.* 2000; 17: 629–635.
86. McNarry MA, Farr C, Middlebrooke A, *et al.* Aerobic function and muscle deoxygenation dynamics during ramp exercise in children. *Med Sci Sports Exerc.* 2015; 47: 1877–1884.
87. Maughan RJ, Shirreffs SM, Leiper JB. Blood sampling. In: Winter EM, Jones AM, Davison RCR, Bromley PD, Mercer TH (eds.) *Sport and physiology testing guidelines. Volume 1: Sport testing.* London: Routledge; 2007. p. 25–29.
88. Newton JL, Robinson S. The distribution of blood lactate and pyruvate during work and recovery. *Fed Proc.* 1965; 24: 590.
89. Williams JR, Armstrong N, Kirby BJ. The influence of the site of sampling and assay medium upon the measurement and interpretation of blood lactate responses to exercise. *J Sports Sci.* 1992; 10: 95–107.
90. Armstrong N, Welsman JR. *Young people and physical activity.* Oxford: Oxford University Press; 1997.
91. Williams JR, Armstrong N. The influence of age and sexual maturation on children's blood lactate responses to exercise. *Pediatr Exerc Sci.* 1991; 3: 111–120.
92. Eriksson BO. Physical training, oxygen supply and muscle metabolism in 11–13-year-old boys. *Acta Physiol Scand.* 1972; 384: 1–48.
93. Armstrong N, Barker AR. New insights in paediatric exercise metabolism. *J Sport Health Sci.* 2012; 1: 18–26.
94. Welsman JR, Armstrong N, Kirby BJ. Serum testosterone is not related to peak $\dot{V}O_2$ and submaximal blood lactate responses in 12–16 year old males. *Pediatr Exerc Sci.* 1994; 6: 120–127.
95. Benson AP, Grassi B, Rossiter HB. A validated model of oxygen uptake and circulatory dynamic interactions at exercise onset in humans. *J Appl Physiol.* 2013; 115: 743–755.
96. Barker AR, Welsman JR, Fulford J, Welford D, Williams CA, Armstrong N. Muscle phosphocreatine and pulmonary oxygen uptake kinetics in children at the onset and offset of moderate intensity exercise. *Eur J Appl Physiol.* 2008; 102: 727–738.
97. Barker AR, Armstrong N. Insights into developmental muscle metabolism through the use of ^{31}P-magnetic resonance spectroscopy: A review. *Pediatr Exerc Sci.* 2010; 22: 350–368.
98. Fawkner SG, Armstrong N. Can we confidently study $\dot{V}O_2$ kinetics in young people? *J Sports Sci Med.* 2007; 6: 277–285.
99. Fawkner SG, Armstrong N. Modelling the $\dot{V}O_2$ kinetic response to moderate intensity exercise in children. *Acta Kinesiol Univ Tartu.* 2002; 7: 80–84.
100. Fawkner SG, Armstrong N. Modelling the $\dot{V}O_2$ kinetic response to heavy intensity exercise in children. *Ergonomics.* 2004; 47: 1517–1527.
101. Lamarra N, Whipp BJ, Ward SA, Wasserman K. Effect of interbreath fluctuations on characterizing gas exchange kinetics. *J Appl Physiol.* 1987; 62: 2003–2012.
102. Fawkner SG, Armstrong N, Potter CR, Welsman JR. Oxygen uptake kinetics in children and adults after the onset of moderate intensity exercise. *J Sports Sci.* 2002; 20: 319–326.
103. Fawkner SG, Armstrong N. The slow component response of $\dot{V}O_2$ to heavy exercise in children. In: Reilly T, Marfell-Jones M (eds.) *Kinanthropometry VIII.* Oxford: Routledge; 2003. p. 105–113.
104. Macek M, Vavra J. The adjustment of oxygen uptake at the onset of exercise: A comparison between pre-pubertal boys and young adults. *In J Sports Med.* 1980; 1: 70–72.
105. Cooper DM, Berry C, Lamarra N, Wassermann K. Kinetics of oxygen uptake and heart rate at onset of exercise in children. *J Appl Physiol.* 1985; 59: 211–217.
106. Barstow TJ, Scheuermann BW. Kinetics; Effects of maturation and aging. In: Jones AM, Poole DC (eds.) *Oxygen uptake kinetics in sport, exercise and medicine.* London: Routledge; 2005. p. 331–352.
107. Hebestreit H, Kriemler S, Hughson RL, Bar-Or O. Kinetics of oxygen uptake at the onset of exercise in boys and men. *J Appl Physiol.* 1998; 85: 1833–1841.
108. Cleuziou C, Lecoq AM, Candau R, Courteix D, Guenon P, Obert P. Kinetics of oxygen uptake at the onset of moderate and heavy exercise in trained and untrained prepubertal children. *Sci Sport.* 2002; 17: 291–296.
109. Williams CA, Carter H, Jones AM, Doust JH. Oxygen uptake kinetics during treadmill running in boys and men. *J Appl Physiol.* 2001; 90: 1700–1706.
110. Leclair E, Berthion S, Borel B, *et al.* Faster pulmonary oxygen uptake kinetics in children vs adults due to enhancements in oxygen delivery and extraction. *Scand J Med Sci Sports.* 2013; 23: 705–712.
111. Armon Y, Cooper DM, Flores R, Zanconato S, Barstow TJ. Oxygen uptake dynamics during high-intensity exercise in children and adults. *J Appl Physiol.* 1991; 70: 841–848.
112. Winlove MA, Jones AM, Welsman JR. Influence of training status and exercise modality on pulmonary O_2 uptake kinetics in pre-pubertal girls. *Eur J Appl Physiol.* 2010; 108: 1169–1179.
113. McNarry MA, Welsman JR, Jones AM. Influence of training status and exercise modality on pulmonary O_2 uptake kinetics in pubertal girls. *Eur J Appl Physiol.* 2011; 111: 621–631.
114. Breese BC, Barker AR, Armstrong N, Jones AM, Williams CA. Effect of baseline metabolic rate on pulmonary O_2 uptake kinetics during very heavy-intensity exercise in boys and men. *Resp Physiol Neurobiol.* 2012; 180: 223–229.
115. Breese BC, Barker AR, Armstrong N, Fulford J, Williams CA. Influence of thigh activation on the $\dot{V}O_2$ slow component in boys and men. *Eur J Appl Physiol.* 2014; 114: 2309–2319.
116. Obert P, Cleziou C, Candau R, Courteix D, Lecoq AM, Guenon P. The slow component of O_2 uptake kinetics during high intensity exercise in trained and untrained prepubertal children. *Int J Sports Med.* 2000; 21: 31–36.
117. Breese BC, Armstrong N, Barker AR, Williams CA. The effect of pedal rate on pulmonary oxygen uptake kinetics during very heavy exercise in trained and untrained teenage boys. *Resp Physiol Neurobiol.* 2011; 177: 149–154.
118. Barker AR, Jones AM, Armstrong N. The influence of priming exercise on oxygen uptake, cardiac output, and muscle oxygenation kinetics during very heavy-intensity exercise in 9–13-year-old boys. *J Appl Physiol.* 2010; 109: 491–500.
119. Barker AR, Trebilcock E, Breese B, Jones AM, Armstrong N. The effect of priming exercise on oxygen uptake kinetics, muscle oxygen delivery and utilisation, muscle activity and exercise tolerance in boys. *Appl Physiol Nutr Metab.* 2014; 39: 308–317.
120. Lai N, Nasca MM, Silva FT, Whipp BJ, Cabrera M. Influence of exercise intensity on pulmonary oxygen uptake kinetics at the onset of exercise and recovery in male adolescents. *Appl Physiol Nutr Metab.* 2008; 33: 107–117.
121. Zanconato S, Cooper DM, Armon Y. Oxygen cost and oxygen uptake dynamics and recovery with 1 min exercise in children and adults. *J Appl Physiol.* 1991; 71: 841–848.
122. Marwood S, Roche D, Garrard M, Unnithan V. Pulmonary oxygen uptake and muscle deoxygenation kinetics during recovery in trained and untrained male adolescents. *Med Sci Sports Exerc.* 2011; 111: 2775–2784.
123. McNarry MA, Welsman JR, Jones AM. Influence of training status and maturity on pulmonary O_2 uptake recovery kinetics following cycle and upper body exercise in girls. *Pediatr Exerc Sci.* 2012; 24: 246–261.
124. Armstrong N, McNarry MA. Aerobic fitness and trainability in healthy youth: Gaps in our knowledge. *Pediatr Exerc Sci.* 2016; 28: 171–177.

CHAPTER 13

Pulmonary oxygen uptake kinetics

Alan R Barker and Neil Armstrong

Introduction

As children grow and mature, the functional capacity of the pulmonary, cardiovascular, and muscle systems are inevitably altered, having a profound impact on measures of aerobic fitness as discussed in Chapter 12. This is usually investigated through the measurement of maximal (or peak) oxygen uptake ($\dot{V}O_2$ max; peak $\dot{V}O_2$), which is considered the single best indicator of aerobic fitness and has an established relationship with aerobic performance[1] and cardiometabolic disease risk[2] in youth. However, children and adolescents rarely exercise close to their maximal metabolic rate, meaning the measurement of $\dot{V}O_2$ max may lack external validity with regard to the 'real world' challenges faced by the oxygen transportation and utilization systems. It is well documented that children's habitual physical activity patterns are characterized by short and rapid transitions to and from a range of submaximal metabolic rates.[3,4] The ability of a child to undertake these activities can be captured in the pulmonary (p) $\dot{V}O_2$ kinetic response to exercise, which reflects the coordinated ability of the pulmonary, cardiovascular, and muscular systems to support oxygen transport and utilization in response to increasing and decreasing energy turnover within the contracting myocytes.

In addition to the practical significance of measuring $p\dot{V}O_2$ kinetics, when appropriately modelled, the $p\dot{V}O_2$ kinetic response to a change in metabolic rate has been shown to provide a non-invasive window into the metabolic activity of the muscle.[5,6] Thus, quantifying the $p\dot{V}O_2$ kinetic adjustment during the transition to and recovery from exercise permits valuable insight into the adjustment of muscle oxidative phosphorylation and by implication the muscle oxygen deficit.[7] The muscle oxygen deficit represents the requirement for substrate-level phosphorylation (phosphocreatine [PCr] breakdown and anaerobic glycolysis) to contribute to the adenosine triphosphate (ATP) turnover in the muscle and is associated with an increase in fatigue-related metabolites (e.g. inorganic phosphate (P_i) and hydrogen ion [H^+]).[8] A slow $p\dot{V}O_2$ kinetic response at exercise onset is linked to an increase in the muscle oxygen deficit and a reduced ability to tolerate exercise.[9] Consequently, documenting the $p\dot{V}O_2$ response to exercise has the potential to advance understanding of the limiting factors of oxidative metabolism and exercise tolerance in children and adolescents.

This chapter outlines how the study of $p\dot{V}O_2$ kinetics has contributed to understanding of the effect of age and sex in altering the adjustment of muscle oxidative metabolism during exercise. It focuses on the factors that limit the $p\dot{V}O_2$ kinetics response to exercise in youth, including regulation by muscle phosphates, muscle oxygen delivery and utilization, and muscle fibre recruitment. Prior to addressing these issues the chapter provides an overview of the phases in the $p\dot{V}O_2$ response to exercise, exercise intensity domains, and methodological issues. The effect of exercise training on the $p\dot{V}O_2$ kinetic response to exercise in youth is addressed in Chapter 34.

Kinetics of oxygen uptake at the mouth and muscle

Since the seminal work of Whipp and colleagues[10] that used advances in gas exchange technology to determine $p\dot{V}O_2$ on a breath-by-breath basis, the $p\dot{V}O_2$ response at the onset of exercise has been described to have three discrete phases (see Figure 13.1a). After a small increase in $p\dot{V}O_2$ within the initial ~20 s of exercise onset (phase I), a single-exponential increase in $p\dot{V}O_2$ is observed (phase II) which reaches a steady-state (phase III) after ~2–3 min. In contrast to this three phase response when $p\dot{V}O_2$ is measured at the mouth or pulmonary level, muscle oxygen consumption ($m\dot{V}O_2$) has been shown to increase immediately at the onset of exercise and to follow a single exponential time course (Figure 13.1b).[11] There is a temporal distortion between the single exponential rise in $p\dot{V}O_2$ and $m\dot{V}O_2$ at the onset of exercise due to the muscle-to-lung transit delay time, meaning a given arteriovenous blood oxygen content difference (a-vO_2 diff) is expressed at the lung with a higher cardiac output ($\dot{Q}$) response.[7,12] Thus the single exponential $m\dot{V}O_2$ response without delay is reflected as a $p\dot{V}O_2$ response with three distinct phases. As the increase in $p\dot{V}O_2$ during phase I is attributable to a rise in $\dot{Q}$ (and hence pulmonary blood flow) at exercise onset and does not reflect a change in tissue oxygen consumption, it is termed the 'cardiodynamic' region.[13,14] The single-exponential rise in $p\dot{V}O_2$ (phase II) starts after the muscle-to-lung transit delay time when a widening of the a-vO_2 diff reaches the lungs, and with the increasing $\dot{Q}$ response, drives $p\dot{V}O_2$ to a new steady-state (phase III).[7,12]

Although at the onset of exercise the kinetics of $m\dot{V}O_2$ and $p\dot{V}O_2$ are temporally dissociated, both computerized simulations[13] and the direct measurement of $m\dot{V}O_2$ during cycling in adults[5,6] have found a ~10% agreement between the time constants (τ) of $m\dot{V}O_2$ and phase II $p\dot{V}O_2$. Due to obvious ethical restrictions, this type of work has not been replicated in children. However, in a series of innovative studies, Rossiter and colleagues[15,16] simultaneously

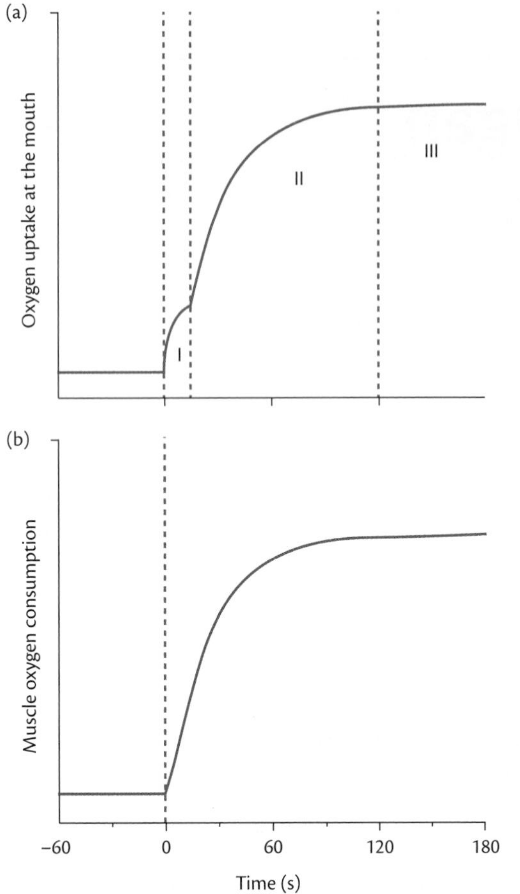

Figure 13.1 Kinetics of oxygen uptake at the mouth and muscle at the onset of moderate intensity exercise.

Schematic of the kinetics of oxygen uptake at the mouth (a) and muscle (b) at the onset of moderate intensity exercise. The muscle oxygen uptake kinetics in (b) are based on the data of Behnke *et al.*[11] The onset of exercise is denoted by the vertical dotted line at 0 s in panels (a) and (b). In A subsequent vertical dotted line depicts the three phases (I, II and III) of the oxygen uptake response. See text for details.

Adapted from Armstrong N, Barker AR. Oxygen uptake kinetics in children and adolescents: a review. Pediatr Exerc Sci. 2009; 21: 130–147.

examined the kinetics of $p\dot{V}O_2$ alongside the kinetics of muscle PCr determined non-invasively using ^{31}phosphorus-magnetic resonance spectroscopy (^{31}PMRS) in adults performing knee-extensor exercise inside the bore of an MR scanner. In this experimental design, muscle PCr kinetics was taken as a surrogate of $m\dot{V}O_2$ dynamics, as predicted by models of metabolic control.[17,18] In agreement with the aforementioned studies using the direct Fick technique, the authors found a close agreement between the kinetics of phase II $p\dot{V}O_2$ and muscle PCr both at the onset and offset of exercise. Given this evidence and the non-invasive nature in which PCr kinetics can be determined using ^{31}PMRS, Barker *et al.*[19] sought to establish whether the underlying $m\dot{V}O_2$ dynamics during exercise are faithfully reflected by the phase II $p\dot{V}O_2$ response in children. Using cycling exercise to determine $p\dot{V}O_2$ kinetics and quadriceps exercise inside the bore of an MR scanner to measure muscle PCr kinetics, the authors found no differences in the phase II $p\dot{V}O_2$ τ and muscle PCr τ both at the onset (PCr 23 ± 5 vs $p\dot{V}O_2$ 23 ± 4 s) and offset (PCr 28 ± 5 vs $p\dot{V}O_2$ 29 ± 5 s) of exercise. Although indirect, these data are in agreement with previous work in healthy adults,[15,16] and suggest that in healthy, young children the dynamics of phase II $p\dot{V}O_2$ reflect the underlying $m\dot{V}O_2$ response.

Exercise intensity domains

At the onset of constant work-rate exercise, the $p\dot{V}O_2$ kinetic response is well-characterized by a three-phase response. However, the temporal- and amplitude-based characteristics of the $p\dot{V}O_2$ response can vary based on the muscle metabolic and blood acid-base profiles observed during exercise. Therefore, different exercise intensity domains have been proposed to reflect a common set of response characteristics in the $p\dot{V}O_2$ response during exercise. Typically, the kinetics of $p\dot{V}O_2$ are classified into four exercise intensity domains (moderate, heavy, very heavy, and severe), the boundaries of which are demarcated by specific parameters of physiological function (Figure 13.2).[7,9,12]

All exercise work-rates that fall below the blood lactate threshold (T_{LAC}) reflect moderate-intensity exercise. In practice T_{LAC} is typically identified using one of its non-invasive equivalents, either the gas exchange threshold (GET) or the ventilatory threshold (T_{VENT}), as this circumvents the requirement for repeated capillary blood samples. Within the moderate-intensity domain the increase in $p\dot{V}O_2$ is characterized, following phase I, by single exponential kinetics which attain a steady-state amplitude within ~2–3 min with an oxygen cost of exercise or 'gain' ($\Delta p\dot{V}O_2/\Delta W$) of ~10 $mL \cdot min^{-1} \cdot W^{-1}$ in healthy participants.[20,21] For exercise work-rates above the T_{LAC} but below $\dot{V}O_2$ max, the rise in $p\dot{V}O_2$ displays unique characteristics based on whether blood lactate accumulation increases and stabilizes (heavy) or rises continuously (very heavy) with time. The upper boundary of the heavy domain is demarcated by the maximal lactate steady state (MLSS),[22] which reflects the highest exercise work-rate that can be sustained at which a balance

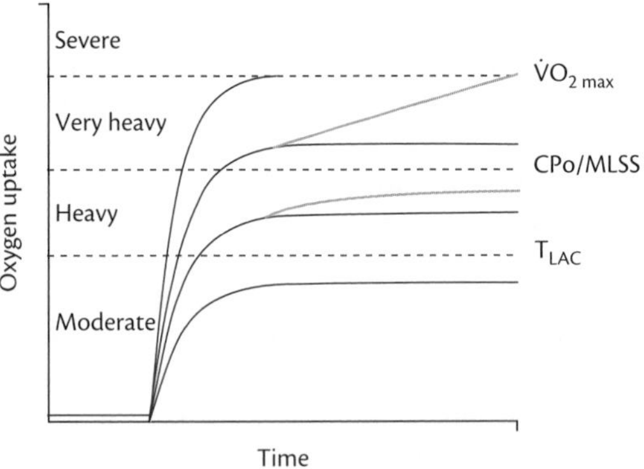

Figure 13.2 Oxygen uptake kinetics at the onset of exercise with respect to exercise intensity domains.

Schematic of the oxygen uptake kinetic response to exercise in relation to exercise intensity domains. Phase I has been omitted for clarity. The boundaries that separate the moderate, heavy, very heavy, and severe exercise domains are shown using the horizontal dotted lines. Where, T_{LAC} is lactate threshold, CPo is critical power, MLSS is maximal lactate steady state, and $\dot{V}O_2$ max is maximal oxygen uptake. The black lines shows the projected $p\dot{V}O_2$ response assuming a constant oxygen cost of exercise that is equivalent to that found during moderate exercise. The additional oxygen cost of exercise when exercising above the T_{LAC} ($p\dot{V}O_2$ slow component) is shown by the grey lines. See text for details.

Adapted from Armstrong N, Barker AR. Oxygen uptake kinetics in children and adolescents: a review. Pediatr Exerc Sci. 2009; 21: 130–147.

between the appearance and removal of lactate within the blood is achieved. In practice, however, many authors use critical power (CPo) to reflect the upper limit of the heavy-intensity domain as it elicits an exercise work-rate very similar but not equal to MLSS.[22,23] Critical power represents the asymptote of the hyperbolic relationship between power output and time to exhaustion and is considered to represent the highest exercise work-rate at which aerobic energy transfer can be achieved without continuous depletion of anaerobic energy stores.[24] For work rates above T_{LAC} but below MLSS/CPo (heavy exercise) $p\dot{V}O_2$ rises with exponential kinetics but is characterized by a delayed and elevated increase in $p\dot{V}O_2$ that may take up to 15 min to reach steady-state.[20,25] The elevated $p\dot{V}O_2$ during exercise above the T_{LAC} represents an additional oxygen cost of exercise (reduced efficiency) compared to that found during moderate intensity exercise such that the 'gain' increases to ~12–14 $mL \cdot min^{-1} \cdot W^{-1}$ in adults.[20,25] This additional increase in $p\dot{V}O_2$ is termed the $p\dot{V}O_2$ slow component and reflects the fatigue processes occurring within the contracting myocytes.[16,26] For exercise work-rates above MLSS/CPo but below $\dot{V}O_2$ max (very heavy exercise), a steady-state in $p\dot{V}O_2$ is not achieved, meaning the $p\dot{V}O_2$ slow component rises rapidly with time and projects towards $\dot{V}O_2$ max, indicating a progressive reduction in exercise efficiency. The closer the work rate is towards $\dot{V}O_2$ max, the smaller the magnitude of the $p\dot{V}O_2$ slow component, such that the $p\dot{V}O_2$ kinetic response follows a single exponential function that is truncated at $\dot{V}O_2$ max within minutes.[7,20] Exercise work-rates which result in exhaustion with a single-exponential $p\dot{V}O_2$ response in the absence of a $p\dot{V}O_2$ slow component are classified as in the severe domain.

It should be noted that there is no universally accepted exercise intensity domain schema within the literature. Although there appears to be agreement with the description of the moderate and heavy domains, for work rates above MLSS/CP alternative schema have been proposed. It has been suggested that the severe intensity domain should represent all exercise work-rates where the participant can sustain exercise with the attainment of $\dot{V}O_2$ max at exhaustion.[27] In this schema, an additional domain has been proposed (extreme) for exercise work-rates where exhaustion occurs prior to achieving $\dot{V}O_2$ max [28] However, as the majority of the paediatric exercise science literature has adopted the terminology illustrated in Figure 13.2 this classification will be adhered to throughout the chapter.

The concept of exercise intensity domains is relatively new in paediatric exercise physiology, as a percentage of $\dot{V}O_2$ max is commonly used to prescribe a given intensity of exercise. However, the impact of exercise intensity on the temporal and amplitude-based features of the $p\dot{V}O_2$ kinetics response to exercise means careful consideration is needed when studying this area. For example, the prescription of a single absolute exercise work-rate (e.g. 150 W) is likely to result in a younger child or a paediatric patient working at a higher percentage of their aerobic power when compared to an older child or age-matched control respectively. Likewise, the prescription of an exercise work-rate relative to $\dot{V}O_2$ max (e.g. 60% $\dot{V}O_2$ max) is likely to result in some participants exercising above, but others below, their T_{LAC}. This is because there is a large variability in the position of the T_{LAC} in relation to $\dot{V}O_2$ max. Indeed, recent evidence, albeit in adults, has shown that prescribing exercise intensities using the domain concept results in markedly less inter-subject variation in gas exchange, heart rate, blood lactate, and perceptual responses when compared to the % $\dot{V}O_2$ max method.[29] Thus the exercise intensity domain concept appears to be superior in allowing the researcher to ensure a similar physiological and perceptual stress across their participants during exercise when compared to the % $\dot{V}O_2$ max approach. Thus when studying $p\dot{V}O_2$ kinetics, the prescribed exercise work-rate should be assigned relative to the physiological variable(s) that identify the domain boundaries for each participant (e.g. % T_{LAC}).

Methodological considerations

Studying the $p\dot{V}O_2$ kinetic response to exercise requires high methodological rigour and this is especially the case in children. Children have a significantly smaller absolute $\dot{V}O_2$ max compared to adults, which compresses the range of metabolic rates within a given exercise intensity domain. This is particularly true for studying $p\dot{V}O_2$ kinetics in the moderate, heavy, and very heavy exercise intensity domains as the T_{LAC} is typically positioned at ~50–60% $\dot{V}O_2$ max in children below 14 years of age.[30,31] To ensure a participant is exercising within the moderate-intensity domain, 80–90% of the T_{LAC} is normally used as the criterion. This may, however, represent a target exercise work-rate of 50 W in a child as young as 9 years of age and only a small amplitude increase in $p\dot{V}O_2$. Critical power is known to occur at ~67–82% $\dot{V}O_2$ max in children and adolescents,[32,33] indicating the absolute difference in exercise intensities between the T_{LAC} and CPo may be small in magnitude, making it difficult to ensure participants are exercising at the same position within the heavy intensity domain. As MLSS/CPo are both time-intensive to establish due to requiring multiple laboratory visits,[32,34] investigators have adopted the delta (Δ) concept which calculates the work rate based on the % difference between the T_{LAC} and $\dot{V}O_2$ max. For example, studies have used 40% Δ or 60% Δ to identify the heavy[35,36] or very heavy[37,38] domains, respectively. However, while the delta concept is certainly superior to prescribing exercise based on % $\dot{V}O_2$ max,[29] it cannot ensure the correct placement of all participants within the correct exercise intensity domain.[39] This is because there is inter-individual variation in the position of MLSS/CPo relative to $\dot{V}O_2$ max.

The $p\dot{V}O_2$ response to exercise in children is considered to have low signal-to-noise properties, caused by their inherently low $p\dot{V}O_2$ amplitude (signal) and the presence of large inter-breath $p\dot{V}O_2$ fluctuations (noise).[40] A $p\dot{V}O_2$ response with low signal-to-noise properties may be problematic as it can mask the identification of the phase II portion of the $p\dot{V}O_2$ response. Therefore, while modelling an exponential function on a $p\dot{V}O_2$ response with low signal-to-noise properties will resolve the phase II τ, its physiological interpretation is complex. This is because the phase II region of the response may be distorted and the resolved τ will have low statistical confidence.[7,41] To uncover the underlying $m\dot{V}O_2$ response within a $p\dot{V}O_2$ profile characterized with low signal-to-noise properties, data filtering and averaging techniques can be used to improve the signal-to-noise ratio and are comprehensively reviewed elsewhere.[7] It is not uncommon for data from up to ten repeat moderate exercise transitions to be time-aligned and averaged to yield a single $p\dot{V}O_2$ kinetic response with suitable signal-to-noise properties to resolve the phase II τ with a level of uncertainly of ~ ±5 s based on the 95% confidence interval (CI).[42] However, in practice this is very time demanding, so it is more common to average the $p\dot{V}O_2$ response using between two and four repeat transitions, especially for exercise within the heavy-intensity domain or above as the $p\dot{V}O_2$ signal is increased.[38,43–45] Some studies have also resorted to using a longer sampling interval to express the $p\dot{V}O_2$ data (e.g. 3 s or 5 s),[46] to improve the signal-to-noise ratio.

A key outcome when measuring $p\dot{V}O_2$ kinetics is to isolate and characterize the phase II portion of the response using an appropriate model. In some cases, the half-time ($t_{0.5}$) has been used to quantify the rate of change in $p\dot{V}O_2$ both at the onset[47] and offset of exercise.[48] However, this method only provides a broad brush characterization of the overall $p\dot{V}O_2$ response dynamics as it is not specific to the phase II part of the response. In contrast, a number of different non-linear regression models have been employed within the paediatric literature and a detailed analysis of them is presented elsewhere.[49,50] The model that has received most use in the paediatric literature is described in equation 13.1:

$$p\dot{V}O_{2\,(t)} = \Delta p\dot{V}O_{2\,ss} \cdot (1 - e^{-(t-TD)/\tau}) \qquad (13.1)$$

where $p\dot{V}O_{2(t)}$, $\Delta p\dot{V}O_{2ss}$, TD, and τ represent the value of $p\dot{V}O_2$ at a given time, the amplitude change in $p\dot{V}O_2$ from baseline to a new steady-state, time delay, and the time constant, respectively.

It is important that when modelling the $p\dot{V}O_2$ response to reflect $m\dot{V}O_2$ the region of interest is the exponential component (phase II), not phase I. Two techniques have been utilized to account for the phase I portion of the $p\dot{V}O_2$ response prior to modelling phase II. Typically, the initial 15–25 s of data from the onset of exercise are deleted from the $p\dot{V}O_2$ profile to remove the influence of phase I from the model fitting window.[10,20,51] In contrast, some authors have elected to model the $p\dot{V}O_2$ response using a double exponential function with independent parameters (τs and TDs) for the phase I and phase II regions, respectively.[52–54] However, given the paucity of data points available within a limited time frame (15–25 s) and the lack of a physiological justification for fitting an exponential function to phase I, it has been recommended that this procedure should be approached with caution.[7,12]

A further utility of the model proposed in equation 13.1 is that the oxygen deficit (substrate level phosphorylation and contribution from oxygen stores) incurred at the onset of moderate intensity exercise can be calculated using the following expression:[10]

$$\text{Oxygen deficit} = \Delta p\dot{V}O_{2\,ss} \cdot p\dot{V}O_2\ \text{MRT} \qquad (13.2)$$

where the MRT (mean response time) is determined by summating the τ and TD parameters from equation 13.1 when fitted from the onset of exercise. The assumption behind this calculation is that steady-state $p\dot{V}O_2$ provides an estimation of the total energetic equivalents required for the exercise task. As such, the emergence of the $p\dot{V}O_2$ slow component during exercise above the T_{LAC} invalidates the calculation of the oxygen deficit using equation 13.2 as the $p\dot{V}O_2$ steady-state may be of delayed onset (heavy) or absent (very heavy).

With the use of data processing and modelling strategies the $p\dot{V}O_2$ kinetic response at the onset of exercise provides a valuable non-invasive window into the dynamics of the underlying $m\dot{V}O_2$ profile and the magnitude of the incurred oxygen deficit. This allows a robust physiological profile to be assembled regarding the interaction between oxidative and non-oxidative metabolism during exercise.

Pulmonary oxygen uptake kinetics: children and adolescents

In contrast to $\dot{V}O_2$ max, few studies have investigated the $p\dot{V}O_2$ kinetic response to exercise in paediatric groups. Furthermore, of the studies that have documented the $p\dot{V}O_2$ kinetic responses in this group, a number of methodological criticisms remain. This relates to prescribing exercise intensity in relation to $\dot{V}O_2$ max,[55] or not using data averaging techniques to yield a phase II τ with an acceptable level of statistical confidence.[56] The kinetic parameters of the $p\dot{V}O_2$ response in the paediatric literature may also have limited physiological meaning as modelling techniques were employed that fail to isolate and characterize the phase II portion of the response.[57,58] As these limitations have been addressed in extensive reviews of this topic,[50,59,60] the following discussion presents a synthesis of methodologically robust studies that have examined the effect of age and sex on the $p\dot{V}O_2$ kinetic response in healthy paediatric groups. A summary of these studies is presented in Table 13.1.

Phase I

Very little is understood about the magnitude and duration of the phase I response during exercise in young people. This is likely due to the inherently low signal-to-noise ratio of the $p\dot{V}O_2$ profile and the short duration of this phase (<25 s) which makes it difficult to study. In addition, the $p\dot{V}O_2$ profile during phase I appears to be sensitive to whether the exercise transition is initiated from rest or baseline pedalling.[10] Consequently, most paediatric exercise physiology researchers assume the duration of phase I to be ~15–25 s and remove this part of the $p\dot{V}O_2$ response from the data set to model phases II and III.[38,42,45,61] However, it is known that the kinetics of phase I is linked to $\dot{Q}$ kinetics (and hence pulmonary blood flow) at the onset of exercise, and when compared to adults, children are known to require a greater increase in $\dot{Q}$ to achieve a given $p\dot{V}O_2$.[62] Thus, it seems reasonable to suggest that the $p\dot{V}O_2$ kinetics of phase I may alter during growth and maturation.

To our knowledge only three studies have investigated the effect of age on phase I $p\dot{V}O_2$ kinetics during moderate-intensity exercise. Cooper and colleagues[63] found no difference in the increase in $p\dot{V}O_2$ during phase I when expressed as a proportion of the $\dot{V}O_2$ steady state between 7- to 10-year-old children and 15–18-year-old adolescents. An assumption in this study was that the duration of phase I was equivalent to 20 s for all participants. By contrast, the same research group found the increase in $p\dot{V}O_2$ during phase I to represent a lower proportion of the $p\dot{V}O_2$ steady state amplitude in 6- to 10-year-old children when compared to 18–33-year-old adults (39 ± 8 vs. 51 ± 11%).[51] However, the duration of phase I was assumed to be 15 s for all participants, which may not be reasonable as the duration of phase I has been reported to remain stable at ~15 s in 9- to 12-year-old boys between ~50–130% $\dot{V}O_2$ max but declines from ~23 to 13 s in 19–27-year-old men over the same exercise intensities.[55] Furthermore, longitudinal data have shown that the duration of phase I increases by ~5 s at the onset of heavy intensity cycling exercise between the ages of 11–13 years.[35]

Moderate-intensity exercise

Initially, it was considered that age and sex do not exert an influence on the $p\dot{V}O_2$ kinetic response to moderate-intensity exercise during growth and maturation. In a seminal study to investigate

Table 13.1 Methodologically robust studies investigating the oxygen uptake kinetic response to exercise in healthy children and adolescents

Study	Design	Sex	Age	*n*	Peak $\dot{V}O_2$ ($mL \cdot kg^{-1} \cdot min^{-1}$)	Modality and intensity	T_n	phase II $\dot{V}O_2$ τ (s)	$\dot{V}O_2$ slow component (%)
Moderate									
Cooper *et al.*[63]	CS	M	10 ± 2	5	40 ± 6	CYC – 75% T_{LAC}	≥6	27 ± 3	–
		M	16 ± 1	5	43 ± 5			24 ± 2	–
		F	9 ± 2	5	37 ± 4			27 ± 4*	–
		F	15 ± 2	5	34 ± 4			32 ± 6*	–
Breese *et al.*[38]	CS	M	13 ± 1	8	~50[a]	CYC – 90% T_{LAC}	2	19 ± 5*	–
		M	26 ± 3	9	~45[a]			30 ± 5*	–
Fawkner *et al.*[42]	CS	M	12 ± 0	12	50 ± 6†	CYC – 80% T_{LAC}	4–10	19 ± 2*	–
		M	21 ± 2	13	50 ± 6†			28 ± 9*	–
		F	12 ± 0	11	44 ± 6†			21 ± 6*	–
		F	22 ± 2	12	41 ± 5†			26 ± 5*	–
Leclair *et al.*[61]	CS	M	10 ± 1	11	43 ± 5	CYC – 90% T_{LAC}	4	12 ± 4*	–
		M	24 ± 4	12	47 ± 6			20 ± 4*	–
Springer *et al.*[51]	CS	M+F	8 ± 1	9	41 ± 9	CYC – 80% T_{LAC}	5	24 ± 5	–
		M+F	28 ± 7	9	45 ± 7			27 ± 4	–
Williams *et al.*[64]	CS	M	12 ± 0	8	52 ± 2	TRE – 80% T_{LAC}	4	10 ± 1	–
		M	30 ± 7	8	57 ± 3			15 ± 3	–
Heavy									
Breese *et al.*[43]	L	M	14 ± 0	14	~50[a]	CYC – 40% Δ	4	25 ± 5*	9 ± 5*
			16 ± 0	14	~53[a]			30 ± 5*	13 ± 4*
Fawkner and Armstrong[69]	CS	M	11 ± 0	25	47 ± 6†	CYC – 40% Δ	4	18 ± 6†	9 ± 4†
		F	11 ± 1	23	39 ± 7†			22 ± 8†	12 ± 6†
Fawkner and Armstrong[35]	L	M	11 ± 0	13	49 ± 6†	CYC – 40% Δ	4	17 ± 5*	9 ± 5*
		M	13 ± 0	13	49 ± 8†			22 ± 5*	14 ± 5*
		F	11 ± 0	9	39 ± 6†			21 ± 8*	10 ± 2*
		F	13 ± 0	9	39 ± 5†			26 ± 8*	16 ± 3*
Williams *et al.*[64]	CS	M	12 ± 0	8	52 ± 2	TRE – 50% Δ	2	15 ± 3*	1 ± 1*
		M	30 ± 7	8	57 ± 3			19 ± 5*	8 ± 1*
Very Heavy									
Breese *et al.*[38]	CS	M	13 ± 1	8	~50[a]	CYC – 60% Δ	4	21 ± 5*	11 ± 4*
		M	26 ± 3	9	~45[a]			34 ± 8*	16 ± 3*
Breese *et al.*[45]	CS	M	11 ± 0	8	51 ± 7	CYC – 60% Δ	3	24 ± 3*	14 ± 7
		M	25 ± 3	8	43 ± 8			36 ± 9*	18 ± 3
Severe									
Hebestreit *et al.*[55]	CS	M	11 ± 1	9	47 ± 6	CYC – 100% $\dot{V}O_2$ max	2	28 ± 5	–
		M	24 ± 3	8	53 ± 7		2	28 ± 4	–
		M	11 ± 1	9	47 ± 6	CYC – 130% $\dot{V}O_2$ max	2	20 ± 4	–
		M	24 ± 3	8	53 ± 6		2	20 ± 6	–

Data are presented as mean ± SD. Where, CS, cross-sectional. L, longitudinal. M, male. F, female. *n*, sample size. CYC, cycling. TRE, treadmill. Δ, delta concept. T_n, number of repeat transitions time aligned and averaged. Phase II $\dot{V}O_2$ τ, time constant of the exponential rise in $\dot{V}O_2$. $\dot{V}O_2$ slow component, magnitude of the $\dot{V}O_2$ slow component expressed as a % of end-exercise $\dot{V}O_2$. UL, unloaded pedalling.

* significant mean difference for age, † significant mean difference for sex. [a] estimated based on mean maximal oxygen uptake and body mass data presented in the paper.

this issue, $p\dot{V}O_2$ kinetics was determined in 7- to 10-year-old children (five male, five female) and 15- to 18-year-old adolescents (five male, five female) at the onset of cycling exercise to 75% T_{LAC}.[63] The authors found no differences between the phase II τ for the younger and older males, but slower $p\dot{V}O_2$ kinetics were evident in the older females compared to the younger group. A significant negative relationship between the phase II τ and $\dot{V}O_2$ max in ratio with body mass ($mL \cdot kg^{-1} \cdot min^{-1}$) was observed in the females, leading the authors to propose that the slower phase II $p\dot{V}O_2$ τ in the older females was related to their reduced aerobic fitness. This conclusion appeared reasonable as, in a later study, the same research group found no evidence of an age-related slowing for the phase II $p\dot{V}O_2$ τ while breathing normoxic (21% oxygen) and hypoxic (15% oxygen) air during moderate-intensity cycling exercise in 6- to 9-year-old children (five males, four females) and 18- to 33-year-old adults (five male, four female).[51] Williams *et al.*[64] extended these findings to treadmill running at 80% T_{LAC}, documenting no significant differences in the phase II $p\dot{V}O_2$ τ in eight 8- to 12-year-old boys and eight adult men (10 ± 3 vs 15 ± 8 s). Interestingly, the boys were found to have a higher oxygen cost of exercise (239 vs 168 $mL \cdot kg^{-1} \cdot km^{-1}$) compared to men, which is consistent with cycling data.[57] An age-related decline in the 'gain' during moderate exercise suggests a progressive improvement in exercise efficiency or the oxygen cost of exercise with age. Interestingly, similar observations have been recorded during studies documenting the steady-state response to submaximal treadmill exercise in prepubertal, pubertal, and adult participants.[65] However, the use of the ratio standard method to express $p\dot{V}O_2$ relative to work rate, running speed, or body mass is not without criticism[66] (interested readers are referred to Chapter 12 for further discussion), and when modelled using multi-level regression within an allometric framework, females but not males appear to become more economical with advancing age.[67]

Based on the results presented in earlier studies[51,63,64], it was considered that the phase II $p\dot{V}O_2$ τ is fully mature in early childhood during moderate-intensity exercise and is sex-independent. To re-examine this notion, Fawkner *et al.*[42] investigated the $p\dot{V}O_2$ kinetic response during moderate-intensity cycling exercise in 11- to 12-year-old children (12 males, 11 females) and 19- to 26-year-old adults (13 males, 12 females). The authors required each participant to complete up to ten repeat exercise transitions so that the 95% CI spanning the phase II $p\dot{V}O_2$ τ was below ± 5 s. Using this robust methodology, the phase II $p\dot{V}O_2$ τ was found to be significantly faster in the boys compared to men (19 ± 2 vs 28 ± 9 s) and in girls than women (21 ± 6 vs 26 ± 5 s) with no evidence of sex differences. The authors also reported no relationship between the phase II $p\dot{V}O_2$ τ and $\dot{V}O_2$ max in the paediatric group, suggesting these parameters of aerobic fitness are independent. In subsequent reviews,[50,59] it has been argued that the failure of previous studies to employ well-defined and adequately powered participant groups, to use appropriate modelling techniques, and to employ data averaging techniques to ensure the phase II $p\dot{V}O_2$ τ has high statistical confidence (95% CI < 5 s) may explain the inter-study discrepancies. Interestingly, recent studies[38,61] support the conclusions of Fawkner *et al.*[42] showing the phase II $p\dot{V}O_2$ τ to be more rapid in prepubertal and adolescent boys compared to men.

Heavy- and very heavy-intensity exercise

Although the heavy- and very heavy-intensity exercise domains are both characterized by the presence of a $p\dot{V}O_2$ slow component, the muscle metabolic, gas exchange, and blood acid-base profiles to these intensity domains are profoundly different.[25,32,68] Within the heavy-exercise domain, a delayed steady-state $p\dot{V}O_2$ slow component is observed, but for very heavy exercise, the $p\dot{V}O_2$ slow component projects towards $\dot{V}O_2$ max under conditions of falling muscle PCr and pH and increasing blood lactate. Thus, the precise placement of a participant within the heavy- or very heavy-exercise domain is essential for meaningful interpretation of the $p\dot{V}O_2$ response kinetics, both within and between participant groups. This issue has yet to be fully accounted for in paediatric studies, and this is likely due to the intense and time-consuming nature of measuring CPo or MLSS, which differentiate the heavy- and very heavy-exercise intensity domains. The delta concept is often used to place a participant within the heavy- or very heavy-intensity domain. This is usually 40% Δ for heavy exercise and 60% Δ for very heavy exercise. One paediatric study has employed 50% Δ[64] which is likely to sit close to the boundary between the heavy- and very heavy-intensity domains. Given this uncertainty, paediatric studies documenting the $p\dot{V}O_2$ response to heavy- and very heavy-intensity exercise will be discussed on a collective basis here.

Two longitudinal studies provide the most robust evidence with regard to the effect of age and sex on the $p\dot{V}O_2$ kinetics response during heavy-intensity exercise.[35,43] The first study was by Fawkner and Armstrong,[35] who examined the $p\dot{V}O_2$ kinetic response during cycling exercise at 40% Δ in a group of 22 prepubertal children (13 boys, nine girls) and re-examined their response 2 years later. Over the 2-year period the phase II $p\dot{V}O_2$ τ was significantly slowed in both the boys (17 ± 5 vs 22 ± 5 s) and girls (21 ± 8 vs 26 ± 8 s). Although a previous report suggested a $p\dot{V}O_2$ slow component may not be manifest in children during exercise above the T_{LAC},[57] a $p\dot{V}O_2$ slow component was observed in all participants and increased in amplitude when expressed as a percentage of end-exercise $p\dot{V}O_2$ over the 2-year period in both boys (9 ± 5 vs 14 ± 5%) and girls (10 ± 2 vs 16 ± 3%). Furthermore, the phase II $p\dot{V}O_2$ amplitude was reduced over the 2-year period, indicating an age-related decrease in the oxygen cost of exercise (i.e. lower gain). A subsequent 2-year longitudinal study[43] from the same research group further demonstrated an increase in the phase II τ (25 ± 5 vs 30 ± 5 s) and $p\dot{V}O_2$ slow component (9 ± 5 vs 13 ± 4%) in adolescent boys between the ages of 14–16 years. These findings during cycling exercise also extend to other modalities, as Williams *et al.*[64] reported 11- to 12-year-old boys to have a faster phase II $p\dot{V}O_2$ τ, lower magnitude of the slow component, and a higher oxygen cost of running during phase II (210 vs 168 $mL \cdot kg^{-1} \cdot km^{-1}$) and at end-exercise (211 vs 182 $mL \cdot kg^{-1} \cdot km^{-1}$) compared to men while running at 50% Δ.

The longitudinal investigation by Fawkner and Armstrong[35] did not find any sex differences in the $p\dot{V}O_2$ kinetic response either at baseline or at 2-years' follow-up, despite a trend for a faster phase II $p\dot{V}O_2$ τ and a reduced $p\dot{V}O_2$ slow component in boys. However, in a subsequent study with a larger sample of prepubertal children (25 boys, 23 girls), girls were characterized by slower phase II $p\dot{V}O_2$ kinetics and a greater relative contribution of the

$p\dot{V}O_2$ slow component to the end-exercise $p\dot{V}O_2$ when compared to boys.[69]

To our knowledge only two studies have examined the effect of age on the $p\dot{V}O_2$ kinetic response to very heavy exercise.[38,45] These studies are consistent with the data for heavy-intensity exercise in that prepubertal[45] or adolescent[38] boys have a more rapid phase II $p\dot{V}O_2$ τ, an increased phase II $p\dot{V}O_2$ 'gain', and a truncated $p\dot{V}O_2$ slow component when compared to men. It is currently unknown whether sex differences exist in the $p\dot{V}O_2$ kinetic response during very heavy exercise.

Severe-intensity exercise

In contrast to moderate, heavy, and very heavy exercise, the tolerable duration of exercise within the severe exercise intensity domain is dramatically reduced such that exhaustion will occur prior to the attainment of $\dot{V}O_2$ max. Unfortunately, very few paediatric data are available within the severe exercise domain to draw any meaningful conclusions. In an interesting study, Hebestreit *et al.*[55] reported $p\dot{V}O_2$ kinetics in nine boys (aged 9–12 years) and eight men (19–27 years) at the onset of cycling exercise set at 100% and 130% $\dot{V}O_2$ max. The intensive nature of the exercise bouts meant that data could only be collected for 120 s and 75 s at 100% and 130% $\dot{V}O_2$ max respectively. Seven boys were able to complete 75 s of exercise in the 130% $\dot{V}O_2$ max condition compared to just two men. No age-related differences were observed for the phase II $p\dot{V}O_2$ τ during exercise. This suggests the reduced ability to tolerate exercise at 130% $\dot{V}O_2$ max in the men was not related to differences in the adjustment of oxidative phosphorylation. However, boys were found to have a higher 'gain' when cycling at 100% $\dot{V}O_2$ max (10.4 vs 8.3 $mL \cdot min^{-1} \cdot W^{-1}$) and 130% (8.6 vs 6.6 $mL \cdot min^{-1} \cdot W^{-1}$) compared to men, which may indicate a greater oxygen contribution during exercise.

Synthesis

It is clear that only a handful of methodologically robust studies have examined the $p\dot{V}O_2$ kinetic response to exercise in healthy children and adolescents. The literature is consistent that during heavy- and very heavy-intensity exercise the phase II $p\dot{V}O_2$ τ is faster, the $p\dot{V}O_2$ slow component is reduced (in some cases almost absent), and the oxygen cost of exercise is elevated in younger children compared to older children or adults. However, the evidence base for moderate-intensity exercise is equivocal. Earlier studies reported a similar phase II $p\dot{V}O_2$ τ between children and adults,[51,63,64] whereas more recent studies consistently show a faster phase II $p\dot{V}O_2$ τ in young people.[38,42,61] Although a robust explanation for this discrepancy is not readily available, two factors require consideration. The first relates to difficulties in determining phase II $p\dot{V}O_2$ τ with acceptable statistical precision in children (95% CI <5 s), which negates the ability to make robust physiological inferences based on the kinetic parameters. The second relates to the possibility of inadequate statistical power to detect differences in the kinetic parameters that biologically are potentially meaningful.

Taken collectively, the data support the notion that the phase II $p\dot{V}O_2$ τ becomes progressively slower with age during the transition from childhood to adulthood. However, the changes during moderate intensity exercise appear to be rather subtle (<5 s) in contrast to heavy- or very heavy-intensity exercise (~15 s), which may account for the inconsistent findings observed during moderate exercise. This age-related slowing of the phase II $p\dot{V}O_2$ τ along with an increased $p\dot{V}O_2$ slow component during exercise above the T_{LAC} suggests the control of oxidative phosphorylation is altered from childhood into adulthood. Thus it is important to consider the physiological mechanism(s) that limit the $p\dot{V}O_2$ kinetic response to exercise and how these factors alter during growth and maturation. Unfortunately, this area of research has received little investigation to date, largely due to ethical restrictions in using invasive techniques (e.g. muscle biopsy) in paediatric groups.

Mechanisms

Although the pulmonary, cardiovascular, and muscular systems all have the potential to alter the $p\dot{V}O_2$ kinetic response to exercise,[70] the clues to the limiting factors of muscle oxidative metabolism can be found in the general equation:

$$3\,ADP + 3\,P_i + NADH + H^+ + \tfrac{1}{2}\,O_2 \rightarrow 3\,ATP + NAD^+ + H_2O \qquad (13.3)$$

where, ADP is adenosine diphosphate, NADH and NAD^+ represent the reduced and oxidized forms of the nicotinamide adenine dinucleotide (NAD) carriers, and H_20 is water.

Accordingly, the factors that have the potential to limit oxidative phosphorylation at exercise onset are: i) the provision of oxygen to the contracting muscle;[71–74] ii) delayed metabolic activation linked to the rise in muscle phosphates (e.g. ADP) released during the hydrolysis of muscle ATP;[75–79] and iii) the availability of NADH, which in turn is related to the flux of metabolic substrate in the form of acetyl units through the tricarboxylic acid cycle, which may be related to the activity of the pyruvate dehydrogenase complex.[80–82] The latter two factors have been termed the 'metabolic inertia' hypothesis, which argues that the rise in oxidative phosphorylation is limited by metabolic factors within the myocyte. Although debate continues as to whether $p\dot{V}O_2$ kinetics are limited due to the ability to deliver or utilize oxygen during exercise,[83] it is likely that an interaction of these factors will ultimately determine the rate of oxidative metabolism,[9,73,84] which is dependent on the muscle fibre type. Thus the following factors will be considered in altering $p\dot{V}O_2$ kinetics during growth and maturation: muscle phosphates, muscle oxygen delivery, and muscle fibre recruitment.

Muscle phosphates

Equation 13.3 indicates that the release of ADP and P_i from the hydrolysis of ATP plays an important role in limiting oxidative phosphorylation. As transportation of ADP into the mitochondrial space is limited,[85] it has been proposed that muscle PCr has an important regulatory role via a shuttle mechanism involving creatine (Cr).[17,18] Known as the PCr-Cr shuttle hypothesis, it is proposed that creatine kinase isoforms in the cytosol and mitochondria enabling the shuttling of a high-energy phosphate bond between the sites of ATP turnover (myofibrils) and synthesis (mitochondria). Faster $p\dot{V}O_2$ kinetics would therefore occur in the presence of a more rapid rise in ADP, which would be reflected by a rapid fall in muscle PCr at exercise onset in order to increase the ADP signal within the inner mitochondrial space.

Indirect support for the PCr-Cr shuttle hypothesis can be found in the close kinetic coupling between the fall in muscle PCr and the rise in phase II $p\dot{V}O_2$ at the onset of moderate-intensity exercise in children[19] and adults.[15,16] Thus, it is reasonable to postulate that an age-related modulation of the muscle phosphate controllers of oxidative metabolism (e.g. PCr and ADP) may explain the more rapid phase II $p\dot{V}O_2$ kinetics measured in children compared to adults. This can be examined based on experimental predictions that muscle PCr kinetics will be faster in muscle with a higher activity of oxidative enzymes, greater mitochondrial density,[86] and a reduced concentration of muscle PCr at rest.[87]

There are reports showing the activity of key oxidative enzymes (e.g. lipoamide dehydrogenase, isocitrate dehydrogenase) taken from the vastus lateralis muscle of 13- to 15-year-olds is higher when compared to adults.[88] Furthermore, a decline in the activity of the fumarase enzyme between pre-, circum-, and postpubertal children has also been reported.[89] However, not all muscle biopsy reports suggest an enhanced muscle oxidative capacity in paediatric muscle. Bell *et al.*[90] found no differences in the relative density of mitochondria in the vastus lateralis muscle of 6-year-old boys and girls when compared to data from young adults in an earlier study. Finally, it is known that the resting concentration of muscle PCr in the rectus femoris muscle progressively increases between the ages of 11 and 16 years in boys,[91] but in the triceps surae muscle is similar between 8- to 13-year-old children and young adults.[92] Thus, the limited muscle metabolic data currently available tentatively suggest that children may have a higher activity of key oxidative enzymes and a lower concentration of PCr when compared to adults. This muscle metabolic profile indirectly supports the experimental predictions[86,87] that the kinetics of muscle PCr at exercise onset are more rapid in children compared to adults; however, direct confirmation of this is required through the measurement of the muscle phosphates during exercise.

A technique that permits the direct measurement of the muscle phosphates at rest and during exercise is ^{31}PMRS. This methodology is ideal for paediatric groups, as the muscle phosphates involved in the control of oxidative phosphorylation (e.g. PCr, P_i, and ATP) and pH can be quantified non-invasively with a high sample resolution (e.g. 1 to 30 s). The application of ^{31}PMRS to study muscle metabolism in youth has been comprehensively reviewed elsewhere[93–95] and is discussed in Chapter 6. Here we will consider how ^{31}PMRS has advanced our understanding of the phosphate regulation of $p\dot{V}O_2$ kinetics in youth.

A study by Barker *et al.*[96] was conducted to test the hypothesis that children have more rapid muscle PCr kinetics than adults. Using ^{31}PMRS, the kinetics of the muscle phosphates and pH during moderate intensity quadriceps exercise were determined in 18 9- to 10-year-old children (eight boys, ten girls) and 16 adults (eight men, eight women). To improve the signal-to-noise ratio for the measures responses, each participant completed between four and ten repeat exercise transitions to a power output that corresponded to 80% of the intracellular pH intracellular threshold,[97] which is equivalent to the T_{LAC}.[98] In conflict with their experimental hypotheses, no age- or sex-related differences in the PCr kinetics τ at the onset (boys: 21 ± 4 s; girls: 24 ± 5 s; men: 26 ± 9 s; women: 24 ± 7 s) or offset (boys: 26 ± 5 s; girls: 29 ± 7 s; men: 23 ± 9 s; women: 29 ± 7 s) of exercise were observed. Furthermore, no age- or sex-related differences were found in the steady-state change of PCr, P_i, and ADP, which are known to be important controllers of muscle oxidative metabolism. Thus, the authors concluded that during moderate-intensity quadriceps exercise, the muscle phosphate regulation of oxidative phosphorylation is fully mature in children as young as 9–10 years of age.

It is interesting to note, however, that age- and sex-related differences in muscle phosphate responses to exercise appear to be dependent on exercise intensity. For example, it has been shown that during incremental exercise, age-related differences in the muscle phosphate and pH dynamics between children and adults only appear when exercise is performed above the intracellular threshold for pH.[99,100] That is, when exercising above the intracellular threshold for pH, children require a lower breakdown in muscle PCr and fall in pH for a given increase in exercise work-rate. Similar findings have also been reported in prepubertal compared to pubertal female swimmers when completing 2 min of calf exercise at 140% (severe) but not 40% (moderate) of maximum.[101] However, it has been reported that despite 13-year-olds (five girls, six boys) having a lower concentration of muscle PCr at rest compared to adults, they do not have more rapid muscle PCr kinetics at the onset of heavy intensity exercise set at 20% Δ.[102] Thus, it appears that the higher the imposed work rate is above the intracellular threshold for pH, the more pronounced the child-adult differences in muscle phosphate responses become. For example, in ^{31}PMRS studies employing either continuous or intermittent exercise protocols where pH falls below rest, children are consistently characterized by a lower fall in muscle PCr to meet the energetic demands of the task.[103–105]

Taken collectively, it appears that the phosphate-linked control of oxidative phosphorylation may be exercise-intensity dependent, with child-adult differences in muscle phosphate dynamics becoming more pronounced when exercise is undertaken above the intracellular threshold for pH.[106] Thus, children are characterized by an enhanced oxidative energy contribution during high-intensity exercise, which reduces the requirement for substrate level phosphorylation (fall in PCr and pH). These findings contribute to an explanation of conflicting data for child-adult differences in $p\dot{V}O_2$ kinetics during moderate-intensity exercise, while children consistently show faster $p\dot{V}O_2$ kinetics during exercise above the T_{LAC}.

Muscle oxygen delivery

Whether or not the delivery of oxygen to the contracting myocyte is the main limiting factor for oxidative phosphorylation has been debated for many years. While reducing muscle oxygen delivery through supine exercise[107] or hypoxic gas inspiration[108] can slow the phase II $p\dot{V}O_2$ τ, interventions that increase oxygen delivery, such as hyperoxia[109] or artificially raising muscle blood flow,[110] do not result in a faster phase II $p\dot{V}O_2$ τ in adults. Thus, although the phase II $p\dot{V}O_2$ τ is sensitive to changes in muscle oxygen delivery, in some cases it may not be limiting. To explain the complex relationship between the phase II $p\dot{V}O_2$ τ and muscle oxygen delivery, a 'tipping point' hypothesis has been proposed (Figure 13.3).[111] The model proposes that for healthy participants exercising in the upright position, phase II $p\dot{V}O_2$ τ is oxygen delivery independent and positioned to the right of the tipping point. In the oxygen delivery independent region phase II $p\dot{V}O_2$ τ is considered to be limited by metabolic factors within the muscle. In contrast, with a reduction in muscle oxygen delivery, possibly related to disease or hypoxic gas inspiration, the kinetics of $p\dot{V}O_2$ become oxygen delivery dependent and are characterized by a slowing of the phase II $p\dot{V}O_2$ τ. In the oxygen delivery dependent region participants are positioned to the left of the tipping point.

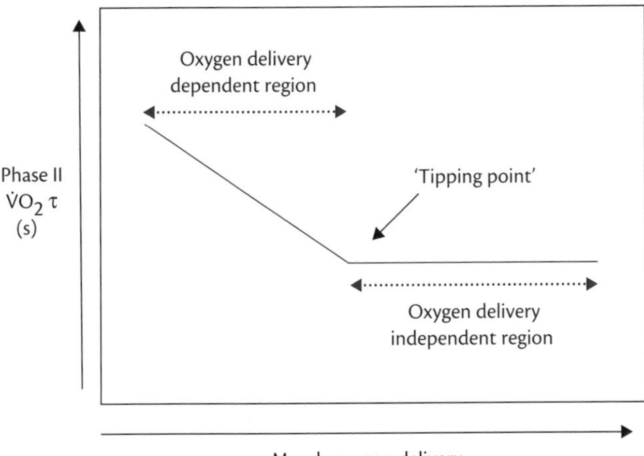

Figure 13.3 The effect of oxygen delivery on phase II oxygen uptake kinetics.
Schematic of the 'tipping point' hypothesis which proposes that the phase II $\dot{V}O_2$ τ can be dependent (oxygen delivery dependent zone) and independent (oxygen delivery independent zone) of oxygen delivery. See text for details.
Adapted from Poole DC, Jones AM. Towards an understanding of the mechanistic bases of $\dot{V}O_2$ kinetics: summary of key points raised in chapters 2–11. In: Jones AM, Poole DC, eds. Oxygen uptake kinetics in sport, exercise and medicine. Oxford: Routledge; 2005: 294–328.

The 'tipping point' hypothesis was developed from experimental data collected on adult and animal investigations. However, data are available which can shed insight as to where paediatric groups are positioned in relation to the tipping point. For example, it is known that paediatric patient groups are likely to reside within the oxygen delivery dependent region of the tipping point. Hebestreit and colleagues[112] have reported young patients with cystic fibrosis (CF) to have slower phase II $p\dot{V}O_2$ τ compared to controls (36.8 ± 13.6 vs 26.4 ± 9.1 s) during semi-supine cycling exercise (see Chapter 27). The authors reported an inverse correlation ($r = -0.69, P = 0.002$) between the phase II $p\dot{V}O_2\tau$ and arterial oxygen saturation measured at the end of the exercise bout in CF patients only, suggesting a mechanistic dependence on muscle oxygen availability. However, correlations were also found between the phase II $p\dot{V}O_2\tau$ and forced expiratory volume in 1 s (FEV_1) ($r = -0.53$, $P = 0.029$) and $\dot{V}O_2$ max ($r = -0.59$, $P = 0.013$) in the CF patients, suggesting respiratory factors and aerobic conditioning may be equally important. Although these data suggest a dependence of phase II $p\dot{V}O_2$ τ on oxygen delivery in a paediatric disease group, it is important to consider if these findings extend to healthy children and adolescents.

In a seminal study, Springer *et al.*[51] found that inspiration of 15% oxygen resulted in a slowing of the phase II $p\dot{V}O_2$ τ during moderate-intensity exercise in 6- to 10-year-old children when compared to normoxic conditions (30 ± 4 vs 24 ± 5 s). Interestingly, a similar slowing of the phase II $p\dot{V}O_2$ τ was also reported in adults (37 ± 10 vs 27 ± 4 s), suggesting that growth and maturation do not alter the adjustment of oxidative metabolism to hypoxia. Although indirect, the slowed $p\dot{V}O_2$ kinetics in children occurred in the presence of slower heart rate kinetics at exercise onset, suggesting a reduction in bulk oxygen delivery. These findings clearly indicate that the phase II $p\dot{V}O_2$ τ in children is sensitive to oxygen delivery and is positioned in the oxygen delivery dependent region when exposed to hypoxia. However, to examine whether $p\dot{V}O_2$ kinetics are limited by oxygen delivery in youth, interventions designed to increase oxygen delivery need be explored.

To provide insights into the limiting factors of $p\dot{V}O_2$ kinetics in youth, Barker *et al.*[36] used 'priming' exercise to increase muscle oxygen delivery in 9- to 13-year-old boys. Participants were asked to perform two repeat bouts of 6 min of cycling exercise at 40% Δ with 6 min of recovery cycling separating the bouts. Priming exercise was found to increase $\dot{Q}$ and oxygenation of the vastus lateralis muscle before and during the second exercise bout. However, despite evidence of increased muscle oxygen delivery, priming exercise did not result in faster phase II $p\dot{V}O_2$ τ in the second exercise bout (bout one: 22 ± 7 vs bout two: 20 ± 4 s; Figure 13.4). Thus, it appears that in healthy boys the phase II $p\dot{V}O_2$ τ is not limited by oxygen availability, at least during heavy-intensity cycling exercise, and is positioned in the oxygen delivery independent region in relation to the tipping point. In contrast, priming exercise did speed the overall $p\dot{V}O_2$ response during bout two by increasing the phase II $p\dot{V}O_2$ amplitude and reducing the $p\dot{V}O_2$ slow component amplitude, which suggests a dependence on muscle oxygen availability. These changes in the $p\dot{V}O_2$ kinetic response to priming exercise have recently been replicated in 10- to 13-year-old boys during cycling at 60% Δ.[46] In addition, this study employed measures of near-infrared spectroscopy (NIRS) derived muscle deoxygenation (HHb), to explore changes in localized oxygen extraction against metabolic rate. Priming exercise was found to blunt the HHb/$p\dot{V}O_2$ ratio at the onset of exercise, indicating less muscle oxygen extraction was required to achieve a change in metabolic rate, likely due to improvements in muscle oxygen delivery. Furthermore, a strong correlation was observed between the change in the phase II $p\dot{V}O_2$ and $p\dot{V}O_2$ slow component amplitudes and the tissue oxygenation

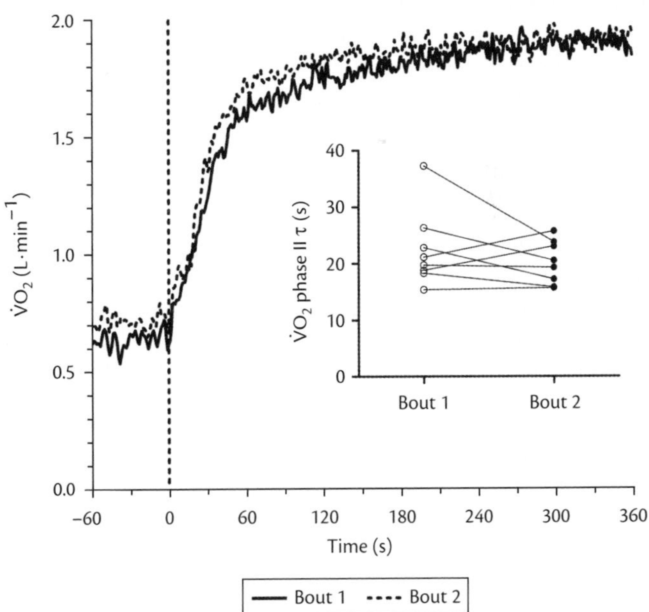

Figure 13.4 Priming exercise and oxygen uptake kinetics in boys.
The effect of priming exercise on the $p\dot{V}O_2$ kinetic response in boys. Bout 1 (control) and bout 2 (primed) were separated by 6 min of unloaded cycling and are shown by the continuous and dotted line respectively. The onset of exercise is illustrated by the vertical dotted line. The figure insert provides the individual phase II $p\dot{V}O_2$ τ, where seven participants had no meaningful change with priming exercise (mean = 1 s, or 3%), whereas one participant with the largest phase II τ, had a 14 s (36%) speeding.
Adapted from Barker AR, Jones AM, Armstrong N. The influence of priming exercise on oxygen uptake, cardiac output, and muscle oxygenation kinetics during very heavy-intensity exercise in 9- to 13-yr-old boys. J Appl Physiol. 2010; 109: 491–500.

index, further highlighting a dependence of these kinetics parameters, but not the phase II $p\dot{V}O_2$ τ on muscle oxygenation.

A study by Lelcair *et al.*,[61] however, suggests that the phase II $p\dot{V}O_2$ τ in youth may be constrained by muscle oxygen delivery during moderate-intensity cycling exercise. Using the vastus lateralis HHb signal measured by NIRS as an indicator of muscle oxygen extraction and phase II $p\dot{V}O_2$ as a surrogate of $m\dot{V}O_2$,[113] the authors were able to estimate the kinetics of muscle capillary blood flow ($\dot{Q}_{cap}$) at the onset of exercise. The MRT for $\dot{Q}_{cap}$ kinetics in children (21 ± 3 s) was strikingly similar to the MRT for $p\dot{V}O_2$ (23 ± 4 s), which the authors interpreted to indicate that $p\dot{V}O_2$ kinetics may be constrained by muscle oxygen delivery. Interestingly, the authors also found a close correspondence between the kinetics of $\dot{Q}_{cap}$ and $p\dot{V}O_2$ in adults (31 ± 5 s vs 33 ± 5 s), which was slower than that reported in children. The notion that muscle blood flow is reduced during exercise from childhood to adulthood is supported by the earlier findings of Koch.[114] Thus, it is reasonable to suggest that capillary blood flow (and thus oxygen delivery) is reduced from childhood to adulthood, and may account for the more rapid phase II $p\dot{V}O_2$ kinetics in children. However Leclair *et al.*[61] also reported children to have more rapid HHb dynamics at the onset of exercise compared to adults (12 ± 1 vs 19 ± 6 s), suggesting more rapid muscle oxygen extraction. Thus, it is possible that a combination of enhanced muscle oxygen delivery and oxygen extraction accounts for the more rapid phase II $p\dot{V}O_2$ kinetics in children compared to adults.

Muscle fibre recruitment

A striking observation is that the age-related changes in the $p\dot{V}O_2$ kinetic response to exercise during growth and maturation have close parallels to studies that have explored the relationship between muscle fibre type and $p\dot{V}O_2$ kinetics in adults.[54,115] The $p\dot{V}O_2$ slow component magnitude is negatively correlated and the phase II $p\dot{V}O_2$ τ is positively correlated with type I muscle fibre distribution during exercise above the T_{LAC}. Furthermore, it is known that muscle with a high proportion of type I fibres has faster $m\dot{V}O_2$ and muscle PCr kinetics.[116,117] Compared to type II muscle fibres, type I fibres have greater activity of oxidative enzymes and mitochondrial content and improved muscle oxygen delivery which are likely to account for the rapid $m\dot{V}O_2$ and PCr kinetics.[118,119] Finally, it is known that ~85% of the magnitude of the $p\dot{V}O_2$ slow component originates from the contracting muscle,[120] and that the slow component phenomenon is related to the activation of less efficient higher-order type II muscle fibres, at the onset of exercise and/or progressively during the exercise bout.[26,121,122] As the $p\dot{V}O_2$ slow component represents a progressive loss of exercise efficiency during exercise, it is considered to reflect the fatigue processes occurring within the myocyte[26] and mirrors the fall in muscle PCr during exercise.[16]

A common hypothesis is that an age-related decline in the expression of type I muscle fibres and their associated properties for oxidative metabolism may underlie the faster $p\dot{V}O_2$ kinetic response in children compared to adults. Data from a review[123] certainly support this contention as the percentage distribution of type I muscle fibres appears to decline from ~58–48% between the ages of 10 and 20 years in boys. However, no clear trend is evident in girls (~50% distribution) and the magnitude of the decline in boys appears relatively modest. It must also be acknowledged that few data are available on muscle fibre type distribution during growth and maturation using clearly defined participant groups. There are, however, robust data showing child-adult differences in muscle energetics during exercise which indirectly support the notion of developmental changes in muscle fibre type recruitment. For example, ^{31}PMRS studies demonstrate children are characterized by a less pronounced fall in muscle PCr and pH and rise in P_i during high-intensity exercise.[99,100] This attenuated accumulation of the fatigue inducing metabolites (e.g. P_i and H^+) during high-intensity exercise in children may alleviate or delay the requirement to recruit additional muscle fibres (presumably type II) during exercise, which in turn may be related to the faster phase II $p\dot{V}O_2$ τ and/or smaller $p\dot{V}O_2$ slow component often found in children compared to adults.

In an attempt to explore further the relationship between muscle activation and $p\dot{V}O_2$ kinetics, Breese *et al.*[38] measured the electrical activity of the vastus lateralis muscle during 6 min of very heavy cycling exercise in boys and men. Consistent with previous reports, the boys had a reduced $p\dot{V}O_2$ slow component compared to adults. However, while the $p\dot{V}O_2$ slow component occurred in the presence of a progressive increase in iEMG between 2–6 min in men, iEMG remained stable in boys over this time frame. This may indicate that the evolution of the $p\dot{V}O_2$ slow component in boys does not depend on a progressive recruitment of motor units. However, no relationship was observed between the magnitude of the $p\dot{V}O_2$ slow component and changes in iEMG in the men or boys, suggesting that changes in muscle activation may not account for the child-adult differences in the magnitude of the $p\dot{V}O_2$ slow component.

The use of iEMG to document changes in muscle activation during exercise has been criticized due to the superficial nature of the measure and that electrodes are typically confined to a single muscle group (e.g. vastus lateralis). To overcome these technical limitations, magnetic resonance imaging (MRI) can be used to quantify the recruitment of superficial and deep muscles by using the transverse relaxation time (T_2) of muscle protons.[124] Using this technique, Breese and colleagues[45] were able document muscle activation patterns across eight thigh muscles in response to 6 min of very heavy exercise in boys and men. Muscle activation patterns were measured at rest, at the onset of the $p\dot{V}O_2$ slow component, and at end exercise. Muscle T_2 increased across all muscles studied during very heavy exercise in boys and men. However, during the $p\dot{V}O_2$ slow component region muscle T_2 increased in the rectus femoris, vastus medialis, and vastus intermedius muscles in boys and the vastus lateralis and adductor magnus muscles in men, suggesting age-related differences in muscle activation patterns during exercise. When the area-weighted average of the T_2 changes was computed to adjust for muscle cross-sectional area, a significant positive relationship was observed with the $p\dot{V}O_2$ slow component in men ($r = 0.92$) but not boys ($r = 0.09$). Assuming changes in muscle T_2 reflect an increase in muscle activation,[122,124] these results suggest that the development of the $p\dot{V}O_2$ slow component in boys may be independent of a progressive activation of muscle fibres and that other factors may be the cause of the progressive loss in exercise efficiency during very heavy exercise in children. Thus, it may be speculated that during the transition from childhood to adulthood, the progressive recruitment of muscle fibres becomes an increasingly important contributor to the development of the $p\dot{V}O_2$ slow component during high-intensity exercise, and may underlie the reduced slow component amplitude reported in child participants.

Recent studies have explored the dependence of the phase II $p\dot{V}O_2$ τ on muscle fibre recruitment during exercise. It is known that muscle fibre recruitment is dependent on both contraction velocity and baseline work rate, such that type II fibres are preferentially recruited at higher contraction velocities or work-rates.[125,126] For example, it has been shown that increasing pedal cadence from 50 to 115 revolutions·min^{-1} during very heavy cycling increases the phase II $\dot{V}O_2$ τ (32 ± 5 vs 42 ± 11 s) in untrained adolescent boys.[37] Furthermore, when a bout of very heavy exercise is immediately preceded by moderate-intensity exercise rather than baseline pedalling, the phase II p$\dot{V}O_2$ τ is lengthened (30 ± 5 vs 19 ± 5 s) in boys.[38] Thus, experimental manipulations which are designed to preferentially recruit high-order type II muscle fibres result in a slowing of the phase II p$\dot{V}O_2$ τ in youth. This, albeit indirectly, suggests that the age-related changes in the phase II p$\dot{V}O_2$ τ may be influenced by alterations in muscle fibre recruitment strategies during exercise. Lastly, it should be noted that although increasing pedal cadence was associated with an increase in the phase II p$\dot{V}O_2$ τ in untrained adolescent boys, no such effect was observed in trained adolescent cyclists.[37] This suggests that cycling training may be associated with alterations in muscle oxidative capacity or muscle fibre recruitment strategies that preserve the p$\dot{V}O_2$ response across a range of exercise intensities.

Conclusions

The p$\dot{V}O_2$ response to exercise provides valuable insights into the control of oxidative phosphorylation and the determinants of exercise tolerance under conditions which reflect the transitory nature of children's physical activity. Recent evidence has shown that when appropriately modelled the phase II p$\dot{V}O_2$ τ provides a close reflection of the underlying muscle metabolic response in children. High methodological rigour is required for analysis of the p$\dot{V}O_2$ kinetic response to exercise in youth, with attention needed to ensure the correct placement of the participant within an exercise intensity domain, that the p$\dot{V}O_2$ profile has sufficient signal-to-noise characteristics, and that physiologically sound models are used to characterize the kinetic response. Of the rigorous studies that have been undertaken, there is compelling evidence that during heavy or very heavy exercise the phase II p$\dot{V}O_2$ τ becomes slower and the magnitude of the p$\dot{V}O_2$ slow component is augmented from childhood to adulthood. However, despite a trend for a faster phase II p$\dot{V}O_2$ τ during moderate-intensity exercise in children, the evidence remains equivocal. The mechanisms underlying this age-related adaptation of oxidative phosphorylation are largely unknown but may be related to modulation of the muscle phosphate controllers of oxidative phosphorylation, muscle oxygen delivery, and utilization and/or muscle fibre type recruitment strategies. In particular, it appears children have a lower requirement for substrate level phosphorylation, have enhanced muscle oxygen delivery and utilization, and recruit fewer higher-order (type II) muscle fibres at the onset and progressively during exercise compared to adults. However, further studies are required to explore the effect of age, sex, biological maturation, and limiting factors on p$\dot{V}O_2$ kinetics in paediatric groups.

Summary

- Studying p$\dot{V}O_2$ kinetics during exercise provides valuable insights into the control of oxidative phosphorylation at the onset and offset of exercise.
- The phase II p$\dot{V}O_2$ time constant provides a non-invasive reflection of m$\dot{V}O_2$ kinetics in young people.
- Children's and adolescents' p$\dot{V}O_2$ kinetic response to exercise should be evaluated with the correct placement of the participant within an established exercise intensity domain.
- Repeat exercise transitions are required to increase the signal-to-noise ratio of the child's p$\dot{V}O_2$ response to exercise.
- Little is known about phase I p$\dot{V}O_2$ kinetics in youth, but sparse data suggest its duration may increase with age.
- There is little consensus regarding the effect of age or sex on the p$\dot{V}O_2$ kinetic response to moderate intensity exercise; however, there is a strong trend for a faster phase II p$\dot{V}O_2$ τ in children.
- During heavy and very heavy exercise there is an age-related slowing of the phase II p$\dot{V}O_2$ time constant and an increase in the p$\dot{V}O_2$ slow component.
- During exercise above the lactate threshold, boys have faster phase II p$\dot{V}O_2$ kinetics and a reduced p$\dot{V}O_2$ slow component amplitude compared to girls.
- Little is known about the p$\dot{V}O_2$kinetic responses to severe exercise.
- The p$\dot{V}O_2$ kinetic response in youth is limited by a combination of factors related to the build-up of muscle phosphates (e.g. ADP), muscle oxygen delivery and utilization, and muscle fibre recruitment.
- Faster p$\dot{V}O_2$ kinetics in young people are likely related to a lower requirement for substrate-level phosphorylation, increased muscle oxygen delivery and utilization, and reduced requirement to recruit high-order muscle fibres (type II) during exercise.

References

1. Nevill A, Rowland T, Goff D, Martel L, Ferrone L. Scaling or normalising maximum oxygen uptake to predict 1-mile run time in boys. *Eur J Appl Physiol.* 2004; 92: 285–288.
2. Ekelund U, Anderssen SA, Froberg K, Sardinha LB, Andersen LB, Brage S. Independent associations of physical activity and cardiorespiratory fitness with metabolic risk factors in children: the European youth heart study. *Diabetologia.* 2007; 50: 1832–1840.
3. Bailey RC, Olson J, Pepper SL, Porszasz J, Barstow TJ, Cooper DM. The level and tempo of children's physical activities: an observational study. *Med Sci Sports Exerc.* 1995; 27: 1033–1041.
4. Baquet G, Stratton G, Van Praagh E, Berthoin S. Improving physical activity assessment in prepubertal children with high-frequency accelerometry monitoring: a methodological issue. *Prev Med.* 2007; 44: 143–147.
5. Grassi B, Poole DC, Richardson RS, Knight DR, Erickson BK, Wagner PD. Muscle O_2 uptake kinetics in humans: implications for metabolic control. *J Appl Physiol.* 1996; 80: 988–998.
6. Krustrup P, Jones AM, Wilkerson DP, Calbet JA, Bangsbo J. Muscular and pulmonary O_2 uptake kinetics during moderate- and high-intensity sub-maximal knee-extensor exercise in humans. *J Physiol.* 2009; 587: 1843–1856.
7. Whipp BJ, Rossiter HB. The kinetics of oxygen uptake: Physiological inferences from the parameters. In: Jones AM, Poole DC (eds.) *Oxygen uptake kinetics in sport, exercise and medicine*. Oxford: Routledge; 2005. p. 62–94.
8. Fitts RH. Cellular mechanisms of muscle fatigue. *Physiol Rev.* 1994; 74: 49–94.
9. Rossiter HB. Exercise: Kinetic considerations for gas exchange. *Compr Physiol.* 2011; 1: 203–244.
10. Whipp BJ, Ward SA, Lamarra N, Davis JA, Wasserman K. Parameters of ventilatory and gas exchange dynamics during exercise. *J Appl Physiol.* 1982; 52: 1506–1513.

11. Behnke BJ, Barstow TJ, Kindig CA, McDonough P, Musch TI, Poole DC. Dynamics of oxygen uptake following exercise onset in rat skeletal muscle. *Respir Physiol Neurobiol.* 2002; 133: 229–239.
12. Whipp BJ, Ward SA, Rossiter HB. Pulmonary O_2 uptake during exercise: conflating muscular and cardiovascular responses. *Med Sci Sports Exerc.* 2005; 37: 1574–1585.
13. Barstow TJ, Lamarra N, Whipp BJ. Modulation of muscle and pulmonary O_2 uptakes by circulatory dynamics during exercise. *J Appl Physiol.* 1990; 68: 979–989.
14. Yoshida T, Yamamoto K, Udo M. Relationship between cardiac output and oxygen uptake at the onset of exercise. *Eur J Appl Physiol Occup Physiol.* 1993; 66: 155–160.
15. Rossiter HB, Ward SA, Doyle VL, Howe FA, Griffiths JR, Whipp BJ. Inferences from pulmonary O_2 uptake with respect to intramuscular [phosphocreatine] kinetics during moderate exercise in humans. *J Physiol.* 1999; 518: 921–932.
16. Rossiter HB, Ward SA, Kowalchuk JM, Howe FA, Griffiths JR, Whipp BJ. Dynamic asymmetry of phosphocreatine concentration and O(2) uptake between the on- and off-transients of moderate- and high-intensity exercise in humans. *J Physiol.* 2002; 541: 991–1002.
17. Mahler M. First-order kinetics of muscle oxygen consumption, and an equivalent proportionality between QO_2 and phosphorylcreatine level. Implications for the control of respiration. *J Gen Physiol.* 1985; 86: 135–165.
18. Meyer RA. A linear model of muscle respiration explains monoexponential phosphocreatine changes. *Am J Physiol Cell Physiol.* 1988; 254: C548–C553.
19. Barker AR, Welsman JR, Fulford J, Welford D, Williams CA, Armstrong N. Muscle phosphocreatine and pulmonary oxygen uptake kinetics in children at the onset and offset of moderate intensity exercise. *Eur J Appl Physiol.* 2008; 102: 727–738.
20. Özyener F, Rossiter HB, Ward SA, Whipp BJ. Influence of exercise intensity on the on- and off-transient kinetics of pulmonary oxygen uptake in humans. *J Physiol.* 2001; 533: 891–902.
21. Burnley M, Doust JH, Carter H, Jones AM. Effects of prior exercise and recovery duration on oxygen uptake kinetics during heavy exercise in humans. *Exp Physiol.* 2001; 86: 417–425.
22. Pringle JS, Jones AM. Maximal lactate steady state, critical power and EMG during cycling. *Eur J Appl Physiol.* 2002; 88: 214–226.
23. Dekerle J, Baron B, Dupont L, Vanvelcenaher J, Pelayo P. Maximal lactate steady state, respiratory compensation threshold and critical power. *Eur J Appl Physiol.* 2003; 89: 281–288.
24. Jones AM, Vanhatalo A, Burnley M, Morton RH, Poole DC. Critical power: implications for determination of VO_2 max and exercise tolerance. *Med Sci Sports Exerc.* 2010; 42: 1876–1890.
25. Poole DC, Ward SA, Gardner GW, Whipp BJ. Metabolic and respiratory profile of the upper limit for prolonged exercise in man. *Ergonomics.* 1988; 31: 1265–1279.
26. Jones AM, Grassi B, Christensen PM, Krustrup P, Bangsbo J, Poole DC. Slow component of VO_2 kinetics: mechanistic bases and practical applications. *Med Sci Sports Exerc.* 2011; 43: 2046–2062.
27. Hill DW, Poole DC, Smith JC. The relationship between power and the time to achieve VO_2 max. *Med Sci Sports Exerc.* 2002; 34: 709–714.
28. Jones AM, Poole DC (eds.) *Oxygen uptake kinetics in sport, exercise and medicine.* Oxford: Routledge; 2005.
29. Lansley KE, Dimenna FJ, Bailey SJ, Jones AM. A 'new' method to normalise exercise intensity. *Int J Sports Med.* 2011; 32: 535–541.
30. Fawkner SG, Armstrong N, Childs DJ, Welsman JR. Reliability of the visually identified ventilatory threshold and v-slope in children. *Pediatr Exer Sci.* 2002; 14: 181–192.
31. Reybrouck T, Weymans M, Stijns H, Knops J, van der Hauwaert L. Ventilatory anaerobic threshold in healthy children. Age and sex differences. *Eur J Appl Physiol Occup Physiol.* 1985; 54: 278–284.
32. Barker AR, Bond B, Toman C, Williams CA, Armstrong N. Critical power in adolescents: physiological bases and assessment using all-out exercise. *Eur J Appl Physiol.* 2011; 112: 1359–1370.
33. Fawkner SG, Armstrong N. Assessment of critical power with children. *Pediatr Exer Sci.* 2002; 14: 259–268.
34. Beneke R, Heck H, Schwarz V, Leithauser R. Maximal lactate steady state during the second decade of age. *Med Sci Sports Exerc.* 1996; 28: 1474–1478.
35. Fawkner SG, Armstrong N. Longitudinal changes in the kinetic response to heavy-intensity exercise in children. *J Appl Physiol.* 2004; 97: 460–466.
36. Barker AR, Jones AM, Armstrong N. The influence of priming exercise on oxygen uptake, cardiac output, and muscle oxygenation kinetics during very heavy-intensity exercise in 9- to 13-yr-old boys. *J Appl Physiol.* 2010; 109: 491–500.
37. Breese BC, Armstrong N, Barker AR, Williams CA. The effect of pedal rate on pulmonary O_2 uptake kinetics during very heavy intensity exercise in trained and untrained teenage boys. *Respir Physiol Neurobiol.* 2011; 177: 149–154.
38. Breese BC, Barker AR, Armstrong N, Jones AM, Williams CA. The effect of baseline metabolic rate on pulmonary O_2 uptake kinetics during very heavy intensity exercise in boys and men. *Respir Physiol Neurobiol.* 2012; 180: 223–229.
39. Fawkner SG, Armstrong N. The slow-component response of VO_2 to heavy intensity exercise in children. In: Reilly T, Marfell-Jones M (eds.) *Kinanthropometry VIII.* London: Routledge; 2003. p. 105–113.
40. Potter CR, Childs DJ, Houghton W, Armstrong N. Breath-to-breath 'noise' in the ventilatory and gas exchange responses of children to exercise. *Eur J Appl Physiol.* 1999; 80: 118–124.
41. Koga S, Shiojiri T, Kondo N. Measuring VO_2 kinetics: the practicalities. In: Jones AM, Poole DC (eds.) *Oxygen uptake kinetics in sport, exercise and medicine.* Oxford: Routledge; 2005. p. 39–61.
42. Fawkner SG, Armstrong N, Potter CR, Welsman JR. Oxygen uptake kinetics in children and adults after the onset of moderate-intensity exercise. *J Sports Sci.* 2002; 20: 319–326.
43. Breese BC, Williams CA, Barker AR, Welsman JR, Fawkner SG, Armstrong N. Longitudinal changes in the oxygen uptake kinetic response to heavy-intensity exercise in 14- to 16-year-old boys. *Pediatr Exerc Sci.* 2010; 22: 69–80.
44. Marwood S, Roche D, Rowland T, Garrard M, Unnithan VB. Faster pulmonary oxygen uptake kinetics in trained versus untrained male adolescents. *Med Sci Sports Exerc.* 2010; 42: 127–134.
45. Breese BC, Barker AR, Armstrong N, Fulford J, Williams CA. Influence of thigh activation on the VO_2 slow component in boys and men. *Eur J Appl Physiol.* 2014; 114: 2309–2319.
46. Barker AR, Trebilcock E, Breese B, Jones AM, Armstrong N. The effect of priming exercise on O_2 uptake kinetics, muscle O_2 delivery and utilization, muscle activity, and exercise tolerance in boys. *Appl Physiol Nutr Metab.* 2014; 39: 308–317.
47. Freedson PS, Gilliam TB, Sady SP, Katch VL. Transient VO_2 characteristics in children at the onset of steady-rate exercise. *Res Q Exerc Sport.* 1981; 52: 167–173.
48. Stevens D, Oades PJ, Armstrong N, Williams CA. Early oxygen uptake recovery following exercise testing in children with chronic chest diseases. *Pediatr Pulmonol.* 2009; 44: 480–488.
49. Fawkner SG, Armstrong N. Can we confidently study VO_2 kinetics in young people. *J Sport Sci Med.* 2007; 6: 277–285.
50. Fawkner S, Armstrong N. Oxygen uptake kinetic response to exercise in children. *Sports Med.* 2003; 33: 651–669.
51. Springer C, Barstow TJ, Wasserman K, Cooper DM. Oxygen uptake and heart rate responses during hypoxic exercise in children and adults. *Med Sci Sports Exerc.* 1991; 23: 71–79.
52. Barstow TJ, Mole PA. Linear and non-linear characteristics of oxygen uptake during heavy exercise. *J Appl Physiol.* 1991; 71: 2099–2106.
53. Williams CA, Carter H, Jones AM, Doust JH. Oxygen uptake kinetics during treadmill running in boys and men. *J Appl Physiol.* 2001; 90: 1700–1706.
54. Barstow TJ, Jones AM, Nguyen PH, Casaburi R. Influence of muscle fiber type and pedal frequency on oxygen uptake kinetics of heavy exercise. *J Appl Physiol.* 1996; 81: 1642–1650.
55. Hebestreit H, Kriemler S, Hughson RL, Bar-Or O. Kinetics of oxygen uptake at the onset of exercise in boys and men. *J Appl Physiol.* 1998; 85: 1833–1841.

56. Obert P, Cleuziou C, Candau R, Courteix D, Lecoq AM, Guenon P. The slow component of O_2 uptake kinetics during high-intensity exercise in trained and untrained prepubertal children. *Int J Sports Med.* 2000; 21: 31–36.
57. Armon Y, Cooper DM, Flores R, Zanconato S, Barstow TJ. Oxygen uptake dynamics during high-intensity exercise in children and adults. *J Appl Physiol.* 1991; 70: 841–848.
58. Zanconato S, Cooper DM, Armon Y. Oxygen cost and oxygen uptake dynamics and recovery with 1 min of exercise in children and adults. *J Appl Physiol.* 1991; 71: 993–998.
59. Armstrong N, Barker AR. Oxygen uptake kinetics in children and adolescents: a review. *Pediatr Exerc Sci.* 2009; 21: 130–147.
60. Barstow TJ, Scheuermann BW. VO_2 kinetics: Effects of maturation and ageing. In: Jones AM, Poole DC (eds.) *Oxygen uptake kinetics in sport, exercise and medicine.* Oxford: Routledge; 2005. p. 331–352.
61. Leclair E, Berthoin S, Borel B, *et al.* Faster pulmonary oxygen uptake kinetics in children vs adults due to enhancements in oxygen delivery and extraction. *Scand J Med Sci Sports.* 2013; 23: 705–712.
62. Turley KR, Wilmore JH. Cardiovascular responses to treadmill and cycle ergometer exercise in children and adults. *J Appl Physiol.* 1997; 83: 948–957.
63. Cooper DM, Berry C, Lamarra N, Wasserman K. Kinetics of oxygen uptake and heart rate at onset of exercise in children. *J Appl Physiol.* 1985; 59: 211–217.
64. Williams CA, Carter H, Jones AM, Doust JH. Oxygen uptake kinetics during treadmill running in boys and men. *J Appl Physiol.* 2001; 90: 1700–1706.
65. Rogers DM, Olson BL, Wilmore JH. Scaling for the VO_2-to-body size relationship among children and adults. *J Appl Physiol.* 1995; 79: 958–967.
66. Welsman JR, Armstrong N. Statistical techniques for interpreting body size-related exercise performance during growth. *Pediatr Exerc Sci.* 2000; 12: 112–127.
67. Welsman JR, Armstrong N. Longitudinal changes in submaximal oxygen uptake in 11- to 13-year-olds. *J Sports Sci.* 2000; 18: 183–189.
68. Jones AM, Wilkerson DP, DiMenna F, Fulford J, Poole DC. Muscle metabolic responses to exercise above and below the 'critical power' assessed using ^{31}P-MRS. *Am J Physiol Regul Integr Comp Physiol.* 2008; 294: R585–R593.
69. Fawkner SG, Armstrong N. Sex differences in the oxygen uptake kinetic response to heavy-intensity exercise in prepubertal children. *Eur J Appl Physiol.* 2004; 93: 210–216.
70. Wasserman K, Hansen J, Sue D, *et al. Principles of exercise testing and interpretation*, 5th ed. Philiadelphia: Lippincott Williams & Wilkins; 2012.
71. MacDonald M, Pedersen PK, Hughson RL. Acceleration of VO_2 kinetics in heavy submaximal exercise by hyperoxia and prior high-intensity exercise. *J Appl Physiol.* 1997; 83: 1318–1325.
72. Hughson RL. Regulation of VO_2 on-kinetics by O_2 delivery. In: Jones AM, Poole DC (eds.) *Oxygen uptake kinetics in sport, exercise and medicine.* Oxford: Routledge; 2005. p. 185–211.
73. Tschakovsky ME, Hughson RL. Interaction of factors determining oxygen uptake at the onset of exercise. *J Appl Physiol.* 1999; 86: 1101–1113.
74. Hughson RL, Shoemaker JK, Tschakovsky ME, Kowalchuk JM. Dependence of muscle VO_2 on blood flow dynamics at onset of forearm exercise. *J Appl Physiol.* 1996; 81: 1619–1626.
75. Meyer RA, Foley JM. Cellular processes intergrating the metabolic response to exercise. In: Rowell LB and Shepherd JT (eds.) *Handbook of physiology, section 12, Exercise: regulation and integration of multiple systems.* Bethesda, MD: American Physiological Society; 1996. p. 841–869.
76. Grassi B. Oxygen uptake kinetics: old and recent lessons from experiments on isolated muscle *in situ*. *Eur J Appl Physiol.* 2003; 90: 242–249.
77. Whipp BJ, Mahler M. Dynamics of pulmonary gas exchange during exercise. In: West JB (ed.) *Pulmonary gas exchange, Vol II.* New York: Academic Press; 1980. p. 33–96.
78. Kindig CA, Howlett RA, Stary CM, Walsh B, Hogan MC. Effects of acute creatine kinase inhibition on metabolism and tension development in isolated single myocytes. *J Appl Physiol.* 2005; 98: 541–549.
79. Rossiter HB, Howe FA, Ward SA. Intramuscular phosphate and pulmonary VO_2 kinetics during exercise: implications for control of skeletal muscle oxygen consumption. In: Jones AM, Poole DC (eds.) *Oxygen uptake kinetics in sport, exercise and medicine.* Oxford: Routledge; 2005. p. 154–184.
80. Timmons JA, Gustafsson T, Sundberg CJ, Jansson E, Greenhaff PL. Muscle acetyl group availability is a major determinant of oxygen deficit in humans during submaximal exercise. *Am J Physiol.* 1998; 274: E377–E380.
81. Timmons JA, Gustafsson T, Sundberg CJ, *et al.* Substrate availability limits human skeletal muscle oxidative ATP regeneration at the onset of ischemic exercise. *J Clin Invest.* 1998; 101: 79–85.
82. Gurd BJ, Peters SJ, Heigenhauser GJ, *et al.* Prior heavy exercise elevates pyruvate dehydrogenase activity and speeds O_2 uptake kinetics during subsequent moderate-intensity exercise in healthy young adults. *J Physiol.* 2006; 577: 985–996.
83. Poole DC, Barstow TJ, McDonough P, Jones AM. Control of oxygen uptake during exercise. *Med Sci Sports Exerc.* 2008; 40: 462–474.
84. Wilson DF. Factors affecting the rate and energetics of mitochondrial oxidative phosphorylation. *Med Sci Sports Exerc.* 1994; 26: 37–43.
85. Grassi B. Delayed metabolic activation of oxidative phosphorylation in skeletal muscle at exercise onset. *Med Sci Sports Exerc.* 2005; 37: 1567–1573.
86. McCully KK, Fielding RA, Evans WJ, Leigh JS, Posner JD. Relationships between in vivo and in vitro measurements of metabolism in young and old human calf muscles. *J Appl Physiol.* 1993; 75: 813–819.
87. Paganini AT, Foley JM, Meyer RA. Linear dependence of muscle phosphocreatine kinetics on oxidative capacity. *Am J Physiol Cell Physiol.* 1997; 272: C501–C510.
88. Haralambie G. Enzyme activities in skeletal muscle of 13–15 years old adolescents. *Bull Europ Physiopath Resp.* 1982; 18: 65–74.
89. Berg A, Kim SS, Keul J. Skeletal muscle enzyme activities in healthy young subjects. *Int J Sports Med.* 1986; 7: 236–239.
90. Bell RD, MacDougall JD, Billeter R, Howald H. Muscle fiber types and morphometric analysis of skeletal muscle in six-year-old children. *Med Sci Sports Exerc.* 1980; 12: 28–31.
91. Eriksson BO. Muscle metabolism in children—a review. *Acta Paediatr Scand Suppl.* 1980; 283: 20–28.
92. Gariod L, Binzoni T, Ferretti G, Le Bas JF, Reutenauer H, Cerretelli P. Standardisation of ^{31}phosphorus-nuclear magnetic resonance spectroscopy determinations of high energy phosphates in humans. *Eur J Appl Physiol Occup Physiol.* 1994; 68: 107–110.
93. Barker AR, Armstrong N. Insights into developmental muscle metabolism through the use of ^{31}P-magnetic resonance spectroscopy: a review. *Pediatr Exerc Sci.* 2010; 22: 350–368.
94. Armstrong N, Barker AR. New insights in paediatric exercise metabolism. *J Sport Health Sci.* 2012; 1: 18–26.
95. Cooper DM, Barstow TJ. Magnetic resonance imaging and spectroscopy in studying exercise in children. *Exerc Sport Sci Rev.* 1996; 24: 475–499.
96. Barker AR, Welsman JR, Fulford J, Welford D, Armstrong N. Muscle phosphocreatine kinetics in children and adults at the onset and offset of moderate-intensity exercise. *J Appl Physiol.* 2008; 105: 446–456.
97. Barker A, Welsman J, Welford D, Fulford J, Williams C, Armstrong N. Reliability of ^{31}P-magnetic resonance spectroscopy during an exhaustive incremental exercise test in children. *Eur J Appl Physiol.* 2006; 98: 556–565.
98. Systrom DM, Kanerek DJ, Kohler SJ, Kazemi H. ^{31}P nuclear magnetic resonance spectroscopy study of the anaerobic threshold in humans. *J Appl Physiol.* 1990; 68: 2060–2066.
99. Barker AR, Welsman JR, Fulford J, Welford D, Armstrong N. Quadriceps muscle energetics during incremental exercise in children and adults. *Med Sci Sports Exerc.* 2010; 42: 1303–1313.

100. Zanconato S, Buchthal S, Barstow TJ, Cooper DM. ^{31}P-magnetic resonance spectroscopy of leg muscle metabolism during exercise in children and adults. *J Appl Physiol.* 1993; 74: 2214–2218.
101. Petersen SR, Gaul CA, Stanton MM, Hanstock CC. Skeletal muscle metabolism during short-term, high-intensity exercise in prepubertal and pubertal girls. *J Appl Physiol.* 1999; 87: 2151–2156.
102. Willcocks RJ, Williams CA, Barker AR, Fulford J, Armstrong N. Age- and sex-related differences in muscle phosphocreatine and oxygenation kinetics during high-intensity exercise in adolescents and adults. *NMR Biomed.* 2010; 23: 569–577.
103. Kappenstein J, Ferrauti A, Runkel B, Fernandez-Fernandez J, Müller K, Zange J. Changes in phosphocreatine concentration of skeletal muscle during high-intensity intermittent exercise in children and adults. *Eur J Appl Physiol.* 2013; 113: 2769–2779.
104. Tonson A, Ratel S, Le Fur Y, Vilmen C, Cozzone PJ, Bendahan D. Muscle energetics changes throughout maturation: a quantitative ^{31}P-MRS analysis. *J Appl Physiol.* 2010; 109: 1769–1778.
105. Willcocks RJ, Fulford J, Armstrong N, Barker AR, Williams CA. Muscle metabolism during fatiguing isometric quadriceps exercise in adolescents and adults. *Appl Physiol Nutr Metab.* 2014; 39: 439–445.
106. Barker AR, Breese BC, Willcocks RJ, Williams CA, Armstrong N. Commentaries on Viewpoint: Do oxidative and anaerobic energy production in exercising muscle change throughout growth and maturation? The importance of exercise intensity when studying developmental energy metabolism. *J Appl Physiol.* 2010; 109: 1565–1566.
107. Koga S, Shiojiri T, Shibasaki M, Kondo N, Fukuba Y, Barstow TJ. Kinetics of oxygen uptake during supine and upright heavy exercise. *J Appl Physiol.* 1999; 87: 253–260.
108. Hughson RL, Kowalchuk JM. Kinetics of oxygen uptake for submaximal exercise in hyperoxia, normoxia, and hypoxia. *Can J Appl Physiol.* 1995; 20: 198–210.
109. Wilkerson DP, Berger NJ, Jones AM. Influence of hyperoxia on pulmonary O_2 uptake kinetics following the onset of exercise in humans. *Respir Physiol Neurobiol.* 2006; 153: 92–106.
110. Grassi B, Hogan MC, Kelley KM, *et al.* Role of convective O_2 delivery in determining VO_2 on-kinetics in canine muscle contracting at peak VO_2. *J Appl Physiol.* 2000; 89: 1293–1301.
111. Poole DC, Jones AM. Towards an understanding of the mechanistic bases of VO_2 kinetics: summary of key points raised in chapters 2–11. In: Jones AM, Poole DC (eds.) *Oxygen uptake kinetics in sport, exercise and medicine.* Oxford: Routledge; 2005. p. 294–328.
112. Hebestreit H, Hebestreit A, Trusen A, Hughson RL. Oxygen uptake kinetics are slowed in cystic fibrosis. *Med Sci Sports Exerc.* 2005; 37: 10–17.
113. Ferreira LF, Townsend DK, Lutjemeier BJ, Barstow TJ. Muscle capillary blood flow kinetics estimated from pulmonary O_2 uptake and near-infrared spectroscopy. *J Appl Physiol.* 2005; 98: 1820–1828.
114. Koch G. Maximal oxygen transport capacity in adolescents aged 12 to 17 years. Effect of growth combined with intensive physcial training. In: Bachl N, Prokop L, Suckert R (eds.) *Current topic in sports medicine.* Wien: Urban & Schwarzenber; 1984. p. 479–497.
115. Pringle JS, Doust JH, Carter H, Tolfrey K, Campbell IT, Jones AM. Oxygen uptake kinetics during moderate, heavy and severe intensity 'submaximal' exercise in humans: the influence of muscle fibre type and capillarisation. *Eur J Appl Physiol.* 2003; 89: 289–300.
116. Kushmerick MJ, Meyer RA, Brown TR. Regulation of oxygen consumption in fast- and slow-twitch muscle. *Am J Physiol.* 1992; 263: C598–C606.
117. Crow MT, Kushmerick MJ. Chemical energetics of slow- and fast-twitch muscles of the mouse. *J Gen Physiol.* 1982; 79: 147–166.
118. Korzeniewski B, Zoladz JA. Factors determining the oxygen consumption rate (VO_2) on-kinetics in skeletal muscles. *Biochem J.* 2004; 379: 703–710.
119. Behnke BJ, McDonough P, Padilla DJ, Musch TI, Poole DC. Oxygen exchange profile in rat muscles of contrasting fibre types. *J Physiol.* 2003; 549: 597–605.
120. Poole DC, Gaesser GA, Hogan MC, Knight DR, Wagner PD. Pulmonary and leg VO_2 during submaximal exercise: implications for muscular efficiency. *J Appl Physiol.* 1992; 72: 805–810.
121. Krustrup P, Soderlund K, Mohr M, Gonzalez-Alonso J, Bangsbo J. Recruitment of fibre types and quadriceps muscle portions during repeated, intense knee-extensor exercise in humans. *Pflugers Arch.* 2004; 449: 56–65.
122. Endo MY, Kobayakawa M, Kinugasa R, *et al.* Thigh muscle activation distribution and pulmonary VO_2 kinetics during moderate, heavy, and very heavy intensity cycling exercise in humans. *Am J Physiol Regul Integr Comp Physiol.* 2007; 293: R812–R820.
123. Jannson E. Age-related fiber type changes in human skeletal muscle. In: Maughan R, Shirreffs S (eds.) *Biochemistry of exercise IX.* Champaign, IL: Human Kinetics; 1996. p. 297–307.
124. Meyer RA, Prior BM. Functional magnetic resonance imaging of muscle. *Exerc Sport Sci Rev.* 2000; 28: 89–92.
125. Sargeant AJ. Neuromuscular determinants of human performance. In: Whipp BJ, Sargeant AJ (eds.) *Physiological determinants of exercise tolerance in humans.* London: Portland Press; 1999. p. 13–28.
126. Henneman E. Recruitment of motor units: the size principle. In: Desmedt J (ed.) *Motor unit types, recruitment and plasticity in health and disease.* Basel: Karger; 1981. p. 26–60.

CHAPTER 14

Temperature regulation

Bareket Falk and Raffy Dotan

Introduction

Humans live in a broad range of environmental conditions, yet can maintain their body temperature within a relatively narrow range (35–41°C). This is achieved behaviourally, technologically, and physiologically. This chapter only deals with the physiological capacity to regulate body temperature, which is essential for maintaining normal physiological function. During exercise, working muscles can increase their metabolic heat production 50-fold or more, while total body heat production may rise as much as 20-fold or more, compared with rest, depending on the working muscle mass and the intensity of exercise. In a hot environment, this heat production places a considerable additional stress on the thermoregulatory system, while in a cold environment, that extra heat may relieve some or all of the incurred cold stress.

Heat is exchanged between the body and the environment via evaporation or via dry heat exchange (radiation, convection, conduction). In a hot environment, physiological means for heat dissipation include sweating, intended to enhance evaporative heat loss, and cutaneous venous dilatation and increased skin blood flow to enhance heat transfer from the body's core to the periphery, and from there to the environment. In the cold, physiological means of heat conservation include metabolic rate increase for enhancing heat production and peripheral vasoconstriction for minimizing heat loss to the environment.

Thermoregulation is affected by environmental conditions as well as by physical and physiological characteristics of the body. In ambient air, environmental factors that affect thermoregulation include air temperature, humidity, velocity, and density, as well as solar or other radiation. Bodily physical factors that can affect evaporative and dry heat exchange include body dimensions, composition, and proportions (e.g. body surface-area-to-mass ratio), while physiological factors include thermal sensitivity of various organ systems, level of acclimatization, aerobic fitness, and hydration state. These factors affect the thermoregulatory response to heat and to cold, although their unique effect in a particular environment is not always clear.

This chapter outlines the physical and physiological changes that take place during growth and maturation and the effects these changes can have on the nature and effectiveness of thermoregulation. The physiological responses to heat stress are discussed in terms of metabolic, circulatory, hormonal, and sweating responses, changes in body temperature, and in terms of heat tolerance. Also discussed is hydration status, which can affect thermoregulatory effectiveness and exercise performance in the heat. The physiological response to cold stress is considered in terms of the metabolic and circulatory responses and their possible influence on the effectiveness of thermoregulation. The discussion does not outline the thermoregulatory response per se, but rather emphasizes the differences in that response between children and adults. Finally, child–adult differences in the acclimatization- and training-induced adaptations to thermal stress are discussed.

Maturation may affect thermoregulation. However, until recently, most studies characterized their participants by chronological age rather than maturational stage. For the purpose of this discussion, the term 'children' is used for girls and boys younger than 10 and 11 years, respectively. When maturational stage is not mentioned, children in this age category are considered 'prepubescents'. The term 'adolescents' is used for older children and, when not specifically mentioned, adolescents are considered 'mid-' or 'late-pubescents'.

Physical and physiological child–adult differences pertinent to thermoregulation

Many of the physical and physiological characteristics that change during growth and maturation affect the body's capacity to dissipate or preserve heat. These changes occur at different rates and both their unique and combined thermoregulatory effects are therefore difficult to quantitatively evaluate. Table 14.1 summarizes these changes and their likely effects on thermoregulation. A short discussion of these changes follows.

Physical differences

Body surface-area-to-mass ratio

Heat transfer between the body and the environment is related to the exposed body surface area (BSA). Metabolic heat production during exercise, on the other hand, is proportional to the active muscle mass, which in turn is related to body mass. The BSA-to-mass ratio of a 10-year-old can be over 30% greater than that of an adult (e.g. 10-year-old boy: 135 cm, 30 kg, BSA = 1.07 m^2, BSA/mass = 356 $cm^2 \cdot kg^{-1}$, vs young adult: 180 cm, 70 kg, BSA = 1.89 m^2, BSA/mass = 269 $cm^2 \cdot kg^{-1}$). During growth and maturation, there is a greater increase in body mass than in BSA. Consequently, the BSA-to-mass ratio decreases.

In a thermoneutral, or warm environment, children's greater BSA-to-mass ratio allows them to rely more on dry heat loss (convection, radiation, conduction) and less on evaporative cooling.[3–6] In the cold, or in extremely hot conditions (when ambient temperatures exceed skin temperature), more heat is exchanged between the body and the environment than under more temperate conditions. In such extreme environments, a greater BSA-to-mass ratio may provide a liability: in very hot environments, the child's greater BSA-to-mass ratio means elevated heat absorption from the

Table 14.1 Physical and physiological changes occurring during growth and maturation and their effect on thermoregulation

Change	Effect on thermoregulation	
	Heat	**Cold**
Physical		
Decreased body-surface-area-to-mass ratio	Reduced heat-gain from the environment (in high heat)	Reduced heat loss to the environment
Increase in adiposity (in females)	Increased thermal insulation – possible impedance of heat loss	Increased thermal insulation – enhanced heat conservation
Increased blood volume and cardiac output relative to surface area	Smaller proportion of blood volume / cardiac output necessary for cutaneous perfusion	
Sweat-gland size increase	Increased sweat-gland output	—
Physiological		
Increased economy of bipedal locomotion (decreased oxygen cost)	Decrease in metabolic heat production per unit body mass in walking/running (not in cycling)	
Increased sweat-gland anaerobic metabolism	Increased sweating rate	—
Cognitive		
Improved perception of actual thermal strain	Possibly, better matching of behaviour to environmental conditions and physiological status	

surroundings. At some point, the child may no longer be able to compensate sufficiently with evaporative cooling. In the cold, on the other hand, children's greater ratio results in a greater heat loss to the environment. At some point, they may no longer be able to compensate sufficiently with their higher metabolic rate or possible greater vasoconstriction.[7]

Body composition

The adipose (fat) and muscle tissues are the most important in terms of thermoregulation. While the former increases insulation, the latter affects heat production.

Overweight/obese individuals may be disadvantaged in terms of heat dissipation. Lower thermoregulatory capacity of obese vs lean children, while walking (4.8 $km \cdot h^{-1}$, 5% grade) in moderate to high heat, was shown by Haymes *et al.*[8,9] More recently, Dougherty *et al.*[10] demonstrated that obese children acclimate more slowly to heat and reach uncompensable heat stress at lower environmental limits, compared with their lean peers. On the other hand, recent comparisons of obese and normal-weight children[11,12] did not demonstrate thermoregulatory disadvantage during 30 min of cycling (50–55% peak oxygen uptake [$\dot{V}O_2$]) in the heat (35°C, 40–45% relative humidity [RH]). That is, the rectal temperature (T_{re}) increase was similar in the obese and non-obese individuals. The authors explained the discrepancy between these and earlier studies by the fact that the latter studies did not match lean and obese individuals for aerobic fitness. Two recent adult studies demonstrated that, as long as exercise intensity and environmental heat stress are low to moderate, excess adipose tissue does not necessarily hinder the thermoregulatory process.[13,14] Apparently, as long as the combined stress is well within thermoregulatory capacity, the potential adverse effects of excess adiposity may not be realized. Thus, it is only when cutaneous blood flow and sweating rate approach their limits that the added insulative capacity of excess adiposity becomes a limiting factor and a heightened risk for heat injury. In cold exposure, however, the extra insulative capacity is generally a definite advantage.

A rarely considered aspect of excess adiposity is the heat-storage capacity of the extra adipose mass. This explains why in limited duration heat and exercise stress (e.g. 30 min, as in Leites *et al.*[11] and Sehl *et al.*[12]) overweight/obese individuals may demonstrate a slower rise in T_{re}.

Although more limited in extent, another aspect of adipose tissue is its own metabolism and heat production, which might add to the thermal stress under hot conditions, but helps in the cold. Brown adipose tissue is mostly active during infancy and brown adipocytes decrease with age.[15] However, in recent years brown adipose tissue was shown to be present and active in both children and most adults. For unclear reasons, brown adipose tissue volume and activity actually increases during puberty, specifically during the later stages of puberty[15] and has thus sparked interest in its potential role in curbing childhood obesity.[16] Cold exposure increases the activity of brown adipose tissue in adults,[17] but this has not been investigated in youth.

Children are characterized by a lower proportion of muscle mass compared with adults.[18] In the heat, this fact might somewhat limit muscular heat production, but in the extreme cold it limits the amount of heat that can be produced by physical exercise to counter heat loss. In passive cold exposure, this lower relative muscle mass can limit the amount of heat that can be produced by shivering.

Blood volume

Relative to body mass, children's blood volume is similar to that of adults.[19] However, due to their greater BSA-to-mass ratio, children's cardiac index (blood volume relative to BSA) is lower than that of adults.[20] This lower cardiac index was suggested as contributing to children's thermoregulatory deficiency because it appears to imply limited cardiac output ($\dot{Q}$) availability for heat dissipation at the skin.[21] However, considering their similar blood volume per body mass and their lower relative muscle mass, we suggest that children are not at a circulatory disadvantage compared with adults. As long as $\dot{Q}$ does not fall below clinical norms (normally, only as a result of cardiac insufficiency), children's lower cardiac index need not be considered a liability. To the contrary, it reflects their greater available BSA, which is highly important for heat dissipation, rather than $\dot{Q}$ insufficiency.

Physiological differences

Metabolic differences

The specific oxygen cost of bipedal locomotion (per unit mass; in walking or running) can be 15–20% higher in children compared with adults for any given locomotive speed,[20,22,23] resulting in higher metabolic heat production. The cost of locomotion decreases during adolescence, as persuasively demonstrated in the Amsterdam Growth, Health, and Fitness Study which followed children from age 13 years to adulthood.[24] The additional energy expenditure is manifested as extra metabolic heat production constituting an added thermoregulatory strain during walking/running in the heat.

In the cold, children's higher locomotive heat production may be advantageous in the short term, but more quickly depletes their energy reserves for long-term exercise when no replenishment is provided.[7]

Circulatory differences

In a landmark study, Turley and Wilmore[25] showed that, compared with adults, children had lower $\dot{Q}$ at any given $\dot{V}O_2$ or exercise intensity. These differences did not significantly change with rising $\dot{V}O_2$ or exercise intensity and were similar in magnitude to those expected at basal or resting conditions. Nevertheless, this finding has been interpreted to imply circulatory and therefore thermoregulatory deficiency on the part of children, particularly during exercise in the heat. When resting $\dot{Q}$ values are subtracted from those observed during exercise, children and adults manifest similar $\dot{Q}$ responses to exercise. We maintain, therefore, that the 'discretionary' $\dot{Q}$ (i.e. that available for exercise and/or thermoregulation, beyond basal/resting demands) is similar in children and adults. In extreme conditions, however, children's greater relative skin surface area and their heavier reliance on dry heat dissipation is a combination that can induce circulatory stress greater than the corresponding one in adults (for more on this, see the section Circulatory responses).

Haemoglobin concentration is lower in boys than in men,[26] which may be construed as compromising circulatory effectiveness, possibly contributing to earlier circulatory insufficiency under high heat stress. This view has never been tested experimentally and we are unaware of any other evidence that supports it. Possibly relevant here is that, being smaller, children also have smaller muscle fibres[27] are likely benefit from shorter diffusion distances, which in turn might compensate for their lower haemoglobin.

Hormonal differences

Several hormones, whose activities change during growth and maturation, and that are associated with physical and sexual development, have been implicated in thermoregulation—particularly in the sweating mechanism. These include testosterone, oestrogen, prolactin, and growth hormone.

As early as 1960, Kawahata[28] argued that testosterone has a sudorific (sweat-causing) effect. He based this argument on the observation of enhanced sweating rate in 70- to 81-year-old men following injections of testosterone propionate. Indeed, androgen receptors were detected on the secretory coils of sweat glands.[29] However, Rees and Shuster[30] could not demonstrate any sudorific effect of testosterone in adult men and women. Thus, they suggested that androgens may initiate, but not maintain, the increase in sweating rate that takes place during maturation.

In women, the menstrual cycle, and particularly the luteal phase, were shown to influence the thermoregulatory response to exercise in the heat, by increasing the temperature thresholds for onset of sweating and cutaneous vasodilation (see Bar-Or[31] for review). Although an oestrogen receptor-related protein was described in human sweat ducts[32], the thermoregulatory differences between the menstrual phases have not been directly linked to any of the hormonal changes (mainly in oestrogen and progesterone) that occur during these phases. Furthermore, it is unknown what if any thermoregulatory effects concentration changes of these hormones may have during maturation.

Prolactin was linked with osmoregulation and is suggested to influence sweat electrolyte concentration in adults[33,34] as well as adolescents.[35] However, its exact influence on sweat gland function and its possible differential role in children and adults is unclear.

Several studies described a reduced local sweating rate in patients with growth hormone (GH) deficiency[36,37] and patients with Laron Syndrome (undetectable or low insulin-like growth factor-1 [IGF-I] levels with normal GH levels).[38] Additionally, GH receptors and binding protein were observed in the human sweat duct.[39,40] The mechanism by which the GH/IGF-I axis may affect sweat-gland function and the possible differential effect of this axis on thermoregulation during growth and maturation need yet to be elucidated.

Finally, basal activity of aldosterone and vasopressin are associated with fluid and electrolyte regulation, but are not known to differ between children, adolescents, and adults.[41] Also, there is no evidence to suggest that sensitivity to these hormones changes during maturation or growth.

Differences in the sweating mechanism

When ambient temperature is equal to, or higher than that of the skin, the only means of heat dissipation is sweat evaporation. A consistent finding at all levels or forms of heat load is that children sweat less than adults not only in absolute terms, but also relative to BSA. Several changes in the sweating mechanism take place during growth and maturation which may explain the observed increase in the sweating response to environmental heat load during this period (see references,[31,42–46] for review).

Three types of sweat glands have been recognized—eccrine, apocrine, and apoeccrine,[47] of which eccrine glands are the most abundant and thermoregulatorily significant. They are smaller in children[48,49] in whom their size is directly related to age ($r = 0.77$) and stature ($r = 0.81$).[48] In vitro experiments in adults demonstrated that a gland's sweating rate was directly related to its size and to its cholinergic sensitivity.[50] Thus, the maturation-related increase in sweat-gland size at least partly explains the greater sweating response to heat stress in adults.

The total number of eccrine glands is determined by the age of 3 years.[51] Consequently, their population density (glands per unit skin area) decreases with subsequent growth.[52,53] Indeed, Wilk *et al.*[54] recently demonstrated a decrease in sweat-gland population density with increasing maturity in adolescent girls exercising in the heat. Thus, the increasing sweating rate during growth and maturation is

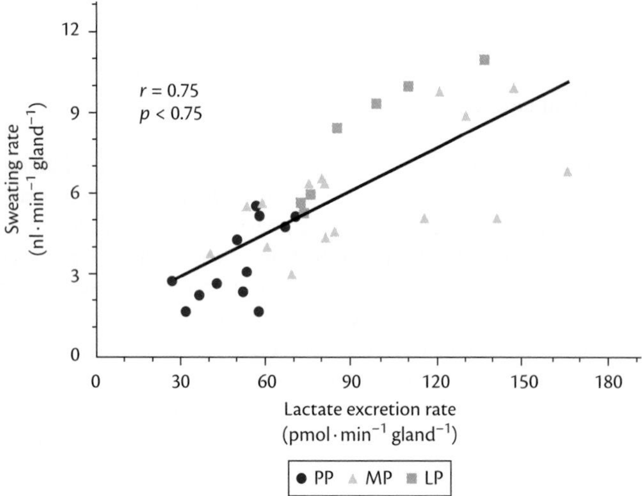

Figure 14.1 The relationship between lactate excretion rate per gland and sweating rate per gland among pre-, mid- and late-pubertal boys (PP, MP, LP, respectively) cycling in the heat (50% $\dot{V}O_2$ max, 42°C, 20% relative humidity).
Modified from Falk B, Bar-Or O, MacDougall JD, McGillis L, Calvert R, Meyer F. Sweat lactate in exercising children and adolescents of varying physical maturity. J Appl Physiol. 1991; 71: 1735–1740.

not attributable to increasing sweat-gland numbers, but rather to their increasing size and productivity.

Sweat production was shown to be directly related to the sweat gland's glycolytic capacity and lactate excretion rate.[55] Indeed, lactate excretion rate has been used as an index of sweat gland metabolism[49,55,56] (Figure 14.1). Much of the observed increase in sweat gland metabolism and sweating rate is a mere reflection of increasing gland size. It is not known to what extent, if any, is the increased sweating rate related to the general rise of glycolytic capacity associated with maturation (e.g. increased glycolytic muscle-enzyme activity,[57] increased anaerobic muscle power[58], etc).

Further research is needed to elucidate and quantify the contribution of sweat gland size and metabolic nature, as well as possible other factors (e.g. hormones), to children's lower sweating rate.

Physiological response to thermal stress

Thermal stress, with or without exercise, is accompanied by changes in body temperature, metabolic, circulatory, and hormonal responses, as well as activation of the sweating mechanism. This section focuses on child-adult differences in the physiological responses to heat and cold stress, and the changes those responses may undergo during growth and maturation. Table 14.2 summarizes the available information on the child-adult differential responses at rest and exercise, in the heat and in the cold. It is clear that there still are wide gaps in our knowledge, especially with regard to cold stress.

The effectiveness of thermoregulation is reflected by heat and cold tolerance, and by the stability of core temperature and the circulatory system, both at rest and while performing various tasks in the heat and cold. The effectiveness of thermoregulation also affects exercise performance. Ultimately, the question is whether or not the gradual change in the physiological response that takes place with growth and maturation also changes heat or cold tolerance. In other words, do the observed child-adult differences in

Table 14.2 Differences in the physiological responses to heat and to cold exposure between children and adults

	Response	In children relative to adults	
		Heat	**Cold**
Body temperature	Rectal	Similar or higher	Similar or lower
	Skin	Higher	Lower
Metabolism	Oxygen uptake	Higher (may be similar during exercise)	Higher
Circulation	Cardiac output	Similar[a]	?
	Stroke volume	Lower	?
	Heart rate	Higher	Lower
	Skin blood flow	Higher	Extremities: lower Torso: likely lower
	Blood pressure	Lower	Lower
Endocrine system	Fluid and electrolyte regulation	Similar or lower	?
	Stress hormones	Similar or lower	?
Sweating rate	Per unit surface area	Lower	—
	Per gland	Lower	—
	Per unit body mass	Similar or lower	—
Fluid regulation	Rate of dehydration	Similar or lower	—

a = Relative to body size and corrected for basal/resting blood flow.
? = Unknown.
— = Not relevant.

physiological responses to heat or cold stresses constitute a thermoregulatory deficiency on the part of children, or do they merely reflect a changing thermoregulatory strategy? This question is central to the discussion in this section.

Physiological response to heat stress

Metabolic response

Children's higher cost of bipedal locomotion implies that, while walking/running at a given speed, children are under a greater metabolic strain than adults. This is the case in both thermoneutral and hot conditions.

The heat stress effect on the metabolic response, at rest or during exercise, is mainly reflected by changes in $\dot{V}O_2$. Most studies, comparing child-adult physiologic responses, typically utilize exercise intensities which provide standardized metabolic loads (i.e. a given percentage of peak $\dot{V}O_2$ and identical environmental conditions). No comparison is normally made with other conditions. Thus, the differential metabolic responses that environmental heat stress may have on children vs adults are difficult to gauge.

Two studies compared the metabolic responses of children vs adults in different environmental conditions. Drinkwater *et al.*[21]

found no $\dot{V}O_2$ changes in prepubertal girls or adult women, following 1-h walking (30% peak $\dot{V}O_2$) in dry (48°C, 10% RH) or humid (35°C, 65% RH) heat, compared with warm conditions (28°C, 45% RH). However, in the second hour of exercise in the hot conditions, a significant $\dot{V}O_2$ rise was observed in the girls, but not in the women, suggesting a differential effect of heat on metabolic rate. Carlson and Le Rossignol[59] observed no $\dot{V}O_2$ effect of heat radiation (black globe temperature of 37 vs 49°C) in 10-year-old boys, nor in adults, cycling for 40 min at 50% peak $\dot{V}O_2$ in humid heat. Thus, it is clear that further research is needed to clarify the metabolic response to heat stress in children and in adolescents and to determine whether this response is different from that in adults.

Circulatory responses

The circulatory response to thermal stress can be reflected by changes in $\dot{Q}$, stroke volume (SV), and heart rate (HR), and by changes in blood pressure and peripheral blood flow. Only limited information on the cardiovascular response to heat stress is available for children and adolescents.

Drinkwater *et al.*[21] had prepubertal girls and young women walk at 30% peak $\dot{V}O_2$ in various environmental heat conditions. The girls' HR was consistently higher than the women's, beyond age-dependent differences. Likewise, Jokinen *et al.*[60] reported that in children younger than 5 years, resting for 10 min in a Finnish sauna (70°C, 20% RH), displayed higher HRs and larger decreases in SV compared with older children, adolescents, and adults. Cardiac output increased in the adults, but not in the children.

On the other hand, Rowland *et al.*[61] reported that exercise tolerance in non-acclimatized prepubertal boys, cycling to exhaustion at 65% $\dot{V}O_2$, max was expectedly lower in the heat (31°C, 56% RH) than in cooler, thermoneutral conditions (20°C, 66% RH). Neither $\dot{Q}$ nor SV differed between the two conditions. In fact, no circulatory insufficiency could be demonstrated in either of the two conditions. Cardiac output rose in the first 10 min, and then remained stable until exhaustion. Notably, however, exhaustion in the hot condition ensued within 30 min, compared with over 40 min in thermoneutral conditions, with similar T_{re} at exhaustion. Similarly, Rivera-Brown *et al.*[62] reported that among heat acclimatized women and prepubertal girls, there was no apparent cardiovascular insufficiency during cycling in humid heat (60% peak $\dot{V}O_2$, 33°C, 55% RH), although the girls stopped or reached termination criteria earlier than the women (~57 vs. 77 min, respectively). Cardiac output increased in the first 10 min of exercise, but stayed stable to the end.

The apparent discrepancy between Drinkwater *et al.*'s[21] findings and those of Rivera-Brown *et al.*'s[62] could be partly explained by the different levels of acclimatization (none vs acclimatized) of the two groups of girls and, possibly, by the rehydration regimens used (none vs sports drink replacement of sweat loss; however, it is not clear that dehydration reached functional significance in Drinkwater *et al.*'s study). Probably the most significant distinction between the two studies, however, was the mode of exercise (i.e. walking vs cycling), an issue which is also relevant in other cross-study comparisons. Treadmill running/walking comparisons of children vs adults are confounded by children's lower bipedal locomotive economy.[20] This means that when walking/running at a given relative exercise intensity (% $\dot{V}O_2$ max), children expend a greater fraction of their energy internally than do adults, and therefore produce relatively more heat which they must dissipate. This, in turn, puts an extra burden on the circulatory/thermoregulatory system which manifests itself by an elevated HR response. In other words, children's responses can be directly compared with adults' in cycling (where no child-adult economy differences exist[63]), but not in treadmill exercise.

Early studies reported higher HRs during exercise in the heat in children vs adults, beyond age-dependent differences.[64] On the other hand, Falk *et al.*[65] reported no difference in the HR response to cycling in the heat (50% peak $\dot{V}O_2$, 42°C, 20% RH) in pre-, mid-, and late-pubertal boys. Similarly, Rivera-Brown *et al.*[62] reported no girl-woman HR differences while cycling in the heat (60% peak $\dot{V}O_2$, 43°C, 55% RH). As discussed, the seemingly discrepant HR responses were, most likely, due to the differences in exercise modes (treadmill vs cycle ergometry).

Skin blood flow was reported to be higher in children than in adults during, or immediately following exercise in the heat, in most studies.[21,64–66] Exceptionally, Rivera-Brown *et al.*[62] did not find a difference in skin blood flow between girls and women exercising in the heat. This discrepancy may be related to the technique used to assess skin blood flow. The latter used the plethysmographic occlusion method, which does not separate skin from muscle blood-flow. Assuming the forearm muscles are inactive, any increase in limb blood flow is assumed to represent an increase in skin blood flow. Shibasaki *et al.*,[66] using the Laser Doppler Flowmetry method, found forearm skin blood flow to be lower in boys while their back and chest skin blood flows were higher than in men during moderate exercise in warm conditions (46% peak $\dot{V}O_2$, 30°C, 45% RH) (Figure 14.2). Thus, it is unclear whether age-related differences in forearm skin blood flow measurements are representative of whole-body cutaneous blood flow differences between children and adults.

Increasing skin blood flow was also demonstrated along the pubertal continuum (pre-, mid-, late-pubertal) in both boys[65] and girls.[67] In support of children's higher cutaneous blood flow, a faster rise in skin temperature (T_{sk}) was observed in 6- to 11-year-old boys compared with adults during heat exposure.[6,68] Furthermore, Shibasaki *et al.*[66] reported that while exercising in the heat, boys had a greater increase of cutaneous blood flow for a given increase in T_{re} than did men. Due to the boys' lower blood pressure (presumably, due to the fall in peripheral resistance that facilitated the increased cutaneous flow), the differences were further pronounced when cutaneous vascular resistance was calculated (dividing skin blood flow by mean arterial pressure). The higher peripheral blood flow means that a greater proportion of $\dot{Q}$ is diverted to the periphery (i.e. skin), potentially imposing an added strain on the cardiovascular system. The higher strain may be partly compensated for by a greater increase in plasma volume, as reported in girls vs women exercising in the heat.[21]

The sometimes reported lower subjective exercise tolerance in children exercising in the heat[21,62,65,69] may be due to maladjustment of the cardiovascular system, resulting in reduced blood flow to the working muscles and/or to the central nervous system. In fact, Jokinen *et al.*[70] reported two cases of vasovagal collapse immediately upon exiting a Finnish sauna (10 min) in children younger than 10 years, but not in older children, adolescents, or adults. The same group[71] also reported extra systoles among children as well as a reversible sinus arrest in a 5-year-old girl during and following 10 min in a sauna. In both cases, the authors emphasized that extreme heat places an added demand on the cardiovascular system in young children. It ought to be emphasized that Jokinen *et al.* studied children's responses to passive sauna exposure (i.e. no exercise). Under

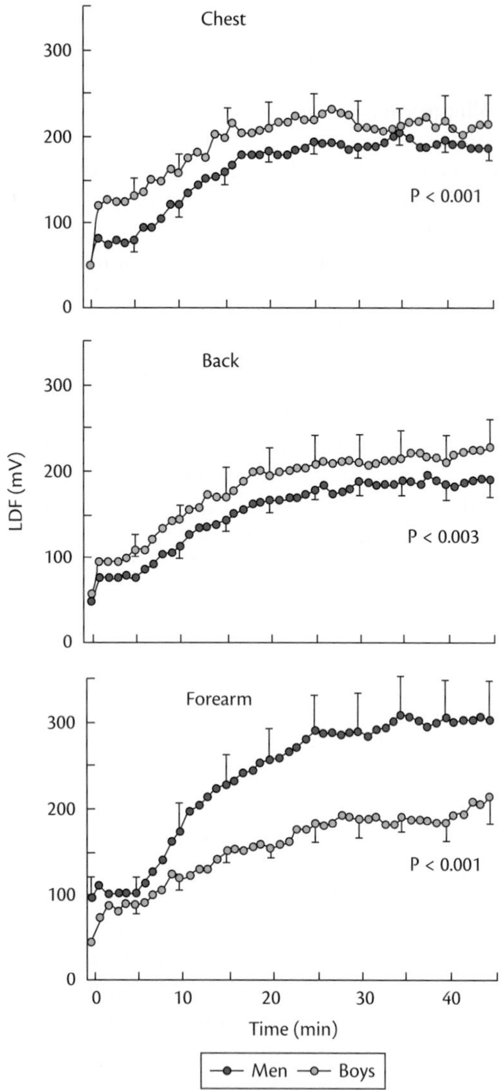

Figure 14.2 Skin blood flow (LDF), as measured by laser Doppler flowmetry, on the chest, back, and forearm of 10- to 11-year-old prepubertal boys and 20- to 25-year-old men cycling in the heat (40% peak $\dot{V}O_2$, 30°C, 45% relative humidity).
p values are for overall effect of age during exercise.
Shibasaki M, Inoue Y, Kondo N, Iwata A. Thermoregulatory responses of prepubertal boys and young men during moderate exercise. Eur J Appl Physiol Occup Physiol. 1997; 75: 212–218.

such conditions, the circulatory system may normally not be pushed to its limits, as exemplified by this group's earlier findings[70] that mean systolic and diastolic blood pressures were unaffected by the sauna exposure, suggesting a good match between the falling peripheral resistance and the rising $\dot{Q}$. However, considering the reported large range of individual cardiovascular responses and the two cases of collapse or other symptoms, it is reasonable to suggest that the responsible factor was individual circulatory maladjustment, rather than a general phenomenon. This emphasizes the need for close supervision under such stressful conditions as sauna exposure.

Hormonal response

The hormonal response to exercise in the heat has traditionally been studied in relation to hormones associated with fluid and electrolyte balance. Few studies have examined this response in children. Increased aldosterone levels were observed in pre- to late-pubertal boys following rest and exercise in the heat.[35,60] This is similar to the response generally described in adults. No change in vasopressin, cortisol, or catecholamines concentration was observed in children following a 10 min exposure to a Finnish sauna, although an increase was observed among adults.[60]

Of the hormones associated with puberty, only prolactin's response to heat stress was investigated in children and adolescents, probably due to its association with osmoregulation. Heat stress, whether accompanied by exercise or not, reportedly results in increased prolactin levels in children and adolescents[35,60] as well as in adults.[33,72] Increased prolactin levels are associated with higher sweat electrolyte concentration in adults[33,34] and adolescent boys.[35] However, its differential influence on sweat gland function in children and adults is unknown. While there has been continued interest in the effect of sex hormones, particularly female sex hormones, on thermoregulation in adults (e.g. Charkoudian and Stachenfeld[73]), there is no such information for youth. Additionally, to the authors' knowledge, aside from prolactin, no study on children/adolescents has examined the relationships between thermal stress and other growth- or maturation-related hormones. Therefore, it is unclear whether and how these hormones may modify the thermoregulatory response and what may be the child-adult differential response.

Sweating response

As mentioned earlier, children's sweating apparatus and pattern is different from that of adults. This is manifested by differences in sweating rates and the sweating response to a given rise in core temperature.

In any given environmental and metabolic load the absolute sweating rate of prepubertal boys is much lower than men's (see Bar-Or[31,42–45] for review), and is still markedly lower relative to BSA.[3,21,28,38,64,66,74–77] Sweating response is also lower relative to a given rise in body temperature (T_{body}) or T_{re}.[76,78] Between boys and men, this difference becomes more evident as exercise intensity or heat stress increase.[45] By contrast, the sweating-rate girl-woman difference is much smaller[21,77] and sometimes non-existent.[38,62]

In an effort to temporally define the observed child-adult differences in sweating rate, Falk *et al.*[79] compared pre-, mid-, and late-pubertal boys, exercising at 50% $\dot{V}O_2$ max in dry heat (42°C, 20% RH). Sweating rate per BSA and per gland increased with physical maturity. Inoue *et al.*[45] suggested that most of the sweating-rate increase takes places at the onset of puberty. This was based on a report by Araki *et al.*[74], who showed sweating rate to increase with age in 7- to 16-year-old boys, especially around 12–13 years of age, corresponding to the onset of puberty. The onset of puberty and the accelerated changes in bodily dimensions and hormonal function are temporally linked. It remains unclear to what extent is the maturation-related sweating rate change[80] due to the hormonal changes, or merely to the dimensional growth that is part and parcel of maturation. Tsuzuki-Hayakawa *et al.*[81] reported that 8 months- to 4.5-year-old boys and girls, resting in a warm and humid environment (35°C, 70% RH), displayed a higher sweating rate compared with their mothers. Thus, the factors governing thermoregulation in very young children may be different than later on, e.g. at the onset of puberty.

Most studies comparing children with adults measured whole body sweating rates, but some investigated specific sites in an attempt to shed light on the seeming discrepancy of children's lower sweating rates.[6,54,66] Site variations did not change the overall picture since, we claim, it is an integral aspect of children's different thermoregulatory strategy of greater dependence on dry heat dissipation and lesser reliance on evaporative cooling. As long as children do not drip their sweat to any appreciable extent (as is often the case with adults), what matters is the cooling power associated with their total sweat volume and not its particular distribution.

Sweating rate per gland can be estimated given the sweating rate and the population density of the heat activated eccrine sweat glands. In line with children's lower observed whole body sweating rate, their calculated sweating rate per gland was also shown to be considerably lower at rest or exercise in the heat.[28,66,75,82] Similarly, Foster *et al.*[82] estimated a three times lower sweating-rate per gland in newborn babies compared with adults, when sweat was induced by an intradermal injection of acetylcholine.

The child–adult differences, described above, were extended by comparing pre-, mid-, and late-pubertal boys who exercised in the heat (50% peak $\dot{V}O_2$, 40°C, 20% RH).[79] Increased sweating rates per unit SA and per gland were observed with increasing maturity (Figure 14.3). Sweating rate was also shown to increase longitudinally, with age, in the same boys in an 18-month follow-up.[80] However, it could not be determined whether the increase was linear, or whether sweating rate changed with the hormonal and physical growth changes that took place during the follow-up period.

Sex-related differences in sweating rate were reported in adults,[83] but corresponding differences are not as clear among children and

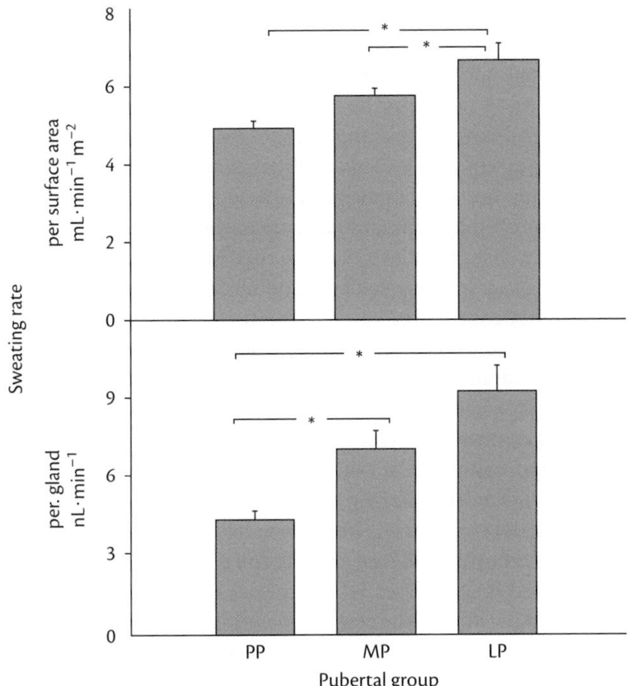

Figure 14.3 Sweating rate per skin surface area and per gland among pre-, mid- and late-pubertal boys (PP, MP, LP, respectively) cycling in the heat (50% $\dot{V}O_2$ max, 42°C, 20% relative humidity).

Falk B, Bar-Or O, MacDougall JD. Thermoregulatory responses of pre-, mid-, and late-pubertal boys to exercise in dry heat. Med Sci Sports Exerc. 1992; 24: 688–694 and Falk B, Bar-Or O, Calvert R, MacDougall JD. Sweat gland response to exercise in the heat among pre-, mid-, and late-pubertal boys. Med Sci Sports Exerc. 1992; 24: 313–319.

adolescents. Several studies reported greater sweating rates in boys compared with girls in response to thermal[28,84] or pharmacological[38] stimuli. However, others reported similar sweating rates, or only tendencies toward higher rates in boys than in girls.[8,9,30,77,85]

Children's maximal sweating rate has not been determined. Rivera-Brown,[62,86] for instance, measured twice the typical reported peak sweating rates in heat acclimatized children (~500 vs 200–300 $mL \cdot m^{-2} \cdot h^{-1}$). However, in many thermally stressful environments the issue might be confounded by sweat dripping. The latter is not normally reported, but experience and anecdotal evidence suggests it frequently occurs in adults, but rarely in children. Compared with late-pubertal girls exercising in the heat, prepubertal girls had a smaller proportion of their skin covered by sweat.[54] This is notable since dripped sweat cannot contribute to evaporative cooling and constitutes a waste for the body's fluid balance.

Bar-Or *et al.*[87] showed (based on comparison with data from an earlier study[88]) that for any given percentage loss of body mass due to sweating, children's T_{re} rose ~50% more than that of adults. This amplified response to fluid loss can be viewed as detrimental to children's thermoregulatory capacity, but may also serve a purpose. Namely, since children appear to rely more on dry rather than evaporative heat dissipation, their greater core temperature response may be viewed as a means to elevate T_{sk}, which in turn, raises the skin-to-air temperature gradient and augments heat dissipation via this channel. This argument is augmented by the observation that, compared with adults, children's sweating response to increasing T_{re} is delayed.[74] High T_{re} is a risk factor for heat injury. However, we have no data on the upper safe T_{re} limit in children vs adults, since studies are ethically never allowed to extend heat stress to presumed dangerous levels. Viewed this way, children's lower sweating rate is not necessarily a disadvantage. Rather, children's lower sweating rate, besides reflecting their different thermoregulatory strategy, also helps them conserve fluids and markedly reduces their susceptibility to the ill effects of fluid loss.

Sweating sensitivity is typically defined as the change in T_{re} necessary to elicit a given sweating response, or the sweating rate associated with each degree of T_{re} rise. Expectedly, under these definitions, children's sensitivity was found lower than that of adults.[74,76] Araki *et al.*[74] demonstrated that during exercise in the heat children began to sweat only when their T_{re} rose 0.7°C, while adults commenced sweating already at a 0.2°C T_{re} rise. Inbar[75,76] demonstrated a lower sweat production per degree rise in T_{re} in 8- to 10-year-old children, compared with adults. Additionally, Wada[89] showed that the sweating response to intra-dermal adrenaline injection rose from prepubertal values and peaked at age 14 years.

It should be pointed out, however, that the definitions of sweating sensitivity are founded on the premise that sweating is the predominant heat dissipating mechanism under all heat stress conditions. Children's seemingly compromised sweating sensitivity should be viewed in light of their different thermoregulatory strategy and the associated negative relationship between T_{sk} and sweating rate. Davies[3] demonstrated that during 60 min of running (~70% $\dot{V}O_2$ max), children dissipated heat comparably via dry and evaporative means, while men relied more on the latter. Thus, the validity of the sweating sensitivity definitions and their underlying premise in the context of child–adult thermoregulatory comparisons should be questioned. As children's 'lower sensitivity' implies some deficiency on their part and is not applicable to child–adult sweating comparisons, it is suggested that 'sweating sensitivity' be replaced by a more neutral term, such as 'sweating quotient'.

Basal or resting metabolism is best correlated with skin surface area in humans and other mammals[90] and that is where heat dissipation takes place. For these reasons, sweating rate has commonly been expressed ('normalized') to BSA. However, exercise-dependent heat production is better correlated with body size and muscle mass. Consequently, as exercise intensity rises, heat production and therefore sweating ought to be increasingly better correlated with body mass and power output. It is thus unfitting to compare sweating rates of vastly differently sized exercising individuals (e.g. children vs. adults) based on BSA alone.

Indeed, when re-calculating published data and relating metabolic loads to sweating rates no clear differences were observed between children and adults (Falk and Dotan, unpublished). Rivera-Brown *et al.*[62] also reported similar sweating rates per unit body mass in prepubertal, acclimatized girls and women, but they were trained and heat acclimatized which might have affected the comparison. On the other hand, Meyer and Bar-Or[91] reported inconsistent findings in reviewing published age-related sweat loss differences, while Araki *et al.*[74] showed lower per-kg sweating rates in children. The available data do not present a clear picture of the relationship between sweating rate and body mass, possibly due to the changing roles of BSA and body mass (or power output) at different stages of growth or maturation and different levels of exertion and environmental conditions. With increasing exercise intensities, sweating rates may be increasingly better related to body mass rather than to BSA. Presumably due to lesser reliance on evaporative cooling, children would still tend to sweat slightly less than adults.

Differences in heat tolerance and body temperature

Theoretically, heat tolerance should be defined as either the highest T_{re} immediately preceding physiological collapse, or that beyond which maintenance of T_{re} and circulatory sufficiency within physiological limits is no longer possible. For ethical and safety reasons, neither criterion can serve in practice. Therefore, various alternatives have been used as criteria for terminating exposure or assessing relative thermal strain. These criteria have been both objective (e.g. T_{re}, T_{body}, total body heat storage) and subjective (e.g. dizziness, high rating of perceived exertion). The ingrained methodological difficulty, when comparing children with adults, is that the appropriateness of these criteria for different age groups is presumed but not necessarily proven or similarly applicable. For example, the subjective exhaustion criterion does not take into account known age-dependent differences in the subjective rating of perceived exertion and possibly motivation, as well. Likewise, using a uniform T_{re} cut-off value does not take into account the possibility alluded to earlier, that critical T_{re} may change with growth or maturation. Moreover, the use of the current formulae for integrated body temperature (T_{body}) and heat-storage may result in an overestimation of these indices in children. Body temperature is calculated in most studies, as a weighted average of T_{re} and T_{sk} (e.g. $0.8T_{re} + 0.2T_{sk}$), based on estimated adult proportions of core vs periphery. Such a formula, even if imprecise, is satisfactory in dimensionally uniform populations. However, since children are smaller and have a relatively larger skin area, their periphery-to-core volume ratio should be higher than that of adults. That is, a higher T_{sk} proportion in the T_{body} and heat storage formulae. These methodological limitations should be borne in mind when considering the results and conclusions of the studies which follow. In light of these difficulties, and since the determining factor in heat tolerance is critical T_{re}, the justification for calculating T_{body} and total heat storage should be questioned in child-adult comparisons.

Studies investigating the thermoregulatory response to exercise in thermoneutral or warm environments, reported similar or even lower T_{re} in children than in adults.[3–5,62,92] In warm conditions (30°C, 45% RH), Shibasaki *et al.*[66] found exercising boys and men to produce a similar rise in T_{re}. This agrees with previous findings comparing girls with women in similar conditions (28°C, 45% RH).[21] This strongly suggests that under thermoneutral or warm conditions, thermoregulatory effectiveness, as reflected by T_{re}, is similar in children and adults.

At high ambient temperatures and, particularly, when accompanied by high humidity, mean body temperature[59,64,81,93] and heat storage per unit body mass[8,9,21] were reported to be higher in children, compared with adults. Two technical reservations to these findings should be raised. Firstly, all mentioned studies used walking, which associated with higher energy cost and heat production, and therefore also with higher heat load in children, compared with adults (see section on Metabolic response. Secondly, the inherent error in weighting T_{re} and T_{sk} for the calculation of T_{body} and heat storage, further adds to overestimating children's objective heat stress.

These problems notwithstanding, we further question the use of these two parameters in cross-age comparisons because the physiological significance of both the T_{body} and the heat storage criteria depend on the thermoregulatory strategy used, which is different in children and adults. A more fundamental question is the preference of using these criteria over T_{re}, which is the ultimate criterion of heat tolerance and thermoregulatory failure. Indeed, when relying on T_{re} and using cycling as the exercise modality, different tolerance outcomes and conclusions are reached. Falk *et al.*[65] found similar T_{re} in children and adolescents of different ages and pubertal stages who cycled in hot, dry conditions (50% $\dot{V}O_2$ max, 42°C, 20% RH). Furthermore, a longitudinal follow-up of these boys did not demonstrate any change in the rate of T_{re} rise.[80] Similarly, no T_{re} differences were observed between boys and men[76] or girls and women[62] cycling in hot conditions.

Ultimately, compromised heat tolerance ought to be reflected in heat-related injuries and fatalities. Inevitably, such adverse events in youths are reported every year (e.g. Gottschalk and Andrish[94]). The question then is whether youths are more vulnerable to heat-related injuries. Experimental data on the relationship between heat and mortality and morbidity in youth are limited for obvious ethical reasons. However, much can be gleaned from epidemiological data. In a recent report,[95] children were deemed uniquely vulnerable to the increased heat stresses by rising global temperatures ('global warming'). Specifically, the authors identified infants (younger than 1 year old) and adolescent football players at particular risk. In a 2011 report on exertional heat-related injuries in the US, Nelson *et al.*[96] reported that youths <19 years of age accounted for almost 50% of ~55 000 emergency room exertional heat-related injury cases, mostly related to sports and recreational exercise. Arguably, <19-year-olds are the largest age group among those engaging in sports and recreational physical activities. Specifically at risk, as highlighted by the authors, are children and adolescents playing football. On the other hand, in study of 457 schoolboys observed

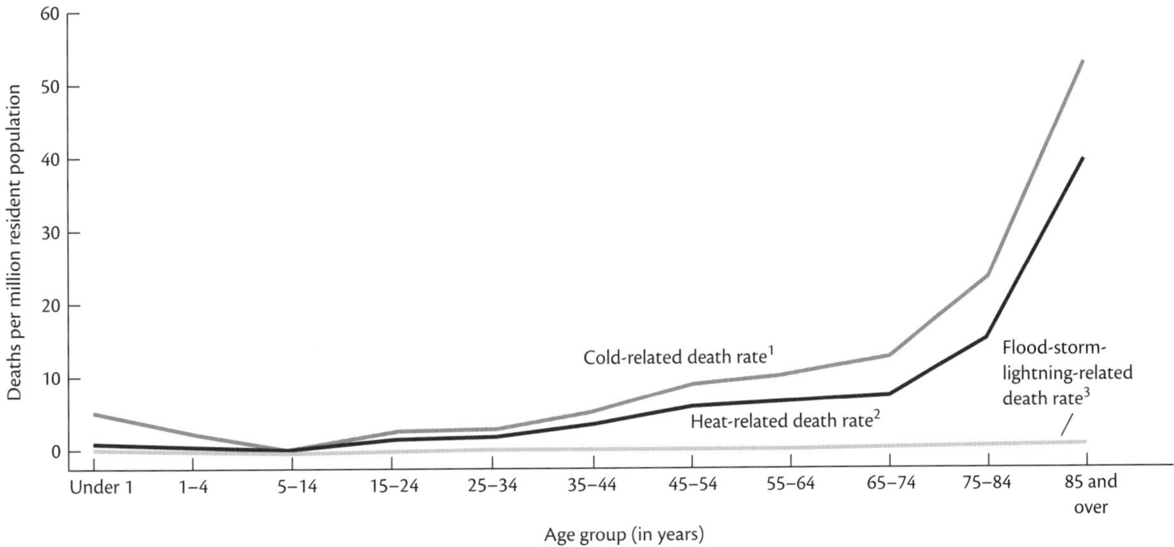
Deaths per million resident population
60
50
40
30
20
10
0
Cold-related death rate[1]
Heat-related death rate[2]
Flood-storm-lightning-related death rate[3]
Under 1
1–4
5–14
15–24
25–34
35–44
45–54
55–64
65–74
75–84
85 and over
Age group (in years)
[1]Deaths attributed to exposure to excessive natural cold (X31) (underlying or contributing cause of death or both), to hypothermia (T68) (contributing cause of death), or to both, according to the International Classification of Diseases, 10th Revision.
[2]Deaths attributed t exposure to excessive natural heat (X30) (underlying or contributing cause of death or both), to heat stroke or sunstroke (T67) (contributing cause of death), or to both accourding to the International Classification of Diseases, 10th Revision.
[3]Deaths attributed to floods (X38), cataclysmic storms (X37), or lightning (X33) (underlying or contributing cause of death or both), according to the International Classification of Diseases, 10th Revision.

Figure 14.4 Death rates for weather-related mortality, by age: United States, 2006–2010.
Berko J, Ingram DD, Saha S, Parker JD. Deaths attributed to heat, cold, and other weather events in the United States, 2006–2010. National Health Statistics Reports. 2014; 30: 1–15.

in outdoor physical education classes in a tropical climate, there was no evidence of heat illness.[97] In only 4.4% of cases did tympanic temperature exceed 38°C, and in 90% of these cases, students did not consume any fluids (see section on Hydration). Despite the fact that no heat illness was observed, the authors concluded that among 5- to 12-year-old schoolboys, poor hydration status, as well as being overweight, may increase the risk of heat illness during outdoor activities in hot climates. The Policy Statement on climatic heat stress and exercising children and adolescents of the American Academy of Pediatric [152] states that, contrary to previous thinking, youths do *not* have lower tolerance for physical exertion in the heat than do adults. In the National Health Statistics report (US Centers for Disease Control and Prevention), Berko *et al.*[98] recently examined all weather-related deaths in the US between 2006 and 2010. The authors reported that there are 2000 such deaths every year and that ~30% of these were related to heat. Importantly, there is a sharp rise in heat-related deaths after age 65, but notably, the lowest rate of such deaths was from less than 1 year of age to approximately 15 years of age, or older (Figure 14.4). These epidemiological data not only refute the notion of higher heat-stress vulnerability prior to puberty, but actually suggest children as having better heat tolerance than any other segment of the population, whether exercise-related or not.

Figure 14.5 schematically depicts our current understanding of thermoregulatory effectiveness, in children vs adults under varying environmental-stress conditions. In thermoneutral and warm conditions, children appear to thermoregulate as effectively as adults.[3,4,21] Under such conditions, children's higher relative skin area allows them to utilize relatively more the dry rather than evaporative heat dissipation venue. However, when heat stress becomes more extreme, Children's thermoregulatory capacity appears to be somewhat deficient compared with adults (references[8,21] vs references[52,64,93,99]). It was suggested that this lower tolerance is largely due to children's relative cardiovascular insufficiency[65,70] (when exercise demands and cutaneous blood flow are increasingly in competition for the finite $\dot{Q}$) and to their more-limited sweating rates.[8,64,77,93]

An exception to the above view and the body of supportive evidence is a study by Inbar *et al.*,[76] in which prepubertal boys, exercising at 41°C (~50% peak $\dot{V}O_2$, 21% RH), reportedly had higher evaporative cooling and better thermoregulation than their adult counterparts. It is difficult to explain these findings. To dissipate their metabolic heat and the relatively greater heat absorbed from the environment under these conditions, children would have to produce sweating rates higher than those of the adults. Such a

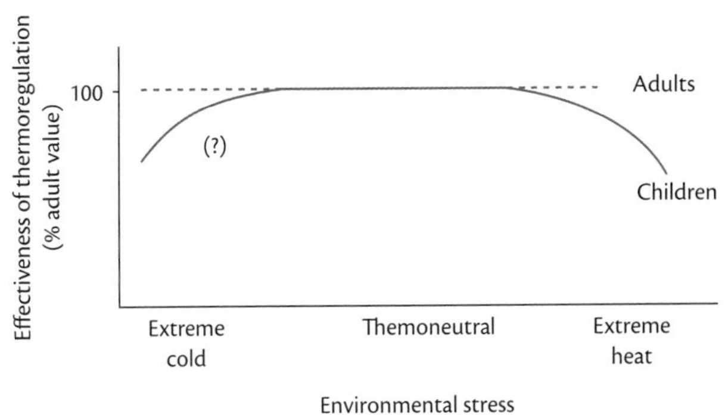
Effectiveness of thermoregulation (% adult value)
100
Adults
(?)
Children
Extreme cold
Themoneutral
Extreme heat
Environmental stress

Figure 14.5 Schematic representation of the effectiveness of thermoregulation among children, compared with adults, in relation to the environmental stress.
Modified from Bar-Or O. Temperature regulation during exercise in children and adolescents. In: Gisolfi CV, Lamb DR, eds. Youth, exercise and sports. Perspectives in exercise science and sports medicine. II. Indianapolis, IN: Benchmark Press; 1989: 335–362.

scenario has not been shown even in trained, heat-acclimatized children,[62,86] while Inbar *et al.*'s boys were neither trained, nor acclimatized. Additional research is needed to support or refute these findings.

Hydration during heat stress

During exercise in the heat, hypohydration may develop, mostly due to fluid losses through sweating. Studies have shown that even when water is available *ad libitum,* neither children,[61,87,100] adolescents,[84,101–109] nor adults[110] sufficiently replace fluid losses. This phenomenon was initially labeled 'voluntary dehydration',[111] although more recently, the term 'involuntary dehydration' has been commonly used. We propose the use of the term 'inadvertent dehydration' as more appropriate. The degree of inadvertent dehydration during exercise in hot conditions appears to be similar in children and adults.[91] Gordon *et al.*[105] recently demonstrated that the knowledge and beliefs about rehydration of adolescent male soccer players did not correspond to their practices. To this end Kavouras *et al.*[104] demonstrated improved hydration status among young adolescent athletes, following a 5-day educational intervention as part of a sports training camp. It included discussions regarding the benefits of hydration and key points for hydration maintenance, as well as the mounting of coloured urine charts in all bathrooms. Endurance running performance was also improved compared with a control group who had no educational intervention. In recent years, the importance of hydration in sports has received wide attention among researchers, as well as the lay media, leading to improved awareness and knowledge among young athletes regarding fluid choices and hydration practices.[103] This may explain the fact that young athletes are recently more often reported as being properly hydrated during training and competition.[112–114]

Chronic hypohydration in children may be present even with no particular exercise regimen.[115,116] In adults, severe hypohydration is linked to poor cognitive performance.[117] In well-nourished young children (7–9 years), several studies consistently demonstrated that fluid consumption improved both memory and attention.[117,118] However, sample sizes in all these studies were relatively small. It is not clear whether improved hydration affects cognitive performance (e.g. decision-making) during exercise, but it was shown to improve the rating of perceived exertion among adolescent athletes.[103]

One way to enhance fluid consumption among children, especially while exercising in the heat, is beverage flavouring.[86,119,120] Additionally, when carbohydrates (~8%) and electrolytes (sodium chloride [NaCl], 15-20 mmol·L^{-1}) are added to the flavoured beverage, as in most commercial sports drinks, fluid consumption is increased by as much as 90% in children.[120–122] In fact, when consuming a flavoured beverage, enriched with carbohydrates and electrolytes, inadvertent dehydration in children appears to be prevented.[86,120,123,112–114] Nevertheless, Wilk *et al.*[124] noted that among 12- to 15-year-old male athletes, a carbohydrate and electrolyte beverage did not prevent dehydration during exercise in the heat. The apparent incongruence between the latter and earlier studies is the higher exercise intensity (65 vs 50–60% $\dot{V}O_2$ max), presumably with more attendant sweating. A much more potent factor appears to be the much shorter rest intervals employed by Wilk *et al.* (5 vs 25 min), which provided much more limited opportunities for fluid consumption. Thus, during training or competition in the heat, it is important not only to encourage fluid consumption to maintain proper hydration status, but also to provide the opportunity to do so.

Following exercise in a hot environment, fluid must be replenished, especially considering that most athletes do not sufficiently hydrate during training or competition. In a series of recent studies, Volterman *et al.* demonstrated, in children, that skim milk consumption following exercise in the heat was more effective in replacing fluid losses than water or a carbohydrate drink.[125] Similarly, a high-protein beverage was more effective than an isocaloric carbohydrate and electrolyte drink, but not more effective than a low-protein beverage.[126] Thus, while carbohydrates and electrolyte solutions appear to be beneficial for fluid retention, particularly during prolonged exercise sessions, it appears that protein-supplemented beverages (or milk) may provide an improved rehydration means during recovery.

The HR rise and SV reduction during steady-rate exercise is directly related to the degree of hypohydration.[127] This places an added strain on the cardiovascular system. The conflicting exercise and thermoregulatory needs may result in reduced skin blood flow[128,129] and be accompanied by lower sweating rates.[128,130] These phenomena were demonstrated in children and adolescents only to a limited extent.[87] The added cardiovascular strain may be greater in children than in adults, due to children's greater reliance on dry heat loss, and the requisite higher cutaneous blood flow.[131,132] As was shown by Bar-Or *et al.*,[100] the same degree of fluid loss (% body mass) will result in a considerably greater T_{re} rise in children than in adults (Figure 14.6). While this seems to be a clear argument for extra attention to fluid replacement in exercising children, it should be stressed (as discussed in the Sweating response section) that children's augmented T_{re}-response to fluid loss may be a means for maximizing the effectiveness of dry heat dissipation.

In spite of the widely reported decrements in physical performance in adults as a result of dehydration, many athletes deliberately dehydrate before competition.[133,134] During youth triathlon competition in a hot, humid climate, Aragon-Vargas *et al.*[108] reported adolescent triathletes to have lost >4% body mass. Walsh *et al.*[135] reported mild dehydration (2% body mass) to result in

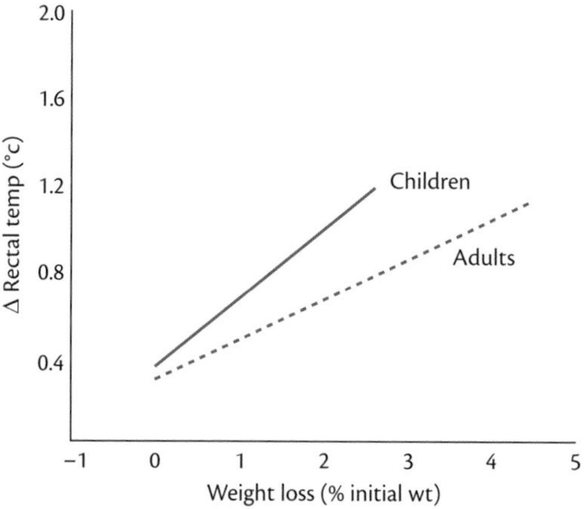

Figure 14.6 The change in rectal temperature in relation to body-mass loss in children and adults.

Bar-Or O. Climate and the exercising child – a review. Int J Sports Med. 1980; 1: 53–65.

performance decrement in adults. In 12- to 15-year-old male basketball players, 2% dehydration was shown to impair performance of basketball skills,[136] although no such decrements in performance were observed among similarly aged, hypohydrated, national-level basketball players.[103] In 10- to 12-year-old children, even a 1% decrease in body mass resulted in reduced aerobic performance (90% $\dot{V}O_2$ max to exhaustion).[137] In adults, carbohydrate and electrolyte solutions were demonstrated to improve performance while exercising in the heat[138] (see Maughan[139] for review). This was also demonstrated among adolescents,[136] but not in children.[140,141] Among adults, it was recently argued that a hypohydration level of up to 3% body mass, does not markedly affect endurance cycling performance in well-trained individuals.[142,143] In view of the inconsistent findings in adults, as well as among youth, further research is needed to better establish critical dehydration limits for performance capacity on the one hand, and heat tolerance and safety on the other. Factors to consider include the levels of fitness, training, and acclimatization, the intensity and type of exercise (e.g. cycling vs walking/running), environmental heat-load level and type (e.g. low-heat/high-humidity, high-heat/low humidity), methods of dehydration and fluid replenishment, and the type of consumed beverage, if any.

A state of hypohydration was also identified in adolescent athletes upon arrival at practice sessions—a condition that was only exaggerated during the ensuing workout.[101,102,104–107,109,144–146] Adolescent judoka, training in a hot and humid environment, were also reported to display hypohydration symptoms during, and even 24 h following, training.[107] Moreover, wrestlers, boxers, judoka, and body builders commonly lose 3–5% of their body mass for 'making weight' before competition.[147] In fact, some wrestlers, mostly in the lightweight categories, lose as much as 10% or more of their body mass before competition.[148] Sansone and Sawyer[149] reported on a 5-year-old boy wrestler who was pressured to lose weight. Although the American National Collegiate Athletic Association (which does not regulate children's sports) adopted rules to eliminate acute weight loss practices,[150] these practices persist.

Once hypohydration sets in it is very difficult to reverse during exercise. Thus, the above findings emphasize the need for sound hydration practices before, during, and following physical activity in children and adolescents, as well as in adults. There are numerous position stands on exercise and fluid replacement in youth,[151–153] but specific recommendations are not much different from those for adults.[153–156] Based on previous research, and acknowledging the large variability in sweating rate during exercise, we recommend that children should initiate fluid consumption even before (20–30 min) training or competition in mild heat. During exercise, fluid consumption should be frequent (every 15–20 min) but in small volumes (2–4 mL · kg-body-mass^{-1}).[157,158] In endurance or prolonged events, longer than ~1 h, and conducted in more extreme heat, that frequency should likely be even higher. Also, to encourage fluid consumption, beverages should be flavoured (especially orange and grape[119]), enriched with carbohydrates (6–8%) and NaCl (18–20 mmol · L^{-1}), cool, and non-carbonated.[120,123,159] Although not necessary for performance enhancements in most sporting events, and therefore not necessarily advocated as fluid replacements in youth,[153,156,160] sports drinks are instrumental in encouraging fluid consumption, water absorption, and retention.[161] Following training or competition, young athletes generally need to compensate for fluid losses not replenished during exercise. Rowland[154] recommended consumption of 4 mL · kg-body-mass^{-1} for each hour of exercise. While Desbrow *et al.*[153] highlight that when recovering between events (e.g. during tournaments), a carbohydrate and electrolyte beverage may be beneficial. In breaks longer than 2 h, milk consumption may be more beneficial.[125,126,153]

It is beyond the scope of this chapter to review the effects of heat stress and hypohydration on exercise performance in youth. For detailed reviews and safety recommendations, the reader is referred to recent publications, including reviews and consensus statements.[154–156,160,162–164]

Physiological response to cold stress

Environmental cold stress not countered by environmental modifications (e.g. seeking shelter, or clothing) results in a peripheral temperature drop, often accompanied by a decrease in T_{re}. To a limited extent this is countered by peripheral vasoconstriction and a rise in basal metabolism. However, in all but borderline cases this is not sufficient by itself. In such cases, preventing or attenuating continued heat loss necessitates further increase of the metabolic rate via piloerection ('goosebumps'), shivering, or exercise. Very few studies have addressed paediatric thermoregulation in cold environments.

Metabolic response to cold stress

In adults, rest or submaximal exercise in the cold is accompanied by a marked increase in $\dot{V}O_2$ as a result of a hormone-mediated rise in basal metabolism, piloerection, shivering, or a decrease in exercise efficiency. Increased $\dot{V}O_2$ was reported in most studies in children, both at rest and during exercise in the cold,[7,78,165–168] although not in all.[169,170] In fact, when compared with adults, the $\dot{V}O_2$ increase was greater in children. Ueda *et al.*[167] commented that the increase in $\dot{V}O_2$ during swimming in cold water (20 and 25°C) in 10- to 12-year-old boys was largely attributed to shivering, although it is unclear how this was measured. This is in line with children's higher subjective sensitivity to cold compared with adults.[7,78] Most studies do not report on shivering or mechanical efficiency. Therefore, it is impossible to determine the mechanisms responsible for the increase in metabolic rate and possible child-adult differences. Nevertheless, in view of children's greater BSA-to-mass ratio, it is expected that at any given cold environment, children would have to elicit a higher metabolic rate to maintain T_{re}.

Children have a basal metabolic rate that can be as much as ~50% higher than that of adults (depending on size; e.g. Wada[90]). However, in response to cold exposure, children do not raise their metabolic rate more than adults[169]. Moreover, children's smaller relative muscle mass (see also the section on Body composition) limits their ability to produce additional heat through shivering, compared with adults. Thus, their higher basal metabolic rate likely does not amount to a considerable advantage in the cold, when heat production needs to increase several fold. There are indications that children's vasoconstriction during cold exposure is greater than adults'.[7] At a certain stage, however, children may no longer be able to compensate via vasoconstriction, or the limited extent to which metabolic heat production could be raised, and would therefore be expected to reach a compromised, hypothermic condition earlier than would adults (e.g. Inoue *et al.*[169]).

Circulatory response to cold stress

Very little is known about the cardiovascular response to cold in children. Lower T_{sk} and faster T_{sk} decrease were reported in children, compared with adults, while resting or exercising in the cold.[7,68,165,169] The authors argue that the lower T_{sk} reflects a greater vasoconstriction in children. However, only two studies actually measured peripheral blood flow in children during cold stress. Wagner *et al.*[165] reported lower finger blood flow in 10- to 13-year-old boys compared with adolescent and adult males, while resting in a cool environment (17°C). More recently, Inoue *et al.*[171] reported that while resting in progressively declining ambient temperature (30→17°C), boys had higher cutaneous vascular conductance (CVC; reciprocal of peripheral resistance) in the trunk, while their fingers' CVC started out higher but decreased more, compared with men. While the boys' trunk CVC findings appear counter-intuitive, it should be noted that both their T_{re} and T_{body} were similar to those of the men. This was likely due to a greater increase in metabolic heat production in the boys, but overall it indicates a similar degree of temperature control. However, even at its lowest (17°C), the cold stress was only mild and the findings do not necessarily reflect what would happen at more extreme conditions. Future studies are needed to determine whether children's vascular response is variably less efficient in some regions (e.g. the trunk) and whether it becomes more consistent and efficient with maturation.

In adults, HR generally decreases in response to cold stress during rest or submaximal exercise, likely due to decreased $\dot{Q}$ with decreasing peripheral demand. In children, several studies,[167,170,172] although not all,[166] also reported decreased HR with lower environmental temperatures. Swimming at 32, 25, and 20°C, 12-year-old boys exhibited decreasing HRs with decreasing temperatures.[167] Mackova *et al.*[170] showed the same effect, in similarly aged boys, cycling at effective temperatures (air temperature, humidity, and movement composite) of 10 and 25°C. Their post-exercise HR decline was faster at the lower temperature. Similarly, 11–12-year-old boys, cycling at 7 and 13°C, displayed lower HRs, compared with 22°C.[172] Following cold exposure, while recovering in a thermoneutral environment, the children's T_{re} continued to decrease and did not increase during the 30 min follow-up. This observation is consistent with the well-described after-drop in T_{re} following cold water immersion.[173] Following exercise in the cold, Walsh and Graham[174] described a similar phenomenon in men and women. Interestingly, the authors state that although T_{sk} was lower in the women (as in children vs adults), no sex-related differences were observed in the rate of T_{re} decrease. In view of the limited number of studies, further research is needed to examine the various issues of children's cardiovascular response to exercise in the cold.

Cold tolerance and body temperature changes

Among 8- to 18-year-olds, swimming in cool water (20.3°C, 30 m·min^{-1}) at a similar speeds, oral temperature was found to decrease more slowly with rising age.[175] That is, in spite of the fact that the younger children swam at higher speeds relative to their size and assumed potential, their rate of cooling was faster than that of the older children. Similarly, Klentrou *et al.*[168] demonstrated a greater drop in T_{re} in smaller, premenarcheal girls, compared with larger, postmenarcheal girls. In both studies, the greater BSA-to-mass ratio was related to the greater drop in body temperature. In fact, it was the BSA-to-mass ratio which explained most of the variance in the T_{re} change (not age or menarcheal status). These results demonstrate the importance of body dimensions, rather than age per se, for thermoregulation in the cold. Additionally, the rate of cooling was inversely related to the level of adiposity, as has more recently been shown by Wakabayashi *et al.*,[176] who investigated in prepubertal children the effect on T_{re} of 23°C water immersion. These results indicate the importance of body dimensions, as well as body adiposity, in maintaining body temperatures in the cold.

The faster cooling rate in the younger children is supported by Inoue *et al.*[169] They compared the thermoregulatory response to a linear decrease in ambient temperature (28→15°C) in prepubertal boys vs young men, at rest. The boys' T_{sk} was lower than the men's, presumably due to greater extent of vasoconstriction. This is in line with other reports of lower T_{sk} in children and adults resting in cool conditions (15–20°C).[68,165] Nevertheless, T_{re} decreased in the boys, while remaining stable in the men.

Different results were reported by Smolander *et al.*,[7] who compared boys' body-temperature responses to those of men, during exercise in a cold environment (5°C). Pre- and early pubescent boys were able to maintain their body temperature as effectively as men while cycling (30% peak $\dot{V}O_2$) in the cold. In fact, the boys' T_{re} even slightly (insignificantly) rose during exercise, compared with the men. The boys' T_{sk} was significantly lower at several sites, indicating a greater peripheral vasoconstriction, than in the men. The authors argued that children are able to maintain their T_{re} during exercise, by increasing metabolic rate and constricting peripheral vessels to a greater extent than adults. This age-related difference was observed when comparing two boys with two men of similar BSA-to-mass ratios. That is, thermoregulatory strategy in the cold is apparently also determined by maturation and not only by body size.

We studied 11- to 12-year-old boys during rest and exercise (50-min rest, 10 min cycle, 50 min rest) in cold (7°C), cool (13°C) and thermoneutral (22°C) conditions.[172] Rectal temperature decreased during the first 50 min of rest and continued to decrease in the subsequent rest period, in spite of the fact that the boys were dressed in sweat-pants and shirts (Figure 14.7). Rectal temperature slightly

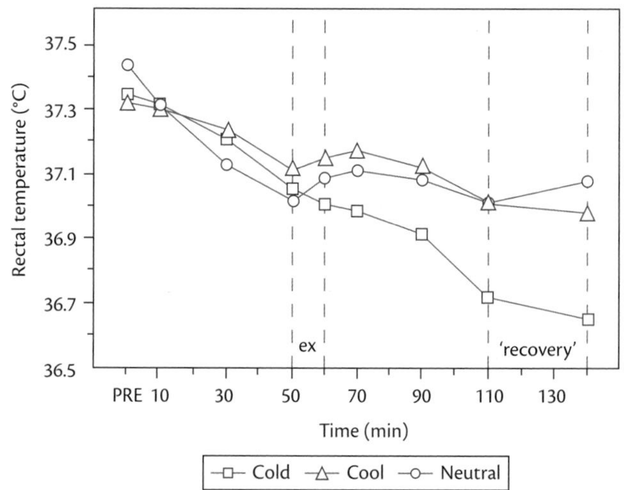

Figure 14.7 Mean rectal temperature in 11- to 12-year-old boys resting and cycling (50 min rest, 10 min cycle, 50 min rest) in a cold (7°C), cool (13°C), and thermoneutral (22°C) environment; ex = exercise.

Modified from Falk B, Bar-Eli M, Dotan R, *et al.* Physiological and cognitive responses to cold exposure in 11–12 year-old boys. Am J Hum Biol. 1997; 9: 39–49.

increased, following the 10 min exercise in the neutral and cool conditions, but not in the cold one. It is interesting to note that T_{re} did not return to pre-exposure levels even after a 30 min re-warming period in thermoneutral conditions (21–23°C). Skin temperature of the exposed hands decreased in the cold and cool environments, while no T_{sk} change was observed in the chest, which was covered by two layers of clothing. While Smolander *et al.*'s[7] boys were able to maintain body temperature, exercising at 5°C and wearing only shorts, our boys were unable to do so at 7°C with more clothing. This seeming discrepancy is likely accounted for by the much longer exercise duration (40 vs 10 min) and much shorter rest duration (20 vs 50 min) in Smolander *et al.*'s study. This observation demonstrates the importance of increasing metabolic rate during cold exposure of children for the maintenance of body temperature. The importance of elevated metabolic rate during exercise in the cold was also demonstrated by the 0.5–0.6°C T_{re} increase in 12-year-old boys exercising at 50% peak $\dot{V}O_2$ for 60 min at effective temperatures of 25 and 10°C.[170]

As is the case with heat tolerance, cold tolerance is reflected in cold-related injuries and fatalities. Limited epidemiological data do not point to a greater rate of cold-related fatalities among children[98] (Figure 14.4). However, the studies described here suggest that during rest in a cold environment, thermoregulatory effectiveness is lower in children than in adults, as schematically illustrated in Figure 14.5. During exercise, children may maintain their T_{re} by markedly increasing their metabolic rate. Doing so, however, may require greater fitness level on the part of children. It has not been established how much more metabolic heat must children produce at any given cold stress to match their cold tolerance with that of adults and how long it could be maintained in prolonged cold exposures.

Adaptation to thermal stress

Repeated exposures to heat stress result in an adaptation to heat, termed 'acclimatization' or 'acclimation', which is clearly evidenced in an array of parameters, both in adults and in children. Repeated cold exposures, on the other hand, result in limited range of adaptations in adults. In children, cold adaptation has not been investigated. Thus, the following section discusses only child-adult differences in heat adaptation. Additionally, physical exercise training, as such, induces adaptations that carry over to better coping with heat stress, but not necessarily with cold.

Heat acclimatization or acclimation

Heat acclimation (a controlled, regimented form of acclimatization) is similar overall in children, adolescents, and adults, although the rate of acclimation may differ. Children and adults were shown to reach a similar acclimation level following a 2-week, three times per week, acclimation protocol of exercise in the heat (43°C, 21% RH).[75] However, children's acclimation rate was slower in the early stages than in adults (Figure 14.8). These findings are in line with the lower levels of acclimation attained by 11- to 16-year-old boys vs men, following an 8-day acclimation regimen of exercise in the heat (48°C, 17% RH).[64]

Proper heat acclimation invariably results in increased sweating rate. This has been demonstrated in both children[75,177] and adults.[178] In adults, five daily exercise sessions in the heat were found to only minimally stimulate sweating adaptation.[179] In children, six sessions at 50% $\dot{V}O_2$ max, 35°C, and 55% RH, over a 2-week period did not have an effect on total sweating rate during the exposures, but exercise sweating rate increased, while resting rate decreased.[180] Inbar,[75] however, did find increased total sweating rate using a similar acclimation protocol, but with higher ambient temperature (43 vs 35°C, 21 vs. 55% RH), which possibly was the determining factor. He also found most of the adaptation to take place during the later acclimation exposures. Thus, the exact nature of children's sweating rate response to different acclimation regimens has not been sufficiently elucidated. It is worth noting, as mentioned earlier, that children who were already well-acclimatized had sweating rates twice as high as those typically reported for children.[62,86] Thus, sweating rate adaptation may be only partly realized in 2 weeks.

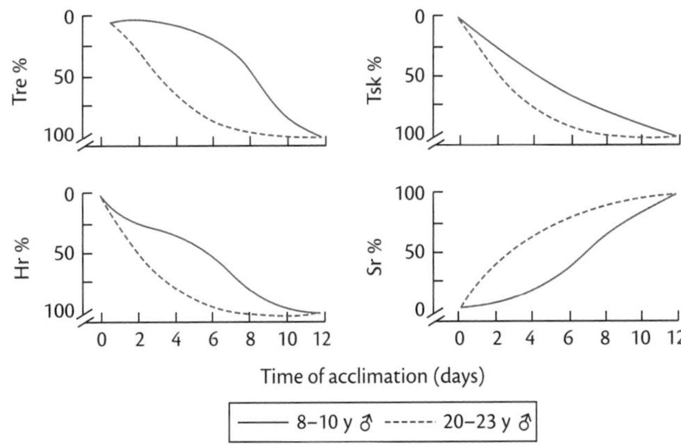

Figure 14.8 Physiological adaptations of 8- to 10-year-old boys and 20- to 23-year-old men during the course of a 2-week heat acclimation regimen (7 exercise sessions at 43°C, 21% RH).

Bar-Or O. Climate and the exercising child – a review. Int J Sports Med. 1980; 1: 53–65; and Bar-Or O. Pediatric sports medicine for the practitioner. New York: Springer-Verlag; 1983.

The time required for heat stress adaptation generally warrants added precaution during the early days of summer or unseasonal heat waves. This is particularly true for children due to their slower initial adaptation and their subjective strain perception, whose rate of decrease was found to be faster than the rate of objective adaptation and faster than in adults.[181] That is, children are less likely to match their behaviour to their actual physiological strain.

Although children appear to respond well to heat-exercise acclimation, other acclimation regimens have been found effective, too.[75,177] For example, exercise in thermoneutral conditions was found as effective as the heat-plus-exercise regimen, in children, but only partly so in adults.[177] Clearly, more research is needed to elucidate the mechanism of children's heat acclimation. Most tested protocols have involved a series of exercise-in-the-heat sessions over 2–3-week periods. In view of the different thermoregulatory strategy utilized by children vs adults (greater reliance on dry heat exchange, less on evaporative cooling), it is intriguing whether the effectiveness of various acclimation protocols will differ between children and adults.

Training-induced adaptations to heat stress

Physical training results in numerous physiological adaptations, some of which bear direct relevance to the thermoregulatory response to heat stress. For example, enhanced cardiovascular function can improve heat tolerance by increasing $\dot{Q}$ and rendering more of it available for cutaneous flow. Presumably, this should be more pronounced in children who rely on cutaneous blood flow to a greater extent and whose $\dot{Q}$ is consequently more heavily strained. However, while the relationship between physical training or aerobic fitness and heat tolerance has been clearly demonstrated in adults, it has not been consistently shown in children.

Peak $\dot{V}O_2$ was associated with enhanced heat tolerance in adults, but Delmarche *et al.*[4] could not demonstrate that relationship in prepubertal boys. Similarly, peak $\dot{V}O_2$ was found to account for only 16% of the variance in the T_{re} response to exercise in the heat among prepubertal boys.[182]

Training studies in children have demonstrated inconsistent effects on the T_{re} response to heat load. Araki *et al.*[68] found no training effect on the T_{re} response to passive heat stress, but Inbar *et al.*[177] observed in 8- to 10-year-old boys that 2-week cycle-training regimens (85% HR max) in hot or thermoneutral conditions, resulted in similarly lower T_{re} and HR responses to exercise in the heat.

Training has been shown to increase sweating rates in adults. Cross-sectional comparisons of trained vs untrained boys, resting in a warm-humid environment (30°C, 70% RH), also showed sweating-rate advantage for the trained boys, at any given T_{re}.[183] However, a 2-week training regimen did not change the sweating rate.[177] Clearly, further research is needed to elucidate the relationship between fitness or training adaptations and the response to heat stress.

Training-induced adaptations to cold stress

Little is known about training-induced adaptations and the thermoregulatory response to cold stress in adults, and even less so in children. We know of no study that investigated children's adaptation to true cold exposure. Two studies explored the effect of training on the response to cool conditions, not far below the thermoneutral zone. During passive rest at 18°C, a smaller drop in T_{re} was observed in trained vs untrained prepubertal boys,[183] while at 20°C, no difference in resting T_{re} response was observed in four prepubertal boys following 40 days of physical training.[68]

Conclusions

During rest and exercise, children appear to thermoregulate as effectively as adults. However, they do so using a different thermoregulatory strategy. Their larger BSA-to-mass ratio allows them to rely more on dry heat dissipation and less on evaporative cooling (sweating). In extreme heat and particularly, in extreme cold, children's higher BSA-to-mass ratio can become a disadvantage relative to adults. Children, like adults, inadvertently dehydrate while exercising in hot conditions and are often hypohydrated, even before training. Importantly, for a given level of hypohydration (% body-mass loss), children's core temperature rises considerably more than adults', possibly putting them at higher risk of heat-related injury. Despite the prevalence of hypohydration and children's likely disadvantage in very high ambient temperatures, there are no epidemiological data to support higher rates of heat-related injuries among children and adolescents than in adults. Most of our understanding of age-related thermoregulatory differences is based on experimental heat exposures. However, children's response to cold stress, particularly circulatory and endocrine response, has been only scantily studied and much remains unclear. Additionally, possible sex-related differences in thermoregulation during childhood, and maturity-related effects, require further research.

Summary

Under most environmental conditions, children's thermoregulatory *effectiveness* is similar to that of adults. However, children's thermoregulation *strategy* is different from adults', resulting in noteworthy differences in physiological responses.

- Under all but extreme heat-stress conditions, children regulate their body temperature as well as adults. By taking advantage of their higher relative surface area, children can afford to sweat less and their reported sweating rates are, accordingly, lower as well. Reports of consistently lower sweating rates in children previously led to regard them as immature or inferior thermoregulators, a notion that is now accepted as a misconception.
- Metabolic, circulatory, and hormonal differences between children and adults may also affect thermoregulation. The metabolic cost of bipedal locomotion is higher in children which places added stress on the thermoregulatory system during heat exposure, but is marginally advantageous in cold conditions. Resting concentrations of testosterone, oestrogen, prolactin, and growth hormone differ between children and adults, which may account for some of the observed differences in sweat-gland function.
- Changes in body temperature, in response to heat or cold stress, are more pronounced in children than in adults. These changes are accompanied by increases in the metabolic cost of exercise that are greater in children than in adults. Relative to exercising adults, children's cardiovascular system appears to be increasingly more strained with rising heat stress, due to the increasing muscle-skin competition on the available cardiac output. This possibly explains the greater subjective heat intolerance sometimes reported in children. Little is understood about children's circulatory response to cold stress, nor about their endocrine response to thermal stress, in general, and to cold stress in particular.
- Inadvertent ('involuntary') dehydration, during exercise in the heat, is common to both children and adults. However, the resulting hypohydration and blood volume loss may put extra strain on children's cardiovascular system due to their greater reliance on cutaneous blood flow. It is not known whether this is the reason for children's greater core temperature (T_{re}) rise for a given level of fluid loss, but their heightened T_{re} response might be regarded as advantageous in producing a greater skin-to-air temperature gradient, congruent with their thermoregulatory strategy. The relative significance of this in the overall thermoregulatory picture is yet to be investigated.
- While exercising in the heat, a degree of inadvertent dehydration may be unavoidable in most voluntary hydration situations. Proper flavouring and temperature of provided beverages can greatly enhance their attractiveness and the effectiveness of any hydration programme.
- Much is yet to be learned about the thermoregulatory response of children and adolescents:

  a. While dimensional changes clearly determine much of the child-adult difference in the thermoregulatory response, the independent contribution of maturation per se must still be elucidated.

b. The determinants of effective acclimation and training-induced thermoregulatory adaptations to heat and particularly to cold are yet little understood.

c. As girl-woman thermoregulatory differences seem more limited than the corresponding male differences, the existence of thermoregulatory sex differences ought to be verified and their determinant factors elucidated.

References

1. Falk B. Temperature regulation. In: Armstrong N, Van Mechelen W (eds.) *Paediatric exercise science and medicine*. New York: Oxford University Press; 2000. p. 223–239.
2. Falk B, Dotan R. Temperature regulation in children. In: Armstrong N, Van Mechelen W (eds.) *Paediatric exercise science and medicine*. New York: Oxford University Press; 2008. p. 309–324.
3. Davies CT. Thermal responses to exercise in children. *Ergonomics*. 1981; 24: 55–61.
4. Delamarche P, Bittel J, Lacour JR, Flandrois R. Thermoregulation at rest and during exercise in prepubertal boys. *Eur J Appl Physiol Occup Physiol*. 1990; 60: 436–440.
5. Gullestad R. Temperature regulation in children during exercise. *Acta Paediatr Scand*. 1975; 64: 257–263.
6. Tochihara Y, Ohnaka T, Nagai Y. Thermal responses of 6- to 8-year-old children during immersion of their legs in a hot water bath. *Appl Human Sci*. 1995; 14: 23–28.
7. Smolander J, Bar-Or O, Korhonen O, Ilmarinen J. Thermoregulation during rest and exercise in the cold in pre- and early pubescent boys and in young men. *J Appl Physiol*. 1992; 72: 1589–1594.
8. Haymes EM, Buskirk ER, Hodgson JL, Lundegren HM, Nicholas WC. Heat tolerance of exercising lean and heavy prepubertal girls. *J Appl Physiol*. 1974; 36: 566–571.
9. Haymes EM, McCormick RJ, Buskirk ER. Heat tolerance of exercising lean and obese prepubertal boys. *J Appl Physiol*. 1975; 39: 457–461.
10. Dougherty KA, Chow M, Kenney WL. Responses of lean and obese boys to repeated summer exercise in the heat bouts. *Med Sci Sports Exerc*. 2009; 41: 279–289.
11. Leites GT, Sehl PL, Cunha Gdos S, Detoni Filho A, Meyer F. Responses of obese and lean girls exercising under heat and thermoneutral conditions. *J Pediatr*. 2013; 162: 1054–1060.
12. Sehl PL, Leites GT, Martins JB, Meyer F. Responses of obese and non-obese boys cycling in the heat. *Int J Sports Med*. 2012; 33: 497–501.
13. Adams JD, Ganio MS, Burchfield JM, *et al*. Effects of obesity on body temperature in otherwise-healthy females when controlling hydration and heat production during exercise in the heat. *Eur J Appl Physiol*. 2015; 115: 167–176.
14. Limbaugh JD, Wimer GS, Long LH, Baird WH. Body fatness, body core temperature, and heat loss during moderate-intensity exercise. *Aviat Space Environ Med*. 2013; 84: 1153–1158.
15. Rogers NH. Brown adipose tissue during puberty and with aging. *Ann Med*. 2015; 47: 142–149.
16. Cypess AM, Haft CR, Laughlin MR, Hu HH. Brown fat in humans: consensus points and experimental guidelines. *Cell metabolism*. 2014; 20: 408–415.
17. Blondin DP, Labbe SM, Tingelstad HC, *et al*. Increased brown adipose tissue oxidative capacity in cold-acclimated humans. *J Clin Endocrinol Metab*. 2014; 99: E438–E446.
18. Malina RM, Bouchard C, Bar-Or O. *Growth, maturation and physical activity*, 2nd ed. Champaign, IL: Human Kinetics: 2004.
19. Graham GR. Blood Volume in Children. *Ann R Coll Surg Engl*. 1963; 33: 149–158.
20. Astrand PO. *Experimental studies of physical work capacity in relation to sex and age*. Copenhagen: Mundsgaard; 1952.
21. Drinkwater BL, Kupprat IC, Denton JE, Crist JL, Horvath SM. Response of prepubertal girls and college women to work in the heat. *J Appl Physiol*. 1977; 43: 1046–1053.
22. Robinson S. Experimental studies of physical fitness in relation to age. *Int Z Angetv Physiol Einschl Arbeitsphysiol*. 1938; 10: 251–323.
23. Unnithan VB, Eston RG. Stride frequency and submaximal treadmill running economy in adults and children. *Pediatr Exerc Sci*. 1990; 2: 149–155.
24. Ariens GA, van Mechelen W, Kemper HC, Twisk JW. The longitudinal development of running economy in males and females aged between 13 and 27 years: the Amsterdam Growth and Health Study. *Eur J Appl Physiol Occup Physiol*. 1997; 76: 214–220.
25. Turley KR, Wilmore JH. Cardiovascular responses to treadmill and cycle ergometer exercise in children and adults. *J Appl Physiol*. 1997; 83: 948–957.
26. Dallman PR, Siimes MA. Percentile curves for hemoglobin and red cell volume in infancy and childhood. *J Pediatr*. 1979; 94: 26–31.
27. Brooke MH, Engel WK. The histographic analysis of human muscle biopsies with regard to fiber types. 4. Children's biopsies. *Neurology*. 1969; 19: 591–605.
28. Kawahata A. Sex differences in sweating. In: Yoshimura H, Ogata K, Itoh S (eds.) *Essential problems in climate physiology*. Kyoto: Nankodo; 1960. p. 169–184.
29. Choudhry R, Hodgins MB, Van der Kwast TH, Brinkmann AO, Boersma WJ. Localization of androgen receptors in human skin by immunohistochemistry: implications for the hormonal regulation of hair growth, sebaceous glands and sweat glands. *J Endocrinol*. 1992; 133: 467–475.
30. Rees J, Shuster S. Pubertal induction of sweat gland activity. *Clin Sci (Lond)*. 1981; 60: 689–692.
31. Bar-Or O. Thermoregulation in females from a life span perspective. In: Bar-Or O, Lamb DR, Clarkson PM (eds.) *Exercise and the female—A life span approach. Perspectives in exercise science and sports medicine. IX*. Traverse City, MI: Cooper Publishing Group; 1996. p. 250–283.
32. Fraser D, Padwick ML, Whitehead M, Coffer A, King RJ. Presence of an oestradiol receptor-related protein in the skin: changes during the normal menstrual cycle. *Br J Obstet Gynaecol*. 1991; 98: 1277–1282.
33. Kaufman FL, Mills DE, Hughson RL, Peake GT. Effects of bromocriptine on sweat gland function during heat acclimatization. *Horm Res*. 1988; 29: 31–38.
34. Robertson MT, Boyajian MJ, Patterson K, Robertson WV. Modulation of the chloride concentration of human sweat by prolactin. *Endocrinology*. 1986; 119: 2439–2444.
35. Falk B, Bar-Or O, MacDougall JD. Aldosterone and prolactin response to exercise in the heat in circumpubertal boys. *J Appl Physiol*. 1991; 71: 1741–1745.
36. Juul A, Main K, Nielsen B, Skakkebaek NE. Decreased sweating in growth hormone deficiency: does it play a role in thermoregulation? *J Pediatr Endocrinol*. 1993; 6: 39–44.
37. Juul A, Hjortskov N, Jepsen LT, *et al*. Growth hormone deficiency and hyperthermia during exercise: a controlled study of sixteen GH-deficient patients. *J Clin Endocrinol Metab*. 1995; 80: 3335–3340.
38. Main K, Nilsson KO, Skakkebaek NE. Influence of sex and growth hormone deficiency on sweating. *Scand J Clin Lab Invest*. 1991; 51: 475–480.
39. Lobie PE, Breipohl W, Lincoln DT, Garcia-Aragon J, Waters MJ. Localization of the growth hormone receptor/binding protein in skin. *J Endocrinol*. 1990; 126: 467–471.
40. Oakes SR, Haynes KM, Waters MJ, Herington AC, Werther GA. Demonstration and localization of growth hormone receptor in human skin and skin fibroblasts. *J Clin Endocrinol Metab*. 1992; 75: 1368–1373.
41. Soldin SJ, Hicks JM. *Pediatric reference ranges*. Washington, DC: AACC Press; 1995.
42. Bar-Or O. Climate and the exercising child—a review. *Int J Sports Med*. 1980; 1: 53–65.
43. Bar-Or O. Temperature regulation during exercise in children and adolescents. In: Gisolfi CV, Lamb DR (eds.) *Youth, exercise and sports. Perspectives in exercise science and sports medicine. II*. Indianapolis, IN: Benchmark Press; 1989. p. 335–362.
44. Falk B. Effects of thermal stress during rest and exercise in the paediatric population. *Sports Med*. 1998; 25: 221–240.

45. Inoue Y, Kuwahara T, Araki T. Maturation- and aging-related changes in heat loss effector function. *J Physiol Anthropol Appl Hum Sci.* 2004; 23: 289–294.
46. Falk B. Physiological and health aspects of exercise in hot and cold climates. In: Bar-Or O (ed.) *The child and adolescent athlete.* Oxford: Blackwell Scientific; 1996. p. 326–352.
47. Sato K, Leidal R, Sato F. Morphology and development of an apoeccrine sweat gland in human axillae. *Am J Physiol.* 1987; 252: R166–R180.
48. Landing BH, Wells TR, Williamson ML. Studies on growth of eccrine sweat glands. In: Cheek DB (ed.) *Human growth: Body composition, cell growth, energy and intelligence.* Philadelphia, PA: Lea & Febiger; 1968. p. 382–394.
49. Wolfe S, Cage G, Epstein M, Tice L, Miller H, Gordon RS, Jr. Metabolic studies of isolated human eccrine sweat glands. *J Clin Invest.* 1970; 49: 1880–1884.
50. Sato K, Sato F. Individual variations in structure and function of human eccrine sweat gland. *Am J Physiol.* 1983; 245: R203–R208.
51. Kuno Y. *Human Perspiration.* Springfield, IL: CC Thomas; 1956.
52. Bar-Or O, Magnusson LI, Buskirk ER. Distribution of heat-activated sweat glands in obese and lean men and women. *Hum Biol.* 1968; 40: 235–248.
53. Szabo G. The number of eccrine sweat glands in human skin. *Advan Biol Skin.* 1962; 3: 1–5.
54. Wilk B, Pender N, Volterman K, Bar-Or O, Timmons BW. Influence of pubertal stage on local sweating patterns of girls exercising in the heat. *Pediatr Exerc Sci.* 2013; 25: 212–220.
55. Falk B, Bar-Or O, MacDougall JD, McGillis L, Calvert R, Meyer F. Sweat lactate in exercising children and adolescents of varying physical maturity. *J Appl Physiol.* 1991; 71: 1735–1740.
56. Fellmann N, Labbe A, Gachon AM, Coudert J. Thermal sweat lactate in cystic fibrosis and in normal children. *Eur J Appl Physiol Occup Physiol.* 1985; 54: 511–516.
57. Eriksson BO, Saltin B. Muscle metabolism during exercise in boys aged 11 to 16 years compared to adults. *Acta Paediatr Belg.* 1974; 28: 257–265.
58. Falk B, Bar-Or O. Longitudinal changes in peak aerobic and anaerobic mechanical power of circumpubertal boys. *Pediatr Exerc Sci.* 1993; 5: 318–331.
59. Carlson JS, Le Rossignol P. Children and adults exercising in hot wet climatic conditions with different levels of radiant heat. *Proceedings of the North American Society of Pediatric Exercise Medicine, ninth annual meeting.* Pittsburgh, PA: 1994.
60. Jokinen E, Valimaki I, Marniemi J, Seppanen A, Irjala K, Simell O. Children in sauna: hormonal adjustments to intensive short thermal stress. *Acta Physiol Scand.* 1991; 142: 437–442.
61. Rowland T, Garrison A, Pober D. Determinants of endurance exercise capacity in the heat in prepubertal boys. *Int J Sports Med.* 2007; 28: 26–32.
62. Rivera-Brown AM, Rowland TW, Ramirez-Marrero FA, Santacana G, Vann A. Exercise tolerance in a hot and humid climate in heat-acclimatized girls and women. *Int J Sports Med.* 2006; 27: 943–950.
63. Rowland TW, Staab JS, Unnithan VB, Rambusch JM, Siconolfi SF. Mechanical efficiency during cycling in prepubertal and adult males. *Int J Sports Med.* 1990; 11: 452–455.
64. Wagner JA, Robinson S, Tzankoff SP, Marino RP. Heat tolerance and acclimatization to work in the heat in relation to age. *J Appl Physiol.* 1972; 33: 616–622.
65. Falk B, Bar-Or O, MacDougall JD. Thermoregulatory responses of pre-, mid-, and late-pubertal boys to exercise in dry heat. *Med Sci Sports Exerc.* 1992; 24: 688–694.
66. Shibasaki M, Inoue Y, Kondo N, Iwata A. Thermoregulatory responses of prepubertal boys and young men during moderate exercise. *Eur J Appl Physiol Occup Physiol.* 1997; 75: 212–218.
67. Brien EK, Wilk B, Iwata M, Bar-Or O. Forearm blood flow in pre/early-, mid, and late-pubertal girls exercising in the heat. *Med Sci Sports Exerc.* 2000; 32: S157.
68. Araki T, Tsujita J, Matsushita K, Hori S. Thermoregulatory responses of prepubertal boys to heat and cold in relation to physical training. *Hum Ergonomics.* 1980; 9: 69–80.
69. Mackie JM. *Physiological responses of twin children to exercise under conditions of heat stress.* Unpublished MSc thesis. University of Waterloo: Canada; 1982.
70. Jokinen E, Valimaki I, Antila K, Seppanen A, Tuominen J. Children in sauna: cardiovascular adjustment. *Pediatrics.* 1990; 86: 282–288.
71. Jokinen E, Valimaki I. Children in sauna: electrocardiographic abnormalities. *Acta Paediatr Scand.* 1991; 80: 370–374.
72. Brisson GR, Audet A, Ledoux M, Matton P, Pellerin-Massicotte J, Peronnet F. Exercise-induced blood prolactin variations in trained adult males: a thermic stress more than an osmotic stress. *Horm Res.* 1986; 23: 200–206.
73. Charkoudian N, Stachenfeld N. Sex hormone effects on autonomic mechanisms of thermoregulation in humans. *Auto Neurosci.* 2015; 196: 75–80.
74. Araki T, Toda Y, Matsushita K, Tsujino A. Age differences in sweating during muscular exercise. *Jap J Fitness Sports Med.* 1979; 28: 239–248.
75. Inbar O. *Acclimatization to dry and hot environments in young adults and children 8–10 years old.* EdD dissertation. New York: Columbia University; 1978.
76. Inbar O, Morris N, Epstein Y, Gass G. Comparison of thermoregulatory responses to exercise in dry heat among prepubertal boys, young adults and older males. *Exp Physiol.* 2004; 89: 691–700.
77. Meyer F, Bar-Or O, MacDougall D, Heigenhauser GJ. Sweat electrolyte loss during exercise in the heat: effects of gender and maturation. *Med Sci Sports Exerc.* 1992; 24: 776–781.
78. Anderson GS, Mekjavic IB. Thermoregulatory responses of circum-pubertal children. *Eur J Appl Physiol Occup Physiol.* 1996; 74: 404–410.
79. Falk B, Bar-Or O, Calvert R, MacDougall JD. Sweat gland response to exercise in the heat among pre-, mid-, and late-pubertal boys. *Med Sci Sports Exerc.* 1992; 24: 313–319.
80. Falk B, Bar-Or O, MacDougall D, Goldsmith C, McGillis L. A longitudinal analysis of the sweating response of pre-, mid- and late-pubertal boys during exercise in the heat. *Am J Hum Biol.* 1992; 4: 527–535.
81. Tsuzuki-Hayakawa K, Tochihara Y, Ohnaka T. Thermoregulation during heat exposure of young children compared to their mothers. *Eur J Appl Physiol Occup Physiol.* 1995; 72: 12–17.
82. Foster KG, Hey EN, Katz G. The response of the sweat glands of the newborn baby to thermal stimuli and to intradermal acetylcholine. *J Physiol.* 1969; 203: 13–29.
83. Shapiro Y, Pandolf KB, Avellini BA, Pimental NA, Goldman RF. Physiological responses of men and women to humid and dry heat. *J Appl Physiol.* 1980; 49: 1–8.
84. Iuliano S, Naughton G, Collier G, Carlson J. Examination of the self-selected fluid intake practices by junior athletes during a simulated duathlon event. *Int J Sport Nutr.* 1998; 8: 10–23.
85. Dill DB, Horvath SM, Van Beaumont W, Gehlsen G, Burrus K. Sweat electrolytes in desert walks. *J Appl Physiol.* 1967; 23: 746–751.
86. Rivera-Brown AM, Gutierrez R, Gutierrez JC, Frontera WR, Bar-Or O. Drink composition, voluntary drinking, and fluid balance in exercising, trained, heat-acclimatized boys. *J Appl Physiol.* 1999; 86: 78–84.
87. Bar-Or O, Dotan R, Inbar O, Rotshtein A, Zonder H. Voluntary hypohydration in 10- to 12-year-old boys. *J Appl Physiol.* 1980; 48: 104–108.
88. Bar-Or O, Harris D, Bergstein V, Buskirk ER. Progressive hypohydration in subjects who vary in adiposity. *Isr J Med Sci.* 1976; 12: 800–803.
89. Wada M. Sudorific action of adrenalin on the human sweat glands and determination of their excitability. *Science.* 1950; 111: 376–377.
90. Kleiber M. *The fire of life.* New York: John Wiley & Sons, Inc: 1961.
91. Meyer F, Bar-Or O. Fluid and electrolyte loss during exercise. The paediatric angle. *Sports Med.* 1994; 18: 4–9.
92. Bittel J, Henane R. Comparison of thermal exchanges in men and women under neutral and hot conditions. *J Physiol.* 1975; 250: 475–489.

93. Sohar E, Shapiro Y, eds. *The physiological reactions of women and children marching during heat: Proceedings of the 1st Israel Physiology and Pharmacology Society Meeting.* (Abstract). 1965; 1: 50.
94. Gottschalk AW, Andrish JT. Epidemiology of sports injury in pediatric athletes. *Sports Med Arthroscop Rev.* 2011; 19: 2–6.
95. Ahdoot S, Pacheco SE, Council On Environmental Health: Global climate change and children's health. *Pediatrics.* 2015; 136: e1468–e1484.
96. Nelson NG, Collins CL, Comstock RD, McKenzie LB. Exertional heat-related injuries treated in emergency departments in the US, 1997–2006. *Am J Prev Med.* 2011; 40: 54–60.
97. Somboonwong J, Sanguanrungsirikul S, Pitayanon C. Heat illness surveillance in schoolboys participating in physical education class in tropical climate: an analytical prospective descriptive study. *BMJ Open.* 2012; 2(4): doi:10.1136/bmjopen-2011-000741
98. Berko J, Ingram DD, Saha S, Parker JD. Deaths attributed to heat, cold, and other weather events in the United States, 2006–2010. *National Health Statistics Reports.* 2014; 30: 1–15.
99. Leppaluoto J. Human thermoregulation in sauna. *Ann Clin Res.* 1988; 20: 240–243.
100. Bar-Or O, Blimkie CJ, Hay JA, MacDougall JD, Ward DS, Wilson WM. Voluntary dehydration and heat intolerance in cystic fibrosis. *Lancet.* 1992; 339(8795): 696–699.
101. Phillips SM, Sykes D, Gibson N. Hydration status andfFluid balance of elite European youth soccer players during consecutive training sessions. *J Sports Sci Med* 2014; 13: 817–822.
102. Yeargin SW, Casa DJ, Judelson DA, *et al.* Thermoregulatory responses and hydration practices in heat-acclimatized adolescents during preseason high school football. *J Athl Train.* 2010; 45: 136–146.
103. Carvalho P, Oliveira B, Barros R, Padrao P, Moreira P, Teixeira VH. Impact of fluid restriction and ad libitum water intake or an 8% carbohydrate-electrolyte beverage on skill performance of elite adolescent basketball players. *Int J Sport Nutr Exerc Metab.* 2011; 21: 214–221.
104. Kavouras SA, Arnaoutis G, Makrillos M, *et al.* Educational intervention on water intake improves hydration status and enhances exercise performance in athletic youth. *Scand J Med Sci Sports.* 2012; 22: 684–689.
105. Gordon RE, Kassier SM, Biggs C. Hydration status and fluid intake of urban, underprivileged South African male adolescent soccer players during training. *J Int Soc Sports Nutr.* 2015; 12: 21.
106. Arnaoutis G, Kavouras SA, Kotsis YP, Tsekouras YE, Makrillos M, Bardis CN. Ad libitum fluid intake does not prevent dehydration in suboptimally hydrated young soccer players during a training session of a summer camp. *Int J Sport Nutr Exerc Metab.* 2013; 23: 245–251.
107. Rivera-Brown AM, De Felix-Davila RA. Hydration status in adolescent judo athletes before and after training in the heat. *Int J Sports Physiol Perform.* 2012; 7: 39–46.
108. Aragon-Vargas LF, Wilk B, Timmons BW, Bar-Or O. Body weight changes in child and adolescent athletes during a triathlon competition. *Eur J Appl Physiol.* 2013; 113: 233–239.
109. Silva RP, Mundel T, Natali AJ, *et al.* Fluid balance of elite Brazilian youth soccer players during consecutive days of training. *J Sports Sci.* 2011; 29: 725–732.
110. Pugh LG, Corbett JL, Johnson RH. Rectal temperatures, weight losses, and sweat rates in marathon running. *J Appl Physiol.* 1967; 23: 347–352.
111. Rothstein A, Adolph EF, Wills JH. Voluntary dehydration. In: Adolph EF (ed.) *Physiology of man in the desert.* New York: Interscience; 1947. p. 254–270.
112. Wilk B, Timmons BW, Bar-Or O. Voluntary fluid intake, hydration status, and aerobic performance of adolescent athletes in the heat. *Appl Physiol Nutr Metab.* 2010; 35: 834–841.
113. Wong SH, Sun FH. Effect of beverage flavor on body hydration in Hong Kong Chinese children exercising in a hot environment. *Pediatr Exerc Sci.* 2014; 26: 177–186.
114. Williams CA, Blackwell J. Hydration status, fluid intake, and electrolyte losses in youth soccer players. *Int J Sports Physiol Perform.* 2012; 7: 367–374.
115. Philip M, Chaimovitz C, Singer A, Golinsky D. Urine osmolality in nursery school children in a hot climate. *Isr J Med Sci.* 1993; 29: 104–106.
116. Bar-David Y, Landau D, Bar-David Z, Pilpel D, Phillip M. Voluntary dehydration among elementary school children living in a hot climate. *Child Ambul Health.* 1998;4: 393–397.
117. Secher M, Ritz P. Hydration and cognitive performance. *J Nutr Health and Aging.* 2012; 16: 325–329.
118. Benton D. Dehydration influences mood and cognition: a plausible hypothesis? *Nutrients.* 2011; 3: 555–573.
119. Meyer F, Bar-Or O, Salsberg A, Passe D. Hypohydration during exercise in children: effect on thirst, drink preferences, and rehydration. *Int J Sport Nutr.* 1994; 4: 22–35.
120. Wilk B, Bar-Or O. Effect of drink flavor and NaCl on voluntary drinking and hydration in boys exercising in the heat. *J Appl Physiol.* 1996; 80: 1112–1117.
121. Bar-Or O, Wilk B. Water and electrolyte replenishment in the exercising child. *Int J Sport Nutr.* 1996; 6: 93–99.
122. Hall EL, Bergeron MF, Brenner JS, Wang X, Ludwig DA. Voluntary fluid intake and core temperature responses in children during exercise in the heat. *Med Sci Sports Exerc.* 2005; 37: S28.
123. Wilk B, Kriemler S, Keller H, Bar-Or O. Consistency in preventing voluntary dehydration in boys who drink a flavored carbohydrate-NaCl beverage during exercise in the heat. *Int J Sport Nutr.* 1998; 8: 1–9.
124. Wilk B, Jae-Hyun L, Bar-Or O. Drink composition, voluntary drinking and aerobic performance in heat-acclimated adolescent male athletes. *Med Sci Sports Exerc.* 2005; 37: S464.
125. Volterman KA, Obeid J, Wilk B, Timmons BW. Effect of milk consumption on rehydration in youth following exercise in the heat. *Appl Physiol Nutr. Metab.* 2014; 39: 1257–1264.
126. Volterman KA, Moore DR, Obeid J, Offord EA, Timmons BW. The effect of post-exercise milk protein intake on rehydration of children. *Pediatr Exerc Sci.* 2015; 28: 286–95.
127. Heaps CL, Gonzalez-Alonso J, Coyle EF. Hypohydration causes cardiovascular drift without reducing blood volume. *Int J Sports Med.* 1994; 15: 74–79.
128. Fortney SM, Wenger CB, Bove JR, Nadel ER. Effect of hyperosmolality on control of blood flow and sweating. *J Appl Physiol.* 1984; 57: 1688–1695.
129. Kenney WL, Tankersley CG, Newswanger DL, Hyde DE, Puhl SM, Turner NL. Age and hypohydration independently influence the peripheral vascular response to heat stress. *J Appl Physiol.* 1990; 68: 1902–1908.
130. Sawka MN, Young AJ, Francesconi RP, Muza SR, Pandolf KB. Thermoregulatory and blood responses during exercise at graded hypohydration levels. *J Appl Physiol.* 1985; 59: 1394–1401.
131. Falk B, Dotan R. Children's thermoregulation during exercise in the heat—a revisit. *Appl Physiol Nutr Metab.* 2008; 33: 420–427.
132. Rowland T. Thermoregulation during exercise in the heat in children: old concepts revisited. *J Appl Physiol.* 2008; 105: 718–724.
133. Webster S, Rutt R, Weltman A. Physiological effects of a weight loss regimen practiced by college wrestlers. *Med Sci Sports Exerc.* 1990; 22: 229–234.
134. Shirreffs SM. The importance of good hydration for work and exercise performance. *Nutr Rev.* 2005; 63: S14–S21.
135. Walsh RM, Noakes TD, Hawley JA, Dennis SC. Impaired high-intensity cycling performance time at low levels of dehydration. *Int J Sports Med.* 1994; 15: 392–398.
136. Dougherty KA, Baker LB, Chow M, Kenney WL. Two percent dehydration impairs and six percent carbohydrate drink improves boys basketball skills. *Med Sci Sports Exerc.* 2006; 38: 1650–1658.

137. Wilk B, Yuxiu H, Bar-Or O. Effect of hypohydration on aerobic performance of boys who exercise in the heat. *Med Sci Sports Exerc.* 2002; 34: S48.
138. Carter J, Jeukendrup AE, Jones DA. The effect of sweetness on the efficacy of carbohydrate supplementation during exercise in the heat. *Can J Appl Physiol.* 2005; 30: 379–391.
139. Maughan RJ. Food and fluid intake during exercise. *Can J Appl Physiol.* 2001; 26: S71–S78.
140. Meyer F, Bar-Or O, MacDougall D, Heigenhauser GJ. Drink composition and the electrolyte balance of children exercising in the heat. *Med Sci Sports Exerc.* 1995; 27: 882–887.
141. Meyer F, Bar-Or O, Wilk B. Children's perceptual responses to ingesting drinks of different compositions during and following exercise in the heat. *Int J Sport Nutr.* 1995; 5: 13–24.
142. Cheung SS, McGarr GW, Mallette MM, *et al.* Separate and combined effects of dehydration and thirst sensation on exercise performance in the heat. *Scand J Med Sci Sports.* 2015; 25(Suppl 1): 104–111.
143. Wall BA, Watson G, Peiffer JJ, Abbiss CR, Siegel R, Laursen PB. Current hydration guidelines are erroneous: dehydration does not impair exercise performance in the heat. *Br J Sports Med.* 2015; 49: 1077–1083.
144. De Felix-Davila RA, Rivera-Brown AM, Lebron LE. Hydration status and sweat electrolyte loss in adolescent judokas training in hot and humid conditions. *Med Sci Sports Exerc.* 2005; 37: S167–S168.
145. Yeargin SW, Casa DJ, Decher NR, O'Connor CB. Incidence and degree of dehydration and attitutdes regarding hydration in children at summer football camp. *Med Sci Sports Exerc.* 2005; 37: S463.
146. Casa DJ, Yeargin SW, Decher NR, McCaffrey M, James CT. Incidence and degree of dehydration and attitudes regarding hydration in adolescents at summer football camp. *Med Sci Sports Exerc.* 2005; 37: S463.
147. Tipton CM, Tcheng TK, Zambraski EJ. Iowa wrestling study: weight classification systems. *Med Sci Sports.* 1976; 8: 101–104.
148. Tipton CM, Tcheng TK. Iowa wrestling study. Weight loss in high school students. *JAMA.* 1970; 214: 1269–1274.
149. Sansone RA, Sawyer R. Weight loss pressure on a 5-year-old wrestler. *Br J Sports Med.* 2005; 39: e2.
150. Oppliger RA, Steen SA, Scott JR. Weight loss practices of college wrestlers. *Int J Sport Nutr Exerc Metab.* 2003; 13: 29–46.
151. American Academy of Pediatrics Committee on Sports Medicine: Climatic heat stress and the exercising child. *Pediatrics.* 1982; 69: 808–809.
152. American Academy of Pediatrics. Committee on Sports Medicine and Fitness. Climatic heat stress and the exercising child and adolescent. *Pediatrics.* 2000; 106: 158–159.
153. Desbrow B, McCormack J, Burke LM, *et al.* Sports Dietitians Australia position statement: sports nutrition for the adolescent athlete. *Int J Sport Nutr Exerc Metab.* 2014; 24: 570–584.
154. Rowland T. Fluid replacement requirements for child athletes. *Sports Med.* 2011; 41: 279–288.
155. Council on Sports Medicine and Fitness and Council on School Health. Policy statement-Climatic heat stress and exercising children and adolescents. *Pediatrics.* 2011; 128: e741-747.
156. Baker LB, Jeukendrup AE. Optimal composition of fluid-replacement beverages. *Comp Physiol.* 2014; 4: 575–620.
157. Anonymous. Position statement on the prevention of thermal injuries during distance running. *Med Sci Sports Exerc.* 1987; 19: 529–533.
158. Anonymous. Position stand on heat and cold illnesses during distance running. *Med Sci Sports Exerc.* 1996; 28: i–x.
159. Horswill CA, Passe DH, Stofan JR, Horn MK, Murray R. Adequacy of fluid ingestion in adolescents and adults during moderate-intensity exercise. *Pediatr Exerc Sci.* 2005; 17: 41–50.
160. Committee on Nutrition and the Council on Sports Medicine and Fitness. Sports drinks and energy drinks for children and adolescents: are they appropriate? *Pediatrics.* 2011; 127:1182–1189.
161. Johnson HL, Nelson RA, Consolazio CF. Effects of electrolyte and nutrient solutions on performance and metabolic balance. *Med Sci Sports Exerc.* 1988; 20: 26–33.
162. Bergeron MF. Hydration and thermal strain during tennis in the heat. *Br J Sports Med.* 2014; 48(Suppl 1): i12–17.
163. Falk B, Dotan R. Temperature regulation and the elite young athlete. *Med Sports Sci.* 2011; 56: 126–149
164. Racinais S, Alonso JM, Coutts AJ, *et al.* Consensus recommendations on training and competing in the heat. *Br J Sports Med.* 2015; 49: 1164–1173.
165. Wagner JA, Robinson S, Marino RP. Age and temperature regulation of humans in neutral and cold environments. *J Appl Physiol.* 1974; 37: 562–565.
166. Marsh ML, Mahon AD, Naftzger LA. *Children's physiological responses to exercise in a cold and neutral temperature. In: Proceedings of the North American Society of Pediatric Medicine Meeting.* Miami, FL: 1992.
167. Ueda T, Choi TH, Kurokawa T. Ratings of perceived exertion in a group of children while swimming at different temperatures. *Ann Physiol Anthropol.* 1994; 13: 23–31.
168. Klentrou P, Cunliffe M, Slack J, *et al.* Temperature regulation during rest and exercise in the cold in premenarcheal and menarcheal girls. *J Appl Physiol.* 2004; 96: 1393–1398.
169. Inoue Y, Araki T, Tsujita J. Thermoregulatory responses of prepubertal boys and young men in changing temperature linearly from 28 to 15 degrees C. *Eur J Appl Physiol Occup Physiol.* 1996; 72: 204–208.
170. Mackova J, Sturmova M, Macek M. Prolonged exercise in prepubertal boys in warm and cold environments. In: Illmarinen J, Valimaki I (eds.) *Children and sports.* Heidelberg: Springer-Verlag; 1984. p. 135–141.
171. Inoue Y, Nakamura S, Yonehiro K, Kuwahara T, Ueda H, Araki T. Regional differences in peripheral vasoconstriction of prepubertal boys. *Eur J Appl Physiol.* 2006; 96: 397–403.
172. Falk B, Bar-Eli M, Dotan R, *et al.* Physiological and cognitive responses to cold exposure in 11–12 year-old boys. *Am J Hum Biol.* 1997; 9: 39–49.
173. Golden F, Tipton M. *Essentials of sea survival.* Champaign, IL: Human Kinetics; 2002.
174. Walsh CA, Graham TE. Male-female responses in various body temperatures during and following exercise in cold air. *Aviat Space Environ Med.* 1986; 57: 966–973.
175. Sloan RE, Keatinge WR. Cooling rates of young people swimming in cold water. *J Appl Physiol.* 1973; 35: 371–375.
176. Wakabayashi H, Kaneda K, Okura M, Nomura T. Insulation and body temperature of prepubescent children wearing a thermal swimsuit during moderate-intensity water exercise. *J Physiol Anthropol.* 2007; 26: 179–183.
177. Inbar O, Bar-Or O, Dotan R, Gutin B. Conditioning versus exercise in heat as methods for acclimatizing 8- to 10-yr-old boys to dry heat. *J Appl Physiol.* 1981; 50: 406–411.
178. Armstrong LE, Maresh CM. The induction and decay of heat acclimatisation in trained athletes. *Sports Med.* 1991; 12: 302–312.
179. Cotter JD, Patterson MJ, Taylor NA. Sweat distribution before and after repeated heat exposure. *Eur J Appl Physiol Occup Physiol.* 1997; 76: 181–186.
180. Wilk B, Bar-Or O. Heat acclimation and sweating pattern in prepubertal boys. (Abstract). *Pediatr Exerc Sci.* 1997; 7: 92.
181. Bar-Or O, Inbar O. Relationship between perceptual and physiological changes during heat acclimatization in 8–10-year-old boys. In: Lavalee H, Shephard RJ (eds.) *Frontiers of activity and child health.* Quebec: Pelican Press; 1977. p. 205–214.
182. Docherty D, Eckerson JD, Hayward JS. Physique and thermoregulation in prepubertal males during exercise in a warm, humid environment. *Am J Phys Anthropol.* 1986; 70: 19–23.
183. Matsushita K, Araki T. The effect of physical training on thermoregulatory responses of pre-adolescent boys to heat and cold. *Jap J Fitness Sports Med.* 1980; 29: 69–74.
184. Bar-Or O. *Pediatric sports medicine for the practitioner.* New York: Springer-Verlag: 1983.

CHAPTER 15

Effort perception

Kevin L Lamb, Gaynor Parfitt, and Roger G Eston

Introduction

Individuals possess a well-developed system for sensing the strain involved in physical effort. Effort perception and perceived exertion are synonymous terms which can be defined as the act of detecting and interpreting the sensations arising from the body during physical exertion.[1] The ability to detect and interpret these sensations has been studied in a wide range of populations in a variety of sporting activities and exercise tasks. The plethora of research activity on perceived exertion in adults in the last 32 years has been the subject of several comprehensive reviews[2–4] and commentaries.[5,6] However, research on the efficacy of using perceived exertion in children is both less extensive and applied. This has been the subject of critical review papers,[7,8] editorials by the authors,[9] and others,[10] and some of the information presented here utilizes material from these manuscripts.

Although there have been over 90 studies incorporating measures of children's perceptions of exercise effort, our understanding of their value to exercise scientists and practitioners remains underdeveloped. For more than two decades researchers have realized that adult-derived methods and applications of the rating of perceived exertion (RPE) notion is not appropriate for use with children. When writing for the first edition of this text, we observed that prior to 2000, most investigators had conducted their research in the same vein as that performed in greater volume on adults, and we appealed for progress in this regard. While we can report that significant progress has been made in the intervening years, even since the second edition of this text in 2008, there remains, regrettably, a lack of consensus in terms of how data should be gathered (which tools and protocols are appropriate) and analysed statistically, making interpretations of validity and reliability quite difficult. Over the last 15 years, existing scales have been refined and new ones have been constructed and promoted across a range of exercise modalities. Arguably, however, their potential for promoting physical activity and its associated health benefits has yet to be exploited. This chapter describes some controversies and advances, and presents the current status of the application of effort perception research in the paediatric exercise domain.

Application and description of traditional adult rating of perceived exertion scales

A description of the most common methods of assessing perceived exertion and how this information is used to assess and regulate the intensity of exercise follows. A variety of scales has been developed in an attempt to assess perceived exertion. The ubiquitous 15-point alpha-numeric RPE Category Scale, developed by Borg in 1970,[11] later revised in 1986,[12] and Borg's lesser-used 12-point Category-Ratio 10 (CR 10) scale,[13] are the most commonly used rating of perceived exertion scales. These scales can be used to assess *overall* feelings of exertion or they can be used to differentiate between respiratory-metabolic ('central') and peripheral ('local') signals of exertion. For example, *differentiated* ratings of perceived exertion may be used to segregate the sensations arising from the upper body and the lower body during cycle ergometry exercise, or during rowing, running, or stepping.

In the traditional 15-point and CR 10 scales, numbers are anchored to verbal expressions. However, in the CR 10 scale the numbers have a fixed relationship to one another. For example, an intensity judgement of 3 would be gauged to be one-third that of 9. On this scale there is a point above 10 (extremely strong, almost maximal) which may be assigned any number in proportion to 10 which describes the proportionate increase in perceived exertion. For example, if the exercise intensity feels 30% harder than ten on the CR 10 Scale, the RPE would be 13. This type of scale has been suggested to reflect the incremental pattern of effort perception in relation to ventilatory drive during exercise.

Estimation and production of exercise effort

It is generally observed that RPE measured during an exercise bout increases as exercise intensity increases. Reviews of studies have confirmed the existence of a strong positive association between RPE and indices of metabolic demand in adults[1–4,14] and children,[7,8] particularly when the exercise stimulus is presented in an incremental fashion. Such relationships have been most frequently observed using the so-called passive *estimation* paradigm. In this way, a rating of perceived exertion is given in response to a request from an exercise scientist or practitioner to indicate how 'hard' the exercise feels. The information is frequently used to compare responses between exercise conditions or after some form of intervention. It may also be used to assist a practitioner or coach to prescribe exercise intensities. For example, a specific exercise intensity (e.g. heart rate (HR), work rate or oxygen uptake ($\dot{V}O_2$)), which is known to coincide with a given RPE, may be prescribed by the practitioner. Alternatively, an active *production* paradigm can be employed whereby the individual is requested to regulate his/her exercise intensity to match specified RPE values (such as 13 or 15 on the 15-point Borg scale). Measures of metabolic demand can then be compared at each RPE-derived exercise intensity and several studies on adults[15–20] and children[21–32] show support for the use of the RPE scale in this way.

Evidence suggests that the accuracy of RPE in estimation and production procedures is improved with practice, although there are surprisingly few studies which have explored this fundamental concept in adults,[16] and only two[30,32] which have attempted to adequately address this issue in children. As this is deemed to be an important area of research by the authors, it is appropriate here to consider some of the issues relating to the process of learning. Consideration of the validity and reliability of an RPE scale for children should not ignore age, reading ability, experience, and conceptual understanding. The latter is a developmental issue, which has been the subject of a review by Groslambert and Mahon.[10] Additionally, a confounding factor recognized by two of the original leading proponents of RPE, Borg[33] and Bar-Or,[34] 40 years ago is the extent to which children's direct experiences of exercise (their exposure to different exercise intensities) influence their perceptions of exertion.[9]

Surprisingly, however, few investigations on perceived exertion in children have incorporated all of these issues into their design. For a child to perceive effort accurately, and then reliably produce a given intensity at a given RPE, it is logical to assume that learning must occur. Implicit in the process of learning is practice (of the skill) and the cognitive ability of the child. According to Piaget's stages of development, children around the age of 7–10 years can understand categorization but find it easier to understand and interpret pictures and symbols rather than words and numbers. Since 2000, investigators have incorporated various symbols to emulate categories of effort and acute fatigue into paediatric versions of an RPE scale. These developments have also recognized the need for verbal descriptors and terminology which are more pertinent to a child's cognitive development, age, and reading ability.

The study of perceived exertion in children: a historical perspective

Oded Bar-Or is credited with being the pioneer of research on perceived exertion in children.[34] In 1975, he presented RPE data on 589 children (aged 7–17 years) at the First International Symposium on Physical Work and Effort, recorded during continuous, incremental cycle ergometry. All six defined age groups reported higher RPEs with increases in power output, though compared with adults, children tended to report a lower RPE for a given relative exercise intensity.

This research acquired a near-definitive status for the next 10 years. With a few exceptions, notably an abstract by Kahle *et al.*[35] that reported an increase in the reproducibility of RPE in healthy girls as they got older, a study by Davies *et al.*,[36] which observed that anorexic girls could use RPE to discriminate between differences in exercise intensity, and Eston's[37] somewhat prescient discussion paper on the potential for using RPE in the secondary school physical education curriculum, there were no further reports in the academic literature until 1986. In that year, there were at least five simultaneous published reports from Canada, England, Japan, and the US.[38–42] With the exception of the paper by Eston,[37] researchers focused on the RPE-objective effort (HR, work rate) relationship in the laboratory setting and in the passive 'estimation' mode, as previously described. From 1990, however, research began to include an active 'production' mode whereby pre-specified RPEs were used to compare objective effort measures in children.[21]

The development of child-specific rating scales

Important advances in the study of effort perception in children have occurred in the last 25 years. Despite recognition that experience of exercise was an important determinant for accurate perception of exercise intensity,[33,34,43] little regard was given to the creation of a more developmentally appropriate scale using meaningful terminology (semantics) and symbols until 1989. In that year, Nystad *et al.*[44] published an illustrated RPE Scale with all the written descriptors removed. Six stick figures depicted various stages of effort for use with a group of 10- to 12-year-old asthmatic children. Despite these attempts to improve the relatively incomprehensible nature of the 6–20 scale, children were still confused by it. The investigators concluded that the children lacked physical experience and awareness of different exercise intensities, and therefore could not understand the concept of perceived exertion.

Following earlier recommendations by Williams *et al.*[24] in 1991 for a more simple 1 to 10 perceived exertion scale, a significant development in the measurement of children's effort perception occurred in 1994 with the publication of two papers which proposed and validated an alternative child-specific rating scale[25,26] (see Table 15.1). Compared to the Borg scale, the Children's Effort Rating Table (CERT) has five fewer possible responses, a range of numbers (1 to 10) more familiar to children (than 6–20), and verbal expressions chosen by children as descriptors of exercise effort. The CERT soon became recognized as a notable advancement in the study of paediatric effort perception[45]. Studies comparing the 6–20 RPE and CERT in children aged 5–10 years[46] during stepping and 8–11 years[26,27,47,48] during cycling exercise provided support for the CERT. The latter study on 69 Chinese children utilized Chinese-translated (Cantonese) versions of both the Borg 6–20 RPE and the CERT, and observed that the validity correlations for CERT, power output, HR, and $\dot{V}O_2$ were consistently higher than those for the 6–20 RPE scale. Leung *et al.*[48] also reported CERT ratings that were more reliable than RPE across two identical continuous, incremental cycling tests.

Table 15.1 Children's effort rating table (CERT)

1	Very, very easy
2	Very easy
3	Easy
4	Just feeling a strain
5	Starting to get hard
6	Getting quite hard
7	Hard
8	Very hard
9	Very, very hard
10	So hard I'm going to stop

Pictorial versions of the Children's Effort Rating Table (CERT)

The CERT initiative for a simplified scale containing more 'developmentally appropriate' numerical and verbal expressions, led to the development of scales which combined numerical and pictorial ratings of perceived exertion. All of these scales depict four to five animated figures, portraying increased states of physical exertion. Like the CERT, the scales have embraced a similar, condensed numerical range and words or expressions which are either identical to (Pictorial-CERT,[29]), abridged from (Cart and Load Effort Rating [CALER])[32], Bug and Bag Effort [BABE])[49], Eston-Parfitt [E-P])[8], or similar in context to the CERT (OMNI[45,50]). The rationale for the development of these scales and their application is described in the following paragraphs.

The principle of presenting a scale that is readily assimilated by children on the basis of their own experiences and stages of development is very important. Accordingly, Figure 15.1 presents a child pulling a cart that is loaded progressively with bricks (CALER scale). The number of bricks in the cart is commensurate with numbers on the scale. The wording was selected from the CERT to accompany some of the categories of effort. In the study by Eston *et al.*,[32] 20 children aged 7–10 years performed four intermittent, incremental active production tests at CALER 2, 5, and 8 over a 4-week period. To reach the specific CALER level the child instructed the experimenter, in the first 2–3 min, to adjust the cycling resistance by adding or taking away weights (not visible to the child). Each bout was 3 min, separated by 2.5 min rest intervals. An increase in power output across trials (44, 65, and 79 W at CALER 2, 5, and 8 respectively), confirmed that the children understood the scale. Analysis between trials indicated that the reliability of the efforts produced improved with practice. This study was the first to apply more than two repeated effort production trials in young children and provides strong evidence that practice improves the reliability of effort perception in children of this age.

A pictorial version of the CERT (PCERT), initially described by Eston and Lamb,[52] has been validated for both estimation and production tasks during stepping exercise in adolescents[29] (see Figure 15.2). The scale depicts a child running up a 45-degree stepped gradient at five stages of exertion, corresponding to CERT ratings of 2, 4, 6, 8, and 10. Yelling first proposed the PCERT at a perceived exertion symposium hosted by the authors and Gunnar Borg in 1999. The scale had immediate appeal and was considered to be a significant improvement on the CERT. To facilitate the development of the PCERT, Yelling *et al.*[29] engaged 48 boys and girls (aged 12–15 years) in a series of play and running activities. Throughout the lessons the children were asked to focus on the exercise sensations of breathlessness, body temperature, and muscle aches. Immediately afterwards, the children were presented with a copy of the CERT in the form of a stepped gradient and five pictorial descriptors and asked to locate the positions which best reflected their own perceptions of effort. The frequency with which the children positioned the visual character at given points along the scale was recorded and the most commonly chosen format was selected, resulting in the pictorial scale.

The validity of the PCERT was determined in a separate group of 48 similarly aged boys and girls in two exercise trials separated by 7–10 days.[29] In trial one, the children completed five 3 min incremental stepping exercise bouts interspersed with 2 min recovery periods. HR and RPE were recorded in the final 15 s of each bout. They observed that perceived exertion increased as exercise intensity increased. This was also reflected by simultaneous significant increases in HR. In trial two, the children were asked to regulate their exercise intensity during four intermittent 4 min bouts of stepping to match randomly assigned ratings of perceived exertion at 3, 5, 7, and 9. Bouts were separated by a 2 min recovery period. The desired step heights and frequency were determined in the first 2 min of the 4 min exercise bout by verbal feedback from the child. HR and power output were recorded in the last 15 s of each bout. The HR and power output produced at each of the four prescribed effort levels were also significantly different. Yelling *et al.*[29] concluded that the children could discriminate between the four different exercise intensities and regulate their exercise intensity according to the four prescribed ratings from the PCERT.

The utility of the PCERT has been augmented by the findings of two rather different studies, one involving an innovative application of the scale in a UK physical education setting,[31] the other a comparison with the Borg Category-Ratio scale among Bulgarian children.[53] The latter study examined the concurrent validity of the PCERT and CR 10 scales during incremental (estimation) laboratory treadmill running in 50 boys and girls aged 10–17 years. The children completed identical trials separated by 1 month, reporting their effort perceptions with one scale in the first trial, and the other scale in the second. The analysis of the associations between effort ratings and physiologic measures ($\dot{V}O_2$, HR, and pulmonary ventilation [$\dot{V}_E$]) revealed significantly higher correlations overall ($r = 0.62$–0.82) for the PCERT than the Borg CR 10 scale ($r = 0.51$–0.71). In the way that the original CERT scale had been shown to be more valid than the 6–20 Borg scale over 20 years ago,[47] these findings lead to the conclusion that the PCERT is more appropriate for estimating exercise effort among such children than the Borg scale.

In the field-based study of Preston and Lamb,[31] 21 boys (aged 13 years) were requested to regulate their exercise outputs during structured (intermittent) physical education activities to match PCERT levels 3, 9, 5, and 7 (in that order). The activity corresponding to PCERT 9 was repeated 1 week later to assess the children's

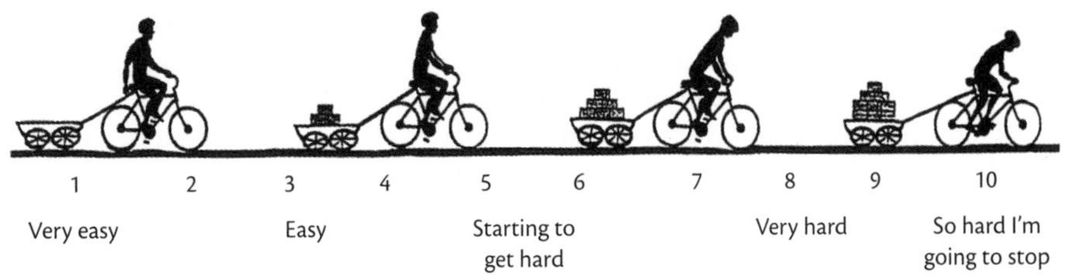

Figure 15.1 Cart and load effort rating (CALER) scale.

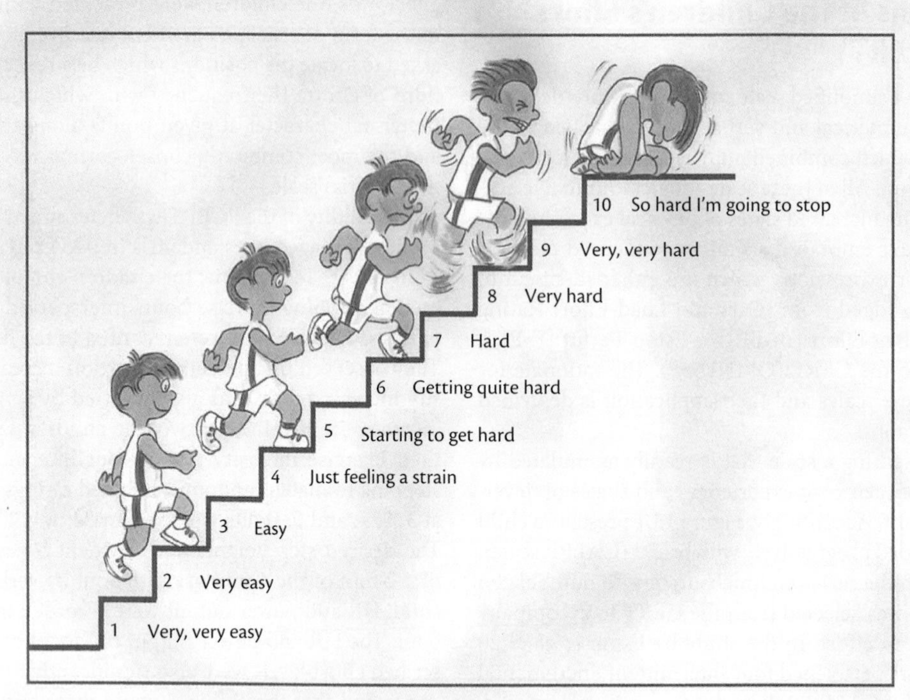

Figure 15.2 The pictorial children's effort rating table (PCERT).

ability to reproduce their exercise efforts. Analysis of HRs recorded during the exercise bouts revealed that the children could distinguish between level 3 ('easy') and level 9 ('very, very hard'), but not so between the other levels. Additionally, while the reliability of effort at PCERT 9 was at best modest overall, some of the children were able to reproduce efforts that were within a relatively narrow range of HRs. These data were encouraging and (still) represent one of the very few attempts there have been to apply effort perception in circumstances of practical, health- or fitness-related value.

A more recent variation on the PCERT addresses the notion that children's perceptions of exercise effort, particularly those of young children, might not rise in a linear fashion with objective markers of effort, such as HR and $\dot{V}O_2$, but that in the later stages of exercise they increase in a curvilinear manner. The E-P scale,[54] based on early empirical observations of Lamb[47] and more recently by Barkley and Roemmich,[55] depicts an ambulatory character (running) at various stages of exertion on a concave slope with a progressively increasing gradient at the higher intensities (see Figure 15.3). Accordingly, the distance between each numbered increment (0 to 10) on the horizontal axis is increasingly reduced in relation to its antecedent. The area under the curve is also shaded progressively from light to dark red from left to right. The validation of the E-P scale was confirmed initially (against HR and $\dot{V}_E$ responses) among 7- to 8-year-olds using a discontinuous incremental cycling protocol to volitional exhaustion,[54] and more recently (against HR, $\dot{V}O_2$, and $\dot{V}_E$) using a discontinuous graded treadmill protocol.[56] In both studies, strong relationships ($R^2 > 0.85$) were observed between the E-P scale ratings and physiological responses, reinforcing our view that such a visual representation of exercise effort might facilitate a young child's understanding of the perceptual framework and thereby his/her ability to provide accurate ratings. Moreover, further evidence of such comprehension can be gleaned from a study in which 7- to 8-year-olds engaged in submaximal production ('perceptually-regulated') paradigms up to E-P scale levels 5 and 7 generated exercise outputs ($\dot{V}O_2$ values) that when extrapolated to the highest intensity (E-P 10), yielded predictions of maximal $\dot{V}O_2$ that were similar to measured values.[57] Similar (unpublished) results were reported recently by Bertelsen[58] during a treadmill estimation paradigm in 8- to 10-year-old children. Such an application of RPE reflects the research among adults (since 2004) which has used estimation and production paradigms successfully to predict this popular measure of cardiorespiratory fitness (see Coquart *et al.*[59] for a review).

OMNI scales

In recognition of the advantages of using a comparatively narrow numerical range to assess perceived exertion, such as that used in the CERT, Robertson[45] proposed the idea of using pictorial descriptors along the scale for assessing perceived exertion in children. As part of a special symposium on effort perception at the European Paediatric Work Physiology Conference in 1997, he presented the idea for a 1 to 10 pictorial scale (now 0 to 10) which would be applicable to variations in race, gender, and health status, hence the term OMNI scale. His original idea was to employ, 'pictorially interfaced cognitive anchoring procedures, eliminating the need for mode-specific maximal exercise tests to establish congruence between stimulus and response ranges'.[45(p35)] However, since then, numerous different pictorial OMNI scales have been validated for various modes of exercise in children—for example, cycling,[50] walking/running,[60] stepping,[61] and resistance exercise.[62]

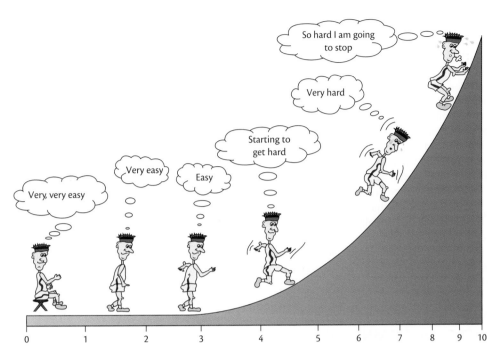

Figure 15.3 Eston-Parfitt (E-P) curvilinear rating of perceived exertion scale.

In the original OMNI scale (see Figure 15.4) validation study,[50] four equal groups of 20 healthy African-American and White boys and girls, aged 8–12 years, performed a continuous, incremental exercise test on a cycle ergometer. Exercise intensities were increased by 25 W every 3 min and RPE, HR, and $\dot{V}O_2$ were monitored in the final minute of each test stage. The authors reported similarly high positive linear associations (r = 0.85–0.94) between HR, $\dot{V}O_2$, and RPE for each gender/race cohort of children. Consequently, this study formed the basis for a succession of subsequent validation studies utilizing various forms of the OMNI in estimation protocols. Fewer studies, however, have focused on the validity of the children's OMNI scales in production mode, although of note are the two involving the cycling[28] and walking/running versions.[60] Robertson *et al.* [28] reported that 8- to 12-year-old boys and girls could use their perceptions of effort during an intermittent cycling protocol to adjust their exercise intensities (i.e. HR and $\dot{V}O_2$) in line with two specified target OMNI values (2 and 6), whereas Groslambert *et al.*[63] observed that younger children (aged 5–7 years) were able to regulate indoor running intensity (HR) over intermittent 300 m distances across three randomly assigned OMNI values (3, 6, and 10). Given their ages and the task at hand, this impressive finding encouraged Groslambert *et al.*[63] to posit that such findings would be of value to physical education teachers and health practitioners who use perceived exertion to prescribe running exercise in children. However, as alluded to earlier, published accounts of such practice are scarce.

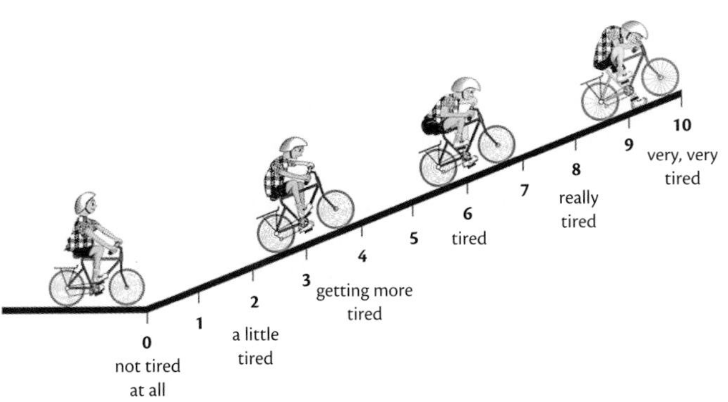

Figure 15.4 Original OMNI perceived exertion scale for children.
Reprinted with permission R. Robertson, personal communication.

Although they were developed independently, there are marked similarities between the PCERT and the OMNI scales. With the exception of the zero starting point on the OMNI scale, there is the same limited range of numbers, a linear gradient and culturally familiar verbal cues derived from common verbal expressions used by the children in the two respective countries (UK and US) to describe their feelings of exertion. With regard to the verbal anchors, it is noteworthy that the original derivation and validation of the CERT was based on children aged 5–9 years of age in the UK, whereas the OMNI was based on children aged 8–12 years of age in the US. Accordingly, such differences in maturational status and cognitive development, in addition to cultural semantics and socioeconomic status, influenced the terminologies that were originally derived for the two scales. Moreover, the common cue throughout the children's OMNI scale is 'tired', the degree of which is indicated by various adverbs: *0—not tired at all, 2—a little tired, 4—getting more tired, 6—tired, 8—really tired, 10—very, very tired*. In the initial validation of the scale, this trunk word appeared 475 times out of a total of 1582 verbal expressions.[50] Conversely, the verbal cues derived for use in the CERT describe degrees of exertion according to various levels of being 'easy' or 'hard' to the extent that the exercise becomes so hard that the child will stop ('so hard I am going to stop'). The appropriateness of the latter term is supported by frequent observations by the authors that young children will often stop exercising when it becomes too uncomfortable. Sometimes, there is little pre-warning of this occurrence.

The connotations of the wording in the two scales are quite distinct. In this regard, the OMNI scale assumes a baseline level of 'tiredness' from the starting point of zero. From a purely semantic and literal perspective, feeling *tired* is a term used to describe a general condition or state of fatigue, weariness, or sleepiness rather than effort. It is not an indication of exertion. Anchoring the scale around the central condition of varying states of 'feeling tired' could be perceived as portraying a negative (unpleasant) perspective on the feelings experienced during physical activity, such as that experienced in children's play. Indeed, feeling tired is a common psychological barrier to engaging in physical activity.[64] We, therefore, feel that the use of this term to describe states of physical exertion is somewhat inapt. It is notable that the more recent adult versions of the OMNI scale developed initially for resistance exercise and later to be re-illustrated for other forms of exercise, utilize the terms 'easy' and 'hard'. In our view, this change of the terminology is better suited for the purpose of rating perceived exertion, for both adults and children.

Independent validation of the pictorial versions of the CERT and OMNI scales

In recognition of the dearth of data for the OMNI walking/running scale[50] and the PCERT scale in young children,[29] Roemmich *et al.*[65] examined the two scales during sub-maximal exercise. In their study, 51 boys and girls aged 11–12 years performed a perceptual estimation paradigm, comprising a five stage incremental treadmill test to elicit about 85% of the HR max. Increases in the PCERT and OMNI scales were correlated with increases in $\dot{V}O_2$ ($r = 0.90$ and $r = 0.92$) and HR ($r = 0.89$ and $r = 0.92$), respectively. There was no difference in the slopes of the PCERT and OMNI scores when regressed against HR or $\dot{V}O_2$. There was also no difference in the percentage of maximal PCERT and OMNI at each exercise stage. In effect, the results showed that the two scales could be used with equal validity. In a later study by the same research group,[55] the validity of the CALER and OMNI scales was confirmed (against HR and $\dot{V}O_2$) among boys aged 9–10 years during an incremental cycle ergometer test to exhaustion. Increases in scores on both scales were associated with increases in $\dot{V}O_2$ ($r = 0.92$ and 0.93) and HR ($r = 0.88$ and 0.89), respectively. These results are not that surprising since the scales utilize basically the same number range. This observation raises the question as to where the child's focus of attention is based. Is it mainly on the number scale, the figures, or equally combined between the two? If attention is focused primarily on the limited number range, it perhaps questions the need for pictorial scales of perceived exertion for children of this age range.

All but one of the pictorial scales considered above have used either a horizontal line or one that has a linear slope. Following earlier suggestions by the authors in the first edition of this text,[52] the aforementioned E-P scale was constructed; its rationale founded on its inherent face validity. It is readily conceivable that a child will recognize from previous learning and experience that the steeper the hill, the more difficult it is to ascend. This may also be helpful in the process of 'anchoring' effort perceptions. Furthermore, as ventilation is a physiological mediator for respiratory-metabolic signals of exertion during endurance exercise, and given that this variable rises in a curvilinear fashion with equal increments in work rate, a curvilinear gradient seems appropriate. Indeed, the study by Barkley and Roemmich[55] showed that the proportions of maximal CALER (75%) and maximal OMNI (74%) were substantially less ($p < 0.001$) than the proportion of HR max (94.5%). In effect, the children's RPE ratings were disproportional to the physiological effort, leading to the authors' conclusion that the upper range of linear scales would benefit from modifications to the verbal descriptors or the slope of their lines.

Methodological issues in children's effort perception research

Anchoring effort perceptions

Whatever scale is used, it is important to provide the child with an understanding of the range of sensations that correspond to categories of effort within the scale. This is known as 'anchoring'. There are three ways by which perceptual anchoring may be accomplished—from memory, by definition, or from actual physical experience. The 'memory' method requires the child to remember the easiest and hardest experiences of exercise and use these as the anchor values on the scale. The 'definition' method involves the experimenter defining the anchors with terms such as 'the lowest effort imaginable' for the low anchor or the 'greatest effort imaginable' as the high anchor. The third method (experience) allows the child to physically experience a range of perceptual anchors. In 2000, Eston and Lamb[52] stated that the experiential method is the preferred of the three methods and recommended that the child should be exposed to a range of intensities that can be used to set the perceptual anchor points at 'low' and 'high' levels. This can be achieved during habituation to the test or exercise procedures. In particular, it was suggested that following a warm-up, the child should be allowed to experience exercise that is perceived as being 'hard' or 'very hard'. To avoid fatigue, a period of time should be allowed to regain full recovery. However, Lamb *et al.*[30] questioned this assertion. In their study, 41 boys and girls aged 11–13 years, randomly assigned to either an experiential anchor group or a non-anchor group, undertook two identical production-only trials (three 3 min cycle ergometer bouts at randomised CERT levels 3, 6, and 8). Before each trial, the anchor group received an experiential exercise trial to provide a frame of reference for their perceived exertions, at levels 2, 1, and 9, in that order. The authors reported slightly better test-retest reproducibility for HR and power output in the non-anchor group, with intraclass correlation (ICC) values ranging from 0.86–0.93 and 0.81–0.95, respectively. Importantly, limits of agreement analysis indicated no marked differences between the two groups in the amount of bias and within-subject error. The implementation of an experiential anchoring protocol therefore, had no positive effect on the reproducibility of the children's ability to self-regulate exercise using prescribed CERT levels. Further research on this theme has not been forthcoming but would seem to be merited.

In her recent overview on the use of perceived exertion in physical education, Lagally[66] reinforced the necessity of anchoring exercise sensations, possibly over the course of several lessons, if it is to be an effective tool. In particular, it was suggested that exercise (experiential) anchoring was desirable given that children have less knowledge of maximal exercise. Although this view was not empirically supported, it was recommended that a means of providing such exercise was via an incremental running protocol conducted as part of their annual fitness testing, which, in principle, would expose them to a range of intensities from low to very high. Alternatively, lessons could be structured with specific activities designed to highlight the spectrum of physical exertion. In addition, teachers could compare their ratings with those of the students regarding the intensity for such activities, and explain any differences that occur.

Intermittent versus continuous exercise protocols

The majority of investigations have typically studied children's perceptions of effort during a passive estimation process (perceptual estimation paradigm) in which ratings recorded from either intermittent or continuous protocols have been correlated against objective measures of physiological strain, such as HR, power output, or $\dot{V}O_2$. Most studies have used a continuous protocol, as with the development and validation of the CERT[25] and the OMNI[50] scales. Fewer studies have applied procedures in which children are requested to regulate (produce) their exercise output to match experimenter-prescribed effort ratings. Of these, it has been most common to compare the objective indicators of effort with *expected* values derived from a previous estimation trial.[21–23,25,28] In this so-called estimation-production paradigm, the ability of children to use perceptions of effort to *actively* self-regulate exercise intensity levels using predetermined RPEs has, in our opinion, been inappropriately compared to their ability to passively appraise exercise intensity from a previous test. It is, therefore, difficult to appraise children's ability to reliably and accurately produce a given objective effort from these studies. For example, in the first full paper published on this theme,[21] it was concluded that overweight children (aged 9–15 years) could discriminate between four work rates based on pre-determined RPE values (7, 10, 13, and 16). However, it was reported that the children produced work rates that were significantly different to expected (or 'criterion') values. It is necessary to point out that these criterion values were derived from a different perceptual process. Similar findings were reported in later studies.[22,23] These observations lead us to recommend that validity studies should focus on either production data only, or estimation data only, and not confound the issue by comparing data derived from a passive perceptual process on one occasion to an active perceptual process on a subsequent occasion.[8] Noble's[67] argument that this involves two dissimilar psychophysical processes is highly pertinent. Furthermore, the disparity between the two psychophysical processes is most likely attenuated by the extent of children's limited perceptual experience. This mismatch has since been recognized as a lack of 'prescription congruence'.[28]

Lamb *et al.*[68] used a production-only paradigm to assess the influence of a continuous and intermittent exercise protocol on the relationship between CERT ratings objective effort in children aged 9–10 years. Common to both groups was the requirement to regulate exercise intensity to match four randomly presented 3 min effort rating levels (3, 5, 7, and 9). The provision of 3 min recovery periods between exercise bouts produced higher relationships between CERT and HR ($r = 0.66$ vs. $r = 0.46$, for the intermittent and continuous protocol, respectively). Heart rates tended to be lower in the discontinuous protocol. These results indicate that children may be more able to use effort ratings to control exercise intensity when the exercise is intermittent, rather than continuous in nature.

The assessment of perceived exertion using a repeat-production paradigm examines a child's ability to discern consistently between different target RPEs while self-regulating exercise intensity.[27,30–32,49,51,68] Studies by Eston and colleagues[32,49,51] are the only ones to apply three or more repeated-effort production trials in young children (7–11 years). The increase in the size of ICCs between paired comparisons of the successive production trials in both studies support the importance of practice. For example, in the 2000 study,[32] the ICCs improved from 0.76 to 0.97 and the overall bias and limits of agreement narrowed from −12 ± 19 W to 0 ± 10 W. These data provide the strongest evidence available to date to demonstrate that practice improves the reliability of effort perception in children of this age.

Much of our understanding of children's effort perceptions has evolved from measuring responses to a situation in which they realize that the exercise is getting progressively harder. Studies which have allowed rest periods between exercise bouts,[32,35,41,69] and thereby reduced the influence of fatigue on effort perceptions, have all been incremental in nature. Few have randomized the order of presentation of workloads.[21,29,39,68] Logically, the 'accuracy' and reliability of effort perceptions and objective markers of effort produced at specified effort ratings will be influenced by test protocol (continuous or intermittent), the order of the load presentation (incremental or random), and the timing of the data collection. Furthermore, future investigations into children's effort perception should not disregard the manner in which the exercise is applied, the duration of the exercise bout, nor the number of practice periods, as these factors seem to have a bearing on the outcome measures.

Effort perception scales: promoting and regulating physical activity levels

Throughout the evolution of child-specific effort perception scales it has been alluded to that they could be valuable as a practical tool for helping physical educators, coaches, or health practitioners, both in the prescription of children's physical activity and in the development of their ability to interpret feelings of exercise and self-regulate their own health-promoting physical activity.[21,23,26,27,30,66,70,71] However, there has been little evidence thus far of this becoming a reality. In the UK, the studies by Yelling and Penny[72] and Preston and Lamb[31] over 10 years ago seem to be the only ones reporting a concerted attempt to integrate a perceived exertion scale (PCERT) into the delivery of structured physical education lessons. Whilst both papers highlighted that the pupils (aged 9–18 years) appeared to grasp the concept of differentiating between physical activity of varying intensity, and were quite reliable at doing so,[31] their rating of activity levels was confounded by problems or complexities, such as their concern with a range of social issues that governed the ratings that they were prepared to give.[72] In effect, and perhaps unsurprising, individual feelings and sensations of physical exertion were not the only (or principal) factors determining their ratings.

More recently, two reports from the US have employed the OMNI walking/running scale in a school setting for monitoring students' exertions during[73] and after[74] the cardiovascular endurance element (the PACER test) of a popular fitness assessment battery. One study involving 80 students (aged 11–12 years) demonstrated, as expected, that OMNI ratings increased as intensity (speed) increased during the incremental, 20 m shuttle-run,[73] whereas the other[74] was concerned with the overall effort exerted during the PACER by a large sample ($n = 792$) of high school boys and girls. In the latter, it was evident that most of the students provided OMNI ratings (greater then 5) immediately after the test that were lower than that equating to 'tired' (6) on the scale, which was a surprise given their task was to run until volitional exhaustion. The authors concluded that, for various reasons, many of the students did not provide a 'true'(maximal) effort during, and/or OMNI response after, the field test of fitness. Notwithstanding these two attempts to use an effort perception scale in a physical education environment, they did not seek to assess its sensitivity to different physical education lessons, or utility as a means of self-regulating exercise within lessons.

Conclusions

As the importance of encouraging physical activity in children is recognized, it makes sense to study the accuracy and reliability of effort perception in this population. While the breadth of research into children's effort perception has expanded over the past 9 years, in particular there has been little progress in examining its oft-stated potential for enhancing their awareness of the range of their exercise capabilities, and the impact that this has on their willingness to engage in health-enhancing activities. In the UK, it has not emerged as a priority worthy of consideration in the National Curriculum for Physical Education, possibly owing to the inertia borne out of traditional teaching, or an insufficient lobby from professionals for its worth. In the US, given the attempts to popularize perceived exertion scales by Bob Robertson and colleagues, perhaps there is optimism here.

Summary

- Effort perception research amongst paediatric populations has been in existence for 30 years, but only since 1994 have exercise scientists endeavoured to develop rating scales that are suited to children's cognitive abilities.
- It is universally recognized that Borg's 6–20 Rating of Perceived Exertion (RPE) scale is unsuitable for use with children of most ages.
- Rating of perceived exertion scales constructed with children in mind have followed the example set by the 1–10 Children's Effort Rating Table (CERT) and typically include words and/or pictures to reflect varying degrees of exercise effort.
- Strong evidence exists to support the validity of paediatric scales against objective indicators of effort (heart rate, oxygen uptake, and power output) when applied via a perceptual estimation paradigm, often involving continuous incremental protocols.
- Studies employing child-specific RPE scales via a production paradigm remain relatively scarce, though the evidence thus far suggests that children can use their understanding of perceived exertion to help them regulate their exercise outputs.
- Some recent evidence suggests that the associations between children's perceived and objective submaximal efforts could provide useful predictions of their cardiorespiratory fitness.
- Research has emerged showing that practice of using the RPE scale has a beneficial effect on the consistency of its application in both estimation and production paradigms.
- The effects of adopting preparatory anchoring techniques on scale application have been virtually overlooked.
- Very few studies have explored the efficacy of using a child scale in a practical (e.g. physical education) setting and the time to consider the external validity of such scales is overdue.

References

1. Noble BJ, Robertson RJ. *Perceived exertion*, Champaign, IL: Human Kinetics; 1996.
2. Carton RL, Rhodes EC. A critical review of the literature on rating scales for perceived exertion. *Sports Med.* 1985; 2: 198–222.
3. Watt B, Grove R. Perceived exertion: antecedents and applications. *Sports Med.* 1993; 15: 225–241.
4. Chen MJ, Fan X, Moe ST. Criterion-related validity of the Borg rating of perceived exertion scale in healthy individuals: A meta-analysis. *J Sports Sci.* 2002; 20: 973–999.
5. Eston, RJ. Use of ratings of perceived exertion in sports. *Int J Sports Phys Perf.* 2009; 7: 175–182.
6. Eston RG. Perceived exertion: Recent advances and novel applications in children and adults. *J Exerc Sci Fit.* 2009; 7: S11–S17.
7. Lamb KL, Eston RG. Effort perception in children. *Sports Med.* 1997; 23: 139–148.
8. Eston RG, Parfitt G. Effort perception. In: Armstrong N (ed.) *Paediatric exercise physiology*. London: Elsevier; 2006. p. 275–297.
9. Eston, RG. What do we really know about children's ability to perceive exertion? Time to consider the bigger picture. *Pediatr Exerc Sci.* 2009; 21: 377–383.
10. Groslambert A, Mahon AD. Perceived exertion: influence of age and cognitive development. *Sports Med.* 2006; 36: 911–928.
11. Borg G. Perceived exertion as an indicator of somatic stress. *J Rehab Med.* 1970; 2: 92–98.
12. Borg G. Psychophysical studies of effort and exertion: some historical, theoretical, and empirical aspects. In: Borg G, Ottoson D (eds.) *The perception of exertion in physical work.* London: MacMillan; 1986. p. 3–14.
13. Borg G. Psychophysical basis of perceived exertion. *Med Sci Sport Exerc.* 1982; 14: 371–381.
14. Pandolf KB. Advances in the study and application of perceived exertion. *Exerc Sport Sci Rev.* 1983; 11: 118–158.
15. Eston RG, Davies BL, Williams JG. Use of perceived effort ratings to control exercise intensity in young healthy adults. *Eur J Appl Physiol Occup Physiol.* 1987; 56: 222–224.
16. Eston RG, Williams JG. Reliability of ratings of perceived effort for regulation of exercise intensity. *Br J Sports Med.* 1988; 22: 153–154.
17. Dunbar CC, Robertson RJ, Baun R, *et al.* The validity of regulating exercise intensity by ratings of perceived exertion. *Med Sci Sport Exerc.* 1992; 24: 94–99.
18. Parfitt G, Eston RG, Connolly DA. Psychological affect at different ratings of perceived exertion in high- and low-active women: a study using a production protocol. *Percept Motor Skills.*1996; 82: 1035–1042.
19. Williams JG, Eston RG. Exercise intensity regulation. In: Eston RG, Reilly T (eds.) *Kinanthropometry and exercise physiology laboratory manual: tests, procedures and data.* London: E and FN Spon; 1996. p. 221–235.
20. Eston RG, Thompson M. Use of ratings of perceived exertion for predicting maximal work rate and prescribing exercise intensity in patients receiving atenolol. *Br J Sports Med.* 1997; 31: 114–119.
21. Ward DS, Bar-Or O. Use of the Borg Scale in exercise prescription for overweight youth. *Can J Sports Sci.* 1990; 15: 120–125.
22. Ward DS, Jackman JD, Galiano FJ. Exercise intensity reproduction: children versus adults. *Pediatr Exerc Sci.* 1991; 3: 209–218.
23. Ward DS, Bar-Or O, Longmuir P, Smith K. Use of ratings of perceived exertion (RPE) to prescribe exercise intensity for wheelchair-bound children and adults. *Pediatr Exerc Sci.* 1995; 7: 94–102.
24. Williams JG, Eston RG, Stretch C. Use of rating of perceived exertion to control exercise intensity in children. *Pediatr Exerc Sci.* 1991; 3: 21–27.

25. Williams JG, Eston RG, Furlong B. CERT: a perceived exertion scale for young children. *Percept Motor Skills.* 1994; 79: 1451–1458.
26. Eston RG, Lamb KL, Bain A, Williams M, Williams JG. Validity of a perceived exertion scale for children: a pilot study. *Percept Motor Skills.* 1994; 78: 691–697.
27. Lamb KL. Exercise regulation during cycle ergometry using the CERT and RPE scales. *Pediatr Exerc Sci.* 1996; 8: 337–350.
28. Robertson RJ, Goss JL, Bell FA, *et al.* Self-regulated cycling using the children's OMNI scale of perceived exertion. *Med Sci Sport Exerc.* 2002; 34: 1168–1175.
29. Yelling M, Lamb K, Swaine IL. Validity of a pictorial perceived exertion scale for effort estimation and effort production during stepping exercise in adolescent children. *Eur Phys Educ Rev.* 2002; 8: 157–175.
30. Lamb KL, Eaves SJ, Hartshorn JE. The effect of experiential anchoring on the reproducibility of exercise regulation in adolescent children. *J Sports Sci.* 2004; 22: 159–165.
31. Preston S, Lamb KL. Perceptually-regulated exercise responses during Physical Education lessons. *J Sports Sci.* 2005; 23: 1214–1215.
32. Eston RG, Campbell L, Lamb KL, Parfitt G. Reliability of effort perception for regulating exercise intensity: a study using the Cart and Load Effort Rating (CALER) scale. *Pediatr Exerc Sci.* 2000; 12: 388–397.
33. Borg G. *Physical work and effort.* Oxford: Pergamon Press; 1977.
34. Bar-Or O. Age-related changes in exercise perception. In: Borg G (ed.) *Physical work and effort.* Oxford: Pergamom Press; 1977. p. 255–266.
35. Kahle C, Ulmer HV, Rummel L. The reproducibility of Borg's RPE scale with female pupils from 7 to 11 years of age. *Pflugers Archiv Eur J Physiol.* 1977; 368: R26 (Abstract).
36. Davies CTM, Fohlin L, Thoren C. Perception of exertion in anorexia nervosa patients. In: Berg K, Eriksson BO (eds.) *Children and exercise IX.* Baltimore, MD: University Park Press; 1980. p. 327–332.
37. Eston RG. A discussion of the concepts: exercise intensity and perceived exertion with reference to the secondary school. *Phys Educ Rev.* 1984; 7; 19–25.
38. Bar-Or O, Reed S. Rating of perceived exertion in adolescents with neuromuscular disease. In: Borg G, Ottoson D (eds.) *The perception of exertion in physical work.* Basingstoke: MacMillan Press; 1986. p. 137–148.
39. Eston RG, Williams JG. Exercise intensity and perceived exertion in adolescent boys. *Br J Sports Med.* 1986; 20: 27–30.
40. Miyashita M, Onedera K, Tabata I. How Borg's RPE scale has been applied to Japanese. In: Borg G, Ottoson D (eds.) *The perception of exertion in physical work.* Basingstoke: MacMillan Press; 1986. p. 27–34.
41. Van Huss WD, Stephens KE, Vogel P, *et al.* Physiological and perceptual responses of elite age group distance runners during progressive intermittent work to exhaustion. In: Weiss M, Gould D (eds.) *The 1984 Olympic Scientific Congress Proceedings, 10.* Champaign, IL: Human Kinetics; 1986. p. 239–246.
42. Ward DS, Blimkie CJR, Bar-Or O. Rating of perceived exertion in obese adolescents. *Med Sci Sport Exerc.* 1986; 18: S72 (Abstract).
43. Bar-Or O, Ward DS. Rating of perceived exertion in children. In: Bar-Or O (ed.) *Advances in pediatric sports sciences.* Champaign, IL: Human Kinetics; 1989. p. 151–168.
44. Nystad W, Oseid S, Mellbye EB. Physical education for asthmatic children: the relationship between changes in heart rate, perceived exertion, and motivation for participation. In: Oseid S, Carlsen K (eds.) *Children and exercise XIII.* Champaign, IL: Human Kinetics; 1989. p. 369–377.
45. Robertson RJ. Perceived exertion in young people: future directions of enquiry. In: Welsman J, Armstrong N, Kirby B (eds.) *Children and exercise XIX volume II.* Exeter: Washington Singer Press; 1997. p. 33–39.
46. Williams JG, Furlong B, MacKintosh C, Hockley TJ. Rating and regulation of exercise intensity in young children. *Med Sci Sport Exerc.* 1993; 25: S8 (Abstract).
47. Lamb KL. Children's ratings of effort during cycle ergometry: an examination of the validity of two effort rating scales. *Pediatr Exerc Sci.* 1995; 7: 407–421.
48. Leung ML, Cheung PK, Leung RW. An assessment of the validity and reliability of two perceived exertion rating scales among Hong Kong children. *Percept Motor Skills.* 2002; 95: 1047–1062.
49. Eston RG, Parfitt G, Shepherd P. Effort perception in children: implications for validity and reliability. In: Papaionnou A, Goudas M, Theodorakis Y (eds.) *Proceedings of 10th World Congress of Sport Psychology.* Skiathos: Christodoulidis; 2001. p. 104–106.
50. Robertson RJ, Goss FL, Boer NF *et al.* Children's OMNI Scale of perceived exertion: mixed gender and race validation. *Med Sci Sport Exerc.* 2000; 32: 452–458.
51. Parfitt G, Shepherd P, Eston RG. Control of exercise intensity using the children's CALER and BABE perceived exertion scales. *J Exerc Sci Fitness.* 2007; 5: 49–55.
52. Eston RG, Lamb KL. Effort perception. In: Armstrong N, Van-Mechelen W (eds.) *Paediatric exercise science and medicine.* Oxford: Oxford University Press; 2000. p. 85–91.
53. Marinov B, Mandadjieva S, Kostianev S. Pictorial and verbal category ratio scales for effort estimation in children. *Child Care Health Dev.* 2008; 34: 35–43.
54. Eston RG, Lambrick DM, Rowlands AV. The perceptual response to exercise of progressively increasing intensity in children aged 7–8 years: Validation of a pictorial curvilinear ratings of perceived exertion scale. *Psychophysiology.* 2009; 46: 843–851.
55. Barkley JE, Roemmich JN. Validity of the CALER and OMNI-bike ratings of perceived exertion. *Med Sci Sport Exerc.* 2008; 40: 760–766.
56. Lambrick DM, Rowlands AV, Eston RG. The perceptual response to treadmill exercise using the Eston-Parfitt scale and marble dropping task in children age 7 to 8 years. *Pediatr Exerc Sci.* 2011; 23: 36–48.
57. Lambrick D. Perceived exertion relationships in adults and children (unpublished Doctoral thesis). Exeter, UK: University of Exeter; 2010.
58. Bertelsen H. Prediction of peak oxygen uptake from submaximal ratings of perceived exertion using the Eston-Parfitt Scale and Children's Effort Rating Table, in children aged 8–10 years (Bachelor's thesis). Wellington, New Zealand: Massey University; 2014.
59. Coquart JB, Garcin M, Parfitt G, Tourny-Chollet C, Eston RG. Prediction of maximal or peak oxygen uptake from ratings of perceived exertion. *Sports Med.* 2014; 44: 563–578.
60. Utter AC, Robertson RJ, Nieman DC, *et al.* Children's OMNI scale of perceived exertion: walking/running evaluation. *Med Sci Sport Exerc.* 2002; 34: 139–144.
61. Robertson RJ, Goss JL, Andreacci JL, *et al.* Validation of the children's OMNI RPE Scale for stepping exercise. *Med Sci Sport Exerc.* 2005; 37: 290–298.
62. Robertson RJ, Goss FL, Andreacci JL, *et al.* Validation of the children's OMNI-Resistance Scale of perceived exertion. *Med Sci Sport Exerc.* 2005; 37: 819–826.
63. Groslambert A, Benoit PM, Grange CC, *et al.* Self-regulated running using perceived exertion in children. *J Sports Med Phys Fitness.* 2005; 45: 20–25.
64. Stankov I, Olds T, Cargo M. Overweight and obese adolescents: what turns them off physical activity. *Int J Behav Nutr Phys Act.* 2012; 9: 53.
65. Roemmich JN, Barkley JE, Epstein LH. Validity of the PCERT and OMNI-walk/run ratings of perceived exertion scales. *Med Sci Sport Exerc.* 2006; 38: 1014–1019.
66. Lagally KM. Using ratings of perceived exertion in physical education. *J Phys Ed Rec Dance.* 2013: 84: 35–39.
67. Noble BJ. Clinical applications of perceived exertion. *Med Sci Sport Exerc.* 1982; 14: 406–411.
68. Lamb KL, Eston RG, Trask S. The effect of discontinuous and continuous testing protocols on effort perception in children. In: Armstrong N, Kirby B, Welsman J (eds.) *Children and exercise XIX.* London: E and FN Spon; 1997. p. 258–264.
69. Ueda T, Kurokawa T. Validity of heart rate and ratings of perceived exertion as indices of exercise intensity in a group of children while swimming. *Eur J Appl Physiol.* 1991; 63: 200–204.
70. Green K, Lamb KL. Health-related exercise, effort perception and physical education. *Eur J Phys Ed.* 2000; 5: 88–103.

71. Robertson, RJ. *Perceived exertion for practitioners,* Champaign, IL: Human Kinetics; 2004.
72. Yelling M, Penny D. Physical activity in Physical Education: pupil activity rating, reason and reality. *Eur J Phys Ed.* 2003; 8: 119–140.
73. Lagally KM, Walker-Smith K. The validity of using ratings of perceived exertion to monitor intensity during physical education classes. *Med Sci Sport Exerc.* 2010; 42(Suppl 1): 60.
74. Smith JD, Holmes PA. Perceived exertion of the PACER in High School students. *Phys Ed.* 2013; 70: 72–88.

PART 2

Exercise medicine

CHAPTER 16

Physical activity, physical fitness, and health

Lauren B Sherar and Sean P Cumming

Introduction

Physical activity (PA) is associated with physical and psychological health during childhood and adolescence. More recently, sedentary behaviour (as defined as sitting and lying during waking hours when there is very low (<1.5 METS) energy expenditure[1]) has also been identified as a unique risk factor for poor health in children and adolescents,[2–3] although perhaps less convincing than the association with moderate to vigorous physical activity (MVPA). Until recent definitions were published, low levels of PA were commonly referred to as 'sedentary'. It is important, however, that clear distinctions are made between these behaviours as evidence indicates that even those meeting guidelines for PA may still accumulate considerable sedentary time,[4] and that these behaviours may independently impact health status.

With regard to children and PA, we live in a world of contrasts. On one hand, children are competing and specializing in sports at increasingly early ages[5] and professional sports teams and National Governing Bodies are investing more resources in the identification and development of young athletes. Teenage world record holders in swimming are commonplace, and many Olympic female gymnasts can be defined as pre- or peri-pubescent. A 13-year-old boy has run the marathon in 2 h and 55 min.

Children and adolescents are also an increasingly popular target for the leisure industry, with many facilities offering child-specific fitness programmes and child-sized exercise equipment. Conversely, there is continued evidence of a global decline in children's PA that can be observed from age of entry into school.[6–7] There is also a general perception that children's freedom to cycle, walk, and play outdoors is being curtailed, and that contemporary lifestyles in developed countries now involve large amounts of activities that entail sitting (e.g. television, playing video games, passive commuting, and more recently using hand-held mobile devices (tablets, smart phones)), which has increased over the past decades.[8–10] Technology will continue to develop, and so we must learn how to embrace it in such a way that does not cause a detriment to children's health. With this in mind, children's participation in PA is a challenge that must be addressed. These contrasts beg the questions: is there a happy medium of physical activity and sedentary behaviour for the child that ensures optimum growth and health[11] (physical, psychological, and behavioural) into adulthood, and to what extent children today are achieving this level.

These questions are difficult to answer. Despite the acceptance that PA is beneficial for children's health, and that there are continued improvements in the quantity and quality of evidence supporting this position, our understanding of this area is still limited. Methodological and conceptual challenges remain, including how to best define and assess PA and sedentary behaviour in children (although considerable advancements have been made),[12] and the need to adopt an interdisciplinary and/or biocultural approach that considers the simultaneous and interactive effects of biological, psychological, and socio-environmental factors and processes.[13] Thus, it remains difficult to distil the available information with a view to establishing absolute recommendations for activity and/or fitness levels that are optimal for health in children.

The lack of a clear evidence-based consensus regarding the optimal levels of PA and sedentary behaviour for enhancing current and future health in children contrasts our equivalent understanding of these associations in adults. In adults, the strength and direction of the associations between PA, fitness, and health are much clearer. In particular, findings from a number of robust, large epidemiological studies show that virtually any increase in PA from a state of very low levels of activity is beneficial to health.[11] We now know that low levels of PA and high amounts of sedentary behaviour are elements of a contemporary lifestyle that impacts significantly, and adversely, upon health.

Given the current epidemic of lifestyle-related chronic diseases, contemporary lifestyles of developed nations have become a matter of concern.[14] The increasing prevalence of inactivity and sedentary behaviour has been documented in both adults[15–16] and children.[17] Secular trends in children's PA mirror those observed in adults, with decreased activity in many different contexts including active transport, physical education, and freedom to play outside. Trends do, however, vary relative to country, culture, or socio-economic status. Furthermore, technological and societal changes have certainly impacted the types of physical activities and sedentary behaviours that children are participating in now compared to previous decades. For example, data from a number of large cross-sectional and longitudinal studies reveal that the types of activities/sedentary behaviours that American youth participate in have changed over the past 40 years. For example, the evidence suggests that between 1971 and 2012 in the US, active commuting, high school physical education, and outdoor play (in 3–12-year-olds) has declined, while sports participation in high school girls has increased. In addition, electronic entertainment and computer use increased during the first decade of the 21st century.[18] This highlights the need for sensitive surveillance systems that can evolve over time to detect secular changes in different types of activity and sedentary behaviours. In summary, despite some improvements in PA, a more general global decline in children's activity levels has undoubtedly contributed to the escalating levels of childhood overweight and obesity.[6]

Declines in children's PA likely stem from social and environmental change, rather than a decreased interest in physical activity or decreased participation in sport. Due to a global investment in health media campaigns, such as Change4Life in the UK and ParticipACTION in Canada, the awareness of the benefits of PA and the detriments of certain sedentary behaviours (such as television watching) are well understood. However, this awareness does not often translate into behaviour change.[19] Opportunities for children to be active are constrained by factors such as school policy or curricula, health and safety fears, parental rules regarding safety and convenience, and a range of other environmental factors.[17]

Although children appear to be becoming less active, there has, until recently, been surprisingly little high-quality evidence to suggest that children's activity and/or fitness levels are so low as to compromise their current or future health.[12,20–21] The increasing use of objective motion sensors—most notably accelerometers—has, however, greatly increased our ability to measure activity levels more accurately, and, thus, more accurate data now clearly suggest that low activity levels are indeed compromising the health of children. This can be seen in terms of higher levels of overweight and obesity,[6,22–24] cardiovascular disease (CVD) risk factors,[25–27] and poor bone health.[28] There are therefore increasingly strong grounds to be very concerned about children's low levels of PA and increase in sedentary behaviour. In this respect, Blair[29] has hypothesized a number of possible relationships between activity levels, health, and stage of life (Figure 16.1), and we have slightly modified it to include sedentary behaviour. (Interested readers are referred to Chapter 17 for detailed discussion of PA and cardiovascular health).

The hypothesized relationships within this model suggest three main beneficial effects which might derive from adequate childhood activity:

- Enhancement of physiological and psychological development during childhood—directly improving childhood health status and quality of life (A).
- Delay in the onset, or retardation of the rate of development of health risk factors—directly improving adult health status (B).
- Improved likelihood of maintaining adequate activity/sedentary behaviour levels into adulthood, thus indirectly enhancing adult health status (C).

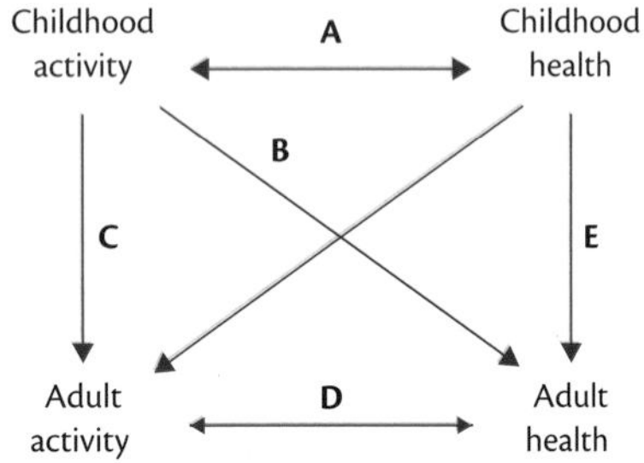

Figure 16.1 Hypothetical relationships between physical activity and health in children and adults.
Organization WH. Report of the commission on ending childhood obesity. Geneva, Switzerland: World Health Organization; 2016.

Considering these possible relations, it is interesting to note that the majority of evidence we have relates to adult activity/sedentary behaviour and adult health (D). Relations between child activity/sedentary behaviour and either child health (A), adult health (B), or adult activity/sedentary behaviour (C) are still relatively weak by comparison. Furthermore, as a cautionary note, it is important to consider that increased PA may also carry a measure of increased health risk through trauma, overuse, or burnout, which must be balanced against the potential benefits.[5]

Defining physical activity, sedentary behaviour, and fitness

Physical activity is a complex behaviour, defined as any bodily movement produced by the skeletal muscles that results in a substantial increase in energy expenditure above resting.[30] Activity behaviour varies within a range of dimensions—frequency (e.g. three times per week), intensity (e.g. light, moderate, vigorous) time/duration (e.g. 30 min) and type/mode (e.g. walking, running). Exercise is a specific type of PA that is planned, structured, repetitive, and results in improvement or maintenance of one or more facets of physical fitness.[30] Finally, the PA context refers to the PA according to identifiable portions of daily life (e.g. leisure-time, occupational/school, transportation-related PA). Physical activity differs from energy expenditure. The global construct representing the exposure variable within the activity-health-fitness paradigm is best defined as 'movement', with two dimensions: PA (the behaviour) and energy expenditure (the physiological response to the behaviour).[31] Regardless of the methods used to measure movement, some form of extrapolation to units of energy expenditure is often required to assess the relationship between movement and health outcomes. Physical activity must also be considered within its sociocultural context if it is to be truly understood.[13]

While the previous decade has seen an increase in research into the impact of sedentary behaviour on health in youth and adults, there have, however, been inconsistencies in the definition of sedentary behaviour used, with the term sedentary commonly being used to describe the absence of some threshold of MVPA. The Sedentary Behaviour Research Network published the definition of sedentary behaviour as any waking behaviour characterized by an energy expenditure ≤1.5 METs while in a sitting or reclining posture. A paradigm shift is underway toward an increasing appreciation of the importance of reducing sedentary behaviour alongside increasing PA in youth.

Because PA and sedentary behaviour are so complex (and variable), they are extremely difficult to measure. Current assessments of PA include, among others, direct observation, PA diaries, qualitative methods (such as interviews and focus groups), recall questionnaires, pedometers, and accelerometers. Direct assessments of energy expenditure include among other methods, calorimetry, labelled isotope methods, and energy intake. No gold-standard method of measuring PA exists which accurately reflects all of its dimensions.[12] When a behaviour is so difficult to assess, it becomes problematic in that a high degree of misclassification of individuals is likely. For example, a questionnaire concentrating on participation in exercise/sports is likely to miss much PA performed through informal play, school, and travel. A child who plays no sport, but who walks to school and participates in housework, can potentially be misclassified as inactive. When assessing relations between

PA levels and other parameters—for example, health status—misclassification in terms of PA will weaken the observed associations and limit the accuracy of estimated dose-response effects.[32]

The strength and limitations of various methods for assessing physical activity[33] and sedentary behaviour[34] are discussed in detail in Chapter 21 and only overviewed in this chapter. Doubly labelled water is considered the 'gold standard' when assessing energy expenditure. However, its practicality is limited by the financial costs required for its use and the need to collect accurate dietary records during the period of study. In the past 15 years accelerometers have become increasingly popular for assessing time spent in PA and/or sedentary. As a result, commercial suppliers have responded by producing a number of different models and greatly increasing the functionality of these measurement tools. Although currently considered the method of choice for assessing PA even in large scale studies, accelerometers remain limited in some ways, as they are impractical when assessing certain activities, such as contact sports (e.g. rugby) or water-based activities (e.g. swimming). The development of accelerometers that simultaneously record movement and heart rate may help address the former of these limitations but still present a problem in terms of assessing PA in contact or water-based sports. Self-report questionnaires are popular due to their feasibility/practicality, low cost, low participant burden, and general acceptance.[35] However, a systematic review of 83 studies of children and adolescents showed substantial discrepancies and only moderate correlations between the common indirect methods of assessing PA in youth and other more robust direct measures.[36]

Self-report methods for recalling intensity, frequency, and duration of bouts of PA are problematic, especially in children who are less time conscious than adults and tend to engage in intermittent and sporadic bouts of PA with varied intensities and inconsistent patterns.[37] Not only is reliability compromised by recall difficulties, but also the validity of measures may be affected in children and adolescents who feel compelled to respond in a socially acceptable manner. Younger children are also more likely to misinterpret questions posed, creating possible content validity problems. However, despite limitations mentioned in assessing volume and intensity of PA, questionnaires can provide important information on type and context of PA and sedentary behaviour. Recent advancements in accelerometry have seen the use of uniaxial, low resolution, epoch level devices replaced with multi-axes, high resolution, waveform sensors. This new generation of accelerometer technologies has the potential, via pattern recognition, to be able to classify the mode/type of PA behaviour and sedentary behaviour. Successfully determining the activity mode would allow for activity-specific energy expenditure prediction equations that should yield increased accuracy of these measurement tools. That said, the widespread use of these rich waveform data will be challenged by the need for advanced signal processing skills and a dearth of published methods and/or normative data. Fortunately, there are key opinion leaders such as the accelerometry group within the National Health and Nutrition Examination Survey (NHANES) and the growing group of accelerometry experts associated with the UK Biobank Physical Activity Monitoring that will help guide the field forward.

Sedentary behaviour or time spent sedentary can be assessed by the previously outlined objective and subjective tools. In brief, accelerometers are limited in their inability to provide contextual information (i.e. setting and type of sedentary behaviour) and also in their ability to distinguish between sitting and standing (the latter not being a true sedentary behaviour see reference[1]). More recently inclinometers have been used to measure sedentary behaviours. Inclinometers assess anatomical position in three planes to assess different postures—lying, sitting, and standing. Technologies to objectively assess sitting/lying include the ActivPal posture sensor and newer generation of accelerometers are incorporating inclinometers into their devices. Lastly, new technologies are becoming more accessible to objectively assess physical location and thus provide some detail on context of activity (see reference[38] for a review of some of these technologies).

In contrast to PA, physical fitness is a set of attributes that people have or achieve that relate to their ability to perform PA.[30,38] Like PA, there are many dimensions of fitness, for example, cardiovascular fitness, strength, flexibility, speed, power, and anaerobic endurance. Many of these dimensions are not only related to performance, but also to health. The component most strongly associated with health is cardiovascular endurance, defined as 'the ability to sustain moderate intensity, whole-body activity for extended time periods'.[39] It can be measured objectively in the laboratory setting using a variety of ergometers (e.g. cycle or treadmill) with or without respiratory gas analysis, or more simply in the field by maximal running tests or submaximal cycle or step tests. Fitness is partly genetically determined, but can be improved by regular appropriate PA. In contrast to PA, fitness can be accurately measured, leading to less misclassification of individuals and observed relations that may be nearer to reality. Both fitness and PA are strongly and independently associated with health in adults, and similar associations can now be observed in children although the associations are often less strong and likely to be confounded by differences in growth and development, especially during adolescence.

Paediatric exercise scientists studying PA and health also need to consider the processes of growth and development. All children are faced with three primary tasks which constitute the business of 'growing up',[13] namely, to grow (changes in body size, physique, and composition), to mature (progress toward a biologically mature state), and to develop (learn culturally appropriate cognitive, emotional, social, and motor behaviours). Although distinct, these processes interact with one another to govern the majority of children's experiences during the first two decades of their life and may confound relations between health, PA, sedentary behaviour, and fitness. Maturity associated variability in physical characteristics (e.g. size, physique, body composition) and functional capacity (e.g. strength, speed, aerobic capacity) have already been documented as predictors of physical and psychological health,[40–41] involvement in PA,[42] sedentary behaviour,[43] training,[44] and sports participation.[40, 45] As a result, researchers interested in examining the health benefits of PA and fitness and the possible detriments of sedentary behaviour in children (particularly adolescents) need to be aware of and (where possible) control for individual variation in growth and maturation.[46]

Physical activity and health

It is clear that young children enjoy and are primed to engage in active play. That is, active play is a time sensitive and biologically determined activity that plays a central role in physical and psychological development.[47] Given a free choice, most young children will play or invent active ways of passing time which involve jumping, dancing, skipping, hopping, chasing, running, climbing, and cycling. Older children might play more organized sports—either formally, in clubs and teams, or informally, in parks and playgrounds. Generally speaking, these forms of play provide a large volume of activity incorporating a wide variety of movements, using many muscle groups, and promoting cardiorespiratory development, muscular strength, muscular endurance, speed, power, and flexibility. These activities also afford the opportunity for children to develop and apply various social and psychological skills (i.e. communication, cooperation, and reasoning), enhancing psychosocial development. In the later teenage years these relatively high levels of active play decline as more sedentary alternatives are chosen. This decline in active play with age is inevitable as play, as an activity, becomes biologically redundant as various developmental milestones are achieved.[48] This decline is also not necessarily problematical, as it is seen in many other animal species. However, if activity levels decline to levels which are too low—and we should remember that adult levels are undoubtedly too low—then this may constitute a problem in the making.

We must therefore ascertain that if children's activity levels decline over the teenage years to such an extent, either their current or future health may be compromised. To determine the validity of this statement, we must scrutinize the evidence relating activity to indicators of health status—or health risk factors—in children.

There is an emerging body of evidence suggesting associations between childhood PA and childhood health are reflected by more favourable overweight/obesity status or a healthier CVD risk profile.[24–25,27] The benefits of PA to physical and psychomotor health have also been documented in early childhood (age 4 years and under), emphasizing the importance of promoting activity from an early age.[49] We should therefore more closely examine the evidence relating to each of the three hypothesized relationships suggested by Figure 16.1.

Overweight and obesity

Childhood overweight and obesity is associated with a host of adverse physical and psychological consequences during childhood and in adulthood.[6,50] A twofold to threefold increase in overweight and obesity prevalence was observed between 1980 and 2000 in children and adolescents in many industrialized countries in the world.[51] Although there is evidence that obesity prevalence may be levelling off in some countries,[52–54] childhood obesity is still well recognized as a global health issue. Adiposity is most commonly measured by body mass index (BMI), waist circumference skinfolds, bioimpedance analysis, and dual-energy X-ray absorptiometry (DEXA).

Clear associations have been reported between children's PA and measures of overweight and obesity;[6,55] however, most studies use BMI as a proxy for fatness and evidence is limited in the early years. The strongest associations are seen in studies where PA has been measured more accurately (e.g. with accelerometers). There appear to be stronger associations between adiposity/waist circumference and MVPA than with total activity[24] and overall sedentary time.[56] However, certain sedentary behaviours such as television watching may be more closely related to obesity, which could be partially explained by the co-existence of unhealthy eating while watching television. For example, a systematic review conducted in 2011[2] of school-age children provided evidence to suggest that watching television for more than 2 $h \cdot day^{-1}$ was associated with unfavourable body composition, in addition to decreased fitness, lowered scores for self-esteem and pro-social behaviour, and decreased academic achievement. However, many of the studies included were cross-sectional and observational which prevent comment on causality.

The limited effectiveness of obesity prevention and treatment programmes (both PA and nutrition based) has been highlighted.[57] A lack of tailoring of interventions to address the needs of specific sub samples of children (e.g. immigrants in industrialized countries, those age 6 years and under, and males) was identified as a particular limitation of these programmes, as was the failure to integrate the strategies for healthy living or use evidence-based strategies.[58] The need to create change at the institutional level (e.g. provide opportunity for competitive and non-competitive forms of PA) and to educate parents about reducing children's use of television, computer games, and hand-held devices (tablets and smart phones) have also been identified as key factors in the fight against childhood obesity.[59] More holistic, multi-dimensional (i.e. PA, psychology, and nutrition based) interventions are probably required in order to achieve real impacts on children's PA levels.

The importance of preventing overweight during adolescence has been highlighted.[60] In a large, prospective study with 55 years of follow-up, being overweight in adolescence predicted a broad range of adverse health effects in adulthood that were independent of adult weight. A review of 32 longitudinal studies tracking adiposity in youth in relation to PA or sedentary behaviour concluded that PA and decreased sedentary behaviour are protective against relative weight and fatness gains over childhood and adolescence.[61] This position is supported by results from large-scale epidemiological studies of European[25] and British youth.[24] However, although obese children are more likely to be obese adults and obesity in adulthood is linked to enhanced adult morbidity,[62] emerging evidence suggests that normal-weight children are also likely to be obese adults and that adult obesity-related morbidity may be more related to obesity accrued in adulthood.[63] This highlights the importance of PA interventions targeting normal-weight as well as overweight/obese children and the importance of maintaining a healthy lifestyle into adulthood. (Interested readers are referred to Chapter 25 for further discussion of obesity and overweight).

Cardiometabolic risk and type 2 diabetes mellitus

Metabolic syndrome has received considerable attention over recent years. The metabolic syndrome components (e.g. abdominal obesity, triglycerides, insulin, HDL-cholesterol, inflammatory markers, etc.) and criteria (e.g. cut-points used to define high-risk values) vary depending on definition used. Whereas the definition and existence of clinical metabolic syndrome in children is debated, clustering of cardiometabolic risk factors can undoubtedly be detected in children.[25,64–65] A study[66] found that half of adolescents in North America presented with one cardiometabolic risk factor and 8.6% had the metabolic syndrome. Prevalence was higher in males (10.8%) than females (6.1%) and in Hispanic (11.2%) and white (8.9%) individuals than in black individuals (4.0%).

The prevalence of type 2 diabetes mellitus (T2DM) is increasing in many countries with the increase in obesity.[67] For example, between 2001 and 2009 there was a 30.5% increase in T2DM in the US in children and adolescents.[68] However, the incidence is still relatively low. Children and adolescents with T2DM are generally characterized by clustering of cardiometabolic risk, hyperglycaemia, obesity, and adverse mental health. Risk factors for T2DM in youth, in addition to obesity, include a family history of diabetes (in particular maternal diabetes during child's gestation), and race/ethnicity (black, Hispanic, American Indian, Asian/Pacific Islander). Findings from the prospective Cardiovascular Risk in Young Finns Study, a study that followed up children 30 years into adulthood, demonstrated that several childhood cardiometabolic risk factors were associated with the risk of subclinical atherosclerosis (ultrasound measures of carotid and brachial arteries) and metabolic syndrome in adulthood.[69] Findings from this prospective study highlight the importance of targeting children and youth. (Readers interested in PA and T2DM are referred to Chapter 23 for further detail).

Physical activity and decreasing sedentary behaviour (in addition to dietary modification) is believed to have an important role in maintaining cardiometabolic health in youth and specifically in the prevention and management of T2DM. Studies of associations between accelerometer-derived MVPA and sedentary time and single CVD risk factors in children[70–72] have reported only weak associations and in many cases evidence is equivocal.

However, studies investigating clustering of CVD risk factors in children have produced stronger associations.[25,73–74] Data derived from the European Heart Study indicate a strong, negative association between PA (measured by accelerometry) and the clustering of CVD risk factors in a sample of over 1700 Estonian, Portuguese, and Danish youth.[25] Time spent in MVPA was 116 min in 9-year-olds and 88 min in 15-year-olds, for the most active (and least at-risk) groups. This suggests that the recommendation of 60 min of moderate PA per day may not be sufficient to prevent the clustering of CVD risk factors in children. In a related study with Danish youth, Brage and colleagues[75] observed an inverse relation between PA and clustered risk, even when potential confounders such as age, sex, maturation, ethnicity, socioeconomic factors, and smoking behaviour were controlled for. An analysis of data from 2527 children and adolescents (6- to 19 years old) from the 2003/04 and 2005/06 waves of the NHANES survey showed that MVPA predicted high cardiometabolic risk after adjusting for sedentary behaviours and other confounders.[76] Further analyses from this dataset showed little difference in the association between MVPA and cardiometabolic risk, when PA was accumulated sporadically (in bouts less than 5 min) or when accumulated in bouts of PA of greater duration (5 min or more).[76]

Emerging data[77–79] show an association between the volume (total accumulated time) of sedentary behaviour and in the pattern (length of bouts and frequency of breaks in sedentary time) in which it is accumulated (such as breaks in sedentary time), and increased cardiometabolic risk in adults. The underlying mechanisms are unknown and likely complex, but are likely connected to changes in lipoprotein lipase activity caused by reduced muscle contractions. Youth spend much of their day sedentary. To date, research is lacking to support an association between objectively assessed overall sedentary time and individual or clustered cardiometabolic risk when adjusted for MVPA. However, certain sedentary behaviours, such as television watching, are likely more detrimental to cardiometabolic health. For example, the aforementioned discussed NHANES paper[76] showed that volume and patterns of sedentary behaviour were not associated with high cardiometabolic risk, after adjusting for accelerometer assessed MVPA. However, high television use (but not high computer use) was a predictor of high cardiometabolic risk (after adjustment for MVPA among other confounders). It was shown that youth who watched ≥4 h of television per day were 2.53 times more likely to have high cardiometabolic risk than those who watched <1 $h \cdot day^{-1}$. Thus in summary, to date there is evidence to suggest that PA (particularly MVPA) is more closely associated with cardiometabolic health in youth when compared to sedentary behaviour, perhaps with the exception of television viewing. However, further prospective studies are required using accurate and objective measures of PA and sedentary behaviour.

Bone health

Osteoporosis and the fractures that are associated with it are largely a feature of old age, and the scale of the problem is certain to grow as life expectancy increases. It is estimated, for example, that the 6.26 million hip fractures currently recorded annually on a worldwide basis will increase fourfold by the year 2050.[80] There is almost a universal consensus that childhood and adolescence are critical periods for reducing the risk of osteoporosis later in life. For example, it has been reported that 60% of the risk of osteoporosis can be explained by the amount of bone mineral acquired by early adulthood.[81] The common method to assess bone health (for research and clinical purposes) is DEXA which generates two-dimensional measures of bone mineral content (BMC, g) and areal bone mineral density ($g \cdot cm^{-2}$). However, DEXA is unable to distinguish between cortical and trabecular bone compartments or to differentiate the specific macrostructures and microstructures that may alter due to PA/sedentary behaviour. However, more recently, imaging techniques such as magnetic resonance imaging, peripheral quantitative computed tomography, and high-resolution computed tomography have been used to assess many aspects of bone structure that contribute to bone strength.[82–84] Peak bone mass, which is achieved in the majority of people by the third decade, is known to be influenced by genetics, PA, nutrition (notably calcium intake), and chronic disease during childhood and adolescence. These factors may have a direct influence on bone, or act indirectly through effects on body composition (i.e. lean mass development), and/or linear growth. There are a number of high-quality interventions and longitudinal studies which provide strong evidence to support a positive effect of PA during the growing years on bone mass accrual in boys and girls. These are summarized in several excellent reviews[84–88] and interested readers are referred to Chapter 18 for a detailed discussion.

Studies indicate that weight-bearing PA in childhood and adolescence is an important predictor of bone geometry, mineral content, and density, while non-weight-bearing activity (such as swimming or cycling) is not.[89] The size of the effect of PA (difference in BMD between the high and low fitness or PA groups) is, typically, between 5 and 15%. Appropriate PA increases peak bone mass somewhat less than one standard deviation, or 7–8%, approximately.[90] This would be sufficient, if maintained into old age, to substantially reduce the risk of osteoporotic fracture.[91] However, more research on the optimal type and volume of PA required for bone health in young people is required. Based on available information[92] it is likely that activities which involve high strains, developed rapidly, and distributed unevenly throughout the movement pattern, may be particularly osteogenic. Thus, activities such as aerobics, dancing, volleyball, basketball, and racket sports may be effective, and need not necessarily be of prolonged duration, as the osteogenic response to such movement appears to saturate after only a few loading cycles.[92]

There is some evidence[93] that PA during the immediate prepubescent and pubescent years may be crucial for maximizing peak bone mass. Data collected from the Avon Longitudinal Study of Parents and Children suggests that that accelerometer assessed PA associated with impacts >4.2 g, such as jumping and running (which further studies suggest requires speeds $>10\,\text{km}\cdot\text{h}^{-1}$) is positively related to hip BMD and structure in adolescents, whereas moderate impact activity (e.g. jogging) is of little benefit. Thus highlighting, the importance of high-impact activity.[94] Further, evidence from the Iowa Bone Development Study[95] suggests that positive associations between objectively assessed PA and bone measures are present during early childhood, well in advance of the onset of peak bone mass and that vigorous PA may be necessary to elicit positive effects.[96] A review of intervention studies suggests beneficial effects of school-based, bone-targeted exercise on bone, and supports the use of brief, jumping-focused interventions to enhance bone development in school age children.

In the light of these observations, intervention strategies to optimize bone development might need to be introduced during childhood. Bed rest and weightlessness studies on bone health in adults[97–98] have led to the suggestion that repeated sedentary behaviour, specifically sitting, could have an adverse direct effect on bone mass through increased bone resorption and decreased stimulation of bone formation.[99] The Healthy Lifestyle in Europe by Nutrition in Adolescence study highlighted the potential importance of sedentary behaviour on bone health. European adolescents from the study self-reported to spend on average $9\,\text{h}\cdot\text{day}^{-1}$ of their waking time sedentary and this self-reported sedentary time was negatively associated with BMC.[100] In confirmation, analysis of data on young people (8–22 years) from the 2005/2006 wave of the NHANES survey[101] showed that self-report time spent in screen-based sedentary behaviours was negatively associated with femoral BMC (males and females) and spinal BMC (females only), this was after adjustment for MVPA. This association was strengthened when self-reported engagement in regular (average five times per week) strengthening exercise (for males) and vigorous playing (for both males and females) were taken into account. Total sitting time and non-screen-based sitting were not associated with bone health.

Questions for future examination include when is the optimal time to introduce PA and reduce sedentary behaviour for the purposes of enhancing bone development, and what dose responses are required to obtain these benefits. Existing studies suggest that prepuberty and the circumpubertal years may be the most opportune time for PA driven enhancements in bone strength in boys and girls;[84] however, this finding is tempered by limited data in older, more mature individuals. A second important question is to be able to tease out how maturation influences the bone's response to PA. This will require longitudinal accurate, objective, and sensitive measures of bone, PA/sedentary behaviour, and biological maturation.

In summary, PA (particularly of a vigorous intensity) is an essential stimulus for bone structure, and has the potential to increase peak bone mass in children and adolescents within the limits set by genetic, hormonal, and nutritional influences. Such enhanced bone mass/structure has considerable potential to reduce risk of osteoporosis and associated fracture in later life, particularly if the increase can be maintained throughout adulthood by increased PA and perhaps, by a reduction in sedentary behaviour.

Psychological health

The psychological benefits of PA are well documented in adult samples,[102–103] and there is growing evidence to suggest that PA may be equally beneficial in children. With an increased prevalence of children presenting psychological problems (an estimated 20% of all children in the UK[104]), there is a need to better understand how PA may be used to prevent and treat psychological problems in children. The majority of research supporting the psychological benefits of PA in children is cross-sectional in design. As such, it is not possible to infer cause and effect relations. Nevertheless, more active children tend to report higher levels of self-esteem, happiness, and life satisfaction,[105] and lower levels of anxiety, depression,[106] stress,[107] and peer victimization.[108] Physical activity, and in particular active play, is also purported to contribute positively towards neural and psychosocial development.[47–48] Consistent with evidence from adult samples, it would appear that the psychological health benefits associated with PA can also be achieved through moderate and low intensity activities such as walking and jogging.[109] Physical activity interventions programmes promoting positive mental health might also be more effective in overweight and/or obese groups. Likewise, over involvement in intense, frequent, sustained bouts of activity can result in 'burnout', a special case of sport withdrawal in which child athletes cease to participate in sport due to chronic stress.[5,110] This is a particular concern for athletes who specialize and compete at an early age.[5] (The overtraining syndrome is addressed in detail in Chapter 38).

More recently, researchers have begun to examine the cognitive benefits of PA and exercise in youth. There is growing evidence to suggest that acute and chronic bouts of PA can benefit numerous aspects of cognition optimizing both learning and performance.[111] These benefits have also been reported in youth with cognitive impairments, such as attention deficient hyperactivity disorder.[112] While the exact mechanisms of these benefits are unclear, advances in brain imaging technology should allow scientists to better understand the various factors and processes that may be involved.

Several recent systematic reviews[113] have highlighted the potentially important link between sedentary behaviour and psychological health in youth. In recent years, a growing number of studies[114] have reported a non-linear association of screen time in youth with depression. Children and adolescents with excessive or no screen time may have higher risk of depression level compared with the occasional or regular screen time, suggesting that appropriate screen time may be associated with lower depression in youth. A recent meta-analysis[113] found that screen time that exceeds $2\,\text{h}\cdot\text{day}^{-1}$ is associated with higher risk of depression, whereas less screen time ($1\,\text{h}\cdot\text{day}^{-1}$) is associated with lower risk of depression. Similar non-linear associations have been found between electronic gaming and prosocial behaviour, life satisfaction, and internalizing and externalizing problems.[115] Emerging evidence suggests a negative association between other facets of psychological health and sedentary behaviours, such as anxiety,[116] hyperactivity/inattention problems, internalizing problems, and low self-esteem;[117] however, more high-quality longitudinal/interventional research is required to confirm findings, determine causality, and to establish possible mediating and moderating variables.

Other health issues

Asthma represents another leading form of chronic illness in children and adolescents. Although acute bouts of strenuous exercise have been identified as triggers for asthmatic attacks, moderate- and low-intensity exercise is often recommended as a complementary therapy in the treatment of asthma. Little is known, however, about the role that PA and sedentary behaviour play in the prevention and treatment of asthma. A cross-sectional study that included over 13 000 US adolescents[118] revealed that sedentary behaviour (>3 h of computer use per day) and being overweight were associated with an increased prevalence of asthma. Surprisingly, levels of PA did not predict incidences of asthma. More recently a systematic review showed swimming training to be well-tolerated in children and adolescents with stable asthma and some evidence of increases in lung function and cardiopulmonary fitness.[119] There also seems to be limited evidence that swimming training caused adverse effects in youth with stable asthma of any severity. However, there is a need for high-quality studies that compare the effects of different types of PA and include follow-up periods to enable potential long-term effects. (Interested readers are referred to Chapter 24 for further discussion).

This chapter has focused on 'apparently healthy children'; however, it is important to acknowledge the importance of PA and sedentary behaviour in all children and youth, including those with childhood disease and those with physical and mental disabilities. These children may have additional challenges to being physically active but also reap unique benefits. (Interested readers are referred to Chapter 28 for further discussion).

From the present dialogue, it is apparent that there is an emerging body of evidence linking PA and sedentary behaviour levels to various health parameters in children.

To gain a more comprehensive understanding of the broader health implications of PA researchers must strive to develop and employ more sophisticated research designs and sensitive measurement tools. Researchers also need to recognize that absence of evidence does not indicate evidence of absence. Likewise, sometimes, such as in the relationship between cognition and habitual PA, positive associations independent of confounders may not be seen.[120] However, an observed lack of a negative impact on academic achievement/cognition of an activity intervention, particularly, school-based interventions, should be seen as an important finding which can be used to leverage important policy change. The failure of many previous studies to identify relations between PA and health parameters may result from limitations associated with research designs, methods, sampling procedures, the types of analysis used, or a failure to control for confounding factors, such as growth and maturation. In other words, subtle relations and effects may exist, but we may not have been able to detect them. Future work needs to concentrate on the pre-school population and special populations.

Physical activity and future health status

Direct effects

It has been argued that degenerative biological processes are initiated during infancy and childhood, manifesting themselves as chronic disease in later life. In fact, there is evidence to suggest that adult health status may be determined, at least in part, by the embryonic environment and/or biological events that occur in utero.[121] It is argued that early biological events trigger a morphological and/or functional change that subsequently becomes a chronic and worsening condition, ultimately leading to overt signs and symptoms, chronic illness, and death. The individual is effectively 'programmed' for susceptibility to a disease through an early biological event. Crucially, the biological event may itself be triggered by an environmental influence (inadequate maternal nutrition, smoking) and it is in this respect that PA may be important. Whereas structured prenatal exercise appears to reduce the risk of having an overweight baby without altering the risk of having an underweight baby,[122] the impact of PA on the child's future health remains unclear. Nevertheless, we have one further argument that PA during the early part of the lifespan is important, despite the fact that morbidity and mortality are features of adult life.

Indirect effects

It seems reasonable to presume that if active children are more likely to be active adults—which enhances health—then childhood PA/sedentary behaviour could indirectly influence adult health. Evidence supporting this contention is, however, limited and weak. The persistence of a behaviour, or attribute, over time is called 'tracking', and refers to the short-, medium-, or long-term maintenance of a rank order position compared to one's peers. Our main concern, therefore, might be whether inactivity and/or high sedentary behaviour in childhood would lead to inactivity and/or high sedentary behaviour in adulthood, and subsequent elevated risk of adult disease.[123] Conversely, we might ask if high activity as a child predicts high activity as an adult.

Levels of tracking through various stages of the lifespan have been comprehensively reviewed.[124–125] Activity tracks at weak to moderate levels during early childhood (0–6 years) to middle childhood[124] and middle childhood through to adolescence,[126] and from adolescence into adulthood.[126] With regards to sedentary behaviour there is evidence of moderate-to-large tracking from early childhood to middle childhood,[124] and moderate tracking from childhood to adolescence.[127] Evidence from longitudinal data suggests that tracking of PA from childhood to adulthood is weak across multiple domains.[128] These studies suggest that prevention and health promotion programmes, targeting both PA and sedentary behaviour, should start early in life. Future studies should assess using validated and objective measures a range of sedentary and PA behaviours. The weak-moderate tracking does suggest that some individuals become more active or less sedentary over time (and vice versa). Identifying these youths and the factors that influence their behaviours will help to inform targeted interventions.

Many factors influence PA levels and patterns from day to day, between seasons of the year, and various life events and transitions. Life events which can disturb activity patterns include changing schools, school-to-work transition, leaving home, moving house, moving to a new neighbourhood, biological and psychological development (especially puberty and adolescence), illness, marriage, and child rearing. Any one of these can significantly affect PA habits, and therefore fluctuations in PA across the lifespan are expected. Linked with this is the fact that individuals' PA interests will change with age. As we grow older, we move from play, through sport, to social and recreational activities and the level of 'background' or lifestyle activity we do—for example, walking to work and housework confounds the whole scenario. We might, therefore, expect tracking coefficients to be only weak or moderate. This finding highlights the importance of encouraging PA across multiple domains.

The methodological and conceptual problems are considerable in our quest to assess the stability of this complex and fundamentally changeable behaviour. Interestingly, evidence suggests[129] that how 'comfortable' a child is about the concept of PA ('psychological readiness') is positively correlated with how active the adult is. For example, physical education grade at the age of 15 years (a measure of competence) is positively associated with psychological readiness to participate in activity at age 30 years. This suggests that encouraging actual and perceived competence in sports and physical recreation—which may not promote higher childhood PA levels—may nevertheless have long-lasting effects on adult attitudes towards activity and subsequently higher adult PA levels.[130] The need to demonstrate competence (in addition to autonomy and relatedness) is, after all, considered one of the basic needs underlying intrinsic motivation.[131]

Prevalence of activity, inactivity, and sedentary behaviour

Whether children are active enough to gain health benefits is one of the important outstanding questions. At this point data remain concerning—and occasionally confusing. A highlight of the 2014 Global Summit on the Physical Activity of Children, was the publication of PA report cards for 15 nations from across five continents. Most countries fared poorly in terms of meeting the PA requirements necessary for promoting and maintaining positive physical health. The reports cards did, however, show substantial variation between, and within, countries in children's PA behaviours and environments (e.g. active play, active transport, physical education provision). Another interesting observation was that across the report cards, grades for active transport positively predicted overall activity; whereas grades for the community and built environment were inversely associated with overall activity.[132] This observation suggests the degree to which various activities or factors may contribute towards overall PA in youth may vary with culture.

Studies conducted on British children have been reviewed[133] and suggest that children seldom participate in PA at a level which would have a cardiovascular training effect, or a health benefit. Sallis[134] examined nine studies and concluded that the average child is sufficiently active to meet the adult recommendations for conditioning activities, with the exception of the average female in mid- to late-adolescence. It has been argued that young children are highly and spontaneously active.[135–136] Simple observation tells us that toddlers are constantly on the move, exploring the environment, playing, and moving apparently for the sheer joy of it.[137] Blair[138] has noted that children are generally fitter and more active than adults, and most of them are active enough to receive important health benefits from their activity.

Data from the recently complied International Children's Accelerometry Database (ICAD)[139] examined accelerometer-assessed PA and time sedentary in 27 637 youth (2.8–18.4 years) from Australia, United States, Europe, and Brazil. Results showed that PA varied (15–20% difference at age 9–10 years, and a 26–28% difference at age 12–13 years) between samples from different countries. Results confirmed the well-documented age- and gender-related decline in PA. Boys were less sedentary and more active than girls at all ages and a decrease of 4.2% was observed each year, due mainly to lower levels of light-intensity PA and greater time spent sedentary. Lastly, only a small proportion of youth (9% of boys and 2% of girls) met the PA guidelines of ≥60 min MVPA on all measured days. However, ≥60 min of MVPA were accumulated on 46% of days for boys and 22% for girls. This highlights the difficulties in ascertaining guideline compliance when observing a short snapshot of time through accelerometry. It should be noted that although ICAD utilized standardized objective measurements of PA and time sedentary, the data utilized were cross-sectional, for the most part non-representative, and limited to the populations/counties included in ICAD.

From the above, it is clear that we have a great deal of conflicting data, but that more precise measurement techniques employed in the more recent (and larger) studies are allowing a better understanding to emerge. We are still not at the stage yet to definitively answer the question if children are active enough to be healthy. However, as obesity levels rise and our environment continues to support low levels of PA and high amounts of sedentary behaviour, the answer for many children is probably 'no'.

Guidelines for physical activity

There are intuitive biological and behavioural arguments in favour of promoting PA to all children. Guidelines reinforce the concept of a health-related threshold, yet the amount and type of PA during childhood which is appropriate for optimal health is probably impossible to ascertain. Relationships between the different dimensions of PA and the different health outcomes will vary, are probably dynamic, and subject to fluctuations depending on age, gender and a broad range of socio-demographic and environmental variables. The concept of a single health-related PA threshold is probably unattainable but perhaps needed when considering simple health promotion messaging.

A number of organizations have advanced PA guidelines for optimizing health and functional capacity in children.[12] The earliest recommendation was presented by the American College of Sports Medicine.[140] Based on adult guidelines, they recommended that children should engage in at least 20 min of vigorous PA each day. Recognizing that children are not simply small adults, the International Conference on Physical Activity Guidelines for Adolescents conducted a systematic review of the available literature to establish empirically based guidelines for physical activity.[141] The panel recommended that all adolescents should i) be active on a daily basis, whether it be through work, play, physical education, sport, or active transport, and ii) engage in at least 20 min of sustained MVPA at least three times per week. In 1997, the Health Education Authority of England commissioned guidelines for activity in children.[142] Recognizing individual differences in fitness and PA levels, the recommendations were that currently active children should achieve a minimum of 60 min of moderate PA per day, whereas less active children should strive for at least 30 min of moderate PA. Children should also engage at least twice per week in activities designed to promote bone growth, flexibility, and strength. These recommendations were restated in the Chief Medical Officer's 2004 report on PA and health in the United Kingdom.[143] The guideline of 60 min MVPA was adopted by a number of leading health organizations, including the World Health Organization (WHO) and the American Heart Association. These criteria also served as the Active Healthy Kid's Global Alliance's benchmark for determining the proportion of youth engaged in acceptable levels of PA in their National Physical Activity Report Cards.[7]

Since 2004 these guidelines and background evidence base have been revisited by many countries. The WHO updated their childhood PA recommendations and now suggest children aged 5–17 years accumulate 60 min of MVPA daily,[6] in addition to everyday physical activities, and that vigorous intensity PA should be incorporated at least three times per week. More recently, a number of countries (e.g. the UK, Canada, and the US) have included a sedentary behaviour recommendation for children and young people and guidelines specific to age ranges (e.g. early years, i.e. under 5 years, capable of walking and not capable of walking, and children and young people, i.e. 5–18 years). The sedentary behaviour guidelines, because of the lack of an evidence base in this area, often lack prescriptive detail (e.g. 'minimise the amount of time spent being sedentary'). Although the Canadians have chosen to include specific sedentary behaviour recommendations (e.g. for children under 2 years, screen time (e.g. TV, computer, electronic games) is not recommended; for children 2–4 years, screen time should be limited to less than 1 $h \cdot day^{-1}$; less is better (readers are referred to[144] for Canadian sedentary behaviour recommendations across the age groups)) in their national guidelines. These recommendations are backed by a small evidence base and a practical rationalization of the risks and benefits of sedentary behaviours. However, the widespread inclusion of sedentary behaviour into country-specific guidelines is indicative of the increased awareness of sedentary behaviour as an independent and important risk factor for health in children and adolescents.

Fitness and health

The majority of evidence supporting associations between fitness and health has been derived from large-scale, cross-sectional population surveys, using multivariate analysis to adjust for potential confounding variables. While such studies have advanced our understanding of this area, the most powerful evidence for causal links between fitness and health come from rarer longitudinal population studies, or from training studies in which changes in the two or more variables can be compared over time. Irrespective of study design, one important distinction between adult and child studies is that the former have the advantage of examining associations between fitness and morbity/mortality, whereas studies with children in this field are restricted to examining risk factors which are more problematical to define and measure. Developing work on the genetics of fitness[145] may improve our understanding of how fitness and health are predetermined and interrelated, and how independent it is of PA level. (The genetics of physical fitness and PA are discussed in Chapter 20).

Numerous adult population studies[146–151] have shown strong and consistent relationships between CV fitness and mortality from CVD and all causes, independent of possible confounding variables. Even more compelling has been evidence from prospective studies[152] which indicate that risk of mortality may be reduced substantially in middle-aged men who improve their fitness over a number of years.

The situation in children is less clear-cut, partly because the outcome measure—'health'—cannot, for obvious reasons, be judged by mortality statistics. Rather, the investigator must rely upon risk factors for CVD, such as high blood pressure, elevated blood lipids, and fatness. However, such risk factors may only account for 50% of eventual coronary mortality and are therefore a relatively crude yardstick for cardiovascular health.[153] Furthermore, as a result of maturation, these biological risk factors are constantly changing throughout adolescence, and may or may not relate to adult values.[154] Despite these limitations, some population studies have shown an independent relation between CV fitness and levels of CVD risk factors.[25,75,155–156] These associations may also emerge in late childhood. For example, a composite risk score for CVD low aerobic fitness (peak $\dot{V}O_2$) has been shown to be associated with an elevated risk for CVD in children aged 8–11 years.[157] Further evidence of a causal relationship between fitness and coronary risk status in children comes from long-term fitness training studies that report concomitant improvements in some, but not all, individual risk factors.[158–159] Again, such benefits may be more evident in those already at greater risk (i.e. overweight/obese youth).[160]

One consistent finding in studies with children is the very strong relationship observed between CV fitness and fatness.[161–163] It is, thus, not surprising that several studies indicate that fatness is a major confounding variable in the relationship between fitness and other CVD risk factors. In at least four population studies,[164–167] robust associations between CV fitness and level of risk were abolished after accounting statistically for body fatness, while one other study[156] reported severely attenuated relationships. It is worth noting that this feature has also been observed in an adult study[168] investigating fitness and coronary risk factors, and so the confounding influence of body fatness on coronary risk does not seem to be confined to paediatric populations. More recent evidence also suggests an association between muscular fitness and fatness that is independent of CV fitness, and may also contribute towards CVD risk factors.[169]

Although cardiovascular and muscular fitness may be associated with elevated CVD risk status in children, these associations may be partly confounded by the level of fatness and/or diet. Thus, any initiatives to improve the health of children should ideally involve measures that simultaneously improve fitness and lower fatness, namely increased PA and dietary control.

Which is more important—physical activity or fitness?

It has been argued[170–172] that physical training adaptations may not be directly related to, nor necessary for, good health. We have discussed the evidence regarding both PA and fitness in relation to health, but the interesting question of whether PA level, or fitness level, is most strongly related to health status continues to remain open for discussion. For example, does an individual who has genetically high fitness, but who is inactive, achieve health benefits from the high fitness level? Conversely, can the genetically low-fit individual gain health benefits through being active? Furthermore, how do individual differences in responsivity to training impact current and future health in youth? These questions are largely unanswered.

It is possible that high fitness, especially cardiorespiratory fitness, is directly related to improved health status. The morphological and functional condition of the heart and circulatory system may lead directly to a reduced risk of, for example, CVD. In this scenario, a genetically high-fit individual would automatically be blessed with better health status. Studies on the association between polymorphisms of the Angiotensin-Converting Enzyme and CV fitness[145] give some credence to this hypothesis. An alternative explanation might be that fitness acts as a marker for high activity (likely of the moderate-vigorous intensity) levels. This activity might not only produce an improved cardiovascular system, but might also promote other biochemical and haemodynamic changes (lower blood pressure, higher HDL cholesterol, lower triglycerides, improved glucose tolerance, modified clotting factors, and post-prandial lipaemia) which are the 'real' mechanisms which promote improved health. What we are considering is, by common understanding, almost a 'spin-off' effect of PA that might be termed 'metabolic fitness'. It is entirely possible that this type of fitness is the true health-related dimension of the generic term 'fitness'.

Physical activity and risks to the child

Physical activity can carry its own inherent risk to both adults and children. Van Mechelen[173] has highlighted the potential for childhood injury when free play in various physical activities is replaced by competitive participation in just one or two sports. Whereas all activities carry increased risk of traumatic (acute) injury, too strong a focus on training for competition in a limited range of activities can result in the additional risk of overuse (chronic) injury. Whereas both types of injury normally heal without permanent disability, the costs must be considered in terms of activity time lost, school time lost, predisposition to re-occurrence, the risk of permanent damage, and the financial cost of treatment. Baxter-Jones *et al.*[174] have reported for elite child athletes an estimated 1-year incidence rate of 40 injuries per 100 children, equating to less than one injury per 1000 h of training. In these elite child athletes, about one-third of injuries were overuse injuries, which were in turn more severe than the traumatic injuries (20 days lay-off vs 13 days respectively). It is equally important to consider the psychological costs associated with overtraining injuries or burnout in competitive sports. Negative experiences during childhood may result in a decreased desire to engage in sport and exercise in adolescence or adulthood, potentially placing the child at greater risk for PA-related illnesses. (Interested readers are referred to Chapter 40 for discussion of overuse injuries).

A growing concern in both youth and adult sports is the risk for concussion and its potential impact on short- and long-term cognitive ability and mental health. While the risk for concussion in youth sports remains comparatively low, there appears to be considerable variance across sports with contact sports generally presenting the greatest level of risk.[175] Nevertheless, a number of initiatives, such as the Centers for Disease Control's 'Heads Up' campaign have been launched in an attempt to educate those involved in the delivery of youth sports on the prevention, recognition, and treatment of concussive injuries in youth sports.[176]

It should be emphasized that all sports and active recreational pursuits carry increased injury risk, yet the risks should be considered relative to the benefits. However, we should not forget the moral issue of when, or at what age or stage of development, a child is capable of making such important judgements. The roles and responsibilities of teachers, parents, sports governing bodies, and coaches in this matter are considerable.

Conclusions

To optimize both physical and psychological health, there is little doubt that children should be encouraged to be and remain physically active through the lifespan and avoid prolonged engagement in sedentary behaviours. It is equally important that children participate in a range of activities that are appropriate to their readiness and developmental level. That said, our understanding of degree to which children need to engage in these activities to obtain these benefits and the various factors, processes, and mechanisms which explain the short- and long-term benefits of PA in youth remain unclear. While recent advances in methods of assessment and analysis have shed new light into this area, it is clear that much continued work needs to be done in order to better understand the complex relationship between PA, sedentary behaviour, and health in youth. Perhaps an even more complex and important question to answer is how we best encourage youth to be and remain physically active through the lifespan. In order to answer this question, it is clear that researchers will need to adopt a more interdisciplinary and/or biocultural approach, considering how biology, psychology, public policy, and the built environment (among other disciplines) interact to explain individual differences in PA and health. Only then will we gain a true understanding of the relationship between PA, sedentary behaviour, and health in youth. This is the challenge for the health scientists and practitioners of the future, and one that must be addressed if we are to solve the problem of inactivity and its health implications.

Summary

- The past two decades have seen a noticeable increase in the quantity and quality of evidence linking physical activity (PA)/ sedentary behaviour/fitness with various health parameters in children.
- That said, our general understanding of how PA and, more recently, sedentary behaviour, impacts on the current or future health of children remain limited. This is most likely due to a number of factors including i) a lack of large scale, longitudinal studies, and randomized control trials, ii) difficulties inherent in measuring health, fitness, sedentary behaviour, and PA over the adolescent period (e.g. naturally occurring shifts in blood pressure, lipids, activity patterns, adiposity), iii) a general failure to control for potential confounders (e.g. growth and maturation), and iv) the potential for individual differences in responsivity to exercise and/or training.
- Given the strong and consistent relations between PA/fitness and health in adults, it is highly likely that ensuring adequate PA and fitness in children will be of ultimate benefit. However, we must be clear that we are basing this judgement largely on limited (but developing) paediatric data, strong adult data, a good measure of common sense, and sound physiological and psychological principles.
- It is intuitively logical that preventive measures, i.e. the fostering of active lifestyles, should begin early in life, and that 'the public health goal of physical education is to prepare children for a lifetime of regular physical activity'.[177] We must not forget that PA is our evolutionary heritage—we have evolved as a species for an active lifestyle, and yet we are now living in an environment which is toxic to PA and embraces sedentary behaviours, where the opportunities for children—and adults—to be physically active are fast disappearing.
- Only enlightened public policy regarding school curricula, school transportation, safe play areas outside of the house, increased licence for children to roam, and enhanced sports opportunities can change this situation for tomorrow's adults.

References

1. Barnes J, Behrens TK, Benden ME, *et al.* Letter to the editor: Standardized use of the terms 'sedentary' and 'sedentary behaviours'. *Appl Physiol Nutr Metab.* 2012; 37: 540–542.
2. Tremblay MS, LeBlanc AG, Kho ME, *et al.* Systematic review of sedentary behaviour and health indicators in school-aged children and youth. *Int J Behav Nutr Phys Act.* 2011; 8: 98.
3. Mitchell JA, Byun W. Sedentary behavior and health outcomes in children and adolescents. *Am J Life Med.* 2013; 8: 173–199.
4. Marshall SJ, Biddle SJH, Sallis JF, McKenzie TL, Conway TL. Clustering of sedentary behaviors and physical activity among youth: A cross-national study. *Pediatr Exerc Sci.* 2002; 14: 401–417.
5. American Academy of Pediatrics. Intensive training and sports specialization in young athletes. *Pediatrics.* 2006; 106: 154–157.
6. World Health Organization. *Report of the commission on ending childhood obesity.* Geneva, Switzerland: World Health Organization; 2016.
7. Tremblay MS, Gonzalez SA, Katzmarzyk PT, *et al.* Physical activity report cards: Active healthy kids global alliance and the lancet physical activity observatory. *J Phys Act Health.* 2015; 12: 297–298.
8. Owen N, Healy GN, Matthews CE, Dunstan DW. Too much sitting: The population health science of sedentary behavior. *Exerc Sport Sci Rev.* 2010; 38: 105–113.
9. Owen N. Ambulatory monitoring and sedentary behaviour: A population-health perspective. *Physiol Meas.* 2012; 33: 1801–1810.
10. Ng SW, Popkin BM. Time use and physical activity: A shift away from movement across the globe. *Obes Rev.* 2012; 13: 659–680.
11. Lee IM. Dose-response relation between physical activity and fitness—even a little is good; more is better. *JAMA.* 2007; 297: 2137–2139.
12. Armstrong N, Welsman JR. The physical activity patterns of European youth with reference to methods of assessment. *Sports Med.* 2006; 36: 1067–1086.
13. Malina RM, Katzmarzyk PT. Physical activity and fitness in an international growth standard for preadolescent and adolescent children. *Food Nutr Bull.* 2006; 27: S295–S313.
14. Department of Health and Social Services. *The health of the nation.* London: H.M.S.O; 1992.
15. Department of Health and Social Services. *Strategy statement on physical activity.* London: Department of Health; 1996.
16. U.S. Department of Health and Human Services. *Physical activity and health: A report of the surgeon general.* Pittsburgh, PA: Department of Health and Human Services, Centers for Disease Control and Prevention, National Center for Chronic Disease Prevention and Health Promotion; 1996
17. Dollman J, Norton K, Norton L. Evidence for secular trends in children's physical activity behaviour. *Br J Sport Med.* 2005; 39: 892–897.
18. Bassett DR, John D, Conger SA, Fitzhugh EC, Coe DP. Trends in physical activity and sedentary behaviors of United States youth. *J Phys Act Health.* 2015; 12: 1102–1111.
19. Croker H, Lucas R, Wardle J. Cluster-randomised trial to evaluate the 'change for life' mass media/social marketing campaign in the UK. *BMC Pub Health.* 2012; 12: 404; doi: 10.1186/1471-2458-12-404
20. Armstrong N, Mechelen WV. Are young people fit and active? In: Biddle SJH, Sallis JF, Cavill N (eds.) *Young and active? Young people and health-enhancing physical activity: Evidence and implications.* London Health Education Authority; 1998. p. 69–97.
21. Harris J, Cale L. A review of children's fitness testing. *Eur Phys Educ Rev.* 2006; 12: 201–225.
22. Ekelund U, Sardhina LB, Anderssen SA, *et al.* Associations between physical activity and body fatness in 9- to 10-year old children: The European Youth Heart Study. *Med Sci Sports Exerc.* 2004; 36: S183.
23. Ekelund U, Sardinha LB, Anderssen SA, *et al.* Associations between objectively assessed physical activity and indicators of body fatness in 9- to 10-year-old European children: A population-based study from 4 distinct regions in Europe (The European Youth Heart Study). *Am J Clin Nutr.* 2004; 80: 584–590.
24. Ness AR, Leary SD, Mattocks C, *et al.* Objectively measured physical activity and fat mass in a large cohort of children. *PLOS Med.* 2007; 4: 476–84.
25. Andersen LB, Harro M, Sardinha LB, *et al.* Physical activity and clustered cardiovascular risk in children: A cross-sectional study (The European Youth Heart Study). *Lancet.* 2006; 368: 299–304.
26. Brage S, Wedderkopp N, Ekelund U, *et al.* Objectively measured physical activity correlates with indices of insulin resistance in Danish children. The European Youth Heart Study (EYHS). *Int J Obesity.* 2004; 28: 1503–1508.
27. Ekelund U, Brage S, Froberg K, *et al.* TV viewing and physical activity are independently associated with metabolic risk in children: The European Youth Heart Study. *PLOS Med.* 2006; 3: 2449–2457.
28. Tobias JH, Steer CD, Mattocks C, Riddoch C, Ness AR. Habitual levels of physical activity influence bone mass in 11-year-old children from the UK: Findings from a large population-based cohort. *J Bone Miner Res.* 2006; 21: S206.
29. Blair SN, Clark DG, Cureton KJ, Powell KE. Exercise and fitness in childhood: Implications for a lifetime of health. In: Gisolfi CV, Lamb DR (eds.) *Perspectives in exercise science and sports medicine.* New York: McGraw-Hill; 1989. p. 401–430.
30. Caspersen CJ, Powell KE, Christenson GM. Physical-activity, exercise, and physical-fitness—definitions and distinctions for health-related research. *Public Health Rep.* 1985; 100: 126–131.
31. Lamonte MJ, Ainsworth BE. Quantifying energy expenditure and physical activity in the context of dose response. *Med Sci Sports Exerc.* 2001; 33: S370–S378.
32. Wareham NJ, Rennie KL. The assessment of physical activity in individuals and populations: Why try to be more precise about how physical activity is assessed? *Int J Obes.* 1998; 22: S30–S38.
33. Rowlands AV. Accelerometer assessment of physical activity in children: An update. *Pediatr Exerc Sci.* 2007; 19: 252–266.
34. Hardy LL, Hills AP, Timperio A, *et al.* A hitchhiker's guide to assessing sedentary behaviour among young people: Deciding what method to use. *J Sci Med Sport.* 2013; 16: 28–35.
35. Kohl HW, Fulton JE, Caspersen CJ. Assessment of physical activity among children and adolescents: A review and synthesis. *Prev Med.* 2000; 31: S54–S76.
36. Adamo KB, Prince SA, Tricco AC, Connor-Gorber S, Tremblay M. A comparison of indirect versus direct measures for assessing physical activity in the pediatric population: A systematic review. *Int J Pediatr Obes.* 2009; 4: 2–27.
37. Bailey RC, Olson J, Pepper SL, *et al.* The level and tempo of childrens physical activities—an observational study. *Med Sci Sports Exerc.* 1995; 27: 1033–1041.
38. Loveday A, Sherar LB, Sanders JP, Sanderson PW, Esliger DW. Technologies that assess the location of physical activity and sedentary behavior: A systematic review. *J Med Internet Res.* 2015; 17: 8.
39. Baranowski T, Bouchard C, Baror O, *et al.* Assessment, prevalence, and cardiovascular benefits of physical-activity and fitness in youth. *Med Sci Sports Exerc.* 1992; 24: S237–S247.
40. Malina RM, Bouchard C, Bar-Or O. *Growth maturation and physical activity.* Champaign, IL: Human Kinetics: 2004.
41. Cumming SP, Standage M, Loney T, *et al.* The mediating role of physical self-concept on relations between biological maturity status and physical activity in adolescent females. *J Adolesc.* 2011; 34: 465–473.
42. Sherar LB, Cumming SP, Eisenmann JC, Baxter-Jones ADG, Malina RM. Adolescent biological maturity and physical activity: Biology meets behavior. *Pediatr Exerc Sci.* 2010; 22: 332–349.
43. Machado Rodrigues AMM, Silva MJCE, Mota J, *et al.* Confounding effect of biologic maturation on sex differences in physical activity and sedentary behavior in adolescents. *Pediatr Exerc Sci.* 2010; 22: 442–453.
44. Bordalo MF, Portal MD, Cader S, *et al.* Comparison of the effect of two sports training methods on the flexibility of rhythmic gymnasts

at different levels of biological maturation. *J Sport Med Phys Fit*. 2015; 55: 457–463.
45. Malina RM, Rogol AD, Cumming SP, Silva MJCE, Figueiredo AJ. Biological maturation of youth athletes: Assessment and implications. *Br J Sport Med*. 2015; 49: 852–859.
46. Baxter-Jones ADG, Eisenmann JC, Sherar LB. Controlling for maturation in pediatric exercise science. *Pediatr Exerc Sci*. 2005; 17: 18–30.
47. Byers JA. The biology of human play. *Child Dev*. 1998; 69: 599–600.
48. Pellegrini AD, Smith PK. Physical activity play: Consensus and debate. *Child Dev*. 1998; 69: 609–610.
49. Timmons BW, LeBlanc AG, Carson V, *et al*. Systematic review of physical activity and health in the early years (aged 0–4 years). *Appl Physiol Nutr Me*. 2012; 37: 773–792.
50. Ebbeling CB, Pawlak DB, Ludwig DS. Childhood obesity: Public-health crisis, common sense cure. *Lancet*. 2002; 360: 473–482.
51. Wang Y, Lobstein T. Worldwide trends in childhood overweight and obesity. *Int J Pediatr Obes*. 2006; 1: 11–25.
52. Bluher S, Meigen C, Gausche R, *et al*. Age-specific stabilization in obesity prevalence in german children: A cross-sectional study from 1999 to 2008. *Int J Pediatr Obes*. 2011; 6: E199–E206.
53. Keane E, Kearney PM, Perry IJ, Kelleher CC, Harrington JM. Trends and prevalence of overweight and obesity in primary school aged children in the Republic of Ireland from 2002–2012: A systematic review. *BMC Pub Health*. 2014; 14: 974.
54. Rokholm B, Baker JL, Sorensen TIA. The levelling off of the obesity epidemic since the year 1999—a review of evidence and perspectives. *Obes Rev*. 2010; 11: 835–846.
55. Jimenez-Pavon D, Kelly J, Reilly JJ. Associations between objectively measured habitual physical activity and adiposity in children and adolescents: Systematic review. *Int J Pediatr Obes*. 2010; 5: 3–18.
56. Ekelund U, Luan JA, Sherar LB, *et al*. Moderate to vigorous physical activity and sedentary time and cardiometabolic risk factors in children and adolescents. *JAMA*. 2012; 307: 704–712.
57. Hung LS, Tidwell DK, Hall ME, *et al*. A meta-analysis of school-based obesity prevention programs demonstrates limited efficacy of decreasing childhood obesity. *Nutr Res*. 2015; 35: 229–240.
58. Stone EJ, McKenzie TL, Welk GJ, Booth ML. Effects of physical activity interventions in youth—review and synthesis. *Am J Prev Med*. 1998; 15: 298–315.
59. Sothern MS. Obesity prevention in children: Physical activity and nutrition. *Nutrition*. 2004; 20: 704–708.
60. Must A, Jacques PF, Dallal GE, Bajema CJ, Dietz WH. Long-term morbidity and mortality of overweight adolescents—a follow-up of the Harvard Growth Study of 1922 to 1935. *New Engl J Med*. 1992; 327: 1350–1355.
61. Must A, Tybor DJ. Physical activity and sedentary behavior: A review of longitudinal studies of weight and adiposity in youth. *Int J Obes*. 2005; 29: S84–S96.
62. Whitlock G, Lewington S, Sherliker P, *et al*. Body-mass index and cause-specific mortality in 900 000 adults: Collaborative analyses of 57 prospective studies. *Lancet*. 2009; 373: 1083–1096.
63. Llewellyn A, Simmonds M, Owen CG, Woolacott N. Childhood obesity as a predictor of morbidity in adulthood: A systematic review and meta-analysis. *Obes Rev*. 2016; 17: 56–67.
64. Andersen LB, Wedderkopp N. Biological cardiovascular risk factors cluster in Danish children and adolescents: The European Youth Heart Study. *Prev Med*. 2003; 37: 363–367.
65. Jackson-Leach R, Lobstein T. Estimated burden of paediatric obesity and co-morbidities in Europe. Part 1. The increase in the prevalence of child obesity in Europe is itself increasing. *Int J Pediatr Obes*. 2006; 1: 26–32.
66. Johnson WD, Kroon JJM, Greenway FL, *et al*. Prevalence of risk factors for metabolic syndrome in adolescents national health and nutrition examination survey (NHANES), 2001–2006. *Arch Pediat Adol Med*. 2009; 163: 371–377.
67. Hsia YF, Neubert AC, Rani F, *et al*. An increase in the prevalence of type 1 and 2 diabetes in children and adolescents: Results from prescription data from a UK general practice database. *Br J Clin Pharmacol*. 2009; 67: 242–249.
68. Dabelea D, Mayer-Davis EJ, Saydah S, *et al*. Prevalence of type 1 and type 2 diabetes among children and adolescents from 2001 to 2009. *JAMA*. 2014; 311: 1778–1786.
69. Juonala M, Viikari JSA, Raitakari OT. Main findings from the prospective cardiovascular risk in young finns study. *Curr Opin Lipidol*. 2013; 24: 57–64.
70. Alpert BS, Wilmore JH. Physical activity and blood pressure in adolescents. *Pediatr Exerc Sci*. 1994; 6: 361–380.
71. Armstrong N, Simons-Morton B. Physical activity and blood lipids in adolescents. *Pediatr Exerc Sci*. 1994; 6: 381–405.
72. Riddoch CJ. Relationships between physical activity and physical health in young people. In: Biddle SJH, Sallis JF (eds.) *Young and active?* London: Health Education Authority; 1998. p. 17–48.
73. Spruyt K, Molfese DL, Gozal D. Sleep duration, sleep regularity, body weight, and metabolic homeostasis in school-aged children. *Pediatrics*. 2011; 127: E345–E502.
74. Sardinha LB, Andersen LB, Anderssen SA, *et al*. Objectively measured time spent sedentary is associated with insulin resistance independent of overall and central body fat in 9- to 10-year-old Portuguese children. *Diabetes Care*. 2008; 31: 569–575.
75. Brage S, Wedderkopp N, Ekelund U, *et al*. Features of the metabolic syndrome are associated with objectively measured physical activity and fitness in Danish children—the European Youth Heart Study. *Diabetes Care*. 2004; 27: 2141–2148.
76. Carson V, Janssen I. Volume, patterns, and types of sedentary behavior and cardio-metabolic health in children and adolescents: A cross-sectional study. *BMC Pub Health*. 2011; 11: 274.
77. Healy GN, Matthews CE, Dunstan DW, Winkler EAH, Owen N. Sedentary time and cardio-metabolic biomarkers in us adults: NHANES 2003–06. *Eur Heart J*. 2011; 32: 590–597.
78. Healy GN, Wijndaele K, Dunstan DW, *et al*. Objectively measured sedentary time, physical activity, and metabolic risk the Australian Diabetes, Obesity and Lifestyle Study (AUSDIAB). *Diabetes Care*. 2008; 31: 369–371.
79. Henson J, Yates T, Biddle SJH, *et al*. Associations of objectively measured sedentary behaviour and physical activity with markers of cardiometabolic health. *Diabetologia*. 2013; 56: 1012–1020.
80. Cooper C, Campion G, Melton LJ. Hip-fractures in the elderly—a worldwide projection. *Osteoporosis Int*. 1992; 2: 285–289.
81. Hui SL, Slemenda CW, Johnston CC. The contribution of bone loss to post menopausal osteoporosis. *Osteoporosis Int*. 1990; 1: 30–34.
82. Theintz G, Buchs B, Rizzoli R, *et al*. Longitudinal monitoring of bone mass accumulation in healthy adolescents—evidence for a marked reduction after 16 years of age at the levels of lumbar spine and femoral neck in female subjects. *J Clin Endocrinol Metab*. 1992; 75: 1060–1065.
83. Lu PW, Brody JN, Ogle GD. Bone mineral density of total body, spine and femoral neck in children and young adults: A cross-sectional and longitudinal study. *J Bone Min Res*. 1994; 9: 1451–1458.
84. Tan VP, Macdonald HM, Kim S, *et al*. Influence of physical activity on bone strength in children and adolescents: A systematic review and narrative synthesis. *J Bone Min Res*. 2014; 29: 2161–2181.
85. Behringer M, Gruetzner S, McCourt M, Mester J. Effects of weight-bearing activities on bone mineral content and density in children and adolescents: A meta-analysis. *J Bone Min Res*. 2014; 29: 467–478.
86. Hind K, Burrows M. Weight-bearing exercise and bone mineral accrual in children and adolescents: A review of controlled trials. *Bone*. 2007; 40: 14–27.
87. MacKelvie KJ, Khan KM, McKay HA. Is there a critical period for bone response to weight-bearing exercise in children and adolescents? A systematic review. *Br J Sport Med*. 2002; 36: 250–257.
88. Ishikawa S, Kim Y, Kang M, Morgan DW. Effects of weight-bearing exercise on bone health in girls: A meta-analysis. *Sports Med*. 2013; 43: 875–892.
89. Grimston SK, Willows ND, Hanley DA. Mechanical loading regime and its relationship to bone-mineral density in children. *Med Sci Sports Exerc*. 1993; 25: 1203–1210.

90. Vuori I. Peak bone mass and physical activity: A short review. *Nutr Rev.* 1996; 54: S11–S14.
91. Rubin K, Schirduan V, Gendreau P, *et al.* Predictors of axial and peripheral bone-mineral density in healthy children and adolescents, with special attention to the role of puberty. *J Pediatr.* 1993; 123: 863–870.
92. Lanyon LE. Using functional loading to influence bone mass and architecture: Objectives, mechanisms, and relationship with estrogen of the mechanically adaptive process in bone. *Bone.* 1996; 18: S37–S43.
93. Morris F, Naughton GA, Gibbs JL, Carlson J, Wark JG. Prospective ten-month exercise intervention in premenarcheal girls: Positive effects on bone and lean mass. *J Bone Min Res.* 1997; 12: 1453–1462.
94. Deere K, Sayers A, Rittweger J, Tobias JH. Habitual levels of high, but not moderate or low, impact activity are positively related to hip bmd and geometry: Results from a population-based study of adolescents. *J Bone Min Res.* 2012; 27: 1887–1895.
95. Janz KF, Burns TL, Torner JC, *et al.* Physical activity and bone measures in young children: The Iowa Bone Development Study. *Pediatrics.* 2001; 107: 1387–1393.
96. Janz KF, Letuchy EM, Burns TL, *et al.* Objectively measured physical activity trajectories predict adolescent bone strength: Iowa Bone Development Study. *Br J Sport Med.* 2014; 48: 1032–1036.
97. Kim H, Iwasaki K, Miyake T, *et al.* Changes in bone turnover markers during 14-day 6 degrees head-down bed rest. *J Bone Min Metab.* 2003; 21: 311–315.
98. Zerwekh JE, Ruml LA, Gottschalk F, Pak CYC. The effects of twelve weeks of bed rest on bone histology, biochemical markers of bone turnover, and calcium homeostasis in eleven normal subjects. *J Bone Min Res.* 1998; 13: 1594–1601.
99. Tremblay MS, Colley RC, Saunders TJ, Healy GN, Owen N. Physiological and health implications of a sedentary lifestyle. *Appl Physiol Nutr Metab.* 2010; 35: 725–740.
100. Moreno LA, Gottrand F, Huybrechts I, *et al.* Nutrition and lifestyle in European adolescents: The HELENA (HEalthy Lifestyle in Europe by Nutrition in Adolescence) study. *Adv Nutr.* 2014; 5: 615s–623s.
101. Chastin SFM, Mandrichenko O, Skelton DA. The frequency of osteogenic activities and the pattern of intermittence between periods of physical activity and sedentary behaviour affects bone mineral content: The cross-sectional NHANES study. *BMC Pub Health.* 2014; 14: 4.
102. Biddle SJH, Mutrie N. *Psychology of physical activity: Determinants, well-being and interventions.* London: Routledge; 2005.
103. Faulkner GEJ, Taylor AH. *Exercise and mental health: Emerging relationships.* London: Routledge; 2005.
104. Mutrie N, Parfitt G. Physical activity and its link with mental, social and moral health in young people. In: Biddle SJH, Sallis JF, Cavill N (eds.) *Young and active.* London: Health Education Authority; 1998. p. 49–68.
105. Stubbe JH, Moor MHM, Boomsma DI, Gues EJC. The association between exercise participation and well-being: A co-twin study. *Prev Med.* 2007; 24: 148–152.
106. Parfitt G, Eston RG. The relationship between children's habitual activity level and psychological well-being. *Acta Paediatr.* 2005; 94: 1791–1797.
107. Yin ZN, Davis CL, Moore JB, Treiber FA. Physical activity buffers the effects of chronic stress on adiposity in youth. *Ann Behav Med.* 2005; 29: 29–36.
108. Storch EA, Milsom VA, DeBraganza N, *et al.* Peer victimization, psychosocial adjustment, and physical activity in overweight and at-risk-for-overweight youth. *J Pediatr Psychol.* 2007; 32: 80–89.
109. Wiles NJ, Haase AM, Lawlor DA, Ness A, Lewis G. Physical activity and depression in adolescents: Cross-sectional findings from the ALSPAC cohort. *Soc Psychiatry Psychiatr Epidemiol.* 2012; 47: 1023–1033.
110. Weinberg RS, Gould D. *Foundations of sport and exercise psychology,* 4th ed. Champaign, IL: Human Kinetics: 2007.
111. Chaddock L, Hillman CH, Pontifex MB, *et al.* Childhood aerobic fitness predicts cognitive performance one year later. *J Sport Sci.* 2012; 30: 421–430.
112. Smith AL, Hoza B, Linnea K, *et al.* Pilot physical activity intervention reduces severity of ADHD symptoms in young children. *J Atten Disord.* 2013; 17: 70–82.
113. Liu M, Wu L, Yao S. Dose–response association of screen time-based sedentary behaviour in children and adolescents and depression: A meta-analysis of observational studies. *Br J of Sports Med.* 2016; 50: 1252–1258.
114. Belanger RE, Akre C, Berchtold A, Michaud PA. A U-shaped association between intensity of internet use and adolescent health. *Pediatrics.* 2011; 127: E330–E335.
115. Przybylski AK. Electronic gaming and psychosocial adjustment. *Pediatrics.* 2014; 134: E716–E722.
116. Teychenne M, Costigan SA, Parker K. The association between sedentary behaviour and risk of anxiety: A systematic review. *BMC Pub Health.* 2015; 15: 513.
117. Suchert V, Hanewinkel R, Isensee B. Sedentary behavior and indicators of mental health in school-aged children and adolescents: A systematic review. *Prev Med.* 2015; 76: 48–57.
118. Everett-Jones S, Merkle SL, Fulton JE, Wheeler LS, Mannino DM. Relationship between asthma, overweight, and physical activity among us high school students. *J of Comm Health.* 2006; 31: 469–478.
119. Beggs S, Foong YC, Le HC, *et al.* Swimming training for asthma in children and adolescents aged 18 years and under. *Paediatr Respir Rev.* 2013; 14: 96–97.
120. Pindus DM, Davis RDM, Hillman CH, *et al.* The relationship of moderate-to-vigorous physical activity to cognitive processing in adolescents: Findings from the ALSPAC birth cohort. *Psychol Res-Psych Fo.* 2015; 79: 715–728.
121. Barker DJP. The fetal and infant origins of adult disease. *Br Med J.* 1990; 301(6761): 1111.
122. Wiebe HW, Boule NG, Chari R, Davenport MH. The effect of supervised prenatal exercise on fetal growth a meta-analysis. *Obstet Gynecol.* 2015; 125: 1185–1194.
123. Riddoch C, Savage JM, Murphy N, Cran GW, Boreham C. Long-term health implications of fitness and physical-activity patterns. *Arch Dis Child.* 1991; 66: 1426–1433.
124. Jones RA, Hinkley T, Okely AD, Salmon J. Tracking physical activity and sedentary behavior in childhood a systematic review. *Am J Prev Med.* 2013; 44: 651–658.
125. Malina RM. Tracking of physical activity across the lifespan. *President's Council on Physical Fitness and Sports Research Digest.* 2001; 3(14): 1–8.
126. Telama R. Tracking of physical activity from childhood to adulthood: A review. *Obesity Facts.* 2009; 2: 187–195.
127. Biddle SJH, Pearson N, Ross GM, Braithwaite R. Tracking of sedentary behaviours of young people: A systematic review. *Prev Med.* 2010; 51: 345–351.
128. Cleland V, Dwyer T, Venn A. Which domains of childhood physical activity predict physical activity in adulthood? A 20-year prospective tracking study. *Br J Sport Med.* 2012; 46: 595–602.
129. Engstrom LM. The process of socialisation into keep-fit activities. *J Sport Sci Med.* 1986; 8: 89–97.
130. Babic MJ, Morgan PJ, Plotnikoff RC, *et al.* Physical activity and physical self-concept in youth: Systematic review and meta-analysis. *Sports Med.* 2014; 44: 1589–1601.
131. Ryan RM, Deci EL. Intrinsic and extrinsic motivations: Classic definitions and new directions. *Contemp Educ Psychol.* 2000; 25: 54–67.
132. Voss C. British Journal of Sports Medicine Blog. *A Global Fail? International Comparisons of Physical Activity of Children and Youth Report Cards.* 24 June, 2014. Available from: http://blogs.bmj.com/bjsm/2014/06/24/a-global-fail-international-comparisons-of-physical-activity-of-children-and-youth-report-cards/. [Cited 2016]
133. Cale L, Almond L. Children's activity levels:A review of studies conducted on British children. *Phys Educ Rev.* 1992; 15: 111–118.

134. Sallis JF. Epidemiology of physical-activity and fitness in children and adolescents. *Crit Rev Food Sci.* 1993; 33: 403–408.
135. Astrand PO. Physical activity and fitness: Evolutionary perspective and trends for the future. In: Bouchard C, Shephard RJ, Stephens T (eds.) *Physical activity, fitness, and health: International proceedings and consensus statement.* Champaign, IL: Human Kinetics; 1994. p. 98–105.
136. Rowland TW. *Exercise and children's health.* Champaign, IL: Human Kinetics Books: 1990.
137. Blair SN, Meredith MD. The exercise-health relationship: Does it apply to children and youth? In: Pate RR, Hohn RC (eds.) *Health and fitness through physical education.* Champaign, IL: Human Kinetics; 1994. p. 11–19.
138. Blair SN. Are american children and youth fit? The need for better data. *Res Q Exerc Sport.* 1992; 63: 120–123.
139. Cooper AR, Goodman A, Page AS, *et al.* Objectively measured physical activity and sedentary time in youth: The International Children's Accelerometry Database (ICAD). *Int J Behav Nutr Phy.* 2015; 12: 113: doi: 10.1186/s12966-015-0274-5
140. American College of Sports Medicine. Physical fitness in children and youth. *Med Sci Sports Exerc.* 1988; 20: 422–423.
141. Sallis JF, Patrick K. Physical activity guidelines for adolescents: A consensus statement. *Pediatr Exerc Sci.* 1988; 6: 302–314.
142. Biddle SJH, Sallis JF, Cavill N. *Young and active? Young people and health-enhancing physical activity—evidence and implications.* London: London Health Education Authority: 1998.
143. Department of Health Physical Activity Health Improvement and Prevention. *At least five a week: Evidence on the impact of physical activity and its relationship to health.* London: Department of Health: 2004.
144. Tremblay MS, Warburton DER, Janssen I, *et al.* New Canadian physical activity guidelines. *Appl Physiol Nutr Metab.* 2011; 36: 36–46.
145. Montgomery HE, Marshall R, Hemingway H, *et al.* Human gene for physical performance. *Nature.* 1998; 393: 221–222.
146. Blair SN, Kohl HW, Paffenbarger RS, *et al.* Physical-fitness and all-cause mortality—a prospective-study of healthy-men and women. *JAMA.* 1989; 262: 2395–2401.
147. Cooper AR, Page A, Fox KR, Misson J. Physical activity patterns in normal, overweight and obese individuals using minute-by-minute accelerometry. *Eur J Clin Nutr.* 2000; 54: 887–894.
148. Farrell SW, Kampert JB, Kohl HW, *et al.* Influences of cardiorespiratory fitness levels and other predictors on cardiovascular disease mortality in men. *Med Sci Sports Exerc.* 1998; 30: 899–905.
149. Gibbons LW, Blair SN, Cooper KH, Smith M. Association between coronary heart-disease risk-factors and physical-fitness in healthy adult women. *Circulation.* 1983; 67: 977–983.
150. Sandvik L, Erikssen J, Thaulow E, *et al.* Physical-fitness as a predictor of mortality among healthy, middle-aged Norwegian men. *New Engl J Med.* 1993; 328: 533–537.
151. Van Saarse J, Noteboom WMP, Vandenbrouke JP. Longevity of men capable of prolonged vigorous physical exercise: A 32-year follow-up of 2259 participants in the dutch eleven cities ice skating tour. *Br Med J.* 1990; 301: 1409–1411.
152. Blair SN, Kohl HW3rd, Barlow CE, *et al.* Changes in physical-fitness and all-cause mortality—a prospective-study of healthy and unhealthy men. *JAMA.* 1995; 273: 1093–1098.
153. Thompson GR, Wilson PW. *Coronary risk factors and their assessment.* London: London Science Press: 1982.
154. Raitakari OT, Porkka KVK, Rasanen L, Ronnemaa T, Viikari JSA. Clustering and 6 year cluster-tracking of serum total cholesterol, HDL-cholesterol and diastolic blood-pressure in children and young-adults—the cardiovascular risk in young finns study. *J Clin Epidemiol.* 1994; 47: 1085–1093.
155. Hofman A, Walter HJ. The association between physical fitness and cardiovascular disease risk factors in children in a five-year follow-up study. *Int J of Epidemiol.* 1989; 18: 830–835.
156. Tell GS, Vellar OD. Physical fitness, physical activity, and cardiovascular disease risk-factors in adolescents—The Oslo Youth Study. *Prev Med.* 1988; 17: 12–24.
157. Dencker M, Thorsson O, Karlsson MK, *et al.* Aerobic fitness related to composite risk factor score for CVD in children. *Circulation.* 2012; 125: E832–E832.
158. Eriksson BO, Koch G. Effect of physical training on hemodynamic response during submaximal and maximal exercise in 11-year-old to 13-year-old boys. *Acta Physiol Scand.* 1973; 87: 27–39.
159. Hansen HS, Froberg K, Hyldebrandt N, Nielsen JR. A controlled-study of 8 months of physical training and reduction of blood pressure in children—The Odense Schoolchild Study. *Br Med J.* 1991; 303: 682–685.
160. Alberga AS, Frappier A, Sigal RJ, Prud'homme D, Kenny GP. A review of randomized controlled trials of aerobic exercise training on fitness and cardiometabolic risk factors in obese adolescents. *Physician Sportsmed.* 2013; 41: 44–57.
161. Boreham CAG, Strain JJ, Twisk JWR, *et al.* Aerobic fitness physical activity and body fatness in adolescents. In: Armstrong N, Kirby B, Welsman JR (eds.) *Children and exercise.* London: E and FN Spon; 1997. p. 69–74.
162. Gutin B, Islam S, Manos T, Cucuzzo N, Smith C, Stachura ME. Relation of percentage of body fat and maximal aerobic capacity to risk-factors for atherosclerosis and diabetes in black and white 7–11-year-old children. *J Pediatr.* 1994; 125: 847–852.
163. Hager RL, Tucker LA, Seljaas GT. Aerobic fitness, blood lipids and body fat in children. *Am J Public Health.* 1995; 85: 1702–1706.
164. Bergstrom E, Hernell O, Persson LA. Endurance running performance in relation to cardiovascular risk indicators in adolescents. *Int J Sports Med.* 1997; 18: 300–307.
165. Fripp RR, Hodgson JL, Kwiterovich PO, *et al.* Aerobic capacity, obesity, and atherosclerotic risk factors in male adolescents. *Pediatrics.* 1985; 75: 813–818.
166. Hansen HS, Hyldebrandt N, Nielsen JR, Froberg K. Blood pressure distribution in a school-age population aged 8–10 years—The Odense Schoolchild Study. *J Hypertens.* 1990; 8: 641–646.
167. Sallis JF, Patterson TL, Buono MJ, Nader PR. Relation of cardiovascular fitness and physical activity to cardiovascular disease risk factors in children and adults. *Am J Epidemiol.* 1988; 127: 933–941.
168. Haddock BL, Hopp HP, Mason JJ, Blix G, Blair SN. Cardiorespiratory fitness and cardiovascular disease risk factors in postmenopausal women. *Med Sci Sports Exerc.* 1998; 30: 893–898.
169. Lavie CJ, McAuley PA, Church TS, Milani RV, Blair SN. Obesity and cardiovascular diseases. *J Am Coll Cardiol.* 2014; 63: 1345–1354.
170. Cureton KJ. Commentary on 'Children and fitness: A public health perspective'. *Res Q.* 1987; 58: 315–320.
171. Haskell WL, Montoye HJ, Orenstein D. Physical-activity and exercise to achieve health related physical-fitness components. *Pub Health Rep.* 1985; 100: 202–212.
172. Seefeldt V, Vogel P. Children and fitness: A public health perspective. *Res Q.* 1987; 58: 331–333.
173. Van Mechelen W. Etiology and prevention of sports injuries in youth. In: Froberg K, Lammert O, Steen Hansen H, Blimkie JR (eds.) *Children and exercise xviii: Exercise and fitness—benefits and risks.* Odense: Odense University Press; 1997. p. 209–227.
174. Baxter-Jones A, Maffulli N, Helms P. Low injury rates in elite athletes. *Arch Dis Child.* 1993; 68: 130–132.
175. Pfister T, Pfister K, Hagel B, Ghali WA, Ronksley PE. The incidence of concussion in youth sports: A systematic review and meta-analysis. *Br J Sport Med.* 2016; 50: 292–297.
176. Covassin T, Elbin RJ, Larson E, Kontos AP. Sex and age differences in depression and baseline sport-related concussion neurocognitive performance and symptoms. *Clin J Sport Med.* 2012; 22: 98–104.
177. Sallis JF, McKenzie TL. Physical education's role in public health. *Res Q Exerc Sport.* 1991; 62: 124–137.

CHAPTER 17

Physical activity, cardiorespiratory fitness, and cardiovascular health

Isabel Ferreira and Jos WR Twisk

Introduction

Cardiovascular disease (CVD) remains one of the greatest causes of adult mortality worldwide. It is now recognized that CVD is partly a paediatric problem given that its onset extends back to childhood, even though clinical symptoms may not become apparent until much later in life. Therefore, from a primary prevention point of view, the extent to which physical activity or physical fitness may deter this process starting already from a young age is of utmost importance. However, in contrast to the large amount of evidence linking adults' physical activity and physical fitness to incident CVD[1,2] and all-cause mortality,[2,3] there is not much evidence linking levels of physical activity or physical fitness in young age to CVD or mortality later in life.[4] Indeed, thus far, no studies have been able to follow children and adolescents to old age to enable the examination of such association prospectively. Because CVD is rare among the young, studies investigating the relationship between physical activity, physical fitness, and cardiovascular health have therefore focused their attention on intermediary pathways linked to *traditional cardiometabolic risk factors*, as illustrated in Figure 17.1. This chapter discusses the evidence across these pathways. In addition, it also covers the associations between physical activity and physical fitness with more direct markers or *early vascular aging*,[5] enabled by the development, over the last two decades, of technology that enables its non-invasive assessment.

In the following, we refer to children if subjects were between the ages of 5 and 12 years, and to adolescents if subjects were between the ages of 13 and 18 years. The term youth is used to cover both the childhood and adolescent periods. The evidence pertaining to physical activity (the behaviour) and also to physical fitness (the attribute, with a genetic component, but also a proxy for [higher intensity] physical activity) will be appraised. Although we recognize that health-related physical fitness is not an unitary concept, but rather consists of several individual components (cardiorespiratory, muscular, motor, metabolic, morphological), typically in studies examining the association with cardiometabolic risk factors, the term 'fitness' refers to aerobic or cardiorespiratory fitness ((CRF) as expressed by direct or indirect measures of maximal oxygen uptake ($\dot{V}O_2$ max).[6]

Physical activity and cardiorespiratory fitness in youth and cardiovascular disease later in life

Paffenbarger *et al.*[4] were the first to investigate, in the Harvard Alumni Study, the relationship between physical activity in relatively

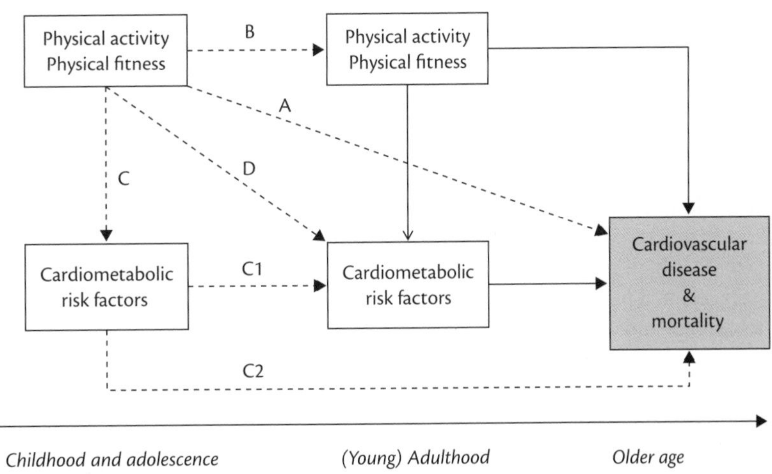

Figure 17.1 Hypothetical pathways linking physical activity and physical fitness in youth to cardiometabolic risk factors and cardiovascular disease throughout life. Paths A to D are explained in detail in the text.

young people and the occurrence of CVD at a later age. In one part of this extensive observational study, physical activity levels during the student period (gathered from university archives) were related to the occurrence of CVD later in life. Male students were divided into three groups according to their physical activity levels: i) athletes, ii) intramural sports play for >5 h · week^{-1}, and iii) intramural sports play for <5 h · week^{-1} (most often none at all) per week. Athletes who discontinued their activity levels after college had a CVD incidence similar to that of alumni classmates who never had been athletes. In fact, alumni who became physically active later in life had the same health benefits as the alumni who were active throughout the whole observation period. Since this classical study, only two other studies have examined associations between childhood/adolescent physical activity with CVD and/or mortality in adulthood.[7,8] In one of these studies, which was confined to women, exercise participation during adolescence was associated with reduced risk of CVD and all-cause mortality in adulthood, independently of adult levels of exercise.[8] The other did not find any such association, but physical activity was operationalized as that performed at work when individuals were 15 years old, which may not be a generalizable measure for contexts other than the one where the study was conducted.[7] However, both studies relied on retrospective recall of adolescent physical activity levels by adult participants.

In contrast to the large amount of evidence linking adults' physical activity and CRF to incident CVD[1,2] and all-cause mortality[2,3] there is thus not much evidence linking physical activity or CRF in young age to CVD or mortality later in life (see path 'A' in Figure 17.1). In fact, Paffenbarger's findings support the view that *maintenance* of a physically active lifestyle *throughout the course of life* may be more important for cardiovascular health than having been active as a child or adolescent per se. But to what extent are physically active children more likely to be physically active adults? In other words, *do physical activity levels in childhood predict physical activity levels in adulthood*?

Tracking of physical activity and cardiorespiratory fitness through childhood and adolescence to adulthood

The extent to which a variable measured at a young age predicts the values of the same variable later in life is called *tracking*. Tracking of physical activity levels through childhood and adolescence to (young) adulthood has been examined in many studies and reviewed elsewhere.[9,10] The overall conclusion is that the level of tracking of physical activity in this period of transition in individuals' life is low to moderate (see path 'B' in Figure 17.1). Some remarks are warranted when interpreting these findings, however.

First, statistically significant tracking coefficients do not mean that the predictive value of a variable measured during childhood or adolescence for its values later in life is high or relevant.[11] Suppose that tracking is calculated for subjects in a particular 'risk' quartile in a longitudinal study with a baseline and a follow-up measurement, and that only 50% of the initial 'high-risk' quartile maintain their position at the follow-up measurement. This would mean that the initial values had 50% predictability, and would be expressed by a very significant odds ratio of five.[12,13] Second, because tracking reflects the relative position of a certain individual within a group over the course of time, a high tracking coefficient does not mean that the level of the variable remains stable over time. It is well known that, in the general population, the level of physical activity tends to decrease from childhood to adolescence[14] and even more so from adolescence to adulthood.[15] Therefore, one could find a high tracking coefficient if all individuals would maintain their *relative position within the group*, even when all individuals in the group had decreased their levels of physical activity (which, from a health perspective, is not a desirable scenario). Third, tracking coefficients are highly influenced by measurement error. This is thought to explain, at least in part, why tracking coefficients for behavioural variables, often assessed through questionnaires and interviews (making them more susceptible to recall and other biases), tend to be lower than tracking coefficients for biological variables, such as CRF, blood lipids and measured body mass index (BMI).[12] Therefore, one would expect that tracking coefficients reported by studies that have used more objective methods to measure physical activity were higher than those reported by studies that have used questionnaires or interviews. However, the number of studies that have examined this is still comparatively small to allow definitive conclusions.[9] Aspects such as different age (and thus, mean levels of physical activity) at baseline and length of follow-up often explain variations in the tracking coefficients reported in the literature.[10] Indeed, a recent examination of the long-term tracking (i.e. from early childhood through adolescence into adulthood) that took measurement error issues into account reported that higher coefficients than those from previous long-term studies were found, and tracking of physical activity was deemed to be moderate or high.[16]

Cardiometabolic risk factors

Because the prevalence and incidence of CVD and related mortality is rather low in paediatric populations, studies investigating the relationship between physical activity, CRF, and cardiovascular health have focused their attention on cardiometabolic risk factors. Traditionally these consist of elevated levels of total body fatness and/or of central fatness, elevated levels of blood pressure (BP), dyslipidaemia (i.e. elevated total or low-density lipoprotein (LDL) cholesterol levels or triglycerides, and/or low levels of high-density lipoprotein (HDL) cholesterol), and impaired glucose metabolism and/or insulin resistance, and more recently, also their clustering.[17]

Physical activity and cardiorespiratory fitness, and cardiometabolic risk factors in youth

The last decades have witnessed an exponential increase in the number of such studies, more often resourcing to objective measures of physical activity, and pooling paediatric cohorts across countries. A wealth of evidence is now available supporting beneficial associations between physical activity and CRF and several cardiometabolic risk factors among the young (see path 'C' in Figure 17.1).

Body fatness

Many cross-sectional studies have shown that higher levels of physical activity and and CRF are both associated with lower levels of total and central fatness. Furthermore, in childhood/adolescence, an agreement exists that these associations are likely stronger for vigorous (VPA) than for light-to-moderate (LMPA) physical activities.[18] Indeed, a recent meta-analysis of 45 observational studies examining the associations between objectively measured physical activity with CRF, body composition, and other cardiometabolic risk factors showed that VPA yielded health benefits above those provided by LMPA for reduced total and central adiposity and improved CRF, while the beneficial associations with other cardiometabolic risk factors did not seem to differ consistently between different physical activity intensities.[19] Because a child or adolescent will have higher total energy expenditure when exercising at a higher intensity than when exercising for the same duration at a lower intensity, it remains unclear whether it is the intensity of physical activity or the total amount (volume) of energy expenditure that accounts for the beneficial effects of physical activity on total and central fatness. There is currently a strong debate regarding this topic. For example, one small study among non-obese children showed that high-intensity training (HIT) improved more risk factors than endurance training (ET).[20] However, another study showed that, in obese children, the health benefits induced by ET or HIT were mostly similar.[21] Because prolonged physical exercise may not match with the typical, mostly intermittent, patterns of children's physical activity, HIT prescription may appeal and be more suitable to children. This contention still needs to be elucidated by well-designed randomized control trials (RCTs) with energy expenditure matched between activities of different intensities. (Interested readers are referred to Chapter 35 where HIT is discussed in detail).

In contrast to observational (mostly cross-sectional) studies showing a strong relationship between physical activity and adiposity, and RCTs showing beneficial changes in BMI (or BMI z-scores) in overweight and obese youth,[22] the effects of physical activity on obesity *prevention* are not that consistent. For instance, a recent meta-analysis of school-based lifestyle interventions showed improvements in children's and adolescents' BMI when physical activity was used in isolation as well as in combination with diet,[23] whereas prior meta-analyses of school-based physical activity controlled trials did not show any appreciable benefit on children's BMI or other measures of body composition.[24,25] The limited success of physical activity in this setting could be explained by the very small improvements in children's physical activity levels induced by the interventions.[26] Another explanation may be that the widely reported cross-sectional associations may not reflect causality, but rather a downstream effect of obesity. The observation, in a prospective study, that increased BMI predicted subsequent declines in physical activity seems to support this reverse causality hypothesis,[27] as do the improvements in body fatness accrued after dietary interventions without additional reductions when combined with aerobic or resistance training.[28] (Interested readers are referred to Chapter 34 and Chapter 36 for detailed discussion of aerobic and resistance training, respectively). In fact, the relationship between physical activity, CRF, and body fatness or obesity is so intricate[29] that it is not clear how to make a distinction between cause and effect (Figure 17.2). This cluster of factors is assumed to constitute a risk factor for CVD on itself, but *what comes first*?

Several longitudinal studies, mostly in adults[30–33] but also in children,[34] have tried to unravel this 'chicken-and-egg' problem. Notably, all reported an inverse association between baseline body fatness and subsequent physical activity, but not between baseline physical activity and body fatness at follow-up. This supports the view that body fatness leads to physical inactivity, but that physical inactivity may not be at the root of subsequent increases in body fatness. A recent Mendelian randomization study confirmed the former but was not able to rule out the reverse, i.e. that lower physical activity may indeed lead to increased adiposity.[35] In other

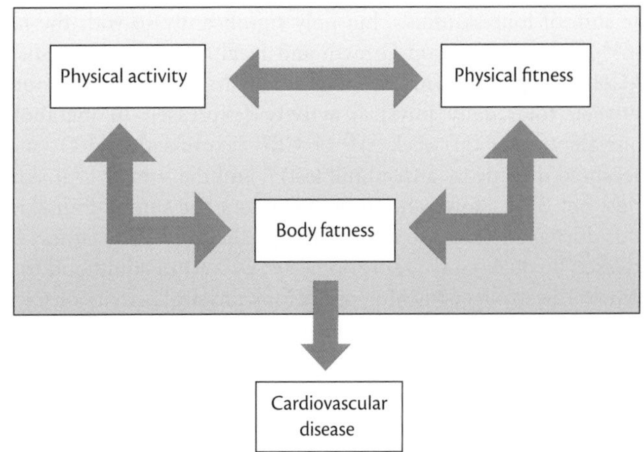

Figure 17.2 The intricate associations between physical activity, cardiorespiratory fitness, and body fatness.

words, the association between physical activity and adiposity may well be bi-directional.[36] From a pathobiological point of view, there is also rationale to support this. Overweight or obesity in children and adolescents is multifactorial but, ultimately, results from an imbalance between energy intake and energy expenditure. Because physical activity accounts for a large portion of energy expenditure in children and adolescents, chronic decreases in physical activity may lead to increases in adiposity. Conversely, the extra energy costs of carrying a greater body mass may result in earlier fatigue during exercise in overweight than in normal-weight children, discouraging them from engaging in that behaviour.[37] Noteworthy, this 'chicken and egg' problem has also been flagged around the physical activity and CRF ($\dot{V}O_2$ max) associations. Attempts to unravel it have also suggested that while both the behaviour (physical activity) and the attribute (CRF) are correlated through childhood to adolescence[38] and through adolescence to adulthood,[39] it may well be that higher CRF leads to higher physical activity instead of, or in addition to, the traditional view that physical activity leads to CRF. Lower CRF is associated with mitochondrial dysfunction, which may impair delivery of aerobic energy at the rate that is required during muscular activity, leading to an earlier accumulation of lactate, and thus muscular discomfort and lower tolerance to continue exercise.[40]

Another problem in the investigation of the physical activity–CRF–fatness relationships is related to the way body fatness has been assessed. Given the ease with which it is measured, BMI has been the most commonly used marker of total body fatness. Strictly, calculated as weight $\cdot$ height^{-2}, BMI is a measure of excess body weight, not adiposity, per se. Body skinfolds discriminate better between fat and lean masses in an individual and are therefore a more sensitive alternative for determining body fatness, especially in youth.[41] Indeed, subjects with high muscle but moderate fat mass (e.g. athletes) will tend to have high BMI but low skinfolds thicknesses. Although both BMI and body skinfolds (usually the sum of two or more) are used as markers of body fatness, they reflect different aspects of body composition. Therefore, analyses with either one or the other can lead to different results, especially if the interest is in the relationship with physical activity and/or CRF. For instance, in the European Youth Heart Study (EYHS), children and adolescent levels of physical activity, as measured by accelerometers, were inversely associated with both the BMI and the sum of four skinfolds, but only significantly so with the latter.[42] In the Amsterdam Growth and Health Longitudinal Study (AGHLS) significant inverse longitudinal associations were found between total daily physical activity (expressed in metabolic equivalents (METs) · week^{-1})[43] or CRF (expressed by $\dot{V}O_2$ max measured directly by a treadmill test)[44] and the sum of four skinfolds, not BMI. Moreover, for both genders, the sum of four skinfolds during adolescence was a better predictor of body fatness (as assessed by dual X-ray absorptiometry; DEXA) in adulthood than BMI.[45] The stronger tracking of BMI (vs physical activity or CRF) from childhood or adolescence to adulthood[12] may thus reflect relatively stronger persistence of body build than of adiposity. Moreover, when BMI is used as indicator of body fatness, the deleterious relationships between physical activity and CRF on the one hand, and body fatness on the other, can be counterbalanced by the beneficial relationships with lean body mass. In the same vein, CRF ($\dot{V}O_2$ max) should be better expressed relative to free fat mass than relative to body mass to avoid collinearity issues when examining associations of CRF with adiposity and other cardiometabolic risk factors.[46]

Blood pressure

Throughout the years the associations of physical activity or CRF with BP in children have not been unequivocal. Early narrative reviews[47,48] and a meta-analysis[49] of observational and intervention studies did not report significant decreases in systolic or diastolic BP among children and adolescents as a result of exercise training. Therefore, by 2004, the American College of Sports Medicine deemed that there was a lack of evidence on the BP-reducing effects of exercise among the young, and it did not advance any recommendations regarding exercise for the prevention or treatment of hypertension in these age groups.[50] It must be noted that BP levels in growing children are also related to the hormonal and body composition changes that characterize puberty and it may therefore be difficult to unveil effects of physical activity in the presence of such changes. Also, most of the earlier studies relied on self-reports of physical activity levels, which could have accounted for the unclear associations. (Interested readers are referred to Chapter 21 for an analysis of methods of assessing physical activity). Indeed, in the EYHS, where physical activity was measured by accelerometers, a significant inverse relationship with both systolic and diastolic BP was observed.[42] In line with these findings, CRF has also been shown to be inversely associated with BP, particularly among overweight adolescents.[51] Earlier reviews had indeed suggested that the effects of exercise interventions on BP could possibly be more visible among those who had already elevated BP[47,48] and/or obesity.[49] This was partly confirmed by recent meta-analyses of RCTs showing significant beneficial effects of exercise on BP among overweight/obese children or adolescents,[52,53] and of school-based lifestyle interventions (including physical activity or diet) among children with the highest systolic BP at baseline.[23] Another meta-analysis examining the effects of (diet and/or physical activity) obesity prevention programmes, showed also significant decreases in both systolic and diastolic BP.[54] These beneficial effects seemed greater when interventions combined diet and physical activity components than when they included diet or physical activity components only, though.[54] Noteworthy, in many of the interventions reviewed, the beneficial effects on BP were not accompanied by improvements in body fatness, suggesting that the BP-lowering effects of lifestyle interventions among the young may, at least in part, be independent of concomitant effects on adiposity.[23,54] Physical activity-related increases in stroke volume and nitric oxide availability, and decreases in resting heart rate, systemic vascular resistance, renal and muscle sympathetic nerve activity, and plasma renin activity are some of the mechanisms possibly explaining the benefits of physical activity on BP in adults.[55] However, the extent to which these mechanisms operate in (growing) children remains poorly understood.

Dyslipidaemia

In an early review, the beneficial associations of physical activity with total-, LDL-, and HDL-cholesterol as well as triglycerides reported by observational studies in school-aged children were deemed weak.[56] A more recent systematic review of mostly RCTs concluded also that the effects of physical activity on blood lipids were mixed,[6] though the RCTs included were small and had been mostly confined to children or adolescents with overweight or obesity or dyslipidaemia. One meta-analysis showed that lifestyle interventions combining exercise and dietary changes among overweight and obese children resulted in improvements in weight and other cardiometabolic risk factors, including blood lipids.[28] Another meta-analysis focused on physical exercise interventions among obese children also found beneficial effects on blood lipid profiles, particularly accruing in response to aerobic exercise.[57] Comparisons between diet-only and diet-plus-exercise interventions among obese youth showed that the addition of exercise to dietary interventions led to greater improvements in levels of HDL-cholesterol, whereas the diet-only interventions caused greater reductions in levels of triglycerides and LDL-cholesterol.[28] A recent review of the effects of childhood obesity *prevention* interventions, i.e. not confined to overweight or obese youth, showed that programmes with diet and/or physical activity components were both effective in improving LDL- and HDL-cholesterol.[58] However, because the majority of the studies reviewed led also to beneficial changes in adiposity, this may indeed be a requirement for meaningful reductions in blood lipids.[58] Another meta-analysis of school-based physical activity programmes showed these to be effective in improving children's and adolescents' blood cholesterol but not BMI, which seems to contradict that contention.[25]

It is known that lipoprotein levels are directly related to the process of atherosclerosis and thereby to the occurrence of CVD. Although total cholesterol is a risk factor for CVD, its atherogenic effect depends merely on the structure of the cholesterol, i.e. on the ratio between LDL- and HDL-cholesterol. It is assumed that LDL may act directly or indirectly to cause endothelial damage, with subsequent proliferation of arterial smooth muscle cells resulting in an accumulation of lipids leading to atherosclerotic plaque formation. HDL, on the other hand, seems to be responsible for carrying cholesterol from peripheral tissues, including the arterial walls, back to the liver where it is metabolized and excreted, and therefore protects against CVD. Besides HDL and LDL, very low-density lipoprotein cholesterol (VLDL) and plasma triglycerides (TG) also need to be considered, although the atherogenic effects of these are not firmly established. During exercise, fatty acids are released from their storage sites to be oxidized for energy production. Several studies suggest that human growth hormone may be responsible for this increased fatty acid mobilization. Growth hormone levels increase sharply with exercise and remain elevated for up to several hours in the recovery period. Other research has suggested that, with exercise, adipose tissue is more sensitive to the actions of the sympathetic nervous system or to the rising levels of circulating catecholamines. Either situation would increase lipid mobilization. It must be noted that lipid profiles of growing children are related to the hormonal changes that characterize puberty and it may therefore be difficult to unveil the effects of physical activity independent of such changes.

Glucose metabolism and insulin resistance

Declines in both physical activity and insulin sensitivity are observed during puberty and are exacerbated by the presence of obesity, which may ultimately lead to type 2 diabetes. The increase in the prevalence of obesity is therefore thought to underlie the alarming increase in the prevalence of type 2 diabetes observed in recent years among the young. Through its beneficial effects on adiposity or, independent of these, increasing physical activity and CRF levels may thus constitute a means to halt insulin resistance and type 2 diabetes. Indeed, both adipose and muscle tissues regulate insulin sensitivity and therefore the extent to which physical activity or CRF and adiposity determine the levels of insulin resistance independent of one another has been an area of research that continues to grow. A systematic review of the experimental and correlational (longitudinal and cross-sectional) literature in children and adolescents reported that most of the studies of physical activity or CRF showed a beneficial relationship with insulin sensitivity.[59] Noteworthy, when examined concurrently, physical activity (of higher intensities) and CRF were both correlated with insulin sensitivity independent of adiposity.[59] Indeed, while systematic reviews and meta-analyses have shown that exercise interventions may lead to only small improvements in children's BMI and body fatness, the effects of physical activity interventions, in particular those with moderate-to-vigorous intensity, have been consistently associated with decreases in fasting glucose and insulin resistance, regardless of changes in BMI or adiposity.[60] Still, a recent meta-analysis examining the effectiveness of aerobic exercise alone on fasting glucose and insulin resistance among children and adolescents with obesity[61] showed stronger beneficial effects than those reported in the previous meta-analysis which was not confined to obese youth.[60] Nevertheless, because only few studies investigated the optimal dose of exercise training without calorie restriction or preferred exercise type (i.e. aerobic vs resistance) for reducing insulin resistance, further investigation of these issues is warranted in the paediatric population.[62]

Metabolic syndrome

The clustering of risk factors, notably (central) obesity, elevated BP, dyslipidaemia (i.e. elevated triglycerides and decreased HDL-cholesterol), and high fasting glucose levels, occurs more often than chance alone would dictate and is currently known as the metabolic syndrome (MetS).[63] Body fatness and a physical inactive or sedentary lifestyle, in the setting of a genetic pre-disposition, are considered its prime aetiological factors.[63] Not surprisingly, the prevalence of the MetS is increasing among the young.[64] The recognition of this phenotype has led to an exponential increase over the past decade in the number of studies of causes and consequences of the MetS (including the development of paediatric definitions),[17,65] though not without many, still on-going, debates and controversies.[66]

The clustering of risk factors,[67] including their association with lower levels of physical activity,[68] was recognized in children long before the new worldwide interest in the phenotype. The main findings of the studies conducted over the past decade are that higher levels of self-reported physical activity are inversely associated with the MetS,[69,70] although not always significantly so.[69] Additionally, when physical activity is measured more objectively (e.g. using accelerometry), the inverse associations are stronger and statistically significant,[71–74] but also attenuated after adjustments for CRF and, to a lesser extent, for body fatness.[72,73] Several initial studies in different cohorts of the EYHS reported an inverse association between CRF and the MetS that was only partially mediated by (but still independent of) body fatness.[75–77] Analyses in a representative sample of US adolescents also reported an inverse association between CRF and the MetS across both sexes and different ethnicities. It is noteworthy that the prevalence of the MetS in the lowest tertile of CRF (~24% in boys and ~17% in girls) was comparable to the overall prevalence of the MetS in the US adult population, while it was practically absent in the highest tertile of fitness (0.1% and 0.9%, respectively).[78] From this same cohort, another report investigating the association between CRF with a risk factor cluster score (not including body weight or adiposity levels) also showed beneficial associations independent of adolescents' weight status.[79] A more recent publication from the EYHS (combining three cohorts), reported that the associations of physical activity and CRF with the MetS were independent of one another, and that obesity only mediated the associations between CRF and the MetS, but not between physical activity and the MetS (excluding the waist circumference trait).[80]

Interestingly, a significant interaction of physical activity with CRF in the associations with the MetS has been also reported, suggesting that the beneficial effects of increasing physical activity levels, in the setting of MetS prevention or regression, may be highest among the less fit.[71] A series of studies all (co-)authored by Eisenman and reviewed by this author, concluded that, in general, body fatness was more strongly associated with the MetS than CRF.[81] Furthermore, while the correlation between body fatness and the MetS remained significant after controlling for CRF, the correlation between CRF and MetS did not remain significant after controlling for body fatness.[81] In addition, the existence of interactions between body fatness and CRF was emphasized in support of the 'fat but fit' theory, such that CRF-related attenuations in the MetS are expectedly greater among the fattest.[81] These conclusions warrant some critical appraisal though. First, they reflect the problems of the intricate physical activity, CRF, and fatness 'triangle' (Figure 17.2), i.e. it is impossible to discern determinant, mediator, and outcome from one another by the cross-sectional designs employed in these studies. Also, assumptions on the associations' directions were unclear and could virtually be any of:

i) physical activity→adiposity→MetS?,

ii) physical activity→CRF→MetS?,

iii) physical fitness→adiposity→MetS?, etc.

Unfortunately, the reader often has to guess. Eisenmann's conclusions were further complicated by methodological problems. Any measure of total body fatness will be highly correlated with a measure of central fatness (i.e. waist circumference), which is a trait of the MetS. Therefore, it is not surprising, as in Eisenmann's studies, to find a stronger association between BMI and the MetS than between CRF and MetS when the waist circumference trait is not excluded from the MetS score.

Combined dietary and exercise interventions can reduce the prevalence of MetS in obese children.[82,83] What the optimal combination is in order to achieve the best results remains unclear, as do issues related to long-term effectiveness and whether preventing or treating childhood MetS should differ, in any meaningful way, from preventing or treating childhood obesity.

Cardiometabolic risk factors in youth and cardiometabolic risk factors or cardiovascular disease in adulthood

The relevancy of the associations observed in childhood or adolescence between physical activity or CRF with cardiometabolic risk factors rests also on the extent to which these factors are associated with their levels later in adulthood (see path 'C1' in Figure 17.1), and thereby, or independently of these, with incident CVD and/or mortality in adulthood (see path C2 in Figure 17.1).

Evidence of the pivotal role of body fatness in the development of other cardiometabolic risk factors in children/adolescents is overwhelming.[84,85] There is also some evidence relating body fatness in youth (measured by BMI) to hypertension, type 2 diabetes, CVD, and all-cause mortality in adulthood (reviewed elsewhere).[86] However, a subsequent systematic review concluded that although there was consistent evidence linking childhood BMI to these outcomes, the adverse effects seemed not to be independent of adult BMI.[87] This has led to the conclusion that obesity in youth does not have 'direct effects' on adult disease and that adult risk can be accounted for, and prevented by, reducing adult BMI only.[87,88] However, adult and childhood BMI are strongly correlated[12,89,90] and, therefore, tracking constitutes an obvious pathway through which childhood BMI is associated with adult disease. In addition, when adjusted for adult BMI, the associations between childhood BMI and adult disease control not only for adult BMI but also for changes in BMI between the two age periods. Moreover, because hypertension, type 2 diabetes, and CVD are interrelated, focus on each of these outcomes separately does not account for competing risks. A recent study accounting for these issues showed that both BMI in early adulthood (21 years of age) and body weight gain thereafter were associated with marked increases in the risk of first occurrence of fatal and nonfatal chronic diseases, including type 2 diabetes mellitus, CVD, and certain cancers in middle-aged and older men.[91] Still, in a large retrospective study, women who were overweight at the age of 10 years but became lean in adulthood did not have a significant increase in the risk of type 2 diabetes as compared with women who were never overweight.[92] Similarly, a large study comprising cohorts across Europe, the US, and Australia showed that persons who were overweight or obese during childhood but who became non-obese as adults had similar risks of hypertension, type 2 diabetes, and dyslipidaemia to those who had a normal BMI throughout.[93] These findings emphasize the reversibility potential of interventions that are able to correct adverse weight trajectories between childhood and adulthood. However, it must be noticed that, as reported by this last study, the portion of obese children who were able to normalize their BMI in adulthood (~25%) is considerably lower than the portion of obese children who remained obese as adults (~75%). This clearly illustrates that, once established, obesity is very hard to 'dismantle'.

Early reports from the Harvard and Pennsylvania Alumni studies showed that mildly raised BP in men (15–29 years) was associated with incident CVD and mortality over the course of 50 years of follow-up.[94,95] Similar findings were reported by the Glasgow Alumni Study (men, ~20 years of age, median follow-up of 41 years).[96] Importantly, a large nationwide cohort study linked both systolic and diastolic BP in late adolescence (mean age of 18.4 years) to incident cardiovascular mortality over a medium follow-up of 24 years.[97] Childhood (mean age of 11.3 years) or adolescent (mean age of 18.3 years) BP[98] or hypertension[102] were also associated with premature death, though this was not observed in another youth cohort.[100] Tracking of BP from childhood to adulthood is moderate, with the magnitude varying depending on age at baseline (higher) and length of follow-up (lower),[101] but higher when measurement error issues are taken into account.[102] Higher BP in adulthood is a major cause of CVD.

In contrast to the links between childhood BMI and BP with incident CVD and mortality in adulthood, no such links have been established between mortality rates and childhood blood lipids[99,100] or MetS/hyperglycaemia.[100] However, levels of blood lipids in youth track strongly to adulthood[12,103] and may thereby lead to increased CVD. Likewise, the MetS, as well as its traits, have been shown to track from childhood/adolescence to adulthood,[104,105] when it is known to raise the risk of CVD and type 2 diabetes.[106]

Altogether, the evidence reviewed (see all 'C' paths in Figure 17.1) suggests that beneficial impacts of physical activity or CRF on youngsters' body fatness and BP, may constitute operative pathways to prevent the risk of incident CVD and mortality.

Physical activity and cardiorespiratory fitness in youth and later-life cardiometabolic risk factors

Despite the large amount of observational and interventional evidence linking lower levels of physical activity to poorer levels of cardiometabolic risk factors among the young, evidence derived from prospective studies through adulthood are comparatively scarce. In a combined effort to address the question as to what extent physical activity or CRF in adolescence are associated with cardiometabolic risk factors in adulthood (see path 'D' in Figure 17.1) analyses were conducted within several on-going longitudinal studies.[107] The general conclusion was that higher CRF, but not higher physical activity levels, during adolescence predicted a healthier cardiometabolic profile in young adulthood.[107] More recently, similar analyses in the Oslo Youth Study have mostly replicated these findings.[108] The beneficial role of adolescent CRF on adult cardiometabolic health has also been shown in a recent large study of Korean adolescents.[109] In all studies physical activity was not measured with objective methods, which could have explained the contrasting results with CRF. We must also note that most studies mentioned here included subjects who grew up in very different circumstances than today's children: those cohort studies were assembled more than 20 years ago, when prevalence of obesity was lower and the environment was less 'obesogenic' than it is nowadays.

Life-course exposures

Assessing the level of physical activity (or any other risk factor) at one time point, or its mean over a relative short period of people's life (e.g. adolescence) may not be the best approach to disclose differences between individuals set on different lifelong trajectories of physical activity despite having similar (mean) levels at that specific time point or period. This could constitute yet another explanation for the not-so-convincing results for physical activity in the studies described in the previous section. Therefore, enabled by its longitudinal design where body fatness, physical activity, and CRF were measured over a 25-year period, the AGHLS compared the *lifecourse* trajectories of these factors between participants with and participants without the MetS at the age of 36 years (Figure 17.3). With this analytical approach it was able to identify late adolescence and the period of transition between adolescence and young adulthood as critical periods in an individual's life when adverse changes in risk factors may be linked to poorer cardiometabolic health later in life.[110] Noteworthy, the more adverse changes in (central) fatness (Figure 17.3, panels A–C) among those with or without the MetS seemed to have preceded the adverse changes in CRF (Figure 17.3, panel D) and physical activity (Figure 17.3, panels E–H). In addition, a striking observation was that, in fact, individuals with the MetS seemed to have accumulated increasingly higher levels of total time spent weekly in physical activities than their peers without the MetS. This apparently counterintuitive observation was explained by the progressive *displacement* of time spent in activities of higher intensity in favour of those with lower intensities. Moreover, the significant differences in CRF (though not in VPA) between individuals with or without the MetS remained even when further adjusted for the increasing levels of body fatness. From a preventive point of view, identification of the critical periods and trigger risk factors across individuals' life (i.e. primarily the increases in total body fatness and a central pattern of fat accumulation during adolescence followed by decreases in physical activity and CRF) have the potential to better inform interventions to break 'chains of risk' that will lead to the greatest lifelong cardiometabolic benefits.

Pre-clinical signs of early vascular aging

The seminal findings from the Pathobiological Determinants of Atherosclerosis in Youth (PDAY) and Bogalusa autopsy studies were key to the revival of the childhood origin of atherosclerosis hypothesis,[111] i.e. that atherosclerosis begins in childhood, progresses asymptomatically through adolescence, and young adulthood into middle-age, when related cardiovascular events start to occur. Indeed, their findings provided the most compelling evidence to that date (1990s) on the adverse influence of modifiable risk factors such as obesity, hypertension, blood lipids, hyperglycaemia, and smoking on atherosclerosis among the young.[112]

With the subsequent development of non-invasive ultrasound imaging methods for the measurement of surrogate markers of atherosclerosis, specifically the intima-media thickness (IMT) of the carotid artery, a new avenue of *pre-clinical* research was soon open and implemented in on-going cohorts studies of (young) adults who had been followed since childhood, such as the Bogalusa Heart Study,[113] the Cardiovascular Risk in Young Fins Study,[114] and also new cohort and clinical studies of children and adolescents.[115] With a special interest in the study of correlations with physical activity and CRF early in life (adolescence), and throughout the course of life, the AGHLS incorporated such measures as well.[116] The arterial protocol of the AGHLS was not confined to measures of carotid IMT but also included structural and functional measures of three large arteries, enabling the assessment of subject's levels of arterial stiffness (using local estimates such as arterial distensibility and compliance coefficients) across the arterial tree.[116] This arterial protocol thus enabled a comprehensive investigation of young adults' arterial properties not only focusing exclusively on the early determinants of atherosclerosis (for as much as reflected by carotid IMT), but also examining the early determinants of arterial stiffness (i.e. arteriosclerosis). Tonometry is yet another method that became popular in the non-invasive assessment of regional arterial stiffness (NB: not atherosclerosis), i.e. over the length of arterial segments (e.g. carotid-to-femoral pulse wave velocity; PWV),[117] which is now considered the reference measure of aortic stiffness.

Atherosclerosis versus arterial stiffness

Although often overlooked, atherosclerosis and arteriosclerosis are pathologically distinct and therefore should be considered as separate disease processes.[118] Indeed, atherosclerosis and arteriosclerosis may share the same risk factors and often (though not always) occur together, but they have distinct pathobiological features. Where atherosclerosis is a gradual, focal, process that leads to impairment of the conduit function of arteries leading to ischaemia or infarction of tissues and organs downstream, arteriosclerosis is a generalized process that reflects the gradual impairment of the cushioning function of arteries, leading to increases in pulse pressure (because hearts ejecting into a stiffer arterial bed must generate higher end-systolic pressures for the same net stroke volume), which in turn may lead to decreases in the arterial volume at the onset of diastole.[119] The main clinical consequences of increased arterial stiffness are thus an increase in the risk of stroke, left ventricular hypertrophy, and decreased coronary perfusion, and, ultimately heart failure.[120] Furthermore, when considering the architecture of the arterial wall, the thickening of the intima layer is an early observation of atherosclerosis, whereas the disruption of the arterial BP load-bearing elastin-collagen network and smooth-muscle cell proliferation into the media layer are hallmarks of arteriosclerosis. However, given that ultrasound imaging of the carotid artery wall does *not* discriminate the intima from the media layers, and that carotid IMT at levels <0.9 mm, as often measured among the young, predominantly reflect adaptive arterial remodelling[121] (mechanism that attempts to restore local haemodynamic conditions to an equilibrium, rather than atherosclerosis per se), early vascular damage among the young is better defined on the basis of arterial stiffness than of carotid IMT measures.[5] Therefore, the next section focuses on the evidence linking physical activity and physical fitness to arterial stiffness among the young.

Physical activity and cardiorespiratory fitness and markers of early vascular aging in youth

Schack-Nielsen *et al.* were the first to examine the associations between physical activity (24 h recall questionnaire) and non-invasively measured levels of arterial stiffness (aortic PWV) in a small sample of 10-year-olds. They reported an inverse association that was independent of other lifestyle risk factors, BMI, and BP.[122] In children of the same age, Reed *et al.* showed the same beneficial and independent associations between CRF and small (though not large) artery compliance.[123] In a larger community-based

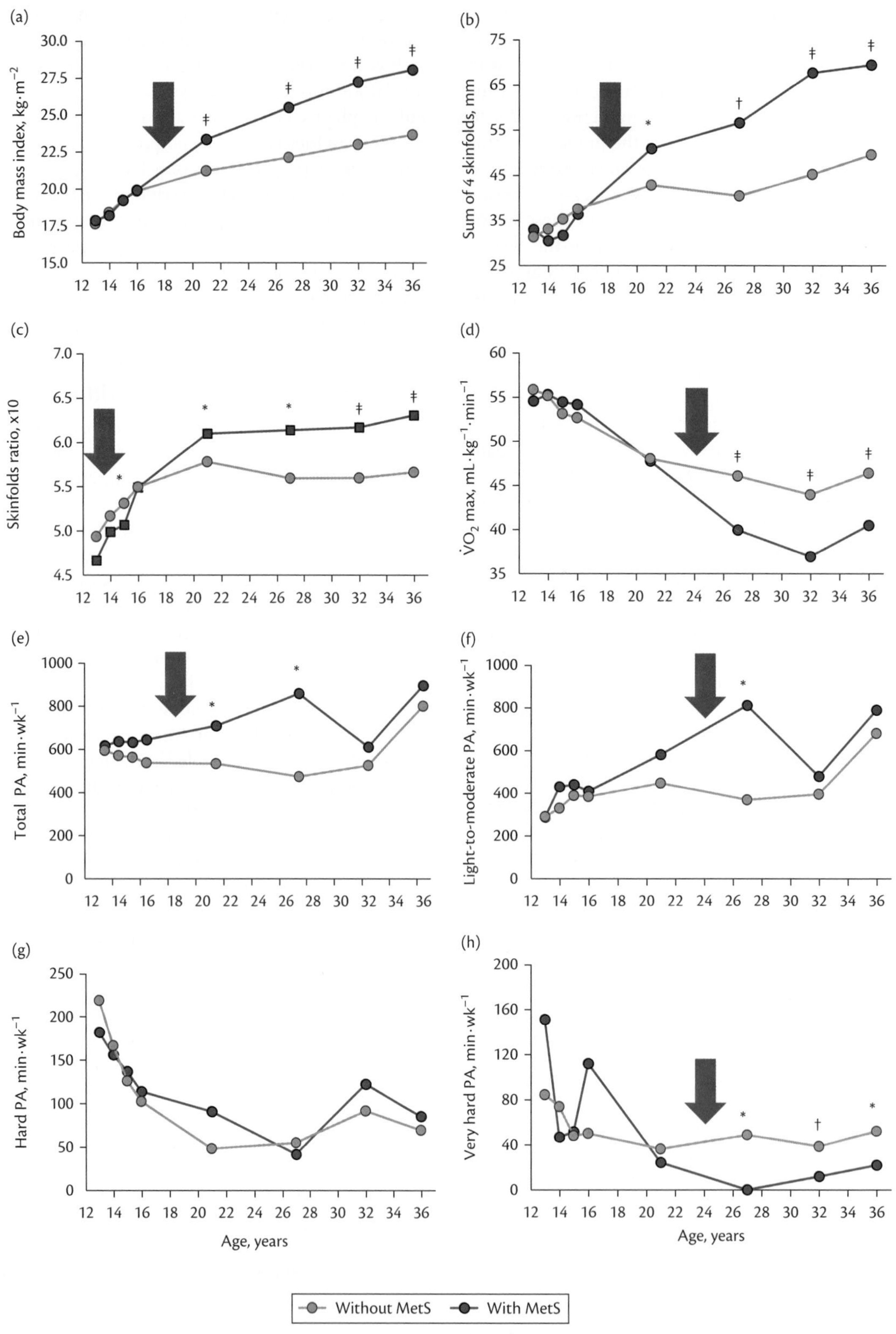

Figure 17.3 Comparisons of the life-course trajectories of (central) fatness, physical activity, and cardiopulmonary fitness between adolescence and adulthood in subjects with and without the Metabolic Syndrome (MetS) at the age of 36 years.

(a) Body mass index (BMI); (b) Sum of 4 skinfolds (i.e. biceps, triceps, subscapular, and suprailiac); (c) Skinfolds ratio (i.e. subscapular + suprailiac/sum of four skinfolds); (d) Cardiorespiratory fitness ($\dot{V}O_2$ max); (e) Total Physical activity (PA); (f) Light- to moderate-intensity PA (i.e. 4–7 METs); (g) High-intensity PA (i.e. 7–10 METs); and (h) Very high-intensity PA (i.e. >10 METs).

*P < 0.05; †P < 01; ‡P < 001 for comparisons between subjects with (n = 38) and without the metabolic syndrome (MetS) (n = 326); Black arrows pinpoint the critical periods.

Ferreira I, Twisk JW, van Mechelen W, Kemper HC, Stehouwer CD. Development of fatness, fitness, and lifestyle from adolescence to the age of 36 years: determinants of the metabolic syndrome in young adults: the Amsterdam Growth and Health Longitudinal Study. Arch Intern Med. 2005; 165: 42–48.

study of over 500 children (mean age of 10 years) physical activity (pedometer counts) and CRF were both associated with lower levels of arterial stiffness (aortic PWV).[124] In contrast, anthropometric and DEXA measures of total and central adiposity were associated with higher levels of arterial stiffness. The associations between CRF and arterial stiffness were attenuated and no longer significant when further adjusted for adiposity, but the association between adiposity and arterial stiffness remained independent of CRF. More recently, MVPA (estimated from accelerometry) was associated with estimates of small, but not large, artery compliance, independently of BMI and BP, in children.[125] Edwards *et al.* found an inverse association between physical activity (estimated from accelerometry) and multiple measures of arterial stiffness (brachial distensibility and aortic PWV) in adolescents and young adults, which persisted after adjustments for BMI and mean BP (brachial distensibility), and were stronger among participants with type 2 diabetes (aortic PWV).[126] In a large sample of children from the PANIC study, physical activity and CRF (beneficially) and total body fatness (adversely) were associated with arterial stiffness (stiffness index), but, in mutually adjusted analyses, only CRF remained independently associated with it.[127] The Danish cohort of the EYHS also reported beneficial associations of physical activity and CRF with carotid stiffness estimates, albeit confined to boys and no longer significant after adjustments for adiposity.[128] However, analysis of physical activity intensity levels during and between childhood and adolescence in this cohort did not find any beneficial association with adolescent carotid stiffness.[129] Accelerometry remains limited in its ability to quantify all physical activities (e.g. swimming and bicycling), thereby underestimating energy expenditure. A subsequent study from the Danish cohort showed that boys who used their bicycle every day had lower arterial stiffness than those who used their bicycle fewer than three times per week. These observations were independent of physical activity levels ascertained by accelerometry and only mildly attenuated by BP and adiposity.[130] In another study, CRF was inversely associated with aortic, but not with carotid stiffness in a large group of adolescents, even after adjustment for BMI, BP, and other risk factors.[131] Noteworthy, increases in aortic stiffness between the ages of 11 and 17 years were smaller among adolescents who were fit at the age of 17 years than peers with the lowest fitness levels.[131]

Although limited by the predominant cross-sectional designs, the findings described here seem to suggest that body fatness mediates the beneficial effects of physical activity on arterial stiffness, whereas the associations between CRF and arterial stiffness may, to some extent, be independent of body fatness. Indeed, adiposity and its metabolic consequences have been consistently linked to impaired arterial function and stiffening among the young.[132,133] Noteworthy, in a RCT, a 3-month regular physical activity programme improved CRF and reduced arterial stiffness (but not carotid IMT) in obese prepubertal children.[134] Reductions in total and abdominal fat as well as in BP were also observed, and could have thus explained the vascular benefits of the exercise programme. Moreover, given its short duration, exercise-related changes in arterial stiffness may have been primarily related to the beneficial changes in BP (which is the primary determinant of arterial stiffness), rather than due to changes in the arterial structure composition.

Physical activity and cardiopulmonary fitness in youth and markers of early vascular aging in adulthood

Several long-term cohort studies that began in childhood have investigated the impact of youth cardiometabolic risk factors on non-invasive markers of atherosclerosis and arterial stiffness in adulthood (reviewed elsewhere).[115] Among these, the AGHLS has been exclusive in providing information on the impact of early life and life course physical activity and CRF. In a first prospective analysis in this cohort, CRF levels during adolescence were not clearly associated with arterial stiffness later in life.[116] Instead, a central pattern of body fat distribution (but not total fatness) during adolescence was independently associated with higher arterial stiffness two decades later.[135] However, changes in physical activity and CRF levels between adolescence and the age of 36 years were inversely associated with stiffness estimates, particularly of the brachial and femoral arteries (i.e. the muscular part of the arterial tree), and for CRF, these were partly independent of (central) fatness and other risk factors.[136] In the Danish cohort of the EYHS, higher youth levels of objectively measured MVPA at the mean age of 15 years were associated with lower arterial stiffness 12 years later. Interestingly, those who maintained a stable level of, or had a small increase in, MVPA minutes from youth to adulthood tended to have the lowest arterial stiffness as adults, independently of other lifestyle factors and BMI.[137]

Life-course exposures

To better understand how the life-course trajectories and cumulative burden of physical activity[138,139] (and other lifestyles), CRF, (central) fatness, BP, and other metabolic risk factors[140] affected arterial stiffness later in life, the AGHLS adopted a life-course model to analyse its 25-year longitudinal exposure data in relation to arterial stiffness in adulthood. The AGHLS's unique design and population enabled the distinction of individuals with roughly the same chronological age (36.5 ± 0.5 years) but with different levels of arterial aging, ruling out any potential cohort effects on such differences. Specifically, 36-year-olds in the lowest sex-specific tertile of the carotid distensibility were considered to have the stiffest arteries (i.e. the early vascular aging phenotype) and those in the middle (T2) and highest tertiles were considered to have intermediate and the least stiff (or more distensible) arteries, respectively (Figure 17.4). By comparison with the international Reference Values for Arterial Measurement Collaboration database,[141] the mean levels of carotid distensibility of the AGHLS' participants in each of the tertiles were equivalent to the mean levels of individuals aged 46, 36, and 27 (in men) and 49, 38, and 30 years (in women).[5] In other words, participants with the stiffest versus least stiff carotid arteries differed by nearly two decades in terms of their arterial age, despite having the same chronological age.[5]

We found that, as compared with individuals with the least stiff arteries, subjects with intermediate and the stiffest carotid arteries at the age of 36 years spent throughout the whole longitudinal period, on average about 25–30 fewer $\text{min} \cdot \text{week}^{-1}$ in VPA (e.g. jogging, cycling, aerobics, and competitive tennis), but not significantly less time in LMPA (e.g. brisk walking).[138] Importantly, the differences in the VPA mean levels between the two groups were independent of other lifestyle risk factors but were explained, to a great extent (by up to ~60%), by the beneficial impact of VPA on fitness, central fatness, and total-to-HDL cholesterol ratio.[138] Trajectory analyses revealed that these differences emerged

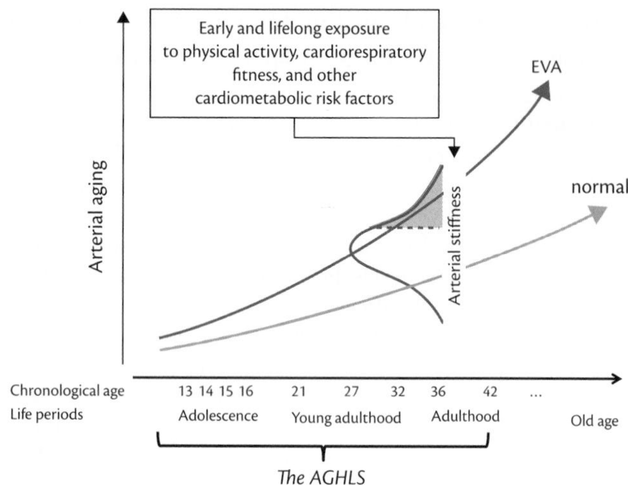

Figure 17.4 Analyses of the early and lifelong exposure to physical activity, cardiorespiratory fitness, and other cardiometabolic risk factors as determinants of early vascular aging in the Amsterdam Growth and Health Longitudinal Study.
EVA is early vascular aging; AGHLS is Amsterdam Growth and Health Longitudinal Study.
Adapted from Ferreira I, van de Laar RJ. Lessons from the Amsterdam Growth and Health Longitudinal Study. In: Nilsson PM, Olsen ME, Laurent S. Early vascular aging (EVA). New directions in cardiovascular protection. Oxford: Academic Press; 2015: 33–44.

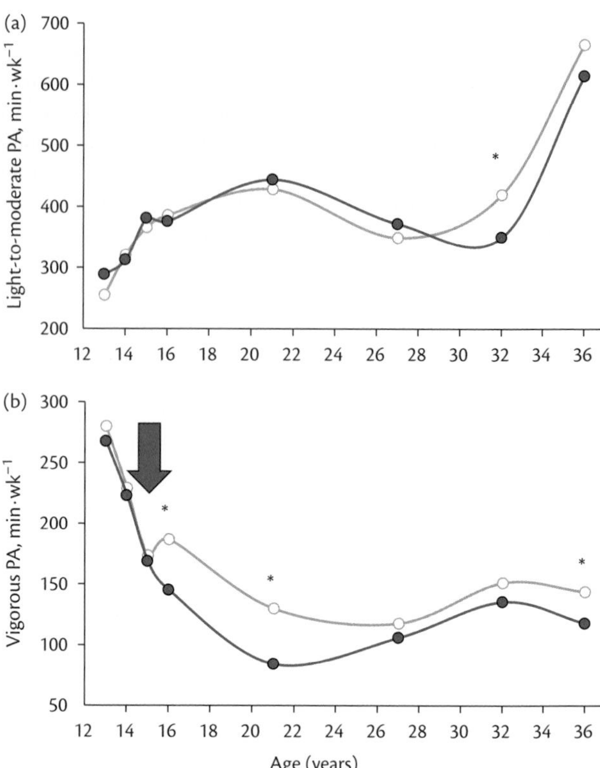

Figure 17.5 Comparison of the life-course trajectories of physical activity between subjects with different carotid stiffness levels at the age of 36 years.
(a) Light to moderate physical activity (PA, 4–7 METs); (b) Vigorous PA (>7 METs); *P < 0.05, for comparisons between subjects with the least stiff and subjects with intermediate and the stiffest arterial levels (defined as belonging to the highest versus middle and lowest tertiles of carotid distensibility categories, respectively); all data were adjusted for sex, height, and time. Arrows pinpoint the critical periods.
van de Laar RJ, Ferreira I, van Mechelen W, Prins MH, Twisk JW, Stehouwer CD. Lifetime vigorous but not light-to-moderate habitual physical activity impacts favorably on carotid stiffness in young adults: the Amsterdam Growth and Health Longitudinal Study. Hypertension. 2010; 55: 33–39.

during late adolescence, persisting thereafter up to the age of 36 years (Figure 17.5).[138] Comparable results were found when participants' vascular aging phenotypes were defined on the basis of compliance estimates of the muscular brachial and femoral arteries.[139]

We also found that those with the stiffest arteries at age 36 years were characterized by greater levels of BP and (central) adiposity from early adolescence compared with those with the least stiff arteries (Figure 17.6, panels A–C).[140] Interestingly, observable differences in CRF (Figure 17.6, panel D) between the adults with different vascular aging phenotypes emerged later in the life-course, when individuals were in their late 20s or early 30s. These differences were to some extent explained by the existent BP and (central) adiposity differences.[140] Taken together, and from a temporal perspective, the AGHLS findings seem to suggest that increases in (central) fatness and blood pressure during adolescence trigger a chain of risks characterized by subsequent lower levels of physical activity and CRF, ultimately leading to early vascular aging. Still, preserving higher levels of physical activity and CRF throughout the life-course may attenuate the adverse impact of those trigger risk factors.

Due to the current interest in sedentary time as a behaviour that usually manifests itself independently of physical activity,[142] and that may carry specific adverse cardiometabolic health impacts, it is perhaps worth mentioning a specific result from the AGHLS. It reported that, as compared with those with the least stiff arteries, subjects with the stiffest arteries at the age of 36 years spent on average about 20 $\text{min}\cdot\text{day}^{-1}$ more watching television (used as marker of sedentary behavior) in the previous 4 years than their peers with the least stiff arteries.[143] This difference was independent of the other lifestyle risk factors, including time spent in VPA, and could only partly be explained (by up to 30%) by the adverse associations of television time with other risk factors (including CRF, fatness, and BP) but remained, to a large extent, independent of these.[143] These observations support the view that (vigorous intensity) physical activity and sedentary behaviours may affect arterial stiffness independently of one another and through specific, though largely unknown, cellular and molecular mechanisms.

Pathobiological mechanisms

There are several possible mechanisms that might explain the association of physical activity in children and young adults with enhanced arterial elasticity. These include increased elastin content of the aortic wall and/or delayed age-related reduction or fraction of elastic lamellae in the arterial wall, reduction in α-adrenergic receptor–mediated vascular tone (i.e. reduced sympathetic nervous system activity), enhanced release of nitric oxide (a vasodilator) via increased shear stress during or immediately after physical activity bouts and/or reduction in plasma endothelin-1 concentrations (a vasoconstrictor secreted by vascular endothelial cells), and reduction of low-grade inflammation, which is a particularly important mechanism in the context of obesity, and for its pivotal link to the aforementioned mechanisms. However, there is an overwhelming lack of studies examining these pathobiological mechanisms in

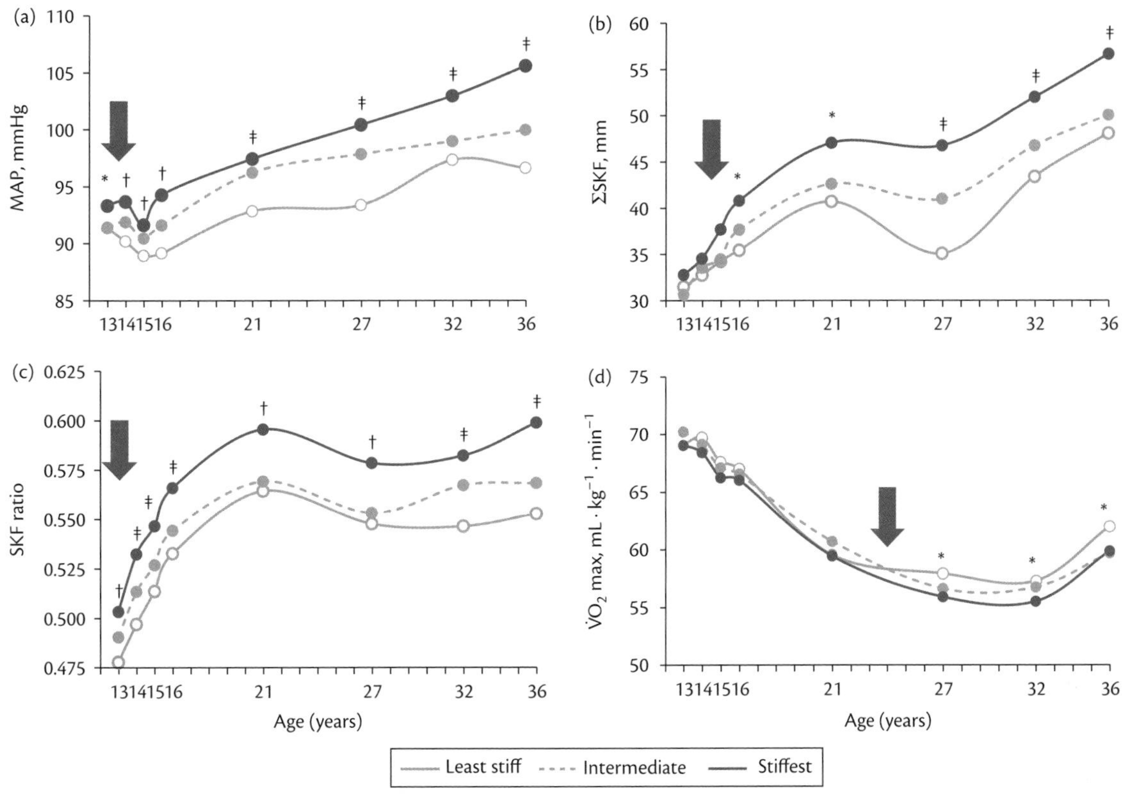

Figure 17.6 Comparison of the life-course trajectories of physical fitness, blood pressure and (central) fatness between subjects with different carotid stiffness levels at the age of 36 years.

(a) Mean arterial pressure (MAP); (b) Sum of 4 skinfolds (ΣSKF, i.e. biceps, triceps, subscapular, and suprailiac); (c) SKF ratio (i.e. subscapular + suprailiac /ΣSKF); and (d) Cardiorespiratory fitness ($\dot{V}O_2$ max). FFM, free fat mass. $^*P < 0.05$; $^{\dagger}P < 0.01$; $^{\ddagger}P < 0.001$, for comparisons between subjects with the stiffest versus the least stiff arteries (defined as belonging to the highest versus lowest tertiles of carotid distensibility, respectively); all data were adjusted for sex and height. Arrows pinpoint the critical periods.

Ferreira I, van de Laar RJ, Prins MH, Twisk JW, Stehouwer CD. Carotid stiffness in young adults: a life-course analysis of its early determinants: the Amsterdam Growth and Health Longitudinal Study. Hypertension. 2012; 59: 54–61.

the context of exercise-induced arterial changes in children. For instance, it is now well established that low-grade inflammation plays a key role in the development of vascular diseases. One of the most commonly measured markers of inflammation (C-reactive protein; CRP) has been linked to arterial changes[144] and obesity[145] in children. However, in contrast to studies in adults, the association between exercise and inflammatory markers in children is inconsistent,[146] and a recent meta-analysis in overweight and obese youths suggested that exercise programmes were not able to mitigate the inflammatory effects of excess body weight.[145] In contrast, a meta-analysis showed beneficial effects of exercise RCTs on flow-mediated dilation (a marker of endothelial function measured also non-invasively by ultrasonography) in overweight and obese children.[147] Clearly, more studies are needed for a better understanding of the interconnectedness of the haemodynamic, cellular, and molecular mechanisms underlying the cardiovascular effects of exercise in the young.

Conclusions

The favourable impact that physical activity and/or CRF during youth have on other cardiometabolic risk factors (mainly obesity, BP, and possibly insulin resistance) seem to constitute the preferential pathways through which related beneficial effects on cardiovascular health later in life can be expected. This holds also true for the associations between physical activity or CRF with markers of arterial aging in children and adolescents, as well as between the cumulative or lifelong exposure levels to lower physical activity and physical fitness levels with those markers in adulthood. Still, according to the evidence available, it is perhaps more important to be active and fit throughout the life-course than to be active or fit only as a child. This sustainability dimension thus needs to be incorporated in preventive measures aiming at the promotion of physical activity among the young as a means to prevent metabolic and cardiovascular diseases later in life.

Summary

- There is no evidence that physical activity (PA) and/or cardiorespiratory fitness (CRF) during childhood and adolescence are related to the occurrence of cardiovascular disease (CVD) in adulthood (see path 'A' in Figure 17.1).
- There is, however, evidence that PA and/or CRF during childhood track into adulthood, albeit moderately so, (see path 'B' in Figure 17.1), and are associated with cardiometabolic risk factors in childhood or adolescence, particularly obesity, blood pressure (BP), insulin resistance, and their clustering (metabolic syndrome) (see path 'C' in Figure 17.1).
- The beneficial effects of PA and CRF on children's and adolescents' cardiometabolic risk factors such as BP and insulin resistance may be, at least in part, independent of any favourable effects on adiposity.

- The association between PA and adiposity is complex, such that excessive energy intake rather than decreases in PA per se seem to be at the root of increases in obesity among the young; increases in obesity do lead to decreases in PA which will contribute to the perpetuation of an unbalanced energy in-energy out vicious cycle throughout the life-course.
- There is a lack of convincing evidence linking PA or physical fitness at a young age with cardiometabolic risk factors in adulthood (see path 'D' in Figure 17.1). Still the strongest evidence linking PA (mostly of higher intensities) and physical fitness at young age with CVD later in life is that along (all) paths C in Figure 17.1.
- The evidence linking obesity and elevated BP to CVD in adulthood and the stronger tracking of these cardiometabolic factors and also their clustering into adulthood (see paths 'C1' and 'C2' in Figure 17.1), support the previous statement.
- The favourable impact that PA and/or CRF may have on other cardiometabolic risk factors (mainly obesity, BP, and possibly insulin resistance) seem to mediate most of their beneficial effects on markers of arterial aging in children and adolescents; the associations with these cardiometabolic risk factors also seem to mediate the beneficial association between the cumulative or lifelong exposure levels to lower PA and CRF levels with markers; the associations with these cardiometabolic risk factors also seem to mediate the beneficial association in adulthood.
- From the evidence available it appears more important to be active and fit throughout the life-course than to be active or fit only as a child.

References

1. Li J, Siegrist J. Physical activity and risk of cardiovascular disease—a meta-analysis of prospective cohort studies. *Int J Environ Res Public Health*. 2012; 9: 391–407.
2. Kodama S, Saito K, Tanaka S, *et al*. Cardiorespiratory fitness as a quantitative predictor of all-cause mortality and cardiovascular events in healthy men and women: a meta-analysis. *JAMA*. 2009; 301: 2024–2035.
3. Samitz G, Egger M, Zwahlen M. Domains of physical activity and all-cause mortality: systematic review and dose-response meta-analysis of cohort studies. *Int J Epidemiol*. 2011; 40: 1382–1400.
4. Paffenbarger RS, Wing AL, Hyde RT. Physical activity as an index of heart attack risk in college alumni. *Am J Epidemiol*. 1978; 108: 161–175.
5. Ferreira I, van de Laar RJ. Lessons from the Amsterdam Growth and Health Longitudinal Study. In: Nilsson PM, Olsen ME, Laurent S (eds.) *Early vascular aging (EVA). New directions in cardiovascular protection*. Oxford: Academic Press; 2015. p. 33–44
6. Janssen I, LeBlanc AG. Systematic review of the health benefits of physical activity and fitness in school-aged children and youth. *Int J Behav Nutr Phys Act*. 2010; 7: 40.
7. Etemadi A, Abnet CC, Kamangar F, *et al*. Impact of body size and physical activity during adolescence and adult life on overall and cause-specific mortality in a large cohort study from Iran. *Eur J Epidemiol*. 2014; 29: 95–109.
8. Nechuta SJ, Shu XO, Yang G, *et al*. Adolescent exercise in association with mortality from all causes, cardiovascular disease, and cancer among middle-aged and older Chinese women. *Cancer Epidemiol Biomarkers Prev*. 2015; 24: 1270–1276.
9. Telama R. Tracking of physical activity from childhood to adulthood: a review. *Obes Facts*. 2009; 2: 187–195.
10. Craigie AM, Lake AA, Kelly SA, Adamson AJ, Mathers JC. Tracking of obesity-related behaviours from childhood to adulthood: A systematic review. *Maturitas*. 2011; 70: 266–284.
11. Twisk JW, Kemper HC, Mellenbergh GJ. Mathematical and analytical aspects of tracking. *Epidemiol Rev*. 1994; 16: 165–183.
12. Twisk JW, Kemper HC, van Mechelen W, Post GB. Tracking of risk factors for coronary heart disease over a 14-year period: a comparison between lifestyle and biologic risk factors with data from the Amsterdam Growth and Health Study. *Am J Epidemiol*. 1997; 145: 888–898.
13. Twisk JW, Kemper HC, van Mechelen W. Tracking of activity and fitness and the relationship with cardiovascular disease risk factors. *Med Sci Sports Exerc*. 2000; 32: 1455–1461.
14. Bélanger M, Gray-Donald K, O'Loughlin J, Paradis G, Hanley J. When adolescents drop the ball. *Am J Prev Med*. 2009; 37: 41–49.
15. Kemper HC, Twisk JW, van Mechelen W. Changes in aerobic fitness in boys and girls over a period of 25 years: data from the Amsterdam Growth And Health Longitudinal Study revisited and extended. *Pediatr Exerc Sci*. 2013; 25: 524–535.
16. Telama R, Yang X, Leskinen E, *et al*. Tracking of physical activity from early childhood through youth into adulthood. *Med Sci Sports Exerc*. 2014; 46: 955–962.
17. Zimmet P, Alberti G, Kaufman F, *et al*. The metabolic syndrome in children and adolescents. *Lancet*. 2007; 369: 2059–2061.
18. Katzmarzyk PT, Barreira TV, Broyles ST, *et al*. Physical activity, sedentary time, and obesity in an international sample of children. *Med Sci Sports Exerc*. 2015; 47: 2062–2069.
19. Gralla MH, McDonald SM, Breneman C. Associations of objectively measured vigorous physical activity with body composition, cardiorespiratory fitness, and cardiometabolic health in youth. A review. *Am J Lifestyle Med*. 2016: doi: 10.1177/1559827615624417 [Epub ahead of print].
20. Buchan DS, Ollis S, Young JD, *et al*. The effects of time and intensity of exercise on novel and established markers of CVD in adolescent youth. *Am J Hum Biol*. 2011; 23: 517–526.
21. Corte de Araujo AC, Roschel H, Picanço AR, *et al*. Similar health benefits of endurance and high-intensity interval training in obese children. *PLOS One*. 2012; 7(8): e42747.
22. Kelley GA, Kelley KS, Pate RR. Effects of exercise on BMI z-score in overweight and obese children and adolescents: a systematic review with meta-analysis. *BMC Pediatr*. 2014; 14: 225.
23. Oosterhoff M, Joore M, Ferreira I. The effects of school-based lifestyle interventions on body mass index and blood pressure: a multivariate multilevel meta-analysis of randomized controlled trials. *Obes Rev* 2016; 17: 1131–1153.
24. Harris KC, Kuramoto LK, Schulzer M, Retallack JE. Effect of school-based physical activity interventions on body mass index in children: a meta-analysis. *CMAJ*. 2009; 180: 719–726.
25. Dobbins M, De Corby K, Robeson P, Husson H, Tirilis D. School-based physical activity programs for promoting physical activity and fitness in children and adolescents aged 6–18. *Cochrane Database Syst Rev*. 2009; 1: CD007651.
26. Metcalf B, Henley W, Wilkin T. Effectiveness of intervention on physical activity of children: systematic review and meta-analysis of controlled trials with objectively measured outcomes (EarlyBird 54). *BMJ*. 2012; 345: e5888.
27. Kimm SY, Glynn NW, Kriska AM, *et al*. Decline in physical activity in black girls and white girls during adolescence. *N Engl J Med*. 2002; 347: 709–715.
28. Ho M, Garnett SP, Baur LA, *et al*. Impact of dietary and exercise interventions on weight change and metabolic outcomes in obese children and adolescents: a systematic review and meta-analysis of randomized trials. *JAMA Pediatr*. 2013; 167: 759–768.
29. Rauner A, Mess F, Woll A. The relationship between physical activity, physical fitness and overweight in adolescents: a systematic review of studies published in or after 2000. *BMC Pediatr*. 2013; 13:19.
30. Bak H, Petersen L, Sørensen TI. Physical activity in relation to development and maintenance of obesity in men with and

without juvenile onset obesity. *Int J Obes Relat Metab Disord.* 2004; 28: 99–104.
31. Petersen L, Schnohr P, Sørensen TI. Longitudinal study of the long-term relation between physical activity and obesity in adults. *Int J Obes Relat Metab Disord.* 2004; 28: 105–112.
32. Ekelund U, Brage S, Besson H, Sharp S, Wareham NJ. Time spent being sedentary and weight gain in healthy adults: reverse or bidirectional causality? *Am J Clin Nutr.* 2008; 88: 612–617.
33. Mortensen LH, Siegler IC, Barefoot JC, Grønbaek M, Sørensen TI. Prospective associations between sedentary lifestyle and BMI in midlife. *Obesity.* 2006; 14: 1462–1471.
34. Metcalf BS, Hosking J, Jeffery AN, Voss LD, Henley W, Wilkin TJ. Fatness leads to inactivity, but inactivity does not lead to fatness: a longitudinal study in children (EarlyBird 45). *Arch Dis Child.* 2011; 96: 942–947.
35. Richmond RC, Davey Smith G, Ness AR, Hoed den M, McMahon G, Timpson NJ. Assessing causality in the association between child adiposity and physical activity levels: a Mendelian randomization analysis. *PLOS Med.* 2014; 11: e1001618.
36. Christiansen E, Swann A, Sørensen TI. Feedback models allowing estimation of thresholds for self-promoting body weight gain. *J Theor Biol.* 2008; 254: 731–736.
37. Shultz SP, Anner J, Hills AP. Paediatric obesity, physical activity and the musculoskeletal system. *Obes Rev.* 2009; 10: 576–582.
38. Baquet G, Twisk JW, Kemper HC, Van Praagh E, Berthoin S. Longitudinal follow-up of fitness during childhood: interaction with physical activity. *Am J Hum Biol.* 2006; 18: 51–58.
39. Kemper H, Koppes LL. Is physical activity important for aerobic power in young males and females? *Med Sport Sci.* 2004; 47: 153–166.
40. Szendroedi J, Roden M. Mitochondrial fitness and insulin sensitivity in humans. *Diabetologia.* 2008; 51: 2155–2167.
41. Freedman DS, Sherry B. The validity of BMI as an indicator of body fatness and risk among children. *Pediatrics.* 2009; 124: S23–S34.
42. Andersen LB, Harro M, Sardinha LB, *et al.* Physical activity and clustered cardiovascular risk in children: a cross-sectional study (The European Youth Heart Study). *Lancet.* 2006; 368: 299–304.
43. Twisk JW, van Mechelen W, Kemper HC, Post GB. The relation between 'long-term exposure' to lifestyle during youth and young adulthood and risk factors for cardiovascular disease at adult age. *J Adolesc Health.* 1997; 20: 309–319.
44. Twisk JW, Kemper HC, van Mechelen W, Post GB, van Lenthe FJ. Body fatness: longitudinal relationship of body mass index and the sum of skinfolds with other risk factors for coronary heart disease. *Int J Obes Relat Metab Disord.* 1998; 22: 915–922.
45. Nooyens AC, Koppes LL, Visscher TL, *et al.* Adolescent skinfold thickness is a better predictor of high body fatness in adults than is body mass index: the Amsterdam Growth and Health Longitudinal Study. *Am J Clin Nutr.* 2007; 85: 1533–1539.
46. Sævarsson ES, Magnusson KT, Sveinsson T, Johannsson E, Arngrímsson SÁ. The association of cardiorespiratory fitness to health independent of adiposity depends upon its expression. *Ann J Hum Biol.* 2015; 43: 229–234.
47. Alpert BS, Wilmore JH. Physical activity and blood pressure in adolescents. *Pediatr Exerc Sci.* 1994; 6: 361–380.
48. Alpert BS. Exercise as a therapy to control hypertension in children. *Int J Sports Med.* 2000; 21: 94–97.
49. Kelley GA, Kelley KS, Tran ZV. The effects of exercise on resting blood pressure in children and adolescents: a meta-analysis of randomized controlled trials. *Prev Cardiol.* 2003; 6: 8–16.
50. Pescatello LS, Franklin BA, Fagard R, Farquhar WB. American College of Sports Medicine Position Stand: exercise and hypertension. *Med Sci Sports Exerc.* 2004; 36: 533–553.
51. Nielsen GA, Andersen LB. The association between high blood pressure, physical fitness, and body mass index in adolescents. *Prev Med.* 2003; 36: 229–234.
52. García-Hermoso A, Saavedra JM, Escalante Y. Effects of exercise on resting blood pressure in obese children: a meta-analysis of randomized controlled trials. *Obes Rev.* 2013; 14: 919–928.
53. Ho M, Garnett SP, Baur L, *et al.* Effectiveness of lifestyle interventions in child obesity: systematic review with meta-analysis. *Pediatrics.* 2012; 130: e1647–1671.
54. Cai L, Wu Y, Wilson RF, Segal JB, Kim MT, Wang Y. Effect of childhood obesity prevention programs on blood pressure: a systematic review and meta-analysis. *Circulation.* 2014; 129: 1832–1839.
55. Sharman JE, La Gerche A, Coombes JS. Exercise and cardiovascular risk in patients with hypertension. *Am J Hypertens.* 2015; 28: 147–158.
56. Strong WB, Malina RM, Blimkie CJ, *et al.* Evidence based physical activity for school-age youth. *J Pediatr.* 2005; 146: 732–737.
57. Escalante Y, Saavedra JM, García-Hermoso A, Domínguez AM. Improvement of the lipid profile with exercise in obese children: a systematic review. *Prev Med.* 2012; 54: 293–301.
58. Cai L, Wu Y, Cheskin LJ, Wilson RF, Wang Y. Effect of childhood obesity prevention programmes on blood lipids: a systematic review and meta-analysis. *Obes Rev.* 2014; 15: 933–944.
59. Berman LJ, Weigensberg MJ, Spruijt-Metz D. Physical activity is related to insulin sensitivity in children and adolescents, independent of adiposity: a review of the literature. *Diabetes Metab Res Rev.* 2012; 28: 395–408.
60. Fedewa MV, Gist NH, Evans EM, Dishman RK. Exercise and insulin resistance in youth: a meta-analysis. *Pediatrics.* 2014; 133: e163–174.
61. García-Hermoso A, Saavedra JM, Escalante Y, Sánchez López M, Martínez-Vizcaíno V. Endocrinology and Adolescence: aerobic exercise reduces insulin resistance markers in obese youth: a meta-analysis of randomized controlled trials. *Eur J Endocrinol.* 2014; 171: R163–R171.
62. Kim Y, Park H. Does regular exercise without weight loss reduce insulin resistance in children and adolescents? *Int J Endocrinol.* 2013; 2013: Article ID 402592.
63. Grundy SM. Metabolic syndrome: connecting and reconciling cardiovascular and diabetes worlds. *J Am Coll Cardiol.* 2006; 47: 1093–1100.
64. Duncan GE, Li SM, Zhou X-H. Prevalence and trends of a metabolic syndrome phenotype among U.S. adolescents, 1999–2000. *Diabetes Care.* 2004; 27: 2438–2443.
65. Jolliffe CJ, Janssen I. Development of age-specific adolescent metabolic syndrome criteria that are linked to the Adult Treatment Panel III and International Diabetes Federation criteria. *J Am Coll Cardiol.* 2007; 49: 891–898.
66. Ford ES, Li C. Defining the metabolic syndrome in children and adolescents: will the real definition please stand up? *J Pediatr.* 2008; 152: 160–164.
67. Webber LS, Voors AW, Srinivasan SR, Frerichs RR, Berenson GS. Occurrence in children of multiple risk factors for coronary artery disease: the Bogalusa heart study. *Prev Med.* 1979; 8: 407–418.
68. Twisk JW, Kemper HC, van Mechelen W, Post GB. Clustering of risk factors for coronary heart disease. The longitudinal relationship with lifestyle. *Ann Epidemiol.* 2001; 11: 157–165.
69. Platat C, Wagner A, Klumpp T, Schweitzer B, Simon C. Relationships of physical activity with metabolic syndrome features and low-grade inflammation in adolescents. *Diabetologia.* 2006; 49: 2078–2085.
70. Kelishadi R, Razaghi EM, Gouya MM, *et al.* Association of physical activity and the metabolic syndrome in children and adolescents: CASPIAN Study. *Horm Res.* 2007; 67: 46–52.
71. Brage S, Wedderkopp N, Ekelund U, *et al.* Features of the metabolic syndrome are associated with objectively measured physical activity and fitness in Danish children: the European Youth Heart Study (EYHS). *Diabetes Care.* 2004; 27: 2141–2148.
72. Rizzo NS, Ruiz JR, Hurtig-Wennlöf A, Ortega FB, Sjöström M. Relationship of physical activity, fitness, and fatness with clustered metabolic risk in children and adolescents: the European youth heart study. *J Pediatr.* 2007; 150: 388–394.
73. Ekelund U, Brage S, Froberg K, *et al.* TV viewing and physical activity are independently associated with metabolic risk in children: the European Youth Heart Study. *PLOS Med.* 2006; 3: e488.
74. Andersen LB, Wedderkopp N, Hansen HS, Cooper AR, Froberg K. Biological cardiovascular risk factors cluster in Danish children

and adolescents: the European Youth Heart Study. *Prev Med.* 2003; 37: 363–367.

75. Andersen LB, Hasselstrom H, Gronfeldt V, Hansen SE, Karsten F. The relationship between physical fitness and clustered risk, and tracking of clustered risk from adolescence to young adulthood: eight years follow-up in the Danish Youth and Sport Study. *Int J Behav Nutr Phys Act.* 2004; 1: 6.
76. Ruiz JR, Ortega FB, Meusel D, Harro M, Pekka O, Sjöström M. Cardiorespiratory fitness is associated with features of metabolic risk factors in children. Should cardiorespiratory fitness be assessed in a European health monitoring system? The European Youth Heart Study. *J Public Health.* 2006; 14: 94–102.
77. Janssen I, Cramp WC. Cardiorespiratory fitness is strongly related to the metabolic syndrome in adolescents. *Diabetes Care.* 2007; 30: 2143–2144.
78. Lobelo F, Pate RR, Dowda M, Liese AD, Daniels SR. Cardiorespiratory fitness and clustered cardiovascular disease risk in US adolescents. *J Adoles Health.* 2010; 47: 352–359.
79. Okosun IS, Boltri JM, Lyn R, Davis-Smith M. Continuous metabolic syndrome risk score, body mass index percentile, and leisure time physical activity in American children. *J Clin Hypertens.* 2010; 12: 636–644.
80. Ekelund U, Anderssen SA, Froberg K, *et al.* Independent associations of physical activity and cardiorespiratory fitness with metabolic risk factors in children: the European youth heart study. *Diabetologia.* 2007; 50: 1832–1840.
81. Eisenmann JC. Aerobic fitness, fatness and the metabolic syndrome in children and adolescents. *Acta Paediatr.* 2007; 96: 1723–1729.
82. Coppen AM, Risser JA, Vash PD. Metabolic syndrome resolution in children and adolescents after 10 weeks of weight loss. *J Cardiometab Syndr.* 2008; 3: 205–210.
83. Reinehr T, Kleber M, Toschke AM. Lifestyle intervention in obese children is associated with a decrease of the metabolic syndrome prevalence. *Atherosclerosis.* 2009; 207: 174–180.
84. Friedemann C, Heneghan C, Mahtani K, Thompson M, Perera R, Ward AM. Cardiovascular disease risk in healthy children and its association with body mass index: systematic review and meta-analysis. *BMJ.* 2012; 345: e4759.
85. Daniels SR. The consequences of childhood overweight and obesity. *Future Child.* 2006; 16: 47–67.
86. Reilly JJ, Kelly J. Long-term impact of overweight and obesity in childhood and adolescence on morbidity and premature mortality in adulthood: systematic review. *Int J Obes.* 2011; 35: 891–898.
87. Park MH, Falconer C, Viner RM, Kinra S. The impact of childhood obesity on morbidity and mortality in adulthood: a systematic review. *Obes Rev.* 2012; 13: 985–1000.
88. Lloyd LJ, Langley-Evans SC, McMullen S. Childhood obesity and adult cardiovascular disease risk: a systematic review. *Int J Obes.* 2010; 34: 18–28.
89. Bayer O, Krüger H, Kries von R, Toschke AM. Factors associated with tracking of BMI: a meta-regression analysis on BMI tracking. *Obesity.* 2011; 19: 1069–1076.
90. Singh AS, Mulder C, Twisk JW, van Mechelen W, Chinapaw MJ. Tracking of childhood overweight into adulthood: a systematic review of the literature. *Obes Rev.* 2008; 9: 474–488.
91. de Mutsert R, Sun Q, Willett WC, Hu FB, van Dam RM. Overweight in early adulthood, adult weight change, and risk of type 2 diabetes, cardiovascular diseases, and certain cancers in men: a cohort study. *Am J Epidemiol.* 2014; 179: 1353–1365.
92. Yeung EH, Zhang C, Louis GMB, Willett WC, Hu FB. Childhood size and life course weight characteristics in association with the risk of incident type 2 diabetes. *Diabetes Care.* 2010; 33: 1364–1369.
93. Juonala M, Magnussen CG, Berenson GS, *et al.* Childhood adiposity, adult adiposity, and cardiovascular risk factors. *N Engl J Med.* 2011; 365: 1876–1885.
94. Paffenbarger RS, Wing AL. Characteristics in youth predisposing to fatal stroke in later years. *Lancet.* 1967; 1: 753–754.
95. Paffenbarger RS, Wing AL. Chronic disease in former college students. X. The effects of single and multiple characteristics on risk of fatal coronary heart disease. *Am J Epidemiol.* 1969; 90: 527–535.
96. McCarron P, Smith GD, Okasha M, McEwen J. Blood pressure in young adulthood and mortality from cardiovascular disease. *Lancet.* 2000; 355: 1430–1431.
97. Sundström J, Neovius M, Tynelius P, Rasmussen F. Association of blood pressure in late adolescence with subsequent mortality: cohort study of Swedish male conscripts. *BMJ.* 2011; 342: d643.
98. Ortega FB, Silventoinen K, Tynelius P, Rasmussen F. Muscular strength in male adolescents and premature death: cohort study of one million participants. *BMJ.* 2012; 345: e7279.
99. Franks PW, Hanson RL, Knowler WC, Sievers ML, Bennett PH, Looker HC. Childhood obesity, other cardiovascular risk factors, and premature death. *N Engl J Med.* 2010; 362: 485–493.
100. Saydah S, Bullard K, Imperatore G, Geiss L. Cardiometabolic risk factors among US adolescents and young adults and risk of early mortality. *Pediatrics.* 2013; 131: e679–e686.
101. Toschke AM, Kohl L, Mansmann U, Kries von R. Meta-analysis of blood pressure tracking from childhood to adulthood and implications for the design of intervention trials. *Acta Paediatr.* 2010; 99: 24–29.
102. Cook NR, Rosner BA, Chen W, Srinivasan SR, Berenson GS. Using the area under the curve to reduce measurement error in predicting young adult blood pressure from childhood measures. *Statist Med.* 2004; 23: 3421–3435.
103. Adams C, Burke V, Beilin LJ. Cholesterol tracking from childhood to adult mid-life in children from the Busselton study. *Acta Paediatr.* 2005; 94: 275–280.
104. Eisenmann JC, Welk GJ, Wickel EE, Blair SN, Aerobics Center Longitudinal Study. Stability of variables associated with the metabolic syndrome from adolescence to adulthood: the Aerobics Center Longitudinal Study. *Am J Hum Biol.* 2004; 16: 690–696.
105. Katzmarzyk PT, Pérusse L, Malina RM, Bergeron J, Després JP, Bouchard C. Stability of indicators of the metabolic syndrome from childhood and adolescence to young adulthood: the Québec Family Study. *J Clin Epidemiol.* 2001; 54: 190–195.
106. Ford ES. Risks for all-cause mortality, cardiovascular disease, and diabetes associated with the metabolic syndrome: a summary of the evidence. *Diabetes Care.* 2005; 28: 1769–1778.
107. Twisk JW, Kemper HC, van Mechelen W. Prediction of cardiovascular disease risk factors later in life by physical activity and physical fitness in youth: general comments and conclusions. *Int J Sports Med.* 2002; 23: S44–S49.
108. Kvaavik E, Klepp K-I, Tell GS, Meyer HE, Batty GD. Physical fitness and physical activity at age 13 years as predictors of cardiovascular disease risk factors at ages 15, 25, 33, and 40 years: extended follow-up of the Oslo Youth Study. *Pediatrics.* 2009; 123: e80–e86.
109. Jekal Y, Kim Y, Yun JE, *et al.* The association of adolescent fatness and fitness with risk factors for adult metabolic syndrome: a 22-year follow-up study. *J Phys Act Health.* 2014; 11: 823–830.
110. Ferreira I, Twisk JW, van Mechelen W, Kemper HC, Stehouwer CD. Development of fatness, fitness, and lifestyle from adolescence to the age of 36 years: determinants of the metabolic syndrome in young adults: the Amsterdam Growth and Health Longitudinal Study. *Arch Intern Med.* 2005; 165: 42–48.
111. Holman RL. Atherosclerosis—a pediatric nutrition problem? *Am J Clin Nutr.* 1961; 9: 565–569.
112. McGill HC, McMahan CA, Gidding SS. Preventing heart disease in the 21st century: implications of the Pathobiological Determinants of Atherosclerosis in Youth (PDAY) study. *Circulation.* 2008; 117: 1216–1227.
113. Li S, Chen W, Srinivasan SR, *et al.* Childhood cardiovascular risk factors and carotid vascular changes in adulthood: the Bogalusa Heart Study. *JAMA.* 2003; 290: 2271–2276.
114. Juonala M, Järvisalo MJ, Mäki-Torkko N, Kähönen M, Viikari JS, Raitakari OT. Risk factors identified in childhood and decreased

carotid artery elasticity in adulthood: the Cardiovascular Risk in Young Finns Study. *Circulation*. 2005; 112: 1486–1493.

115. Magnussen CG, Smith KJ, Juonala M. What the long term cohort studies that began in childhood have taught us about the origins of coronary heart disease. *Curr Cardiovasc Risk Rep*. 2014; 8: 373.
116. Ferreira I, Twisk JW, van Mechelen W, Kemper HC, Stehouwer CD. Current and adolescent levels of cardiopulmonary fitness are related to large artery properties at age 36: the Amsterdam Growth and Health Longitudinal Study. *Eur J Clin Invest*. 2002; 32: 723–731.
117. Laurent S, Cockcroft J, Van Bortel L, *et al*. Expert consensus document on arterial stiffness: methodological issues and clinical applications. *Eur Heart J*. 2006; 27: 2588–2605.
118. Pickering G. Arteriosclerosis and atherosclerosis. The need for clear thinking. *Am J Med*. 1963; 34: 7–18.
119. Nichols WW, O'Rourke MF, Vlachopoulos C. *McDonald's blood flow in arteries: theoretical, experimental and clinical principles*, 6th ed. Boca Raton, FL: Taylor Francis Group; 2011.
120. Stehouwer CD, Henry RMA, Ferreira I. Arterial stiffness in diabetes and the metabolic syndrome: a pathway to cardiovascular disease. *Diabetologia*. 2008; 51: 527–539.
121. Ferreira I, Beijers HJ, Schouten F, Smulders YM, Twisk JW, Stehouwer CD. Clustering of metabolic syndrome traits is associated with maladaptive carotid remodeling and stiffening: a 6-year longitudinal study. *Hypertension*. 2012; 60: 542–549.
122. Schack-Nielsen L, Mølgaard C, Larsen D, Martyn C, Michaelsen KF. Arterial stiffness in 10-year-old children: current and early determinants. *Br J Nutr*. 2005; 94: 1004–1011.
123. Reed KE, Warburton DR, Lewanczuk RZ, *et al*. Arterial compliance in young children: the role of aerobic fitness. *Eur J Cardiovasc Prev Rehabil*. 2005; 12: 492–497.
124. Sakuragi S, Abhayaratna K, Gravenmaker KJ, *et al*. Influence of adiposity and physical activity on arterial stiffness in healthy children: the lifestyle of our kids study. *Hypertension*. 2009; 53: 611–616.
125. Nettlefold L, McKay HA, Naylor P-J, Bredin SD, Warburton DE. The relationship between objectively measured physical activity, sedentary time, and vascular health in children. *Am J Hypertens*. 2012; 25: 914–919.
126. Edwards NM, Daniels SR, Claytor RP, *et al*. Physical activity is independently associated with multiple measures of arterial stiffness in adolescents and young adults. *Metab Clin Exp*. 2012; 61: 869–872.
127. Veijalainen A, Tompuri T, Haapala EA, Associations of cardiorespiratory fitness, physical activity, and adiposity with arterial stiffness in children. *Scand J Med Sci Sports*. 2016; 26: 943–950. doi:10.1111/sms.12523
128. Ried-Larsen M, Grøntved A, Froberg K, Ekelund U, Andersen LB. Physical activity intensity and subclinical atherosclerosis in Danish adolescents: the European Youth Heart Study. *Scand J Med Sci Sports*. 2013; 23: e168–177.
129. Ried-Larsen M, Grøntved A, Møller NC, Larsen KT, Froberg K, Andersen LB. Associations between objectively measured physical activity intensity in childhood and measures of subclinical cardiovascular disease in adolescence: prospective observations from the European Youth Heart Study. *Br J Sports Med*. 2014; 48: 1502–1507.
130. Ried-Larsen M, Grøntved A, Østergaard L, *et al*. Associations between bicycling and carotid arterial stiffness in adolescents: The European Youth Heart Study. *Scand J Med Sci Sports*. 2015; 25: 661–669.
131. Pahkala K, Laitinen TT, Heinonen OJ, *et al*. Association of fitness with vascular intima-media thickness and elasticity in adolescence. *Pediatrics*. 2013; 132: e77–84.
132. Whincup PH, Gilg JA, Donald AE, *et al*. Arterial distensibility in adolescents: the influence of adiposity, the metabolic syndrome, and classic risk factors. *Circulation*. 2005; 112: 1789–1797.
133. Cote AT, Harris KC, Panagiotopoulos C, Sandor GGS, Devlin AM. Childhood obesity and cardiovascular dysfunction. *J Am Coll Cardiol*. 2013; 62: 1309–1319.
134. Farpour-Lambert NJ, Aggoun Y, Marchand LM, Martin XE, Herrmann FR, Beghetti M. Physical activity reduces systemic blood pressure and improves early markers of atherosclerosis in pre-pubertal obese children. *J Am Coll Cardiol*. 2009; 54: 2396–2406.
135. Ferreira I, Twisk JW, van Mechelen W, Kemper HC, Seidell JC, Stehouwer CD. Current and adolescent body fatness and fat distribution: relationships with carotid intima-media thickness and large artery stiffness at the age of 36 years. *J Hypertens*. 2004; 22: 145–155.
136. Ferreira I, Twisk JW, Stehouwer CD, van Mechelen W, Kemper HC. Longitudinal changes in VO_2 max: associations with carotid IMT and arterial stiffness. *Med Sci Sports Exerc*. 2003; 35: 1670–1678.
137. Ried-Larsen M, Grøntved A, Kristensen PL, Froberg K, Andersen LB. Moderate and vigorous physical activity from adolescence to adulthood and subclinical atherosclerosis in adulthood: prospective observations from the European Youth Heart Study. *Br J Sports Med*. 2015; 49: 107–112.
138. van de Laar RJ, Ferreira I, van Mechelen W, Prins MH, Twisk JW, Stehouwer CD. Habitual physical activity and peripheral arterial compliance in young adults: the Amsterdam Growth and Health Longitudinal Study. *Am J Hypertens*. 2011; 24: 200–208.
139. van de Laar RJ, Ferreira I, van Mechelen W, Prins MH, Twisk JW, Stehouwer CD. Lifetime vigorous but not light-to-moderate habitual physical activity impacts favorably on carotid stiffness in young adults: the Amsterdam Growth and Health Longitudinal Study. *Hypertension*. 2010; 55: 33–39.
140. Ferreira I, van de Laar RJ, Prins MH, Twisk JW, Stehouwer CD. Carotid stiffness in young adults: a life-course analysis of its early determinants: the Amsterdam Growth and Health Longitudinal Study. *Hypertension*. 2012; 59: 54–61.
141. Engelen L, Bossuyt J, Ferreira I, *et al*. Reference values for local arterial stiffness. Part A: carotid artery. *J Hypertens*. 2015; 33: 1981–1996.
142. Pearson N, Braithwaite RE, Biddle SJ, van Sluijs EM, Atkin AJ. Associations between sedentary behaviour and physical activity in children and adolescents: a meta-analysis. *Obes Rev*. 2014; 15: 666–675.
143. van de Laar RJ, Stehouwer CD, Prins MH, van Mechelen W, Twisk JW, Ferreira I. Self-reported time spent watching television is associated with arterial stiffness in young adults: the Amsterdam Growth and Health Longitudinal Study. *Br J Sports Med*. 2014; 48: 256–264.
144. Järvisalo MJ, Harmoinen A, Hakanen M, *et al*. Elevated serum C-reactive protein levels and early arterial changes in healthy children. *Arterioscler Thromb Vasc Biol*. 2002; 22: 1323–1328.
145. García-Hermoso A, Sánchez López M, Escalante Y, Saavedra JM, Martínez-Vizcaíno V. Exercise-based interventions and C-reactive protein in overweight and obese youths: a meta-analysis of randomized controlled trials. *Pediatr Res*. 2016; 79: 522–527.
146. Thomas NE, Williams DR. Inflammatory factors, physical activity, and physical fitness in young people. *Scand J Med Sci Sports*. 2008; 18: 543–556.
147. Dias KA, Green DJ, Ingul CB, Pavey TG, Coombes JS. Exercise and vascular function in child obesity: A meta-analysis. *Pediatrics*. 2015; 136: e648–e659.

CHAPTER 18

Physical activity and bone health

Han CG Kemper and Rômulo A Fernandes

Introduction

The skeleton is generally thought of as a passive structure. When bone is formed and calcified, the structure remains stable; even after death the remains of the skeleton can be found in graves hundreds to thousands of years later. Contrary to this belief, bone is a vital, dynamic connective tissue, which can grow and continuously adapt its structure to its function.[1] To fulfil this structure-function relation adequately, bone is continuously being broken down and rebuilt in a process that is called 'bone remodelling'.

Bone mass increases at the same rate during growth and development in boys and girls, but at the beginning of puberty a sexual dimorphism occurs and bone mass increases faster in boys than girls. Maximal bone mass is reached in the late teens and early twenties. Thereafter it gradually declines. This decrease is accelerated in women after the menopause (Figure 18.1).

The average woman has a higher risk of osteoporosis than the average man for at least two reasons. Firstly, women reach a lower maximal bone mass in their youth, and secondly, women lose bone at a higher rate after menopause. This decrease in bone density leaves elderly individuals, particularly females, at risk for exaggerated bone thinning, or osteoporosis, with subsequent disability and death from bone fractures.

This chapter reviews i) the different methods to measure bone mass, ii) the growth and development of bone mass during childhood and adolescence, iii) the effects of physical activity (PA) and exercise on physical fitness and bone health during youth, and iv) the most effective exercise regimens to strengthen the bone.

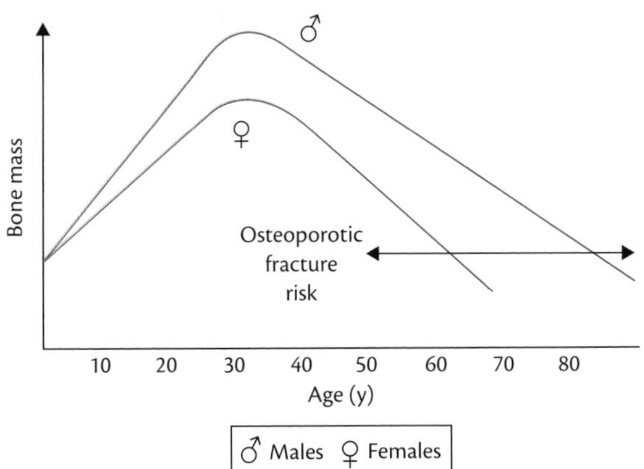

Figure 18.1 The development of bone mass in males and females with age.
The osteoporotic fracture risk is usually reached at an earlier age in females than in males.
Kemper HCG. Skeletal development during childhood and adolescence and the effects of physical activity. Pediatr Exerc Sci. 2000; 12: 198–216.

Although primarily considered a disorder of the elderly, emerging evidence suggests the antecedents of osteoporosis are established during childhood and adolescence. A complex interplay of genetic, environmental, hormonal, and behavioural factors determine skeletal development.[2]

Because bone mass predicts fracture risk and peak bone mass, knowledge about bone mass can help us to understand the impact of PA as one of the important lifestyle factors during youth for prevention of osteoporosis at older age.[3] Strategies that optimize bone strength and maximize peak bone mass are therefore required to counter the deleterious effects of age-related bone loss and the anticipated global epidemic in osteoporosis.[4–6]

Growth of bone

Physical growth and development have been extensively investigated from prenatal growth to birth, and from postnatal growth to adulthood by many longitudinal studies from all over the world. In 1955, JM Tanner published the first edition of his book *Growth at Adolescence*,[7] followed in 1981 by *A History of the Study of Human Growth*.[8] Since then, both books have been regarded as cornerstone publications on human growth and development. The methods that are used in general to measure growth changes are mainly based on simple anthropometric measurements of the total body (body height, body mass) or of body segments (trunk height, limb lengths). Also breadth measurements (shoulder, hip, wrist, and knee), circumferences (head, trunk, hip, waist, and limbs) and skinfold measurements at different sites of the body are applied according to standard methods.[9] All of these measurements estimate different dimensions of the body, but do not take into consideration changes in the composition of these body parts.

Radiographic methods are used to indicate calcified cartilage and ossified bone and to estimate skeletal maturation. Different methods have been developed to assess the rate of maturation or biological age from X-rays at wrist and knee. From a comparison of skeletal age with calendar age the child can be characterized as an early or late maturer.[10]

In recent years new methods have been developed to measure the bone mass by energy absorption from gamma radiation by calcium in the bone. The methods mostly described in the literature are single photon absorptiometry (SPA), dual photon absorptiometry (DPA), dual energy X-ray absorptiometry (DEXA), and quantitative computed tomography (QCT).

In the reviewed literature bone mass is measured in different parts of the human skeleton, such as the arm, hip, spine, and heel, or in the total body mass. The details of method and place of measurement will only be mentioned here if necessary, and if they have important consequences for the interpretation of the outcomes.

Since not much is known about the natural development of bone mass during youth, the literature will be reviewed on i) the changes in bone mass during prepubertal, circumpubertal, and postpubertal development, ii) the differences in bone development between boys and girls, and iii) the point of time at which the maximal amount of bone mass, or peak bone mineral density (PBMD), is reached.

Most BMD studies are aimed at prevention and retardation of bone loss in postmenopausal women. An important question remains as to whether it is possible to increase the bone mass during the growing years by exercise in order to attain higher maximal bone mass at young adult age.[11] There are to date several experimental studies published that have investigated the effects of PA programmes on bone health in youth.

Methods of measurement of bone mass

Anthropometrics

Von Döbeln[12] proposed a measure for estimation of skeletal weight from body height and four breadth measurements (left and right femur condyli and radio-ulnar width). This method provides satisfactory data as long as it is used for estimating total weight of bone mass in comparison with estimates of muscle and fat mass estimated by skinfolds and circumferences, in combination with body height and weight. In the Netherlands, this concept is used to correct the body weight to body height relationship; the Dutch Heart Foundation constructed a reference scale (for ideal body weight) based on the Quetelet Index or Body Mass Index (BMI; $kg \cdot m^{-2}$) that included the possibility of calculating the ideal body weight, taking the breadth of the femur condyle into consideration. However, this is a misuse of the skeletal component of this algorithm, because an adjustment is made for the least variable of the three component models of body composition, with lean and fat mass being the other components.

Radiographics

In November 1895, the German physicist Wilhelm Conrad Röntgen discovered gamma radiation and demonstrated a radiogram showing the bones of his own hand. He called this X radiation. The anatomist Albert von Kölliker connected Röntgen's name to this kind of radiation. Since then, X-rays have been widely used in medicine for detection of infectious diseases, pathologic neoplasmata, and traumatology.

Another field in radiographics is its use as a measure of biological age with respect to skeletal growth and development. Skeletal maturation begins as a process when rudiments of bones appear during embryonic life and is completed when skeletal form becomes comparatively stable in young adulthood. During maturation there are increases in the types and numbers of specialized cells, including cartilage and fibrous tissue cells that form part of a bone.[13] Roche *et al.*[14] in their longitudinal study used the knee joint as bones of interest for determination of skeletal maturation (the Roche-Wainer-Thissen method, or RWT). However, most assessments of skeletal maturity are made from radiographs of the hand-wrist, because this site has considerable advantages over other parts of the skeleton. These advantages stem from the little irradiation required, the ease of radiographic positioning, and the large number of bones included in the area. Therefore, the RWT method using the knee joint as a biological indicator for growth was extended with the hand-wrist method. In Europe in 1975, Tanner *et al.*[15] published their Tanner-Whitehouse (TW2) method for the determination of growth, also using X-ray photographs of the left hand and including 20 bones of the hand and wrist.

All these skeletal maturity scales are used to estimate the developmental or biological age of children, correcting for children who mature faster or slower than the average child with the same calendar age (interested readers are referred to Chapter 1 for discussion of the assessment of biological maturity using skeletal age and other methods of assessment). In paediatrics it can be used to predict adult height of children (mostly girls) who are expected to end up very tall, and where there is a consideration of intervention in their growth by using hormones to close their endplates earlier.

Dual energy X-ray absorptiometry

Radiographs cannot easily quantify changes in bone density, because 30% of it has to be lost before it can be detected by X-ray. However, recent technical advances have made it possible to measure bone mass by energy absorption from gamma radiation in the bone. Dual energy X-ray absorptiometry (DEXA) remains the most widely used method of assessing bone density, which has been indicated as important tool in the complex diagnosis of osteoporosis in the paediatric population.[16] Dual energy X-ray absorptiometry is the preferred method because scanning time is shorter than with DPA. Additionally, resolution has been improved, and measurements can be made of the lumbar spine, femoral neck, forearm, and of the total body.

From the DEXA method, two measures are calculated: the bone mineral content (BMC) and the BMD. The BMC is the total amount of minerals in the selected bone in grams, and the BMD is the amount of grams of bone mineral divided by the area of the selected bone ($g \cdot cm^{-2}$). However, the BMD is not a real measure of bone density ($g \cdot cm^{-3}$), and is therefore called area density, or areal BMD. In growth, bones not only increase their area, but also their volume. These size changes influence the areal BMD. Therefore, attempts have been made to estimate the volume of the bone of interest and to correct for this bone size effect by an additional measure of bone mineral apparent density (BMAD).[17] In fact, the DEXA technique does not provide actual information about bone morphology and architecture, but significant advances in computational software have permitted it to estimate some bone geometric properties in adolescents, such as subperiosteal width and endocortical diameter.[18]

Quantitative computed tomography

Quantitative computed tomography systems have been adapted for estimation of bone mineral content, allowing cortical bone to be separated from trabecular bone. Furthermore, it provides us with a true measure of total, cortical, or trabecular bone mineral volumetric density ($mg \cdot mm^{-3}$). However, the equipment is more expensive, and exposes patients to high radiation doses. A peripheral QCT system is another alternative method to assess bone morphology and architecture, in which the scan time is fast and produces low radiation exposure to the patient.[16] On the other hand, the main limitations in the use of the peripheral QCT are still based in the absence of standardized methods to the technique.[16]

Quantitative ultrasound

Ultrasound measurements have been available since the 1980s, and have the potential for widespread clinical applications because they do not use radiation. Quantitative ultrasound measurements are made to assess broadband ultrasound attenuation (BUA in $dB \cdot MHz^{-1}$) and SOS (speed of sound in $m \cdot s^{-1}$). One of the advantages is that it not only gives a quantitative measure of bone (mass) but also a qualitative aspect (structure). The validity of ultrasound for bone measurement has, however, still to be proven.

Mechanisms of bone formation

Movement is the result of electric impulses being passed from the central nervous system to the skeletal muscles. These muscles contract in order to move body parts with respect to each other (arms, legs, head, and trunk) and/or the whole body with respect to the surroundings (e.g. walking, cycling, and swimming). Exercise is not necessarily dynamic and sometimes muscles contract without causing movements but still increase their tension, e.g. static exercises such as standing, active sitting, or pushing against a wall.

Both the duration and intensity of exercise play a role in the physical load placed on the body. Low-intensity, long-lasting exercise increases ventilation and circulation to meet oxygen demand for delivering energy to the active muscles. This is important for better capillarization and oxygen delivery to the muscle. High-intensity, short-lasting exercise is important for the development of muscle and bone mass. Results show that the key factor affecting bone health is not the duration of exercise but the intensity of the forces that act upon the bones. Weight-bearing activities, such as walking, running, and dancing, have more effect on bone health of the legs and vertebrae of the lower back than have swimming and cycling, although all activities need approximately the same amount of energy when performed for identical lengths of time. This difference in effect on bone health is in contrast to the effects of these activities on the lungs, heart, and circulation: if performed with the same intensity and duration, swimming has the same effect as running on the oxygen transport system.

Two different mechanisms seem to act on bone mass. Firstly, there are central hormonal factors, such as oestrogen production. Then there are local mechanical factors, such as the muscle forces exerted on the bones of the skeleton during contraction, as well as the forces of gravity that act on the entire body during standing and other weight-bearing activities.[19]

Central hormonal factors maintain serum calcium concentrations within a limited range. Calcium is one of the most common ions in the human body, and almost 99% of body calcium is deposited in the skeleton. Oestrogens suppress the activity of osteoclasts, the bone resorbing cells, and thus help to maintain bone mass. During exercise, serum concentrations of testosterone and oestrogen are elevated, influencing calcium homeostasis and the activity of osteoclasts and osteoblasts. Hormonal replacement therapy in women after the menopause makes use of this action of oestrogen.

The local mechanical forces of exercise cause i) stress on the bone and calcium accumulation on the concave side of the bending bone, and ii) microtraumata, which are removed by osteoclasts and repaired by osteoblasts.

The supposed mechanisms behind the local mechanical forces are as follows:

First, during flexion the bone acts like a piezo-electric crystal while accumulating calcium at the concave (= negatively loaded) side.

Secondly, mechanical demands, occurring by overload, are sensed in the bone by osteocytes via strain-derived flows of interstitial fluid. They stimulate the osteoclasts in removing the damaged structures and at the same time the osteoblasts repair the structure of the bone matrix.[20]

In the case of excessive damage, or too-often damaged bone, the process of repairing falls behind the process of removal and micro-fracture will occur. When the mechanical load falls below the fracture intensity, remodelling activities are stimulated and result in bone hypertrophy.

Remodelling of the bone after a change in mechanical load by weight-bearing activities (including experiments with added extra weights) has been proved in experimental studies in a great number of animals.[21]

Moreover, in some of these experiments it has been shown that the effects are proportional to the intensity of the (extra) load. The amount of hypertrophy seems also to depend on the difference between the extra load and the load to the bone before the extra load was added.

Not much is known about the interaction between central hormonal and local mechanical factors. However, PA leads to an increase of serum oestrogen levels, which diminishes the sensitivity of the bone for the parathyroid hormone and the activity of the osteoclasts. Therefore, when bone mass thus increases, more calcium (Ca^{2+}) and phosphorus (P) are resorbed from the blood. Subsequently, this lowering of Ca^{2+} and P concentrations in the blood stimulates the parathyroid hormone; the latter inhibits vitamin D production, stimulates calcium absorption, and decreases calcium secretion.

As long as the forces exerted on the bones remain weaker than those needed to cause a macro-fracture (referred to as the fracture limit), this remodelling process is able to adapt the bone to the external biomechanical stress and bring about bone thickening (hypertrophy). During long periods of inactivity, such as prolonged bed rest, the bone becomes atrophic as a result of relatively higher osteoclast activity compared to osteoblast activity. The central hormonal system and the local mechanical system interact to optimize the function of the skeletal system. In the case of exercise, mechanical factors seem to be most important for affecting bone mass.

Animal experiments[22] in an ulna-model of roosters have shown that loading of bone a few times (four times) a day can prevent bone loss, and that high frequency of loading (36 per day) results in an optimal increase in bone mass. Bone mass is not further increased by increasing the daily frequency of bone loading to 360 or even 1800 times per day. This suggests that bone tissue rapidly becomes desensitized to prolonged exercise. Others have replicated these findings.[23] Rats that were trained to jump multiple times increased tibial and femoral bone mass, but the anabolic response saturated after about 40 loading cycles. The results of both experiments are illustrated in Figure 18.2.

Therefore, in humans short bursts of explosive exercise, such as skipping, stair climbing, and jumping, are supposedly more

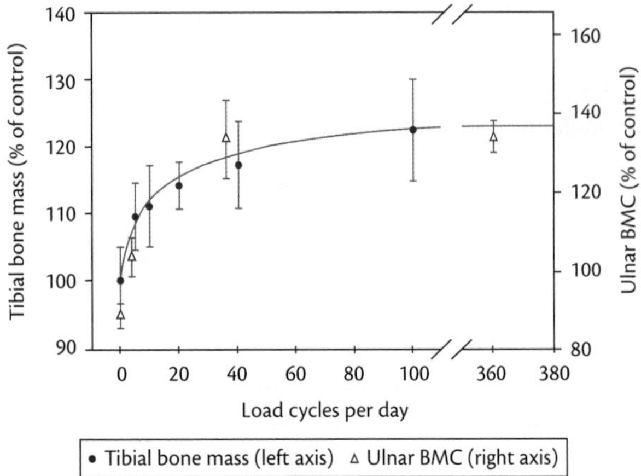

Figure 18.2 Bone mass in roosters and rats. Experiments in animals (roosters and rats) show that loading bones at a frequency of more than 40 load cycles per day is an optimal rate to increase bone mass.
(open triangles tibia of roosters, Rubin *et al.*[22] and closed circles ulna of rats, Umemura *et al.*[23]). [after Turner[24], with permission].

effective for bone development, than more popular forms of exercise such as walking, jogging, bicycling, and swimming.

Bone, therefore, appears to react best to exercise that is characterized by a pattern of unexpected and irregular high dynamic loads, with a relatively low frequency and short duration.[24] Turner formulated three rules, stating that i) bone adaptation is driven by dynamic, rather than static, loading, ii) only a short duration of mechanical loading is necessary to initiate an adaptive response; extending the loading duration has a diminishing effect on further bone adaptation, and iii) bone cells accommodate to a customary mechanical loading environment, making them less responsive to routine loading signals.

Exercise for bone development is different to endurance exercise aimed at enhancing aerobic function; the latter consists of long duration (or high frequency) and low intensity. For comparison, Figure 18.3 shows an example of a typical and effective exercise for loading bone (skipping) and an effective exercise for loading the oxygen transport system (jogging). Extrapolated from the results of animal studies, skipping for 1 min a day (six times for 10 s) seems effective for maintaining bone mass, whereas jogging for 1 h a day (i.e. two times 30 min) is more effective for the development of the oxygen transport system. Exercise that is effective in maintaining bone mass is of shorter duration than endurance exercise.[25]

From the available data on exercise regimens, Turner and Robling[26] constructed an osteoporotic index (OI) including intensity of load upon bone (times body weight), multiplied by the number of loading cycles, multiplied by the number of days per week. The OI increased by 30% if the number of $d \cdot week^{-1}$ increased from one to five, and as much as 50% if daily exercise is divided into two shorter sessions separated by at least 8 h; an increase of loading cycles from 150 to 600 resulted in a 20% increase.

Natural course of bone mass development

Although Figure 18.1 outlines the general course of bone mass, not much is known about the exact timing of the age at which the maximal amount of bone mass is developed. Therefore, we first review the literature about bone development in boys and girls before puberty. Secondly, we make an estimate about the importance of the pubertal period in the total development of bone mass. Thirdly, we provide answers regarding the age at which maximal or PBMD occurs in males and females.

Development of bone density before puberty

Six cross-sectional studies[27–32] and one longitudinal study[33] conclude that between boys and girls there is no significant difference between the BMD of the radius and the lumbar spine. This indicates that the development of BMD before puberty is not dependent on steroids.

Although there is a trend for a gradual increase from birth to puberty in bone mass, despite information from seven reviewed publications, it is not possible to make a quantitative estimation of the proportional contribution of this time window to the total (adult) bone mass. Before puberty there is no difference in BMD between boys and girls. Sex differences on bone growth still constitute an open line of research[34], but even when observing similar bone development, some experimental evidence shows that before puberty, boys' skeletons seem more responsive to exercise interventions than that of girls'.[35–36]

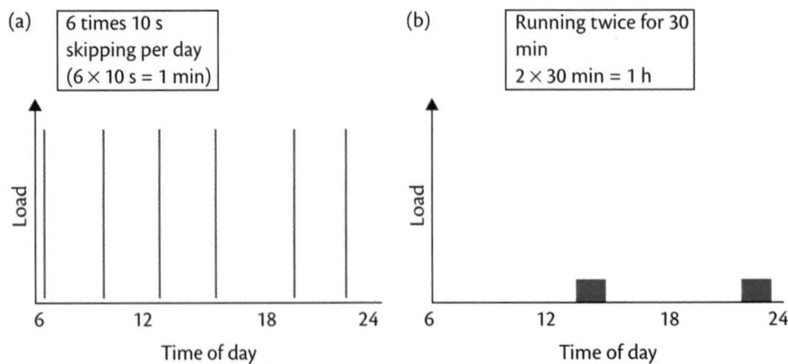

Figure 18.3 Comparison of two types of exercise with different effects on the musculo-skeletal and the cardiorespiratory system.
Short explosive exercise (a), such as skipping six times a day for 10 s (total exercise time per day 60 s), is effective for bone and muscle strength, whereas low-intensity exercise (b) of long duration, such as jogging two times a day for 30 min (total exercise time 60 min), is more effective for the development of the oxygen transport system.
Kemper HCG. Skeletal development during childhood and adolescence and the effects of physical activity. Pediatr Exerc Sci. 2000; 12: 198–216.

Development of bone density during puberty

Puberty is a relative short period of 3–5 years, and is very important for the development of bone mass. Six cross-sectional studies[27–32] report increases between 17% and 70% of BMD in girls, and between 11% and 75% in boys, compared to total adult values. The high variation in these results can be attributed to several factors:

i) Differences in the classification of puberty;

ii) Confounding factors such as nutritional and/or activity patterns that are different for the populations studied;

iii) The possible influence of early or late maturation, where early maturation coincides with a relative but longer exposition to sex-specific hormones than late maturation, i.e. oestrogen levels in girls and testosterone levels in boys seem to be related to bone mass development.

These cross-sectional data suggest that during the pubertal years boys and girls add between 50–75% to total bone mass of the lumbar spine, and 30% to the radial bone mass.[37]

However, Bailey *et al.*[38] reported that the BMD changes should be interpreted with caution because of the methods used. Determination of BMD by projectional methods like DEXA provide areal densities ($g \cdot cm^{-2}$) which are confounded by the previously mentioned size changes accompanying growth. Consequently, calculated volumetric BMD percentage increases are substantially less than the corresponding area BMD value increases. This dimensional consideration explains why Gilsanz *et al.*[27] showed the lowest increase (15%); as they used the QCT method to measure BMD, their results are in line with this method, which provides real volumetric BMDs.

As the literature reports that around 50% of BMD is accreted during puberty, and considering that the DEXA method is used to measure these changes, we must allow for some doubt in the interpretation of these data. In contrast, the only study with QCT methodology reports a 15% volume BMD increase in pubertal girls, which seems to be a more realistic value.

The most convincing data regarding the normal pattern of bone mineral accrual around the ages 8–18 years come from the University of Saskatchewan Pediatric Bone Mineral Accrual study.[39] The authors measured bone mineral content in 200 boys and girls annually for 7 years at four anatomical regions (lumbar spine, femoral neck, proximal femur, and total body). The velocity curves showed that the bone mineral accrual occurs ~18 months earlier in girls than in boys and is 20% less in magnitude. The former is of clinical interest, because the dissociation between peak linear growth and peak bone mineral accrual may constitute a period of relative bone fragility during the 4 years around peak height velocity (PHV). In fact, it is not clear whether higher bone mass/density values prevent fracture risk in paediatric populations.[40,41] However, a multicentre American study monitored 1470 children and adolescents (aged 6–17 years) annually for 6 years and identified that fracture risk was significantly higher in subjects having a skeletal age of 10–14 years compared to adolescents ≥15 years.[40] In targeting the prevention of fractures in adolescents, coaches and physical education teachers should pay special attention to this period of relative bone fragility during puberty, in which there is a temporary imbalance between bone acquisition and muscle mass development.

Age at which maximal bone mass is reached (peak bone mineral density)

Most of the anatomical structures and physiological functions, such as muscle mass, cardiorespiratory functions, immune system, and central nervous system, show a typical pattern of growth and decline over time. This pattern is characterized by a steep increase during the growth period until the age of 20 years, followed by a plateau, and then a gradual decline during aging (see Figure 18.4).[42] This pattern implies that there is a point or period in time where the human functions reach their maximal capacities. The question remains if there is a similar pattern observable in the development of bone mass, and if so, at what point in time of life PBMD occurs.

Twelve cross-sectional studies have recorded age on reaching PBMD, seven on girls and five on both boys and girls. They report on an age period of reaching PBMD, in girls between 16 and 23 years, and in boys between 16 and 25 years. However, it is important to note that, in principle, a cross-sectional design is not adequate to indicate individual changes over time. It also has methodological constraints (such as cohort effects, secular trends, etc.). With these flaws in mind the results of six of these cross-sectional studies that feature acceptable methodology and sufficient information from the publication are taken into account.[27–29,33,43,44]

Five longitudinal studies have investigated the development of BMD and PBMD; all of the studies used female subjects. From a methodological point of view, the quality of three studies can be questioned seriously,[47–49] as they tend to confirm the cross-sectional results that PBMD occurs before age 20 years. However, two high-quality studies in women, from Davies *et al.*[45] (with a follow up of 4 years) and from Recker *et al.*[46] (with a follow up of 5 years), provide data that show clearly the age of PBMD is reached much later than 20 years; lumbar, radial, and total BMD reach their highest values around the age of 30 years.

The estimated age at PBMD of three low-quality[47–49] and two high-quality[45,46] longitudinal studies ranged from 17 to <20 years in low-quality studies, while PBMD ranged from >26 to 29 years in high-quality studies. In general, low-quality cross-sectional studies tend to establish PBMD in females between 16 and 25 years of age, where the high-quality longitudinal investigations establish

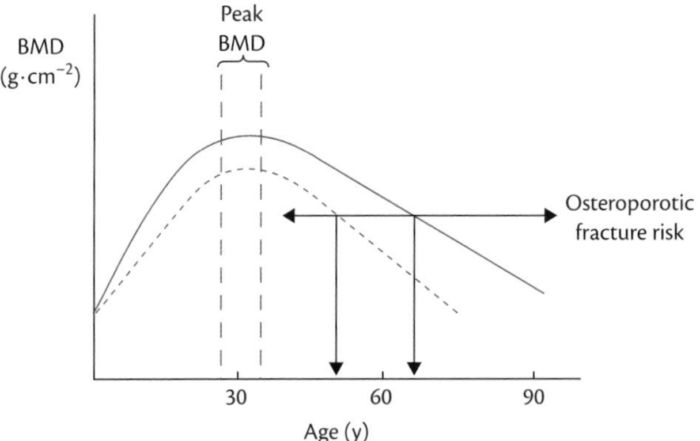

Figure 18.4 The possible effects of lifetime exercise on the developmental curve of bone mineral density.

The average curve of inactive people (interrupted line) is shifted to the top-right (solid line) resulting in a higher bone mineral density of any age and crossing the osteoporotic limit at a later age.

Kemper HCG. Skeletal development during childhood and adolescence and the effects of physical activity. Pediatr Exerc Sci. 2000; 12: 198–216.

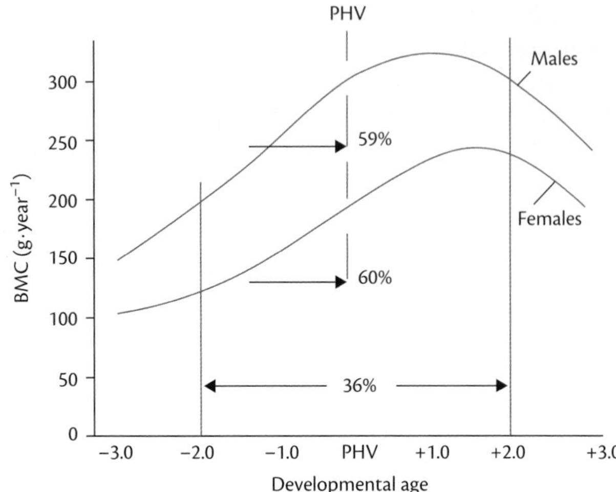

Figure 18.5 Total body bone mineral content (BMC) velocity curves of boys and girls aligned around 4 years of age at peak height velocity (PHV).
Bailey DA. The Saskatchewan Pediatric Bone Mineral Accrual Study: Bone Mineral Acquisition during the growing years. Int J Sports Med. 1997; 18: S191–S195.

PBMD in females much later, around the age of 30 years. A Dutch study published in 2010 grouped cross-sectional and longitudinal datasets of 501 Caucasian subjects aged 13–29 years. Using a robust statistical model, the Dutch study identified that PBMD occurred at 20 and 23 years in girls and boys, respectively.[50] On the other hand, it is not clear the actual burden of longitudinal and cross-sectional data in the PBMD created, as well as if the PBMD data generated are similar to the cross-sectional studies previous published.[27,28,29,33,43,44] Therefore, because longitudinal data are more valid to detect age changes, it is more likely that PBMD in females does not occur in the late teens, but rather in the mid- to late twenties.

To investigate how bone mineral at clinically important sites proceeds in relation to maturation and size in youth, distance and velocity curves were developed for body height and BMC for both boys and girls, based on data from the Saskatchewan Pediatric Bone Mineral Accrual Study.[51] Study participants were measured every 6 months during a follow-up of 6 years (see Figure 18.5). In both boys and girls, over 35% of total body BMC was laid down during the 4-year circumpubertal period. This result is 30% greater than cross-sectional estimates,[51] which demonstrates the 'blunting' of values that occurs when cross-sectional data are used to represent longitudinal change.[52]

A subsequent report from this longitudinal study determined the amount of calcium that was added to the skeleton during the rapid growth period. To meet the demands of the skeleton during time, a mean dietary calcium intake of approximately 1100 $mg \cdot day^{-1}$ for boys at age 14 years, and of 850 $mg \cdot day^{-1}$ for girls at age 12.5 years, would be required. These values are comparable to the current recommended dietary allowances for calcium of between 900–1200 $mg \cdot day^{-1}$ for both boys and girls during puberty.

Effects of physical activity and physical fitness on bone mass

Physical fitness (including neuro-motor and cardiorespiratory fitness) is often used as a proxy measure of PA. However, in theory, physical fitness is the result of both genetic and environmental influences. For most physical fitness parameters, the genetic component is responsible for about 60–80% of the variance, (e.g. maximal aerobic power, maximal muscle force, flexibility). Physical activity is only one of several environmental factors that can modify physical fitness. Therefore, this chapter does not discuss the relationship between bone health and physical fitness.

Randomized controlled trials

Longitudinal studies that include interventions with extra PA are indispensable to prove that bone mass can be influenced by the daily PA pattern of the subjects involved. The majority of these so called randomized controlled trials (RCTs) are done in females older than 45 years in order to prevent postmenarcheal bone loss osteoporosis. On the other hand, over the last few years, the number of RCTs analysing the effect of interventions in physical education classes on bone tissue have become more common, leading to relevant findings about this issue.

In a meta-analysis the effects of exercise training programmes in pre- and postmenopausal women on BMD of the lumbar spine (LS) and the femoral neck (FN) were studied by Wolff *et al.*[53] The study treatment effect was defined as the difference between the % change in BMD per year in the training and the control group. Seventeen articles were included. The summary treatment effects were in premenopausal women 0.9% (95% CI: 0.4–1.4) in LS and 0.9% (0.3–1.5), and in postmenopausal women 0.9 (0.4–1.3) in LS and 1.0 (0.4–1.5) in FN. It showed that exercise prevented almost 1% BMD loss per year in both pre- and postmenopausal women. The separate analysis for endurance and strength training type did not reveal large differences. The main reasons for this are twofold: i) the small number of studies with specific strength training, and ii) the endurance programmes also may have included exercises with high strains.

The number of RCT studies in young subjects has increased in the last few years,[54–62] but the development of this type of study remains rare, which denotes a significant lack in the literature due the significant impact of ethnic/racial characteristics in the development of bone tissue.[40]

The Margulies[54] study of 268 male military recruits between the ages of 18–21 years who followed an intensive training programme of 8 h per day, had no control group, and the period of follow-up was relatively short (14 weeks). More importantly, however, about 40% of the subjects could not comply because of stress fractures. In 1998, Bradney *et al.*[55] published a study in prepubertal boys comparing an 8-month, three times per week, 30 min programme consisting of weight-bearing exercise with a control group matched for age, height, weight, and BMD. The increase in BMD was site specific, and twice that in controls in lumbar spine, legs, and total body. In the Copenhagen School Child Intervention Study, Hasselstrom *et al.*[56] demonstrated in 6- to 8-year-old boys (n = 297) and girls (n = 265) that different intensities (measured with accelerometers), the daily amount, and effort levels of PA are all associated with significantly higher forearm and calcaneal BMD.

Gleeson *et al.*[57] performed a 1-year, three times per week weight-training programme of 30 min duration, with an intensity of 60% of the one repetition maximum in 34 postpubertal women (24–46 years). They compared the bone density in the lumbar spine and the calcaneus with 38 controls. No changes in either group were found in BMD. Blimkie *et al.*[58] also found non-significant changes in younger postpubertal girls (14–18 years) following a weight-training programme over a shorter period of 26 weeks.

Morris *et al.*[59] performed a 10-month intervention in premenarcheal girls where high-impact strength-building exercise showed a significant increase at all four bone sites of interest (proximal femur, neck of femur, lumbar spine, and total body). This increase was accompanied by better physical fitness, including decrease in fat mass, gain in lean mass, shoulder, knee, and grip strength.

Heinonen *et al.*[61] compared the effects of a 9-month step aerobics intervention on BMD in pre-and postmenarcheal girls. Significantly more bone gain (in the lumbar spine and femoral neck BMD) was found between exercisers and controls, but only in the premenarcheal group.

A 2-year prospective controlled exercise intervention trial was performed with ninety-nine 7- to 9-year-old girls from the Pediatric Osteoporosis Prevention Study. This study evaluated a school curriculum-based training programme (5 days with 40 min versus 2 days 30 min per week) and showed that the annual gain in BMC, areal BMD, and bone size of lumbar spine, femoral neck, and legs was greater in the intervention group than in the controls.[62]

A study from Witzke *et al.*[63] in postpubescent girls intervening using a progressive programme of plyometric jumps over a period of 9 months also did not show significant BMC at hip and spine, although knee extensor strength was improved.

McKay *et al.*[60] randomized healthy third- and fourth-grade children (mean age 8.9 years) from ten different primary schools into exercise and control groups. The groups consisted of both boys and girls. The exercise groups performed tuck jumps, hopping, and skipping for 10–20 min within school physical education classes, three times weekly. After an 8-month intervention, the exercise group showed a significantly greater change in proximal femur and trochanter BMD compared to the control classes.

More recently, RCTs have been carried out in school environments, targeting the beneficial effects of physical education classes. Weeks *et al.*[34] implemented an 8-month intervention protocol (twice weekly; 10 min of directed jumping activities [~300 jumps per session]) during physical education classes where pubertal and postpubertal boys and girls were organized into an exercise group and a control group. The exercise group (n = 43) performed activities during the warm-up, while the control group (n = 38) performed regular warm-up and stretching activities. After the warm-up activities, both groups performed the same regular physical education class. The proposed intervention improved indices of bone strength in both sexes of the exercise group.

A 9-month intervention was also performed, in which two additional physical education classes were added to the exercise group (45 min each with at least 10 min of jumping activities [n = 224]). The control group performed three classes per week (n = 67). Both groups involved prepubertal and early pubertal boys and girls.[35] In both sexes, BMC and BMD in different sites (whole body, femoral neck, and lumbar spine) were noted in the exercise group (5–8%), mainly in prepubertal subjects. Another study identified the beneficial impacts of a school-based exercise intervention performed during seven months. Groups were split into exercise and control groups. The exercise group performed 10 min of jumps. The control group performed 10 min of stretching. Both groups performed these activities 3 days per week. Improvements in hip BMC were observed 7 years after the end of the exercise protocol.[64] Finally, 6 years of physical exercise intervention is capable of improving both bone mass and skeletal architecture in adolescents.[65]

The outcome of the reviewed studies seems to vary depending on the maturity level of the adolescents. Studies in pre-and early pubescent children report significant increases in BMC and BMD, where studies with postpubertal adolescents report no significant difference in bone mineral between control and intervention groups. Conversely, it is noteworthy that in postpubertal adolescents, even without modifications in BMD and BMC values, geometrical properties of the bone can improve via weight-bearing physical exercise, such as soccer practice.[18]

The results of three prospective exercise intervention studies in pre- and pubertal girls and boys are illustrated in Figure 18.6.

Systematic review of randomized controlled trials

Recently a systematic review was published where 22 randomized and non-randomized controlled trials were evaluated on the effects on bone mineral accrual in children and adolescents.[66] All nine early pubertal trials reported positive effects, measured as a mean increase over 6 months (0.9–4.9%), and six prepubertal trials measured 1.1–5.5, and two pubertal trials measured 0.3–1.9%.

Long-term effects of physical activity

Non 'true' experimental results are available from the Amsterdam Growth and Health Longitudinal Study.[67] About 200 boys and 200 girls were measured longitudinally from age 13–27 years. In follow-up, six measurements were taken of habitual PA and nutritional intake. At age 27 years, the BMD of the lumbar region was measured by DEXA. The longitudinal information of weight-bearing activity and calcium intake were considered over three periods: the adolescent period from 13–18 years, the period between 13–22 years, and the total period between the ages of 13–27 years.

Results of multiple regression analysis showed that in both sexes weight-bearing activity and body mass were significantly positive contributors in the prediction of BMD at age 27 years. Calcium intake never appeared to be a significant predictor of BMD in any of the three periods. From these results we conclude that BMD in the lumbar spine at age 27 years may be influenced by body mass and a high level of weight-bearing PA carried out during youth.

The PA data were scored in two different ways in order to determine the most important factor in determining BMD in youth. Firstly, the total weekly energy expenditure of all weight-bearing activities (expressed as the number of weight bearing METs per week) was calculated. This was followed by creating a score using the ground reaction forces of weight-bearing activities as multiples of body weight, irrespective of the frequency and the duration of the activity, i.e. giving a weighted peak strain score. These scores are comparable with the bone loading history questionnaire from Dolan *et al.*,[68] which proved to be a reproducible and valid measure of bone loading exposure in premenopausal women.

The two different habitual PA scores were again calculated for each subject over three time periods: the adolescent period (four annual measurements between ages 13–17 years), the young adult period (two measurements between ages 17–22 years), and the adult period (two measurements between ages 22–27 years).

Linear regression analysis was performed to analyse the relation between BMD at age 28 years and the PA scores over three foregoing periods. The PA scores were entered in the regression model

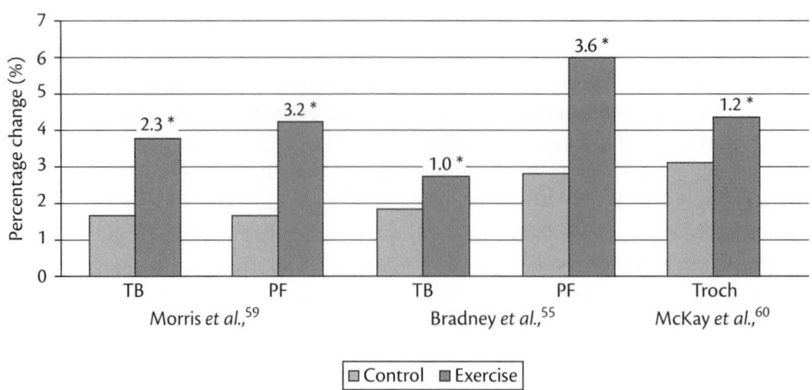

Figure 18.6 Results of three prospective exercise intervention studies in pre- and early pubertal youth.

Data for girls (Morris *et al.*)[59], boys (Bradney *et al.*)[55] and both girls and boys (McKay *et al.*[60]). Differences in percentage change between exercise and control groups are given in numbers. [after Kahn *et al.*,[52] with permission].

as independent variables, and gender was added to the model as a covariate. In Figure 18.7, the standard regression coefficients of lumbar BMD are given for the MET score and the peak strain score, and for the three different periods.

The results show that during the three periods over which the PA scores were taken, the peak score and the MET score were similar in the BMD measurement in the young adult period; the peak strain score of PA became more important. For this biomechanical component of PA, the explained variance of BMD increased from 2% during adolescence to 13% in adulthood. For the PA energetic score, the explained variance decreased from 6% during adolescence to 1% in adulthood for both sexes.[69] These data strongly support the validity of the results of animal studies when considering possible similarities in human subjects.

In fact, a recent review[36] identifies that there is evidence supporting the idea that skeletal gains resulting from exercise during growth are maintained during adulthood, lowering fracture risk and preventing osteoporosis. However, it is important to note that many studies included in this review applied cross-sectional or retrospective designs. The preventive effect of peak strain, however, has to be confirmed in youth using true experimental designs, since the significant differences in BMD can still be explained by self-selection of PA levels during the growing years.[70]

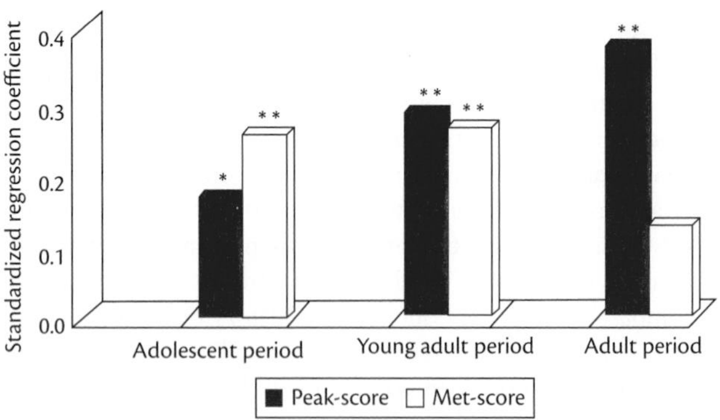

Figure 18.7 The relationship of bone mineral density in the lumbar spine at age 27 years with energetic physical activity (MET) score and peak strain physical activity (peak) score during three different preceding periods in 182 males and females from the Amsterdam Growth and Health Longitudinal Study.

$^*p < 0.05$; $^{**}p < 0.01$.

Groothausen J, Siemer H, Kemper HCG, Twisk JWR, Welten DC. Influence of peak strain on lumbar bone mineral density: an analysis of physical activity in young males and females. Pediatr Exerc Sci. 1997; 9: 159–173.

Importance of physical activity in puberty

Results from Mirwald *et al.*[71] comparing active subjects (top quartile) with inactive subjects (bottom quartile) suggest that a modifiable lifestyle factor like PA plays a role in the optimization of bone mineral acquisition at the lumbar spine in boys and girls during the adolescent growth spurt. This was confirmed by Debar *et al.*,[72] who applied a health plan-based lifestyle intervention designed to improve diet and increase PA in 14- to 16-year-old girls; it included behavioural interventions (bimonthly group meetings, quarterly coaching telephone calls, and weekly self-monitoring). After one year, the girls in the intervention group had significantly higher BMD in the lumbar spine and femoral neck compared with controls, and this improvement was maintained during the second year. A cross-sectional study of tennis and squash female players[73] showed that training started in puberty is maximally beneficial for mineralization of the bone of the playing arm. This training effect on BMD also remained in adulthood (age 21–30 years) after 4 years of stopping training.[74,75] Good maintenance of high-impact activity-induced bone gain in an 8-month follow-up of a randomized control trial was also reported.

Physical activities undertaken in childhood, particularly weight-bearing activities that apply large forces, quickly show optimal benefits to bone mass, size, and structure. Evidence is accumulating that benefits persist well beyond cessation of the activity.[76]

Physical exercise, inflammation, and bone mass

Over the last few decades, comprehension of the mechanisms underlying the protective effect to human health generated by the regular practice of exercise has increased. It is currently well documented that inflammatory markers are related to the development of many diseases,[77] and that PA at moderate intensity has a potential anti-inflammatory action.[78,79] In fact, bone formation is also affected by inflammatory status, and long periods of higher inflammation could be harmful to skeletal formation.[80] This is due to pro-inflammatory markers, i.e. tumour necrosis factor-α, interleukin-6, and interleukin 1, participating in osteoclast differentiation and bone reabsorption.[80] For instance, although mechanical loading stimulates bone formation, a large variety of pro-inflammatory markers (including tumor necrosis factor-α and interleukin-6) are increasingly released in the body as obesity increases.[77,80] Studies have documented a negative relationship between bone variables and abdominal obesity.[80,81]

Prolonged PA at moderate intensity has anti-inflammatory effects, but it is important to note that prolonged intense physical exercise stimulates pro-inflammatory activity.[78,79] Physical exercise, depending on combinations of frequency, intensity, and duration can assume either anabolic or catabolic effects.[79] In male adolescent wrestlers, the acute effect of a single, very high-intensity exercise session significantly increased the concentration of inflammatory markers and decreased IGF-I concentrations.[82] After 5 weeks of a very high amount of physical exercise in prepubertal and early pubertal males, inflammation markers increased, while IGF-I and IGF-I binding protein 3 decreased significantly.[83] On the other hand, IL-6 produced during physical exercise by muscle contraction has beneficial effects to the organism, such as increased lipolysis and fat oxidation, despite IL-6 being an inflammatory marker.[78] Therefore, although inflammation promoted by physical exercise can be potentially harmful to the growth hormone-IGF-I axis, all the physiological actions of some inflammatory markers produced by physical exercise remain unclear. This issue encourages further research.[78]

Conclusions

Skeletal growth and development in children and adolescents of both sexes are strongly affected by maturational events, as well as lifestyle factors like nutrition and PA. A prolonged engagement in weight-bearing physical exercise seems relevant in the promotion of bone health in children and adolescents. Although evidence has increased in the last few years regarding the osteogenic effects related to physical exercise practice in children and adolescents, doubts related to the interrelationship between PA and gender, hormones, and pubertal stage still remain.

Summary

- Bone mass increases rapidly during growth and development. The mechanism seems to be dependent on three factors: centrally regulated hormonal factors, locally determined mechanical factors, and the interaction between hormonal and mechanical factors.
- The quantitative increase of bone mineral density (BMD) during growth, measured by energy absorption methods such as dual photon absorptiometry, single photon absorptiometry, and dual energy X-ray absorptiometry, probably gives an overestimation; these measures do not take into consideration differences in dimensional growth and bone architecture of the bones in question.
- Before the age of puberty (~12 years in girls and ~13 years in boys) no significant differences in BMD between boys and girls are observed.
- During the pubertal growth spurt the increase in bone mineral content (BMC), on average, is 35% of total BMC increase. The fact that as much BMC is gained during the four adolescent growing years as most people will lose during all adult life is clinically significant.
- Investigations longitudinally measuring BMD indicate that boys and girls reach their peak BMD in the late 20s, not in the late teens. In both sexes the greatest change in BMC per year occurs 1–2 years after peak height velocity.
- There are at least two exercise-related strategies to prevent osteoporosis (Figure 18.7). The first is to increase bone accrual during youth by increasing the amount of exercise in order to achieve a greater peak bone mass. The second is to ensure that adults maintain a physically active lifestyle through old age, thus minimizing bone loss during aging. In this way, exercise postpones the age at which the osteoporotic fracture limit is reached (Figure 18.4).
- Experimental studies show significant effects of weight-bearing activity and high-impact strength training programmes on the site-specific BMD in both pre- and circumpubertal boys and girls. The earlier a child starts with physical exercise the more bone is accumulated.
- School-based exercise interventions seem effective in the promotion of bone health in both boys and girls, independent of the maturational status.
- A preventive effect of weight-bearing activities on the peak bone mineral density (PBMD) is also shown in the Amsterdam Growth and Health Longitudinal study: both 27-year-old males and females with relative high levels of peak strain weight-bearing PA patterns during the foregoing 15 years show significantly higher PBMD in their lumbar spine than their inactive counterparts.
- Further research is needed to establish the most effective type of exercise intervention for increasing bone mass and the most effective health plan-based lifestyle intervention in true experimental studies that are aimed at the possibility to increase daily physical activity patterns in both sexes in order to attain optimal maximal bone mass at young adult age.
- Taking into account the inflammatory response to physical exercise, the most profitable combination of intensity, frequency, and duration targeting bone health in paediatric populations is not yet completely clear.

References

1. Kemper HCG. *My e-motions*. Maarssen: Elsevier Publishers; 2004.
2. Farr JN, Laddu DR, Going SB. Exercise, hormones, and skeletal adaptations during childhood and adolescence. *Pediatr Exerc Sci.* 2014; 26: 384–391.
3. Warden SJ, Fuchs RK, Castillo AB, Nelson IR, Turner CH. Exercise when young provides lifelong benefits to bone structure and strength. *J Bone Miner Res.* 2007; 2: 251–259.
4. Bachrach LK. Acquisition of optimal bone mass in childhood and adolescence. *Trends Endocrinol Metab.* 2001; 12: 22–28.
5. Slemenda C. Prevention of hip fractures: Risk modification *Am J Med.* 1997; 2: 65S–73S.
6. Magarey AM, Boulton TJ, Chatterton BE, Schultz C, Nordin BE, Cockington RA. Bone growth from 11 to 17 years: Relationship to growth, gender and changes with pubertal stages including timing of menarche. *Acta Paediatr.* 1999; 88: 139–146.
7. Tanner JM. *Growth at adolescence.* Oxford: Blackwell; 1955.
8. Tanner JM. *A history of the study of human growth.* London: Cambridge University Press: 1981.
9. Weiner JS, Lourie J. *Human biology, a guide to field methods IBP handbook no.9.* Oxford: Blackwell; 1969.
10. Falkner F, Tanner JM. *Human growth, part 1, 2 and 3.* New York: Plenum Press; 1979.

11. Snow-Harter C, Marcus R. Exercise, bone mineral density and osteoporosis. *Exerc Sport Sci Rev.* 1991; 19: 351–388.
12. Döbeln W von. Anthropometric determination of fat-free body weight. *Acta Med Scand.* 1959; 165: 37–42.
13. Roche AF, Chumlea WC, Thissen D. *Assessing the skeletal maturity of the hand-wrist: Fels Method.* Springfield, IL: CC Thomas; 1988.
14. Roche AF, Wainer H, Thissen D. *Skeletal maturity: The knee joint as a biological indicator.* New York: Plenum; 1975.
15. Tanner JM, Whitehouse RH, Marshall WA, Healy MJR, Goldstein H. *Assessment of skeletal maturity and prediction of adult height (TW2 method).* London: Academic Press; 1975.
16. Ma NS, Gordon CM. Pediatric osteoporosis: where are we now? *J Pediatr.* 2012; 161: 983–990.
17. Sievänen H, Kannus P, Nieminen V, Heinonen, A, Oja P, Vuori, I. Estimation of various mechanical characteristics of human bones using DEXA: Methodology and precision. *Bone.* 1996; 18: 173–175.
18. Ferry B, Lespessailles E, Rochcongar P, Duclos M, Courteix D. Bone health during late adolescence: effects of an 8-month training program on bone geometry in female athletes. *Joint Bone Spine.* 2013; 80: 57–63.
19. Smith EL, Raab DM. Osteoporosis and physical activity. *Acta Med Scand.* 1986; 711: 149S–156S.
20. Burger EH, Klein-Nulend J. Mechanotransduction in bone-role of the lacuno-canalicular network. *FASEB J.* 1999; 13: 101S–112S.
21. Lanyon LE. Using functional loading to influence bone mass and architecture: Objectives, mechanism, and relationship with estrogen of the mechanically adaptive process in bone. *Bone.* 1996; 18: 37S–43S.
22. Rubin CT, Lanyon LE. Regulation of bone formation by applied dynamic loads. *J Bone Joint Surg.* 1984; 66: 397–402.
23. Umemura Y, Ishiko T, Yamauchi T, Kurono M, Mashiko S. Five jumps per day increase bone mass and breaking force in rats. *J Bone Miner Res.* 1997; 12: 1480–1485.
24. Turner CH. Three rules for bone adaptation to mechanical stimuli. *Bone.* 1998; 23: 399–407.
25. Kemper HCG. Skeletal development during childhood and adolescence and the effects of physical activity. *Pediatr Exerc Sci.* 2000; 12: 198–216.
26. Turner CH, Robling AG. Designing exercise regimens to increase bone strength. *Exerc Sport Sci Rev.* 2003; 31: 45–50.
27. Gilsanz V, Gibbons DT, Roe TF, Carlson M. Vertebral bone density in children: Effect of puberty. *Radiology.* 1988; 166: 847–850.
28. Glastre C, Braillon P, David L, Cochat P, Meunier PJ, Delmas PD. Measurement of bone mineral content of the lumbar spine by dual energy X-ray absorptiometry in normal children: correlations with growth parameters. *J Clin Endocrinol Metab.* 1990; 70: 1330–1333.
29. Gordon CL, Halton JM, Atkinson SA, Webber CE. The contributions of growth and puberty to peak bone mass. *Growth Dev Aging.* 1991; 55: 257–262.
30. Southard RN, Morris JD, Hayes JR, Torch M., Sommer A. Bone mass in healthy children: Measurement with quantitative DXA. *Radiology.* 1991; 79: 735–738.
31. Bonjour JF, Theintz G, Buchs B, Slosman D, Rizzoli R. Critical years and stages of puberty for spinal and femoral bone mass accumulation during adolescence. *J Clin Endocrinol Metab.* 1991; 73: 555–563.
32. Geusens P. Cantatore F, Nijs J, Proesmans W, Emma F, Dequeker J. Heterogeneity of growth of bone in children at the spine, radius and total skeleton. *Growth Dev Aging.* 1991; 55: 249–256.
33. Theintz G, Buchs B, Rizolli R, *et al.* Longitudinal monitoring of bone mass accumulation in healthy adolescents: Evidence for a marked reduction after 16 years of age at the levels of lumbar spine and femoral neck in female subjects. *J Clin Endocrinol Metab.* 1992; 75: 1060–1066.
34. Weeks BK, Young CM, Beck BR. Eight months of regular in-school jumping improves indices of bone strength in adolescent boys and Girls: the POWER PE study. *J Bone Miner Res.* 2008; 23: 1002–1011.
35. Meyer U, Romann M, Zahner L, *et al.* Effect of a general school-based physical activity intervention on bone mineral content and density: a cluster-randomized controlled trial. *Bone.* 2011; 48: 792–797.
36. Karlsson MK, Rosengren BE. Training and bone—from health to injury. *Scand J Med Sci Sports.* 2012; 22: e15–e23.
37. Grimston SK, Morrison K, Harder JA, Hanley DA. Bone mineral density during puberty in Western Canadian children. *J Bone Min Res.* 1992; 19: 85–96.
38. Bailey DA, Drinkwater D, Faulkner R, McKay H. Proximal femur bone mineral changes in growing children: Dimensional considerations. *Pediatr Exerc Sci.* 1993; 5: 388.
39. Bailey DA, Martin AD, McKay HA. Calcium accretion in girls and boys during puberty: a longitudinal analysis. *J Bone Miner Res.* 2000; 15: 2245–2250.
40. Wren TA, Shepherd JA, Kalkwarf HJ, *et al.* Racial disparity in fracture risk between white and nonwhite children in the United States. *J Pediatr.* 2012; 161: 1035–1040.
41. Löfgren B, Dencker M, Nilsson JÅ, Karlsson MK. A 4-year exercise program in children increases bone mass without increasing fracture risk. *Pediatrics.* 2012; 129: e1468–e1476.
42. Kemper HCG, Binkhorst RA. Exercise and the physiological consequences of the aging process. In: Schroots JJF (ed.) *Aging, health and competence.* Amsterdam: Elsevier; 1996. p. 109–126.
43. Buchanan JR, Meyers C, Lloyd T, Greer RB. Early vertebral trabecular bone loss in normal premenopausal women. *J Bone Miner Res.* 1998; 3: 445–449.
44. Rico H, Revilla M, Hernandez ER, Villa LF, Alvarez del Buergo L. Sex differences in the acquisition of total bone mineral mass peak assessed through dual energy X-ray absorptiometry. *Calcif Tissue Int.* 1992; 51: 251–254.
45. Davies KM, Recker RR, Stegman MR, Heaney RP, Kimmel DB, Leist J. Third decade bone gain in women. In: Cohn DV, Glorieux FH, Martin TJ (eds.) *Calcium regulation and bone metabolism.* Amsterdam: Elsevier Sciences; 1990. p. 1497–1500.
46. Recker RR, Davies KM, Hinders SM, Heaney RP, Stegman RP, Kimmel DB. Bone gain in young adult women. *JAMA.* 1992; 268: 2403–2408.
47. Riggs BL, Melton J. Involutional osteoporosis. *N Eng J Med.* 1986; 413: 1676–1686.
48. Moen S, Sanborn C, Bonnick S, Keizer H, Gench B, DiMarco N. Longitudinal lumbar bone mineral density changes in adolescent female runners. *Med Sci Sports Exerc.* 1992; 38: S12–S24.
49. Slemenda CW, Miller JZ, Hui, LS, Reister TK, Johnston CC. Role of physical activity in the development of skeletal mass in children. *J Bone Miner Res.* 1991; 6: 1227–1233.
50. Boot AM, de Ridder MA, van der Sluis IM, van Slobbe I, Krenning EP, Keizer-Schrama SM. Peak bone mineral density, lean body mass and fractures. *Bone.* 2010; 46: 336–341.
51. Bailey DA. The Saskatchewan Pediatric Bone Mineral Accrual Andy: Bone Mineral Acquisition during the growing years. *Int J Sports Med.* 1997; 18: S191–S195.
52. Kahn K, McKay H, Kannus P, Bailey D, Wark J, Bennell K. *Physical activity and bone health.* Champaign, IL: Human Kinetics; 2001.
53. Wolff I, Croonenberg II, Kemper HCG, Kostense PJ, Twisk JWR. The effect of exercise training programs on the bone mass: A meta-analysis of published controlled trials in pre- and postmenopausal women. *Osteoporos Int.* 1999; 9: 1–12.
54. Margulies JY, Simkin A, Leichter I, *et al.* Effect of intensive physical activity on the bone mineral density content in power limbs of young adults. *J Bone Joint Surg.* 1986; 68: 1090–1093.
55. Bradney M, Pearce G, Naughton G, *et al.* Moderate exercise during growth in prepubertal boys: changes in bone mass, size, volumetric density and bone strength: a controlled prospective study. *J Bone Miner Res.* 1998; 13: 1814–1821.
56. Hasselstrom H, Karlsson KM, Hansen SE, Gronfeldt V, Froberg K, Andersen B. Peripheral bone mineral density and different intensities of physical activity in children 6–8 years old: The Copenhagen School Child Intervention Study. *Calcif Tissue Int.* 2007; 80: 31–38.
57. Gleeson PB, Protas EJ, LeBlanc AD, Schneider VS, Evans HJ. Effects of weight lifting on bone mineral density in premenopausal women. *J Bone Miner Res.* 1990; 5: 153–158.
58. Blimkie CJ, Rice S, Webber J, Martin Levy D, Parker D. Bone density, physical activity, fitness, antropometry, gynaecologic, endocrine and

nutrition status in adolescent girls. In: J Coudert and E von Praagh (eds.) *Pediatric Work Physiology*. Paris: Masson; 1993. p. 201–204.
59. Morris FL, Naughton GA, Gibbs JL, Carlson JS, Wark JD. Positive effects on bone and lean mass. *J Bone Miner Res*. 1997; 12: 1453–1462.
60. McKay HA, Petit MA, Schutz RW. Augmented trochanteric bone mineral density after modified physical education classes: A randomized school-based exercise intervention in prepubertal and early pubertal children. *J Pediatr*. 2000; 136: 156–162.
61. Heinonen A, Sievanen H, Kannus P. High impact exercise and bones of growing girls: A 9-months controlled trial. *Osteoporos Int*. 2000; 11: 1010–1017.
62. Linden C, Ahlborg HG, Besjakov J, Gardsel, P, Karlsson MK. A school curriculm-based exercise program increases bone mineral accrual and bone size in prepubertal girls: Two-year data from the Pediatric Osteoporosis Prevention (POP) Study. *J Bone Miner Res*. 2006; 6: 829–835.
63. Witzke KA, Snow CM. Effects of plyometric jump training on bone mass in adolescent girls. *Med Sci Sports Exerc*. 2000; 32: 1051–1057.
64. Gunter K, Baxter-Jones AD, Mirwald RL, *et al*. Impact exercise increases BMC during growth: an 8-year longitudinal study. *J Bone Miner Res*. 2008; 23: 986–993.
65. Detter F, Rosengren BE, Dencker M, Lorentzon M, Nilsson JÅ, Karlsson MK. A 6-year exercise program improves skeletal traits without affecting fracture risk: a prospective controlled study in 2621 children. *J Bone Miner Res*. 2014; 29: 1325–1336.
66. Hind K, Burrows M. Weight-bearing exercise and bone mineral accrual in children and adolescents: A review of controlled trials. *Bone*. 2007; 40: 14–27.
67. Welten DC, Kemper HCG, Post GB, *et al*. Weight-bearing activity during youth is a more important factor for peak bone mass than calcium intake. *J Bone Miner Res*. 1994; 9: 1029–1096.
68. Dolan SH, Williams DP, Ainsworth BE, Shaw JM. Development and reproducibility of the bone loading history questionnaire. *Med Sci Sports Exerc*. 2006; 38: 1121–1131.
69. Groothausen J, Siemer H, Kemper HCG, Twisk JWR, Welten DC. Influence of peak strain on lumbar bone minral density: an analysis physical activity in young males and females. *Pediatr Exerc Sci*. 1997; 9: 159–173.
70. Kemper HCG. Amsterdam Growth and Health Longitudinal Study (AGHLS). A 23-year follow-up from teenager to adult about lifestyle and Health. *Med Sport Sci*. 2004; 47: 5–20.
71. Mirwald RL, Bailey DA, McKay H, Crocker PE. Physical activity and bone mineral acquisition at the lumbar spine during the adolescent growth spurt. (Programme abstract). *First International Conference on Children's Bone Health, Maastricht*. 1999. p. 57.
72. Debar L, Ritenbauch C, Aickin M, *et al*. A health plan-based lifestyle intervention increases bone mineral density in adolescent girls *Arch Pediatr Adolesc Med*. 2006; 160: 1269–1276.
73. Kannus P, Haapasalo H, Sankelo M, *et al*. Effect of starting age of physical activity on bone mass in the dominant arm of tennis and squash players. *Ann Intern Med*. 1995; 123: 27–31.
74. Kontulainen S, Kannus P, Haapsalo H, *et al*. Changes in bone mineral content with decreased training in competitive young adult tennis players and controls: a prospective 4-year follow-up. *Med Sci Sports Exerc*. 1999; 31: 640–652.
75. Heinonen A, Kannus P, Oja P. Good maintenance of high-impact activity-induced bone gain by voluntary, unsupervised exercises: An 8-month follow up of a randomised control trial. *J Bone Miner Res*. 1999; 14: 125–128.
76. Gunther KB, Almstedt HC, Janz KF. Physical activity in childhood may be the key to optimizing lifespan skeletl health. *Exerc Sport Sci Rev*. 2012; 49: 13–21.
77. Huang PL. eNOS, metabolic syndrome and cardiovascular disease. *Trends Endocrinol Metab*. 2009; 20: 295–302.
78. Pedersen BK. Muscular interleukin-6 and its role as an energy sensor. *Med Sci Sports Exerc*. 2012; 44: 392–396.
79. Eliakim A, Nemet D. Interval training and the GH-IGF-I axis—a new look into an old training regimen. *J Pediatr Endocrinol Metab*. 2012; 25: 815–821.
80. Cao JJ. Effects of obesity on bone metabolism. *J Orthop Surg Res*. 2011; 6: 30.
81. Júnior IF, Cardoso JR, Christofaro DG, Codogno JS, de Moraes AC, Fernandes RA. The relationship between visceral fat thickness and bone mineral density in sedentary obese children and adolescents. *BMC Pediatr*. 2013; 13: 37.
82. Nemet D, Oh Y, Kim HS, Hill M, Cooper DM. Effect of intense exercise on inflammatory cytokines and growth mediators in adolescent boys. *Pediatrics*. 2002; 110: 681–689.
83. Scheett TP, Nemet D, Stoppani J, Maresh CM, Newcomb R, Cooper DM. The effect of endurance-type exercise training on growth mediators and inflammatory cytokines in pre-pubertal and early pubertal males. *Pediatr Res*. 2002; 52: 491–497.

CHAPTER 19

Sport, physical activity, and other health behaviours

Stewart G Trost and Barbara Joschtel

Introduction

Millions of children worldwide are involved in organized sports. In the United States alone, an estimated 44 million children are involved in school and community sports programmes.[1] National survey data from the US, Canada, Australia, and the United Kingdom suggest that between 50% and 80% of young people participate on at least one school or community-based sports team annually.[2–5]

Sports participation has long been thought to provide children and adolescents with a pro-social environment that fosters basic values such as fair play, competitiveness, and achievement.[6] It is also widely believed that participation in organized sports offers protection against the negative social influences that can lead to problem behaviour and experimentation with tobacco, alcohol, and illicit drugs.[6] Most youth sports programmes are offered during 'at-risk' times (after school and weekends), thus limiting participants' opportunities to engage in risky health behaviours, and participation in school-sponsored sport programmes is often made contingent upon following rules and regulations that overtly discourage health risk behaviours such as experimentation with alcohol and drugs. Sports participation may also promote positive youth development and avoidance of certain health risk behaviours by improving social skills and enhancing self-esteem.[6,7] In 2003, the United Nations Interagency Task Force on Sport for Development and Peace endorsed sport as a forum to learn skills such as discipline, confidence, and leadership; sport was also identified as an ideal behaviour setting to teaching core principles such as tolerance, cooperation, and respect.[7] Additionally, the Task Force officially recognized the opportunity to participate and enjoy sport and play as a basic human right that must be promoted and supported.[7]

A related issue that has received an increasing amount of research attention over the last two decades is the question of whether a health-promoting behaviour such as physical activity (PA) 'clusters' with other health-promoting behaviours in youth.[8–10] The existence of such clustering implies that favourable status or change in one behaviour (e.g. regular PA) is associated with favourable status or change in others (e.g. healthy eating, tobacco use, experimentation with illicit drugs).

This chapter summarizes the research literature pertaining to the relationships between sports participation, PA, and selected health risk behaviours in children and adolescents. It examines health risk behaviours including tobacco use (cigarettes and smokeless tobacco), alcohol consumption, illicit drug use, anabolic steroid use, dietary practices (fruit and vegetable intake, eating breakfast, consumption of foods high in saturated fat), inappropriate weight control practices, sexual activity, and violent behaviour.

Searches of the peer-reviewed scientific literature were conducted using several electronic databases, including PubMed, SPORT Discus, Web of Science, ERIC, and Embase. Key words used for the search were: children, teenagers, youth, adolescents, exercise, sports, sport participation, physical activity, violence, alcohol, cigarette smoking, tobacco use, smokeless tobacco, sexual risk, diet, eating habits, drug use, substance use, and anabolic steroids. Searches were supplemented by direct examination of reference lists of recovered articles. No limitations were imposed as to publication date or country of origin, except that the article had to be published in the English language. Studies were included if they involved children and/or adolescents and provided a measure of association between sports or PA participation and a specific health behaviour (e.g. correlation coefficient, beta coefficient, prevalence contrast, odds ratio). We did not include experimental or interventional studies in which sport or PA was used a treatment for substance abuse or problem behaviour. The majority of studies included participants aged 18 years or younger, although studies including young adults were included if they contributed to the breadth of the topic. A total of 10 391 unique citations were identified through the search process and screened on the basis of title and abstract. Of these, 203 full-text articles were assessed for eligibility. A total of 138 articles, inclusive of studies reviewed in the previous edition, met the inclusionary criteria. Studies examining the relationship between youth sports participation and other health behaviours are summarized in Table 19.1. Studies examining the relationship between PA and other health behaviours are summarized in Table 19.2.

Sports participation and other health behaviours

Cigarette smoking

A significant number of studies have examined the relationship between sports participation and cigarette smoking. Forty-five studies investigating the association between sports participation and cigarette smoking met the inclusionary criteria. Of this number, 21 studies analysed data from nationally representative samples. Of these 21, 18 studies reported sports participation to decrease the risk of cigarette smoking,[11–28] two studies reported

Table 19.1 Summary of studies examining the association between sports participation and other health behaviours

Study	Design	Sample	Health behaviours examined									Relationship
			CIG	SN	ALC	DRG	AS	DIET	WCP	SEX	VL	
Aaron[55]	L	N = 405 Age = 12–16 y USA	✓		✓						✓	←CIG, ↑ALC(B), ←VL
Abrams[32]	XC	N = 1549 Grades 6, 8, 10, 12 USA	✓	✓								↓CIG, ←SN
Adachi-Mejia[33]	L	N = 2048 Age = 16–21 y USA	✓									↓CIG
Adachi-Mejia[11]	XC	N = 3646 Age = 13–18 y USA	✓									↓CIG
Adachi-Mejia[34]	XC	N = 6522 Age = 10–14 y USA	✓		✓							↓CIG, ←ALC
Baumert[35]	XC	N = 6849 Grades 9–12 USA	✓	✓	✓	✓		✓				↓CIG, ←SN, ←ALC, ↓DRG, ↑DIET
Bedendo[31]	XC	N = 1 872 Age = 14–18 y Brazil	✓		✓							←CIG, ↑ALC
Beebe[52]	XC	N = 134 Age = 13–19 y US	✓		✓	✓						←CIG, ←ALC, ←DRUG
Buckley[75]	XC	N = 3403 Boys 12th grade USA					✓					↑AS
Buhrman[53]	XC	N = 857 Girls Grades 9–12 Canada	✓		✓							←CIG, ↓ALC
Burton[114]	XC	N = 169 Age = 14–15 y UK									✓	←VL
Carr[72]	XC	N = 1713 grades 10–12 USA			✓							←ALC
Castrucci[12]	XC	N = 16 357 Grades 9–12 USA	✓	✓								↓CIG, ↑SN
Cerkez[70]	XC	N = 1015 Age = 17–18 Bosnia and Herzegovina			✓							↓ALC(B)
Crissey[90]	XC	N = 7214 Girls Age = 12–18 y USA							✓			↑WCP

Table 19.1 Continued

Study	Design	Sample	Health behaviours examined									Relationship
			CIG	SN	ALC	DRG	AS	DIET	WCP	SEX	VL	
Croll[87]	XC	N = 4746 Age = 11–18 y USA						✓				↑DIET
Davies[69]	XC	N = 296 Age = 14–15 y UK			✓							↑ALC(B)
Davis[54]	XC	N = 1200 Boys Grades 9–12 USA	✓	✓								←CIG, ↑SN
de Bruin[92]	XC	N = 140 Girls Age = 13–18 y Netherlands							✓			↑WCP
Dever[59]	XC	N = 36 514 8 sequential cohorts of 8th- and 10th-grade students from MTF USA			✓	✓						↑ALC(b), ↓DRUG(g)
Diehl[36]	XC	1138 Elite German athletes compared to national health survey Germany	✓		✓	✓						↓CIG, ↑ALC, ↓DRUG
Dodge[76]	L	N = 15 000 Grades 7–12 Add Health USA					✓					↑AS(B)
Donato[71]	XC	N = 696 boys Age = 17–19 y Italy			✓							↓ALC
Dunn[13]	XC	N = 16 343 Grades 9–12 2009 CDC YRBS USA	✓	✓	✓	✓						↓CIG, ↑SN(B), ↑ALC, ↑DRUG(G)
DuRant[79]	XC	N = 12 272 Grades 9–12 1991 CDC YRBS USA					✓					←AS
Elliot[77]	XC	N = 7544 Girls Grades 9–12 2003 CDC YRBS USA					✓					↓AS
Escobedo[14]	XC	N = 11 248 Grades 9–12 1990 CDC YRBS USA	✓									↓CIG
Endresen[110]	L	N = 477 boys Age = 11–13 at time 0 Norway									✓	↑VL

(continued)

Table 19.1 Continued

Study	Design	Sample	Health behaviours examined									Relationship
			CIG	SN	ALC	DRG	AS	DIET	WCP	SEX	VL	
Ferron[15]	XC	N = 9268 Age = 15–20 y France	✓		✓	✓				✓		↓CIG, ↓ALC, ↓DRUG, ↓SEX
Fite[111]	XC	N = 89 Age = 9–12 y USA									✓	↑VL
Forman[74]	XC	N = 1117 Males National survey controls USA				✓						↓DRUG
Fortes[93]	XC	N = 942 Age = 10–19 y Brazil							✓			↑WCP
Garcia-Rodriguez[37]	XC	N = 2841 Age 12–16 y Spain	✓									↓CIG(B)
Gardner[116]	L	N = 1344 Age = 9–12 year at time 0 USA									✓	←VL
Garry[51]	XC	N = 4346 Grades 6–8 USA	✓	✓	✓	✓	✓		✓		✓	↑CIG, ←SN, ↑ALC, ↑DRG, ←AS, ←WCP, ↑VL
Geisner[65]	XC	N = 653 High-school seniors USA			✓				✓			↑ALC, ↑WCP
Giannakopoulos[38]	XC	N = 2008 Age = 12–17 y Greek	✓									↓CIG
Gomes[99]	XC	N = 248 Age = 13–18 y Portugal							✓			↓WCP
Grossbard[66]	XC	N = 2123 Age = 17–19 y USA			✓					✓		↑ALC, ↑SEX
Guevremont[29]	XC	N = 3202 Age = 14–17 y Canada	✓		✓	✓						↑CIG, ↑ALC, ↑DRUG
Habel[106]	XC	N = 10 487 Grades 6–12 USA								✓		↑SEX
Halldorsson[64]	XC	N = 10 992 Age = 13–16 y Iceland			✓							↓ALC
Harrison[39]	XC	N = 50 168 9th-grade students USA	✓		✓	✓		✓		✓		↓CIG, ↓ALC, ↓DRUG, ↑DIET, ↓SEX

Table 19.1 Continued

Study	Design	Sample	Health behaviours examined									Relationship
			CIG	SN	ALC	DRG	AS	DIET	WCP	SEX	VL	
Herbrich[94]	XC	52 Ballet dancers 44 Age-matched controls Age = 13–20 y Germany							✓			↑WLC
Hoffmann[60]	L	N = 9893 Grades 10–12 USA			✓							↑ALC
Holmen[40]	XC	N = 6811 Age = 12–19 y Norway	✓									↓CIG
Jiang[109]	L	N = 13 236 Grades 7–13 Add Health USA									✓	←VL
Kreager[108]	L	N = 6397 Boys Grades 7–12 USA									✓	↑VL
Krentz[95]	XC	N = 96 Elite athletes N = 96 controls Mean age = 14 y Germany							✓			↑WCP
Kristjansson[16]	XC	N = 7430 Age = 14–16 y Iceland	✓									↓CIG
Kulig[17]	XC	N = 15 142 Grades 9–12 1999 CDC YRBS USA	✓		✓	✓	✓			✓		↓CIG, ←ALC, ↓DRUG(B), ←AS, ↓SEX
Larson[41]	XC	N = 4746 Age = 11–18 y USA	✓									↓CIG
Levin[113]	XC	N = 2436 Grades 9–12 USA									✓	↑VL (contact sports)
Lee[42]	L	N = 766 Age = 15 year at time 0 USA	✓		✓	✓						↓CIG, ↑ALC, ↓DRUG
Linville[112]	XC	N = 235 Grades 8–12 USA									✓	↑VL(g)
Lisha[61]	L	N = 8179 Age = 9–18 y USA			✓	✓						↑ALC, ↓DRUG
Lorang[86]	XC	N = 4231 Grades 9–12 USA					✓					↑AS

(continued)

Table 19.1 Continued

Study	Design	Sample	Health behaviours examined									Relationship
			CIG	SN	ALC	DRG	AS	DIET	WCP	SEX	VL	
Maïano[96]	XC	N = 335 Age = 11–18 y France							✓			↑WCP
Martinsen[97]	XC	N = 677 Elite sport N = 421 Controls Grades 9–12 Norway							✓			↑WCP
Martinsen[43]	XC	N = 677 Elite sport N = 421 Controls Grades 9–12 Norway	✓	✓	✓							↓CIG, ↓SN, ↓ALC
Mattila[44]	XC	N = 16 746 Median age = 19 y Male conscripts Finland	✓	✓								↓CIG, ↑SN
Mays[18]	XC	N = 311 Age = 13–21 y USA	✓									↓CIG with non-smoking peers ↑CIG with smoking peers
Mays[62]	XC	N = 13 956 Grades 9–12 2005 CDC YRBS USA			✓							↑ALC
Mays[63]	L	N = 8271 Grades 7–12 at time 0 USA			✓							↑ALC
Mays[67]	XC	N = 378 Grades 9–12 USA			✓							↑ALC
Melnick[19]	XC	N = 16 262 Grades 9–12 1997 CDC YRBS USA	✓	✓								↓CIG, ↑SN
Metzger[45]	L	N = 1140 Grades 9–10 at time 0 USA	✓									↓CIG(B)
Michaud[20]	XC	N = 7428 Age 16–20 y Switzerland	✓		✓	✓			✓			↓CIG(g), ←ALC, ←DRUG, ←WCP
Miller[80]	XC	N = 16 183 Grades 9–12 1997 CDC YRBS USA					✓					←AS
Miller[103]	XC	N = 611 Age = 13–16 USA								✓		↓SEX(G)

Table 19.1 Continued

Study	Design	Sample	Health behaviours examined									Relationship
			CIG	SN	ALC	DRG	AS	DIET	WCP	SEX	VL	
Miller[102]	XC	N = 16 262 1997 grades 9–12 USA								✓		PA ↓SEX(G), ↑SEX(B) SP ↓SEX(G-W), ↑SEX(B-AA), ↓SEX(B-W)
Miller[104]	L	N = 699 Age = 12–17 y USA								✓		↓SEX(w)
Miller[115]	XC	N = 608 Age = 12–17 y USA									✓	←VL
Monthuy-Blanc[101]	XC	43 Basketball players 52 Ballet dancers 49 Non-athlete controls France							✓			←WCP
Naylor[46]	XC	N = 1515 Grades 9–12 USA	✓	✓	✓	✓	✓					↓CIG, ←SN, ←ALC, ↓DRUG, ←AS
Nelson[21]	L	N = 11 957 Grades 7–12 Add Health USA	✓		✓	✓				✓	✓	↓CIG, ↓DRUG, ←ALC, ↓SEX, ↓VL
Oler[50]	XC	N = 823 Grades 9–12 USA	✓	✓	✓	✓						↓CIG, ←SN, ←ALC, ↓DRUG(B)
Page[22]	XC	N = 12 272 Grades 9–12 1991 CDC YRBS USA	✓	✓	✓	✓	✓			✓	✓	↓CIG, ↑SN(b), ←ALC, ↓DRUG, ↑AS(b), ↓VL, ↓SEX
Pate[23]	XC	N = 14 221 Grades 9–12 1997 CDC YRBS USA	✓	✓	✓	✓	✓	✓	✓	✓	✓	↓CIG(B), ↓CIG(G-W), ↑DIET, ←ALC, ↑SN(G), ↓DRUG(W–H), ↑DRUG(AA), ↑AS (G-H), ↓AS(G-W), ↓SEX(G), ↑SEX(B-AA), ↓WCP(B), ↓VL(W), ↑VL(G-H)
Rainey[47]	XC	N = 7846 Grades 9–12 USA	✓	✓	✓							↓CIG, ←SN, ↑ALC
Rodriguez[48]	L	N = 1098 9th grade at time 0 USA	✓									↓CIG
Rosendahl[100]	XC	576 High-school athletes 291 Non-athlete controls Germany							✓			↓WCP
Sabo[105]	XC	N = 699 Age = 13–16 USA								✓		↓SEX(G)

(continued)

Table 19.1 Continued

Study	Design	Sample	Health behaviours examined									Relationship
			CIG	SN	ALC	DRG	AS	DIET	WCP	SEX	VL	
Scott[81]	XC	N = 4722 Grades 7–12 USA					✓					↑AS(B)
Sekulic[49]	XC	N = 1032 Age = 17–18 y Bosnia and Herzegovina	✓		✓							↑CIG(B), ←ALC, ←DRUG
Smith[107]	XC	N = 1071 Grades 9–12 USA								✓		↑SEX
Sussman[58]	XC	N = 1193 7th-grade students USA		✓								↑SN(G)
Taliaferro[24]	XC	Sequential analyses of the 1998, 2001, 2003, 2005, 2007 CDC YRBS N = 13 601–15 349 USA	✓	✓	✓	✓	✓	✓	✓	✓	✓	↓CIG(B), ↓CIG(G-W), ↑SN(B), ↑ALC(B) ↓DRUG(B-W), ↓DRUG(G-W), ←AS(B), ↓AS(G) ↑DIET (B), ↑DIET(G-W), ↑WCP(B), ↑SEX(B-AA-H), ↓SEX(G), ↓VL(G), ↓VL(B)
Tanner[82]	XC	N = 6 930 Grades 9–12 USA					✓					↑AS
Taub[98]	XC	110 athletes 112 non-athletes Grades 9–12 USA							✓			↑WCP
Terry-McElrath[25]	L	N = 11 741 High-school seniors Followed up to age 26 y USA	✓		✓	✓						↓CIG, ↑ALC, ↓DRUG
Terry-McElrath[26]	XC	289 503 middle school students, and 363 708 high-school students USA	✓	✓	✓	✓	✓					↑SN, ↑AS, ↓CIG, ↓DRUG, ↑ALC
Thorlindsson[78]	XC	N = 11 031 Mean age = 17.7 y Iceland					✓					↓AS
Thorlindsson[73]	XC	Icelandic youth 12–15 year two random samples N = 456 and N = 358 Iceland				✓						↓DRUG
Thorlindsson[27]	XC	N = 1200 Age = 15–16 y Iceland	✓		✓							↓CIG, ↓ALC

Table 19.1 Continued

Study	Design	Sample	Health behaviours examined									Relationship
			CIG	SN	ALC	DRG	AS	DIET	WCP	SEX	VL	
Van den Berg[83]	L	N = 2516 Grades 7–12 at time 0 USA					✓					↑AS(G)
Veliz[30]	XC	N = 21 049 Grades 8 and 10 MTF Study USA	✓		✓	✓						↑CIG(CS), ↓CIG(NC), ↑ALC, ↑DRUG(CS)
Vertalino[84]	XC	N = 4746 Grades 7–12 USA					✓		✓			↑AS, ↑WCP
Wetherill[68]	XC	N = 2247 High-school seniors USA			✓					✓		↑ALC, ↑SEX
Wichstrom[28]	L	N = 3251 Age = 13–19 year at time 0 Norway	✓		✓	✓						↓CIG, ↑ALC, ↑DRUG
Windsor[85]	XC	N = 901 Grades 9–12 USA					✓					↑AS(B)

↑ = Positive association, ↓ Inverse association, ← No evidence of an association, B = boys, G = girls, W = White, AA = African-American, H = Hispanic.

a positive association,[29,30] and one study reported no evidence of an association.[31] Seven studies evaluated the association between sports participation and cigarette smoking using data from the CDC Youth Risk Behaviour Survey (YRBS).

Escobedo *et al.*[14] examined the relationship between participation in school sports and cigarette smoking among high-school students completing the 1990 YRBS. After adjustments for age, sex, race/ethnicity, and academic performance, students reporting participation in three or more sports teams in the previous 12 months were 2.5 times less likely than non-participants to be classified as regular smokers. Analysing data from the 1991 YRBS, Page *et al.*[22] reported male and female sports participants to be 25–40% less likely than their non-sporting peers to try cigarette smoking, smoke cigarettes in the past 30 days, or smoke cigarettes regularly. These associations remained statistically significant after controlling for age, sex, and race/ethnicity. Pate *et al.*[23] assessed the relationship between sports participation and cigarette smoking in high-school students completing the 1997 YRBS. After controlling for age, race/ethnicity, and PA performed outside of sport, students reporting participation in one or more sports teams during the previous 12 months were 1.2 to 1.3 times less likely than non-participants to report smoking in the past 30 days. Melnick *et al.*[19] also examined the relationship between sports participation and cigarette smoking in the 1997 YRBS data. Not only did the authors confirm the protective effects of sports participation, they provided evidence of a dose-response relationship between the level of sports participation and cigarette smoking. After controlling for age, race/ethnicity, parental education, and type of residence, students reporting moderate (one to two teams in the past year) and high (three or more teams in the past year) levels of sports participation were 25–32% and 39–42% less likely than their non-sporting counterparts to report regular smoking.

Kulig *et al.*[17] analysed data from the 1999 YRBS to determine if the relationship between sports participation and cigarette smoking was moderated by PA status. Students reporting involvement in one or more sporting teams in the past year *and* participation in vigorous PA three or more times per week were 1.4 times less likely to smoke cigarettes in the past 30 days than non-active, non-sport participants. Participation in team sports in the absence of regular vigorous PA, or regular vigorous PA in the absence of team sports participation did not significantly reduce the risk of cigarette smoking. Dunn[13] examined the association between sports participation and cigarette smoking using data from the 2009 YRBS. Students who participated in school or community-based sports were 1.2 to 1.7 times less likely to report recent cigarette use or regular smoking than non-sports participants. Finally, Taliaferro *et al.*[24] analysed data from six consecutive YRBS surveys administered between 1999 and 2007. Participation in school or community-based sports was consistently inversely associated with cigarette smoking.

Twenty-four studies investigated the association between sports participation and cigarette smoking in samples of youth from a single school, school district, or geographical region. Of these 24, 19 studies reported sports participation to be protective of cigarette smoking,[32–50] one study reported a positive association,[51] and four studies reported no evidence of an association.[52–55] Eight studies employed longitudinal study designs to explore the impact of sports

Table 19.2 Summary of studies examining the association between physical activity and other health behaviours

Study	Design	Sample	Health behaviours examined									Relationship
			CIG	SN	ALC	DRG	AS	DIET	WCP	SEX	VL	
Aarnio[117]	XC	N = 3254 Finnish twins Age 16 y Finland	✓		✓			✓				↓CIG, ↓ALC, ↑DIET
Aarnio[118]	L	N = 5028 Finnish twins Age = 16–18 y Finland	✓		✓			✓				↓CIG, ←ALC, ↑DIET
Aaron[55]	L	N = 405 Age = 12–16 y USA	✓		✓						✓	↓CIG(G), ↑ALC(B), ←VL
Al-Hazzaa[146]	XC	N = 2822 Age = 15–19 y Saudi Arabia						✓				↑DIET
Ali[119]	L	N = 13 171 Grades 7–12 USA	✓									↓CIG(W)
Audrain-McGovern[126]	L	N = 1384 Age = 14–18 y USA	✓	✓								↓CIG, ←SN
Audrain-McGovern[125]	L	N = 1356 Age = 14–18 y USA	✓									↓CIG
Charilaou[120]	XC	N = 1390 Grades 7–12 Cyprus	✓									↓CIG
Cohen[136]	XC	N = 318 Grades 9–12 Canada	✓					✓				←CIG, ↑DIET
Coulson[127]	XC	N = 932 Grades 8–10 UK	✓					✓				↓CIG, ↑DIET
D'Elio[137]	XC	N = 303 Grades 4–5 African-American USA	✓		✓							←CIG, ←ALC
Demissie[152]	XC	N = 16 343 Grades 9–12 2009 CDC YRBS USA									✓	↑VL(B), ↓VL(G)
Dunn[13]	XC	N = 16 343 Grades 9–12 2009 CDC YRBS USA	✓	✓	✓	✓						↓CIG, ←SN, ↓ALC, ↑DRUG(G)
DuRant[79]	XC	N = 12 272 Grades 9–12 1991 CDC YRBS USA					✓					↑AS (strength training)
Durksen[147]	XC	N = 330 Age = 9–17 y Canada						✓				↑DIET

Table 19.2 Continued

Study	Design	Sample	Health behaviours examined									Relationship
			CIG	SN	ALC	DRG	AS	DIET	WCP	SEX	VL	
Easton[128]	XC	N = 2410 Grades 9–12 Hungary	✓									↓CIG
Faulkner[142]	XC	N = 257 Grades 9–10 Canada			✓							↑ALC(b)
French[148]	XC	N = 1492 Grades 7–10 USA						✓	✓			↑DIET, ↑WCP
García[129]	XC	N = 344 Age 12–16 y Spain	✓									↓CIG
Karvonen[140]	L	N = 3175 Age 16–18 y Finland		✓								↑SN
Kirkcaldy[130]	XC	N = 988 Age = 14–18 y Germany	✓		✓	✓						↓CIG, ↓ALC, ↓DRUG
Kokkevi[144]	XC	N = 18 430 16-year-olds European school survey alcohol and other drugs 6 European countries					✓					↑AS
Korhonen[141]	L	N = 4240 Finnish twin cohort 1870 twin pairs 16 y Finland			✓	✓						↓ALC(g), ↓DRUG
Kovacs[131]	XC	N = 881 Age = 14–18 y Hungary	✓		✓	✓						↓CIG, ↑ALC, ↓DRUG
Larson[41]	XC	N = 4746 Age = 11–18 y USA	✓									↓CIG
Leatherdale[132]	XC	N = 25 560 Grades 9–12 Canada	✓									↓CIG
Lowry[145]	XC	N = 11 429 Grades 9–12 2010 CDC NYPANS USA						✓				↑DIET
Middleman[91]	XC	N = 3055 Grades 9–12 USA							✓			↑WCP(g)
Miller[102]	XC	N = 16 262 1997 grades 9–12 USA								✓		↓SEX(g), ↑SEX(m)
Moreno-Murcia[133]	XC	N = 472 Age = 16–20 y Spain	✓		✓							↓CIG(b), ↓ALC(b)

(continued)

Table 19.2 Continued

Study	Design	Sample	Health behaviours examined									Relationship
			CIG	SN	ALC	DRG	AS	DIET	WCP	SEX	VL	
Nelson[21]	L	N = 11 957 Grades 7–12 Add Health USA	✓		✓	✓				✓	✓	↓CIG, ↓DRUG, ↓ALC, ↓SEX, ←VL
Paavola[138]	L	N = 903 Age 15 year at time 0 Finland	✓		✓							←CIG, ↓ALC
Pate[121]	XC	N = 4293 Grades 9–12 1990 CDC YRBS USA	✓		✓	✓		✓			✓	↓CIG, ↓ALC(G), ↓DRUG, ↑DIET(W-H), ←VL
Peltzer[123]	XC	N = 24 593 8 African Countries Age = 13–15 y	✓		✓	✓						←CIG, ↑ALC, ←DRUG
Raitakari[122]	L	N = 961 Age = 12, 15, 18 at time 0 Finland	✓					✓				↓CIG, ↑DIET
Robinson[143]	XC	N = 1447 10th-grade students USA				✓						←DRUG
Rosenberg[149]	XC	N = 878 Age = 11–15 y USA						✓				←DIET
Tao[135]	XC	N = 5433 Grades 9–12 China	✓									↑CIG
Thorlindsson[78]	XC	N = 11 031 Mean age = 17.7 y Iceland					✓					↑AS
Valois[139]	XC	N = 374 Age = 10–13 y USA	✓									←CIG
Vissers[150]	XC	N = 1 317 Age = 9–10 y UK						✓				←DIET
Vuori[124]	XC	N = 1670 9th-grade students Finland	✓	✓	✓	✓				✓		←CIG, ←SN, ←ALC, ↓DRUG, ←SEX
Winnail[134]	XC	N = 3 437 Grades 9–12 South Carolina YRBS USA	✓	✓		✓						↓CIG(B-W), ↓SN(B-W), ↓SN(G-AA), ↓DRUG(B-W)

↑ = Positive association, ↓ Inverse association, ← No evidence of an association, B = boys, G = girls, W = White, AA = African-American, H = Hispanic.

participation on subsequent cigarette smoking.[21,25,28,33,42,45,48,55] With the exception of one study,[55] all of them found youth sport participation to be protective of smoking during late adolescence or early adulthood.

Rodriguez and Audrain-McGovern[48] followed a cohort of approximately 1500 high-school students from the ninth through eleventh (ages approximately 14–17 years) grade. Using general growth mixture modelling, the authors identified four distinct trajectories of sports involvement—decreasing participation, erratic participation, consistently high participation, and consistently low participation. Students exhibiting a decreasing sports participation profile were three times more likely than students with consistently high sports participation to be smokers in the eleventh grade. Nelson and Gordon-Larsen[21] analysed data from the US National Longitudinal Study of Adolescent Health to examine the association between organized sport participation and cigarette smoking. Adolescents with a high frequency of sports participation were approximately 20% less likely than non-participants to report smoking five or more cigarettes in the previous month.

Adachi-Mejia *et al.*[33] examined the effects of sports participation at ages 9 and 14 years on cigarette smoking 7 years later, at ages 16 and 21 years. After controlling for age, sex, parental education, peer smoking status, parental smoking status, rebelliousness, school performance, and exposure to smoking in movies, non-sport participants were almost twice as likely to be established smokers as sport participants. Lee *et al.*[42] analysed data from the National Institute of Child Health and Human Development Study of Early Child Care and Youth Development. After controlling for socio-demographic factors, unsupervised time with peers, impulsivity, prior smoking status, and involvement in other organized activities, greater participation in sports at age 15 years predicted lower levels of cigarette smoking by the end of high school. Metzger *et al.*[45] examined the relationship between sports participation and cigarette smoking in a cohort of 1040 ninth and tenth grade students. After controlling for baseline peer problems and involvement in other school activities, boys' participation in team sports at baseline predicted lower levels of cigarette smoking at 15- and 24-months follow-up. No association was observed among girls.

Terry-McElrath *et al.*[25] analysed data from the US Monitoring the Future Study to explore the relationship between high school sports participation and cigarette smoking during early adulthood. At age 18 years, greater sports participation was associated with lower cigarette smoking, with subsequent increases in sports participation related to significant decreases in cigarette smoking at age 21/22 years and 25/26 years, respectively.

Wichstrom *et al.*[28] examined the association between adolescent sports participation and cigarette smoking during early adulthood in a population-based cohort of Norwegian high-school students. Students involved in team sports at baseline exhibited significantly lower growth in cigarette smoking rates during early adulthood than non-sports participants.

Smokeless tobacco

Smokeless tobacco (chewing tobacco, dipping tobacco, snuff) is associated with several serious health conditions including periodontal disease, nicotine addiction, and cancers of the mouth, throat and digestive system. Because smokeless tobacco use is considered socially acceptable and often encouraged in sports such as baseball and ice hockey, the relationship between sports participation and smokeless tobacco use is a serious concern for health authorities and sports officials.[56,57]

Seventeen studies examining the association between sports participation and smokeless tobacco met the inclusionary criteria. Of these 17, seven studies analysed data from nationally representative samples.[12,13,19,22–24,26] All seven studies reported sports participation to be positively associated with smokeless tobacco use. No longitudinal studies were identified. Five of the seven population-based studies used data from the CDC YRBS.[13,19,22–24]

Page *et al.*[22] examined the association between sports participation and smokeless tobacco use in high-school students completing the 1991 YRBS. Boys reporting participation in one or two sports teams in the previous year were 1.3 times more likely than non-participants to report smokeless tobacco use in the past month. Melnick *et al.*[19] examined the association between sports participation and smokeless tobacco use in high-school students completing the 1997 YRBS. Among males, sports participants were 1.4 times more likely than non-participants to report smokeless tobacco use in the last 30 days. Among females, sports participants were 1.8 times more likely than non-participants to report smokeless tobacco use. Notably, the risk of smokeless tobacco use increased with level of sport involvement. Compared to non-participants, the odds of smokeless tobacco use among males and females reporting participation in three or more sports teams was 1.6 and 3.2 greater, respectively. Pate *et al.*[23] also explored the relationship between sports participation and smokeless tobacco using the 1997 YRBS data. In conflict with the findings of other YRBS studies, sports participation was only positively associated with smokeless tobacco use among older girls (grades 11 and 12). No association was observed in boys and younger girls. Dunn[13] examined the association between sports participation and smokeless tobacco using data from the 2009 YRBS. Males reporting participation in two or more sports in the previous year were 1.25 times more likely to report smokeless tobacco use in the past 30 days. Finally, Taliaferro *et al.*[24] analysed data from six consecutive YRBS surveys administered between 1999 and 2007. Among boys, sports participation was consistently associated with greater smokeless tobacco use. Among girls, sports participation was consistently protective for smokeless tobacco use, but only among white and Hispanic girls.

Findings from two other national surveys further support the notion that sports participation increases the risk of smokeless tobacco use in adolescents. Castrucci *et al.*[12] contrasted smokeless tobacco use in sports participants and non-participants in a nationally representative sample of US high-school students. Sports participants were approximately twice as likely as non-participants to report current use of chew or snuff. Analysing data from the US Monitoring the Future Study, Terry-McElrath *et al.*[26] examined the relationship between school sports participation and smokeless tobacco use in nationally representative cross-sectional samples of eighth, tenth, and twelfth grade students (approximately 12, 15, and 18 years, respectively). After controlling for gender, race/ethnicity, parent education, and other substance use outcomes, the authors observed a weak, but positive, association between sports participation and smokeless tobacco use.

Ten studies investigated the association between sports participation and smokeless tobacco use in samples of youth from a single school, school district, or geographical region. Of these ten, three studies reported a positive association,[44,54,58] one study reported an inverse or protective association,[43] and six studies reported no evidence of an association.[32,35,46,47,50,51]

Davis *et al.*[54] examined the association between sports participation and smokeless tobacco use in 1200 high school males from northwest Louisiana. After controlling for race, grade point average, and sports intensity, athletes were significantly more likely than non-athletes to use chewing tobacco or snuff. On average, the rate of smokeless tobacco use was approximately 1.5 times higher among athletes than non-athletes. Sussman *et al.*[58] examined the predictors of smokeless tobacco use in two successive cohorts of seventh-grade students (age approximately 13 years) residing in the Los Angeles metropolitan area. Cross-sectional analyses of data collected during the participants' seventh- and eighth-grade years showed sports participation to be unrelated to experimentation with smokeless tobacco use. However, among girls in the second cohort, sports participation in the seventh grade was significantly associated with smokeless tobacco use in the eighth grade. Seventeen percent of the girls who reported participation in four or more competitive sports reported having tried smokeless tobacco, compared with 8.5% of girls who participated in three or fewer competitive sports over the same period.

Mattila *et al.*[44] examined the relationships between sport activity, type of sport, and smokeless tobacco use in a sample of 16 746 Finnish male conscripts (median age 19 years). Males reporting regular participation in competitive team sports were more than ten times as likely as non-active males to report current smokeless tobacco use. When examined by type of sport, ice hockey and weight lifting were positively associated with smokeless tobacco use, while cycling and skiing were inversely associated. Martinsen and Sundgot-Borgen[43] contrasted smokeless tobacco use among Norwegian students attending elite sport high schools and randomly selected controls. In conflict with the other studies, a higher percentage of control students (31.1%) compared with athletes (16.6%) reported smokeless tobacco use.

Alcohol use

The association between sports participation and alcohol use in children and adolescents has been scrutinized in numerous studies and population health surveys. The results of these investigations have been far from consistent. While some studies report a protective inverse relationship between sports participation and alcohol use, others have found sports participants to be at significantly greater risk for alcohol use.

Forty-three studies investigating the association between sports participation and alcohol use met the inclusionary criteria. Of this number, 22 analysed data from nationally representative samples of youth. Of these 22, 15 studies reported sports participation to be positively associated with alcohol use,[13,24–31,42,59–63] three studies reported an inverse association,[15,21,64] and four studies reported no evidence of an association.[17,20,22,23]

Twenty-one studies investigated the association between sports participation and alcohol use in samples of youth from a single school, school district, or geographical region. Of these 21, nine studies reported sports participation to significantly increase the risk of alcohol use,[34,36,47,51,55,65–69] five studies reported an inverse association,[39,43,53,70,71] and seven studies reported no evidence of an association.[34,35,46,49,50,52,72] Eight studies employed a longitudinal study design to examine the relationship between youth sports participation and subsequent alcohol use.[21,25,28,42,55,60,61,63] Seven of them reported a positive association between sports participation and alcohol use.[25,28,42,55,60,61,63]

Hoffman[60] investigated the effects of sports participation on alcohol use in adolescents participating in the National Education Longitudinal Study. Among both males and females, a positive association was observed between sports participation and alcohol use. For every 1% increase in sports participation there was an 8% increase in the risk of alcohol use. Lisha *et al.*[61] analysed data from over 8000 youth participating in the National Survey of Parents and Youth. Sports participation at age 14 years was associated with increased alcohol use at age 18 years. Lee *et al.*[42] analysed longitudinal data from the National Institute of Child Health and Human Development Study on Early Child Care and Youth Development. Participants reporting participation in sports at age 15 years were 1.2 times more likely to report alcohol use at the end of high school than non-participants.

Using data from the US National Longitudinal Study of Adolescent Health, Nelson and Gordon-Larsen[21] evaluated the association between sports participation and the use of alcohol. Adolescents with a high frequency of sports participation were significantly less likely than non-sporting adolescents to report being drunk at least once in the past year; however, no association was observed for being drunk more than once a month, or driving when drunk. An analysis of the same data by Mays *et al.*[63] yielded opposing findings. Using latent growth modelling, participation in school sports alone during adolescence was associated with faster than average acceleration in problem alcohol use during the 6-year follow-up. Terry-McElrath *et al.*[25] analysed data from the US Monitoring the Future Study to explore the relationship between high school sports participation and alcohol use during early adulthood. Sports participation at age 18 years was associated with higher alcohol use at age 21/22 years and 25/26 years, respectively. Wichstrom *et al.*[28] examined the association between adolescent sports participation and alcohol use during early adulthood in a population-based cohort of Norwegian high-school students. Students involved in team sports during adolescence exhibited significantly greater growth in alcohol intoxication rates during early adulthood than non-sports participants.

Illegal drug use

Illicit drugs are pharmacological or chemical agents that are considered illegal to use, possess, or sell without appropriate authority. Well-known examples of illicit drugs include marijuana, cocaine, heroin, amphetamines, barbiturates, PCP, LSD, and the inhalation of glues/solvents. Participation in youth sports is frequently cited as a deterrent to experimentation with drugs; however, a surprisingly modest number of empirical studies have evaluated the relationship between sports participation and illicit drug use in children or adolescents.

Twenty-five studies investigating the association between sports participation and illegal drug use met the inclusion criteria. Of this number, 17 studies analysed data from nationally representative samples of youth. Of these 17, 11 studies reported sports participation to decrease the risk of illegal drug use,[15,17,21,22,24–26,42,59,61,73] five studies reported a positive association between sports participation and illegal drug use,[13,23,28–30] and one study reported no evidence of an association.[20]

Although the majority of studies conducted in nationally representative samples reported sports participation to be protective against illegal drug use, the direction and strength of the association tended to vary by gender and race/ethnicity. As an example, Pate *et al.*[23] assessed the relationship between sports participation and illicit drug use in US high-school students participating in the 1997 YRBS. Among male students, participation in school- or community-based sports was protective against marijuana use in whites and Hispanics, but not in African-Americans. Sports participation significantly reduced the risk of cocaine and other illicit drug use (LSD, PCP, ecstasy, mushrooms, speed, ice, heroin) in white males, but it increased the risk of use of these substances in African-American and Hispanic males. Among female students, sports participation was protective against cocaine and other illicit drugs regardless of race/ethnicity. However, only white female sports participants were at significantly decreased risk for marijuana use and sniffing glue or paint.

Additionally, the association between sports participation and illegal drug use appears to be at least partially dependent on the type of sport played. Veliz *et al.*[30] examined the association between sports participation and illegal drug use in high-school students participating in the US Monitoring the Future Study. Adolescents who participated in contact sports were at a significantly greater risk of illegal drug use in the past month than non-sports participants. In contrast, adolescents who participated in non-contact sports had a reduced risk of illegal drug use compared to non-sport participants.

Eight studies investigated the association between sports participation and illegal drug use in samples of youth from a single school, school district, or geographical region.[35,36,39,46,50–52,74] Of these eight, six studies reported sports participation to be protective of illegal drug use,[35,36,39,46,50,74] one study reported a positive association,[51] and one study reported no evidence of an association.[52] Five studies employed longitudinal study designs.[21,25,28,42,61] Of these five, four studies reported sports participation to be protective of illegal drug use[21,25,42,61] and one study reported sports participants to be a greater risk for illegal drug use.[28]

Using data from the US National Longitudinal Study of Adolescent Health, Nelson and Gordon-Larsen[21] evaluated the association between sports participation and use of alcohol. Adolescents reporting a high frequency of sports participation with parents or regular use of sport and recreation centres were significantly less likely than non-sporting adolescents to report marijuana or other illegal drug use. Lisha *et al.*[61] analysed data from over 8000 youth participating in the National Survey of Parents and Youth. Sports participation at age 14 years was related to decreased rates of illegal drug use at age 18 years. Lee *et al.*[42] analysed longitudinal data from the National Institute of Child Health and Human Development Study on Early Child Care and Youth Development. Participants reporting participation in sports at age 15 years were 25% less likely to report marijuana use at the end of high school than non-participants. Terry-McElrath *et al.*[25] explored the relationship between high school sports participation and illegal drug use among students participating in the US Monitoring the Future Study. Greater sports participation at age 18 years was associated with lower illegal drug use, with subsequent increases in sports participation related to significant decreases in drug use at age 21/22 years and 25/26 years, respectively. Wichstrom *et al.*[28] examined the association between adolescent sports participation and marijuana use during early adulthood in a population-based cohort of Norwegian high-school students. In conflict with the other longitudinal studies, students involved in team sports at baseline exhibited significantly greater growth in marijuana use during early adulthood than non-sports participants.

Anabolic steroid use

Population health surveys conducted in the United States suggest that the prevalence of steroid use among adolescent youth is small yet significant. In 2013, the prevalence of anabolic steroid use without a prescription among US high-school students was 4.0% and 2.2% in males and females, respectively.[5] Although illegal and associated with numerous short- and long-term health risks, anabolic steroids are used by some athletes to enhance athletic performance, including those involved in high school sports. Thus, the association between youth sports participation and steroid use has been scrutinized in several studies (interested readers are referred to Chapter 49 for further discussion of drug use in sport). The results of these studies, however, have been inconsistent with the strength and direction of the reported associations varying by sex and race/ethnicity.

Nineteen studies investigating the association between sports participation and anabolic steroid use met our inclusionary criteria. Of this number, 11 studies analysed data from nationally representative samples of youth. Of these 11, five studies reported sports participation to be positively associated with anabolic steroid use,[22,23,26,75,76] three studies reported an inverse association,[24,77,78] and three studies reported no evidence of an association.[17,79,80]

Several studies contrasted anabolic steroid use among high school sports participants and non-participants completing the CDC YRBS. Using data from the 1991 YRBS, DuRant *et al.*[79] assessed the relationship between steroid use and sports participation. After controlling for age, sex, academic performance, other drug use, and region of the country, students who participated on a sports team were more likely than non-participants to report steroid use; however, this association did not reach statistical significance. Page *et al.*[22] also examined the relationship between the level of sports participation and steroid use among high-school students participating in the YRBS. Male students participating in three or more sports teams were nearly twice as likely as non-participants to report ever using steroids. No association was observed among female students. Analysing data from the 1997 YRBS, Pate *et al.* [23] reported sports participation to be positively associated with steroid use, but only among African-American males. Elliot *et al.*[77] used data from the 2003 YRBS survey to evaluate the relationship between school-sponsored sports participation and anabolic steroid use in high school girls. After adjusting for grade level and race/ethnicity, team sports participants were nearly two times less likely to be steroid users than non-participants. Finally, Taliaferro *et al.*[24] analysed data from six consecutive YRBS surveys administered between 1999 and 2007. Among boys, sports participation was consistently unrelated to anabolic steroid use. Among girls, however, sports participation was consistently protective for anabolic steroid use, but only among white girls.

Eight studies investigated the association between sports participation and anabolic steroid use in samples of youth from a single school, school district, or geographical region. Of these eight, six studies reported sports participation to significantly increase the risk of anabolic steroid use[81–86] and two studies reported no evidence of an association.[46,51] No studies reporting an inverse association between sports participation and anabolic steroid use were located. No longitudinal studies meeting the inclusionary criteria were identified.

Dietary practices

The question of whether participation in youth sports promotes healthy eating in children and adolescents has not been studied extensively. Just five studies investigating the association between sports participation and dietary practices met the inclusion criteria.[23,24,35,39,87] All five reported sports participation to be positively associated with healthy eating. Of the five studies identified, two analysed data from nationally representative samples of youth.[23,24] Both reported sport participation to have a positive influence of dietary practices; however, the strength and direction of the associations varied by gender and race/ethnicity. No longitudinal studies meeting the inclusionary criteria were identified.

Pate *et al.*[23] evaluated the relationship between school and community sports participation and dietary behaviours in high-school students completing the 1997 YRBS. After controlling for grade level, race/ethnicity, and non-sport PA level, male sports participants were significantly more likely to report recent consumption of fruits and vegetables than non-participants. Female sports participants were more likely to report recent consumption of salad or vegetables than non-participants. A positive association was also observed for sports participation and consumption of fruit or fruit juice, although this association was only significant among white females. Taliaferro *et al.*[24] analysed data from six consecutive YRBS surveys administered between 1999 and 2007. Among males, sports participation was consistently and positively associated with daily fruit and vegetable consumption, although the association for vegetable consumption was strongest among white and Hispanic students. Among females, sports participation was consistently and positively associated with daily fruit and vegetable consumption, with these associations being consistently stronger among white and Hispanic females.

Three studies investigated the association between sports participation and dietary practices in samples of youth from a single school, school district, or geographical region.[35,39,87] All three reported sports participation to be associated with healthful dietary practices. Baumert *et al.*[35] examined the relationship between sports participation and dietary intake in high-school students from a single county in the southern United States. Compared to non-participants, sport participants were significantly more likely to report consuming breakfast, fruits and vegetables, and one serving from the dairy food group on a daily basis. They were also less likely to add salt to their foods. No differences were found in reported consumption of red meats, fried foods, and snack foods. Croll *et al.*[87] contrasted the eating behaviours of adolescents participating in weight-related and power team sports and non-sports participants. For both males and females, participation in weight-related and power team sports was associated with eating breakfast more frequently and significantly higher intakes of protein, calcium, iron, and zinc. Harrison *et al.*[39] examined the association between sports participation and healthful eating practices in just over 50 000 ninth grade students (approximately age 14) in Minnesota. Students reporting participation in school sports were 1.4 to 2.1 times more likely than non-participants to report consumption of five or more fruits and vegetables and three or more glasses of milk on the day before the survey.

Inappropriate weight-control practices

There is evidence to suggest that those who participate in sports in which leanness is emphasized, such as ballet or gymnastics, are more likely to diet inappropriately or have eating disorders such as bulimia and anorexia nervosa.[88] Others have recognized that, owing to the rules of their sport, certain athletes are subject to a particular pressure to maintain a low body weight[89] (interested readers are referred to Chapter 47 and Chapter 50 for further discussion).

Eighteen studies investigating the association between sports participation and inappropriate weight control practices met the inclusion criteria. Of this number, five studies analysed data from nationally representative samples of youth.[20,23,24,90,91] Of these five, two studies reported sports participation to be positively associated with inappropriate weight control practices,[24,90] two studies reported an inverse or protective association,[23,91] and one study reported no evidence of an association.[20]

In an analysis of the 1993 YRBS data for the state of Massachusetts, Middleman and colleagues[91] found no association between high school sports participation and weight loss behaviours, including use of vomiting or diet pills to lose weight. In fact, young girls (younger than 16 years) involved in sports were less likely to report trying to lose weight than non-athletes. Pate *et al.*[23] assessed the relationship between sports participation and inappropriate weight loss practices in US high-school students completing the 1997 YRBS. After controlling for grade level, race/ethnicity, and non-sport PA, female sports participants were approximately 1.3 times less likely than non-participants to report trying to lose weight. However, female sport participants were not significantly more likely than non-participants to report use of vomiting, laxatives, or pills to lose weight. Sports participation was not associated with inappropriate weight loss practices in males. Taliaferro *et al.*[24] analysed data from six consecutive YRBS surveys administered between 1999 and 2007. Across all survey years, sports participants were significantly less likely to report trying to lose weight than non-sports participants. However, male sports participants were consistently more likely than their non-sporting counterparts to report vomiting or using laxatives or pills to lose weight. Among females, sports participation was not associated with vomiting or using laxative or pills to lose weight.

Michaud *et al.*[20] investigated the relationship between sports participation and inappropriate weight control practices in a nationally-representative sample of Swiss adolescents. Students reporting sports participation exhibited similar levels of body satisfaction, plans to lose weight, and frequency of dieting than non-sport participants. Crissey *et al.*[90] explored the relationship between sport participation and weight-loss strategies among adolescent girls participating in the National Longitudinal Study of Adolescent Health. Girls reporting participation in feminine sports (majority of participants female) were 65% more likely to report that they were trying to lose weight than non-sport participants. Furthermore, girls participating in feminine sports were more than twice as likely as non-participants to report using both diet and exercise to lose weight in the past 7 days.

Thirteen studies investigated the association between sports participation and inappropriate weight control practices in samples of youth from a single school, school district, or geographical region. Of these 13, nine studies reported sports participation to significantly increase the risk of inappropriate weight control practices,[65,84,92–98] two studies reported an inverse or protective association,[99,100] and two studies reported no evidence of an association.[51,101]

Sexual risk behaviours

There has been considerable interest in assessing whether sports participation is associated with avoidance of sexual risk behaviours in adolescents. The available evidence, although limited, suggests that sports participation is protective against sexual risk behaviours in female adolescents. However, among adolescent males, the evidence related to sport participation and sexual risk behaviours is inconsistent.

Fifteen studies investigating the association between sports participation and sexual risk behaviours met the inclusion criteria. Of this number, seven studies analysed data from nationally representative samples of youth. Of these seven, four studies reported sports participation to be inversely associated with sexual risk behaviours,[15,17,21,22] while three studies reported both positive and negative associations.[23,24,102]

Several authors have evaluated the relationship between youth sports participation and sexual risk behaviours using data from the CDC YRBS. Using data from the 1991 YRBS, Page *et al.*[22] examined the association between school and community sports participation and sexual risk behaviour. Compared to non-participants, girls reporting participation on one or two sports teams were 1.7 times less likely to have not ever had a sexually transmitted disease, and 1.5 times less likely to have not been pregnant. Among males, there was no relationship between sports participation and sexual risk behaviour. Among high-school students who had reported sexual intercourse, sports participants were significantly less likely than non-participants to have had multiple partners and were more likely than non-participants to use a condom the last time they had sexual intercourse.

Using data from the 1997 YRBS, Miller *et al.*[102] examined the association between team sports participation and sexual risk behaviours. Sexual risk was measured using the Sexual Risk Scale which included six dichotomous items related to adolescent sexual risk—intercourse prior to age 15 years, failure to use birth control at the most recent sexual intercourse, use of alcohol or drugs at most recent sexual intercourse, multiple lifetime sex partners, multiple recent sex partners, and involvement in a past pregnancy. Participants were classified as at-risk if they responded affirmatively to one or more of the six items. Girls who reported participation in team sports were significantly less likely than their non-sporting counterparts to engage in sexual risk. The protective effects of sports participation were stronger among white and Hispanic girls than African-American and Asian/Pacific Islander girls. In contrast to girls, boys reporting participation in team sports were significantly more likely than non-participants to engage in risky sexual behaviour. However, when sexual risk was examined by race/ethnicity, sports participation was associated with a significantly lower risk among white boys, significantly higher risk for African-American boys, with no association observed among Hispanic or Asian/Pacific Islander boys.

Kulig *et al.*[17] examined the association between team sports participation and sexual risk behaviours using data from the 1999 YRBS. After controlling for grade and race/ethnicity, female sports participants classified as physically active had a significantly reduced risk of ever having had intercourse, having had four or more sexual partners in their lifetime or in the three previous months, and having been pregnant than girls not active or participating in team sports. Sports participation was not associated with sexual risk behaviours in male students

Eight studies investigated the association between sports participation and sexual risk behaviour in samples of youth from a single school, school district, or geographical region. Of these eight, four studies reported sports participation to reduce the risk of sexual risk behaviours,[39,103–105] while four studies reported a positive association between sports participation and sexual risk behaviours.[66,68,106,107] Two studies employed longitudinal study designs to characterize the relationship between youth sports participation and sexual risk behaviours. Both reported an inverse or protective association in female sports participants, but not male participants.[21,104]

Miller *et al.*[104] longitudinally examined the effects of sports participation on sexual behaviour in a sample of 611 Western New York adolescents. The authors observed the relationship between sports participation and sexual behaviour to be highly gender specific. Whereas male sport participants were more likely than non-participants to report sexual activity, female sport participants were significantly less likely than non-participants to report sexual activity. These findings remained intact after controlling for race, age, socioeconomic status, quality of family relations, and participation in other extracurricular activities. Nelson and Gordon-Larsen[21] analysed data from the US National Longitudinal Study of Adolescent Health to examine the association between organized sport and sexual risk behaviours. Adolescents reporting a high frequency of sports participation with parents were 30% less likely than sedentary adolescents to report using no birth control during their most recent sexual intercourse.

Violence

The notion that participation in sports can deter delinquent behaviours in adolescent youth has motivated a number of authors to examine the association between sports participation and behaviours that contribute to violence (i.e. carrying a weapon or being in a physical fight). Fifteen studies investigating the association between sports participation and violence met the inclusion criteria. Of this number, six studies analysed data from nationally representative samples of youth. Of these six, three studies reported sports participation to be inversely associated with violent behaviours,[21,22,24] one study reported a positive association,[108] one study reported both protective and risk associations,[23] and one study reported no evidence of an association.[109]

The available evidence suggests that the relationship between sports participation and violence-related behaviours in youth is moderated by gender and race/ethnicity. Pate *et al.*[23] assessed the relationship between sports participation and violence in high-school students completing the 1997 YRBS. Among male students, participation in school- or community-based sports significantly decreased the likelihood of carrying a weapon in white students, but increased the likelihood of carrying a weapon in African-American students. Sports participation was not associated with weapon carrying in Hispanic males. Among female students, sports participation decreased the likelihood of carrying a weapon in white students, but increased the likelihood of carrying a weapon in Hispanic students. Sports participation was not associated with weapon carrying in African-American females. Sports participation was not associated with the risk of physical fighting in both genders.

Nine studies investigated the association between sports participation and violence in samples of youth from a single school, school district, or geographical region. Of these nine, five studies reported a positive association between sports participation and violent behaviour,[51,110–113] while four studies reported no evidence of an association.[55,114–116] Four studies employed longitudinal study designs. Of these four, one study reported sports participation to significantly increase the risk of violence,[108] one study reported an inverse association,[21] and two studies reported no evidence of an association.[55,109]

Aaron *et al.*[55] contrasted the cumulative frequency of weapon carrying in high school sports participants and non-participants. Over the 3-year follow-up period, a higher proportion of sports participants reported carrying a weapon (32%) than non-sport participants (25%); however, this difference was not statistically significant. Nelson and Gordon-Larsen[21] analysed data from the US National Longitudinal Study of Adolescent Health to examine the association between sports participation and violent behaviour. Adolescents with a high frequency of sports participation with parents were 12% less likely than sedentary adolescents to engage in one or more violent behaviours such as being in a serious physical fight, seriously injuring another person, participating in a group fight, using a weapon, or stabbing someone in the past year. No association was observed among adolescents reporting a high frequency of sports participation at school or neighbourhood recreation centres. Jiang *et al.*[109] analysed data from the US National Longitudinal Study of Adolescent Health to explore the relationship between extracurricular activities and the risk of youth violence. After controlling for socio-demographic factors, parental control, parental monitoring, and participation in other extracurricular activities, participation in sports was not associated with the risk of adolescent violence. Kreager *et al.*[108] utilized data from the US National Longitudinal Study of Adolescent Health to explore the relationship between sports participation and the risk of serious fighting in male adolescents. Participation in general sport was not associated with the risk of serious fighting. However, when examined on a sport-specific basis, males participating in football and wrestling were 1.41 and 1.45 times more likely to report being in a serious fight than non-sports participants. Participation in basketball, baseball, tennis, or other sports demonstrated no relationship with the risk of serious fighting.

Physical activity and other health behaviours

Cigarette smoking

A smaller but significant number of studies have evaluated the relationship between PA participation and cigarette smoking in children and adolescents. Twenty-six studies investigating the association between PA and cigarette smoking met the inclusion criteria. Of this number, ten studies analysed data from nationally representative samples of youth. Of these ten, eight studies reported PA to be inversely associated with cigarette smoking,[13,21,117–122] while two studies reported no evidence of an association.[123,124]

Seventeen studies investigated the association between PA and cigarette smoking in samples of youth from a single school, school district, or geographical region. Of these 17, 12 studies reported physical activity to be inversely associated with cigarette smoking,[41,55,125–134] one study reported a positive association,[135] and four reported no evidence of an association.[136–139] Six studies employed longitudinal study designs to examine the relationship between PA and cigarette smoking. All six reported PA to be inversely associated with cigarette smoking.[21,55,118,119,122,126]

Raitakari *et al.*[122] prospectively examined the association between PA and cigarette smoking in a representative sample of Finnish youth aged 12–18 years. Participants who remained sedentary over the 6-year follow-up period were significantly more likely than their active counterparts to either begin smoking or smoke on a daily basis.

Aaron *et al.*[55] longitudinally examined the relationship between PA and cigarette smoking in a small cohort of US high-school students. A significant inverse association was observed among females for PA and smoking. The percentage of females initiating cigarette use was significantly lower among those reporting high levels of PA (10%) compared to those reporting low or moderate participation in PA (22–23%). No association was found between PA and cigarette smoking in males.

Aarnio *et al.*[118] longitudinally evaluated the association between smoking status and PA in a population representative sample of Finnish twins. Male adolescents who were classified as regular smokers were 80% less likely than non-smokers to be persistent exercisers between the ages of 16 and 18.5 years. Similarly, female adolescents classified as regular smokers were 48% less likely than non-smokers to be persistent exercisers between the ages of 16 and 18.5 years. Nelson and Gordon-Larsen[21] analysed data from the US National Longitudinal Study of Adolescent Health to examine the association between PA and cigarette smoking. Adolescents who reported five or more bouts of moderate-to-vigorous intensity PA per week were 22% less likely than low-active adolescents to report smoking five or more cigarettes in the previous month. Analysing the same data, Ali *et al.*[119] reported PA participation to be protective of cigarette smoking. Their analysis indicated that one additional weekly occurrence of exercise was associated with a 0.3% decline in the probability of being a smoker, and a 4.1% reduction in the number of cigarettes smoked by a smoker during a month.

Audrain-McGovern *et al.*[126] examined the relationship between PA participation in cigarette smoking in a cohort of approximately 1400 high-school students progressing from the ninth to the twelfth grades. Using general growth mixture modelling, the authors identified five distinct PA trajectories—stable higher PA, decreased PA, stable regular PA, curvilinear PA, and stable low PA. Students exhibiting a decreased-PA profile were 3.3 times more likely than students with consistently higher levels of PA to be smokers in the tenth grade. Only 3% of the adolescents belonging to the stable higher-PA trajectory were regular smokers in grade 12, whereas 17% of adolescents belonging to the stable low-PA trajectory, and 27% of the adolescents belonging to the decreasing pattern of PA trajectory smoked regularly in grade 12.

Smokeless tobacco

Perhaps because smokeless tobacco use is more closely linked with participation in selected sports, the association between PA participation and smokeless tobacco use has received relatively little research attention. Just five studies investigating the association between PA and smokeless tobacco use met the inclusion criteria.[13,124,126,134,140] Of these five, three studies analysed data from nationally representative samples of youth.[13,124,140] Of these three, one study reported PA to be positively associated with smokeless tobacco use,[140] while two studies reported no evidence of an association.[13,124] Only one study employed a longitudinal study design.[126]

Karvonen *et al.*[140] assessed the relationship between PA participation and smokeless tobacco use in three population-representative samples of Finnish adolescents aged 16–18 years. After controlling for socioeconomic status, participation in PA was positively associated with smokeless tobacco use, but only among boys living in urban areas. Winnail *et al.*[134] assessed the relationship between PA level and smokeless tobacco use among high-school students completing the 1993 South Carolina YRBS. Among white males and African-American females, students with low and moderate levels of PA were significantly more likely than those with high levels of PA to report smokeless tobacco use in the previous 30 days. Among white females and African-American males, low and moderate levels of PA were associated with decreased risk of smokeless tobacco use compared to those with high levels of PA; however, none of these associations reached statistical significance.

Dunn[13] investigated the relationship between PA participation and smokeless tobacco use using data from the 2009 YRBS. High-school students reporting recreational PA on 5 or more days per week were 17–20% less likely to report smokeless tobacco use in the past month than those reporting no PA. However, the association was not statistically significant. Vuori *et al.*[124] examined the association between PA and smokeless tobacco use in a nationally-representative sample of Finnish 15-year-olds. Neither leisure time PA nor participation in moderate- to vigorous-intensity PA was related to smokeless tobacco use.

Audrain-McGovern *et al.*[126] followed a cohort of approximately 1400 high-school students from the ninth to the twelfth grade. Using general growth mixture modelling, the authors identified five distinct PA trajectories—stable higher PA, decreased PA, stable regular PA, curvilinear PA, and stable low PA. Ten percent of the adolescents belonging to the stable higher PA group were smokeless tobacco users in grade 12, whereas 32% of the adolescents belonging to the decreasing pattern of PA reported smokeless tobacco use in grade 12.

Alcohol use

Inconsistent findings have emerged from studies investigating the relationship between PA participation and alcohol use in children and adolescents. Fifteen studies investigating the association between PA and alcohol use met the inclusion criteria. Of this number, eight studies analysed data from nationally representative samples of youth.[13,21,117,118,121,123,124,141] Of these eight, five studies reported PA to be inversely associated with alcohol use,[13,21,117,121,141] one study reported a positive association,[123] and two studies reported no evidence of an association.[118,124]

Seven studies investigated the association between PA and alcohol use in samples of youth from a single school, school district, or geographical region.[55,130,131,133,137,138,142] Of these seven, three studies reported PA to be positively associated with alcohol use,[118,131,142] three studies reported an inverse association,[130,133,138] and one study reported no evidence of an association.[137] Four studies employed longitudinal study designs.[21,55,118,141] Of these four, two studies reported PA to be inversely associated with alcohol use,[21,141] one study reported a positive association,[55] and one study reported no evidence of an association.[118]

Aaron *et al.*[55] prospectively examined the relationship between leisure time PA and alcohol use in high-school students in a single city in the north-eastern US. The percentage of males initiating alcohol use was significantly higher among those reporting both moderate and high levels of PA (42–48%) compared to those reporting low participation in PA (24%). No association was found between PA and alcohol use in females.

Aarnio *et al.*[118] longitudinally evaluated the association between alcohol use and PA in a population representative same of Finnish twins. Male and females reporting heavy alcohol use were less likely to be classified as persistent exercisers than non-users; however, the association was not statistically significant. In an extended follow-up of the Finnish twin cohort (mean age 24.4 years), women who were persistently inactive between the ages of 16 and 18.5 years were 4.4 times more likely to report weekly intoxication than those were persistently active during this period. Among men, there was no relationship between PA between the ages of 16 and 18.5 years and subsequent alcohol use. In the US National Longitudinal Study of Adolescent Health, adolescents reporting five or more moderate to vigorous bouts of PA per week were 16–28% less likely than low-active adolescents to report being drunk more than once per month or driving while drunk in the previous year.[21]

Illegal drug use

Compared to the number of studies focused on sport, fewer investigations have examined the association between PA and illegal drug use. Ten studies investigating the association between PA and illegal drug use met the inclusion criteria. Of this number, six studies analysed data from nationally representative samples of youth.[13,21,121,123,124,141] Of these six, three studies reported PA to be inversely associated with illegal drug use,[21,121,141] two studies reported a positive association,[13,124] and one study reported no evidence of an association.[123]

Pate *et al.*[121] examined the relationship between PA status and illicit drug use in high-school students completing the 1990 YRBS. After controlling for grade level, sex, and race, students classified as physically active were significantly less likely to report using cocaine and marijuana in the 30 days preceding the survey. Dunn[13] investigated the relationship between PA participation and illegal drug use using data from the 2009 YRBS. Female high-school students reporting 1–4 days of recreational PA per week were 1.23 times more likely to report marijuana use in the past month than females reporting no PA. Recreational PA was not associated with marijuana use among males. Peltzer[123] examined the association between PA and illicit drug use in 13- to 15-year-olds from nationally representative samples from eight African countries. Leisure time PA was not associated with illicit drug use. Vuori *et al.*[124] examined the association between PA and cannabis use in a nationally representative sample of Finnish 15-year-olds. Leisure time PA, but not moderate to vigorous PA was positively associated with cannabis use.

Four studies investigated the association between PA and illegal drug use in samples of youth from a single school, school district, or geographical region.[130,131,134,143] Of these four, three studies reported PA to be inversely associated with illegal drug use,[130,131,134] and one study reported no evidence of an association.[143] Two studies employed longitudinal study designs.[21,141] Both reported PA to be inversely associated with illegal drug use.

In their analysis of data from the National Longitudinal Study of Adolescent Health, Nelson and Gordan-Larson[21] found physically active adolescents to be 27% less likely than their less active counterparts to report using illegal drugs in the previous year. Korhonen *et al.*[141] longitudinally evaluated the association between PA in late adolescence and illegal drug use in young adulthood in a population representative cohort of Finnish twins. Persistently inactive men and women were 3.75 times more likely to report regular drug use than more active men and women. In 20 of the 25 pairs discordant for PA and drug use, it was the less active co-twin who reported regular drug use.

Anabolic steroid use

Few studies have formally evaluated the association between PA participation and anabolic steroid use in children and adolescents. Just three studies met the inclusion criteria.[78,79,144] All three reported PA participation to significantly increase the risk of anabolic steroid use.

DuRant *et al.*[79] assessed the relationship between steroid use and strength training using data from the 1991 YRBS. After controlling for age, sex, academic performance, other drug use, and region of the country, students who engaged in strength training were more likely to report lifetime steroid use than students who did not engage in strength training. Kokkevi *et al.*[144] examined the relationship between PA and anabolic steroid use in 18 430 16-year-old high-school students from six European countries (Bulgaria, Croatia, Cyprus, Greece, the Slovak Republic, and the UK). After controlling for gender, deviant behaviour, cigarette smoking, alcohol consumption, other drug use, and country of origin, adolescents reporting anabolic steroid use were 1.4 times more likely than non-users to report exercise almost daily. Thorlindsson and Halldorsson[78] investigated the use of anabolic steroids in a nationally representative sample of Icelandic high-school students. Informal or fitness sports participation, but not organized sports participation, significantly increased the risk of anabolic steroid use. After controlling for school, parenting practices, school behavioural problems, illegal substance use, and tobacco and alcohol use, high-school students reporting participation in recreational exercise or fitness on four or more occasions per week were 2.7 times more likely to use anabolic steroids than those who do not participate in formal sports.

Dietary practices

Compared to sports participation, the relationship between PA and healthy dietary practices has been studied somewhat more extensively. Twelve studies investigating the association between PA and dietary practices met the inclusion criteria. Of these studies, five analysed data from nationally representative samples of youth.[117,118,121,122,145] All five studies reported PA to have a positive influence on dietary practices.

Pate *et al.*[121] analysed data from the national 1990 YRBS to determine if physically active adolescents were more likely than their low-active counterparts to report consumption of fruit or vegetables on the previous day. After adjustment for age group, sex, and race, students who did not eat vegetables on the previous day were almost twice as likely to be low active than students who reported eating at least one serving of vegetables. Among the Hispanic and white subgroups, students who ate no fruit on the previous day were 2.3 and 3.1 times, respectively, more likely to be low active than those who ate one or more servings of fruit on the previous day.

Using data from the 2010 National Youth Physical Activity and Nutrition Study, Lowry *et al.*[145] examined the association between PA and dietary behaviours in a nationally representative sample of US high-school students in grades 9 through 12. Students who participated in the recommended 60 min of daily PA were more than twice as likely to eat two or more servings of fruits per day and three or more servings of vegetables per day as non-active students.

Seven studies investigated the association between PA and dietary practices in samples of youth from a single school, school district, or geographical region.[127,136,146–150] Of these seven, five studies reported PA participation to be associated with healthful dietary practices[127,136,146–148] and two studies reported no evidence of an association.[149,150] Notably, the two studies reporting no association used a motion sensor to objectively measure PA behaviour (interested readers are referred to Chapter 21 for for an analysis of methods of assessing PA).

Two longitudinal studies examining the relationship between PA and dietary practices met the inclusionary criteria. Both found PA to be positively associated with healthful dietary practices. Raitakari *et al.*[122] tracked the health-related behaviours of 961 Finnish adolescents, aged 12–18 years. Comparing the constantly active to the constantly low active, it was found that the low active young males consumed significantly more saturated fat and had a lower polyunsaturated to saturated fat ratio than the active males. Aarnio *et al.*[118] prospectively evaluated the relationship between habitual PA and dietary practices in a representative cohort of Finnish twins. Males reporting eating breakfast only once a week were just over 60% less likely to be persistently physically active between the ages of 16 and 18.5 years. Among females, persistent PA was associated with eating breakfast regularly; however, the association was somewhat weaker than that observed among males.

Inappropriate weight-loss practices

Just two studies investigating the association between PA and inappropriate weight control practices met the inclusion criteria. One study reported participation in PA to be positively associated with inappropriate weight-control practices,[148] while the other reported no evidence of an association.[91] French *et al.*[148] collected data from 708 males and 786 females in grades seven through ten from a suburban school district in the mid-western US. A 21-item eating-disorder checklist was developed for the study, based on previous research and DSM-III-R criteria for eating disorders. The number of affirmative responses constituted a risk score for eating disorders. Physical activity was measured using a 28-item checklist of activities. Principal components analysis resulted in three categories of sport activities: leisure or outdoor sports, conditioning sports, and atypical sports. Among males, atypical sports participation (e.g. bowling, aerobics, and softball) was a significant predictor of the risk score for eating disorders. Among females, all three categories of PA (conditioning sports, leisure sports, and atypical sports) were significant predictors of the risk score for eating disorders.

In their analysis of YRBS data from the state of Massachusetts, Middleman *et al.*[91] reported participation in vigorous exercise, stretching, and strength-promoting exercises to be associated with trying to lose weight among females and trying to gain weight in males. However, there were no indications that PA was associated with inappropriate weight-gain or weight-loss behaviours.

Sexual risk behaviours

Four studies investigating the association between PA and sexual risk behaviours met the inclusion criteria.[21,102,121,124] Of this number, one study reported PA to reduce the risk of sexual risk behaviours,[21] one study reported both positive and inverse associations,[102] and two studies reported evidence of no association.[121,124] All four studies analysed data from nationally representative samples of youth.

Vuori *et al.*[124] examined the association between PA and sexual risk taking in a nationally representative sample of Finnish 15-year-olds. Neither leisure time PA nor moderate to vigorous PA were associated with risky sexual behaviour. Pate *et al.*[121] examined the relationship between PA status and sexual activity in high-school students completing the 1990 YRBS. In unadjusted analyses, students classified as low active were significantly more likely than active students to report having one or more sexual partners in the previous 3 months. However, no association was observed between PA and sexual activity after controlling for age group, gender, and race/ethnicity. Using data from the 1997 YRBS, Miller *et al.*[102] examined the association between PA participation and sexual risk behaviours. Sexual risk was measured using the Sexual Risk Scale, which includes six dichotomous items related to adolescent sexual risk—intercourse prior to age 15 years, failure to use birth control at the most recent sexual intercourse, use of alcohol or drugs at most recent sexual intercourse, multiple lifetime sex partners, multiple recent sex partners, and involvement in a past pregnancy. Participants were classified as at-risk if they responded affirmatively to one or more of the six items. Girls who reported exercising vigorously 3 or more days per week were 16% less likely than their non-exercising counterparts to engage in sexual risk. In contrast, boys reporting regular vigorous intensity exercise were 19% more likely than non-exercisers to engage in risky sexual behaviour. Nelson and Gordon-Larsen[21] analysed data for the US National Longitudinal Study of Adolescent Health to examine the association between PA participation and sexual activity. Adolescents reporting five or more bouts of moderate-to-vigorous PA per week were significantly less likely than low active adolescents to report having sexual intercourse in the previous year and 13% less likely to report using no birth control in their most recent sexual intercourse.

Violence

Four studies investigating the association between PA and violence met the inclusion criteria.[55,121,151,152] Of these, one study reported PA to be positively associated with violence (in males only),[152] and three studies reported evidence of no association.[21,55,121]

Two studies employed longitudinal study designs. Aaron *et al.*[55] contrasted the prevalence of weapon carrying in high-school students reporting low, medium, and high levels of leisure time PA. Boys were significantly more likely than girls to report carrying a weapon in the previous 30 days; however, within gender groups, the prevalence of weapon carrying was similar across the three PA groups. Pate *et al.*[121] examined PA participation and the relative odds of being injured in a physical fight in a nationally representative sample of US high-school students. After controlling for age, sex, and race/ethnicity, no association was found between PA level and injury from physical fighting. Nelson and Gordon-Larsen[21] analysed data from the US National Longitudinal Study of Adolescent Health to examine the association between PA participation and violent behaviour. Participation in moderate to vigorous PA on 5 or more days per week was not associated with violent behaviours, such as being in a serious physical fight, seriously injuring another person, participating in a group fight, using a weapon, or stabbing someone in the past year. Demissie *et al.*[152] examined the association between PA and violence-related behaviours among US high-school students participating in the 2009 YRBS. After controlling for grade level, race/ethnicity, and other violence-related behaviours, males reporting being in a physical fight on or off school property were approximately 30% more likely to accumulate 60 min of PA daily than those not involved in a fight. Physical activity was not associated with violence-related behaviours among females.

Table 19.3 Summary of the associations between specific health behaviours and participation in sport and physical activity

Health behaviour*	Sports participation	Physical activity
Cigarette smoking	− −	− −
Smokeless tobacco	+	?
Alcohol use	+	− +
Illegal drugs	−	−
Anabolic steroids	+	?
Improper dietary practices	−	−
Improper weight control practices	+	?
Sexual activity	− +	− +
Violence	− +	?

* Note that each health behaviour is presented as a health-*compromising* behaviour. A negative (−) association indicates that sports participants and/or physically active individuals are *less* likely to engage in that behaviour. A positive (+) association indicates that sports participants and/or physically active individuals are *more* likely to engage in that behaviour. (− −) repeatedly documented inverse association; (−) weak or mixed evidence of an inverse association; (↔) evidence of no association; (+) weak or mixed evidence of a positive association; (+ +) repeatedly documented evidence of a positive association; (− +) evidence to support both a positive and negative association; (?) insufficient data available.

Conclusions

This chapter compiles the scientific evidence pertaining to the relationship between sports and/or PA and nine health behaviours associated with significant morbidity and mortality in children and adolescents. The findings for each health behaviour are summarized in Table 19.3.

Summary

- The available evidence suggests that participation in sport is protective against cigarette smoking, illegal drug use, unhealthy dietary practices, and sexual activity. However, only the evidence related to cigarette smoking could be regarded as consistent.
- For alcohol use, illegal drug use, sexual activity, and violence, the reported associations varied by gender, race/ethnicity, and type of sport.
- On the negative side, participation in sport appears to increase the risk for smokeless tobacco use, anabolic steroid use, inappropriate weight-loss practices, and for some population subgroups, violence and problematic sexual behaviour.
- Although fewer studies have investigated the relationship between physical activity (PA) and other health behaviours, there is evidence that regular PA is protective against cigarette smoking, illegal drug use, and improper dietary practices.

- Regular PA may protect one against smokeless tobacco use, improper weight-control practices, and violent behaviour, but more evidence is needed before more definite conclusions can be made about these health behaviours.
- For alcohol consumption, there is evidence that regular PA both increases and decreases the risk of alcohol consumption.
- No clear conclusions could be made regarding the impact of PA participation on anabolic steroid use in youth.
- Considerable caution should be exercised in interpreting the evidence, as the literature is still mostly comprised of cross-sectional studies. However, a number of longitudinal studies exploring the influence of sports participation and/or PA and substance use and other health behaviours have emerged since the last review.

References

1. National Council on Youth Sports. *Report on trends and participation in organised youth sports*. Stuart, FL: National Council of Youth Sports; 2008.
2. Clark W. Kids' sports. *Can Soc Trends*. 2008; 85: 54-61.
3. Schranz N, Olds T, Cliff D, *et al*. Results from Australia's 2014 Report Card on Physical Activity for Children and Youth. *J Phys Act Health*. 2014; 11: 21–25.
4. Sport and Recreation Alliance. *Sport in the UK: Facts and figures*. London: Sport and Recreation Alliance; 2014.
5. Centers for Disease Control and Prevention. *2013 Youth risk behaviour survey*. Available from: http://www.cdc.gov/healthyyouth/data/yrbs/index.htm. Accessed 8/1/2016.
6. Poinsett A, Ewing ME, Seefeldt V, Brown TP. *The role of sports in youth development: Report of a meeting convened by Carnegie Corporation of New York*. 18 March 1996. New York: Carnegie Corporation of New York; 1996.
7. United Nations. Sport for development and peace: Towards achieving the millennium development goals. Report from the United Nations Inter-Agency Task Force on Sport for Development and Peace. New York: United Nations Office on Sport for Development and Peace; 2003.
8. Boone-Heinonen J, Gordon-Larsen P, Adair LS. Obesogenic clusters: multidimensional adolescent obesity-related behaviours in the US. *Ann Behav Med*. 2008; 36: 217–230.
9. Cuenca-Garcia M, Huybrechts I, Ruiz JR, *et al*. Clustering of multiple lifestyle behaviours and health-related fitness in European adolescents. *J Nutr Educ Behav*. 2013; 45: 549–557.
10. Burke V, Milligan RA, Beilin LJ, *et al*. Clustering of health-related behaviours among 18-year-old Australians. *Prev Med*. 1997; 26: 724–733.
11. Adachi-Mejia AM, Carlos HA, Berke EM, Tanski SE, Sargent JD. A comparison of individual versus community influences on youth smoking behaviours: a cross-sectional observational study. *BMJ Open*. 2012; 2(5): doi: 10.1136/bmjopen-2011-000767.
12. Castrucci BC, Gerlach KK, Kaufman NJ, Orleans CT. Tobacco use and cessation behaviour among adolescents participating in organized sports. *Am J Health Behav*. 2004; 28: 63–71.
13. Dunn MS. Association between physical activity and substance use behaviours among high school students participating in the 2009 Youth Risk Behaviour Survey. *Psychol Rep*. 2014; 114: 675–685.
14. Escobedo LG, Marcus SE, Holtzman D, Giovino GA. Sports participation, age at smoking initiation, and the risk of smoking among US high school students. *JAMA*. 1993; 269: 1391–1395.
15. Ferron C, Narring F, Cauderay M, Michaud PA. Sport activity in adolescence: associations with health perceptions and experimental behaviours. *Health Educ Res*. 1999; 14: 225–233.
16. Kristjansson AL, Sigfusdottir ID, Allegrante JP, Helgason AR. Social correlates of cigarette smoking among Icelandic adolescents: a population-based cross-sectional study. *BMC Public Health*. 2008; 8: 86.
17. Kulig K, Brener ND, McManus T. Sexual activity and substance use among adolescents by category of physical activity plus team sports participation. *Arch Pediatr Adolesc Med*. 2003; 157: 905–912.
18. Mays D, Luta G, Walker LR, Tercyak KP. Exposure to peers who smoke moderates the association between sports participation and cigarette smoking behaviour among non-white adolescents. *Addict Behav*. 2012; 37: 1114–1121.
19. Melnick MJ, Miller KE, Sabo DF, Farrell MP, Barnes GM. Tobacco use among high school athletes and nonathletes: results of the 1997 Youth Risk Behaviour Survey. *Adolescence*. 2001; 36: 727–747.
20. Michaud PA, Jeannin A, Suris JC. Correlates of extracurricular sport participation among Swiss adolescents. *Eur J Pediatr*. 2006; 165: 546–555.
21. Nelson MC, Gordon-Larsen P. Physical activity and sedentary behaviour patterns are associated with selected adolescent health risk behaviours. *Pediatrics*. 2006; 117: 1281–1290.
22. Page RM, Hammermeister J, Scanlan A, Gilbert L. Is school sports participation a protective factor against adolescent health risk behaviours? *J Health Educ*. 1998; 29: 186–192.
23. Pate RR, Trost SG, Levin S, Dowda M. Sports participation and health-related behaviours among US youth. *Arch Pediatr Adolesc Med*. 2000; 154: 904–911.
24. Taliaferro LA, Rienzo BA, Donovan KA. Relationships between youth sport participation and selected health risk behaviours from 1999 to 2007. *J Sch Health*. 2010; 80: 399–410.
25. Terry-McElrath YM, O'Malley PM. Substance use and exercise participation among young adults: parallel trajectories in a national cohort-sequential study. *Addiction*. 2011; 106: 1855–1865.
26. Terry-McElrath YM, O'Malley PM, Johnston LD. Exercise and substance use among American youth, 1991-2009. *Am J Prev Med*. 2011; 40: 530–540.
27. Thorlindsson T, Vilhjalmsson R, Valgeirsson G. Sport participation and perceived health status: a study of adolescents. *Soc Sci Med*. 1990; 31: 551–556.
28. Wichstrom T, Wichstrom L. Does sports participation during adolescence prevent later alcohol, tobacco and cannabis use? *Addiction*. 2009; 104: 138–149.
29. Guevremont A, Findlay L, Kohen D. Organized extracurricular activities: are in-school and out-of-school activities associated with different outcomes for Canadian youth? *J Sch Health*. 2014; 84: 317–325.
30. Veliz PT, Boyd CJ, McCabe SE. Competitive sport involvement and substance use among adolescents: a nationwide study. *Subst Use Misuse*. 2015; 50: 156–165.
31. Bedendo A, Noto AR. Sports practices related to alcohol and tobacco use among high school students. *Revista Brasileira de Psiquiatria*. 2015; 37: 99–105.
32. Abrams K, Skolnik N, Diamond JJ. Patterns and correlates of tobacco use among suburban Philadelphia 6th- through 12th-grade students. *Fam Med*. 1999; 31: 128–132.
33. Adachi-Mejia AM, Primack BA, Beach ML, *et al*. Influence of movie smoking exposure and team sports participation on established smoking. *Arch Pediatr Adolesc Med*. 2009; 163: 638–643.
34. Adachi-Mejia AM, Gibson Chambers JJ, Li Z, Sargent JD. The relative roles of types of extracurricular activity on smoking and drinking initiation among tweens. *Acad Pediatr*. 2014; 14: 271–278.
35. Baumert PW, Jr., Henderson JM, Thompson NJ. Health risk behaviours of adolescent participants in organized sports. *J Adolesc Health*. 1998; 22: 460–465.
36. Diehl K, Thiel A, Zipfel S, Mayer J, Schneider S. Substance use among elite adolescent athletes: findings from the GOAL Study. *Scand J Med Sci Sports*. 2014; 24: 250–258.
37. Garcia-Rodriguez O, Suarez-Vazquez R, Secades-Villa R, Fernandez-Hermida JR. Smoking risk factors and gender differences among Spanish high school students. *J Drug Educ*. 2010; 40: 143–156.
38. Giannakopoulos G, Panagiotakos D, Mihas C, Tountas Y. Adolescent smoking and health-related behaviours: interrelations in a Greek school-based sample. *Child Care Health Dev*. 2009; 35: 164–170.

39. Harrison PA, Narayan G. Differences in behaviour, psychological factors, and environmental factors associated with participation in school sports and other activities in adolescence. *J Sch Health*. 2003; 73: 113–120.
40. Holmen TL, Barrett-Connor E, Clausen J, Holmen J, and Bjermer L. (2002). Physical exercise, sports, and lung function in smoking versus nonsmoking adolescents. *Eur Respir J*, 19: 8–15.
41. Larson NI, Story M, Perry CL, Neumark-Sztainer D, Hannan PJ. Are diet and physical activity patterns related to cigarette smoking in adolescents? Findings from Project EAT. *Prev Chronic Dis*. 2007; 4: A51.
42. Lee KTH, Vandell DL. Out-of-School Time and Adolescent Substance Use. *J Adolesc Health*. 2015; 57: 523–529.
43. Martinsen M, Sundgot-Borgen J. Adolescent elite athletes' cigarette smoking, use of snus, and alcohol. *Scand J Med Sci Sports*. 2014; 24: 439–446.
44. Mattila VM, Raisamo S, Pihlajamaki H, Mantysaari M, Rimpela A. Sports activity and the use of cigarettes and snus among young males in Finland in 1999-2010. *BMC Public Health*. 2012; 12: 230.
45. Metzger A, Dawes N, Mermelstein R, Wakschlag L. Longitudinal modeling of adolescents' activity involvement, problem peer associations, and youth smoking. *J Appl Dev Psychol*. 2011; 32: 1–9.
46. Naylor AH, Gardner D, Zaichkowsky L. Drug use patterns among high school athletes and nonathletes. *Adolescence*. 2001; 36: 627–639.
47. Rainey CJ, McKeown RE, Sargent RG, Valois RF. Patterns of tobacco and alcohol use among sedentary, exercising, nonathletic, and athletic youth. *J Sch Health*. 1996; 66: 27–32.
48. Rodriguez D, Audrain-McGovern J. Team sport participation and smoking: analysis with general growth mixture modeling. *J Pediatr Psychol*. 2004; 29: 299–308.
49. Sekulic D, Ostojic M, Ostojic Z, Hajdarevic B, Ostojic L. Substance abuse prevalence and its relation to scholastic achievement and sport factors: an analysis among adolescents of the Herzegovina-Neretva Canton in Bosnia and Herzegovina. *BMC Pub Health*. 2012; 12: 274.
50. Oler MJ, Mainous AG, 3rd, Martin CA, *et al*. Depression, suicidal ideation, and substance use among adolescents. Are athletes at less risk? *Arch Fam Med*. 1994; 3: 781–785.
51. Garry JP, Morrissey SL. Team sports participation and risk-taking behaviours among a biracial middle school population. *Clin J Sport Med*. 2000; 10: 185–190.
52. Beebe LA, Vesely SK, Oman RF, Tolma E, Aspy CB, Rodine S. Protective assets for non-use of alcohol, tobacco and other drugs among urban American Indian youth in Oklahoma. *Matern Child Health J*. 2008; 12(Suppl 1): 82–90.
53. Buhrman HE. Athletics and Deviance: An examination of the relationship between athletic participation and deviant behaviour of high school girls. *Rev Sport Leisure*. 1977; 2: 17–35.
54. Davis TC, Arnold C, Nandy I, *et al*. Tobacco use among male high school athletes. *J Adolesc Health*. 1997; 21: 97–101.
55. Aaron DJ, Dearwater SR, Anderson R, Olsen T, Kriska AM, Laporte RE. Physical activity and the initiation of high-risk health behaviours in adolescents. *Med Sci Sports Exerc*. 1995; 27: 1639–1645.
56. Rolandsson M, Hugoson A. Factors associated with snuffing habits among ice-hockey-playing boys. *Swed Dent J*. 2001; 25: 145–154.
57. Walsh MM, Ellison J, Hilton JF, Chesney M, Ernster VL. Spit (smokeless) tobacco use by high school baseball athletes in California. *Tob Control*. 2000; 9(Suppl 2): 32–39.
58. Sussman S, Holt L, Dent CW, *et al*. Activity involvement, risk-taking, demographic variables, and other drug use: prediction of trying smokeless tobacco. *NCI Monogr*. 1989; 8: 57–62.
59. Dever BV, Schulenberg JE, Dworkin JB, O'Malley PM, Kloska DD, Bachman JG. Predicting risk-taking with and without substance use: the effects of parental monitoring, school bonding, and sports participation. *Prev Sci*. 2012; 13: 605–615.
60. Hoffmann JP. Extracurricular activities, athletic participation, and adolescent alcohol use: gender-differentiated and school-contextual effects. *J Health Soc Behav*. 2006; 47: 275–290.
61. Lisha NE, Crano WD, Delucchi KL. Participation in Team Sports and Alcohol and Marijuana Use Initiation Trajectories. *J Drug Issues*. 2014; 44: 83–93.
62. Mays D, Thompson NJ. Alcohol-related risk behaviours and sports participation among adolescents: an analysis of 2005 Youth Risk Behaviour Survey data. *J Adolesc Health*. 2009; 44: 87–89.
63. Mays D, Depadilla L, Thompson NJ, Kushner HI, Windle M. Sports participation and problem alcohol use: a multi-wave national sample of adolescents. *Am J Prev Med*. 2010; 38: 491–498.
64. Halldorsson V, Thorlindsson T, Sigfusdottir ID. Adolescent sport participation and alcohol use: The importance of sport organization and the wider social context. *Int Rev Sociol Sport*. 2014; 49: 311–330.
65. Geisner IM, Grossbard J, Tollison S, Larimer ME. Differences between athletes and non-athletes in risk and health behaviours in graduating high-school seniors. *J Child Adolesc Subst Abuse*. 2012; 21: 156–166.
66. Grossbard JR, Lee CM, Neighbors C, Hendershot CS, Larimer ME. Alcohol and risky sex in athletes and nonathletes: what roles do sex motives play? *J Stud Alcohol Drugs*. 2007; 68: 566–574.
67. Mays D, Thompson N, Kushner HI, Mays DF2nd, Farmer D, Windle M. Sports-specific factors, perceived peer drinking, and alcohol-related behaviours among adolescents participating in school-based sports in Southwest Georgia. *Addict Behav*. 2010; 35: 235–241.
68. Wetherill RR, Fromme K. Alcohol use, sexual activity, and perceived risk in high school athletes and non-athletes. *J Adolesc Health*. 2007; 41: 294–301.
69. Davies FM, Foxall GR. Involvement in sport and intention to consume alcohol: An exploratory study of UK adolescents. *J Appl Social Psychol*. 2011; 41: 2284–2311.
70. Cerkez I, Culjak Z, Zenic N, Sekulic D, Kondric M. Harmful alcohol drinking among adolescents: The influence of sport participation, religiosity, and parental factors. *J Child Adolesc Subst Abuse*. 2015; 24: 94–101.
71. Donato F, Assanelli D, Marconi M, Corsini C, Rosa G, Monarca S. Alcohol consumption among high school students and young athletes in north Italy. *Rev Epidemiol Sante Publique*. 1994; 42: 198–206.
72. Carr CN, Kennedy SR, Dimick KM. Alcohol use among high school athletes: A comparison of alcohol use and intoxication in male and female high school athletes and non-athletes. *J Alcohol Drug Educat*. 1990; 36: 39–43.
73. Thorlindsson T. Sport participation, smoking, and drug and alcohol use among Icelandic youth. *Soc Sport J*. 1989; 6: 136.
74. Forman ES, Dekker AH, Javors JR, Davison DT. High-risk behaviours in teenage male athletes. *Clin J Sport Med*. 1995; 5: 36–42.
75. Buckley WE, Yesalis CE, 3rd, Friedl KE, Anderson WA, Streit AL, Wright JE. Estimated prevalence of anabolic steroid use among male high school seniors. *JAMA*. 1988; 260: 3441–3445.
76. Dodge TL, Jaccard JJ. The effect of high school sports participation on the use of performance-enhancing substances in young adulthood. *J Adolesc Health*. 2006; 39: 367–373.
77. Elliot DL, Cheong J, Moe EL, Goldberg L. Cross-sectional study of female students reporting anabolic steroid use. *Arch Pediatr Adolesc Med*. 2007; 161: 572–577.
78. Thorlindsson T, Halldorsson V. Sport and use of anabolic androgenic steroids among Icelandic high school students: a critical test of three perspectives. *Subst Abuse Treat Prev Policy*. 2010; 5: doi 10.1186/1747-597x-5-32
79. DuRant RH, Escobedo LG, Heath GW. Anabolic-steroid use, strength training, and multiple drug use among adolescents in the United States. *Pediatrics*. 1995; 96: 23–28.
80. Miller KE, Hoffman JH, Barnes GM, Sabo D, Melnick MJ, Farrell MP. Adolescent anabolic steroid use, gender, physical activity, and other problem behaviours. *Subst Use Misuse*. 2005; 40: 1637–1657.
81. Scott DM, Wagner JC, Barlow TW. Anabolic steroid use among adolescents in Nebraska schools. *Am J Health Syst Pharm*. 1996; 53: 2068–2072.
82. Tanner SM, Miller DW, Alongi C. Anabolic steroid use by adolescents: prevalence, motives, and knowledge of risks. *Clin J Sport Med*. 1995; 5: 108–115.
83. vandenBerg P, Neumark-Sztainer D, Cafri G, Wall M. Steroid use among adolescents: longitudinal findings from Project EAT. *Pediatrics*. 2007; 119: 476–486.

84. Vertalino M, Eisenberg ME, Story M, Neumark-Sztainer D. Participation in weight-related sports is associated with higher use of unhealthful weight-control behaviours and steroid use. *J Am Diet Assoc*. 2007; 107: 434–440.
85. Windsor R, Dumitru D. Prevalence of anabolic steroid use by male and female adolescents. *Med Sci Sports Exerc*. 1989; 21: 494–497.
86. Lorang M, Callahan B, Cummins KM, Achar S, Brown SA. Anabolic androgenic steroid use in teens: Prevalence, demographics, and perception of effects. *J Child Adolesc Subst Abuse*. 2011; 20: 358–369.
87. Croll JK, Neumark-Sztainer D, Story M, Wall M, Perry C, Harnack L. Adolescents involved in weight-related and power team sports have better eating patterns and nutrient intakes than non-sport-involved adolescents. *J Am Diet Assoc*. 2006; 106: 709–717.
88. Ponton LE. A review of eating disorders in adolescents. *Adolesc Psychiatry*. 1995; 20: 267–285.
89. Thiel A, Gottfried H, Hesse FW. Subclinical eating disorders in male athletes. A study of the low weight category in rowers and wrestlers. *Acta Psychiatr Scand*. 1993; 88: 259–265.
90. Crissey SR, Honea JC. The relationship between athletic participation and perceptions of body size and weight control in adolescent girls: The role of sport type. *Soc Sport J*. 2006; 23: 248–272.
91. Middleman AB, Vazquez I, Durant RH. Eating patterns, physical activity, and attempts to change weight among adolescents. *J Adolesc Health*. 1998; 22: 37–42.
92. de Bruin AP, Woertman L, Bakker FC, Oudejans RRD. Weight-related sport motives and girls' body image, weight control behaviours, and self-esteem. *Sex Roles*. 2009; 60: 628–641.
93. Fortes LdS, Kakeshita IS, Almeida SS, Gomes AR, Ferreira MEC. Eating behaviours in youths: A comparison between female and male athletes and non-athletes. *Scand J Med Sci Sports*. 2014; 24: e62–e68.
94. Herbrich L, Pfeiffer E, Lehmkuhl U, Schneider N. Anorexia athletica in pre-professional ballet dancers. *J Sports Sci*. 2011; 29: 1115–1123.
95. Krentz EM, Warschburger P. Sports-related correlates of disordered eating in aesthetic sports. *Psychol Sport Exerc*. 2011; 12: 375–382.
96. Maïano C, Morin AJS, Lanfranchi MC, Therme P. Body-related sport and exercise motives and disturbed eating attitudes and behaviours in adolescents. *Eur Eating Disorders Rev*. 2015; 23: 277–286.
97. Martinsen M, Sundgot-Borgen J. Higher prevalence of eating disorders among adolescent elite athletes than controls. *Med Sci Sports Exerc*. 2013; 45: 1188–1197.
98. Taub DE, Blinde EM. Eating disorders among adolescent female athletes: influence of athletic participation and sport team membership. *Adolescence*. 1992; 27: 833–848.
99. Gomes R, Goncalves S, Costa J. Exercise, eating disordered behaviours and psychological well-being: a study with Portuguese adolescents. *Revista Latinoamericana De Psicologia*. 2015; 47: 66–74.
100. Rosendahl J, Bormann B, Aschenbrenner K, Aschenbrenner F, Strauss B. Dieting and disordered eating in German high school athletes and non-athletes. *Scand J Med Sci Sports*. 2009; 19: 731–739.
101. Monthuy-Blanc J, Maiano C, Therme P. Prevalence of eating disorders symptoms in nonelite ballet dancers and basketball players: An exploratory and controlled study among French adolescent girls. *Rev Epidemiol Sante Publique*. 2010; 58: 415–424.
102. Miller KE, Barnes GM, Melnick MJ, Sabo DF, Farrell MP. Gender and racial/ethnic differences in predicting adolescent sexual risk: athletic participation versus exercise. *J Health Soc Behav*. 2002; 43: 436–450.
103. Miller KE, Sabo DF, Farrell MP, Barnes GM, Melnick MJ. Athletic participation and sexual behaviour in adolescents: the different worlds of boys and girls. *J Health Soc Behav*. 1998; 39: 108–123.
104. Miller KE, Farrell MP, Barnes GM, Melnick MJ, Sabo D. Gender/racial differences in jock identity, dating, and adolescent sexual risk. *J Youth Adolesc*. 2005; 34: 123–136.
105. Sabo DF, Miller KE, Farrell MP, Melnick MJ, Barnes GM. High school athletic participation, sexual behaviour and adolescent pregnancy: a regional study. *J Adolesc Health*. 1999; 25: 207–216.
106. Habel MA, Dittus PJ, De Rosa CJ, Chung EQ, Kerndt PR. Daily participation in sports and students' sexual activity. *Perspect Sex Reprod Health*. 2010; 42: 244–250.
107. Smith EA, Caldwell LL. Participation in high-school sports and adolescent sexual activity. *Pediatr Exerc Sci*. 1994; 6: 69–74.
108. Kreager DA. Unnecessary roughness? School sports, peer networks, and male adolescent violence. *Am SocRev*. 2007; 72: 705–724.
109. Jiang X, Peterson RD. Beyond participation: the association between school extracurricular activities and involvement in violence across generations of immigration. *J Youth Adolesc*. 2012; 41: 362–378.
110. Endresen IM, Olweus D. Participation in power sports and antisocial involvement in preadolescent and adolescent boys. *J Child Psychol Psychiatry*. 2005; 46: 468–478.
111. Fite PJ, Vitulano M. Proactive and Reactive Aggression and Physical Activity. *J Psychopath Behav Assess*. 2011; 33: 11–18.
112. Linville DC, Huebner AJ. The analysis of extracurricular activities and their relationship to youth violence. *J Youth Adolesc*. 2005; 34: 483–492.
113. Levin DS, Smith EA, Caldwell LL, Kimbrough J. Violence and high school sports participation. *Pediatr Exerc Sci*. 1995; 7: 379–388.
114. Burton JM, Marshall LA. Protective factors for youth considered at risk of criminal behaviour: does participation in extracurricular activities help? *Crim Behav Ment Health*. 2005; 15: 46–64.
115. Miller KE, Melnick MJ, Farrell MP, Sabo DF, Barnes GM. Jocks, gender, binge drinking, and adolescent violence. *J Interpers Violence*. 2006; 21: 105–120.
116. Gardner M, Roth J, Brooks-Gunn J. Sports participation and juvenile delinquency: the role of the peer context among adolescent boys and girls with varied histories of problem behaviour. *Dev Psychol*. 2009; 45: 341–353.
117. Aarnio M, Kujala UM, Kaprio J. Associations of health-related behaviours, school type and health status to physical activity patterns in 16-year-old boys and girls. *Scand J Soc Med*. 1997; 25: 156–167.
118. Aarnio M, Winter T, Kujala U, Kaprio J. Associations of health related behaviour, social relationships, and health status with persistent physical activity and inactivity: a study of Finnish adolescent twins. *Br J Sports Med*. 2002; 36: 360–364.
119. Ali MM, Amialchuk A, Heller LR. The influence of physical activity on cigarette smoking among adolescents: evidence from Add Health. *Nicotine Tob Res*. 2015; 17: 539–545.
120. Charilaou M, Karekla M, Constantinou M, Price S. Relationship between physical activity and type of smoking behaviour among adolescents and young adults in Cyprus. *Nicotine Tob Res*. 2009; 11: 969–976.
121. Pate RR, Heath GW, Dowda M, Trost SG. Associations between physical activity and other health behaviours in a representative sample of US adolescents. *Am J Public Health*. 1996; 86: 1577–1581.
122. Raitakari OT, Porkka KV, Taimela S, Telama R, Rasanen L, Viikari JS. Effects of persistent physical activity and inactivity on coronary risk factors in children and young adults. The Cardiovascular Risk in Young Finns Study. *Am J Epidemiol*. 1994; 140: 195–205.
123. Peltzer K. Leisure time physical activity and sedentary behaviour and substance use among in-school adolescents in eight African countries. *Int J Behav Med*. 2010; 17: 271–278.
124. Vuori MT, Kannas LK, Villberg J, Ojala SA, Tynjala JA, Valimaa RS. Is physical activity associated with low-risk health behaviours among 15-year-old adolescents in Finland? *Scand J Public Health*. 2012; 40: 61–68.
125. Audrain-McGovern J, Rodriguez D. All physical activity may not be associated with a lower likelihood of adolescent smoking uptake. *Addict Behav*. 2015; 51: 177–183.
126. Audrain-McGovern J, Rodriguez D, Rodgers K, Cuevas J, Sass J. Longitudinal variation in adolescent physical activity patterns and the emergence of tobacco use. *J Pediatr Psychol*. 2012; 37: 622–633.
127. Coulson NS, Eiser C, Eiser JR. Diet, smoking and exercise: interrelationships between adolescent health behaviours. *Child Care Health Dev*. 1997; 23: 207–216.
128. Easton A, Kiss E. Covariates of current cigarette smoking among secondary school students in Budapest, Hungary, 1999. *Health Educ Res*. 2005; 20: 92–100.

129. García PLR, Villalba FJL, Miñarro PAL, Cantó EG. Physical exercise, energy expenditure and tobacco consumption in adolescents from Murcia (Spain). *Archivos Argentinos de Pediatria*. 2014; 12: 12–18 + e12–e18.
130. Kirkcaldy BD, Shephard RJ, Siefen RG. The relationship between physical activity and self-image and problem behaviour among adolescents. *Soc Psychiatry Psychiatr Epidemiol*. 2002; 37: 544–550.
131. Kovacs E, Piko BF, Keresztes N. The interacting role of physical activity and diet control in Hungarian adolescents' substance use and psychological health. *Subst Use Misuse*. 2014; 49: 1278–1286.
132. Leatherdale ST, Wong SL, Manske SR, Colditz GA. Susceptibility to smoking and its association with physical activity, BMI, and weight concerns among youth. *Nicotine Tob Res*. 2008; 10: 499–505.
133. Moreno-Murcia JA, Hellin P, Gonzalez-Cutre D, Martinez-Galindo C. Influence of perceived sport competence and body attractiveness on physical activity and other healthy lifestyle habits in adolescents. *Span J Psychol*. 2011; 14: 282–292.
134. Winnail SD, Valois RF, McKeown RE, Saunders RP, Pate RR. Relationship between physical activity level and cigarette, smokeless tobacco, and marijuana use among public high school adolescents. *J Sch Health*. 1995; 65: 438–442.
135. Tao FB, Xu ML, Kim SD, Sun Y, Su PY, Huang K. Physical activity might not be the protective factor for health risk behaviours and psychopathological symptoms in adolescents. *J Paediatr Child Health*. 2007; 43: 762–767.
136. Cohen B, Evers S, Manske S, Bercovitz K, Edward HG. Smoking, physical activity and breakfast consumption among secondary school students in a southwestern Ontario community. *Can J Public Health*. 2003; 94: 41–44.
137. D'Elio MA, Mundt DJ, Bush PJ, Iannotti RJ. Healthful behaviours: do they protect African-American, urban preadolescents from abusable substance use? *Am J Health Promot*. 1993; 7: 354–363.
138. Paavola M, Vartiainen E, Haukkala A. Smoking, alcohol use, and physical activity: a 13-year longitudinal study ranging from adolescence into adulthood. *J Adolesc Health*. 2004; 35: 238–244.
139. Valois RF, Dowda M, Trost S, Weinrich M, Felton G, Pate RR. Cigarette smoking experimentation among rural fifth grade students. *Am J Health Behav*. 22: 101–7.
140. Karvonen JS, Rimpelä AH, Rimpelä M. Do sports clubs promote snuff use? Trends among Finnish boys between 1981 and 1991. *Health Educ Res*. 1995; 10: 147–154.
141. Korhonen T, Kujala UM, Rose RJ, Kaprio J. Physical activity in adolescence as a predictor of alcohol and illicit drug use in early adulthood: a longitudinal population-based twin study. *Twin Res Hum Genet*. 2009; 12: 261–268.
142. Faulkner RA, Slattery CM. The relationship of physical activity to alcohol consumption in youth, 15–16 years of age. *Can J Public Health*. 1990; 81: 168–169.
143. Robinson TN, Killen JD, Taylor CB, *et al*. Perspectives on adolescent substance use. A defined population study. *JAMA*. 1987; 258: 2072–2076.
144. Kokkevi A, Fotiou A, Chileva A, Nociar A, Miller P. Daily exercise and anabolic steroids use in adolescents: a cross-national European study. *Subst Use Misuse*. 2008; 43: 2053–2065.
145. Lowry R, Michael S, Demissie Z, Kann L, Galuska DA. Associations of physical activity and sedentary behaviours with dietary behaviours among US high school students *J Obes*. 2015: doi 10.1155/2015/876524
146. Al-Hazzaa HM, Al-Sobayel HI, Abahussain NA, Qahwaji DM, Alahmadi MA, Musaiger AO. Association of dietary habits with levels of physical activity and screen time among adolescents living in Saudi Arabia. *J Hum Nutr Diet*. 2014; 27(Suppl 2): 204–213.
147. Durksen A, Downs S, Mollard R, Forbes L, Ball GD, McGavock J. The association between time spent in vigorous physical activity and dietary patterns in adolescents: a cross-sectional study. *J Phys Act Health*. 2015; 12: 208–215.
148. French SA, Perry CL, Leon GR, Fulkerson JA. Food preferences, eating patterns, and physical activity among adolescents: correlates of eating disorders symptoms. *J Adolesc Health*. 1994; 15: 286–294.
149. Rosenberg DE, Norman GJ, Sallis JF, Calfas KJ, Patrick K. Covariation of adolescent physical activity and dietary behaviours over 12 months. *J Adolesc Health*. 2007; 41: 472–478.
150. Vissers PA, Jones AP, van Sluijs EM, *et al*. Association between diet and physical activity and sedentary behaviours in 9–10-year-old British White children. *Pub Health*. 2013; 127: 231–240.
151. Laska MN, Pasch KE, Lust K, Story M, Ehlinger E. Latent class analysis of lifestyle characteristics and health risk behaviours among college youth. *Prev Sci*. 2009; 10: 376–386.
152. Demissie Z, Lowry R, Eaton DK, Hertz MF, Lee SM. Associations of school violence with physical activity among U.S. high school students. *J Phys Act Health*. 2014; 11: 705–711.

CHAPTER 20

Genetics of physical activity and physical fitness

Nienke M Schutte, Meike Bartels, and Eco JC de Geus

Introduction

Individual differences

Regular physical activity (PA) and physical fitness are key contributors to children's health.[1] In addition, lower levels of physical fitness measured in childhood and adolescence are associated with cardiovascular risk factors such as hypercholesterolaemia or hypertension in adulthood.[2,3] Despite this, the majority of youth do not engage in regular PA at the recommended level.[4,5] Traditionally, the individual differences in physically active lifestyles of children and adolescents have been explained by environmental and social factors, such as low socioeconomic status (of the parents), health beliefs, and support by peers and family.[6–9] However, as is the case for many human (behavioural) traits,[10] another major source of variation in PA is innate biological differences.

The contribution of genes to the differences in PA has been under study for many decades, since the first heritability study by Kaprio *et al.*[11] was published in 1981 on a large sample of adult male twins. Twin and family studies provide the ability to calculate the relative importance of genetic and environmental factors to the observed individual differences. Evidence of familial aggregation of a behavioural trait can be found when this specific trait occurs more often in members of a family than can be readily accounted for by chance. A twin design exploits the known differences in genetic similarity in monozygotic and dizygotic twins (or siblings) to separate genetic effects (the heritability) from other factors that are shared by family members (e.g. family or school environment).

Studying the heritable components of a trait like PA is referred to as quantitative genetics. Whereas these family and twin studies provide a starting point in exploring the effects of genetic and environmental factors on a phenotype, molecular genetic studies aim to detect the genes underlying the heritability. Studies in animals are used to identify the genetic mechanisms underlying PA by means of selective breeding and (fine) mapping of genomic regions. Progress in molecular genetics makes it feasible to collect and analyse human DNA on a large scale.

A major determinant of a physically active lifestyle may be physical fitness.[12,13] Especially in late childhood and adolescence, the trainability of an individual may play a key role in the maintenance of PA behaviour as people may gravitate towards leisure time activities that they are good at. Performing better in physical activities or exercise than others, or achieving gains in performance more rapidly when exposed to comparable training regimes, will lead to feelings of competence. Vice versa, lower levels of trainability or gains in performance might lead to disappointment. Of note, indicators of physical fitness that are responsive to PA and exercise, such as cardiorespiratory fitness, muscle strength, and motor control, are heritable traits themselves.

This chapter briefly introduces the principles of family, twin, animal, and molecular genetic studies, followed by an overview of published studies on the quantitative genetics and molecular genetic findings for PA, exercise behaviour, and physical fitness.

The principles of family, twin, animal, and molecular genetic studies

Family studies

Familial aggregation is seen when the occurrence of the trait among relatives is substantially higher than that among non-relatives.[14] For quantitative traits (i.e. continuous traits: the trait has a quantitative value), such as the amount of PA, familial aggregation can be investigated by computing correlations among relatives such as siblings, parents and their offspring, grandparents and grandchildren, nieces, etc., depending on the extent of the pedigrees from which data are available. Most family studies report sibling and parent-offspring correlations. Siblings among each other, and parents and their offspring, share on average half of their genes. They also share a household, the neighbourhood, and various other aspects of belonging to the same family (the so-called shared environment). Therefore, evidence of familial aggregation may be due to shared exposure to a risk factor, due to genetic factors, or result from a mixture of both. Thus, this familial resemblance includes both genetic and shared environmental sources of covariance. If the effect of shared environment can be assumed zero, the familial resemblance in the trait can be ascribed to genetic factors and can be used to estimate its heritability. When familial environmental factors influence the trait of interest as well, familial resemblance only provides us with an indication of the upper value of the traits' heritability.

Twin studies

A more powerful design to disentangle the relative importance of environmental and genetic influences on a trait or behaviour is the classical twin design. This design compares the intra-pair resemblance between two types of sibling relationships; genetically identical twins or monozygotic (MZ) twins, a result of division of

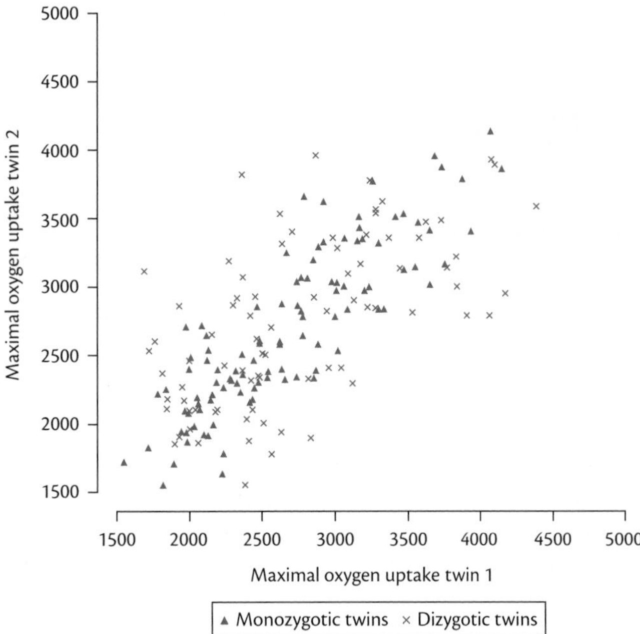

Figure 20.1 Intrapair resemblance in pairs of MZ and DZ twins for maximal oxygen uptake (mL·min^{-1}).

a single fertilized egg during an early stage in embryonic development, and non-identical twins or dizygotic (DZ) twins, resulting from two separate fertilized eggs. Consequently, MZ twins are genetically identical and the difference between the twins is due to person-specific environmental factors: i.e. experiences that one of the twins has and the co-twin does not. Dizygotic twins share on average 50% of their genetic make-up. If MZ-resemblance for the trait of interest is higher than DZ-resemblance, this constitutes evidence for genetic influences (referred to as 'A') on the trait. Figure 20.1 shows a scatterplot of the cardiorespiratory fitness of MZ and DZ twins in which the scores of Twin 1 are plotted against his/her co-twin (Twin 2). This figure shows clearly that MZ twins (triangles) resemble each other more than DZ twins.

Twin studies decompose all phenotypic variance of the trait of interest in sources of genetic influences (A), shared environmental influences (influences shared with other family members e.g. upbringing; referred to as 'C') and person-specific influences (influences that are unique to the individual; referred to as 'E'). An important assumption is that the shared environmental effects are independent of zygosity (and thus equal for both MZ and DZ twins). Thus, the correlation between MZ twins (r_{MZ}) comprises A + C, whereas the DZ twin correlation (r_{DZ}) is an estimate of ½A + C. Following from this, a simple formula by Falconer[15] computes the relative contribution of genetic influences (A) to the total variance, as twice the difference in MZ/DZ resemblance:

$$\text{heritability} = 2(r_{MZ} - r_{DZ})$$

An alternative to this simple formula is the use of structural equation modelling to obtain a more precise estimate of heritability. In contrast to familial aggregation studies that cannot separate genetic and familial environmental sources of covariance, the classic twin design can separate how much of the variance in a trait is due to genetic effects (the heritability; A) and how much appears to be due to shared environmental effects (the shared environment; C).

Animal studies

Artificial selection practices in animals have long provided proof of genetic influences on phenotypes. For example, farmers started to selectively interbreed cattle that produce the most milk to increase production in offspring generations. The increased milk production in the offspring provides evidence of this trait being influenced by genetic factors and can be used to estimate its heritability. With regard to PA, Swallow *et al.*[16] used selective breeding to create four lines of mice with high activity levels: ten generations of selective breeding of voluntary wheel-running behaviour resulted in an increase of approximately 75% in activity level compared with mice from control lines. Mice from the four selected lines ran significantly more than mice from the control lines after ten generations.[16]

Another way to show heritability of a trait is measuring this trait in different strains of inbred mice, growing up in identical environments. Systematically mating brothers and sisters for 20 consecutive generations results in isogenic (genetically identical strains) groups of mice, allowing the mean of the trait to be compared across different strains. With regard to daily wheel running, Lightfoot *et al.*[17] detected significant inter-strain differences in 13 strains of inbred mice, which suggests that genetic background indeed plays a role in determining spontaneous daily wheel running activity in mouse strains.

Molecular genetic studies

After establishing heritability of a trait, the next step is to identify the genomic regions that contribute to the heritable trait variation. For quantitative traits it is likely that heritability reflects the additive effects of thousands of genetic variants in a manifold of different genes. Molecular genetic studies, such as linkage analysis and association studies, provide an opportunity to localize genetic variants and confirm their association with the trait of interest.

Linkage analysis examines whether specific genetic markers, positioned strategically across the entire genome segregate jointly with traits in clusters of related individuals. The markers that are linked to the genomic region that influences the trait will be seen to segregate more frequently with the occurrence of this trait. The genomic region carrying such markers is likely to harbour causative genetic variants for the trait. Genetic linkage can easily be demonstrated in breeding experiments in mice, when two mice that differ genetically for a trait of interest are crossed (parental line) and the segregation of genetic markers can be followed in each of the offspring, along with phenotypic characteristics.

Genes (in genomic regions) of interest found in these animal studies can provide the first clues for conducting association studies in both animals and humans. Alternatively, candidate genes can be selected, based on known or inferred biological function that make it plausible that they may predispose to the trait of interest. Association studies are similar to traditional epidemiological approaches in which an a priori hypothesis between exposure to a given factor, in this case, a genotype at a given locus, and trait is formulated: candidate gene studies test the association of quantitative traits with the frequency of specific genetic variants in low-scoring and high-scoring individuals on a quantitative trait.

Quantitative genetics of physical activity and exercise behaviour

Since the first twin study[11] on the heritability of PA, several studies provided evidence for genetic influences on PA. A number of studies measured total PA objectively with accelerometers, in a respiration chamber, or with the doubly labelled water method. However, most twin and family studies used PA questionnaires (self-report) to quantify total PA. Surveys are a more convenient tool for epidemiological-scaled research, even though the correlation with accelerometry or doubly labelled water varies to a great extent.[18] The phenotypes used in these survey studies often captured rather different constructs: some measured sport participation specifically, with a questionnaire that included items such as: 'Do you participate in (moderate to vigorous) sports regularly?' Others questionnaires used an activity record, in which subjects were asked to note the energy expenditure of the dominant activity every 15 min using a list of categorized activities.

When discussing twin and family studies of PA, a distinction will be made between PA due to all possible sources (i.e. total PA) and PA due to sports participation in leisure time (i.e. voluntary exercise behaviour). However, this distinction is not always clear. A large part of total PA is classified as light-intensity PA and will be due to transportation (walking, cycling, standing), light work, or household activities. Moderate- to vigorous-intensity physical activities (MVPA) are more ambiguous and may often include voluntary sports activities in leisure time. Therefore, studies reporting MVPA will be discussed together with studies on voluntary exercise behaviour.

All twin and family studies on the heritability of total PA in childhood or adolescent samples are summarized in Table 20.1, ranked by age. All twin and family studies on the heritability of MVPA or voluntary exercise behaviour are summarized in Table 20.2.

Total physical activity

The heritability estimates found in 11 family studies include both genetic and familial environmental sources of variance, and are therefore listed in a separate column in Table 20.1.

Especially in younger children (up until the age of 11 years), accelerometers or doubly labelled water were used to quantify PA.[19–24] The family studies by Cai *et al.*[20] and Butte *et al.*[19] were largest in sample size and reported moderate to high estimates of familial aggregation. In addition, Saudino and Zapfe[23] showed that 31% of the variation in total PA in 2-year-old twins could be explained by genetic factors. The twin studies by Franks *et al.*[22] and Fisher *et al.*[21] did not report significant genetic factors. This may be because the sample size was modest, and the study could have been underpowered to find small genetic influences. Indeed, the MZ correlations in the study by Fisher *et al.*[21] were slightly higher than DZ correlations. A more robust finding is the substantial part (35–73%) of the variance in PA in these twins that could be attributed to shared environmental factors.

Five studies reported heritability estimates of PA measured by surveys.[25–29] The mean age in these studies was 13–17 years, indicating that self-report of PA is feasible in adolescence. The heritability estimates range from 6% for work-related PA[29] to 63% for leisure time PA.[26]

Table 20.1 Heritability of physical activity behaviour: an overview of twin and family studies

Children's age (y) Mean (±SD)		Reference	Sample	Instrument	Phenotype	Familial aggregation	A	C
2	(±.1)	Saudino and Zapfe[23]	144 MZ pairs/168 DZ pairs	Accelerometer	TPA		31%	55%
7	(±1)	Franks *et al.*[22]	62 MZ pairs/38 DZ pairs	Doubly labeled water	PAEE[ab]		41%	35%
				Doubly labeled water	PAEE[abc]		0%	69%
				Doubly labeled water	PAL[ab]		0%	65%
8	(±.4)	Wood *et al.*[24]	150 MZ pairs/113 DZ pairs	Accelerometer	TPA		35%	40%
11	(±.2)	Butte *et al.*[19]	319 families	Accelerometer	TPA[ab]	60%		
11	(±4)	Cai *et al.*[20]	319 families	Accelerometer	TPA[ab]	55%		
					LPA[ab]	46%		
					MPA[ab]	49%		
11	(±1)	Fisher *et al.*[21]	57 MZ pairs/60 DZ pairs	Accelerometer	TPA		0%	73%
13	(±4)	de Chaves *et al.*[25]	260 families	Baecke questionnaire	TPA[abd]	24%		
14	(±3)	Perusse *et al.*[27]	375 families; 55 MZ pairs/ 56 DZ pairs	3-day activity record	TPA[abd]		29%	0%
14	(±3)	Santos *et al.*[28]	339 families	Baecke questionnaire	TPA[ab]	23%		
16	(±4)	Seabra *et al.*[29]	2375 families	Baecke questionnaire	TPA[abd]	23%		
					WPA[abd]	6%		
					LTPA[abd]	25%		
17	(±6)	Maia *et al.*[26]	203 MZ pairs/208 DZ pairs	Baecke questionnaire	LTPA		63%/32%[e]	0%/38%[e]

A = variance explained by genetic factors; C = variance explained by shared environmental factors; TPA = Total Physical Activity; PAEE = Physical Activity Energy Expenditure; PAL = Physical Activity Level; LPA = Low Physical Activity; MPA = Moderate Physical Activity; WPA = Work Physical Activity; LTPA = Leisure Time Physical Activity.
[a] Adjusted for age; [b] Adjusted for sex; [c] Adjusted for body weight; [d] Adjusted for SES; [e] boys/girls.

Table 20.2 Heritability of exercise behaviour: an overview of twin and family studies

Children's age (y) Mean (±SD)		Reference	Sample	Instrument	Phenotype	Familial aggregation	A	C
7	(±0.3)	Huppertz *et al.*[30]	648 MZ pairs/1320 DZ pairs	Multiple survey items	EB		24%/22%[d]	71%/22%[d]
10	(±0.3)	Huppertz *et al.*[30]	620 MZ pairs/1141 DZ pairs	Multiple survey items	EB		66%/16%[d]	25%/72%[d]
11	(±4)	Cai *et al.*[20]	319 families	Accelerometer	VPA[ab]	18%		
11	(±1)	Fisher *et al.*[21]	57 MZ pairs/60 DZ pairs	Accelerometer	MVPA[ab]		0%	61%
12	(±0.4)	Huppertz *et al.*[30]	1540 MZ pairs/2746 DZ pairs	Multiple survey items	EB		38%/36%[d]	50%/50%[d]
12	(±1)	White *et al.*[31]	72 MZ pairs/76 DZ pairs	3-day activity record	MVPA		0%/0%[d]	66%/33%[d]
13/14		Stubbe *et al.*[32]	276 MZ pairs/370 DZ pairs	Multiple survey items	EB		0%	84%
14	(±3)	Perusse *et al.*[27]	375 families; 55 MZ pairs/ 56 DZ pairs	3-day activity record	MVPA[abc]		0%	12%
14	(±0.3)	van der Aa *et al.*[86]	554 MZ pairs/948 DZ pairs	Multiple survey items	EB		85%/38%[d]	0%/46%[d]
15		Beunen & Thomis[87]	43 MZ pairs/61 DZ pairs	Single survey item	EB		83%/44%	0%/54%[d]
15/16		Stubbe *et al.*[32]	321 MZ pairs/442 DZ pairs	Multiple survey items	EB		0%	78%
16	(±0.6)	van der Aa *et al.*[86]	662 MZ pairs/969 DZ pairs	Multiple survey items	EB		80%	0%
16	(±1)	de Moor *et al.*[34]	1736 families; 656 MZ pairs/1628 DZ pairs	Multiple survey items	EB		42%/36%[d]	44%/52%[d]
16	(±0.1)	Aaltonen *et al.*[88]	769 MZ pairs/1743 DZ pairs	Single survey item	EB		52%/52%[d]	19%/24%[d]
16	(±4)	Seabra *et al.*[89]	2375 families	Baecke questionnaire	EB[abc]	19%		
16	(±4)	Seabra *et al.*[29]	2375 families	Baecke questionnaire	EB[abc]	50–60%		
17	(±2)	Boomsma *et al.*[90]	44 MZ pairs/46 DZ pairs	Single survey item	EB		64%	0%
17	(±6)	Maia *et al.*[26]	203 MZ pairs/208 DZ pairs	Baecke questionnaire	EB		68%/40%[d]	20%/28%[d]
17	(±2)	de Geus *et al.*[33]	69 MZ pairs/88 DZ pairs	Multiple survey items	MVPA[a]		79%	0%
17	(±0.1)	Aaltonen *et al.*[88]	724 MZ pairs/1614 DZ pairs	Single survey item	EB		44%/50%[d]	24%/26%[d]
17/18		Stubbe *et al.*[32]	248 MZ pairs/395 DZ pairs	Multiple survey items	EB		36%	47%
18	(±2)	Koopmans *et al.*[91]	1593 families: 578 MZ pairs/1000 DZ pairs	Single survey item	EB		45%	44%
18	(±0.7)	van der Aa *et al.*[86]	488 MZ pairs/747 DZ pairs	Multiple survey items	EB		72%	0%

A = variance explained by genetic factors; C = variance explained by shared environmental factors; EB = Voluntary Exercise Behaviour; VPA = Vigorous Physical Activity; MVPA = Moderate to Vigorous Physical Activity.
[a] Adjusted for age; [b] Adjusted for sex; [c] Adjusted for SES; [d] boys/girls.

Voluntary exercise behaviour

Sixteen twin and/or family studies reported heritability estimates for voluntary exercise behaviour or MVPA. Heritability estimates vary widely, ranging from 0–85%. Possible sources of this variation are differences in the age, differences in measurement instrument, and sample size. The age of all studies shown in Table 20.2 ranges from four[19,20] to 25 years.[26] Up to 12 years of age, heritability estimates are low to moderate.[21,30,31] In adolescence, heritability estimates of voluntary exercise behaviour are moderate to high, with the exception of two studies in which heritability estimates are low or zero.[32] Nevertheless, the importance of shared environmental factors seems to decrease in adolescence, whereas genetic effects become more prominent in explaining individual differences in voluntary exercise behaviour. In adults, heritability of voluntary exercise behaviour levels off to ~40%.[33,34] The changing genetic architecture of voluntary exercise behaviour across the life span has been described before.[32,35] The notion that shared environmental factors play a greater role in childhood than adolescence can be explained by the important role of parents. They provide children with the opportunity to become active by providing transportation to exercise activities, giving exercise activities priority over other leisure time activities, and offering motivation and encouragement to exercise.

Two studies employed accelerometers (i.e. Actiwatch or Actigraph) to quantify MVPA in children (~11-year-olds).[20,21] The heritability estimates were low, but Fisher *et al.*[21] demonstrated significant influences of shared environmental factors (61%). Two studies used prospective 3-day activity recording, which may be more accurate then retrospective surveys, and reported heritability estimates of 0%.[27,31] However, the majority of the studies specifically measured voluntary exercise behaviour by starting their surveys with questions similar to 'Do you participate in sports regularly?' These studies generally found evidence of significant genetic influences. Finally, by comparing the heritability estimates of voluntary exercise behaviour (Table 20.2) with the estimates for total PA (Table 20.1), we can conclude that the part of the variation in adolescents that can be attributed to genes appears higher in voluntary exercise behaviour compared to total PA. It is important to note that such a finding could be driven in part by higher measurement error in self-reported total PA than in self-reported voluntary exercise behaviour. Conscious planning of exercise activities is easier to recall than how much energy is spent on activities at school or commuting. This might introduce more measurement error in self-reported total PA surveys, which will inflate the unique environmental contribution to the variance in this trait. Consequently, the relative genetic contribution to the total variance decreases, i.e. the heritability.

Molecular genetic findings for physical activity and exercise behaviour

Studies with spontaneous wheel-running inbred mice strains and selective breeding in mice for high voluntary wheel-running activity resulted in numerous genomic regions that were associated with PA in mice. For instance, Lightfoot *et al.*[36] identified four genomic regions that were associated with the distance, duration, and speed of voluntary wheel-running on chromosomes 9 and 13, with the genomic locus for running speed (on chromosome 9) accounting for the largest percentage of phenotypic variance. The research group led by Garland found even more loci to be associated with these phenotypes,[37,38] but the only overlap they reported were loci close to the *TYR* gene on chromosome 7 coding for tyrosinase, a precursor for the neurotransmitter dopamine, found be involved in voluntary movement and reward.[39]

In spite of the evidence for a contribution of heritable factors to PA from twin and family studies, surprisingly little work has been done to identify the actual genes contributing to the heritability of PA and exercise behaviour in humans. Even fewer candidate gene studies have specifically addressed PA in children. Lorentzon *et al.*[40] found that in a sample of 97 healthy Caucasian girls (mean age 16.9 years) the A986S polymorphism in the calcium sensor receptor gene (*CASR*) was significantly associated with self-reported PA level. This *CASR* gene is involved in the regulation of calcium homeostasis and bone resorption. Calcium receptor gene mRNA is also expressed in the hypothalamus of the rat brain, a region that has been associated with regulating motivation. In 7-year-old boys, self-reported PA level was associated with the Gln223Arg polymorphism in the leptin receptor (*LEPR*) gene,[41] known to regulate food intake and energy balance.[42] Physical activity measured for 3 days with an Actiwatch accelerometer in 10-year-olds was associated with variants within the Melanocortin 4 Receptor Gene (*MC4R*),[43] a gene associated with weight-related phenotypes. Two studies in 15- and 16-year-old children did not find a significant association of a common variant in the *FTO* gene (rs9939609) and self-reported PA, as well as PA objectively measured with Actigraphs.[44,45]

Candidate genes suffer from the shortcoming that they are based on our current biological knowledge. A more agnostic and open study design to find genetic variants associated with a trait of interest is a genome wide association (GWA) study. Using millions of measured or imputed single nucleotide polymorphism (SNP) markers, the entire genome is searched for SNP variants that occur more frequently in people with higher levels of the trait of interest, compared to people with lower trait level. However, no GWA study in children has been conducted to date. The only GWA study conducted on exercise behaviour (in leisure time) published by de Moor *et al.*[46] was entirely based on an adult sample. In 1644 unrelated Dutch and 978 unrelated American adults of European ancestry several novel variants were associated with exercise behaviour, mainly in the *PAPSS2* gene. The effect sizes were small, such that these variants did not contribute much to the heritability of exercise behaviour and would not have reached significance according to current GWA standards.[47] In hindsight, lessons learned from GWA studies on other complex traits make it likely that this study on exercise behaviour was underpowered to detect the many small genetic effects causing heritability.[48] Meta-analyses across a total sample size of tens of thousands of individuals will be needed for successful detection of the association of specific genetic variants with a physically active lifestyle.

Quantitative genetics of physical fitness

Physical fitness can be defined as a set of components that influence exercise ability and performance in sports,[49] such as endurance capacity, muscle strength, and motor control. A good index of endurance capacity is maximal oxygen uptake ($\dot{V}O_2$ max), which is the highest rate of oxygen consumption during maximal intensity exercise performed until exhaustion.[50] Direct measurement of oxygen consumption during the climax of the maximal graded exercise test is the golden standard for measuring $\dot{V}O_2$ max. Maximal oxygen uptake measurement may not always be feasible in large-scale epidemiological studies as it requires time and laboratory equipment which might not be available in every clinical setting or gym. In addition, maximal exercise requires strenuous PA from the participant, which cannot be attained by or poses a health risk for some subgroups, e.g. overweight individuals or patients suffering from cardiovascular or respiratory disease. This might explain the limited number of twin and family studies on the heritability of $\dot{V}O_2$ max. Fortunately, physical fitness also entails static and explosive muscle strength, flexibility, speed, and coordination of limb movements, etc.[49] As these traits are fairly easy to measure, the number of publications on the heritability of these phenotypes is considerably higher. Herein we discuss twin and family studies on $\dot{V}O_2$ max, as well as the heritability studies on other fitness phenotypes.

Maximal oxygen uptake

Only four studies report an estimate of the heritability of $\dot{V}O_2$ max in children (Table 20.3). Two studies in 10-year-olds show heritability estimates of 85% for girls and 95% for a mixed sample.[51,52] The resemblance in male twins in the study by Maes *et al.*[52] could be explained by shared environmental influences. All four studies had rather small sample sizes and lacked power to discriminate between genetic and shared environmental influences. Two larger studies report heritability estimates in 15- and 17-year-olds and show estimates of 35–60%.[53,54] The study by Lortie *et al.*[53] submitted their subjects to a submaximal exercise protocol that halted

Table 20.3 Heritability of maximum oxygen uptake: an overview of twin and family studies

Children's age (y) Mean (±SD)		Reference	Sample	$\dot{V}O_2$ max test mode	A	C
10		Maes *et al.*[52]	43 MZ pairs/61 DZ pairs	Maximal exercise test on cycle ergometer	0%/85%	66%/0%
10	(±2)	Klissouras *et al.*[51]	15 MZ pairs/10 DZ pairs	Maximal exercise test on treadmill	93%	–[a]
15	(±3)	Lortie *et al.*[53]	223 sibling pairs/594 parent-offspring pairs	Submaximal exercise test on cycle ergometer	35–40%	–[a]
17	(±1)	Schutte *et al.*[54]	115 MZ pairs/105 DZ pairs	Maximal exercise test on cycle ergometer	55–60%	0%

A = variance explained by genetic factors; C = variance explained by shared environmental factors.
[a] Not estimated. $\dot{V}O_2$ max is maximal oxygen uptake.

at a predetermined point that was less than the maximal exercise capability of the individual, and used extrapolation of the heart rate (HR)/$\dot{V}O_2$ curve to the predicted HR max (220-age) to estimate VO_2 max. This might have introduced more error and an increase in environmental factors (E) and subsequently, reduced the heritability estimate. Two family studies were not included in Table 20.3, as they did not report an estimate of the heritability or familial aggregation. Montoye and Gayle[55] reported significant familial correlations for $\dot{V}O_2$ max in 70 brother pairs and 93 father-son pairs of 0.36 and 0.21 (age 10–69 years). In addition, in 39 sibling pairs and 96 parent-offspring pairs (mean age was 16 years in children and 43 years in parents) Lesage *et al.*[56] found these correlations to be 0.14 and 0.06. Altogether, these results point towards evidence of genetic effects on $\dot{V}O_2$ max, but the extent to which genes contribute to the variance seen in this phenotype is not clear. Inter-individual variation in growth and maturation might affect the heritability estimates of $\dot{V}O_2$ max.[57] A recent meta-analysis of studies in young adults (<30 years) found heritability estimates of 59% (in $mL \cdot min^{-1}$) and 72% (in $mL \cdot kg^{-1} \cdot min^{-1}$),[54] suggesting that $\dot{V}O_2$ max is a heritable trait at least when adulthood is reached. (The heritability of $\dot{V}O_2$ max is discussed further in Chapter 31.)

Other fitness phenotypes

Numerous tests exist for measuring physical fitness, so discussion is limited here to the fitness tests that are most used throughout the literature; i.e. the handgrip strength test, the vertical jump test, flexibility, and balance. The execution of these tests is more or less similar in most studies as they are all included in the Eurofit Physical Fitness Test Battery.[58] Table 20.4 summarizes all twin and family studies that report an estimate of the heritability of these fitness tasks. Although the heritability estimates range from 0–96%, the data in Table 20.4 suggest that a large part of the individual differences in these fitness tasks can be explained by genetic factors.

For vertical jump, seven studies, including one longitudinal study,[59] report heritability estimates in children. Although sample sizes are small for most studies, on average more than half of the variation in vertical jump performance can be explained by genetics. Whereas in all twin studies, the shared environmental factors could be fixed at zero, one exception reported a significant contribution of shared environmental influences to vertical jump performance in boys at age 16 years.[59] A meta-analysis of all twin studies found a weighted heritability estimate of 49% in children and young adults.[60]

Eight studies reported heritability estimates and familial aggregation of handgrip strength, ranging from 8 to 88%. The lowest estimates were reported by Szopa[61] with genetic factors stronger for boys (21–40%) than for girls (0–20%).[61] The contribution of shared environmental factors is 0% in all twin studies, except for the study by Isen *et al.*,[62] who found a small effect of shared environmental factors in girls (5%). However, despite the impressive sample size, this effect was not significant.

Flexibility is commonly measured with the sit-and-reach test. Five studies report on the heritability of flexibility, all providing moderate to high estimates of familial aggregation[63] and heritability,[52,60,64] except for the study by Chatterjee and Das.[65] The age range of the participants in this study was rather large (10–27 years) and the sample size very small. When correcting for age, the heritability estimate increased to 50%.[65]

Balance seems less heritable, with estimates ranging from 24–46%.[52,60,66,67] Balance is considered mainly a performance-related fitness component, whereas the other fitness phenotypes are regarded as health related.[49] These moderate heritability estimates and the absence of shared environmental factors suggest that most of the variance can be explained by person-specific environmental factors.

Molecular genetic findings for physical fitness

Every year since 2000, a review has been published with an update on the human gene map for performance and health-related phenotypes (the first review was by Rankinen *et al.*[68], and at the time of writing this chapter the last update was in 2015[69]). Although gene findings techniques are available and are subject to improvement every day, study outcomes in the field of exercise ability and sports performance are not easily obtainable, as they involve laboratory equipment, a significant amount of time (training studies), well-characterized cohorts, and, of course, willing subjects. Therefore, it is challenging to collect sufficient data to be well-powered for gene finding studies (which require large sample sizes) or to replicate earlier findings.

Two of the most studied polymorphisms in adults are the R577X variation in the *ACTN3* gene and the I/D polymorphism in the angiotensin-converting enzyme (*ACE*) gene.[70,71] This latter gene was one of the first genes to be associated with physical performance in humans.[72] Angiotensin-converting enzyme plays a role in the regulation of blood pressure and has been linked to exercise related phenotypes in human adults. The *ACTN3* gene seems to influence the performance of fast skeletal muscle fibres and *ACTN3* XX homozygotes may have modestly lower skeletal muscle strength in comparison with R-allele carriers.[73] Other candidate genes studied have focused on insulin-like growth factor-1 (IGF-I)

Table 20.4 Heritability of vertical jump, handgrip strength, flexibility and balance: an overview of twin and family studies

Phenotype	Age children: Range or Mean (±SD)		Reference	Sample	Familial aggregation	A	C
Vertical jump	3–10		Szopa[61]	347 families[a]	25%		–
	6–12		Malina & Mueller[92]	215 sibling pairs		22%	–[b]
	10	(±0.3)	Maes *et al.*[52]/Beunen *et al.*[59]	43 MZ pairs/61 DZ pairs		47%/78%[c]	0%
	11		Beunen *et al.*[59]	91–105 twin pairs		47%/79%[c]	0%
	12		Beunen *et al.*[59]	91–105 twin pairs		59%/92%[c]	0%
	13		Beunen *et al.*[59]	91–105 twin pairs		85%/77%[c]	0%
	14		Beunen *et al.*[59]	91–105 twin pairs		74%	0%
	11–17		Szopa[61]	347 families[a]	56%		–
	15		Beunen *et al.*[59]	91–105 twin pairs		63%/91%[c]	0%
	15		Chatterjee & Das[65]	30 MZ pairs/24 DZ pairs		71%	–[b]
	16		Beunen *et al.*[59]	91–105 twin pairs		0%/82%[c]	65%/0%[c]
	17	(±1.2)	Schutte *et al.*[60]	116 MZ pairs/111 DZ pairs		49%	0%
	18		Beunen *et al.*[59]	91–105 twin pairs		63%/78%[c]	0%
	11–25		Kovar[93]	17 MZ pairs/13 DZ pairs		83%–96%	–[b]
Handgrip strength	3–10		Szopa[61]	347 families[a]	8%–29%		–
	6–12		Malina & Mueller[92]	215 sibling pairs		44%–58%	–[b]
	12	(±0.4)	Isen *et al.*[62]	788 MZ pairs/466 DZ pairs		88%/79%[c]	0%/5%[c]
	12	(±5.5)	Katzmarzyk *et al.*[63]	205 families	48%		–
	10–15		Okuda *et al.*[64]	90 MZ pairs/68 DZ pairs		77%	0%
	9–17		Venerando & Milani–Comparetti[94]	24 MZ pairs/24 DZ pairs		32%–50%	–[b]
	11–17		Szopa[61]	347 families[a]	9%–14%		–
	17	(±1.2)	Schutte *et al.*[60]	116 MZ pairs/111 DZ pairs		59%	0%
	11–25		Kovar[93]	17 MZ pairs/13 DZ pairs		35%–63%	–[b]
Flexibility	10	(±0.3)	Maes *et al.*[52]	43 MZ pairs/61 DZ pairs		38%/50%[c]	0%
	12	(±5.5)	Katzmarzyk *et al.*[63]	205 families	64%		–
	10–15		Okuda *et al.*[64]	90 MZ pairs/68 DZ pairs		55%	0%
	16	(±4.5)	Chatterjee & Das[65]	30 MZ pairs/24 DZ pairs		18%	–[b]
	17	(±1.2)	Schutte *et al.*[60]	116 MZ pairs/111 DZ pairs		77%	0%
Balance	10	(±0.3)	Maes *et al.*[52]	43 MZ pairs/61 DZ pairs		46%	0%
	15	(±2.1)	Williams & Gross[67]	22 MZ pairs/41 DZ pairs		27%	–[b]
	14–18		Vandenberg[66]	40 MZ pairs/30 DZ pairs		24%	–[b]
	17	(±1.2)	Schutte *et al.*[60]	116 MZ pairs/111 DZ pairs		38%	0%

A = variance explained by genetic factors; C = variance explained by shared environmental factors.

[a] Of which 94 sons and 87 daughters in the 3–10 age group and 120 sons and 143 daughters in the 11–17 age group;

[b] Not estimated; [c] boys/girls. The study by Beunen *et al.*[59] is a longitudinal study.

and myostatin-related genes and genes involved in inflammatory factors. Unfortunately, studies in children are limited. Nevertheless, already in childhood, most indices of physical fitness are heritable traits. It is plausible that the same genetic variants that influence exercise ability and sport performance in adults also explain the heritability of these phenotypes in children. However, the increase of bone mass and muscular development during childhood and adolescents can point towards the influence of other more age-specific genetic variants during this period.

Genes and environment

Future exploration of the genetic mechanisms underlying PA, exercise ability, and physical fitness should more prominently model possible gene-environment interplay. The effect of an environmental exposure on an individual may depend on his or her genotype. Conversely, the effects of a specific genetic variant may be dependent on the environment. The effect of genetic variants can be amplified during or after being exposed to specific environmental factors. New previously 'dormant' genetic variants may become expressed due to exposure to environmental factors, whereas 'active' genetic variants may become suppressed by them. These (heritable) changes in gene expression are also known as epigenetics. Classic twin studies typically assume the gene-environment (GxE) interaction to be negligible, as the design (estimating A, C, and E) cannot discriminate between the main effects of genes and their interaction. When applying the classical twin model, interactions between genetic factors and the shared environment will result in an overestimation of the main effects of genes, whereas interactions between genetic factors and the unique environment will result in an underestimation of the main effects of genes. Fortunately, when (multiple) measures of environmental factors are collected, GxE interaction terms can be included in heritability modelling, thereby improving the accuracy of the heritability estimate.[74] Gene-environment interaction can also be incorporated in candidate gene studies[75] and even GWA.[76,77]

Gene-environment interaction is also clearly manifested in physical fitness. Individuals differ to a great extent in their response to a standardized training protocol, and this may be due to genetic variation. Bouchard demonstrated this effect in families in the HERITAGE Study,[78] by submitting more than 200 families to a 20-week exercise programme. Large individual differences in trainability were seen for several performance phenotypes. Data from this study indicate that the training-induced changes in $\dot{V}O_2$ max, several skeletal muscle phenotypes, resting HR, resting blood pressure, and other risk markers for cardiovascular diseases could for a large part be explained by genetics.[79–84]

Whereas the family environment, either as a main effect or in interaction with the genotype, is important to initiate PA and exercise (e.g. children rely on the financial support and willingness of their parents to organize transportation to sport clubs[85]), innate exercise ability and trainability might be important determinants of the maintenance of PA and exercise behaviour in adolescence. Especially in adolescence, being a 'natural' in sports or showing large gains during training will give young individuals a sense of competence and will boost their self-confidence, particularly when the exercise is performed in a competitive and comparative context. In this scenario, the heritability of exercise behaviour can partly be explained by genes coding for exercise ability. In addition, positive feedback on sport performance by family and peers will enhance these feelings of mastery and aid in the maintenance of exercise behaviour.

Implications for paediatrics

The evidence that the variance in PA, exercise, and physical fitness is under substantial genetic control does not mean that it is impossible to increase the amount of PA and exercise or to improve sports performance in children and adolescents. These findings should, however, contribute to the acknowledgment that the substantial range in PA and physical fitness in population-based samples of children and adolescents will *not* be erased by exercise intervention. We argue that this should never be a goal to begin with, as intervention is about shifting the mean of the distribution towards a more favourable value, not about reducing its variance.

To encourage adolescents to stay active, the innate individual differences can be used as a starting point. Children may experience rather different 'gains' when exercising or adopting a physically active lifestyle. By being good at sports some adolescents may gain self-esteem, whereas others who are less successful at sports but greatly enjoy the activity or its social aspects reap a different benefit. Acknowledgement of these differences in gains may aid in abandoning population-based strategies and moving towards personalized or family-based intervention strategies. Information on the source of individual differences at different time points during childhood and adolescence can inform type and timing of the optimal intervention approaches. To achieve the same aim of optimizing the appetitive aspects that are specific for that individual and generating realistic person-specific goals, different genotypes may require entirely different PA or exercise programmes.

Conclusions

Within the last few decades, there have been significant advances in discovering the genetic characteristics of PA, exercise, and physical fitness. Because of the rapid increase in knowledge of genomics and the enhanced technological aids for prolonged PA recordings in large-scale samples, even greater progress is probable in the coming decade. This progress will lead to better understanding of the genetic and environmental determinants of PA and physical fitness in the young, which in turn will expand the capability to improve paediatric health.

Summary

- Twin and family studies provide the ability to estimate the relative importance of genetic and environmental factors to the observed individual differences.
- Heritability estimates of physical activity and exercise behaviour vary widely, depending on sample size and measurement instrument, but the importance of shared environmental factors seems to decrease in adolescence, whereas genetic effects become more prominent in explaining individual differences.
- Most physical fitness traits are highly heritable; no evidence of shared environmental influences is reported.
- Gene-finding studies for physical activity and exercise behaviour in children are scarce, but several weight-related genes (*LEPR* and *MC4R*) have been found to be associated with physical activity.
- Although studies in children are limited, several studies in adults provide evidence of genes coding for physical fitness, such as *ACE* and *ACTN3*.
- Knowledge of the source of individual differences at different time points during childhood and adolescence can significantly contribute to the choice of exercise interventions.

References

1. Janssen I, Leblanc AG. Systematic review of the health benefits of physical activity and fitness in school-aged children and youth. *Int J Behav Nutr Phys Act*. 2010; 7: 40–55.
2. Ortega FB, Ruiz JR, Castillo MJ, Sjostrom M. Physical fitness in childhood and adolescence: a powerful marker of health. *Int J Obes (Lond)*. 2008; 32: 1–11.
3. Wedderkopp N, Froberg K, Hansen H, Riddoch C, Andersen L. Cardiovascular risk factors cluster in children and adolescents with low

physical fitness: The European Youth Heart Study (EYHS). *Pediatr Exerc Sci*. 2003; 15: 419–429.
4. Martinez-Gonzalez MA, Martinez JA, Hu FB, Gibney MJ, Kearney J. Physical inactivity, sedentary lifestyle and obesity in the European Union. *Int J Obes Relat Metab Disord*. 1999; 23: 1192–1201.
5. Troiano RP, Berrigan D, Dodd KW, Masse LC, Tilert T, McDowell M. Physical activity in the United States measured by accelerometer. *Med Sci Sports Exerc*. 2008; 40: 181–188.
6. Bergstrom E, Hernell O, Persson LA. Cardiovascular risk indicators cluster in girls from families of low socio-economic status. *Acta Paediatr*. 1996; 85: 1083–1090.
7. Dishman RK, Sallis JF, Orenstein DR. The determinants of physical activity and exercise. *Public Health Rep*. 1985; 100: 158–171.
8. Drenowatz C, Eisenmann JC, Pfeiffer KA, Welk G, Heelan K, Gentile D, *et al*. Influence of socio-economic status on habitual physical activity and sedentary behavior in 8- to 11-year old children. *BMC Public Health*. 2010; 10: 214.
9. Sallis JF, Prochaska JJ, Taylor WC. A review of correlates of physical activity of children and adolescents. *Med Sci Sports Exerc*. 2000; 32: 963–975.
10. Polderman TJ, Benyamin B, de Leeuw CA, *et al*. Meta-analysis of the heritability of human traits based on fifty years of twin studies. *Nat Genet*. 2015; 47: 702–709.
11. Kaprio J, Koskenvuo M, Sarna S. Cigarette smoking, use of alcohol, and leisure-time physical activity among same-sexed adult male twins. *Prog Clin Biol Res*. 1981; 69: 37–46.
12. Bryan A, Hutchison KE, Seals DR, Allen DL. A transdisciplinary model integrating genetic, physiological, and psychological correlates of voluntary exercise. *Health Psychol*. 2007; 26: 30–39.
13. de Geus E, de Moor M. A genetic perspective on the association between exercise and mental health. *Mental Health Phys Act*. 2008; 1: 53–61.
14. Liang KY, Beaty TH. Statistical designs for familial aggregation. *Stat Methods Med Res*. 2000; 9: 543–562.
15. Falconer D. *Introduction to quantitative genetics*. Edinburgh and London: Oliver and Boyd; 1960.
16. Swallow JG, Carter PA, Garland T, Jr. Artificial selection for increased wheel-running behavior in house mice. *Behav Genet*. 1998; 28: 227–237.
17. Lightfoot JT, Turner MJ, Daves M, Vordermark A, Kleeberger SR. Genetic influence on daily wheel running activity level. *Physiol Genomics*. 2004; 19: 270–276.
18. Chinapaw MJ, Mokkink LB, van Poppel MN, van MW, Terwee CB. Physical activity questionnaires for youth: a systematic review of measurement properties. *Sports Med*. 2010; 40: 539–563.
19. Butte NF, Cai G, Cole SA, Comuzzie AG. Viva la Familia Study: genetic and environmental contributions to childhood obesity and its comorbidities in the Hispanic population. *Am J Clin Nutr*. 2006; 84: 646–654.
20. Cai G, Cole SA, Butte N, Bacino C, Diego V, Tan K, *et al*. A quantitative trait locus on chromosome 18q for physical activity and dietary intake in Hispanic children. *Obesity (Silver Spring)*. 2006; 14: 1596–1604.
21. Fisher A, van Jaarsveld CH, Llewellyn CH, Wardle J. Environmental influences on children's physical activity: quantitative estimates using a twin design. *PLOS One*. 2010; 5: e10110.
22. Franks PW, Ravussin E, Hanson RL, *et al*. Habitual physical activity in children: the role of genes and the environment. *Am J Clin Nutr*. 2005; 82: 901–908.
23. Saudino KJ, Zapfe JA. Genetic influences on activity level in early childhood: do situations matter? *Child Dev*. 2008; 79: 930–943.
24. Wood AC, Rijsdijk F, Saudino KJ, Asherson P, Kuntsi J. High heritability for a composite index of children's activity level measures. *Behav Genet*. 2008; 38: 266–276.
25. de Chaves RN, Baxter-Jones A, Santos D, *et al*. Clustering of body composition, blood pressure and physical activity in Portuguese families. *Ann Hum Biol*. 2014; 41: 159–167.
26. Maia JA, Thomis M, Beunen G. Genetic factors in physical activity levels: a twin study. *Am J Prev Med*. 2002; 23(Suppl): 87–91.
27. Perusse L, Tremblay A, Leblanc C, Bouchard C. Genetic and environmental influences on level of habitual physical activity and exercise participation. *Am J Epidemiol*. 1989; 129: 1012–1022.
28. Santos DM, Katzmarzyk PT, Diego VP, Blangero J, Souza MC, Freitas DL, *et al*. Genotype by sex and genotype by age interactions with sedentary behavior: the Portuguese Healthy Family Study. *PLOS One*. 2014; 9: e110025.
29. Seabra AF, Mendonca DM, Goring HH, Thomis MA, Maia JA. Genetic influences of sports participation in Portuguese families. *Eur J Sport Sci*. 2014; 14: 510–517.
30. Huppertz C, Bartels M, van Beijsterveldt CE, Boomsma DI, Hudziak JJ, de Geus EJ. Effect of shared environmental factors on exercise behavior from age 7 to 12 years. *Med Sci Sports Exerc*. 2012; 44: 2025–2032.
31. White E, Slane JD, Klump KL, Burt SA, Pivarnik J. Sex differences in genetic and environmental influences on percent body fatness and physical activity. *J Phys Act Health*. 2014; 11: 1187–1193.
32. Stubbe JH, Boomsma DI, de Geus EJ. Sports participation during adolescence: a shift from environmental to genetic factors. *Med Sci Sports Exerc*. 2005; 37: 563–570.
33. de Geus EJ, Boomsma DI, Snieder H. Genetic correlation of exercise with heart rate and respiratory sinus arrhythmia. *Med Sci Sports Exerc*. 2003; 35: 1287–1295.
34. De Moor MH, Willemsen G, Rebollo-Mesa I, Stubbe JH, de Geus EJ, Boomsma DI. Exercise participation in adolescents and their parents: evidence for genetic and generation specific environmental effects. *Behav Genet*. 2011; 41: 211–222.
35. Stubbe J, de Geus E. Genetics of Exercise Behavior. In: Kim YK (ed.) *Handbook of behavior genetics*. New York: Springer Science and Business Media; 2009. p. 343–358.
36. Lightfoot JT, Turner MJ, Pomp D, Kleeberger SR, Leamy LJ. Quantitative trait loci for physical activity traits in mice. *Physiol Genomics*. 2008; 32: 401–408.
37. Kelly SA, Nehrenberg DL, Peirce JL, *et al*. Genetic architecture of voluntary exercise in an advanced intercross line of mice. *Physiol Genomics*. 2010; 42: 190–200.
38. Nehrenberg DL, Wang S, Hannon RM, Garland T, Jr., Pomp D. QTL underlying voluntary exercise in mice: interactions with the 'mini muscle' locus and sex. *J Hered*. 2010; 101: 42–53.
39. Rhodes JS, Gammie SC, Garland T, Jr. Neurobiology of mice selected for high voluntary wheel-running activity. *Integr Comp Biol*. 2005; 45: 438–455.
40. Lorentzon M, Lorentzon R, Lerner UH, Nordstrom P. Calcium sensing receptor gene polymorphism, circulating calcium concentrations and bone mineral density in healthy adolescent girls. *Eur J Endocrinol*. 2001; 144: 257–261.
41. Richert L, Chevalley T, Manen D, Bonjour JP, Rizzoli R, Ferrari S. Bone mass in prepubertal boys is associated with a Gln223Arg amino acid substitution in the leptin receptor. *J Clin Endocrinol Metab*. 2007; 92: 4380–4386.
42. Elmquist JK, Maratos-Flier E, Saper CB, Flier JS. Unraveling the central nervous system pathways underlying responses to leptin. *Nat Neurosci*. 1998; 1: 445–450.
43. Cole SA, Butte NF, Voruganti VS, *et al*. Evidence that multiple genetic variants of MC4R play a functional role in the regulation of energy expenditure and appetite in Hispanic children. *Am J Clin Nutr*. 2010; 91: 191–199.
44. Hakanen M, Raitakari OT, Lehtimaki T, Peltonen N, Pahkala K, Sillanmaki L, *et al*. FTO genotype is associated with body mass index after the age of seven years but not with energy intake or leisure-time physical activity. *J Clin Endocrinol Metab*. 2009; 94: 1281–1287.
45. Liu G, Zhu H, Lagou V, Gutin B, *et al*. FTO variant rs9939609 is associated with body mass index and waist circumference, but not with energy intake or physical activity in European and African-American youth. *BMC Med Genet*. 2010; 11: 57.
46. De Moor MH, Liu YJ, Boomsma DI, *et al*. Genome-wide association study of exercise behavior in Dutch and American adults. *Med Sci Sports Exerc*. 2009; 41: 1887–1895.

47. Clarke GM, Anderson CA, Pettersson FH, Cardon LR, Morris AP, Zondervan KT. Basic statistical analysis in genetic case-control studies. *Nat Protoc.* 2011; 6: 121–133.
48. Klein RJ. Power analysis for genome-wide association studies. *BMC Genet.* 2007; 8: 58.
49. Caspersen CJ, Powell KE, Christenson GM. Physical activity, exercise, and physical fitness: definitions and distinctions for health-related research. *Public Health Rep.* 1985; 100: 126–131.
50. Kenney W, Wilmore J, Costill D. *Physiology of sport and exercise.* Champaign, IL: Human Kinetics; 2012.
51. Klissouras V. Heritability of adaptive variation. *J Appl Physiol.* 1971; 31: 338–344.
52. Maes HH, Beunen GP, Vlietinck RF, *et al.* Inheritance of physical fitness in 10-year-old twins and their parents. *Med Sci Sports Exerc.* 1996; 28: 1479–1491.
53. Lortie G, Bouchard C, Leblanc C, *et al.* Familial similarity in aerobic power. *Hum Biol.* 1982; 54: 801–812.
54. Schutte NM, Nederend I, Hudziak JJ, Bartels M, de Geus EJ. A twin-sibling study and meta-analysis on the heritability of maximal oxygen consumption. *Physiol Genomics.* 2016; 48: 210–219.
55. Montoye HJ, Gayle R. Familial relationships in maximal oxygen uptake. *Hum Biol.* 1978; 50: 241–249.
56. Lesage R, Simoneau JA, Jobin J, Leblanc J, Bouchard C. Familial resemblance in maximal heart rate, blood lactate and aerobic power. *Hum Hered. 1985;* 35: 182–189.
57. Armstrong N. Aerobic fitness of children and adolescents. *J Pediatr (Rio J).* 2006; 82: 406–408.
58. Council of Europe Committee for the development of sport. *Eurofit: handbook for the EUROFIT tests of physical fitness.* Rome: Committee for the development of sport; 1988.
59. Beunen G, Thomis M, Peeters M, Maes H, Claessens A, Vlietinck R. Genetics of strength and power characteristics in children and adolescents. *Pediatr Exerc Sci.* 2003; 15: 128–138.
60. Schutte NM, Nederend I, Hudziak JJ, de Geus EJ, Bartels M. Differences in adolescent physical fitness: A multivariate approach and meta-analysis. *Behav Genet.* 2016; 46: 217–227.
61. Szopa J. Familial studies on genetic determination of some manifestations of muscular strength in man. *Genetica Polonica.* 1982; 28: 65–78.
62. Isen J, McGue M, Iacono W. Genetic influences on the development of grip strength in adolescence. *Am J Phys Anthropol.* 2014; 154: 189–200.
63. Katzmarzyk PT, Gledhill N, Perusse L, Bouchard C. Familial aggregation of 7-year changes in musculoskeletal fitness. *J Gerontol A Biol Sci Med Sci.* 2001; 56: B497–B502.
64. Okuda E, Horii D, Kano T. Genetic and environmental effects on physical fitness and motor performance. *Int J Sport Health Sci.* 2005; 3: 1–9.
65. Chatterjee S, Das N. Physical and motor fitness in twins. *Jpn J Physiol.* 1995; 45: 519–534.
66. Vandenberg SG. The Hereditary Abilities Study: Hereditary Components in a Psychological Test Battery. *Am J Hum Genet.* 1962; 14: 220–237.
67. Williams LR, Gross JB. Heritability of motor skill. *Acta Genet Med Gemellol (Roma).* 1980; 29: 127–136.
68. Rankinen T, Perusse L, Rauramaa R, Rivera MA, Wolfarth B, Bouchard C. The human gene map for performance and health-related fitness phenotypes. *Med Sci Sports Exerc.* 2001; 33: 855–867.
69. Loos RJ, Hagberg JM, Pérusse L, *et al.* Advances in exercise, fitness, and performance genomics in 2014. *Med Sci Sports Exerc.* 2015; 47: 1105–1112.
70. MacArthur DG, North KN. The ACTN3 gene and human performance. In: Bouchard C, Hoffman E (eds.) *Genetic and molecular aspects of sport performance.* West Sussex: Wiley-Blackwell; 2011. p. 204–214.
71. Skipworth JRA, Puhucheary ZA, Rawal J, Montgomery HE. The ACE gene and performance. In: Bouchard C, Hoffman E (eds.) *Genetic and molecular aspects of sport performance.* West Sussex: Wiley-Blackwell; 2011. p. 195–203.
72. Montgomery HE, Marshall R, Hemingway H, *et al.* Human gene for physical performance. *Nature.* 1998; 393: 221–222.
73. Yang N, MacArthur DG, Gulbin JP, *et al.* ACTN3 genotype is associated with human elite athletic performance. *Am J Hum Genet.* 2003; 73: 627–631.
74. Purcell S. Variance components models for gene-environment interaction in twin analysis. *Twin Res.* 2002; 5: 554–571.
75. Dick DM, Agrawal A, Keller MC, *et al.* Candidate gene-environment interaction research: reflections and recommendations. *Perspect Psychol Sci.* 2015; 10: 37–59.
76. Thomas D. Methods for investigating gene-environment interactions in candidate pathway and genome-wide association studies. *Annu Rev Public Health.* 2010; 31: 21–36.
77. Winham SJ, Biernacka JM. Gene-environment interactions in genome-wide association studies: current approaches and new directions. *J Child Psychol Psychiatry.* 2013; 54: 1120–1134.
78. Bouchard C, Leon AS, Rao DC, Skinner JS, Wilmore JH, Gagnon J. The HERITAGE family study. Aims, design, and measurement protocol. *Med Sci Sports Exerc.* 1995; 27: 721–729.
79. An P, Pérusse L, Rankinen T, *et al.* Familial aggregation of exercise heart rate and blood pressure in response to 20 weeks of endurance training: the HERITAGE family study. *Int J Sports Med.* 2003; 24: 57–62.
80. Bouchard C, An P, Rice T, *et al.* Familial aggregation of $\dot{V}O_2$ max response to exercise training: results from the HERITAGE Family Study. *J Appl Physiol.* 1999; 87: 1003–1008.
81. Hong Y, Rice T, Gagnon J, *et al.* Familiality of triglyceride and LPL response to exercise training: the HERITAGE study. *Med Sci Sports Exerc.* 2000; 32: 1438–1444.
82. Pérusse L, Rice T, Province MA, *et al.* Familial aggregation of amount and distribution of subcutaneous fat and their responses to exercise training in the HERITAGE family study. *Obes Res.* 2000; 8: 140–150.
83. Rice T, Despres JP, Pérusse L, *et al.* Familial aggregation of blood lipid response to exercise training in the health, risk factors, exercise training, and genetics (HERITAGE) Family Study. *Circulation.* 2002; 105: 1904–1908.
84. Rico-Sanz J, Rankinen T, Joanisse DR, *et al.* Familial resemblance for muscle phenotypes in the HERITAGE Family Study. *Med Sci Sports Exerc.* 2003; 35: 1360–1366.
85. Beets MW, Cardinal BJ, Alderman BL. Parental social support and the physical activity-related behaviors of youth: a review. *Health Educ Behav.* 2010; 37: 621–644.
86. van der Aa N, de Geus EJ, van Beijsterveldt TC, Boomsma DI, Bartels M. Genetic Influences on individual differences in exercise behavior during adolescence. *Int J Pediatr.* 2010; 2010: 138345.
87. Beunen G, Thomis M. Genetic determinants of sports participation and daily physical activity. *Int J Obes Relat Metab Disord.* 1999; 23(Suppl): S55–S63.
88. Aaltonen S, Ortega-Alonso A, Kujala UM, Kaprio J. Genetic and environmental influences on longitudinal changes in leisure-time physical activity from adolescence to young adulthood. *Twin Res Hum Genet.* 2013; 16: 535–543.
89. Seabra AF, Mendonca DM, Goring HH, Thomis MA, Maia JA. Genetic and environmental factors in familial clustering in physical activity. *Eur J Epidemiol.* 2008; 23: 205–211.
90. Boomsma DI, van den Bree MB, Orlebeke JF, Molenaar PC. Resemblances of parents and twins in sports participation and heart rate. *Behav Genet.* 1989; 19: 123–141.
91. Koopmans J, van Doornen L, Boomsma D. Smoking and sports participation. In: Goldbourt U, de Faire U, Berg K (eds.) *Genetic factors in coronary heart disease.* Dordrecht: Springer Science and Business Media; 1994. p. 217–235.
92. Malina RM, Mueller WH. Genetic and environmental influences on the strength and motor performance of Philadelphia school children. *Hum Biol.* 1981; 53: 163–179.
93. Kovar R. Genetic analysis of motor performance. *J Sports Med Phys Fitness.* 1976; 16: 205–208.
94. Venerando A, Milani-Comparetti M. Twin studies in sport and physical performance. *Acta Genet Med Gemellol (Roma).* 1970; 19: 80–82.

CHAPTER 21

The assessment of physical activity

Maria Hildebrand and Ulf Ekelund

Introduction

Physical activity (PA) is one of the most important lifestyle factors for improving public health and disease prevention in humans.[1,2] Accurate measurement of PA is important for several reasons when examining this behaviour in observational and experimental studies in free-living individuals. This includes examining dose-response relationships between PA and various health outcomes, monitoring the effect of interventions in experimental studies, making cross-cultural comparisons, and determining levels, pattern, and trends in PA in surveillance systems.[3] An imprecise measure of PA will attenuate the true effect, thus underestimating or masking the true association between the exposure and outcome.

Despite much progress in the assessment of PA, substantial limitations related to measurement accuracy still exist. These limitations are amplified in young people and some are unique for this age group as young people's PA is different from adults due to alterations in physiology and changes during natural growth and development, as well as the nature of their PA pattern. Young people's PA tends to be irregular and of more variable intensity than that of adults, as well as being less organized activity, and characterized by intermittent movements with variable intensities, sometimes with PA bouts only lasting a few seconds.[4] In addition, the strength of the relationship between PA and health varies considerably and it may be weaker in young people than in adults and therefore more difficult to establish.[2] This could possibly be explained by a longer lifetime of exposure in adults, with more time for disease to develop. Subsequently, this has consequences for the assessment of PA and for the interpretation of PA data in young people. Although many methodological considerations can be generalized between adults and young people, the assessment of PA in young people is not synonymous with that in adults and should be considered separately.

This chapter presents the assessment and interpretation of PA in young people in three main sections. The first describes definitions of various terminologies and measurement metrics frequently used in the field of PA research. The next section describes the methods used to measure PA and summarizes advantages, limitations, and issues surrounding data analysis and the interpretation of PA data from each method. Finally, it offers some practical advice for choosing the right assessment method.

Key concepts in measuring physical activity

Physical activity is a complex behaviour comprising numerous terms associated with bodily movement such as clapping, jumping, or running. Physical activity, exercise, and physical fitness are often used interchangeably, although they are not synonymous and it is therefore important to define terms often used in PA research.

Definitions and dimensions of physical activity

For clarity this chapter uses definitions and terms of PA as defined by Caspersen *et al.*[5] *Physical activity* is 'any bodily movement produced by skeletal muscles that result in energy expenditure'. *Exercise* is 'a subset of physical activity that is planned, structured, and repetitive and has as a final or an intermediate objective the improvement or maintenance of physical fitness'. Hence, exercise is only a minor part of PA. *Physical fitness* is 'a set of attributes either health- or skill-related which can be measured with a specific test, for example a maximum oxygen uptake test'.

Physical activity is often divided into different dimensions, the most common being *frequency, duration*, and *intensity*, which together make up the total volume of PA. *Frequency* is the number of PA bouts during a specific period and *duration* is the time of participation in a single bout of PA. *Intensity* is the physiological effort involved in performing PA and can be defined in absolute terms (e.g. in METs; see section on Physical activity outcomes) and relative terms (e.g. maximal heart rate [HR]), and it can sometimes be normalized for different body sizes.[6] Two other important dimensions of PA are *type/mode*, which refers to the specific PA being performed, and *domain* of PA, which is the context in which the PA takes place, e.g. at home, school, school break time, and during sports or leisure time. Finally, in this chapter habitual PA is defined as the assessment of the usual PA carried out in normal daily life in every domain and in any dimension. It is not possible to measure habitual PA directly so it must be estimated by the measurement of free-living PA for a defined period.

The word sedentary originates from the Latin word *sedere*, which means to sit. *Sedentary behaviour* and *sedentary time* are often used interchangeably and are defined as a distinct class of waking behaviour in a seated or reclined posture with an energy expenditure ≤1.5 METs.[7] The same posture allocation can serve many different types of sedentary behaviour, including sitting at school or sitting watching TV, while other types of sitting activities with a higher metabolic rate (e.g. cycling and rowing) are appropriately defined as physical activities. A detailed review of different assessment methods for sedentary behaviour in young people is available elsewhere.[8]

Measurement metrics of physical activity

Physical activity can be expressed in a variety of different metrics, which can be grouped into two main categories: the estimation of energy expenditure, and other quantifying metrics of PA (e.g. total steps or intensity of PA).

Energy expenditure outcomes

Energy expenditure is often measured in joules (J) or kilocalories (kcal) typically expressed per day. *Total energy expenditure* (TEE) is the total amount of energy required by an individual, and is commonly divided into *basal metabolic rate* (BMR), *resting energy expenditure* (REE), *thermic effect of feeding* (TEF), or *diet-induced thermogenesis* (DIT), and *physical activity energy expenditure* (PAEE).[9] Basal metabolic rate (BMR) is the amount of energy required to sustain the functioning of vital organs, such as blood circulation and respiration, measured in a post-absorptive state (at least 12 h after the last meal) immediately after waking in a thermoneutral environment.[10] Relative energy expenditure is the amount of energy required at rest and is not subject to such a rigorous protocol as when measuring BMR. Relative energy expenditure is often slightly higher (10–20%) than BMR because of increased energy expenditure due to food intake or PA.[9] Thermic effect of feeding or DIT is the increment in energy expenditure above BMR associated with the cost of absorption and processing of food for storage, and is largely determined by the amount and composition of the food consumed. Physical activity energy expenditure is the amount of energy required to carry out PA, and is usually calculated as PAEE = TEE-BMR or PAEE = (0.9*TEE)-BMR to account for the TEF (commonly assumed to be approximately 10% of the TEE).[10] *Physical activity intensity* (PAI) is equal to PAEE per unit of time (e.g. $J \cdot min^{-1}$), while *Physical activity level* (PAL) is calculated as PAL = TEE/RMR.

Physical activity energy expenditure is the most variable component of TEE, and is strongly influenced by body weight and movement efficiency, and may therefore not be reflective of the energy cost of the activity.[9] This is an important issue in children as PA measured as body movement by accelerometry decreases with age,[11,12] while absolute PAEE increases as a function of greater body weight.[13] Physical activity energy expenditure is also greater in the obese than the normal-weight child, even if he/she has a lower level of PA.[14] Consequently, it is necessary to normalize PAEE for body size when making comparisons between individuals with different body sizes and several approaches exist, including simple models such as scaling PAEE for body weight (e.g. $J \cdot kg^{-1}$), and more complex power function models using allometric scaling.[15] However, even if PAEE is normalized by body size, other factors such as gender and age can still influence PAEE, and perhaps scaling PAEE by fat-free mass is more appropriate as it may account for sex differences in body composition.[14]

Physical activity outcomes

Most measurement methods for PA can be expressed in not just one, but various outcomes. For example, PA can be expressed as time spent physically active (e.g. $min \cdot day^{-1}$), total counts/steps, duration of bouts of PA, and mode of PA.

In general, the most common measures of interest are intensity of PA (i.e. sedentary, light, moderate, and vigorous) and time spent in these intensities. A MET is a widely used absolute physiological term for expressing the intensity and is the multiples of REE, where the traditionally accepted value for 1 MET is 3.5 $mLO_2 \cdot kg^{-1} \cdot min^{-1}$ for adults. In children, the adult value for one MET is not appropriate to use since REE expressed in relation to body weight is substantially higher than in adults (4–7 $mLO_2 \cdot kg^{-1} \cdot min^{-1}$). It is therefore difficult to identify a single accepted value for one MET across a wide age range.[15,16] Nevertheless, public health recommendations on PA intensity are often expressed as METs and in general, moderate intensity PA refers to 3 to 6 METs,[17] which correspond to ~40–55% of maximal oxygen uptake or ~60–70% of maximal HR in adolescents.[18] Further, in PA research, it is common to differentiate between an individual that is *sedentary*, i.e. engaging in a large amount of daily sedentary behaviour, and an individual that is *physically inactive*, i.e. not meeting the recommended dose of PA according to public health recommendations.[19]

How active are young people?

The current PA recommendation for young people is 60 min of at least moderate-intensity activity every day,[20] and various studies have sought to determine whether young people are achieving these recommendations. The answer to this question at least partly depends on the assessment method and subsequent interpretation of the PA data. Most results using an objective measure, such as the accelerometer, indicate that the prevalence of young people's PA level according to these recommendations are low,[21–23] but there is some disparity. However, it is generally agreed that the overweight are less active than the lean,[24,25] boys are more active than girls, and PA decreases with age.[11,12] Different methods of measurement and analyses are not always comparable, which makes comparisons about PA levels across studies and populations challenging.

Reliability, validity, accuracy, and responsiveness of physical activity assessment methods

Reliability, validity, accuracy, and responsiveness are important concepts for all types of assessment methods and should be considered when using a method or reading a scientific paper. These concepts are closely linked to each other and sometimes overlap. All assessment methods have a small or large degree of measurement error; although, by performing validation and reliability studies these errors are better understood, and hence become limited.

Reliability

Reliability refers to the consistency of the method and is the degree to which a method is free of random error (i.e. error by chance).[26] A reliable method must give the same results under different conditions in which it is likely to be used, and it is a requirement for validity. Reliability is often calculated as the intra-class coefficient (ICC) or the Kappa test (non-parametric).[27] There are different types of reliability, since random error can be due to i) the method itself, ii) the tester using the method, and/or iii) the behaviour being assessed. *Intra-class reliability (test-retest reliability)* refers to the comparison of repeated measurements using the same instrument to the same population. For example, Scott *et al.*[28] asked adolescents to complete a single-item PA questionnaire on two occasions separated by 2 weeks, and the ICC between the measurements was 0.75. Hence, the authors concluded that the test-retest reliability

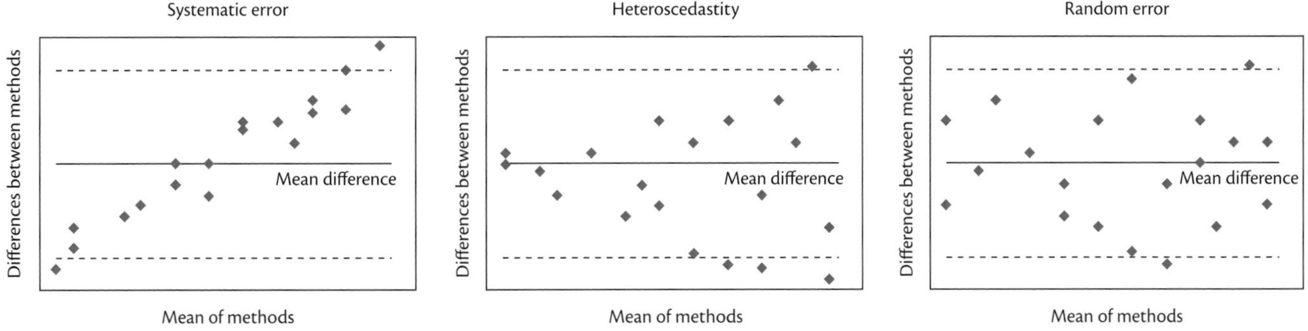

Figure 21.1 Graphical representation of error.

Systematic error; error that is not due to chance but is introduced by biases in the measurement method, or by human factors. The error may have a directional bias dependent on x-values. Heteroscedasticity; when the error at each x-value is not the same and is therefore greater at some x-values than others are. Random or non-differential error; the distribution of measurement errors is randomly distributed and usually results in a dilution of association.

of the questionnaire was acceptable. The *intra-rater reliability* is related to the consistency of observations made by the same tester on different occasions, while *inter-rater reliability* is the degree to which different testers agree when measuring the same behaviour. This is relevant to methods such as direct observation and interviews, where several testers perform the assessments.

With objective methods, for example, the accelerometer, there is often variation between the outputs of different monitors of the same brand and model *(inter-instrument reliability)* and this can be tested using a standard mechanical calibration procedure or by having the participants wear multiple monitors during physical activity. Other important considerations for a reliable estimate of habitual PA are days of monitoring, seasonality, school terms, school holidays, and climate.[29] Therefore, a single measurement occasion may not adequately reflect young people's habitual PA as there may be considerable intra-individual variation.

Validity

Validity refers to the degree the method measures what it is intended to measure, in other words, the accuracy of the method, and there are several types of validity.[26] *Concurrent validity*, which is a type of *criterion validity*, can be determined by comparing a specific assessment method with an already established method ('a gold standard') that is administered about the same time. For example, Lee *et al.*[30] examined the concurrent validity of the pedometer function in four activity monitors by comparing the monitors' step counts with manually counted steps. It is of great importance to choose a suitable criterion method. Otherwise, the concurrent validity is of little value. If comparison with a criterion method is not possible, the specific method can be compared to another method that is believed to measure the same exposure of interest. This is then called *convergent validity*, which is a sub-group under *construct validity*.[31] In validation studies, even if the two methods should measure the same exposure, the methods should be without correlated errors. Hence, validation of a questionnaire against an activity diary or an accelerometer against another accelerometer may therefore not be the preferred option, and can result in an unreasonably high correlation.

Validation studies of PA assessment methods are normally conducted in i) a controlled environment on a treadmill or during various 'lifestyle' activities, ii) a semi-controlled environment, e.g. school break, or iii) a free-living environment. Large differences in PA are likely to be present between age groups, populations, and ethnic groups, meaning that the population chosen for a validation study should be as representative as possible to where the technique is to be applied. However, it is not feasible to have a validation study for every population and therefore many studies use healthy and limited populations due to convenience, the expensive nature of criterion methods, and time-constraints. These factors should all be considered when choosing an assessment method as, for example, a method valid for use in lean children may not be suitable for assessing the same exposure in obese children.[13]

Correlation coefficients are the traditional outcome variable used in validation studies. However, they might be misleading and perhaps do not allow for investigation of direction of error, systematic bias, or heteroscedasticity.[32] Preferably, Bland-Altman plots with limits of agreement should be used to define the magnitude of the bias and to estimate heteroscedasticity in comparative studies. The main types of error experienced in validation studies are displayed graphically in Bland-Altman plots (Figure 21.1).

Accuracy and responsiveness

Accuracy is a measure of how close the data are to the actual true value, while responsiveness refers to the method's capability of capturing changes over time, and both validity and reliability are prerequisites. For example, a method used for classifying individuals as inactive or physically active may not be suited to identify changes in PA levels after an intervention. The responsiveness of a method depends on the methods' *sensitivity* and *specificity*. *Sensitivity* refers to the method's ability to detect changes, while *specificity* refers to the method's ability to measure no change, when no change has occurred.[26]

Methods of physical activity assessment

Assessment methods for free-living PA can be divided into two groups; subjective and objective methods. Subjective methods such as questionnaires, interviews, and activity diaries may be influenced by opinion and perception from the participant, investigator, or both. Objective methods record a physiological or biomechanical parameter to estimate PA or energy expenditure, and are not influenced by opinion or perception, but instead are susceptible to measurement error. Characteristics of the most common assessment methods are shown in Table 21.1.

Table 21.1 Characteristics of commonly used assessment methods for physical activity

	DLW	Indirect calorimetry	Direct observation	Questionnaires	Accelerometry	Inclinometers	Pedometers	Combined HR and movement
Measured dimensions of PA	Total PA	Intensity, duration, FREQ	All	All	Intensity, duration, FREQ	Duration, FREQ	Total PA	Intensity, duration, FREQ
Outcome	TEE	PAEE, intensity	Min in PA type, domain or intensity	Min in PA type, domain or intensity	g $(m \cdot s^{-2})$ or counts	Min per postures	Steps	HR/min, PAEE
Measurement period	7–14 days	A few hours	Short, a few hours	1 day to habitual	1–14 days	1–7 days	1–14 days	1–14 days
Suited for:								
free-living sedentary behavior	No	No	Yes	Yes	Yes	Yes	No	Yes
estimation of EE	Yes	Yes	No	No	Yes	No	No	Yes

DLW, doubly labelled water; FREQ, frequency; HR, heart rate; TEE, total energy expenditure; EE, energy expenditure; PA, physical activity.

Criterion methods

Doubly labelled water (DLW) and calorimetry are often considered as criterion methods for assessing TEE and PAEE. Both these objective methods derive their estimates of physiological energy expenditure from oxygen consumption and/or carbon dioxide production, but from different sources. Direct observation may be a more practical criterion measure for PA since in theory it can measure all dimensions of PA.

Doubly labelled water

The DLW method was developed in the late 1940s by Lifson *et al.*,[33] but it was not until about 35 years ago that it became used to assess daily energy expenditure in humans.[34] The DLW method has been described in detail elsewhere.[35] In summary, water labelled with known amounts of the stable isotopes deuterium (^2H) and ^{18}O are ingested orally and after a few hours the isotopes are distributed throughout the body water pool. The ^2H-isotope is eliminated from the body as water in perspiration and urine, and ^{18}O as both water and carbon dioxide (CO_2) in expired air. The difference in elimination rates between the two isotopes is therefore a measure of CO_2 production, which is proportional to energy expenditure. This method requires collection of urine or saliva samples, usually daily over 7–14 days consecutively, barely disrupting daily life. The levels of isotopes in the samples are measured using high-precision mass spectrometry, and from these estimates, TEE is calculated. The amount of energy used for activity (PAEE) can be estimated by subtracting the measured or predicted REE or BMR from TEE.

The advantage of this method is that it provides a non-invasive, safe measurement that does not affect the individual's behaviour. With a high accuracy to measure TEE, the DLW method is undoubtedly the gold-standard for the assessment of free-living energy expenditure over a prolonged time period in humans.[10] Despite the advantages in using this method, it is usually limited to smaller samples due to the high cost of isotopes and analyses. In addition, the method only provides information about the total amount of energy expenditure (i.e. TEE), and does not capture hourly or daily patterns of PA, including duration, intensity, and frequency.

Calorimetry

Direct and indirect room calorimetry are able to provide very accurate estimates of energy expenditure, but unfortunately in unnatural environments and at high cost. Direct room calorimetry uses the heat transfer from the body to the environment and the latter uses the measurement of all expired gases to calculate energy expenditure. Detailed descriptions of these methods are available elsewhere.[36] Both methods are unsuitable for the assessment of habitual PA in young people as they require confinement to a metabolic chamber.[37] However, metabolic chambers are appropriate for validating energy expenditure equations from accelerometry or HR, even for young children.[38,39]

Indirect calorimetry using a stationary or portable measurement system is more feasible and is frequently the criterion method when validating HR monitors, pedometers, and accelerometers in laboratory and free-living settings for a limited period. Indirect calorimetry uses standard equations to predict energy expenditure from oxygen consumption and carbon dioxide production. A facemask, mouthpiece, or hood covering the head collects the expired air, and a stationed system next to the individual or a portable system mounted on the individual's body analyses the respiratory gases. Portable indirect calorimetry systems are lightweight and have been used successfully during structured laboratory activities with young children.[40,41] However, the equipment is still too cumbersome to use during prolonged periods and therefore the method is not suited to measure habitual PA.

Direct observation

Direct observation is the most applied method for assessing patterns of PA and is sometimes considered as the gold standard for PA assessment in children.[42] A trained observer will watch the participants using one of many observational systems available to record PA in time intervals, e.g. every minute, and these systems have been reviewed elsewhere.[42,43] Direct observation is suitable for assessment of PA and sedentary behaviours in controlled environments, such as during school break-times, and can provide detailed information about all dimensions of PA.[19] Direct observation has been shown to provide a valid estimate for absolute intensity in free-living adults compared to indirect calorimetry.[44] However, it could be argued that this method is not suited for assessing PA intensity due to the subjective nature of classification, especially at the mid-ranges of intensity levels, as well as the variable intensity bouts only lasting a few seconds in children. Other limitations with this method include the substantial investigator burden which makes it unsuitable for the assessment of free-living PA, the invasion of the individual's privacy, and reactivity to the method, which can consequently result in altered behaviour (Hawthorne effect).

Subjective methods

Subjective assessment methods such as questionnaires, diaries, logs, or recalls are the most widely used method for measuring different sedentary behaviours, in addition to PA.[45] Data are often collected retrospectively and are influenced by the individual's cognitive function and recall.

Questionnaires

Questionnaires are arguably the cheapest and simplest method of assessing PA in a large number of people in a short time. They can either be self-reported or interviews and can assess all dimensions of PA and sedentary behaviour. While some questionnaires are short, others are long, detailed, and time-consuming for the respondent.[6] In general, questionnaires can be categorized into three different types: global, recall, and quantitative questionnaires.

Types of questionnaires

A global questionnaire usually consists of one to four items and is very quick for the respondent to answer. In general, these questionnaires tend to inquire about PA over a long period (e.g. 1 year) which reduces errors due to season and day of the week. A global questionnaire does not provide any quantification of PA, but aims to classify individuals into two or more categories of activity (e.g. inactive and active), and is often used for epidemiological studies or as screening tools.[46] A recall questionnaire generally includes 5–15 items and can be used to stratify individuals into finer categories of PA, in addition to quantify PA. These types of questionnaires are often used in descriptive epidemiology, surveillance studies, but also in intervention studies to detect changes in PA.[6] Quantitative questionnaires usually consist of 15–60 items aimed to capture detailed information on PA and sedentary behaviour in various domains and according to several dimensions. From these measures, it is possible to derive variables on patterns of PA and energy expenditure over a lifetime, to examine the relationship with different health outcomes. It is often used for aetiological studies.[45]

Advantages and limitations

Questionnaires can accurately determine the type of PA, are practical to use in large samples, are low cost, can (in theory) capture all dimensions of PA, and are often used to assess specific sedentary behaviours such as TV-viewing or screen-time. They can be used to adequately rank or categorize PA levels, and possibly even assess some aspects of moderate to vigorous physical activity (MVPA).[47] However, questionnaires have limited ability to quantify total volume of PA and PAEE accurately and may therefore mask or distort the true underlying relationship between PA and health.[48] Questionnaires for children have lower accuracy than questionnaires for adolescents.[8,47]

Collection of PA and sedentary behaviour is a highly complex cognitive task and therefore prone to *recall bias*. This can either be intentional (*social desirability bias*) or accidental false recall, missed recall, or differential reporting accuracy of different intensities, dimensions, and domains of activity.[49] The subjective classification of intensity is a problem with all subjective methods and may lead to misclassification, and contributing to the large variation in error in individual estimates of energy expenditure. Participation in discrete activities is generally more accurately recalled by self-report methods as the individual has made a conscious decision to carry out that activity in a defined period. However, habitual PA is much more difficult to capture accurately with subjective methods. In addition, some questionnaires do not include questions about sedentary and light-intensity activities, or behaviours that are spontaneous and of short duration.[50] As a result, the methods suffer from a floor effect, in other words, the lowest score available is too high for the most sedentary individuals.

Subjective methods are, as opposed to objective methods, usually developed for specific groups and are therefore age and culturally specific. Questionnaires developed for adults may not be suited for young people. In addition, children below 10–12 years of age are less likely to provide accurate self-report data and therefore parental or teacher-reported questionnaires are often used. However, recollection of children's PA is difficult for adults[51] and neither a parent nor teacher will be able to constantly monitor any one child for elongated periods.

The PA output from a questionnaire is subject to substantial interpolation and assumption; consequently, it is best to use the data as raw as possible. Even if it is not recommended to estimate PAEE or activity intensity using a questionnaire, especially in young children as far too many assumptions need to be made, a comprehensive children's compendium providing the energy cost for a wide variety of activities is available,[52] making it possible to assign intensity levels to self-reported PA. However, many of the values in the compendium are based on data from adults due to the low number of studies examining activity energy expenditure in young people, and therefore caution is warranted using these values.

Activity diaries

Activity diaries are inexpensive, can be used in large sample sizes, and can provide detailed information about PA. Unlike questionnaires that are retrospective, an activity diary requires the respondent to continuously record the activity or the intensity of the activity being carried out in specific time segments of the day, for example every 15 min. This methodology is therefore sometimes referred to as ecological momentary assessment (EMA), referring to real-world and real-time data collection.[53] Data can be collected with paper and pen, but electronic devices such as mobile phones are becoming more common to use, and the method has been successfully used in children as young as 9 years old.[54] However, caution should be taken, as children might be unlikely to cope as well as adults with the task of accurately completing a diary. The method can provide detailed information about patterns of PA, sedentary behaviour, and energy expenditure, and it can assess other aspects of PA, including with whom PA is undertaken and emotions associated with the activity.

Activity diaries are valid to assess PAEE and EE in adolescents,[55] levels of PA compared to accelerometer,[51,56] and also PA type. However, these instruments are associated with high participant burden, which may limit compliance, and they may affect habitual behaviour (Hawthorne effect). In addition, the method only assesses PA in pre-determined time segments and inevitably, short-term activities may be omitted or misclassified. Nonetheless, recall periods shorter than 15 min have been found to be too cumbersome with low compliance.[57] One way to increase compliance among adolescents can be by using cell phone-based diaries,[54] although reluctance to provide an answer while engaging in physical activities, especially more intense activities, still exists.[53]

Objective methods

Objective measurement methods such as accelerometers and HR monitors are not influenced by the individual's self-assessment of PA, and may thus be less prone to recall and social desirability bias. It is becoming more common to assess both PA and sedentary time with accelerometry, even in large-scale epidemiological studies.

Accelerometry

Acceleration is a change in velocity and can be measured by small, lightweight, and portable devices that record movement of the body segment to which it is attached. The acceleration produced during movement is proportional to the net internal muscular forces used and therefore the acceleration can be used as an estimate of the energy cost of the movement.[58] The monitor can provide detailed information about the frequency, duration, and intensity of PA.[59,60] Uniaxial accelerometers measure acceleration in one direction, biaxial in two directions, while tri-axial measures the acceleration in three directions. The underlying technical specifications have been comprehensively described elsewhere.[60,61]

Advantages and limitations

Accelerometers provide detailed information about patterns of PA, are easy to wear, and not too expensive to be used with large sample sizes.[62] In general, accelerometers can provide a reasonably accurate assessment of ambulatory activities, including time spent in different intensities.[40,63,64] Compared to DLW, the accelerometer shows a larger variability in output and is less accurate in predicting energy expenditure.[64,65] Energy expenditure is often underestimated due to external work and the monitor's inadequate capability to capture PA with little or no movement of the body segment where the monitor is attached. Despite that the accelerometer is often the tool of choice for measuring PA, there are several issues associated with data processing that need to be considered for the user.

Monitor placement

Since movement varies between body segments, the output from an accelerometer placed at, for example, the hip and the wrist is not directly comparable, even for the same activity type.[40,66,67] A hip placement is commonly used, as this is the closest place to the centre of gravity of the body. However, recently there has been a shift towards a wrist placement since it has numerous advantages, including greater user acceptability among individuals, leading to greater compliance, less loss of data, and the ability to measure upper body movement.

Wear time, valid days, and epoch length

In general, the accelerometer is worn during waking hours, and is removed for sleeping, and for showering and swimming if the monitor is not waterproof. Normally the monitor should be worn for 4 to 7 continuous days, including both weekdays and weekends,[68,69] since PA patterns differ between week and weekend days.[70] In addition, a minimum of 10 $h \cdot day^{-1}$ of registered movement is required to reflect the entire day.[62] Data when the monitor is not worn can be excluded by deleting data consisting of continuous zeros. The number of zeros chosen may increase with age due to the sporadic and frequent nature of young children's PA. The minimum number of continuous zeros to discount time as not worn is likely to be about 10 min in young children, probably increasing to about 20 min in adolescents.[71] However, protocols vary between studies, and this can have substantial impact on PA and sedentary outcomes.[72,73]

The output from an accelerometer is usually summed over a period, called an epoch. In general, the shortest epoch possible should be used. In children, it is recommended to use an epoch of 1–10 s.[74]

Accelerometer output

Choosing the most accurate and appropriate method for the interpretation of accelerometry data is possibly one of the biggest challenges facing researchers, due to the multitude and variety of published methods.[75] The primary outcome from an accelerometer is acceleration expressed as units of gravity (g, where $1\ g = 9.81\ m \cdot s^{-2}$). However, older versions of accelerometers only provided data expressed in 'counts' or '$counts \cdot min^{-1}$' and therefore the majority of studies express their data in this unit. A 'count' is an arbitrary value that is not comparable between monitor brands and influenced by filtering procedures and the amplitude and frequency of acceleration.[76,77] Activity $counts \cdot min^{-1}$ can be translated into time spent in different intensities (i.e. sedentary, light, moderate, and vigorous intensity) and energy expenditure by using cut-points that are equivalent to different PA intensities. The vast majority of calibration studies conducted to derive energy expenditure prediction equations and intensity cut-points from accelerometer counts have measured oxygen consumption during treadmill walking and running and/or a combination of lifestyle activities performed in the laboratory.[78] However, specific activities performed during a limited time in a laboratory may not accurately reflect all activities performed during free-living and when used in the field, equations derived during flat treadmill activity tend to underestimate PAEE. Therefore, calibration studies have also been performed during free-living activities to be generalizable to the full range of activities encountered in daily life. Nonetheless, the included activities in any calibration study will affect the relationship between accelerometer counts and energy expenditure, which has resulted in a wide variety of published intensity cut-points, affecting the comparability between studies. For example, in youth and for one specific accelerometer, the upper limits for sedentary activities range from 100–1100 $counts \cdot min^{-1}$ [79,80] and the lower cut-points for moderate intensity activity from 615–3581 $counts \cdot min^{-1}$.[80,81] When used in the same population, the diverse cut-points can give substantially different results regarding activity level and estimates of energy expenditure.[82–85] Unfortunately, there is no consensus on which cut-points expressed in counts to use and consequently, the field of accelerometry has been fragmented by inconsistency in data calibration and the conversion of accelerometer raw output into counts.

Novel methods

Advances in technology and memory capacity make it possible for the newest versions of accelerometers to provide their output in raw acceleration data at a high frequency. This allows increased control over data processing and in theory enables comparisons between acceleration data regardless of monitor brands. By increasing the number of acceleration samples per minute, more sophisticated analytical approaches have been applied to several aspects of PA monitoring. This includes identification of different types of PA through machine learning algorithms[86] and the use of neural networks to estimate both type of PA and energy expenditure.[87] However, computational complexity and the need for a large number of annotated examples of activities limit current feasibility of the method, and a repository of available calibration data collected from representative samples is needed to facilitate the development of algorithms that can be applied in population-based studies.

Pedometers

Pedometers are small, lightweight, portable monitors, which can provide an estimate of the number of steps taken, or mileage walked over a period. In general, an electronic pedometer consists of a horizontal spring-suspended lever arm that moves with the vertical acceleration of the hips during ambulation, while newer versions often involve an accelerometer with a horizontal beam and a piezoelectric crystal.[88]

Several studies have systematically examined the use and validity of pedometers PA research with young people.[89–91] The two main advantages of pedometers are an objective measure of step counts and low cost. Correlations between pedometer step counts and oxygen uptake are generally good,[92] and comparative studies of different pedometer brands show good accuracy at faster speeds, generally above 80 $m \cdot min^{-1}$, but less accuracy in capturing steps during low walking speeds.[93] Pedometer data will not necessarily be comparable across different age groups due to insensitivity to gait differences, such as stride length. Other limitations include that the monitors are only able to assess ambulatory activity accurately and do not record horizontal or upper body movement, and they may be susceptible to noise during activities such as cycling or driving on uneven surfaces.

Unlike accelerometers, pedometers usually give an overall estimate of the total number of steps, and can therefore not assess intensity, duration, or frequency of PA. Consequently, pedometers are suitable for measuring and comparing levels of walking in large-scale studies when limitations in resources prevent the use of other more advanced objective methods. Additionally, pedometers can be a successful motivational tool in intervention studies with adolescents.[94,95]

Inclinometers

Inclinometers are small, lightweight, uniaxial accelerometers, normally worn on the anterior mid-line of the thigh, and have recently received increased attention as a suitable assessment method for assessing duration of sedentary time in addition to PA.[96,97] The device uses accelerometer-derived information to assess thigh orientation with respect to gravity to determine time spent in different posture allocation, including lying/sitting, standing, postural changes (sit-to-stand), and PA-related acceleration. The advantages of inclinometers are that they provide a valid and reliable measurement of time spent in different body positions and are usable in all age groups, including young children.[96,97] Limitations of inclinometers include an inability to distinguish between lying and sitting, accurately categorizing postures apart from those standardized (e.g. crawling or kneeling),[98] expensive to use, and an inability to provide contextual information. In addition, postural misclassification of sitting as standing has been reported,[96] possibly explained by the set degree used by the proprietary algorithms to distinguish between the horizontal and vertical position of the thigh.

Heart rate monitoring

Traditional HR monitors are portable and non-restraining devices, generally watches, which display and record HR from a chest-band transmitter. Newer HR monitors have the ability to store minute-by-minute data for over a week while not displaying HR, hence reducing the chance of altered behaviour due to measurement effect. The method relies on the linear relationship between HR and energy expenditure during PA and can predict PAEE or determine time spent physically active, with heartbeats per min above a certain level, both in controlled and free-living settings.[99] Heart rate data have not been anywhere as prolific as the use of movement sensors such as the accelerometer, which is most likely due to the complex individual calibration needed and a higher proportion of missing and erroneous data.

The relationship between HR and energy expenditure is relatively linear during MVPA, but unfortunately not during sedentary and low intensity activities. This is due to differences in stroke volume and factors other than body movements affecting HR without an increase in energy expenditure, including age, emotions, food intake, or medications.[99] In addition, there is a substantial inter-individual variance for the relationship between HR and energy expenditure in terms of slope, intercept, and curve characteristics due to variation in resting HR, stroke volume and cardiorespiratory fitness.[100] To overcome some of these problems individual calibration is generally necessary and traditionally this is derived in a laboratory environment and then applied to predict PAEE in a free-living situation. One common method for individual calibration is the use of a HR FLEX point. Above this threshold, a linear equation is used to estimate energy expenditure from HR data, while below the HR FLEX point, the relationship between HR and energy expenditure is more variable, and the average of several HR values obtained during rest is used for estimating energy expenditure. Compared to DLW and indirect calorimetry, studies in young people show that this method has acceptable accuracy on group level, although not on an individual level.[101,102] Individual calibration in the laboratory is time consuming and may still not be valid to assess free-living PAEE, as the choice of activities in the protocol will affect the accuracy of the prediction. In situations where indirect calorimetry is not feasible as a calibration procedure, step-tests with a standard workload can be used for a simple individual calibration.[103]

Other limitations with this method are the lag of the HR response to bodily movement and prolonged elevation in combination with intermittent activity patterns, which may affect assessment of sporadic free-living PA in young people. Further, the HR data can be affected by electrical interference from household devices or a bad connection with the skin, leading to missing or spurious data. Therefore, in order to avoid large measurement errors, 'cleaning' of

HR data, including the identification of erroneous data points and their subsequent deletion or interpolation, is necessary.[59]

Combined methods

There is an emerging generation of new methods of assessing PA and energy expenditure, often able to measure and combine accelerometry with a physiological parameter using one device. The most common being the combined HR and movement sensors. Accelerometry can accurately assess PA at lower intensities of PA, as it has the ability to determine whether someone is moving or not. However, accelerometers have significant limitations during certain activities, since they can only measure acceleration of the body part they are attached to. Heart rate monitoring is accurate during higher intensities, but has limitations at lower-intensity levels. To improve the accuracy of predicted PAEE from combined movement and HR sensing, branched modelling techniques have been developed to account for the limitations in accuracy of the two methods when used separately. A detailed account of this method is available elsewhere,[104] but briefly, PAEE from separate accelerometry and HR equations are weighted in four different weightings for HR and acceleration, depending on the level of HR and activity counts. The combination of HR and accelerometry has been shown to be more accurate than either method used alone in controlled environments in children.[105] However, free-living studies have shown poorer accuracy in measuring PAEE compared to DLW.[106]

It is logical that combined parameters would capture more variance in activity than one alone. However, the increase in accuracy must be considered in relation to extra costs and feasibility of these new technologies. Currently, the high cost of some of these methods inhibits their use for large-scale epidemiological studies, but they can nevertheless provide very interesting information on body positioning and are useful in clinical populations. Novel methods are now also being used for assessing additional aspects of PA, such as where the PA takes place, and potential environmental determinants of PA, including the use of global positioning systems to map movement, environmental characteristics, and even determinants of PA.[107]

How to choose the right measurement method

Because of the diversity in available methods for the assessment of PA, choosing the most appropriate method for any given study is a complex process. It is generally easier to assess PA in a specific domain with a short time-frame, e.g. school break time PA can quite easily be assessed with direct observation. However, despite the importance of studies carried out in controlled and short-term environments for the improvement and optimization of data collection and analysis techniques, these studies are not often directly applicable to the assessment of habitual PA.

When choosing a method a multitude of factors need to be considered, not only validity, reliability, accuracy, and responsiveness. Several previous reviews have examined this in detail.[6,19,47,74] First, no single method is able to assess all specific dimensions of PA. Therefore, the choice of an appropriate assessment method depends on the research question and the dimensions of PA required for addressing the research question. Other aspects affecting the choice of method include sample size, budget and resources, personnel available, time limitations, special subject characteristics to be considered (e.g. age, cognitive capacity etc.), and participant burden. Unfortunately, there is a negative relationship between the accuracy and the feasibility and ease of use of a method. This relationship is demonstrated in Figure 21.2. However, this is just an illustration of the relationship, which is not necessary linear.

Online toolkits have been developed to aid the choice of the most appropriate assessment method for a specific research question or

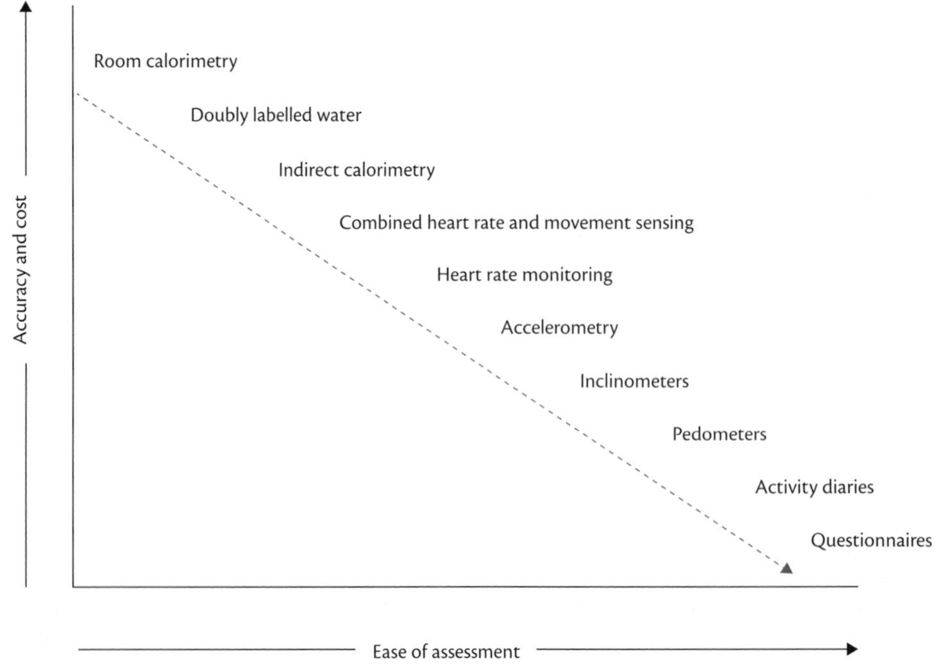

Figure 21.2 The accuracy of an assessment method is inversely associated with the cost and ease of assessment.

study (http://dapa-toolkit.mrc.ac.uk/choosing-a-method/physical-activity/index.php).

Conclusions

Physical activity is a complex human behaviour comprising several dimensions. To be able to understand the relationship between PA and health, accurate assessment methods for PA are essential. Subjective methods are often easy to use and cost-effective. However, they are prone to several limitations and are not able to provide accurate estimates of PAEE or PA intensity. Objective methods provide a reasonably accurate quantification of intensity, frequency, duration, and PAEE. When choosing a method for assessing PA several factors need to be considered, including validity, reliability, accuracy, and responsiveness, as well as the purpose of the study, the population being studied, and the outcome of interest.

Summary

- Physical activity (PA) is a complex human behaviour comprising several dimensions, including intensity, frequency, duration, type/mode, and domain.
- Physical activity outcomes can be divided into two main categories: the estimation of energy expenditure, and other quantifying metrics of PA.
- A reliable method must give the same results under the different conditions in which it is likely used, and it is a requirement for validity.
- Validity refers to the degree the method measures what it is intended to measure, in other words, the accuracy of the method. Accuracy of the PA measurement refers to the degree to which a measurement represents the true value.
- Objective methods, especially accelerometry, are currently the methods with the greatest potential of accurately assessing PA and PAEE in epidemiological PA research.
- Subjective methods are able to assess type of PA, and possibly sports and vigorous activities, to rank PA levels but are not able to give accurate estimates of PAEE or PA intensity.
- Subjective methods are not recommended in preference to an objective method if quantification of intensity, frequency, duration, and PAEE is the primary purpose of the study.
- The validity, reliability, accuracy, and responsiveness of available measurement methods must be carefully considered with regard to the PA variable of interest and the specific population studied.

References

1. Ekelund U, Ward HA, Norat T, *et al.* Physical activity and all-cause mortality across levels of overall and abdominal adiposity in European men and women: the European Prospective Investigation into Cancer and Nutrition Study (EPIC). *Am J Clin Nutr.* 2015; 10: 613–621.
2. Janssen I, LeBlanc AG. Systematic review of the health benefits of physical activity and fitness in school-aged children and youth. *Int J Behav Nutr Phys Act.* 2010; 7: 40.
3. Wareham NJ, Rennie KL. The assessment of physical activity in individuals and populations: why try to be more precise about how physical activity is assessed? *Int J Obes Relat Metab Disord.* 1998; 22(Suppl 2): S30–S38.
4. Hoos MB, Kuipers H, Gerver WJ, Westerterp KR. Physical activity pattern of children assessed by triaxial accelerometry. *Eur J Clin Nutr.* 2004; 58: 1425–1428.
5. Caspersen CJ, Powell KE, Christenson GM. Physical activity, exercise, and physical fitness: definitions and distinctions for health-related research. *Public Health Rep.* 1985; 100: 126–131.
6. Strath SJ, Kaminsky LA, Ainsworth BE, *et al.* Guide to the assessment of physical activity: Clinical and research applications: a scientific statement from the American Heart Association. *Circulation.* 2013; 128: 2259–2279.
7. Sedentary Behaviour Research Network. Letter to the editor: standardized use of the terms 'sedentary' and 'sedentary behaviours'. *Appl Physiol Nutr Metab.* 2012; 37: 540–542.
8. Lubans DR, Hesketh K, Cliff DP, *et al.* A systematic review of the validity and reliability of sedentary behaviour measures used with children and adolescents. *Obes Rev.* 2011; 12: 781–799.
9. Butte NF, Ekelund U, Westerterp KR. Assessing physical activity using wearable monitors: measures of physical activity. *Med Sci Sports Exerc.* 2012; 44(Suppl 1): S5–S12.
10. Westerterp KR. Physical activity and physical activity induced energy expenditure in humans: measurement, determinants, and effects. *Front Physiol.* 2013; 4: 90.
11. Basterfield L, Reilly JK, Pearce MS, *et al.* Longitudinal associations between sports participation, body composition and physical activity from childhood to adolescence. *J Sci Med Sport.* 2015; 18: 178–82.
12. Harding SK, Page AS, Falconer C, Cooper AR. Longitudinal changes in sedentary time and physical activity during adolescence. *Int J Behav Nutr Phys Act.* 2015; 12: 44.
13. Ekelund U, Yngve A, Brage S, Westerterp K, Sjostrom M. Body movement and physical activity energy expenditure in children and adolescents: how to adjust for differences in body size and age. *Am J Clin Nutr.* 2004; 79: 851–856.
14. Ekelund U, Aman J, Yngve A, *et al.* Physical activity but not energy expenditure is reduced in obese adolescents: a case-control study. *Am J Clin Nutr.* 2002; 76: 935–941.
15. McMurray RG, Butte NF, Crouter SE, *et al.* Exploring metrics to express energy expenditure of physical activity in youth. *PLOS One.* 2015; doi: 10.1371/journal.pone.0130869
16. Harrell JS, McMurray RG, Baggett CD, *et al.* Energy costs of physical activities in children and adolescents. *Med Sci Sports Exerc.* 2005; 37: 329–336.
17. Ainsworth BE, Haskell WL, Whitt MC, *et al.* Compendium of physical activities: an update of activity codes and MET intensities. *Med Sci Sports Exerc.* 2000; 32(Suppl): 498–504.
18. Ekelund U, Poortvliet E, Yngve A, *et al.* Heart rate as an indicator of the intensity of physical activity in human adolescents. *Eur J Appl Physiol.* 2001; 85: 244–249.
19. Hardy LL, Hills AP, Timperio A, *et al.* A hitchhiker's guide to assessing sedentary behaviour among young people: deciding what method to use. *J Sci Med Sport.* 2013; 16: 28–35.
20. Warburton DE, Charlesworth S, Ivey A, Nettlefold L, Bredin SS. A systematic review of the evidence for Canada's Physical Activity Guidelines for Adults. *Int J Behav Nutr Phys Act.* 2010; 7: 39.
21. Anderssen SA, Hansen BH, Kolle E, *et al.* Fysisk aktivitet blant voksne og eldre i Norge. Resultater fra en kartlegging i 2008 og 2009. Oslo: Helsedirektoratet; 2009.
22. Cooper AR, Goodman A, Page AS, *et al.* Objectively measured physical activity and sedentary time in youth: the International children's accelerometry database (ICAD). *Int J Behav Nutr Phys Act.* 2015; 12: 113.
23. Verloigne M, Van Lippewelde W, Maes L, *et al.* Levels of physical activity and sedentary time among 10- to 12-year-old boys and girls across 5 European countries using accelerometers: an observational study within the ENERGY-project. *Int J Behav Nutr Phys Act.* 2012; 9: 34.

24. Ekelund U, Luan J, Sherar LB, *et al.* Moderate to vigorous physical activity and sedentary time and cardiometabolic risk factors in children and adolescents. *JAMA*. 2012; 30: 704–712.
25. Katzmarzyk PT, Barreira TV, Broyles ST, *et al.* Physical activity, sedentary time, and obesity in an international sample of children. *Med Sci Sports Exerc.* 2015; 47: 2062–2069.
26. Thomas JR, Nelson JK, Silverman SJ. *Research methods in physical activity*, 6th ed. Champaign, IL: Human Kinetics; 2011.
27. Atkinson G, Nevill AM. Statistical methods for assessing measurement error (reliability) in variables relevant to sports medicine. *Sports Med.* 1998; 26: 217–238.
28. Scott JJ, Morgan PJ, Plotnikoff RC, Lubans DR. Reliability and validity of a single-item physical activity measure for adolescents. *J Paediatr Child Health.* 2015; 51: 787–793.
29. Rich C, Griffiths LJ, Dezateux C. Seasonal variation in accelerometer-determined sedentary behaviour and physical activity in children: a review. *Int J Behav Nutr Phys Act.* 2012; 9: 49.
30. Lee JA, Williams SM, Brown DD, Laurson KR. Concurrent validation of the Actigraph gt3x +, Polar Active accelerometer, Omron HJ-720 and Yamax Digiwalker SW-701 pedometer step counts in lab-based and free-living settings. *J Sports Sci.* 2015; 33: 991–1000.
31. Macfarlane DJ, Lee CC, Ho EY, Chan KL, Chan D. Convergent validity of six methods to assess physical activity in daily life. *J Appl Physiol.* 2006; 101: 1328–1334.
32. Bland JM, Altman DG. Applying the right statistics: analyses of measurement studies. *Ultrasound Obstet Gynecol.* 2003; 22: 85–93.
33. Lifson N, Gordon GB, McClintock R. Measurement of total carbon dioxide production by means of D2O18. *J Appl Physiol.* 1955; 7: 704–710.
34. Schoeller DA, van Santen E. Measurement of energy expenditure in humans by doubly labeled water method. *J Appl Physiol Respir Environ Exerc Physiol.* 1982; 53: 955–959.
35. Park J, Kazuko IT, Kim E, Kim J, Yoon J. Estimating free-living human energy expenditure: Practical aspects of the doubly labeled water method and its applications. *Nutr Res Pract.* 2014; 8: 241–248.
36. Murgatroyd PR, Shetty PS, Prentice AM. Techniques for the measurement of human energy expenditure: a practical guide. *Int J Obes Relat Metab Disord.* 1993; 17: 549–568.
37. Levine JA. Measurement of energy expenditure. *Public Health Nutr.* 2005; 8: 1123–1132.
38. Butte NF, Wong WW, Hopkinson JM, *et al.* Energy requirements derived from total energy expenditure and energy deposition during the first 2 years of life. *Am J Clin Nutr.* 2000; 72: 1558–1569.
39. Janssen X, Cliff DP, Reilly JJ, *et al.* Validation and calibration of the activPAL for estimating METs and physical activity in 4–6 year olds. *J Sci Med Sport.* 2014; 17: 602–606.
40. Ekblom O, Nyberg G, Bak EE, Ekelund U, Marcus C. Validity and comparability of a wrist-worn accelerometer in children. *J Phys Act Health.* 2012; 9: 389–393.
41. Pate RR, Almeida MJ, McIver KL, Pfeiffer KA, Dowda M. Validation and calibration of an accelerometer in preschool children. *Obesity (Silver Spring).* 2006; 14: 2000–2006.
42. Sirard JR, Pate RR. Physical activity assessment in children and adolescents. *Sports Med.* 2001; 31: 439–454.
43. Oliver M, Schofield GM, Kolt GS. Physical activity in preschoolers: understanding prevalence and measurement issues. *Sports Med.* 2007; 37: 1045–1070.
44. Lyden K, Petruski N, Mix S, Staudenmayer J, Freedson P. Direct observation is a valid criterion for estimating physical activity and sedentary behavior. *J Phys Act Health.* 2014; 11: 860–863.
45. Warren JM, Ekelund U, Besson H, *et al.* Assessment of physical activity—a review of methodologies with reference to epidemiological research: a report of the exercise physiology section of the European Association of Cardiovascular Prevention and Rehabilitation. *Eur J Cardiovasc Prev Rehabil.* 2010; 17: 127–139.
46. Milton K, Clemes S, Bull F. Can a single question provide an accurate measure of physical activity? *Br J Sports Med.* 2013; 47: 44–48.
47. Chinapaw MJ, Mokkink LB, van Poppel MN, van Mechelen W, Terwee CB. Physical activity questionnaires for youth: a systematic review of measurement properties. *Sports Med.* 2010; 40: 539–563.
48. Celis-Morales CA, Perez-Bravo F, Ibanez L, *et al.* Objective vs. self-reported physical activity and sedentary time: effects of measurement method on relationships with risk biomarkers. *PLOS One.* 2012; doi: 10.1371/journal.pone.0036345
49. Sallis JF, Saelens BE. Assessment of physical activity by self-report: status, limitations, and future directions. *Res Q Exerc Sport.* 2000; 71(2 Suppl): S1–S14.
50. Tudor-Locke CE, Myers AM. Challenges and opportunities for measuring physical activity in sedentary adults. *Sports Med.* 2001; 31: 91–100.
51. Bringolf-Isler B, Mader U, Ruch N, *et al.* Measuring and validating physical activity and sedentary behavior comparing a parental questionnaire to accelerometer data and diaries. *Pediatr Exerc Sci.* 2012; 24: 229–245.
52. Ridley K, Ainsworth BE, Olds TS. Development of a compendium of energy expenditures for youth. *Int J Behav Nutr Phys Act.* 2008; 5: 45.
53. Marszalek J, Morgulec-Adamowicz N, Rutkowska I, Kosmol A. Using ecological momentary assessment to evaluate current physical activity. *Biomed Res Int.* 2014; 2014: 915172.
54. Dunton GF, Liao Y, Intille SS, Spruijt-Metz D, Pentz M. Investigating children's physical activity and sedentary behavior using ecological momentary assessment with mobile phones. *Obesity (Silver Spring).* 2011; 19: 1205–1212.
55. Machado-Rodrigues AM, Figueiredo AJ, Mota J, *et al.* Concurrent validation of estimated activity energy expenditure using a 3-day diary and accelerometry in adolescents. *Scand J Med Sci Sports.* 2012; 22: 259–264.
56. Wickel EE, Welk GJ, Eisenmann JC. Concurrent validation of the Bouchard Diary with an accelerometry-based monitor. *Med Sci Sports Exerc.* 2006; 38: 373–379.
57. Bratteby LE, Sandhagen B, Fan H, Samuelson G. A 7-day activity diary for assessment of daily energy expenditure validated by the doubly labelled water method in adolescents. *Eur J Clin Nutr.* 1997; 51: 585–591.
58. Kavanagh JJ, Menz HB. Accelerometry: a technique for quantifying movement patterns during walking. *Gait Posture.* 2008; 28: 1–15.
59. Corder K, Ekelund U, Steele RM, Wareham NJ, Brage S. Assessment of physical activity in youth. *J Appl Physiol.* 2008; 105: 977–987.
60. Chen KY, Bassett DR, Jr. The technology of accelerometry-based activity monitors: current and future. *Med Sci Sports Exerc.* 2005; 37(11 Suppl): S490–S500.
61. John D, Freedson P. ActiGraph and Actical physical activity monitors: a peek under the hood. *Med Sci Sports Exerc.* 2012; 44(1 Suppl 1): S86–S89.
62. Matthews CE, Hagstromer M, Pober DM, Bowles HR. Best practices for using physical activity monitors in population-based research. *Med Sci Sports Exerc.* 2012; 44(Suppl 1): S68–S76.
63. Phillips LR, Parfitt G, Rowlands AV. Calibration of the GENEA accelerometer for assessment of physical activity intensity in children. *J Sci Med Sport.* 2013; 16: 124–128.
64. Plasqui G, Bonomi AG, Westerterp KR. Daily physical activity assessment with accelerometers: new insights and validation studies. *Obes Rev.* 2013; 14: 451–462.
65. Plasqui G, Westerterp KR. Physical activity assessment with accelerometers: an evaluation against doubly labeled water. *Obesity (Silver Spring).* 2007; 15: 2371–2379.
66. Routen AC, Upton D, Edwards MG, Peters DM. Discrepancies in accelerometer-measured physical activity in children due to cut-point non-equivalence and placement site. *J Sports Sci.* 2012; 30: 1303–1310.
67. Hildebrand M, van Hees VT, Hansen BH, Ekelund U. Age-group comparability of raw accelerometer output from wrist- and hip-worn monitors. *Med Sci Sports Exerc.* 2014; 46: 1816–1824.
68. Cain KL, Sallis JF, Conway TL, Van DD, Calhoon L. Using accelerometers in youth physical activity studies: a review of methods. *J Phys Act Health.* 2013; 10: 437–450.

69. Byun W, Beets MW, Pate RR. Sedentary behavior in preschoolers: how many days of accelerometer monitoring is needed? *Int J Environ Res Public Health*. 2015; 12: 13148–13161.
70. Comte M, Hobin E, Majumdar SR, *et al*. Patterns of weekday and weekend physical activity in youth in 2 Canadian provinces. *Appl Physiol Nutr Metab*. 2013; 38: 115–119.
71. Janssen X, Basterfield L, Parkinson KN, *et al*. Objective measurement of sedentary behavior: impact of non-wear time rules on changes in sedentary time. *BMC Public Health*. 2015;15: 504.
72. Chinapaw MJ, de Niet M, Verloigne M, *et al*. From sedentary time to sedentary patterns: accelerometer data reduction decisions in youth. *PLoS One*. 2014; 9: e111205. doi: 10.1371/journal.pone.0111205
73. Toftager M, Kristensen PL, Oliver M, *et al*. Accelerometer data reduction in adolescents: effects on sample retention and bias. *Int J Behav Nutr Phys Act*. 2013; 10: 140.
74. Rowlands AV. Accelerometer assessment of physical activity in children: an update. *Pediatr Exerc Sci*. 2007; 19: 252–266.
75. Kim Y, Beets MW, Welk GJ. Everything you wanted to know about selecting the 'right' Actigraph accelerometer cut-points for youth, but ... : a systematic review. *J Sci Med Sport*. 2012; 15: 311–321.
76. Matthew CE. Calibration of accelerometer output for adults. *Med Sci Sports Exerc*. 2005; 37(11 Suppl): S512–S522.
77. Reilly JJ, Penpraze V, Hislop J, *et al*. Objective measurement of physical activity and sedentary behaviour: review with new data. *Arch Dis Child*. 2008; 93: 614–619.
78. Welk GJ. Principles of design and analyses for the calibration of accelerometry-based activity monitors. *Med Sci Sports Exerc*. 2005; 37(11 Suppl): S501–S511.
79. Treuth MS, Schmitz K, Catellier DJ, *et al*. Defining accelerometer thresholds for activity intensities in adolescent girls. *Med Sci Sports Exerc*. 2004; 36: 1259–1266.
80. Puyau MR, Adolph AL, Vohra FA, Zakeri I, Butte NF. Prediction of activity energy expenditure using accelerometers in children. *Med Sci Sports Exerc*. 2004; 36: 1625–1631.
81. Mattocks C, Leary S, Ness A, *et al*. Calibration of an accelerometer during free-living activities in children. *Int J Pediatr Obes*. 2007; 2: 218–226.
82. Lyden K, Kozey SL, Staudenmeyer JW, Freedson PS. A comprehensive evaluation of commonly used accelerometer energy expenditure and MET prediction equations. *Eur J Appl Physiol*. 2011; 111: 187–201.
83. van Cauwenberghe E, Labarque V, Trost SG, De Bourdeaudhuij I, Cardon G. Calibration and comparison of accelerometer cut points in preschool children. *Int J Pediatr Obes*. 2011; 6: e582–e589.
84. Trost SG, Loprinzi PD, Moore R, Pfeiffer KA. Comparison of accelerometer cut points for predicting activity intensity in youth. *Med Sci Sports Exerc*. 2011; 43: 1360–1368.
85. Alhassan S, Lyden K, Howe C, *et al*. Accuracy of accelerometer regression models in predicting energy expenditure and METs in children and youth. *Pediatr Exerc Sci*. 2012; 24: 519–536.
86. Ellis K, Kerr J, Godbole S, Staudenmayer J, Lanckriet G. Hip and Wrist Accelerometer Algorithms for Free-Living Behavior Classification. *Med Sci Sports Exerc*. 2016; 48: 937–940.
87. Trost SG, Wong WK, Pfeiffer KA, Zheng Y. Artificial neural networks to predict activity type and energy expenditure in youth. *Med Sci Sports Exerc*. 2012; 44: 1801–1809.
88. Schneider PL, Crouter S, Bassett DR. Pedometer measures of free-living physical activity: comparison of 13 models. *Med Sci Sports Exerc*. 2004; 36: 331–335.
89. Beets MW, Morgan CF, Banda JA, *et al*. Convergent validity of pedometer and accelerometer estimates of moderate-to-vigorous physical activity of youth. *J Phys Act Health*. 2011; 8 (Suppl 2): S295–S305.
90. Clemes SA, Biddle SJ. The use of pedometers for monitoring physical activity in children and adolescents: measurement considerations. *J Phys Act Health*. 2013; 10: 249–262.
91. Tudor-Locke C, McClain JJ, Hart TL, Sisson SB, Washington TL. Pedometry methods for assessing free-living youth. *Res Q Exerc Sport*. 2009; 80: 175–184.
92. Saunders TJ, Gray CE, Borghese MM, *et al*. Validity of SC-StepRx pedometer-derived moderate and vigorous physical activity during treadmill walking and running in a heterogeneous sample of children and youth. *BMC Public Health*. 2014; 14: 519.
93. Beets MW, Patton MM, Edwards S. The accuracy of pedometer steps and time during walking in children. *Med Sci Sports Exerc*. 2005; 37: 513–520.
94. Lee LL, Kuo YC, Fanaw D, Perng SJ, Juang IF. The effect of an intervention combining self-efficacy theory and pedometers on promoting physical activity among adolescents. *J Clin Nurs*. 2012; 21: 914–922.
95. Lubans DR, Morgan PJ, Tudor-Locke C. A systematic review of studies using pedometers to promote physical activity among youth. *Prev Med*. 2009; 48: 307–315.
96. Davies G, Reilly JJ, McGowan AJ, *et al*. Validity, practical utility, and reliability of the activPAL in preschool children. *Med Sci Sports Exerc*. 2012; 44: 761–768.
97. Dowd KP, Harrington DM, Donnelly AE. Criterion and concurrent validity of the activPAL professional physical activity monitor in adolescent females. *PLOS One*. 2012; 7: e47633.
98. Janssen X, Cliff DP, Reilly JJ, *et al*. Validation of activPAL defined sedentary time and breaks in sedentary time in 4- to 6-year-olds. *Pediatr Exerc Sci*. 2014; 26: 110–117.
99. Shephard RJ, Aoyagi Y. Measurement of human energy expenditure, with particular reference to field studies: an historical perspective. *Eur J Appl Physiol*. 2012; 112: 2785–2815.
100. Leonard WR. Measuring human energy expenditure: what have we learned from the flex-heart rate method? *Am J Hum Biol*. 2003; 15: 479–489.
101. Emons HJ, Groenenboom DC, Westerterp KR, Saris WH. Comparison of heart rate monitoring combined with indirect calorimetry and the doubly labelled water ($2H_2{}^{18}O$) method for the measurement of energy expenditure in children. *Eur J Appl Physiol Occup Physiol*. 1992; 65: 99–103.
102. Livingstone MB, Coward WA, Prentice AM, *et al*. Daily energy expenditure in free-living children: comparison of heart-rate monitoring with the doubly labeled water ($2H_2{}^{18}O$) method. *Am J Clin Nutr*. 1992; 56: 343–352.
103. Brage S, Ekelund U, Brage N, *et al*. Hierarchy of individual calibration levels for heart rate and accelerometry to measure physical activity. *J Appl Physiol*. 2007; 103: 682–692.
104. Brage S, Brage N, Franks PW, *et al*. Branched equation modeling of simultaneous accelerometry and heart rate monitoring improves estimate of directly measured physical activity energy expenditure. *J Appl Physiol*. 2004; 96: 343–351.
105. Corder K, Brage S, Wareham NJ, Ekelund U. Comparison of PAEE from combined and separate heart rate and movement models in children. *Med Sci Sports Exerc*. 2005; 37: 1761–1767.
106. Campbell N, Prapavessis H, Gray C, *et al*. The Actiheart in adolescents: a doubly labelled water validation. *Pediatr Exerc Sci*. 2012; 24: 589–602.
107. Burgi R, Tomatis L, Murer K, de Bruin ED. Localization of physical activity in primary school children using accelerometry and global positionings. *PLOS One*. 2015; 10: e0142223.

CHAPTER 22

Systematic promotion of physical activity

Stef Kremers, Ree M Meertens, and Robert AC Ruiter

Introduction

It is widely acknowledged that physical activity (PA) has a positive impact on the physiological and psychological health of young people. This leads us to consider the question of how we can promote such a lifestyle. This chapter presents a general approach for the theory- and evidence-based development of health promotion interventions. We illustrate this approach with examples concerning the promotion of PA among young people.

Planned health promotion

Promoting a healthy lifestyle can be challenging. At first glance, prescribing lifestyle changes seems only to require informing or educating those who need to change about the benefits of physical activity on health and well-being. However, despite the fact that most people understand this in principle, they may perceive exercise as unenjoyable or too expensive, there may be barriers to exercise (e.g. lack of time, distance to the gym), and work and family environments may not be supportive of a physically active lifestyle. Therefore, a broad approach is needed to support these lifestyle changes, and regulations and policies may be needed to make these changes easier. In addition to information, people need motivation and social support to change their lifestyles. This kind of broad approach is known as 'health promotion'.

Health promotion is defined as 'any planned combination of educational, political, regulatory, and organisational supports for actions and conditions of living conducive to the health of individuals, groups, or communities'.[1] Health promotion objectives are i) primary prevention, ii) early detection and treatment (secondary prevention), and iii) patient care and support (tertiary prevention). Health promotion strategies include i) legislation and regulations designed to enforce behaviour change, ii) the provision of non-compulsory services, and iii) education that focuses on encouraging and helping people to change their behaviour of their own accord. Generally, health promotion is most effective when it involves several mutually reinforcing strategies, and when it affects different levels of society.[2,3]

When developing health promotion programmes, the objectives, target population, intervention methods and applications, useful media, etc., must all be identified. Importantly, these decisions cannot be made without careful analysis of the health problem, the behavioural and environmental factors affecting this problem, and the options for intervention and behaviour change. Without a planned and systematic approach, there is a risk of addressing a health problem that is not relevant, or developing an intervention that addresses irrelevant factors or target groups. Figure 22.1 depicts a general planning and evaluation model for the development of health promotion programmes.[1,4]

The first phase in the planning process addresses the social and epidemiological diagnosis of the health problem. This phase should make clear whether the health problem is linked to individual and social perceptions of quality of life, whether the assumed problem has serious individual and social consequences, and whether it relates to other health problems. This phase should also reveal which people or institutions are involved.

The second planning phase includes the diagnosis of the behavioural, social, and environmental factors that are linked to the health problem of interest. This phase should reveal whether the health problem is linked to specific behaviours, and if it is, to whose behaviours. This phase should also make clear whether reduction of the health problem needs an environmental change, and if so, the decision-makers who are responsible for environmental change should be identified.

The third phase of the model examines the determinants of the behavioural and environmental conditions that are linked to health status or quality-of-life concerns. It also identifies the factors that must be changed to initiate and sustain the process of behavioural and environmental change. There are three categories of factors that apply to individual behaviour. Predisposing factors also apply, and this refers to cognitive antecedents that provide a rationale or motivation for behaviour (e.g. knowledge, attitudes, values, and goal priorities). Enabling factors, i.e. factors that can facilitate or hinder the desired behaviours, as well as environmental changes (e.g. skills, financial and human resources, cultural barriers) must also be taken into consideration. Lastly, reinforcing factors, which, following a behaviour, enhance its persistence or repetition (e.g. availability of resources, social approval, rules, or laws) must also be acknowledged.

The fourth phase, intervention development, addresses the analysis of the possible usefulness of (components of) health promotion and other potential interventions (resources, regulations). This phase may include i) the assessment of the usefulness of current health promotion interventions, ii) the development and small-scale evaluation of new interventions or intervention components,

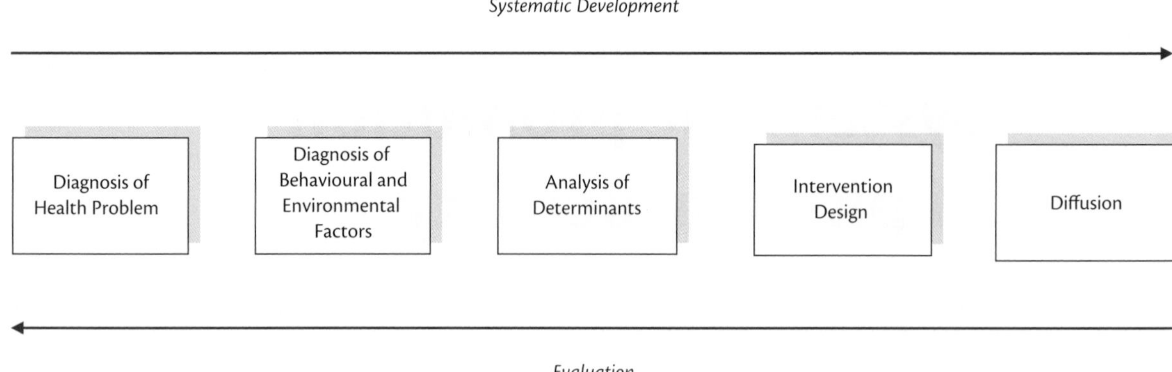

Figure 22.1 Evidence-based development of health promotion.

and iii) a diagnosis of the political, regulatory, and organizational factors that may facilitate or hinder the development and widespread implementation of a health promotion intervention.

The fifth planning phase addresses the diffusion of an intervention programme. This phase includes the diagnosis of the factors that are linked to the adoption, actual implementation, and institutionalization of a health promotion programme, and the launching of activities to enhance widespread programme diffusion. It is important to take the (im)possibilities of the future diffusion process into account in the development of the health promotion programme, as otherwise there is the risk of developing a programme that will never be used on a large scale.

Subsequent phases of the model all refer to the evaluation of the process, impact, and outcomes of the health promotion programme, resulting in feedback and adjustment. The core evaluation question—whether a programme results in a reduction of the health problem—often cannot be answered because of a delay between behaviour change and observable effects on health status (e.g. PA and cardiovascular diseases). Generally, a change of behaviour is the best possible indication of the effectiveness of health promotion programmes.[5] The next section discusses each of the phases in theory- and evidence-based development of health promotion interventions to increase PA amongst children and adolescents.

Health promotion and physical activity

Problems and problem-causing factors

Premature death is strongly related to chronic diseases such as heart disease, cancers, stroke, and diabetes. Lifestyle factors like smoking, alcohol abuse, improper diet, and physical inactivity all play an important role in the aetiology of these chronic diseases. Epidemiological studies have demonstrated that, together with smoking, physical inactivity is the most important independent risk factor for the leading causes of death in Western society.[6,7] Consequently, it is generally accepted that a physically active lifestyle has enormous direct and indirect health advantages for both adults and adolescents.[8–12] Individual and populational public health status will both benefit from a physically active lifestyle. Estimates by Lee and colleagues[7] showed that worldwide, physical inactivity causes 6% of the burden of disease from coronary heart disease, 7% of type 2 diabetes, 10% of breast cancer, and 10% of colon cancer. Inactivity causes 9% of premature mortality. If inactivity was decreased by 10%, more than 533 000 deaths could be averted every year.

Young children seem to have a naturally physically active lifestyle. They play, jump, cycle, and run throughout the day. When they grow older, most children in Western society participate in school-based physical education, organized sports, and leisure time activities in which they are physically active.

Although young people seem to be fairly physically active, many in Western society gradually develop an inactive lifestyle during secondary school years, partly because of a combination of daily activities such as homework, screen time, part-time jobs, and social events.[13–16] According to the Health Behaviour in School Aged Children survey data from 41 countries and regions across North America and Europe, less than half of the youth population currently meet the recommended daily 60 min of moderate- to vigorous-intensity physical activity (MVPA).[17] Boys consistently report higher levels of PA than girls and PA tends to decline with increasing age.

Childhood sedentary behaviour plays a specific role in the current obesity epidemic.[18–20] Parallel increases in the time spent participating in sedentary behaviours and the increase of obesity suggest a causal relation between the two,[21] and some prospective studies in children have shown positive relationships.[22–24] Screen-viewing behaviour,[25] including television viewing[26–28] and computer use,[29,30] has been identified as key sedentary behaviour in this age group.[31] Most European youngsters spend approximately 3–4 h on screen-viewing each day, with boys spending approximately 0.5 $h \cdot day^{-1}$ more on screen-viewing than girls.[32]

Determinants of physical activity

Theory

An analysis of cognitive determinants of behaviour illustrates the differences between young people's exercise behaviour. Various traditional social-psychological models predicting goal-oriented behaviour can be applied to health-related behaviours. Although these models include a broad range of variables, there are four general categories of core cognitive antecedents of health behaviours:[33,34]

i) *Attitude*: beliefs and evaluations about advantages and disadvantages (e.g. health risks) of behaviour; also referred to as outcome expectations, resulting in an overall evaluation of a specific health behaviour.

ii) *Perceived social influences*: injunctive social norms (i.e. perceptions of which behaviors are typically approved or disapproved), descriptive social norms (i.e. behaviours based on mimicking what others actually do), and perceived direct social pressures (i.e. perceptions of direct social sanctions and rewards for behaviour).

iii) *Self-efficacy*: perceptions of one's own capability to successfully perform a particular behaviour; also referred to as perceived behavioural control.

iv) *Preparation for action*: how people are able, or are prompted to plan how, to enact their intentions amidst competing everyday priorities.

The four types of cognitions follow from theoretical approaches, such as the Theory of Planned Behavior,[35] that have defined motivation as a linear quantitative construct. It can be expressed on a continuum from very low to very high. In the last decade, however, an increasing number of studies have shown that it is more the quality of motivation, rather than the quantity of motivation, that predicts engagement in (and maintenance of) PA.[36] Such studies typically draw from the tenets of the self-determination theory (SDT)[37,38] as a theoretical framework. Self-Determination Theory proposes that the regulation of human behaviour can either be autonomous, controlled, or amotivated. On a decreasing motivational quality scale from self-determined (autonomous) to extrinsically controlled, the categories are intrinsic regulation, integrated regulation, identified regulation, introjected regulation, and external regulation. Intrinsic regulation can be seen as the most desirable and self-determined (autonomous) type of motivation. Applied to child PA, intrinsic motivation occurs if a child engages in PA for the fun and inherent pleasure it provides. Integrated regulation is a form of controlled motivation, and describes when PA is controlled by outcomes other than personal enjoyment (e.g. health benefits). Integrated regulation activity is still autonomous motivation, however, and is considered to be related to important personal norms and values. Identified regulation occurs when a child believes that putting an effort into PA will lead to a certain personally valued outcome, such as health benefits or feeling more fit. Introjected regulation occurs if a child imposes an external pressure on to himself, for example, by taking part in physical education classes to avoid feelings of guilt. Extrinsic regulation of PA takes place when a child engages in the behaviour because of external rewards or punishment that are perceived to be linked to the behaviour. Amotivation is a state in which motivation is absent and a person lacks any intention to show the desired behaviour.[38] Approaching the study of determinants of PA in young people from a self-determination point of view has improved our understanding of the main cognitive drivers of PA.[39–46]

In addition to the cognitive factors that determine motivation to participate in PA, environmental influences can be especially relevant to children and adolescents because their behavioural choices are less autonomous.[47] Specific recommendations for research on the determinants of PA in youth have emphasized the need to examine environmental influences at different levels (e.g. home, neighbourhood, school)[48,49] to better inform the development of interventions attempting to improve youth PA levels.[50,51]

Different classifications of possible environmental determinants of health behaviours have been proposed,[52–56] all of them showing great overlap and similarities. A conceptual framework that is frequently used is the ANalysis Grid for Environments Linked to Obesity (ANGELO).[57] This framework was specifically developed to conceptualize 'obesogenic' environments (i.e. environments that promote excessive energy intake and low levels of PA), enabling the identification of specific areas and settings to be targeted by intervention programmes. The ANGELO framework divides the variety in types of environmental determinants into four distinct types of influence: physical (what is available), economic (what are the costs), political (what are the rules), and sociocultural (what is the social and cultural background). In addition, two levels of influence are distinguished: micro-environmental settings and macro-environmental sectors. Individuals interact with the environment in multiple micro-environmental settings, including schools, workplaces, homes, and neighbourhoods, which are, in turn, influenced by broader macro-environments, including health systems, governments, and the food industry. When types and levels of environment are crossed, a grid is formed that comprises four types of environment on one axis and two sizes of environment on the other.

The Environmental Research framework for weight gain prevention (EnRG)

It has been suggested that an integrated approach to the study of determinants of PA, in which social-psychological models are combined with ecological models of health behaviour, would improve our knowledge regarding the causal mechanisms that underlie behaviour.[58] The Environmental Research framework for weight Gain prevention (EnRG) (Figure 22.2) is an example of such an integrated framework that describes how environmental influences impact on individual behaviour. Three main propositions from the model refer to i) dual-processes, ii) person-environment interactions, and iii) interactions between types and levels of environmental influences.

Dual processes

In the EnRG framework, environmental influences (as defined in ANGELO) are hypothesized to affect dietary intake and PA both indirectly and directly, reflecting the dual-process view. The indirect causal mechanism reflects the mediating role of intrapersonal behaviour-specific cognitions and the direct influence reflects the automatic, unconscious, influence of the environment on behaviour. For example, the friends of a certain child may be willing to go out and play on a sunny day. The child's perception of his friends' plans and the likelihood that they would want him to play along (subjective norm) may determine the child's intention to play outside. This intention could, in turn, predict actual outside play on this particular occasion. This process, where the child's cognitive energy used in considering PA reflects cognitive mediation of environmental influences, is an example of an indirect environment-behaviour route. Seeing his/her friends play outside may however also evoke automatic responses in the child. A child may immediately respond to seeing friends by going outside, without spending cognitive energy on it. In this case, friends playing outside serve as an environmental cue that leads to relatively immediate and automatic responses.

Person-environment interactions

The EnRG hypothesizes that intrapersonal factors interact with the environment in order to determine its obesogenicity. To gain more insight into environment-behaviour relations, it is essential to explore the more complex interactions involved in the mechanisms

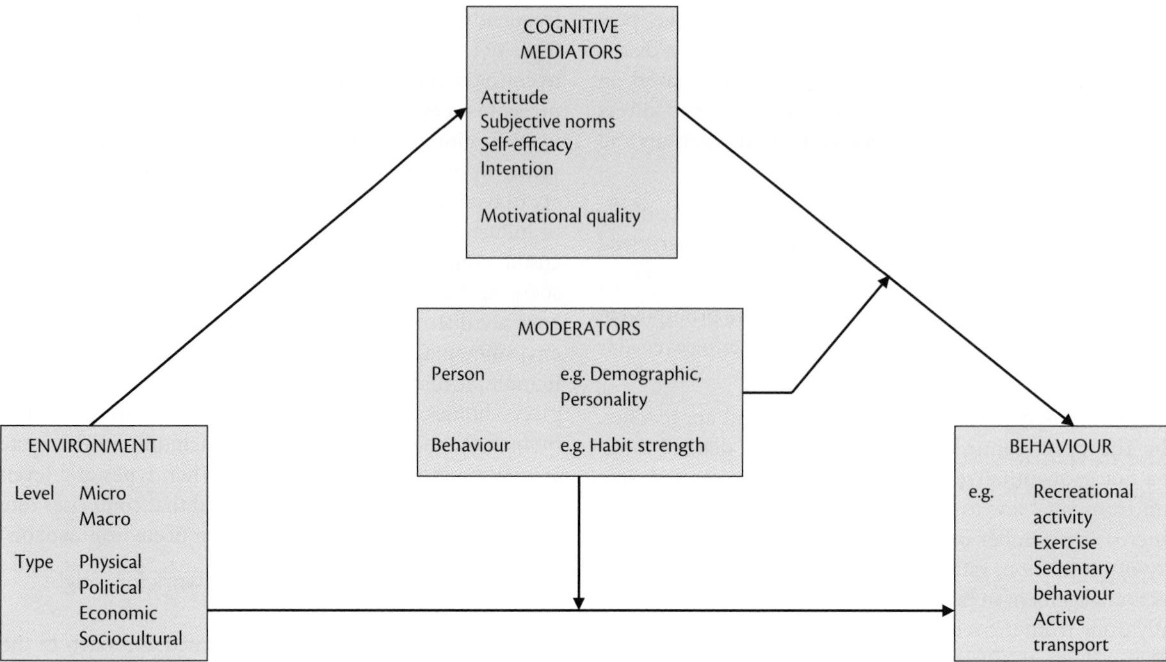

Figure 22.2 Environmental and cognitive determinants of physical activity.
Adapted from Kremers SPJ, De Bruijn GJ, Visscher TLS, Van Mechelen W, De Vries NK, Brug J. Environmental influences on energy balance-related behaviors: A dual-process view. Int J Behav Nutr Phys Act. 2006: 3; 9; and Kremers SP. Theory and practice in the study of influences on energy balance-related behaviors. Patient Educ Couns. 2010; 79: 291–298.

underlying behavioural decision making. Distinct types of personal factors (e.g. demographic factors, personality, and habit strength) are postulated to moderate the causal path from environment to behaviour (i.e. inducing either the automatic or the cognitively mediated environment-behaviour relation). Habit strength might be a very important concept in this respect. Once learned, a child's walking, running, and jumping would seem to be unconscious behaviours.[59] In line with this observation, Triandis[60] posited that deliberate decisions to act become irrelevant in guiding behaviour when the behaviour has been performed repeatedly in the past. Repeated behaviours may be largely determined by habit rather than by reasoned action. When habits are formed, subsequent behaviour is associated with, and automatically triggered by, specific environmental cues that normally precede the action.[59] In the example of the child playing with his/her friends, he/she may thus be more likely to respond in an automatic, direct way to friends playing outside when the behaviour occurs often. The first time friends were observed at play, the child is likely to have put cognitive energy into the decision to join them. But when the process has been repeated multiple times, with satisfactory consequences, habit strength has increased and the process becomes more automatic.

Interactions between types and levels of environmental influences

A third important proposition of EnRG is the possibility of interactions between types and levels of environmental influences. Behaviour cannot be viewed in isolation, but rather takes place at different ecological levels, and it is the combined influence of these ecological levels that determines individual decision making, forming a complex system.[34] This is in line with an ecological 'systems' view of environmental influences on human behaviour.[61,62] Ecological models propose an interaction between the environment and the individual, as well as interaction between elements within the environment.[63,64] Conceptually, this means environmental influences on PA cannot be generalized, but are person- and situation-specific.[65]

Childcare and similar facilities (e.g. pre-school, kindergarten, day care) could play an important role in promoting PA.[66] An example of an environmental determinant of PA at childcare is childcare staff behaviour, which has been found to be important for shaping children's PA level.[67] Increased PA has further been linked to for instance the availability of play equipment and PA opportunities,[68,69] a 'natural' environment,[70] smaller group size,[71,72] child-initiated instead of staff-initiated play,[72] and prompts by peers.[67] Although the interaction between types of environment has been proposed in ecological models of human development, it has rarely been examined in the field of PA in children. Gubbels *et al.*[67] examined the influence of social and physical environmental factors on PA at childcare, and whether there was an interaction between both. Moderation analyses showed that the positive influence of activity opportunities (physical environment) on outdoor PA was only present when children were engaged in an activity together with multiple peers (social environment). Children playing alone or with one other child seemed unaffected by the presence of activity opportunities. Among older children, a study of the influence of the neighbourhood environment on PA showed that among children with parents with high responsibility towards their child's PA, functionality of the neighbourhood was related to more outside play; however, this was not the case in children with parents with low responsibility towards their child's PA level.[73]

The EnRG hypothesizes higher-order moderation processes,[34,58] thus implying that factors at higher, more distal levels can moderate the impact of factors at a lower level.[62] As a result, a factor at a higher level forms the context in which proximal parenting processes operate. For example, in the home environment, the emotional climate in which a child is raised (the parenting style of the parents) may thus function as a contextual higher-order moderator of the impact of PA-specific parenting practices, such as setting rules regarding television and computer screen time. There is some early evidence regarding the relationship between general parenting styles and specific parenting practices from the field of research on child dietary behaviour[74,75] and weight,[76] but this kind of evidence is lacking to date for PA. The studies mentioned provide some evidence that general parenting style sets the context in which specific parenting practices are performed, but evidence is needed from the field of PA in order to optimally inform intervention development.

Systematic development of physical activity-promoting interventions

Theory

The phase following the need assessment addresses the development of a health promotion programme. In this stage insights from theory and research have to be translated into methods and strategies. A shift must be made from *explaining* behaviour to *changing* behaviour. There is no such thing as a *magic bullet*: no intervention method is universally effective.[77] Intervention programmes have to be tailored very carefully to the behaviour, behavioural determinants, and target population(s). The process of intervention design includes several steps,[78] in which the Intervention Mapping protocol[79] has proven to be a helpful tool (Figure 22.3).

Intervention Mapping (IM) is a systematic process that explicates a series of six steps for the development of health promotion programmes based on theory, empirical evidence, and additional research. The steps are followed in an iterative way, i.e. programme planners are moving back and forth throughout the process. Intervention Mapping enables health promoters to create feasible and effective programmes. Thus, IM should be viewed as a specific elaboration and route planner for operationalizing systematic health promotion. A brief introduction to the steps is introduced, and interested readers are referred to Peters[80] and Kok.[81]

Step one assesses the health problem under scrutiny in order to correctly plan the intervention. Figure 22.1 describes the first three

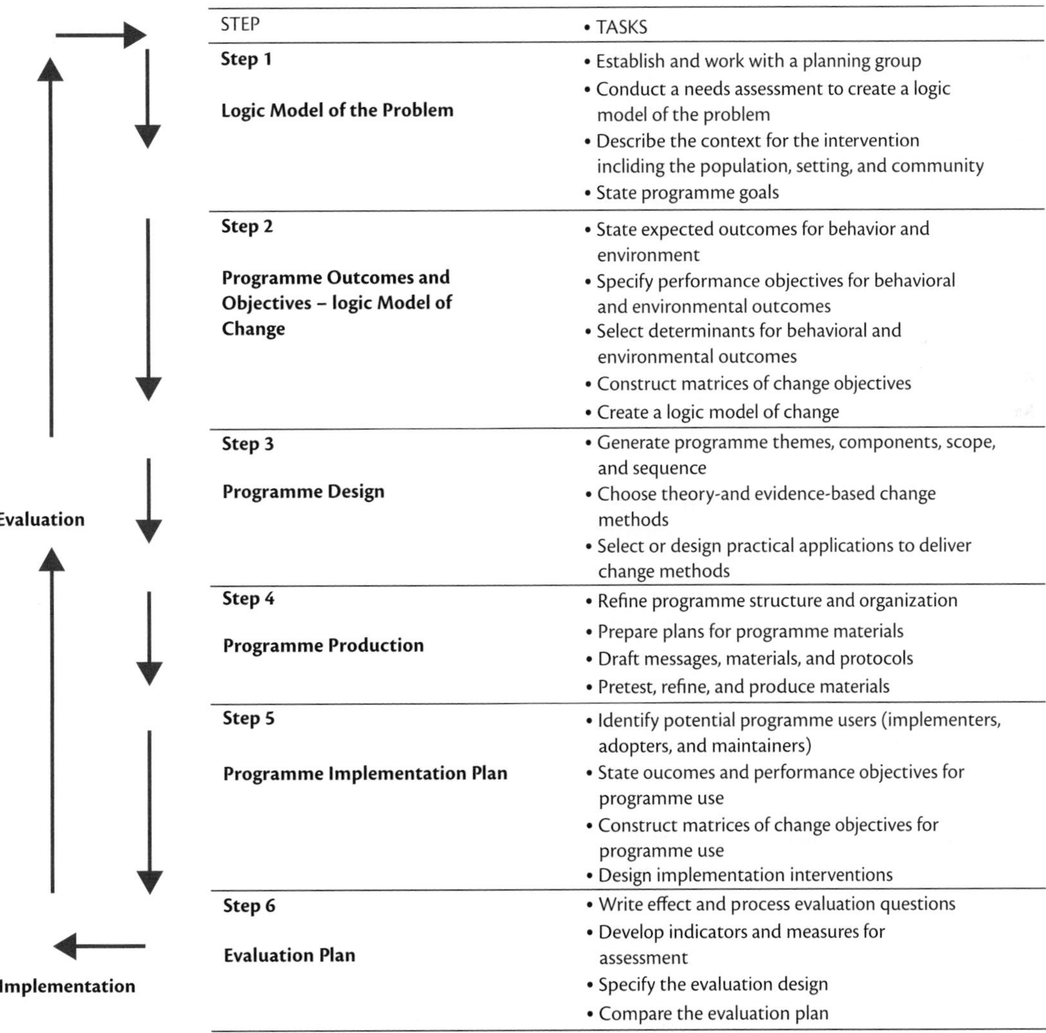

STEP	• TASKS
Step 1 **Logic Model of the Problem**	• Establish and work with a planning group • Conduct a needs assessment to create a logic model of the problem • Describe the context for the intervention incliding the population, setting, and community • State programme goals
Step 2 **Programme Outcomes and Objectives – logic Model of Change**	• State expected outcomes for behavior and environment • Specify performance objectives for behavioral and environmental outcomes • Select determinants for behavioral and environmental outcomes • Construct matrices of change objectives • Create a logic model of change
Step 3 **Programme Design**	• Generate programme themes, components, scope, and sequence • Choose theory-and evidence-based change methods • Select or design practical applications to deliver change methods
Step 4 **Programme Production**	• Refine programme structure and organization • Prepare plans for programme materials • Draft messages, materials, and protocols • Pretest, refine, and produce materials
Step 5 **Programme Implementation Plan**	• Identify potential programme users (implementers, adopters, and maintainers) • State oucomes and performance objectives for programme use • Construct matrices of change objectives for programme use • Design implementation interventions
Step 6 **Evaluation Plan**	• Write effect and process evaluation questions • Develop indicators and measures for assessment • Specify the evaluation design • Compare the evaluation plan

Figure 22.3 Intervention Mapping.

Adapted from Bartholomew Eldredge LK, Markham C, Ruiter RAC, Fernández ME, Kok G, Parcel GS. Planning health promotion programs; an Intervention Mapping approach, 4th ed. Hoboken NJ: Wiley; 2016.

phases of the planning and evaluation model for the development of health promotion interventions. In addition, previous experiences, mooted potential solutions are assessed, and important internal and external players are identified.[79]

Step two of IM reduces the behaviours and environmental conditions identified as causing the problem. At this stage, the target groups (which includes the key intermediaries) are identified, which then allows the planner to formulate performance objectives. These objectives specify the specific behaviours and protocols which must be adopted in order for the target groups to realize the behavioural and environmental outcomes. Determinants of the specific performance objectives of individuals and environmental agents are identified. Finally, the performance objectives are merged with these determinants, which results in matrices enabling the identification of the proximal programme objectives (i.e. statements on what must be learned by the programme participants, or what must be changed in the environment in order to facilitate behaviour change). The end products of step two are matrices for each target population, listing performance objectives, determinants, and proximal programme objectives.

In step three of IM, proximal programme objectives are linked to theory-based behaviour change methods and the practical applications thereof. A theoretical method is a change technique derived from theory and research to realize a programme objective. An application is the translation of that method to the specific intervention context. For instance, a theoretical method for attitude change to motivate screen-time reduction is self-reevaluation. A practical application that reflects this theoretical method could be an exercise in which a child compares his/her image as a sedentary person to a possible image of him/herself as an active person. An important task in this step is to identify the conditions or parameters that qualify the effectiveness of theoretical methods. These conditions must be met when translating theoretical methods into practical applications.[82] The widely applied method of modelling, for instance, is only effective when the model is reinforced (rewarded). Additionally, observers must pay attention, have sufficient self-efficacy and skills, identify with the model, and perceive a coping model instead of a mastery model.[79] The efficacy of using healthy models in an intervention to promote PA will thus highly depend on the way that it is operationalized in the programme.

Step four in IM gives specific guidance for designing a coherent intervention programme that conveys the intent and form of the behaviour change methods outlined in step three. In this step, the programme materials are designed and drafted, taking into account the context in which the programme will be used, and its scope. These materials are then pretested and pilot tested before being finally produced.

Step five in IM involves the adoption and implementation plan for the health promotion programme defined in step four. A linkage system is developed in order to connect the developers with those who put the intervention into motion. Next, proximal programme objectives are set with regard to the adoption and implementation of the intervention. Accordingly, a project plan is written to promote programme sustainability following first-time use.

Finally, in step six of IM, a follow-up plan is prepared to evaluate the success or failure of the programme, and to what extent. Effect and process evaluations are designed to assess the programme's success in reaching the programme objectives and the behavioural and determinants levels, as well as the completeness and fidelity of programme implementation, respectively.

Evidence

Explanations and descriptions of how data and theories are applied in health promotion interventions are rare. Few programme developers have provided details regarding the underlying rationale for the components of the intervention, the theoretical background, or behaviour-change methodology (e.g. see reference[83]). Consequently, other researchers and practitioners have little knowledge about the efficacy of specific teaching methods or approaches with regard to the promotion of healthy behaviours.[84] Reviews do provide some insight in the effectiveness of programmes promoting PA, especially those in the school setting, although their evaluation design could be improved in order to better contribute to theory development.[85–88] School-based interventions are often planned around increasing duration, frequency, and/or intensity of physical education lessons,[89] and most also indicate that the school environment provides adequate possibilities to positively influence PA levels in youth.[86,87,90] Schools also provide a captive audience, which makes them excellent settings for health promotion activities for children.[91] This kind of setting can positively affect the potential impact of an intervention. Most school-based PA interventions focus solely on the school setting,[92–95] whereas it could be argued that school is only one setting of influence.[96] Various studies have indicated that interactions taking place in different ecological settings (e.g. home environment or local neighbourhood) are more likely to change health behaviours.[29,65,97] Therefore, PA interventions that apply a comprehensive, or 'integral' approach,[98] i.e. focus on school or child-care settings as well as on local neighbourhoods and the home environment, are most likely to create sustained effects.[99] Such comprehensive interventions may, for example, aim to create PA-friendly school environments by creating a supportive physical environment (e.g. safe routes to school, improved aesthetics of neighbourhood playgrounds, and active schoolyards) accompanied by a supportive social environment (e.g. provision of active family games, parental support to walk to school, and facilitative teacher practices in schoolyards). The synergy of implementing changes at multiple types and levels of influences is presumed to affect PA in youth favourably.[97]

Implementation and diffusion of health promotion interventions

Theory

Implementation of a prevention programme is an essential part of the health promotion planning process. Underestimating diffusion and adoption barriers is one of the major causes of ineffectiveness in health promotion. While the need for information about individual behaviour determinants is commonly accepted, the need for information about institutional 'behaviour' determinants (such as organizational adoption of a prevention programme) is not widely recognized. Consequently, due to lack of information about behaviour determinants, many expensive programmes are never adequately applied in the contexts where they are most likely to be effective.

The diffusion of a health promotion programme can be described as a process consisting of four phases: dissemination, adoption, implementation, and maintenance.[100,101] Dissemination concerns the transfer of information about the programme to potential users. This phase involves the selection of communication channels and systems that facilitate the diffusion of the programme to a target population. Adoption refers to potential users' intention to use the programme. This phase includes a diagnosis of the target population with regard to their needs, values, and attitudes, as well as their perception of programme attributes and adoption barriers. These may include things like the relative advantage of the programme, its fit with the target population, its complexity, and the observability of programme outcomes. This phase also includes identifying ways to encourage adoption of the programme and ways to overcome perceived barriers. Implementation refers to the actual use of the programme. The major focus in this phase is on the enhancement of adopters' self-efficacy and skills, and on encouraging trial programme implementation. Maintenance or continuation succeeds initial implementation. This phase refers to the stage in which the programme has become current practice and in which the allocation of recourses is routinely made.[102]

According to Orlandi and colleagues,[103] many health promotion innovations have failed because of 'the gap that is frequently left unfilled between the point where innovation-development ends and diffusion planning begins', as if innovation-development barriers and diffusion barriers were aspects of unrelated problems. To bridge this gap, Orlandi and colleagues stressed the need for a *linkage system* between the resource system that develops and promotes the intervention (e.g. a Health Education Authority), and the user system that is supposed to adopt the intervention (e.g. sports organizations, schools). Such a liaison group should include representatives of the user system, representatives of the resource system, and a change agent facilitating the collaboration. Diffusion of the innovation may be carried out by any of the members of this liaison group. The essential point is that the innovation-development process and the diffusion planning process have been developed through co-operation, to improve the fit between innovation and user, to attune intervention innovations to practical possibilities and constraints, and to facilitate widespread implementation.

The development of a diffusion strategy can be based on a planning process that is similar to the planning of health-promotion programmes. A diffusion strategy should be based on insights in the determinants of potential users' decisions regarding the adoption, implementation, and continuation of a health-promoting programme. These determinants can be measured with the same kind of protocol as is used in the determinants of behaviour analyses, using the same kind of theories.[78] A diffusion strategy should further be based on useful theoretical methods and theory-based strategies.[104]

Diffusion of school-based programmes to promote physical activity

Social Cognitive Theory[105] provides a valuable framework for the development of interventions to stimulate the diffusion of school-based health-promotion programmes.[106,107] A strategy for the diffusion of a school-based programme to promote PA may be that teachers and administrators are aware of the programme, view the programme favourably, and communicate with colleagues about the programme. Useful methods to reach these objectives are personal communication from opinion leaders and the reference to models showing teachers successfully using the programme, e.g. through video or role-model stories in newsletters. An adoption strategy can focus on the advantages of the PA programme in terms of outcomes, expectancies, and social reinforcements. Useful methods to reach these objectives are modelling (e.g. peer model stories in written material), incentives, and social contracting, e.g. through a newsletter. An implementation strategy could focus on the reinforcement of teachers' skills and their self-efficacy to use the exercise programme with acceptable completeness, fidelity, and proficiency. Data from other implementation studies have shown the importance of in-service training.[108] Methods to reach these objectives are direct modelling and guided enactment through live workshop training, and symbolic modelling through online video training. The objectives of a continuation strategy may include teachers and administrators receiving positive feedback and reinforcement on the use of the PA programme after 1 year, and therefore being motivated to continue using it.[109] These objectives may be accomplished by means of various kinds of incentives (social, monetary, status, and self-evaluation incentives). In addition, online implementation support systems can be designed in such a way that they align with the most influential contextual matters in relation the establishment and sustainability of the promotion of PA in schools. Thus, in addition to personal professional support, online support systems can substantially support school coordinators and teachers. For example, systems can provide access to intervention and implementation materials and manuals, and feature video excerpts demonstrating best practices.

Conclusions

When developing programmes to promote PA among young people, programme objectives, intervention methods, applications, and dissemination strategies must all be taken into consideration. Importantly, these decisions cannot be made without careful analysis of the behavioural and environmental determinants of the physical (in)activity of the target population. If these decisions and analyses are made using a careful and systematic approach, chances of developing effective and sustainable interventions are substantially increased.

Summary

- From a public health perspective the promotion of physical activity (PA) has many benefits.
- Inactivity is a risk factor for multi-causal, lifestyle-related chronic disease, and a physically active lifestyle helps to maintain body weight.
- Physical activity-promoting programmes should be based on a systematic approach combining empirical findings, theoretical insights, and practical considerations.
- Successful health-promotion interventions to increase PA typically consist of strategies to improve intra-personal determinants of PA, as well as environmental strategies that facilitate PA-positive behaviour, assist in breaking unhealthy habits, or sustain healthy ones.
- The Intervention Mapping protocol is a helpful tool in the systematic development, implementation, diffusion, and evaluation of interventions aimed at the promotion of PA in young people.

References

1. Green LW, Kreuter MW. *Health promotion planning: an educational and environmental approach*. Mountain View: Mayfield: 1991.
2. De Leeuw ED. *The sane revolution. Health promotion: backgrounds, scope, prospects*. Van Gorcum, Assen: 1989.
3. Milio N. Strategies for health promoting policy: a study of four national case studies. *Health Promot Int*. 1988; 3: 307–311.
4. Kok GJ. Quality of planning as decisive determinant of health education. *Hygie*. 1992; 11: 5–8.
5. Tones K, Tilford S, Robinson YK. *Health education: effectiveness and efficiency*. London: Chapman; 1990.
6. Pate RR, Pratt M, Blair SN, *et al.* Physical activity and public health. A recommendation from the Centers for Disease Control and Prevention and the American College of Sports Medicine. *JAMA*. 1995; 273: 402–407.
7. Lee IM, Shiroma EJ, Lobelo F, *et al.* Effect of physical inactivity on major non-communicable diseases worldwide: an analysis of burden of disease and life expectancy. *Lancet*. 2012; 380: 219–229.
8. Tell GS, Vellar OD. Physical fitness, physical activity, and cardiovascular disease risk factors in adolescents: the Olso study. *Prev Med*. 1988; 17: 12–24.
9. World Cancer Research Fund/American Institute for Cancer Research. *Food, nutrition, physical activity, and the prevention of cancer: A global perspective*. Washington DC: AICR; 2007.
10. NIH Consensus development panel and physical activity and cardiovascular health. Physical activity and cardiovascular health. *JAMA*. 1996; 276: 241–246.
11. Suter E, Hawes MR. Relationship of physical activity, body fat, diet, and blood lipid profile in youth 10–15 yr. *Med Sci Sports Exerc*. 1993; 25: 748–754.
12. Bauer UE, Briss PA, Goodman RA, Bowman BA. Prevention of chronic disease in the 21st century: elimination of the leading preventable causes of premature death and disability in the USA. *Lancet*. 2014; 384: 45–52.
13. Robinson TN, Hammer LD, Killen LD, *et al.* Does television viewing increase obesity and reduce physical activity in adolescents? *Prev Med*. 1993; 19: 541–551.
14. van Mechelen W, Kemper H. Habitual physical activity in longitudinal perspective. In: Kemper HCG (ed.) *The Amsterdam Growth Study: a longitudinal analysis of health, fitness, and lifestyle*. Champaign, IL: Human Kinetics; 1995. p. 135–159.
15. Kelder SH, Perry CL, Klepp K-I. Community-wide youth exercise promotion: long term outcomes of the Minnesota Heart Health Program and the Class of 1989 study. *J School Health*. 1993; 63: 218–223.
16. Gortmaker SL, Dietz WH, Cheung LWY. Inactivity, diet and the fattening of America. *J Am Diet Assoc*. 1990; 90: 1247–1255.
17. Currie C, Nic Gabhainn S, Godeau E, International HBSC Network Coordinating Committee. The Health Behaviour in School-aged Children: WHO Collaborative Cross-National (HBSC) study: origins, concept, history and development 1982–2008. *Int J Public Health*. 2009; 54(Suppl 2): 131–139.
18. World Health Organization/UN Food and Agriculture Organization. *Diet, nutrition and the prevention of chronic diseases: Report of a joint WHO/FAO expert consultation*. 28 January–1 February 2002, Geneva, Switzerland; 2002.
19. Pearson N, Braithwaite RE, Biddle SJH, van Sluijs EMF, Atkin AJ. Associations between sedentary behaviour and physical activity in children and adolescents: a meta-analysis. *Obes Rev*. 2014; 15: 666–675.
20. Saunders TJ, Chaput JP, Tremblay MS. Sedentary behaviour as an emerging risk factor for cardiometabolic diseases in children and youth. *Can J Diabetes*. 2014; 38: 53–61.
21. Rennie KL, Johnson L, Jebb SA. Behavioural determinants of obesity. *Best Pract Res Clin Endocrin Met*. 2005; 19: 343–358.
22. Parsons TJ, Power C, Logan S, Summerbell CD. Childhood predictors of adult obesity: a systematic review. *Int J Obes*. 1999; 23: S1–S107.
23. Hill JO, Wyatt HR, Melanson EL. Genetic and environmental contributions to obesity. *Med Clin North Am*. 2000; 84: 333–345.
24. Hancox RJ, Milne BJ, Poulton R. Association between child and adolescent television viewing and adult health: a longitudinal birth cohort study. *Lancet*. 2004; 364: 257–262.
25. He M, Irwin JD, Sangster Bouck LM, Tucker P, Pollett GL. Screen-viewing behaviors among preschoolers. Parents' perceptions. *Am J Prev Med*. 2005; 29: 120–125.
26. Dietz W, Gortmaker S. Do we fatten our children at the television set? *Pediatr*. 1985; 75: 807–812.
27. Gortmaker S, Sobol A, Peterson K, Colditz G, Dietz W. Television viewing as a cause of increasing obesity among children in the United States, 1986–1990. *Arch Pediatr Adolesc Med*. 1996; 150: 356–362.
28. Crespo C, Smit E, Troiano R, Bartlett S, Macera C, Andersen R. Television watching, energy intake, and obesity in US children: Results from the third National Health and Nutrition Examination Survey, 1988–1994. *Arch Pediatr Adolesc Med*. 2001; 155: 360–365.
29. Attewell P, Suazo-Garcia B, Battle J. Computers and young children: social benefit or social problem? *Soc Forces*. 2003; 82: 277–296.
30. Stettler N, Signer TM, Suster PM. Electronic games and environmental factors associated with childhood obesity in Switzerland. *Obes Res*. 2004; 12: 896–903.
31. Marshall SJ, Gorely T, Biddle SJ. A descriptive epidemiology of screen-based media use in youth: a review and critique. *J Adolesc*. 2006; 29: 333–349.
32. Fernández-Alvira JM, De Bourdeaudhuij I, Singh AS, *et al.* Clustering of energy balance-related behaviors and parental education in European children: the ENERGY-project. *Int J Behav Nutr Phys Act*. 2013; 10: 5.
33. Abraham C, Sheeran P, Johnston M. From health beliefs to self-regulation: theoretical advances in the psychology of action control. *Psychol Health*. 1998; 13: 569–591.
34. Kremers SP. Theory and practice in the study of influences on energy balance-related behaviors. *Patient Educ Couns*. 2010; 79: 291–298.
35. Ajzen I. *Attitude, personality and behavior*. Milton Keynes: Open University Press; 1988.
36. Wasserkampf A, Silva MN, Santos IC, *et al.* Short- and long-term theory-based predictors of physical activity in women who participated in a weight-management program. *Health Educ Res*. 2014; 29: 941–952.
37. Deci EL, Ryan RM. A motivational approach to self: Integration in personality. In R. Dienstbier (ed.) *Nebraska symposium on motivation: Perspectives on motivation. Vol. 38*. Lincoln, NE: University Of Nebraska Press; 1991. p. 237–288.
38. Deci EL, Ryan RM. The 'what' and 'why' of goal pursuits: Human needs and the self-determination of behavior. *Psychol Inquiry*. 2000; 11: 227–268.
39. Sebire SJ, Jago R, Fox KR, Edwards M, Thompson JL. Testing a self-determination theory model of children's physical activity motivation: a cross-sectional study. *Int J Behav Nutr Phys Act*. 2013; 10: 111.
40. Gillison FB, Standage M, Skevington SM. Motivation and body-related factors as discriminators of change in adolescents' exercise behavior profiles. *J Adolesc Health*. 2011; 48: 44–51.
41. Verloigne M, De Bourdeaudhuij I, Tanghe A, *et al.* Self-determined motivation towards physical activity in adolescents treated for obesity: an observational study. *Int J Behav Nutr Phys Act*. 2011; 8: 97.
42. Chatzisarantis N, Hagger M. Effects of an intervention based on self-determination theory on selfreported leisure-time physical activity participation. *Psychol Health*. 2009; 24: 29–48.
43. Haerens L, Kirk D, Cardon G, De Bourdeaudhuij I, Vansteenkiste M. Motivational profiles for secondary school physical education and its relationship to the adoption of a physically active lifestyle among university students. *Eur Phys Educ Rev*. 2010; 16: 117–139.
44. Lim BS, Wang CKJ. Perceived autonomy support, behavioural regulations in physical education and physical activity intention. *Psychol Sport Exerc*. 2009; 10: 52–60.
45. McDavid L, Cox AE, Amorose AJ. The relative roles of physical education teachers and parents in adolescents' leisure-time physical activity motivation and behavior. *Psychol Sport Exerc*. 2012; 13: 99–107.

46. Taylor IM, Ntoumanis N, Standage M, Spray CM. Motivational predictors of physical education students' effort, exercise intentions, and leisure-time physical activity: a multilevel linear growth analysis. *J Sport Exerc Psychol.* 2010; 32: 99–120.
47. Nutbeam D, Aar L, Catford J. Understanding children's health behaviour: the implications for health promotion for young people. *Soc Sci Med.* 1989; 29: 317–325.
48. Kohl HWIII, Hobbs KE. Development of physical activity behaviors among children and adolescents. *Pediatrics.* 1998; 101: 549–554.
49. Sallis JF, Simons-Morton BG, Stone EJ, *et al.* Determinants of physical activity and interventions in youth. *Med Sci Sports Exerc.* 1992; 24: S248–S257.
50. Brug J, Oenema A, Ferreira I. Theory, evidence and Intervention Mapping to improve behavioral nutrition and physical activity interventions. *Int J Behav Nutr Phys Act.* 2005; 2: doi:10.1186/1479-5868-2-2
51. Baranowski T, Cullen KW, Nicklas T, Thompson D, Baranowski J. Are current health behavioral change models helpful in guiding prevention of weight gain efforts? *Obes Res.* 2003; 11: S23–S43.
52. French SA, Story M, Jeffery RW. Environmental influences on eating and physical activity. *Annu Rev Public Health.* 2001; 22: 309–335.
53. Story M, Neumark-Sztainer D, French S. Individual and environmental influences on adolescent eating behaviors. *J Am Diet Assoc.* 2002; 102: S40–S51.
54. Owen N, Leslie E, Salmon J, Fotheringham MJ. Environmental determinants of physical activity and sedentary behavior. *Exerc Sport Sci Rev.* 2000; 28: 153–158.
55. Flay BR, Petraitis J. The theory of triadic influence: a new theory of health behavior with implications for preventive interventions. *Adv Med Soc.* 1994; 4: 4–19.
56. Kumanyika S, Jeffery RW, Morabia A, Ritenbaugh C, Antipatis VJ. Obesity prevention: the case for action. *Int J Obes.* 2002; 26: 425–436.
57. Swinburn B, Egger G, Raza F. Dissecting obesogenic environments: the development and application of a framework for identifying and prioritizing environmental interventions for obesity. *Prev Med.* 1999; 29: 563–570.
58. Kremers SPJ, De Bruijn GJ, Visscher TLS, Van Mechelen W, De Vries NK, Brug J. Environmental influences on energy balance-related behaviors: A dual-process view. *Int J Behav Nutr Phys Act.* 2006; 3: 9.
59. Aarts H, Paulussen T, Schaalma H. Physical exercise habit: on the conceptualization and formation of habitual health behaviours. *Health Educ Res.* 1997; 12: 363–374.
60. Triandis HC. *Interpersonal behavior.* Monterey, CA: Brooks/Cole; 1977.
61. Friedman SL, Wachs TD. *Measuring environment across the life span. Emerging methods and concepts.* Washington, DC: American Psychological Association; 1999.
62. Wachs TD. Celebrating complexity: Conceptualization and assessment of the environment. In: Friedman SL, Wachs TD (eds.) *Measuring environment across the life span: emerging methods and concepts.* Washington DC: American Psychological Association; 1999. p. 357–392.
63. Kok G, Gottlieb NH, Commers M, Smerecnik C. The ecological approach in health promotion programs: A decade later. *Am J Health Promot.* 2008; 22: 437–442.
64. Spence JC, Lee RE. Toward a comprehensive model of physical activity. *Psychol Sport Exerc.* 2003; 4: 7–24.
65. Gubbels JS, Van Kann DHH, de Vries NK, Thijs C, Kremers SPJ. The next step in health behavior research: the need for ecological moderation analyses—an application to diet and physical activity at childcare. International *J Behav Nutr Phys Act.* 2014; 11: 52.
66. Larson N, Ward DS, Neelon SB, Story M. What role can child-care settings play in obesity prevention? A review of the evidence and call for research efforts. *J Am Diet Assoc.* 2011; 111: 1343–1362.
67. Gubbels JS, Kremers SP, van Kann DH, *et al.* Interaction between physical environment, social environment, and child characteristics in determining physical activity at child care. *Health Psychol.* 2011; 30: 84–90.
68. Bower JK, Hales DP, Tate DF, Rubin DA, Benjamin SE, Ward DS. The childcare environment and children's physical activity. *Am J Prev Med.* 2008; 34: 23–29.
69. Gubbels JS, van Kann DH, Jansen MW. Play equipment, physical activity opportunities, and children's activity levels at childcare. *J Environ Public Health.* 2012; 2012: 326520.
70. Boldemann C, Blennow M, Dal H, *et al.* Impact of preschool environment upon children's physical activity and sun exposure. *Prev Med.* 2006; 42: 301–308.
71. Cardon G, van Cauwenberghe E, Labarque V, Haerens L, de Bourdeaudhuij I. The contribution of preschool playground factors in explaining children's physical activity during recess. *Int J Behav Nutr Phys Act.* 2008, 5: 11.
72. Brown WH, Pfeiffer KA, McIver KL, Dowda M, Addy CL, Pate RR. Social and environmental factors associated with preschoolers' nonsedentary physical activity. *Child Dev.* 2009; 80: 45–58.
73. Remmers T, Van Kann D, Gubbels J, *et al.* Moderators of the longitudinal relationship between the perceived physical environment and outside play in children: the KOALA birth cohort study. *Int J Behav Nutr Phys Act.* 2014; 11: 150.
74. Sleddens EF, Kremers SP, Stafleu A, *et al.* Food parenting practices and child dietary behavior. Prospective relations and the moderating role of general parenting. *Appetite.* 2014; 79: 42–50.
75. Rodenburg G, Kremers SP, Oenema A, *et al.* Associations of parental feeding styles with child snacking behaviour and weight in the context of general parenting. *Public Health Nutr.* 2014; 17: 960–969.
76. Tung HJ, Yeh MC. Parenting style and child-feeding behaviour in predicting children's weight status change in Taiwan. *Public Health Nutr.* 2014; 17: 970–978.
77. Mullen PD, Green LW, Persinger G. Clinical trials for patient education for chronic conditions: a comparative meta-analysis of intervention types. *Prev Med.* 1985; 14: 753–781.
78. Kok G, Schaalma H, De Vries H, Parcel G, Paulussen T. Social psychology and health education. In: Stroebe W, Hewstone M (eds.) *European review of social psychology, vol. 7.* Chichester: Wiley; 1996. p. 201–240.
79. Bartholomew Eldredge LK, Markham C, Ruiter RAC, Fernández ME, Kok G, Parcel GS. *Planning health promotion programs; an Intervention Mapping approach,* 4th ed. Hoboken, NJ: Wiley; 2016.
80. Peters GJY. A practical guide to effective behavior change: how to identify what to change in the first place. *Eur Health Psychol.* 2014; 16: 142–155.
81. Kok G. A practical guide to effective behavior change: How to apply theory- and evidence-based behavior change methods in an intervention. *Eur Health Psychol.* 2014; 16: 156–170.
82. Schaalma H, Kok, G. Decoding health education interventions: The times are a-changin'. *Psychol Health.* 2009; 24: 5–9.
83. Singh AS, Chin A Paw MJM, Kremers SPJ, Visscher TLS, Brug J, van Mechelen W. Design of the Dutch Obesity Intervention in Teenagers (NRG-DOiT): Systematic development, implementation and evaluation of a school-based intervention aimed at prevention of excessive weight gain in adolescents. *BMC Public Health.* 2006; 6: 304.
84. Kremers SPJ, Visscher TLS, Brug J, *et al.* Netherlands Research programme weight gain prevention (NHF-NRG): rationale, objectives and strategies. *Eur J Clin Nutr.* 2005; 59: 498–507.
85. Kremers SPJ, De Bruijn GJ, Droomers M, Van Lenthe F, Brug J. Moderators of environmental intervention effects on diet and activity in youth. *Am J Prev Med.* 2007; 32, 163–172.
86. Dobbins M, Husson H, DeCorby K, LaRocca R. School-based physical activity programs for promoting physical activity and fitness in children and adolescents aged 6 to 18. *Cochrane Database Syst Rev.* doi: 10.1002/14651858.CD007651.pub2
87. Kriemler S, Meyer U, Martin E, van Sluijs E, Andersen L, Martin B. Effect of school-based interventions on physical activity and fitness in children and adolescents: a review of reviews and systematic update. *Br J Sports Med.* 2011; 45: 923–930.

88. McGoey T, Root Z, Bruner MW, Law B. Evaluation of physical activity interventions in children via the reach, efficacy/effectiveness, adoption, implementation, and maintenance (RE-AIM) framework: A systematic review of randomized and non-randomized trials. *Prev Med.* 2016; 82: 8–19.
89. Kahn EB, Ramsey LT, Brownson RC, *et al.* The effectiveness of interventions to promote physical activity: a systematic review. *Am J Prev Med.* 2002; 22: S73–S107.
90. De Bruijn GJ, Kremers S, Wendel-Vos W, Van Lenthe F, Brug J. Environmental interventions on physical activity in youth. In: Brug J, Van Lenthe F (eds.) *Environmental determinants and interventions for physical activity, nutrition and smoking: A review.* Zoetermeer: Speed-Print BV; 2005. p. 78–106.
91. Story M, Nanney M, Schwartz M. Schools and obesity prevention: creating school environments and policies to promote healthy eating and physical activity. *Milbank Q.* 2009; 87: 71–100.
92. Broekhuizen K, Scholten A-M, de Vries S. The value of (pre)school playgrounds for children's physical activity level: a systematic review. *Int J Behav Nutr Phys Act.* 2014; 11: 59.
93. Escalante Y, García-Hermoso A, Backx K, Saavedra JM. Playground designs to increase physical activity levels during school recess: A systematic review. *Health Educ Behav.* 2014; 41: 138–144.
94. Ridgers N, Salmon J, Parrish A, Stanley R, Okely A. Physical activity during school recess: a systematic review. *Am J Prev Med.* 2012; 43: 320–328.
95. Parrish A, Okely A, Stanley R, Ridgers N. The effect of school recess interventions on physical activity: a systematic review. *Sports Med.* 2013; 43: 287–299.
96. Sallis JF, Cervero RB, Ascher W, Henderson KA, Kraft MK, Kerr J. An ecological approach to creating active living communities. *Ann Rev Pub Health.* 2006; 27: 297–322.
97. Van Kann, DHH, Jansen MWJ, de Vries SI, de Vries NK, Kremers SPJ. Active Living: development and quasi-experimental evaluation of a school-centered physical activity intervention for primary school children. *BMC Public Health.* 2015; 15: 1315.
98. van Koperen MT, van der Kleij RM, Renders CC, *et al.* Design of CIAO, a research program to support the development of an integrated approach to prevent overweight and obesity in the Netherlands. *BMC Obes.* 2014; 1: 5.
99. Flynn MA, McNeil DA, Maloff B, *et al.* Reducing obesity and related chronic disease risk in children and youth: a synthesis of evidence with 'best practice' recommendations. *Obes Rev.* 2006; 7(Suppl 1): 7–66.
100. Oldenburg B, Hardcastle D, Kok G. Diffusion of innovations. In: Glanz K, Lewis FM, Rimer BK (eds.) *Health behavior and health education: theory, research and practice*, 2nd ed. San Francisco: Jossey-Bass; 1997. p. 270–286.
101. Koorts H, Gillison F. Mixed method evaluation of a community-based physical activity program using the RE-AIM framework: practical application in a real-world setting. *BMC Public Health.* 2015; 15: 1102.
102. Miles MB, Louis KS. Research on institutionalization: a reflective review. In: Miles MB, Ekholm M, Vandenberghe R (eds.) *Lasting school improvement: exploring the process of institutionalization.* Leuven: ACCO; 1987. p. 25–44.
103. Orlandi MA, Landers C, Weston R, Haley N. Diffusion of health promotion innovations. In: Glanz K, Lewis FM, Rimer BK (eds.) *Health behavior and health education: theory, research and practice.* San Francisco: Jossey-Bass; 1990. p. 288–313.
104. Tabak RG, Khoong EC, Chambers DA, Brownson RC. Bridging research and practice: models for dissemination and implementation research. *Am J Prev Med.* 2012; 43: 337–350.
105. Bandura A. *Social foundation of thought and action: a social cognitive theory.* Englewood Cliffs, NJ: Prentice-Hall; 1986.
106. Parcel G, Taylor WC, Brink SG, Gottlieb NH, Enquist KE, Eriksen MP. Translating theory into practice: intervention strategies for the diffusion of a health promotion innovation. *Fam Comm Health.* 1989; 12: 1–13.
107. Parcel G, Erikson MP, Lovato CY, Gottlieb NH, Brink SG, Green LW. The diffusion of school-based tobacco-use prevention programmes; project description and baseline data. *Health Educ Res.* 1989; 4, 111–124.
108. Joyce B, Showers B. *Student achievement through staff development.* New York: Longman; 1988.
109. Langford R, Bonell C, Jones H, Campbell R. Obesity prevention and the Health promoting Schools framework: essential components and barriers to success. *Int J Behav Nutr Phys Act.* 2015; 13: 15.

CHAPTER 23

Exercise, physical activity, and diabetes mellitus

Edgar GAH van Mil

Introduction

Definition of diabetes mellitus

The term diabetes mellitus describes a complex metabolic disorder characterized by chronic hyperglycaemia resulting from defects in insulin secretion, insulin action, or both. Inadequate insulin secretion and/or diminished tissue responses to insulin in the complex pathways of hormone action result in deficient insulin action on target tissues, which leads to abnormalities of carbohydrate, fat, and protein metabolism. Impaired insulin secretion and/or action may coexist in the same patient.

While the aetiology of diabetes is heterogeneous, most cases of diabetes can be classified into three broad aetiopathogenetic categories: i) type 1 diabetes mellitus (T1DM), which is characterized by an absolute deficiency of insulin secretion; ii) type 2 diabetes mellitus (T2DM), which results from a combination of resistance to insulin action and an inadequate compensatory insulin secretory response, and; iii) monogenetic forms of diabetes.[1]

Diagnostic criteria for diabetes mellitus in childhood and adolescence

Diagnostic criteria for diabetes are based on blood glucose measurement and the presence or absence of symptoms as shown in Box 23.1.

Box 23.1 Diagnostic criteria for diabetes

- Symptoms of diabetes plus casual plasma glucose concentration > 11.1 mmol·L^{-1} (200 mg·dL^{-1})*. Casual is defined as any time of day without regard to time since the last meal.

  Or

- Fasting plasma glucose > 7.0 mmol·L^{-1} (126 mg·dL^{-1})#. Fasting is defined as no caloric intake for at least 8 h.

  Or

- 2-h post-load glucose ≥ (11.1 mmol·L^{-1} or 200 mg·dL^{-1}) during an oral glucose tolerance test (OGTT). The test should be performed as described by the World Health Organization, using a glucose load containing the equivalent of 75 g anhydrous glucose dissolved in water or 1.75 g·kg^{-1} of body weight to a maximum of 75 g.

* Corresponding value > 10.0 mmol·L^{-1} for venous whole blood and
\# corresponding value > 6.3 mmol·L^{-1} for venous whole blood.

Classification of diabetes mellitus

The aetiological classification recommended by the American Diabetes Association (ADA)[2] and the World Health Organization (WHO) expert committee[3] defines three groups as shown in Box 23.2.

The differentiation between T1DM, T2DM, and monogenetic diabetes has important implications for both therapeutic decisions and educational approaches. Type 1 diabetes mellitus accounts for more than 90% of childhood and adolescent diabetes, with annual incidence rates from 0.1–37.4 per 100 000, depending on the country. However, with the increasing prevalence of childhood obesity, T2DM is becoming more common in youth.[4] This chapter focuses on T1DM, which remains the most common form of diabetes in young people in many populations, especially those of Caucasian background.

The aetiology and incidence of type 1 diabetes mellitus

Type 1 diabetes mellitus is associated with deficient insulin secretion. The beta cells of the pancreas are largely destroyed. Insulin secretory responses to standard glucose tolerance tests are markedly reduced or absent. C-peptide responses are used instead of insulin to check beta cell capacity when the diabetic is already receiving exogenous insulin. Type 1A diabetes mellitus refers to immune-related T-lymphocyte-mediated diabetes mellitus, which results in destruction of the beta cells of the pancreas, and features anti-islet autoantibodies. Genetic factors are involved, although there is no recognizable pattern of inheritance. The risk of diabetes to an identical twin of a patient with T1DM is about 36%. For a sibling, the risk is approximately 4% by the age of 20 years and 9.6% by the age of 60 years, compared with 0.5% for the general population. The human leukocyte antigen (HLA) region, also known as the human major histocompatibility complex (MHC), influences T1DM susceptibility, especially in Europe.

Box 23.2 Classification of diabetes

i) Type 1 (T1DM)

B-cell destruction, usually leading to absolute insulin deficiency

Autoimmune

Idiopathic

ii) Type 2 (T2DM)

May range from predominantly insulin resistance with relative deficiency to a predominantly secretory defect with or without insulin resistance

iii) Other specific types

Genetic defects of B-cell function (e.g. Maturity Onset Diabetes of the Young; MODY)

Genetic defects in insulin action

Diseases of the exocrine pancreas

Endocrinopathies

Drug or chemical induced

Infections-related

Uncommon forms of immune-mediated diabetes

Other genetic syndromes sometimes associated with diabetes

Many countries have reported a rise in incidence of T1DM with a disproportionately greater increase in those younger than 5 years.[1] However, in Japan, the incidence of T1DM is extremely low, at 1.5–2.0 per 100 000, and has a different and unique HLA association compared with Caucasians.

The clinical spectrum of type 1 diabetes mellitus

The presentation

Diabetes in children usually presents with characteristic symptoms such as polyuria, polydipsia, blurring of vision, and body weight loss, in association with glycosuria and ketonuria. In its most severe form, ketoacidosis may develop and lead to cerebral oedema, and in the absence of effective treatment, death. Diabetes ketoacidosis remains the main cause of death in young T1DM.[5]

The management of type 1 diabetes mellitus

The aims

The main aim is to render as normal a lifestyle as possible to the diabetic, by four main targets of management: obtaining good metabolic control, preventing long-term complications, promoting social competence, and promoting self-esteem.[6] The main challenges are that the patient must receive insulin subcutaneously and there must be attention given to lifestyle.[7] The young person with diabetes also faces a number of hurdles, mainly in the form of complications. Complications can be divided into acute and chronic. The acute complications include hypoglycaemia and diabetic ketoacidosis. The chronic complications are the triopathy of retinopathy, nephropathy, and neuropathy. Although the chronic complications may not affect the young person with diabetes, nevertheless, the control of the diabetes during this time may have impact on the development of such complications in later life. The Diabetes Control and Complications Trial (DCCT)[8] established criteria to be achieved, which will lead to the prevention, at least in part, of the triopathy of complications. In this well-controlled DCCT study, the research group concluded that intensive therapy effectively delays the onset and slows the progression of diabetic retinopathy, nephropathy, and neuropathy. Intensive therapy included delivery of insulin by an external pump or three or more daily insulin injections. This resulted in maintaining blood glucose concentrations close to the normal range in addition to glycosylated haemoglobin. The major side-effect was a two to threefold increase in severe hypoglycaemia. In a thoughtful article, Watkins[9] considered the advantages and disadvantages of conclusions of the DCCT. The price of achieving excellent control will almost certainly result in more frequent insulin injections and a greater risk of hypoglycaemia. The choice of intensive therapy is sometimes difficult, although it is necessary for long-term health. Such intensive regimens are even more daunting when the child is faced with exercise and sport. Many find that intensive insulin therapy helps with glucose management during physical activity (PA), because it allows for frequent changes in insulin dosages, particularly if an insulin pump is used. Intensive insulin therapy attempts to mimic the natural pattern of insulin secretion. The major problems in the management of T1DM are that no matter how intensive the regimen, it is impossible to mimic the physiological state and the second-to-second control of blood glucose by the normal pancreas.

The main aims in the management of a child or teenager with diabetes are:

- The diet should have sufficient calories balanced among protein, fat, and carbohydrate to result in normal growth and body weight.
- The diet has to be regimented in that the patient must eat on a regular basis, sometimes including snacking between meals, in order to prevent hypoglycaemia.

The insulin regimen should be such that it achieves the goals of DCCT, within the tolerance of the young person and/or parents.

Practical aspects

To achieve these aims requires a considerable amount of education of the young patient and the parents. What can be achieved will be dependent on the age of the patient; the younger the patient, the more management will fall on the parents. The patient should be taught the core concepts of diabetes mellitus, the self-monitoring of blood glucose levels and their interpretation, and the practicalities of self-injection of insulin. The patient should fully understand the warning symptoms of hypoglycaemia, how to prevent it, and how to take action should symptoms occur. Hypoglycaemia will be covered more extensively when PA and sport are considered. The patient (and parents) should also be aware of possible situations which may lead to ketoacidosis, and know what regimens to employ when the patient becomes ill for other reasons (most often an infective illness). The psychological aspects of diabetes are not to be ignored. The impact of diabetes can lead to emotional reactions, including anger, grief, depression, anxiety, and denial. Many children maintain some endogenous insulin secretion for some time just after the diagnosis, which creates an extra challenge for metabolic control.

The adolescent with diabetes presents with other special problems. The secretion of sex hormones and an increased secretion of growth hormone in a pulsatile fashion leads to growth spurts and initiation of secondary sex characteristics, creating a temporary state of insulin resistance. The impact of new social interest will lead to changes in lifestyle and feelings of independence sometimes amounting to rebelliousness. Eating disorders may occur at this age.[10] This will result in increased dosage of insulin, but may also lead to deterioration in control due to all the quoted factors. So-called 'brittle diabetes' is common in this age group, where the diabetic experiences wild swings in blood sugar with frequent hypoglycaemic attacks and ketoacidosis. The period of adolescence with all its physiological and psychological changes may be responsible, although the behavioural disturbances are often behind the 'brittleness'.[11]

The insulin regimen in childhood diabetes offers several choices. In the younger child, a two- or three-dose insulin regimen is still common. This will usually consist of a mixture of soluble insulin and intermediate acting insulin before breakfast, and this is repeated in the evening. This is conveniently given in cartridges by the pen system in a 'pre-mix' of insulin, where the ratio of the soluble and intermediate can be varied.

Another regimen suitable for young children with a stable feeding pattern is a combination of pre-mix insulin before breakfast, short-acting insulin at dinner time, and long-acting insulin before bedtime. Parents and patients will be instructed to vary the dose depending on a number of factors, including the prevailing blood glucose, and other factors such as intercurrent illness, PA, etc. The preferable regimen is the intensive therapy regime, either by pen or by insulin pump. The pen regimen is to administer short-acting insulin prior to meals and long-acting insulin in the evening. The pump regimen contains a pre-set insulin programme delivering a constant infusion of insulin in the subcutaneous compartment, completed by short insulin infusions prior to carbohydrate ingestion. This usually offers better control and better mimics the physiological situation. It also confers greater flexibility and is very suited to a busy adolescent, especially one involved in sport. Currently, the newest pumps are suitable for connection to glucose sensors in order to deliver automatic insulin stops in case of hypoglycaemia. The combination of pump and sensor is also referred to as continuous glucose monitoring (CGM), which provides constant feedback about the glucose levels within the interstitial fluid and blood, and thereby delivers an excellent learning tool for patients, parents, and care keepers to understand the influences of food, stress, illness, or activities.[12]

Hypoglycaemia

As hypoglycaemia is a significant problem in the exercising diabetic, this section covers it in detail. It is also the most feared acute complication in the insulin dependent diabetic, creating havoc with lifestyle. Insulin therapies, no matter how sophisticated the regimen, cannot mimic the physiological state. If the blood runs high to avoid hypoglycaemia, then the feared chronic complications are an ever-present worry. In the normal subject hypoglycaemia (blood glucose $<2.5\ \text{mmol} \cdot \text{L}^{-1}$) is prevented by inhibition of insulin secretion, secretion of counter-regulatory hormones, in particular adrenaline and glucagon, and by neural influences.[13]

The main symptoms of hypoglycaemia are a combination of the effects on the brain and catecholamines. Palpitations (tachycardia), sweating, hunger, and shaking are early warning symptoms. In mild hypoglycaemia, double vision, difficulty in concentrating, and slurring of the speech occur. Moderate cases present with confusion and behavioural changes. In severe cases, the patient can become unconscious with fits and neurological deficits such as haemiplegia.[14] The major precipitating factors are insufficient carbohydrate at meals, delayed meals, over-dosage with insulin, and PA, especially severe.

There are other problems with which the diabetic must contend. Loss of awareness of hypoglycaemia is a worrying development, probably due to loss of neurohumoral responses to repeated hypoglycaemia in the past.[15] There is, however, evidence that hypoglycaemic awareness can be restored by scrupulous hypoglycaemic avoidance.[16] Preventative actions include frequent snacking, end reduced bedtime long-acting insulin after vigorous intensity, or sustained PA on the evening after. Excess alcohol should be avoided. Both patient and doctor should be educated.

The importance of physical activity for the diabetic patient

Physical activity

The insulin dependent diabetic must face PA with disordered or even absent insulin secretion, as well as other potential problems relating to complications, including disordered autonomic function. Physical activity may be divided into two categories:

i) Random and recreational PA. This will certainly be the category the young child with diabetes will inevitably be involved in. This will include the normal activity of the young child, but on occasion will involve somewhat more extensive PA, e.g. an outing, a sports day etc. According to the American Department of Health and Human Services 'Healthy People 2010' recommendations, 'young people should participate in at least 60 $\text{min} \cdot \text{day}^{-1}$ of moderate intensity physical activity for most days of the week'. Or, according to the ISPAD guidelines, 'all patients with diabetes should be given the opportunity to benefit from the many effects of physical activity'.[17]

ii) Sport and training. Children from about the age of 6 years, sometimes even younger, begin to participate in organized sport, such as running, gymnastics, football, hockey, swimming, etc. This will include some training, but usually not involving more than 2–3 $\text{h} \cdot \text{week}^{-1}$. When the subject reaches 11 or 12 years of age, training might increase and intensify, and continue into adolescence and teenage years.

Philosophy of involvement of diabetics in sport

It may be argued that because of potential risks, children and teenagers with diabetes should not be involved in sport. Certainly life without sport and training will be a more sedate and less complicated existence. In one study maximal oxygen uptake ($\dot{V}O_2$ max) measurements in young subjects with T1DM were decreased compared to healthy controls,[18] but other studies have been unable to confirm this finding.[19,20] Increased PA in Brazilian children and adolescents was associated with the best glucose control.[21]

Michael Hall, Chairman of the Board of Trustees of the British Diabetic Association, wrote[22] that diabetics should not be sheltered from the normal activities of mankind, and should be able to undertake a full range of sporting activities. He quoted outstanding athletes in many sports who are diabetic and who have reached the highest levels. He found it regrettable that some sports bodies treat diabetics as disabled, and that diabetics have been refused entry to some events. There is an International Diabetes Athletes' Association which caters for diabetics in sport.

Diabetic athletes should be treasured, since they function as role models for children and teenagers. One international organization pays tribute to these 'ambassadors in sports' (www.diabetes-exercise.org). Fortunately, a Belgium study, using 24 h continuous heart-rate monitoring, showed that the majority of diabetic children and teenagers meet the guidelines for PA and compare favourably with their healthy peers,[23] and it has also been suggested that most US children with T1DM attain at least 30 min of daily PA.[24]

Safety, however, must be the watchword, and a complete understanding by the parents or the patient as to how to control his/her diabetes is essential. Most sports have safety standards so that training is supervised, and it is vital that a coach or attendant is informed that the athlete is a diabetic.

Regular PA will improve the health of the insulin-dependent diabetic in the following ways:

- Increased cardiorespiratory fitness
- Increased insulin sensitivity
- Increased/maintained muscle mass-to-fat ratio with better weight control
- Reduction in serum lipids
- Decline in resting heart rate and blood pressure
- Improved quality of life
- Diminished glycaemic response to a meal, and a reduction in daily insulin needs

A positive association between glycaemic control and aerobic fitness or reported PA exists in youth with T1DM, suggesting that either increased aerobic capacity may improve metabolic control, or that glycaemic control maximizes aerobic capacity.[25] Adolescents with T1DM improve cardiorespiratory endurance and muscle strength at least as much as their non-diabetic peers after aerobic training.[26] Moreover, sports participation among high school students has been associated with multiple positive health behaviours, including fruit and vegetable consumption and reduced cigarette smoking.[27] Indeed, the goal of regular PA should be to increase insulin sensitivity and to improve the overall cardiovascular and psychosocial profile of the child with T1DM, regardless of any putative benefits to blood glucose management.[17] However, diabetics will respond to PA differently from normal subjects, particularly with respect to glucose homeostasis.

The effect of physical activity on the patient with type 1 diabetes mellitus

Blood glucose responses to PA vary in subjects with diabetes. This does not mean that the response cannot be anticipated. The blood glucose response to 60 min of intermittent PA is reproducible in a child if the timing of exercise, amount of insulin, and the pre-exercise meal remain consistent.[28] In healthy children glucose production increases with exercise intensity as the muscle glucose uptake raises.

The normal person

In order to understand the problems facing the insulin-dependent diabetic, knowledge of glucose homeostasis during PA in the normal subject is required. During PA insulin falls and the counter-regulatory hormones glucagon and catecholamines rise. The glucagon:insulin molar ratio appears critical to glucose output from the liver, and a very small amount of insulin is all that is necessary to control glucose uptake.[29] Furthermore, non-insulin-dependent glucose uptake by muscle increases by the translocation of the insulin-sensitive glucose transporter (GLUT)-4 receptors to the cell surface.[30] Carbohydrate is stored as glycogen in muscle and liver, and fatty acids are stored, mainly as triglycerides, in adipose tissue. Protein may also be used as a fuel, but to a lesser extent.[31] Physical activity in the normal subject is usually accompanied by euglycaemia. Therefore, in exercise, the glucose output from the liver matches the glucose uptake by muscle. As a result of precise autonomic and endocrine regulation, blood glucose levels remain stable under most exercise conditions.[32]

At relatively low energy levels, up to 50% of $\dot{V}O_2$ max, fat (free fatty acids and muscle triglycerides) is the main source of fuel, completed by a mixture of muscle glycogen and blood glucose derived from liver glycogen. Similar effects have been demonstrated in trained individuals. Trained athletes have increased utilization of lipids compared to untrained individuals. However, as exercise intensity increases, carbohydrate (muscle glycogen and plasma glucose-derived liver glycogen) becomes the main source of fuel. In adults, the plasma glucose concentration is tightly regulated in PA up to 60% of $\dot{V}O_2$ max, with the increment of uptake precisely matched by that of production. During heavy exercise, blood glucose utilization may be as great as 1.5 $g \cdot min^{-1}$, and this fuel source must be continuously replaced at an equal rate or hypoglycaemia will ensue. During such exercise, insulin secretion is inhibited by B-cell a-adrenergic receptor activation. It is suggested that catecholamine response is the primary regulator for the up to eight-fold increase in glucose production during intense exercise (above 80% $\dot{V}O_2$ max).[33] This leads to hyperglycaemia with accompanying hyperinsulinemia after brief intense exercise to exhaustion and persists up to 60 min of recovery.

Depletion of carbohydrate stores in muscle are the main causes of fatigue in athletes. The liver has only 2–3 h of storage glycogen to meet the needs of a person exercising at high intensity.[34] Children have even lower endogenous carbohydrate stores. Even a single bout of PA can increase glucose uptake into skeletal muscle tissue for at least 16 h post-exercise in healthy and in diabetic subjects.[35] Feeding on a high-carbohydrate diet (70% of energy intake as carbohydrate) enabled runners who were training for 2 $h \cdot day^{-1}$ to maintain muscle glycogen levels.[36] A dietary carbohydrate intake of 500–600 g may be necessary to ensure adequate glycogen resynthesis.[37] The conclusion must be that in athletes who are competing in prolonged events at a high energy level, increased dietary intake of carbohydrate is essential. The athlete who is also training frequently and for prolonged times must ensure that sufficient carbohydrate is ingested between training times to ensure adequate stores of glycogen in muscle and liver, otherwise fatigue will result.

Carbohydrate feeding during prolonged PA has been shown to enhance performance.[38] This probably works to spare muscle glycogen thus delaying fatigue.[39] Alternatively, it may improve performance by maintaining blood glucose at a critical point in endurance exercise, when liver and glycogen levels are low and the uptake of glucose by skeletal muscle is increased.[40]

Physical training enhances insulin stimulated glucose disposal in proportion to the improvement in physical fitness.[41] This appears to be mediated through increases in blood flow, GLUT-4 expression, and glycogen synthase activity.[42] The increased insulin sensitivity is seen in participants in aerobic events, but not in participants in anaerobic events.[43]

Physical activity can influence intestinal absorption of fluids and glucose. Gastric emptying may be affected by PA, the process being inhibited.[44] In post-absorptive humans, splanchnic blood flow decreases during supine and upright PA.[45] Hypoxia to mucosal cells affects sugar absorption, leading to the conclusion that intense PA will also have this effect due to diminished blood flow.[46]

The person with type 1 diabetes mellitus

Several characteristics of exercise may strongly influence the development of exercise hypoglycaemia. Among them, duration and intensity of the exercise, physical training, and diet prior to the exercise are major determinants.[47]

The key problem is that the insulin-dependent diabetic does not have the normal insulin response to PA. Peripheral insulin concentrations are tightly related by the injective therapy as well as to the site of injections and the time elapsed since the last administration. To repeat, insulin levels fall to low levels in normal subjects during PA. The diabetic has a very significant problem in mimicking this, and indeed injected insulin often rises in the blood during PA in the diabetic.[48] This is caused by more rapid absorption of the injected insulin particularly if the insulin is injected into the exercising part of the body.[49]A rise in body temperature and increased blood flow in subcutaneous tissue and skeletal muscle have been demonstrated to be causally related to the increased insulin concentrations during sports.[50] This rapid absorption is more marked when the insulin is given shortly before the PA, than if given 60–90 mins before the PA. Physical activity does not appear to alter insulin glargine (long-acting insulin) absorption rate.[51]

The inappropriately elevated insulin levels during PA will have undesirable effects by inhibiting hepatic glucose output and by enhancing peripheral glucose uptake and stimulating glucose uptake by exercising muscle, usually within 20–60 min after the onset of exercise.[52] This process is also called over-insulinization. Lastly, during PA there is a dramatic increase in non-insulin-mediated glucose uptake that considerably reduces the need for circulating insulin levels.[53] Contradictory to what one might think, glucose oxidation during 60 min of moderate- to vigorous-intensity PA is lower in diabetic adolescent boys than in age- and weight-matched controls,[54] possibly because of a decreased insulin sensitivity.[55] Gluconeogenesis is also impaired. Counter-regulatory responses, such as glucagon, can be deficient in the diabetic. These changes inevitably lead to hypoglycaemia during PA. Within 45 min of vigorous intensity PA performed 2 h after a standard meal and their usual insulin dose, hypoglycaemia will develop. A reduction of 30–50% in bolus insulin delivery reduces the likelihood of developing hypoglycaemia in these patients.[25] On the other hand, if counter-regulatory responses are intact, a further decline in blood glucose for at least 2 h after PA was seen in adult cyclists, who ended with an intense cycling sprint at maximal intensity after moderate intensity exercise.[56] For children as well, typical for sports and play are repeated short periods of intensive activity, alternated by periods of rest or low-intensity activities, which are associated with a lesser fall in blood glucose levels when compared to continuous moderate intensity physical activities (40% of $\dot{V}O_2$ max).[57] Prolonged exercise (>90 min), however, will always require a greater reduction of insulin, often up to 80% of normal.

Post-exercise hypoglycaemia can also be encountered up to several hours after exercise and even the following day.[58] In T1DM adolescents the hypoglycaemia was found to be biphasic: increased glucose requirements during and shortly after exercise and again 7–11 h or even up to 24 h after exercise.[59] This is probably due to increased glucose uptake and glycogen synthesis in the previously exercised muscle groups. In addition, severe post-exercise late-onset hypoglycaemia (i.e. up to 36 h after exercise) may be particularly relevant in physically active children, possibly because proper insulin and nutritional strategies are not adopted, while muscle and liver glycogen stores are being replaced.

Strategies to limit the possibility of hypoglycaemia caused by PA are shown in Box 23.3.

Box 23.3 Strategies to limit the possibility of hypoglycaemia caused by physical activity

Before physical activity

- avoid or correct for hyperglycaemia or ketonuria.
- inform staff or supporters in hypoglycaemia procedures such as dextrose and glucagon injection.
- determine the timing, mode, duration, and intensity of exercise.
- eat a carbohydrate meal 1–3 h prior to exercise.
- assess metabolic control.
  - if blood glucose <5.0 mmol·L^{-1} and levels are decreasing, extra carbohydrates may be needed.
  - if blood glucose 5–13.9 mmol·L^{-1}, extra carbohydrates may not be needed, depending on the duration of exercise and individual response to exercise.
  - if blood glucose is >14 mmol·L^{-1} and urine or blood ketones are present, delay exercise until normalized with insulin administration.
  - if the activity is aerobic, estimate energy expenditure and determine if insulin or additional carbohydrate will be needed based on peak insulin activity.
  - if insulin dose is to be adjusted for long-duration and/or moderate- to high-intensity exercise, try a 50% pre-meal insulin dose reduction 1 h prior to exercise. Dosages can be altered on subsequent exercise days, based on the measured individual response. Insulin should be injected into a site distal to the exercising muscle and into subcutaneous tissue; an abdominal site is ideal.
  - if carbohydrate is to be increased, try 1 g·kg^{-1}(body mass)·h^{-1} moderate- to vigorous-intensity exercise performed during peak insulin activity and less carbohydrate as the time since insulin injection increases. The amount of carbohydrate can be altered on subsequent exercise days, based on the measured insulin responses. The total dose of

carbohydrate should be divided equally and consumed at 20 min intervals.

- if the exercise is anaerobic or occurring during heat or accompanied by competition stress, an increase in insulin may be needed.
- consider fluid intake to maintain hydration (~250 mL 20 min prior to exercise).

During physical activity

- monitor blood glucose every 30 min.
- continue fluid intake (250 mL every 20–30 min).
- if required, consume carbohydrate at 20–30 min intervals.

After physical activity

- monitor blood glucose, including overnight, if amount of physical activity is not habitual.
- consider adjusting insulin therapy to decrease immediate and delayed insulin action.
- consider consuming additional slow-acting carbohydrate to protect against post-exercise late onset hypoglycaemia.

Practical guidelines are adapted from Riddell *et al.*[53]

The Diabetes Research in Children Network Study Group[60] demonstrated that 22% of the T1DM teenagers developed hypoglycaemia overnight after an afternoon exercise session on the treadmill. The exercise session consisted of 15 min walking on a treadmill at a heart rate of ~140 beats·min^{-1}, followed by a 5 min rest period. This cycle was repeated three more times, for a total intervention time of 75 min. Besides the significant hypoglycaemias, the mean glucose level at 6 a.m. was lower on an exercise day compared to a sedentary day. Furthermore, the glucose level before the bedtime snack was a predictor of overnight hypoglycaemia: hypoglycaemia was uncommon if the glucose level was above 7.2 mmol L^{-1}. Another study demonstrated that when exercising children maintained their basal insulin infusion rates during unplanned activity, they typically developed late-onset post-exercise hypoglycaemia during sleep, even though hypoglycaemia did not occur during PA. Even when basal insulin rates were omitted during PA, six of ten patients still had nocturnal hypoglycaemia.[61] Reductions in nocturnal basal insulin rates and proper bedtime snacks seem the most logical approach. A complex carbohydrate (e.g. uncooked corn starch), or a mixed snack containing fat and protein may help spread the gastrointestinal uptake during the night.[62]

Should PA be undertaken during a state of severe insulin deficiency exercise-induced ketoacidosis can occur. During exercise under such circumstances, peripheral glucose utilization is impaired and hepatic glucose output is enhanced as is lipolysis.[63]

The type of PA will make differences. Low- to moderate-intensity exercise especially for longish spells increases the risk of hypoglycaemia.[64] In very high-intensity exercise (>80% of $\dot{V}O_2$ max), blood glucose levels rise, as in healthy individuals, possibly by counter-acting hormones such as catecholamines, growth hormone, and cortisol.[65] Also after a short period of intense exercise, hyperglycaemia remains, but only as long as there are elevations in counter-regulatory hormones (i.e. 30–60 min).[66] As stated earlier, this is a physiological response and one could argue whether the insulin therapy should be adapted to it. Furthermore, since hypoglycaemia will be encountered in aerobic exercise especially if prolonged, it has even been suggested to counter the exercise-mediated fall in glycaemia with a 10 s maximal sprint[56] or to favour intermittent high-intensity compared to continuous moderate-intensity exercise.[67]

Compared to aerobic training, resistance training does not seem to have such a strong effect on metabolic control,[68] whereas anaerobic training may give a dramatic rise in blood glucose, due to the release of the counter-acting hormones. Since the increase usually only lasts 30–60 min and may be followed by hypoglycaemia, it is again not advised to adapt insulin therapy to it.[69]

The time of the day on which PA is performed can make a difference. Physical activity before insulin administration in the morning is associated with a low risk of hypoglycaemia, since circulating insulin levels are low and liver and muscle glycogen stores are full.[64] Sprinting can be a useful strategy to prevent hypoglycaemia.[70] To a lesser extent, age, gender, level of metabolic control, and level of aerobic fitness also contribute.

The insulin-dependent diabetic may also have gastrointestinal motor dysfunction. This can include gastric motor dysfunction, known as gastroparesis, with significant delay in stomach emptying.[71] This can result in delay of emptying of meals and enhancing the possibility of hypoglycaemia during PA.

In addition, the blunted neuro-hormonal response to PA that is known in diabetes appears to be exponentially increased by previous exercise performance or by antecedent hypoglycaemic episodes. Lastly, in individuals with poor metabolic control, PA can increase the risk of hyperglycaemia and ketoacidosis, causing dehydration and acidosis, both of which impair exercise performance.[69]

Strategies to optimize performance and prevent complications in type 1 diabetes mellitus

An exact prescription for the exercising young diabetic cannot be made. However, if major precautions and preparations are taken, then the acute problems of severe hypoglycaemia can be largely prevented. Probably the childhood diabetic athlete who undertakes regular training and competition is more likely to be well educated in actions, and will, therefore, be safer than the child who undertakes occasional and variable exercise. There is extensive literature in this field.[63,72–74] Additionally, there are publications that specifically cover the diabetic child athlete.[54,63,75] Diet and insulin therapy management remain the two main important strategies possible in patients with T1DM practising sports in order to minimize the occurrence of sports-related adverse events. Since children mostly perform spontaneous exercise, it is not always possible to anticipate the need to decrease. In these instances, carbohydrate ingestion is a valuable option.

Pre-exercise assessment

Education of the patient and the parents is essential, especially if the patient is very young. No young diabetic should embark on sport and exercise without having substantial awareness of the problems and how to overcome these problems. This can be appropriately undertaken by a doctor experienced in diabetes management, a specialist diabetic nurse, a dietician, and possibly also an exercise physiologist who can advise on the energy requirements of the type of exercise.

The patient should be trained to have the following competences:

i) self-monitoring of blood levels;

ii) monitoring of ketone levels in urine or blood;

iii) knowledge of dietary factors; and

iv) awareness of the symptoms of hypoglycaemia, methods of prevention, and how to treat it.

The patient should preferably be on intensive insulin therapy, either by pen or by pump. Although possibly not introducing better control, the flexibility afforded is a major advantage. Until now no significant advantages have been found for subjects with pump treatment.[61]

If the child participates in regular physical training for a sport, the club, coach, or teacher must be informed. Often a doctor is involved in the sport.[76] The diabetic should wear identification showing that he/she is a diabetic. Those supervising the training should be aware of the symptoms of hypoglycaemia and the treatment required.

It is generally recommended that the patient should have a full medical assessment prior to undertaking high-intensity exercise, in order to identify complicating factors such as vascular disease, microangiopathy, nephropathy, and neuropathy. Significant disease may preclude some sports, or require a modified approach to exercise. It is, however, unlikely that a young diabetic will have such significant disease. The so-called 'brittle' diabetic or someone with psychological problems should be cautious about involvement in highly demanding sports.

Prior to physical activity

Before a diabetic child begins any type of PA, the type of exercise should be assessed. It may be regularly recurring, for example, training 1–2 h of swimming, football, athletics, etc. The diabetic may, therefore, have a standard regime. In these cases, total daily insulin administration is often already reduced, leading to a greater reliance on lipid oxidation.[77] Alternatively, the exercise may be unusual, e.g. a sports day with several intermittent events. If the exercise is prolonged and aerobic, there is probably greater danger of hypoglycaemia than if the exercise is short and anaerobic.

The patient should already be well and replete in carbohydrate stores. A meal should be taken about 3–4 h before exercise. The meal should have a large carbohydrate component with mainly complex 'slowly absorbable' carbohydrates (at least 60%, but if long-lasting aerobic exercise is programmed, it should reach 70%).

Short-acting insulin should preferably be used, since long-acting insulin would normally have been taken the prior evening. The dose should be taken prior to a meal and a reduction in dosage is essential. This reduction varies by 30–50%, but will depend on the type of exercise and the previous experience of the patient concerning insulin dosage. Flexible insulin dosing regimens, especially for pump users, will help reduce the risk of exercise-induced nocturnal hypoglycaemia. The insulin should not be injected into an exercising extremity; thus an abdominal site is usually preferable. This will prevent rapid absorption of insulin. Pre-meal insulin may be reduced by 30–50%, and in case of more prolonged exercise the dose might be reduced up to 90%. Because it is impossible to predict the exact insulin reduction needed, individuals should use records of previous experiences as a guideline and always have additional carbohydrates available. Importantly, a well-organized plan should be developed and conveyed to the child's coaches, teachers, friends, guardians, and siblings.[53] Metabolic control should be assessed. If the blood glucose is $<5\ \text{mmol}\cdot\text{L}^{-1}$, extra calories prior to exercise will be required. If the blood glucose is $>15\ \text{mmol}\cdot\text{L}^{-1}$, measure urinary ketones, and if positive, take more insulin, and delay exercise until blood glucose is satisfactory and urinary ketones are negative. Be aware that psychological stress before a match may also induce hyperglycaemia. The adrenal response underlying this phenomenon may require corrective insulin administration.[33] Also warm and humid environments may elevate blood glucose levels. Therefore, it is advisable to check blood sugar 1 h before and 30 min before any activity, in order to identify a trend in blood sugar concentration. For instance, a blood glucose level of $5.5\ \text{mmol}\cdot\text{L}^{-1}$ may be considered safe at one time, but potentially dangerous if the previous value was $10\ \text{mmol}\cdot\text{L}^{-1}$. If low, a sugary drink of 15 g of simple chain molecules could be used.

During physical activity

As a general rule, $1\text{–}1.5\ \text{g carbohydrate}\cdot\text{kg}^{-1}(\text{body mass})\cdot\text{h}^{-1}$ should be consumed during exercise performed during peak insulin action. When the same exercise is performed 2.5 and 4 h after insulin administration, then required carbohydrate intake will be 0.5 and $0.25\ \text{g}\cdot\text{kg}^{-1}$, respectively.[78]

If the exercise is prolonged, then further monitoring of blood may be required. This will obviously be awkward and will lose time in a prolonged marathon type event, but in a training situation it should be possible. The use of more muscles for aerobic exercise or weight-bearing activities is likely to lead to a greater drop in blood glucose. The convenience of continuous glucose monitoring devices (e.g. Guardian RT, Medtronic) and insulin pump therapy may be ideal for youth. If the exercise is prolonged >30 min, supplemental rapidly absorbable carbohydrate (15~40 g) should be taken every 30 min. This can be made up in drinks, as fluid replacement is also essential. During a moderate-intensity exercise session of 55–60% of $\dot{V}O_2$ max for 60 min T1DM adolescents were able to maintain the blood glucose concentration with 8–10% carbohydrate drinks.[79] When stomach upset causes delayed gastric absorption, isotonic beverages containing less than 8% glucose are good alternatives.[69] Should the subject experience symptoms of hypoglycaemia he/she should inform someone else, and take absorbable carbohydrate. Exercise can then be continued when the subject has recovered. Should severe hypoglycaemia occur and if oral administration is impossible (35–45 g of oral glucose), then intravenous glucose and/or intramuscular 1 mg of glucagon will be required.

However, to prevent strong fluctuations in blood glucose, frequent self-monitoring of blood sugar, information about the exercise, insulin administration, and carbohydrate intake should be recorded in an exercise training log that also documents the type, timeline, and duration of the exercise protocol. Logging this personal experience may help reaching near-normal blood glucose concentration during PA. Hyperglycaemia is associated with increased rating of perceived exertion and a shift from lipid to carbohydrate oxidation,[80] while hypoglycaemia has been related to poor sport performance and cognitive function.[81] Therefore, a euglycaemic to slightly hyperglycaemic state seems to give optimal aerobic and endurance capapcity.[82]

After physical activity

The main problem is delayed hypoglycaemia and a reduction in insulin dosage may be required, and possibly increased caloric intake for 12–14 h after the activity. For patients experiencing post-exercise late-onset hypoglycaemia during the night, a complex carbohydrate (uncooked starch) or a mixed snack containing fat and protein may be particularly beneficial at bedtime. It is also useful having somewhat higher target glucose levels at bedtime on days of intense exercise, especially for those who receive a pre-breakfast dose of glargine insulin. Physical activity may exacerbate abnormalities detected in patients with diabetic neuropathy, such as maximal cardiac capacity and output, decreased cardiovascular rate to response to physical exercise, orthostatic hypotension, impaired sweating, and impaired gastrointestinal function.[83–85]

Although in many countries alcohol is prohibited before adulthood, alcohol is often used among students in all-day tournaments. As alcohol inhibits gluconeogenesis, it impairs the counter-regulatory effect in case of a hypoglycaemia.[86]

Other points

It should be emphasized that exact prescriptions are impossible. Campaigne *et al.*[87] concluded that general recommendations on how to adjust insulin or diet before PA are difficult to give. Individualized recommendations for treatment modification appear most appropriate. As in athletes without diabetes, the athlete with T1DM with hypoglycaemia will dramatically lower his exercise performance and increase the rating of perceived exertion. Hyperglycaemic athletes may already be dehydrated, thereby impairing performance,[53] Furthermore, hyperglycaemia has been associated with the reduced ability to secrete beta-endorphins during exercise.[80]

Sport specific training advice can be found at:

- Diabetes Exercise and Sports Association (www.diabetes-exercise.org), an international organization that provides guidance and networking between novices, health professionals, and experienced diabetic athletes.
- www.runsweet.com where a combination of contributions from sportsmen and sportswomen are interspersed with expert advice.
- www.Ispad.org, an international society for paediatric and adolescent diabetes that aims to promote clinical and basic science, research, education, and advocacy in childhood and adolescent diabetes

Short-acting insulin analogues and basal insulins

Tuominen *et al*[88] found that a short-acting insulin analogue [Lys (B28) Pro (B29)] peaked earlier than human insulin and postprandial blood glucose was lower. Exercise-induced hypoglycaemia was also 2.2 times greater during early exercise, but 46% less during late exercise. They concluded that as PA is usually not performed until 2–3 h after a meal, short-acting insulin analogues may be more feasible than soluble human insulin. This also means that there is a high risk of hypoglycaemia during PA 2–3 h after injection. For rapid-acting insulin analogues, the risk already comes up 40 min after injection. Furthermore, PA can strongly increase blood flow through skin, thereby increasing glucose and insulin delivery to skeletal muscle and rapid-acting insulin absorption rate.[49,51] A general rule is to reduce rapid-acting analogues prior to PA lasting longer than 30 min.

Basal insulins (Neutral Protamine Hagedorn [NPH], glargine or detemir) given once daily in the evening are often split in half, with one dose in the evening and a lower, second dose in the morning by 20–50% to compensate for the increased activity.[17]

New technologies leading to more possibilities in monitoring and adapting to the effects of physical activity in type 1 diabetes mellitus

Patients using insulin pumps, and especially patients who participate in contact sports, often disconnect from the pump, sometimes for up to 2 h. New insulin-pump technology, such as CGM, uses an automatic pump that stops when hypoglycaemia is detected by the sensor,[89] or that can even predict trends, preventing hypoglycaemia from occurring.[90] Indeed, for prevention and early detection of exercise-induced hypoglycaemia, CGM has proven to be a valuable tool.[77]

Conclusions

Diabetes mellitus is a complex metabolic disorder characterized by chronic hyperglycaemia resulting from defects in insulin secretion, insulin action, or both. The main goal is to render as normal a lifestyle as possible to the diabetic, by four main targets of management: obtaining good metabolic control, preventing long-term complications, promoting social competence, and promoting self-esteem. Physical activity is an essential tool for each of these goals and therefore the child with diabetes should be able to undertake a full range of sporting activities. At the same time, PA is a direct risk for hypoglycaemia, the most feared complication. Knowledge of strategies that limit the possibility of hypoglycaemia caused by PA, while at the same time optimize performance, is vital (see Box 23.3).

Summary

- Diabetes mellitus is a group of metabolic diseases characterized by chronic hyperglycaemia, resulting from defects in insulin secretion, insulin action, or both, leading to insufficient action of insulin on target tissue.
- Several forms of diabetes mellitus can be identified, each with their specific clinical characterization and treatment. The general aim, especially for type 1 diabetes mellitus (T1DM), is as normal a lifestyle as possible using four main targets of management: obtaining good metabolic control, preventing long-term complications, promoting social competence, and promoting self-worth.
- Intensive insulin therapy attempts to mimic the natural pattern of insulin secretion, effectively delays the late complications of T1DM, and is the treatment of choice, especially for the child who is involved in sports or intensive exercise regimens.
- Hypoglycaemia remains a significant problem in the exercising diabetic. During PA there is a dramatic increase in non-insulin-mediated glucose uptake, which reduces the need for circulating insulin levels.
- Post-exercise hypoglycaemia in adolescents has a biphasic character with increased glucose requirements shortly after and 7–11 h after exercise, although late-onset hypoglycaemia is known to occur up to 36 h post-exercise due to increased insulin sensitivity.
- Do not inject the insulin in a site that will be involved in muscular activity.
- On the other hand, hyperglycaemia can occur during high-intensity exercise, but may also be related to pre-competition psychological stress.

- The exact prescription cannot be made, but diet and insulin therapy management remain the two most important strategies possible in patients with T1DM practising sports, in order to minimize the occurrence of sports-related adverse events.
- Discuss the percentage reduction in insulin before exercise.
- The pump needs to be disconnected or a temporary lowering of the basal rate at least 90 min before starting exercise.
- Any exercise is dangerous and should be avoided if pre-exercise blood glucose levels are high (>14 $mmol \cdot L^{-1}$) with ketonuria (small or more)/ ketonaemia (>0.5 $mmol \cdot L^{-1}$). Give approximately 0.05 $U \cdot kg^{-1}$ or 5% of total daily dose (including all meal bolus doses and basal insulin/basal rate in pump) and postpone exercise until ketones have cleared.
- Consume up to 1.0–1.5 g of carbohydrate $\cdot kg^{-1}$(body mass) $\cdot h^{-1}$ of strenuous or longer-duration exercise when circulating insulin levels are high, if pre-exercise insulin doses are not decreased.
- Meals with high content of carbohydrates should be consumed shortly after the exercise event, taking advantage of the period of heightened insulin sensitivity to help replenish glycogen content and limit post-exercise hypoglycaemia.
- Dehydration is a risk unless sugar-free fluids also are consumed.
- Measure blood glucose before going to bed and decrease bedtime basal insulin (or pump basal) by 10–20% after an afternoon or evening exercise session if the exercise was more intense than usual or was an activity not performed regularly.
- Short sprints added to aerobic training can minimize the risk of hypoglycaemia
- Extra carbohydrate after the activity is often the best option to prevent post-exercise hypoglycaemia when short-duration and high-intensity anaerobic activities are performed.
- A mixture between aerobic and anaerobic exercise (soccer, cycling, jogging, and swimming) will typically require extra carbohydrate before, possibly during, and often after the activity.
- The rise in blood glucose after intense exercise may be prevented by giving a small additional dose of rapid-acting insulin at half-time or immediately after the exercise is finished—for example, a 50% correction bolus when blood glucose levels are >15 $mmol \cdot L^{-1}$.
- Risk of post-exercise nocturnal hypoglycaemia is high, and particular care should be taken if bedtime blood glucose level is <7.0 $mmol \cdot L^{-1}$ (125 $mg \cdot dL^{-1}$) with Neutral Protamine Hagedorn (NPH) basal insulin. With basal analogues, the bedtime glucose level can be slightly lower without a substantial risk of night-time hypoglycaemia, but no specific value is a guarantee that hypoglyacemia will be avoided.
- A diabetes care plan containing written advice about exercise and sports should be provided for carers/teachers.
- Continuous glucose monitoring may have a role in helping to avoid hypoglycaemia during and after exercise.
- New pump technologies such as low-glucose suspend and programmed low-glucose management may also be useful in the future.

References

1. Craig ME, Jefferies C, Dabelea D, Balde N, Seth A, Donaghue KC. ISPAD Clinical Practice Consensus Guidelines 2014. Definition, epidemiology, and classification of diabetes in children and adolescents. *Pediatr Diabetes*. 2014; 15(Suppl 20): 4–17.
2. American Diabetes Association. Diagnosis and classification of diabetes mellitus. *Diabetes Care*. 2014; 37(Suppl 1): S81–S90.
3. Alberti KG, Zimmet PZ. Definition, diagnosis and classification of diabetes mellitus and its complications. Part 1: diagnosis and classification of diabetes mellitus provisional report of a WHO consultation. *Diabetic Med*. 1998; 15: 539–553.
4. Zeitler P, Fu J, Tandon N, *et al*. ISPAD Clinical Practice Consensus Guidelines 2014. Type 2 diabetes in the child and adolescent. *Pediatr Diabetes*. 2014; 15(Suppl 20): 26–46.
5. Wolfsdorf JI, Allgrove J, Craig ME, *et al*. ISPAD Clinical Practice Consensus Guidelines 2014. Diabetic ketoacidosis and hyperglycemic hyperosmolar state. *Pediatr Diabetes*. 2014; 15(Suppl 20): 154–179.
6. Silverstein J, Klingensmith G, Copeland K, *et al*. Care of children and adolescents with type 1 diabetes: a statement of the American Diabetes Association. *Diabetes Care*. 2005; 28: 186–212.
7. Swift PG, Skinner TC, de Beaufort CE, *et al*. Target setting in intensive insulin management is associated with metabolic control: the Hvidoere childhood diabetes study group centre differences study 2005. *Pediatr Diabetes*. 2010; 11: 271–278.
8. Gautier JF, Beressi JP, Leblanc H, Vexiau P, Passa P. Are the implications of the Diabetes Control and Complications Trial (DCCT) feasible in daily clinical practice? *Diabetes Metab*. 1996; 22: 415–419.
9. Watkins PJ. DCCT: the ecstasy and the agony. *Q J Med*. 1994; 87: 315–316.
10. Garvey KC, Telo GH, Needleman JS, Forbes P, Finkelstein JA, Laffel LM. Health care transition in young adults with type 1 diabetes: perspectives of adult endocrinologists in the US. *Diabetes Care*. 2016; 39: 190–197.
11. Bertuzzi F, Verzaro R, Provenzano V, Ricordi C. Brittle type 1 diabetes mellitus. *Curr Med Chem*. 2007; 14: 1739–1744.
12. Castle JR, Jacobs PG. Nonadjunctive use of continuous glucose monitoring for diabetes treatment decisions. *J Diabetes Sci Technol*. 2016; 10: 1169–73.
13. Frier BM. Lawrence Lecture. Hypoglycaemia and diabetes. *Diabetic Med*. 1986; 3: 513–525.
14. Watkins PJ. ABC of diabetes: practical problems. *BMJ*. 1982; 285(6345): 866–867.
15. Ryder RE, Owens DR, Hayes TM, Ghatei MA, Bloom SR. Unawareness of hypoglycaemia and inadequate hypoglycaemic counterregulation: no causal relation with diabetic autonomic neuropathy. *BMJ*. 1990; 301(6755): 783–787.
16. Cranston I, Lomas J, Maran A, Macdonald I, Amiel SA. Restoration of hypoglycaemia awareness in patients with long-duration insulin-dependent diabetes. *Lancet*. 1994; 344(8918): 283–287.
17. Robertson K, Riddell MC, Guinhouya BC, *et al*. ISPAD Clinical Practice Consensus Guidelines 2014. Exercise in children and adolescents with diabetes. *Pediatr Diabetes*. 2014; 15(Suppl 20): 203–223.
18. Komatsu WR, Gabbay MA, Castro ML, *et al*. Aerobic exercise capacity in normal adolescents and those with type 1 diabetes mellitus. *Pediatr Diabetes*. 2005; 6: 145–149.
19. Adolfsson P, Nilsson S, Albertsson-Wikland K, Lindblad B. Hormonal response during physical exercise of different intensities in adolescents with type 1 diabetes and healthy controls. *Pediatr Diabetes*. 2012; 13: 587–596.
20. Cuenca-Garcia M, Jago R, Shield JP, Burren CP. How does physical activity and fitness influence glycaemic control in young people with Type 1 diabetes? *Diabetic Med*. 2012; 29: e369–376.
21. Miculis CP, De Campos W, da Silva Boguszweski MC. Correlation between glycemic control and physical activity level in adolescents and children with type 1 diabetes. *J Phys Act Health*. 2015; 12: 232–237.
22. Hall M. Sport and diabetes. *Br J Sports Med*. 1997; 31: 3.

23. Massin MM, Lebrethon MC, Rocour D, Gerard P, Bourguignon JP. Patterns of physical activity determined by heart rate monitoring among diabetic children. *Arch Dis Child*. 2005; 90: 1223–1226.
24. Raile K, Kapellen T, Schweiger A, *et al*. Physical activity and competitive sports in children and adolescents with type 1 diabetes. *Diabetes Care*. 1999; 22: 1904–1905.
25. Sackey AH, Jefferson IG. Physical activity and glycaemic control in children with diabetes mellitus. *Diabetic Med*. 1996; 13: 789–793.
26. Mosher PE, Nash MS, Perry AC, LaPerriere AR, Goldberg RB. Aerobic circuit exercise training: effect on adolescents with well-controlled insulin-dependent diabetes mellitus. *Arch Phys Med Rehab*. 1998; 79: 652–657.
27. Pate RR, Trost SG, Levin S, Dowda M. Sports participation and health-related behaviors among US youth. *Arch Pediatr Adolesc Med*. 2000; 154: 904–911.
28. Temple MY, Bar-Or O, Riddell MC. The reliability and repeatability of the blood glucose response to prolonged exercise in adolescent boys with IDDM. *Diabetes Care*. 1995; 18: 326–332.
29. Wasserman DH, Vranic M. Interaction between insulin and counterregulatory hormones in control of substrate utilization in health and diabetes during exercise. *Diabetes Metab Rev*. 1986; 1: 359–384.
30. Thorell A, Hirshman MF, Nygren J, *et al*. Exercise and insulin cause GLUT-4 translocation in human skeletal muscle. *Am J Physiol*. 1999; 277: E733–E741.
31. Cahill GF, Jr. Starvation in man. *N Eng J Med*. 1970; 282: 668–675.
32. Riddell M, Perkins BA. Exercise and glucose metabolism in persons with diabetes mellitus: perspectives on the role for continuous glucose monitoring. *J Diabetes Sci Technol*. 2009; 3: 914–923.
33. Marliss EB, Vranic M. Intense exercise has unique effects on both insulin release and its roles in glucoregulation: implications for diabetes. *Diabetes*. 2002; 51(Suppl 1): S271–S283.
34. Maughan RJ. Nutritional aspects of endurance exercise in humans. *Proc Nutr Soc*. 1994; 53: 181–188.
35. Borghouts LB, Keizer HA. Exercise and insulin sensitivity: a review. *Int J Sports Med*. 2000; 21: 1–12.
36. Costill DL. Carbohydrates for exercise: dietary demands for optimal performance. *Int J Sports Med*. 1988; 9: 1–18.
37. Coyle EF. Timing and method of increased carbohydrate intake to cope with heavy training, competition and recovery. *J Sports Sci*. 1991; 9: 29–51.
38. Wilber RL, Moffatt RJ. Influence of carbohydrate ingestion on blood glucose and performance in runners. *Int J Sport Nutr*. 1992; 2: 317–327.
39. Hargreaves M, Costill DL, Coggan A, Fink WJ, Nishibata I. Effect of carbohydrate feedings on muscle glycogen utilization and exercise performance. *Med Sci Sports Exerc*. 1984; 16: 219–222.
40. Coyle EF, Hagberg JM, Hurley BF, Martin WH, Ehsani AA, Holloszy JO. Carbohydrate feeding during prolonged strenuous exercise can delay fatigue. *J Appl Physiol Resp Environ Exerc Physiol*. 1983; 55: 230–235.
41. Soman VR, Koivisto VA, Deibert D, Felig P, DeFronzo RA. Increased insulin sensitivity and insulin binding to monocytes after physical training. *N Eng J Med*. 1979; 301: 1200–1204.
42. Ebeling P, Bourey R, Koranyi L, *et al*. Mechanism of enhanced insulin sensitivity in athletes. Increased blood flow, muscle glucose transport protein (GLUT-4) concentration, and glycogen synthase activity. *J Clin Invest*. 1993; 92: 1623–1631.
43. Yki-Jarvinen H, Koivisto VA. Effects of body composition on insulin sensitivity. *Diabetes*. 1983; 32: 965–969.
44. Costill DL, Saltin B. Factors limiting gastric emptying during rest and exercise. *J Appl Physiol*. 1974; 37: 679–683.
45. Rowell LB, Blackmon JR, Bruce RA. Indocyanine green clearance and estimated hepatic blood flow during mild to maximal exercise in upright man. *J Clin Invest*. 1964; 43: 1677–1690.
46. Darlington WA, Quastel JH. Absorption of sugars from isolated surviving intestine. *Arch Biochem Biophys*. 1953; 43: 194–207.
47. Giannini C, de Giorgis T, Mohn A, Chiarelli F. Role of physical exercise in children and adolescents with diabetes mellitus. *J Pediatr Endocrin Met*. 2007; 20: 173–184.
48. Berger M, Halban PA, Assal JP, Offord RE, Vranic M, Renold AE. Pharmacokinetics of subcutaneously injected tritiated insulin: effects of exercise. *Diabetes*. 1979; 28(Suppl 1): 53–57.
49. Koivisto VA, Felig P. Effects of leg exercise on insulin absorption in diabetic patients. *N Eng J Med*. 1978; 298: 79–83.
50. Zinman B, Murray FT, Vranic M, *et al*. Glucoregulation during moderate exercise in insulin treated diabetics. *J Clin Endocrinol Metab*. 1977; 45: 641–652.
51. Peter R, Luzio SD, Dunseath G, *et al*. Effects of exercise on the absorption of insulin glargine in patients with type 1 diabetes. *Diabetes Care*. 2005; 28: 560–565.
52. Riddell MC, Bar-Or O, Ayub BV, Calvert RE, Heigenhauser GJ. Glucose ingestion matched with total carbohydrate utilization attenuates hypoglycemia during exercise in adolescents with IDDM. *Int J Sport Nutr*. 1999; 9: 24–34.
53. Riddell MC, Iscoe KE. Physical activity, sport, and pediatric diabetes. *Pediatr Diabetes*. 2006; 7: 60–70.
54. Riddell MC, Bar-Or O, Hollidge-Horvat M, Schwarcz HP, Heigenhauser GJ. Glucose ingestion and substrate utilization during exercise in boys with IDDM. *J Appl Physiol*. 2000; 88: 1239–1246.
55. Timmons BW, Bar-Or O, Riddell MC. Energy substrate utilization during prolonged exercise with and without carbohydrate intake in preadolescent and adolescent girls. *J Appl Physiol*. 2007; 103: 995–1000.
56. Bussau VA, Ferreira LD, Jones TW, Fournier PA. The 10-s maximal sprint: a novel approach to counter an exercise-mediated fall in glycemia in individuals with type 1 diabetes. *Diabetes Care*. 2006; 29: 601–606.
57. Guelfi KJ, Jones TW, Fournier PA. The decline in blood glucose levels is less with intermittent high-intensity compared with moderate exercise in individuals with type 1 diabetes. *Diabetes Care*. 2005; 28: 1289–1294.
58. MacDonald MJ. Postexercise late-onset hypoglycemia in insulin-dependent diabetic patients. *Diabetes Care*. 1987; 10: 584–588.
59. McMahon SK, Ferreira LD, Ratnam N, *et al*. Glucose requirements to maintain euglycemia after moderate-intensity afternoon exercise in adolescents with type 1 diabetes are increased in a biphasic manner. *J Clin Endocrin Metab*. 2007; 92: 963–968.
60. Tsalikian E, Mauras N, Beck RW, *et al*. Impact of exercise on overnight glycemic control in children with type 1 diabetes mellitus. *J Pediatr*. 2005; 147: 528–534.
61. Admon G, Weinstein Y, Falk B, *et al*. Exercise with and without an insulin pump among children and adolescents with type 1 diabetes mellitus. *Pediatrics*. 2005; 116: e348–e355.
62. Kalergis M, Schiffrin A, Gougeon R, Jones PJ, Yale JF. Impact of bedtime snack composition on prevention of nocturnal hypoglycemia in adults with type 1 diabetes undergoing intensive insulin management using lispro insulin before meals: a randomized, placebo-controlled, crossover trial. *Diabetes Care*. 2003; 26: 9–15.
63. Horton ES. Exercise and diabetes mellitus. *Med Clin N Am*. 1988; 72: 1301–1321.
64. Ruegemer JJ, Squires RW, Marsh HM, *et al*. Differences between prebreakfast and late afternoon glycemic responses to exercise in IDDM patients. *Diabetes Care*. 1990; 13: 104–110.
65. Purdon C, Brousson M, Nyveen SL, *et al*. The roles of insulin and catecholamines in the glucoregulatory response during intense exercise and early recovery in insulin-dependent diabetic and control subjects. *J Clin Endocrin Met*. 1993; 76: 566–573.
66. Sigal RJ, Purdon C, Fisher SJ, Halter JB, Vranic M, Marliss EB. Hyperinsulinemia prevents prolonged hyperglycemia after intense exercise in insulin-dependent diabetic subjects. *J Clin Endocrin Metab*. 1994; 79: 1049–1057.
67. Guelfi KJ, Ratnam N, Smythe GA, Jones TW, Fournier PA. Effect of intermittent high-intensity compared with continuous moderate exercise on glucose production and utilization in individuals with type 1 diabetes. *Am J Physiol Endocr Metab*. 2007; 292: E865–E870.

68. Ramalho AC, de Lourdes Lima M, Nunes F, *et al.* The effect of resistance versus aerobic training on metabolic control in patients with type-1 diabetes mellitus. *Diabetes Res Clin Prac.* 2006; 72: 271–276.
69. Robertson K, Adolfsson P, Riddell MC, Scheiner G, Hanas R. Exercise in children and adolescents with diabetes. *Pediatr Diabetes.* 2008; 9: 65–77.
70. Davey RJ, Paramalingam N, Retterath AJ, *et al.* Antecedent hypoglycaemia does not diminish the glycaemia-increasing effect and glucoregulatory responses of a 10 s sprint in people with type 1 diabetes. *Diabetologia.* 2014; 57: 1111–1118.
71. Horowitz M, Dent J. Disordered gastric emptying: mechanical basis, assessment and treatment. *Bailliere Clin Gastr.* 1991; 5: 371–407.
72. Choi KL, Chisholm DJ. Exercise and insulin-dependent diabetes mellitus (IDDM): benefits and pitfalls. *Aust N Zeal J Med.* 1996; 26: 827–833.
73. Fahey PJ, Stallkamp ET, Kwatra S. The athlete with type I diabetes: managing insulin, diet and exercise. *Am Fam Physician.* 1996; 53: 1611–1624.
74. Landry GL, Allen DB. Diabetes mellitus and exercise. *Clin Sports Med.* 1992; 11: 403–418.
75. Dorchy H, Poortmans J. Sport and the diabetic child. *Sports Med.* 1989; 7: 248–262.
76. Jimenez CC. Diabetes and exercise: the role of the athletic trainer. *J Athl Train.* 1997; 32: 339–343.
77. Pasieka AM, Nikoletos N, Riddell MC. Advances in exercise, physical activity, and diabetes mellitus. *Diabetes Technol Ther.* 2016; 18(Suppl 1): S76–S85.
78. Huttunen NP, Kaar ML, Knip M, Mustonen A, Puukka R, Akerblom HK. Physical fitness of children and adolescents with insulin-dependent diabetes mellitus. *Ann Clin Res.* 1984; 16: 1–5.
79. Perrone C, Laitano O, Meyer F. Effect of carbohydrate ingestion on the glycemic response of type 1 diabetic adolescents during exercise. *Diabetes Care.* 2005; 28: 2537–2538.
80. Wanke T, Auinger M, Formanek D, *et al.* Defective endogenous opioid response to exercise in type I diabetic patients. *Metabolism.* 1996; 45: 137–142.
81. Kelly D, Hamilton JK, Riddell MC. Blood glucose levels and performance in a sports cAMP for adolescents with type 1 diabetes mellitus: a field study. *Int J Pediatr.* 2010; 2010: doi: 10.1155/2010/216167
82. Heyman E, Briard D, Gratas-Delamarche A, Delamarche P, De Kerdanet M. Normal physical working capacity in prepubertal children with type 1 diabetes compared with healthy controls. *Acta Paediatr.* 2005; 94: 1389–1394.
83. Colhoun HM, Francis DP, Rubens MB, Underwood SR, Fuller JH. The association of heart-rate variability with cardiovascular risk factors and coronary artery calcification: a study in type 1 diabetic patients and the general population. *Diabetes Care.* 2001; 24: 1108–1114.
84. Hilsted J, Galbo H, Christensen NJ. Impaired cardiovascular responses to graded exercise in diabetic autonomic neuropathy. *Diabetes.* 1979; 28: 313–319.
85. Margonato A, Gerundini P, Vicedomini G, Gilardi MC, Pozza G, Fazio F. Abnormal cardiovascular response to exercise in young asymptomatic diabetic patients with retinopathy. *Am Heart J.* 1986; 112: 554–560.
86. Turner BC, Jenkins E, Kerr D, Sherwin RS, Cavan DA. The effect of evening alcohol consumption on next-morning glucose control in type 1 diabetes. *Diabetes Care.* 2001; 24: 1888–1893.
87. Campaigne BN, Wallberg-Henriksson H, Gunnarsson R. Glucose and insulin responses in relation to insulin dose and caloric intake 12 h after acute physical exercise in men with IDDM. *Diabetes Care.* 1987; 10: 716–721.
88. Tuominen JA, Karonen SL, Melamies L, Bolli G, Koivisto VA. Exercise-induced hypoglycaemia in IDDM patients treated with a short-acting insulin analogue. *Diabetologia.* 1995; 38: 106–111.
89. Garg S, Brazg RL, Bailey TS, *et al.* Reduction in duration of hypoglycemia by automatic suspension of insulin delivery: the in-clinic ASPIRE study. *Diabetes Technol Ther.* 2012; 14: 205–209.
90. Danne T, Tsioli C, Kordonouri O, *et al.* The PILGRIM study: in silico modeling of a predictive low glucose management system and feasibility in youth with type 1 diabetes during exercise. *Diabetes Technol Ther.* 2014; 16: 338–347.

CHAPTER 24

Exercise, physical activity, and asthma

Helge Hebestreit, Susi Kriemler, and Thomas Radtke

Introduction

'Asthma is a chronic inflammatory disorder associated with variable airflow obstruction and bronchial hyperresponsiveness. It presents with recurrent episodes of wheeze, cough, shortness of breath, and chest tightness'.[1]

Information on the prevalence of asthma in children and adolescents is dependent on the diagnostic criteria used. In a study in Denmark, the prevalence of asthma in 8- to 10-year-old children, as diagnosed by their general practitioner or during a medical assessment of children who were selected based on a screening interview and monitoring of peak flow, was 6.6%.[2] In an survey of 12-year-old children,[3] a history of asthma was reported in 16.8% of children in New Zealand, while other countries showed lower prevalence (South Africa: 11.5%, Sweden: 4.0%, Wales: 12.0%). In another epidemiological study surveying 12–15-year-old children in Australia, England, Germany, and New Zealand, 20–27% of the participants experienced wheezing during the past 12 months, and 4–12% reported more than three episodes per year.[4] Thus, the prevalence of asthma in childhood and adolescence varies among countries and can be estimated to be somewhere between 5 and 20%. Over time, there seems to be increasing asthma prevalence in western countries.[5,6] There is a growing body of literature that implicates lifestyle change, specifically decreased physical activity (PA), as a contributor to the increase in asthma prevalence and severity.[7,8]

One of the characteristics of asthma is that the bronchial system is hyperresponsive to a variety of triggers. These stimuli include airway infections, exposure to allergens or air pollutants, inhalation of dry and cold air, and exercise. Thus, exercise-induced asthma (EIA) is a feature of asthma and may affect any patient with asthma, provided that the exercise is of a sufficient intensity and duration.[9] Therefore, knowledge about the interrelationships between asthma and exercise is of major importance when dealing with a physically active paediatric population.

This chapter reviews the existing data on exercise capacity and PA of children with asthma. The mechanisms underlying pathologic responses to exercise in these children are summarized. Most of the information provided in this chapter is valid not only for children, but also for adults.

Exercise-induced asthma

Children at risk

Exercise-induced asthma may affect any child diagnosed with asthma, but also children with a history of bronchopulmonary dysplasia, a diagnosis of hay fever, or cystic fibrosis.[10,11] There are also children and adolescents suffering from EIA, who do not exhibit any of the risk factors for asthma. It has been suggested that some 10% of adolescent athletes suffer from EIA, many of them without being recognized.[12]

Symptoms of exercise-induced asthma

In most patients, EIA leads to coughing, wheezing, and shortness of breath shortly following exercise.[13] However, rather than reporting these typical respiratory symptoms, some patients complain following exercise about chest discomfort, nausea, or stomach ache. In children, symptoms usually resolve within 10–90 min following cessation of exercise, although some may experience a progressive worsening of bronchoconstriction.

Pathophysiology of exercise-induced bronchoconstriction

It has long been recognized that children with asthma are less likely to experience an attack when exercising in a warm and humid environment than when inhaling cold and dry air. Based on this observation, it was suggested that either heat loss from the respiratory epithelium and/or loss of water might trigger the bronchoconstriction.[14] Based on subsequent studies, the role of airway cooling/drying during exercise and/or rewarming of the bronchi after cessation of exertion is now generally accepted as the major mechanism responsible for EIA.[15,16] However, even if the respiratory heat loss is controlled for, the likelihood and severity of EIA is influenced by exercise intensity (low vs high) and exercise mode (swimming vs running).[17] Whether these latter findings indicate that airway cooling/drying/rewarming are not the exclusive pathogenic triggers responsible for EIA remains a matter of debate, as facial cooling may augment bronchial constriction.[18] Furthermore, recurrent hyperventilation with thermal and/or osmotic stress to the airway epithelium and/or inhalation of toxins such as chlorine from swimming pools have been associated with epithelial damage and eosinophilic and/or neutrophilic airway inflammation predisposing to exercise-induced bronchoconstriction.[16]

The exact pathway linking airway cooling/rewarming/drying to bronchial obstruction is not yet completely understood.[15] The following mechanisms have been suggested:

i) The cooling of the bronchial wall stimulates the parasympathetic system which then leads to a bronchoconstriction.[19]

ii) The cooling of the airways or the increase in bronchial surface osmolality paralleling airway drying triggers the release of neutrophil chemotactic factor of anaphylaxis, histamine, and/or leukotrienes, which then initiate a bronchoconstriction.[20,21] Restitution of vagal tone following exercise and the decrease in adrenaline levels may then lead to bronchoconstriction.[22]

iii) The rewarming of the airways following exercise induces either a contraction of smooth airway muscles, or a hyperaemia and swelling of the bronchial mucosa.[15,23]

Late response

Several studies have suggested that a considerable number of patients suffering from EIA experience a second fall in pulmonary function parameters several hours after the first exercise-induced airway narrowing has resolved.[24,25] These 'late responses' are reported to begin 2–4 h following the exercise challenge, peak between 4–8 h, and resolve after 12–24 h. There are, however, some studies that could not detect a significant exercise-induced late response compared to a placebo visit.[26,27] The authors attributed the reports of late asthmatic responses following exercise to the increased spontaneous within-day variation of pulmonary mechanics in children with asthma.[26,27]

Refractory period

In patients with EIA, a second bout of exercise 1–2 h following a first exercise task may induce less bronchial obstruction than a task of similar exercise intensity and duration, which is administered without a preceding exercise.[28] This reduced responsiveness is referred to as 'refractory period' and may occur even if the first challenge did not induce a significant bronchial narrowing, or was performed with other muscle groups than the subsequent exercise.[29] Refractoriness can be induced by continuous submaximal exercise, but also by intermittent sprints.[30,31]

It is important to stress that only about 40–60% of all patients with EIA show a refractory period.[32] In those patients who do exhibit this phenomenon the most effective exercise protocol seems to vary among individuals. Therefore, asthma patients who wish to utilize the refractory period to prevent EIA during training and competition should be counselled to try several exercise procedures and to select the most effective routine.

The mechanisms underlying the refractory period are not yet understood. It has been suggested that mast cells might be depleted from mediators, including histamine, with the first exercise challenge and that the replenishment of the stores takes up to 2 h.[33] Another explanation put forward is that prostaglandins, possibly type E_2, are released with the initial exercise bout and prevent a bronchial obstruction with a subsequent exercise challenge.[34] A third hypothesis is based on the assumption that a second exercise task induces less airway cooling than the first task.[35]

Diagnosing exercise-induced asthma

Exercise-induced asthma should be suspected if a patient complains about shortness of breath, wheezing, or cough during or following exercise. In children or adolescents who complain about chest pain with exercise, EIA should also be suspected.[36]

In patients diagnosed to have asthma, a history of exercise-related symptoms typical for EIA justifies a medical treatment without further evaluation.[15] Only if the improvement with medication is less than expected is a further evaluation including an exercise challenge necessary.

Children and adolescents who have no established diagnosis of asthma should be tested for impairment of resting pulmonary functions. If this test reveals bronchial obstruction that is markedly improved with inhalation of ß-adrenergic drugs, asthma as the cause for the exercise-related symptoms can be assumed. Unless required by national or international sports and anti-doping agencies such as Olympic committees to allow anti-asthma medications in training and competition, no further testing is necessary to establish the diagnosis if an adequate treatment leads to satisfactory results. In all other cases, a standardized challenge to prove bronchial hyperresponsiveness is recommended.

Physical activity and exercise capacity of children and adolescents with asthma or exercise-induced asthma

Acute asthmatic attacks are often triggered by exercise.[37] It would, therefore, not be surprising if children with asthma were less active than their peers. Astonishingly relatively little information is available on this issue. Children with untreated or poorly controlled asthma appear to be less fit and less physically active than their peers.[38,39] In children with known asthma both reduced[39] and normal[40] habitual PA has been reported. However, most children with asthma are probably as active as healthy children, if effectively treated.

Most[41–43], but not all[44], studies have shown that children with asthma have a decreased short-term and endurance exercise capacity, compared to healthy controls. The different findings between studies might reflect, in part, differences in disease severity.[42,43] Mechanisms limiting exercise capacity in asthmatic patients could be an increase in end-expiratory lung volume with exercise which results in increased work for ventilation, limitation of minute ventilation,[45] and a disturbance of the ventilation-perfusion relationship in the lung.[46] However, the latter mechanisms should lead to oxygen desaturation with exercise, which is rarely seen in patients with asthma.[23]

Since there is increasing evidence that a reduced level of PA in children with asthma is a more important predictor of low aerobic fitness than disease severity,[44,47] reduced aerobic fitness in a child with asthma should be primarily 'treated' with education and conditioning. Moreover, in a trained state, an asthmatic child's minute ventilation will be lower for any given exercise, making the stimulus for EIA less severe. Thus, regular exercise can reduce the likelihood of an EIA response. An adjustment of medication might also be necessary in some cases.

Exercise-related benefits to children with asthma

Several studies have evaluated the benefits of increased PA in children and adolescents with asthma.[48] In general, the effects are more pronounced in patients with severe disease compared to those with moderately severe asthma. Patients with mild asthma may not benefit from specific exercise programmes more than healthy children.

While many studies[48,49] showed an improvement in aerobic fitness or psychological variables in structured and supervised training programmes, some,[49] but not all,[50] observed a beneficial effect from a home-based unsupervised exercise programme. It might therefore be reasonable to refer those patients with moderate to severe asthma who might benefit from exercise rehabilitation to a structured programme. Possibly, the advantage of a structured exercise programme might be related to the effects of education[51] in addition to a more regular and intense physical training.

Improvements in fitness

Regular exercise training is effective in enhancing aerobic and anaerobic fitness and motor coordination in children with asthma.[42,48,51–53] The mechanisms underlying these improvements most probably act via the training effects also observed in healthy children, but may also invoke a more comfortable feeling for the children with asthma and their parents when the child engages in physical activities.

Psychological benefits

Children with asthma show disturbances in their psychological development which might be improved via an exercise programme.[54] Specifically, positive effects have been shown for ego structure, body image, social development, and concentration capacity.[54]

It should also be kept in mind that children with asthma strongly value the ability to engage in physical activities. For example, when 71 children aged 9 to 11 years were asked, 'How do you know when you are healthy'? 46% of all responses referred to activity or other physical/functional abilities.[55] In contrast, only 9% of the responses related to the absence of asthma-specific symptoms. In other words, many children with asthma consider PA as an integral part of daily life. To them, being allowed to exercise means to be normal.

Reduction in asthma symptoms and exercise-induced asthma

Large randomized, controlled trials on the effects of regular exercise on asthma morbidity are missing in children. However, some data available from relatively short exercise programmes with duration of 2–6 months suggest that physical conditioning may reduce the frequency of asthma symptoms, hospitalizations, emergency room visits, and school absenteeism.[56,57] The effects of an exercise programme on EIA are less clear. While Fitch *et al.*[58] did not see any change in the severity of EIA after a 3-month-long running training, Svenonius *et al.*[49] and Henrikson and Nielsen[59] found a significant improvement in EIA following combined land-based and swimming interval training for 3–4 months and 6 weeks training, respectively. At least part of the improvements in hyperresponsiveness observed in the latter two studies might be attributed to the fact that the exercise challenge to determine EIA was not adjusted for the improvements in physical fitness with training. Thus, the relative intensity of the exercise was lower for the post-training tests, compared to the pre-training challenge that might have been paralleled by lower minute ventilation.

Does regular exercise reduce airway inflammation?

To the authors' knowledge, only one randomized controlled study has assessed the effects of a physical conditioning programme on airway inflammation in children with asthma.[60] In this study, exhaled nitric oxide, a marker of airway inflammation, was significantly reduced after 8 weeks of video game exercises, but not after 8 weeks of treadmill exercise. This suggests that it was the exercise itself that led to the reduced inflammation. Yet, data from a mouse model of asthma shows that regular exercise may reduce airway inflammation.[61]

Can physical training cause asthma?

Several studies on adult elite athletes have shown that the prevalence of EIA is considerably increased in elite swimmers and endurance athletes engaging in winter sports.[62,63] Possibly, the inhalation of chemical irritants such as chlorine and/or of large amounts of cold, dry air triggers airway inflammation in these athletes, which results in bronchial hyperresponsiveness and EIA. When the training load is reduced the process might be reversed and symptoms may cease.[64] Although in elite athletes allergic disease predisposes to EIA, it is generally assumed that the mechanism underlying EIA in many swimmers and cross-country skiers is distinct from that in allergic asthma.

Compared with the adult literature, few data are available in children. However, one study assessed the risk of children to develop asthma relative to the number of sports played and the concentration of air pollutants in their community.[65] It was shown that children playing three or more sports exposed to ozone had a higher risk of developing asthma, compared with less active children or active children living in low-ozone communities. On the other hand, there is some evidence that regular PA in general might prevent the development of asthma,[66] and that physical inactivity may trigger it.[7]

Exercise testing in children with asthma or suspected exercise-induced asthma

Indications

As pointed out, exercise testing might be helpful to establish the diagnosis of EIA. Furthermore, once a treatment for EIA has been started, the effectiveness of that therapy can be assessed using a follow-up exercise test.

In addition, exercise testing in patients with asthma or EIA can serve several other purposes. The diagnosis of asthma is based on the patient's medical history, physical examination, and, last but not least, laboratory tests.[1,67] Therefore, when asthma is suspected but cannot be proven otherwise, an exercise test may help to establish the diagnosis by demonstrating a hyperresponsive airway system. The same objective can, however, be met with provocation tests using other triggers, such as hyperventilation with room air or cold air, inhalation of hypertonic saline or mannitol, or histamine/metacholine provocation. It should be kept in mind that most of these tests, including an exercise challenge, have a sensitivity to diagnose asthma of about 40–60%.[68–71] The specificity is generally somewhat higher (around 80–90%). Exercise testing has been used as a screening tool for asthma in epidemiological research.[3] A relatively low sensitivity and a poor stability of the bronchial responses over time, however, debase its value for this purpose.[72]

i) Several studies have shown that children who are not known to have asthma, but who show a pathological fall in pulmonary function parameters following an exercise challenge, are at high risk to develop clinically recognizable asthma during the subsequent years.[69] Therefore, exercise testing could be used to screen for children at risk to develop asthma. To date, however, a pathological airway response to an exercise test without any other signs of respiratory disease would not result in any treatment, so this indication for an exercise test is hypothetical.

ii) Many children with asthma and their parents are afraid of EIA. The patient and her/his parents might be convinced during an exercise test that exercise can be safe even when intensity is maximal. Furthermore, the appropriate behaviour before, during, and after exercise can be practised to prevent EIA.

iii) In children with significant asthma, decreased fitness might be suspected. Exercise testing can provide quantitative measures of fitness and may thereby help to document the deficit and to follow up changes during an exercise intervention.

Who should not be tested?

Exercise testing in asthmatic patients always includes the risk of severe exercise-induced bronchoconstriction. In most exercise tests, this pathological response is actually striven for. Since the decrease in pulmonary functions is larger in patients with a bronchial obstruction prior to the test, a patient should not be subjected to an exercise test if the patient's baseline forced expiratory volume in 1 s (FEV_1) is below 50–60% of predicted.[73] No exercise testing should be performed during infections and in times of high seasonal allergen exposure. Furthermore, health conditions other than pulmonary impairment, such as cardiovascular or neuromuscular diseases, should also be considered.[74]

Preparation before the test and safety procedures

Based on the purpose of the exercise test, the child should discontinue bronchodilators such as cromoglycate sodium or short-acting ß-adrenergic drugs prior to testing.[73] Long-acting ß-mimetic drugs should be discontinued for up to 48 h. Four hours before the exercise test, the child should refrain from any strenuous activities and should not ingest large amounts of food. After arrival at the laboratory, the patient should be seen by a physician to obtain a recent medical history and to perform a physical examination. A test of pulmonary functions at rest is mandatory to estimate the risks of an exercise test and to reconsider the indication. A resting ECG might be considered, unless congenital conduction abnormalities can be excluded from an older ECG. The exercise test should then be explained in detail to the child and parents and, at least, verbal consent should be obtained. Experimental conditions including temperature and humidity should be noted.

During the exercise challenge, at least power output on the cycle ergometer or slope and speed of the belt on the treadmill, heart rate (HR), and breath sounds should be monitored. In patients with unclear respiratory disease or severe asthma, it is recommended to further monitor ECG, blood pressure, oxygen saturation (SaO_2), minute ventilation, end tidal PCO_2, and oxygen uptake. Based on these latter parameters, a list of situations has been compiled in which an exercise test should be terminated (Box 24.1).[75,76]

Box 24.1 Reasons to terminate an exercise test in children

Reasons for exercise test termination

- Patient request.
- Diagnostic findings have been established.
- Failure of monitoring equipment.
- Cardiac arrhythmias precipitated or aggravated by the exercise test.
- Myocardial ischaemia on ECG (ST segment depression or elevation >0.3 mV).
- Progressive decrease in systolic blood pressure.
- Significant respiratory distress.
- Rise in end tidal PCO_2 of more than 10 torr or exceeding 55 torr.
- Drop in SaO_2 of more than 10% or below 85%.

Based on Cropp[75] and Washington *et al.*[76]

Conducting the exercise challenge

Mode of exercise

Early studies indicated that the most effective exercise challenge to induce EIA was a run outdoors. However, recent research shows that treadmill running is as effective as free running in triggering EIA, if climatic conditions and exercise intensity are controlled for.[74] Since there are concerns with the standardization of an exercise challenge outdoors as well as with monitoring and safety, usually a laboratory-based exercise test is used to test for EIA.

Although some studies indicate that cycling is less effective than treadmill running in triggering an EIA,[77] others suggest that the asthmatic response to various land-based exercises might be of equal magnitude, provided that the volume, temperature, and humidity of the inspired air are similar among challenges.[78,79] Thus, treadmill and cycle ergometer are suitable and recommended for an exercise challenge.[73]

Duration and intensity of exercise

It is generally agreed that an exercise of 6–10 min duration and at an intensity severe enough to raise HR to at least 85% of predicted maximum (i.e. ~170 beats $\cdot$ min^{-1} in children and adolescents) or oxygen uptake to 60–80% of maximum is most suitable to induce EIA.[15,73] Using shorter duration exercise, but supramaximal exercise intensities, might also be effective to induce EIA.[80] However, an exercise of longer duration (and lower intensity) may result in a false negative test, because the subject may run through the temporary EIA. A study evaluated the exercise load in relationship to EIA severity in 9- to 17-year-old youth with asthma and found that treadmill tests at 85% and 95% of calculated maximal HR (HRmax) resulted in truly different decreases in FEV_1. The decrease in FEV_1 was 25% at 95% HRmax and 9% at 85% HRmax, resulting in a diagnosis of EIA (10% decrement in FEV_1) in 9 of 20 participants at 85% HRmax, whereas all 20 participants had decreases greater than 10% at 95% HRmax. This study underlines the necessity for high-exercise intensity triggering high minute ventilation.[81] The required exercise intensity is usually achieved employing exercise

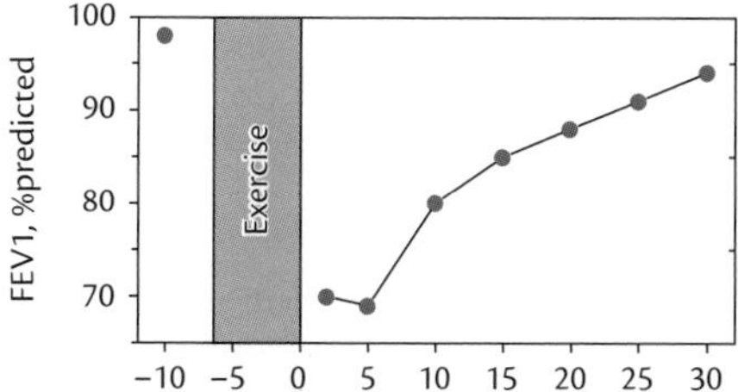

Figure 24.1 Pulmonary function response (change in forced expiratory volume in 1 s, percentage predicted) to an exercise challenge test in a child with exercise-induced asthma.

intensities on the cycle ergometer of 2–2.5 $W \cdot kg^{-1}$ body weight, but may be higher in well-trained children and adolescents. Due to developmental changes in running economy, the optimal speed and slope during a treadmill challenge are less easy to predict.

Criteria to identify exercise-induced asthma with an exercise challenge

In order to detect EIA, pulmonary functions are assessed before the exercise challenge, immediately afterwards and thereafter in 5 min intervals until 30 min after exercise.[73]

Although many different parameters derived from pulmonary function testing have been used to diagnose EIA, FEV_1 is most commonly employed.[73] Post-exercise FEV_1 is expressed as a percentage of pre-exercise values. A fall below 90% is often considered indicative for EIA.[73] Some authors also use 85% as a criterion for EIA, especially when field testing is used.[82] A typical pulmonary function response (change in FEV_1% predicted) to an exercise challenge test (cycling for 6 min with a heart rate of 180–186 beats.min^{-1} after the first minute) in a child with EIA is shown in Figure 24.1.

Reliability of bronchial responsiveness to a standardized exercise challenge

Intraclass correlation coefficients for the fall in FEV_1 with treadmill exercise while breathing dry air were reported to be 0.57.[83] The reliability, as described by the coefficient of variation (CV) is higher in subjects with a fall in FEV_1 > 20% (CV 26%) than in subjects with a fall in FEV_1 < 20% (CV 81%).[84] This moderate reliability limits the information from repeated testing of one individual in order to assess the effectiveness of medication in preventing EIA.

Prevention of exercise-induced asthma and exercise counselling

Based on the reported benefits of exercise and PA for patients suffering from asthma or EIA, every physician should try to enable a child with asthma to engage in as much PA as possible. The following section summarizes different approaches and principles that might be adopted to minimize exercise-related risks for the child with asthma (see also Box 24.2). The average daily doses of various drugs[85] used to control asthma are summarized in Table 24.1.

Control of asthma

During periods of airway inflammation, patients with asthma respond to an exercise challenge with a larger than usual fall in pulmonary function parameters. Long-term treatment of asthmatic patients with inhaled steroids such as budesonide or fluticasone propionate may decrease the hyperresponsiveness of the bronchi to a variety of stimuli, including exercise,[86,87] thereby lowering the frequency or severity of EIA. Long acting $ß_2$-adrenoceptor agonists such as salmeterol or formoterol may help to reduce the risk of EIA in patients who are not symptom free with inhaled steroids alone.[88–91] Of note, ATS guidelines discourage inhalative cortico-steroids on demand and highly discourage the daily use of long acting $ß_2$-adrenoceptor agonists as single therapy in EIA.[91] Leukotriene antagonists are also effective in reducing EIA.[92]

Box 24.2 Recommendations to reduce the risk of exercise-induced asthma in patients with asthma

Recommendations

- Control asthma (use anti-inflammatory drugs whenever bronchodilators are necessary on several days per week).
- Prefer swimming over running or cycling (note that swimming in pools with chlorinated water may lead to an asthmatic attack in some patients).
- Stop exercise during a period of severely reduced airway patency.
- Closely monitor exercise after inhalation of allergens.
- Do not exercise at high ozone levels (above 180 ppm) or in an environment with a high concentration of allergens.
- Warm up before exercise.
- Inhale ß2-adrenergic agonists or cromolyn nebulisers 10–20 min before exercise.
- Wear a face mask in cold weather (prevents heat/water loss from bronchial system).
- In case of EIA, use ß2 adrenergic agonists.

Select the least asthmogenic activity

Inhaling cold and dry air while exercising increases the risk for severe bronchial obstruction. Therefore, children with asthma are sometimes advised not to participate in winter sports activities. Using the precautions outlined in this section, such as wearing a face mask, properly administered medications, and monitoring of peak flow, exercise in cold weather can be safe for children with asthma.[93] However, if the physician is asked to provide an activity recommendation he should emphasize swimming, since EIA is less common during swimming than during land-based activities. However, this recommendation does not apply to those few patients who experience bronchoconstriction when swimming in chlorinated water.

Select the right time to exercise

In patients with EIA, pulmonary function at rest is related to the exercise-induced fall in pulmonary functions.[94] Therefore, exercise should be avoided in times of bronchial obstruction. Although monitoring peak expiratory flow rate (PEFR) is not the best method to detect airway narrowing, in children with unstable asthma it is recommended to measure PEFR before engaging in PA. If PEFR is below 80% of the child´s average PEFR, short-acting ß-mimetic drugs should be administered and exercise should be postponed until PEFR has improved.

Table 24.1 Examples of commonly used drugs in the treatment of bronchial asthma

Drug	Children 6–11 years Daily dose (mcg)			Adults and adolescents ≥12 years Daily dose (mcg)		
Inhaled corticosteroids						
	Low	**Moderate**	**High**	**Low**	**Moderate**	**High**
Budesonide, dry powder inhaler	100–200	>200–400	>400	200–400	>400–800	>800
Budesonide, nebulizer	250–500	>500–1000	>1000	–	–	–
Cromoglycate sodium						
Fluticasone, dry powder	100–200	>200–400	>400	100–200	>200–500	>500
Inhaled ß-adrenergic agonists						
Salbutamol nebulizer	100–200 10–15 min before exercise, treatment of asthma attack 200–400 (preferred: autohaler or spacer)					
Formoterol	9–24 in two doses					
Salmeterol	100 in two doses					

Adapted from Global Initiative For Asthma. Global Strategy For Asthma Management And Prevention. http://www.ginasthma.org, 2015. Accessed at 26th January 2016.

The exercise-induced bronchial response is enhanced for several days after inhalation of allergens.[95] Avoiding allergens for 1 month has been shown to reduce the risk for EIA.[96] For practical reasons, however, this recommendation can rarely be implemented. It should, however be emphasized that exercising in an environment with a high allergen concentration, dust, or ozone may trigger EIA. For instance, the hazard ratio was six for new-onset asthma or EIA for children who participate in team sports in high ambient ozone.[97]

Prevention of exercise-induced asthma shortly before and during exercise

A specific warm-up might be effective in some patients to lower the risk for EIA during the subsequent 2h.[30–32] Although a warm-up consisting of variable high-intensity exercise, as opposed to continuous high- or low-intensity exercise, appears to be the most effective strategy to attenuate EIA,[91,98] the optimal pattern and efficacy of a warm-up protocol should be determined individually.

Several substances, such as sodium cromoglycate sodium 20 mg, nedocromil sodium 4 mg, ipatropium bromide 80 µg, and $ß_2$-adrenoceptor agonists such as salbutamol 0.2–0.4 mg or formoterol 6 (–12 µg) administered 10–20 min prior to exercise have been shown to offer protection against EIA.[99-102] ß-adrenergic agonists seem to be more effective compared to cromoglycate or ipatropium bromide.[103] Using the same absolute dose, spacers do not improve the effect of cromoglycate or nedocromil.[104]

Based on the finding that an asthmatic attack with exercise most likely results from cooling and/or fluid loss of the bronchial system, the use of face masks has been recommended in cold or dry air, but the evidence is brittle due to high risk of bias and imprecision of the studies.[91]

Treatment of exercise-induced asthma

Once EIA has developed, it can be treated successfully with nebulized short-acting ß-adrenoceptor agonists such as terbutaline sulphate or salbutamol.[105] For patients with EIA who continue to have symptoms despite using an inhaled short-acting ß-adrenoceptor agonist SABA before exercise, or who require inhaled SABA daily or more frequently, the daily administration of inhaled corticosteroids or of a leukotriene receptor antagonist is indicated.[91] Formoterol, one of the long acting $ß_2$-adrenoceptor agonists, may also be used, but only as an add-on to inhaled steroids.

Anti-doping rules and exercise-induced asthma

Until a few years ago, all ß-adrenoceptor agonists were on the World Anti-Doping Association's (WADA) prohibited list and athletes were required to obtain a therapeutic use exemption certificate to use some of them in inhaled form, but with most being banned entirely. Since 2013, WADA has allowed inhaled salmeterol (no dose limit), salbutamol (up to 1600 micro-grams per 24 h) and formoterol (up to 54 micro-grams per 24 h). Inhaled steroids are permitted provided an athlete has a declaration of use certificate, whereas all oral and injected ß-adrenoceptor agonists and steroids are prohibited, unless an athlete has a therapeutic use exemption certificate. These rules continue to be adapted and should be checked each year at the WADA (www.wada-ama.org) and at the national level. (Interested readers are referred to Chapter 49 for further discussion).

Conclusions

Provided that the child with asthma and her or his parents are well educated and trained in the management of EIA, that the disease is treated adequately, and that the methods to prevent bronchoconstriction with exercise are consequently employed, exercise can be safe. Under these conditions, nearly every child with asthma can engage in all types of physical activities[106] and may even be successful at the very elite level of competitive athletics, for example, the Olympic games.[107]

Summary

- The incidence of asthma in children varies among countries and can be estimated to range between 5% and 20%. Exercise-induced asthma (EIA) attacks may occur in any patient with asthma and in some children without this diagnosis.
- Typical symptoms of EIA include cough, chest tightness, and shortness of breath shortly after exercise.

- The pathophysiology of EIA is not fully understood but airway cooling and drying with increased ventilation during exercise, and airway re-warming after exercise play an important role. Lifestyle with a lack of physical activity may also play a role.[23]
- The diagnosis of EIA is based on the typical history and may be verified by an exercise challenge. Typically, a drop in forced expiratory volume in 1 s exceeding 10% from baseline is regarded as diagnostic.
- Regular exercise may increase fitness and psychological well-being in children with asthma. Furthermore, moderate exercise may also have a beneficial effect on airway inflammation in patients with asthma.
- With proper education and (pharmaco-) therapy, exercise can be safe in children with asthma. Even more, individuals with asthma can successfully participate in competitive sports at a very high level. In this case, anti-doping rules should be regularly checked.

References

1. Papadopoulos NG, Arakawa H, Carlsen KH, *et al.* International consensus on (ICON) pediatric asthma. *Allergy*. 2012; 67: 976–997.
2. Prahl P, Christiansen P, Hjuler I, Kaae HH. Prevalence of asthma in Danish children aged 8–10 years. *Acta Paediatr*. 1997; 86: 1110–1113.
3. Burr ML, Limb ES, Andrae S, Barry DM, Nagel F. Childhood asthma in four countries: a comparative survey. *Int J Epidemiol*. 1994; 23: 341–347.
4. Pearce N, Weiland S, Keil U, *et al.* Self-reported prevalence of asthma symptoms in children in Australia, England, Germany and New Zealand: an international comparison using the ISAAC protocol. *Eur Respir J*. 1993; 6: 1455–1461.
5. Brozek G, Lawson J, Szumilas D, Zejda J. Increasing prevalence of asthma, respiratory symptoms, and allergic diseases: Four repeated surveys from 1993–2014. *Respir Med*. 2015; 109: 982–990.
6. Robertson CF, Heycock E, Bishop J, *et al.* Prevalence of asthma in Melbourne schoolchildren: changes over 26 years. *BMJ*. 1991; 302: 1116–1118.
7. Lucas SR, Platts-Mills TA. Physical activity and exercise in asthma: relevance to etiology and treatment. *J Allergy Clin Immunol*. 2005; 115: 928–934.
8. Huovinen E, Kaprio J, Laitinen LA, Koskenvuo M. Social predictors of adult asthma: a co-twin case-control study. *Thorax*. 2001; 56: 234–236.
9. McFadden ER, Jr. Exercise-induced asthma. Assessment of current etiologic concepts. *Chest*. 1987; 91: 151S–157S.
10. Bader D, Ramos AD, Lew CD, *et al.* Childhood sequelae of infant lung disease: exercise and pulmonary function abnormalities after bronchopulmonary dysplasia. *J Pediatr*. 1987; 110: 693–699.
11. Silverman M, Hobbs FD, Gordon IR, Carswell F. Cystic fibrosis, atopy, and airways lability. *Arch Dis Child*. 1978; 53: 873–877.
12. Rupp NT, Guill MF, Brudno DS. Unrecognized exercise-induced bronchospasm in adolescent athletes. *Am J Dis Child*. 1992; 146: 941–944.
13. Storms WW. Exercise-induced asthma: diagnosis and treatment for the recreational or elite athlete. *Med Sci Sports Exerc*. 1999; 31: S33–S38.
14. Chen WY, Horton DJ. Heat and water loss from the airways and exercise-induced asthma. *Respiration*. 1977; 34: 305–313.
15. McFadden ER, Jr., Gilbert IA. Exercise-induced asthma. *N Engl J Med*. 1994; 330: 1362–1367.
16. Del Giacco SR, Firinu D, Bjermer L, Carlsen KH. Exercise and asthma: an overview. *Eur Clin Respir J*. 2015; 2: 27984.
17. Noviski N, Bar-Yishay E, Gur I, Godfrey S. Exercise intensity determines and climatic conditions modify the severity of exercise-induced asthma. *Am Rev Respir Dis*. 1987; 136: 592–594.
18. Zeitoun M, Wilk B, Matsuzaka A, *et al.* Facial cooling enhances exercise-induced bronchoconstriction in asthmatic children. *Med Sci Sports Exerc*. 2004; 36: 767–771.
19. McNally JF, Jr., Enright P, Hirsch JE, Souhrada JF. The attenuation of exercise-induced bronchoconstriction by oropharyngeal anesthesia. *Am Rev Respir Dis*. 1979; 119: 247–252.
20. Anderson SD. Is there a unifying hypothesis for exercise-induced asthma? *J Allergy Clin Immunol*. 1984; 73: 660–665.
21. Kikawa Y, Hosoi S, Inoue Y, *et al.* Exercise-induced urinary excretion of leukotriene E4 in children with atopic asthma. *Pediatr Res*. 1991; 29: 455–459.
22. White SW, Pitsillides KF, Parsons GH, *et al.* Coronary-bronchial blood flow and airway dimensions in exercise-induced syndromes. *Clin Exp Pharmacol Physiol*. 2001; 28: 472–478.
23. Lemanske R, Henke KG. Exercise-induced asthma: In: Gisolfi CV, Lamb DR (eds.) *Youth, exercise, and sport. Perspectives in exercise science and sports medicine*. Indianapolis, IN: Benchmark Press; 1989. p. 465–511.
24. Koh YY, Lim HS, Min KU. Airway responsiveness to allergen is increased 24 hours after exercise challenge. *J Allergy Clin Immunol*. 1994; 94: 507–516.
25. Speelberg B, Panis EA, Bijl D, van Herwaarden CL, Bruynzeel PL. Late asthmatic responses after exercise challenge are reproducible. *J Allergy Clin Immunol*. 1991; 87: 1128–1137.
26. Boner AL, Vallone G, Chiesa M, *et al.* Reproducibility of late phase pulmonary response to exercise and its relationship to bronchial hyperreactivity in children with chronic asthma. *Pediatr Pulmonol*. 1992; 14: 156–159.
27. Hofstra WB, Sterk PJ, Neijens HJ, *et al.* Occurrence of a late response to exercise in asthmatic children: multiple regression approach using time-matched baseline and histamine control days. *Eur Respir J*. 1996; 9: 1348–1355.
28. Hamielec CM, Manning PJ, O'Byrne PM. Exercise refractoriness after histamine inhalation in asthmatic subjects. *Am Rev Respir Dis*. 1988; 138: 794–798.
29. Wilson BA, Bar-Or O, Seed LG. Effects of humid air breathing during arm or treadmill exercise on exercise-induced bronchoconstriction and refractoriness. *Am Rev Respir Dis*. 1990; 142: 349–352.
30. Reiff DB, Choudry NB, Pride NB, Ind PW. The effect of prolonged submaximal warm-up exercise on exercise-induced asthma. *Am Rev Respir Dis*. 1989; 139: 479–484.
31. Schnall RP, Landau LI. Protective effects of repeated short sprints in exercise-induced asthma. *Thorax*. 1980; 35: 828–832.
32. Lin CC, Wu JL, Huang WC, Lin CY. A bronchial response comparison of exercise and methacholine in asthmatic subjects. *J Asthma*. 1991; 28: 31–40.
33. Ben-Dov I, Bar-Yishay E, Godfrey S. Refractory period after exercise-induced asthma unexplained by respiratory heat loss. *Am Rev Respir Dis*. 1982; 125: 530–534.
34. Wilson BA, Bar-Or O, O'Byrne PM. The effects of indomethacin on refractoriness following exercise both with and without a bronchoconstrictor response. *Eur Respir J*. 1994; 7: 2174–2178.
35. Gilbert IA, Fouke JM, McFadden ER, Jr. The effect of repetitive exercise on airway temperatures. *Am Rev Respir Dis*. 1990; 142: 826–831.
36. Wiens L, Sabath R, Ewing L, *et al.* Chest pain in otherwise healthy children and adolescents is frequently caused by exercise-induced asthma. *Pediatrics*. 1992; 90: 350–353.
37. Sarafino EP, Paterson ME, Murphy EL. Age and the impacts of triggers in childhood asthma. *J Asthma*. 1998; 35: 213–217.
38. Vahlkvist S, Pedersen S. Fitness, daily activity and body composition in children with newly diagnosed, untreated asthma. *Allergy*. 2009; 64: 1649–1655.
39. Siersted HC, Boldsen J, Hansen HS, Mostgaard G, Hyldebrandt N. Population-based study of risk factors for underdiagnosis of asthma in adolescence: Odense schoolchild study. *BMJ*. 1998; 316: 651–655; discussion: 655–656.
40. Groth SW, Rhee H, Kitzman H. Relationships among obesity, physical activity and sedentary behavior in young adolescents with and without lifetime asthma. *J Asthma*. 2015; 19: 1–6.
41. Counil FP, Varray A, Karila C, *et al.* Wingate test performance in children with asthma: aerobic or anaerobic limitation? *Med Sci Sports Exerc*. 1997; 29: 430–435.

42. Ludwick SK, Jones JW, Jones TK, Fukuhara JT, Strunk RC. Normalization of cardiopulmonary endurance in severely asthmatic children after bicycle ergometry therapy. *J Pediatr*. 1986; 109: 446–451.
43. Strunk RC, Mrazek DA, Fukuhara JT, *et al*. Cardiovascular fitness in children with asthma correlates with psychologic functioning of the child. *Pediatrics*. 1989; 84: 460–464.
44. Santuz P, Baraldi E, Filippone M, Zacchello F. Exercise performance in children with asthma: is it different from that of healthy controls? *Eur Respir J*. 1997; 10: 1254–1260.
45. Kiers A, van der Mark TW, Woldring MG, Peset R. Determination of the functional residual capacity during exercise. *Ergonomics*. 1980; 23: 955–959.
46. Freyschuss U, Hedlin G, Hedenstierna G. Ventilation-perfusion relationships during exercise-induced asthma in children. *Am Rev Respir Dis*. 1984; 130: 888–894.
47. Garfinkel SK, Kesten S, Chapman KR, Rebuck AS. Physiologic and nonphysiologic determinants of aerobic fitness in mild to moderate asthma. *Am Rev Respir Dis*. 1992; 145: 741–745.
48. Wanrooij VH, Willeboordse M, Dompeling E, van de Kant KD. Exercise training in children with asthma: a systematic review. *Br J Sports Med*. 2014; 48: 1024–1031.
49. Svenonius E, Kautto R, Arborelius MJr. Improvement after training of children with exercise-induced asthma. *Acta Paediatr Scand*. 1983; 72: 23–30.
50. Holzer FJ, Schnall R, Landau LI. The effect of a home exercise programme in children with cystic fibrosis and asthma. *Aust Paediatr J*. 1984; 20: 297–301.
51. Perrin JM, MacLean WE, Jr., Gortmaker SL, Asher KN. Improving the psychological status of children with asthma: a randomized controlled trial. *J Dev Behav Pediatr*. 1992; 13: 241–247.
52. Counil FP, Varray A, Matecki S, *et al*. Training of aerobic and anaerobic fitness in children with asthma. *J Pediatr*. 2003; 142: 179–184.
53. Matsumoto I, Araki H, Tsuda K, *et al*. Effects of swimming training on aerobic capacity and exercise induced bronchoconstriction in children with bronchial asthma. *Thorax*. 1999; 54: 196–201.
54. Engstrom I, Fallstrom K, Karlberg E, Sten G, Bjure J. Psychological and respiratory physiological effects of a physical exercise programme on boys with severe asthma. *Acta Paediatr Scand*. 1991; 80: 1058–1065.
55. Kieckhefer GM. The meaning of health to 9-, 10-, and 11-year-old children with chronic asthma. *J Asthma*. 1988; 25: 325–333.
56. Huang SW, Veiga R, Sila U, Reed E, Hines S. The effect of swimming in asthmatic children—participants in a swimming program in the city of Baltimore. *J Asthma*. 1989; 26: 117–121.
57. Szentagothai K, Gyene I, Szocska M, Osvath P. Physical exercise program for children with bronchial asthma. *Pediatr Pulmonol*. 1987; 3: 166–172.
58. Fitch KD, Blitvich JD, Morton AR. The effect of running training on exercise-induced asthma. *Ann Allergy*. 1986; 57: 90–94.
59. Henriksen JM, Nielsen TT. Effect of physical training on exercise-induced bronchoconstriction. *Acta Paediatr Scand*. 1983; 72: 31–36.
60. Gomes EL, Carvalho CR, Peixoto-Souza FS, *et al*. Active Video Game Exercise Training Improves the Clinical Control of Asthma in Children: Randomized Controlled Trial. *PLOS One*. 2015; 10: e0135433. doi: 10.1371/journal.pone.0135433
61. Luks V, Burkett A, Turner L, Pakhale S. Effect of physical training on airway inflammation in animal models of asthma: a systematic review. *BMC Pulm Med*. 2013; 13: 24.
62. Helenius I, Haahtela T. Allergy and asthma in elite summer sport athletes. *J Allergy Clin Immunol*. 2000; 106: 444–452.
63. Weiler JM, Ryan EJ, 3rd. Asthma in United States Olympic athletes who participated in the 1998 Olympic winter games. *J Allergy Clin Immunol*. 2000; 106: 267–271.
64. Helenius I, Rytila P, Sarna S, *et al*. Effect of continuing or finishing high-level sports on airway inflammation, bronchial hyperresponsiveness, and asthma: a 5-year prospective follow-up study of 42 highly trained swimmers. *J Allergy Clin Immunol*. 2002; 109: 962–968.
65. McConnell R, Berhane K, Gilliland F, *et al*. Asthma in exercising children exposed to ozone: a cohort study. *Lancet*. 2002; 359: 386–391.
66. Eijkemans M, Mommers M, Draaisma JM, Thijs C, Prins MH. Physical activity and asthma: a systematic review and meta-analysis. *PlOS One*. 2012; 7: e50775.
67. Weiler JM, Anderson SD, Randolph C, *et al*. Pathogenesis, prevalence, diagnosis, and management of exercise-induced bronchoconstriction: a practice parameter. *Ann Allergy Asthma Immunol*. 2010; 105: S1–S47.
68. Foresi A, Corbo GM, Valente S. Airway responsiveness to exercise and ultrasonically nebulized distilled water in children: relationship to clinical and functional characteristics. *Respiration*. 1988; 53: 205–213.
69. Jones A, Bowen M. Screening for childhood asthma using an exercise test. *Br J Gen Pract*. 1994; 44: 127–131.
70. Ponsonby AL, Couper D, Dwyer T, Carmichael A, Wood-Baker R. Exercise-induced bronchial hyperresponsiveness and parental ISAAC questionnaire responses. *Eur Respir J*. 1996; 9: 1356–1362.
71. West JV, Robertson CF, Roberts R, Olinsky A. Evaluation of bronchial responsiveness to exercise in children as an objective measure of asthma in epidemiological surveys. *Thorax*. 1996; 51: 590–595.
72. Powell CV, White RD, Primhak RA. Longitudinal study of free running exercise challenge: reproducibility. *Arch Dis Child*. 1996; 74: 108–114.
73. Crapo RO, Casaburi R, Coates AL, *et al*. Guidelines for methacholine and exercise challenge testing—1999. *Am J Respir Crit Care Med*. 2000; 161: 309–329.
74. Garcia de la Rubia S, Pajaron-Fernandez MJ, Sanchez-Solis M, *et al*. Exercise-induced asthma in children: a comparative study of free and treadmill running. *Ann Allergy Asthma Immunol*. 1998; 80: 232–236.
75. Cropp GJA. Exercise bronchoprovocation test—standardization of procedures and evaluation of response. *J Allergy Clin Immun*. 1979; 64: 627–633.
76. Washington RL, Bricker JT, Alpert BS, *et al*. Guidelines for exercise testing in the pediatric age group. From the Committee on Atherosclerosis and Hypertension in Children, Council on Cardiovascular Disease in the Young, the American Heart Association. *Circulation*. 1994; 90: 2166–2179.
77. Fitch KD. Comparative aspects of available exercise systems. *Pediatrics*. 1975; 56: 904–907.
78. Bundgaard A, Ingemann-Hansen T, Schmidt A, Halkjaer-Kristensen J. Exercise-induced asthma after walking, running and cycling. *Scand J Clin Lab Invest*. 1982; 42: 15–18.
79. Kilham H, Tooley M, Silverman M. Running, walking, and hyperventilation causing asthma in children. *Thorax*. 1979; 34: 582–586.
80. Inbar O, Alvarez DX, Lyons HA. Exercise-induced asthma—a comparison between two modes of exercise stress. *Eur J Respir Dis*. 1981; 62: 160–167.
81. Carlsen KH, Engh G, Mork M. Exercise-induced bronchoconstriction depends on exercise load. *Respir Med*. 2000; 94: 750–755.
82. Haby MM, Anderson SD, Peat JK, *et al*. An exercise challenge protocol for epidemiological studies of asthma in children: comparison with histamine challenge. *Eur Respir J*. 1994; 7: 43–49.
83. Hofstra WB, Sont JK, Sterk PJ, *et al*. Sample size estimation in studies monitoring exercise-induced bronchoconstriction in asthmatic children. *Thorax*. 1997; 52: 739–741.
84. Eggleston PA, Guerrant JL. A standardized method of evaluating exercise-induced asthma. *J Allergy Clin Immunol*. 1976; 58: 414–425.
85. Global Initiative For Asthma. Global Strategy For Asthma Management And Prevention. Available from: http://www.ginasthma.org. [Accessed 26 January 2016].
86. Vathenen AS, Knox AJ, Wisniewski A, Tattersfield AE. Effect of inhaled budesonide on bronchial reactivity to histamine, exercise, and eucapnic dry air hyperventilation in patients with asthma. *Thorax*. 1991; 46: 811–816.
87. Pedersen S, Hansen OR. Budesonide treatment of moderate and severe asthma in children: a dose-response study. *J Allergy Clin Immunol*. 1995; 95: 29–33.

88. Adkins JC, McTavish D. Salmeterol. A review of its pharmacological properties and clinical efficacy in the management of children with asthma. *Drugs*. 1997; 54: 331–354.
89. de Benedictis FM, Tuteri G, Pazzelli P, *et al.* Salmeterol in exercise-induced bronchoconstriction in asthmatic children: comparison of two doses. *Eur Respir J*. 1996; 9: 2099–2103.
90. Daugbjerg P, Nielsen KG, Skov M, Bisgaard H. Duration of action of formoterol and salbutamol dry-powder inhalation in prevention of exercise-induced asthma in children. *Acta Paediatr*. 1996; 85: 684–687.
91. Parsons JP, Hallstrand TS, Mastronarde JG, *et al.* An official American Thoracic Society clinical practice guideline: exercise-induced bronchoconstriction. *Am J Respir Crit Care Med*. 2013; 187: 1016–1027.
92. Leff JA, Busse WW, Pearlman D, *et al.* Montelukast, a leukotriene-receptor antagonist, for the treatment of mild asthma and exercise-induced bronchoconstriction. *N Engl J Med*. 1998; 339: 147–152.
93. Silvers W, Morrison M, Wiener M. Asthma ski day: cold air sports safe with peak flow monitoring. *Ann Allergy*. 1994; 73: 105–108.
94. Nolan P. Clinical features predictive of exercise-induced asthma in children. *Respirology*. 1996; 1: 201–205.
95. Mussaffi H, Springer C, Godfrey S. Increased bronchial responsiveness to exercise and histamine after allergen challenge in children with asthma. *J Allergy Clin Immunol*. 1986; 77: 48–52.
96. Benckhuijsen J, van den Bos JW, van Velzen E, de Bruijn R, Aalbers R. Differences in the effect of allergen avoidance on bronchial hyperresponsiveness as measured by methacholine, adenosine 5′-monophosphate, and exercise in asthmatic children. *Pediatr Pulmonol*. 1996; 22: 147–153.
97. Islam T, Berhane K, McConnell R, *et al.* Glutathione-S-transferase (GST) P1, GSTM1, exercise, ozone and asthma incidence in school children. *Thorax*. 2009; 64: 197–202.
98. Stickland MK, Rowe BH, Spooner CH, Vandermeer B, Dryden DM. Effect of warm-up exercise on exercise-induced bronchoconstriction. *Med Sci Sports Exerc*. 2012; 44: 383–391.
99. Ben-Dov I, Bar-Yishay E, Godfrey S. Heterogeneity in the response of asthmatic patients to pre-exercise treatment with cromolyn sodium. *Am Rev Respir Dis*. 1983; 127: 113–116.
100. Boner AL, Antolini I, Andreoli A, De Stefano G, Sette L. Comparison of the effects of inhaled calcium antagonist verapamil, sodium cromoglycate and ipratropium bromide on exercise-induced bronchoconstriction in children with asthma. *Eur J Pediatr*. 1987; 146: 408–411.
101. Ferrari M, Balestreri F, Baratieri S, *et al.* Evidence of the rapid protective effect of formoterol dry-powder inhalation against exercise-induced bronchospasm in athletes with asthma. *Respiration*. 2000; 67: 510–513.
102. Novembre E, Frongia GF, Veneruso G, Vierucci A. Inhibition of exercise-induced-asthma (EIA) by nedocromil sodium and sodium cromoglycate in children. *Pediatric allergy and immunology: official publication of the European Society of Pediatric Allergy and Immunology*. 1994; 5: 107–110.
103. Svenonius E, Arborelius MJr, Wiberg R, Ekberg P. Prevention of exercise-induced asthma by drugs inhaled from metered aerosols. *Allergy*. 1988; 43: 252–257.
104. Comis A, Valletta EA, Sette L, Andreoli A, Boner AL. Comparison of nedocromil sodium and sodium cromoglycate administered by pressurized aerosol, with and without a spacer device in exercise-induced asthma in children. *Eur Respir J*. 1993; 6: 523–526.
105. dos Santos JM, Costa H, Stahl E, Wiren JE. Bricanyl Turbuhaler and Ventolin Rotahaler in exercise-induced asthma in children. *Allergy*. 1991; 46: 203–205.
106. Bundgaard A. Exercise and the asthmatic. *Sports Med*. 1985; 2: 254–266.
107. Wilber RL, Rundell KW, Szmedra L, *et al.* Incidence of exercise-induced bronchospasm in Olympic winter sport athletes. *Med Sci Sports Exerc*. 2000; 32: 732–737.

CHAPTER 25

Exercise, physical activity, eating and weight disorders

Andrew P Hills, Steven J Street, and Nuala M Byrne

Introduction

Obesity has been described in various ways, including as 'one of today's most blatantly visible—yet most neglected—public health problems'.[1–4] The term 'globesity' has been coined to refer to the overweight and obesity epidemic, as well as its impact on both developed and developing societies. The high prevalence of overweight and obesity in industrialized nations is well documented; however, both are now also commonplace in low- to middle-income countries undergoing economic and nutrition transition.[3,5–8] In recent decades, overweight and obesity have increased substantially and are impacting younger children.[3,9,10] Recent projections suggest that about a third of youth in developed countries such as Australia will be overweight or obese by 2025.[11]

Obesity is a chronic condition which is the result of a persistent energy imbalance, typically a combination of reduced levels of energy expenditure and higher than necessary energy intake. Over time, the energy imbalance contributes to excess weight gain characterized by unhealthy levels of body fat. However, issues associated with diet and exercise are not limited to obesity, but are contributing factors across a broad spectrum of weight disorders encompassing obesity at one extreme and frank eating disorders such as anorexia nervosa at the other end. Sadly, in addition to those individuals who are obese or suffer from anorexia nervosa, many others display disordered eating and activity behaviours.

A wide range of factors or determinants contribute to the spectrum of common eating and weight disorders and provide numerous challenges for both youngsters and responsible adults.[12–15] At one extreme, some individuals appear to be preoccupied with body size, shape, weight, and fatness[16,17] while others appear to be resolved to their higher level of body fat.[18] Diet and exercise are the primary strategies used to alter body size and shape[13,19,20] although it is important to consider the potential consequences if diet and/or exercise are abused, e.g. in individuals whose primary motivation for physical change is for cosmetic rather than health reasons. More specifically, it is important to identify unhealthy modifications to diet and/or exercise. Furthermore, are there potential consequences for children and adolescents if the diet and exercise practices of their parents are inappropriate? Similarly, do diet and exercise behaviours differ according to ethnic background?

A low level of body fat is considered a 'desirable' physical characteristic for most sports, particularly where the transfer of body weight and aesthetics is important.[13,21,22] Not surprisingly, many athletes train to attain a body size and shape they perceive as 'ideal' for their chosen activity area and that they believe to be consistent with maximal performance. When unrealistic adjustments are made to body composition through inappropriate diet and exercise behaviours in an attempt to meet a desired size or shape, poor health outcomes may result.[13,23]

Consistent with the weight-related challenges facing a proportion of the young athletic population, the rising prevalence of overweight and obesity in many settings has seen the propensity for a proportion of the adult population to explore avenues to reduce body fat.[24] Unfortunately, some of the weight-conscious adult population who perceive themselves as being fat and desire to be slimmer may already be 'normal' weight or even underweight. To what extent are similar concerns influencing the weight control practices of those in younger age groups? In short, we must identify what we know of the eating, exercise, and weight-related behaviours of children and adolescents. Furthermore, we must also identify the role of medical practitioners, other health professionals, and parents in this important area.

As for adults, the weight-control practices of children and adolescents appear to reflect a heightened concern with body image.[16,25–28] The potential consequences of maintenance of inappropriate weight control practices in young people are serious, and include disordered eating practices,[12,29–31] growth retardation, delayed menarche, amenorrhoea, osteoporosis, and psychological disturbances.[15,22,32,33] The commonly employed weight control practices, dietary modification, and exercise, are pervasive[17] and not limited to the female population.[34] While all health professionals have a role to play in the area, medical practitioners who are widely consulted and held in such high esteem by the general public are potentially best placed to identify problems in children and adolescents in their care.[13,21] This chapter provides an overview of the range of factors contributing to inappropriate eating and activity behaviours, with a particular focus on the formative years of childhood and adolescence.

A central concern: fear of fatness

A pervasive preference for leanness in Western society has resulted in body fatness being stigmatized in many settings with a consequent social and psychological burden for many young people.[35,36] Paradoxically, this preference for leanness coexists with an escalating prevalence of obesity in many societies.

When extreme levels of physical activity (PA) and dietary restriction are undertaken to achieve a low level of body fatness, the net result is a proliferation of poor diets, high levels of exercise, body image disturbances including weight dissatisfaction, and the potential for an increase in frank eating disorders.[12,13,22] For example, dieting practices in adolescent girls and boys can play a role in the development of eating and weight disorders, including obesity.[37–41] Sadly, there is also evidence that dieting is not restricted to overweight adolescents, but is also practised by prepubertal children,[42] including those who are normal weight or underweight.[43,44] It is also commonplace for those who diet with periods of dietary restraint to regain weight because of reactionary episodes of excessive or inappropriate energy intake.[45] If such practices are repeated and associated with adverse psychological effects, this may include the contribution to clinical eating disorders.[46]

Some have suggested that being female is consistent with a preoccupation with weight, generally feeling too fat and often wishing to weigh less.[47] The perception of fatness and the fear of being overweight may be more powerful determinants of eating behaviour in many women than weight per se. If the fear of fatness is commonplace in many adult women, and it is important to determine at what age this begins, and what the potential implications are for young people. It is critical for youngsters to be protected from extraneous pressures to lose weight.[40] Where a change in body composition is necessary, this change should be achieved through a sensible approach to nutrition and exercise along with an appreciation of the salience of individual differences in body size and shape. Health professionals, educators, and parents have a major responsibility to be supportive in this area, including being vigilant during the formative years.

Eating and weight disorders

The term 'eating disorder' has traditionally been limited to three conditions: anorexia, bulimia nervosa, and binge eating disorder. Despite obesity having many similarities with the frank eating disorders, it has not commonly been described as an eating disorder.[48] It may be correct to reference obesity in many individuals as an eating and weight disorder, particularly given that approximately 30% of obese adults seeking treatment for their weight disorder may have binge eating disorder.[49] Another common feature of the eating and weight disorders in many individuals is a lack of self-esteem.[24]

There are conflicting reports of the extent of eating and weight disorders in different populations[16], but data suggest that eating-disordered behaviour has increased, particularly in boys.[34,50] Some of the confusion also relates to the contribution of predisposing genetic and environmental factors and the level of associated psychological ill health.[51] This may be due to the use of different approaches to define the conditions. A number of studies have referenced the difficulty to clearly define the boundaries between normality and abnormality regarding body weight and eating behaviour in athletic populations,[12,13,22,23] and this perhaps may also be true of the wider population. Despite acknowledgement of an increased awareness of eating and weight disorders, the common perception is that a relatively small number of individuals meet the strict criteria for frank eating disorders classified according to DSM-5 criteria. However, significantly more individuals display subclinical eating behaviours, including a preoccupation with weight and food, crash diets, fasting, binge eating, and purging behaviours. Of note is that in many groups, including athletes, it may be difficult to distinguish a conscientious and potentially over-zealous desire to follow eating and activity guidelines from disordered eating.[13,22,23]

Contrasting scenarios: overnutrition and physical inactivity, undernutrition and excessive physical activity

Both overnutrition and undernutrition may lead to impaired health and predispose an individual to an increased risk of an eating or weight disorder. Overnutrition and physical inactivity characterize the most common prescription for increased body fatness, often with low levels of physical fitness. The second scenario distinguishes individuals who combine attempts to reduce body weight (generally with the view to reducing body fatness) with heavy physical training. Consistent with this situation, concern has often been expressed for the health status of young people who participate in sport and PA where size, shape, and aesthetics are paramount, particularly in gymnastics and dance. Similar concerns exist for endurance athletes such as swimmers and runners who engage in heavy training over an extended period and often persist with inappropriate energy intake.[13,15,16,21,22,52] (Readers interested in eating disorders and disordered eating in young athletes are referred to Chapter 47 for further discussion).

Obesity

Obesity is increasingly recognized as a complex and multi-factorial condition. The term bio-psycho-social has been coined to reference the condition and its psychosocial, anatomical, and metabolic adaptations. The numerous interrelated causes of obesity may include overnutrition, physical inactivity, a genetic predisposition, psychologically determined eating disorders, and a host of social factors.[53–55] A number of studies have reported a systematic global increase in obesity prevalence.[9,10] The specific causes of the increase in obesity at the population level (i.e. increased intake alone, or decreased PA, or both) are contentious.[56,57] However, there is good evidence that lower levels of PA in all settings[58] have occurred coincident with an increase in sedentary behaviours.

There is increasing evidence for the protective effect of regular PA and exercise for health, including against the accumulation of excess body fat and assistance in long-term weight control.[2,59–62] A higher prevalence of obesity is common in groups whose spontaneous, habitual, and occupational activity have decreased. In contrast, there is a low incidence of obesity in athletic populations. Appropriate levels of body weight and adiposity are related to good health, and excess body fatness is associated with cardiorespiratory, articular, metabolic, locomotor, social, and psychological complications.[63–71] One of the most unfortunate consequences of the global obesity epidemic is that the serious health consequences once limited to adults are increasingly prevalent in obese children and adolescents.[72–76]

Treatment and management

Appropriate management of childhood obesity is critical as excess body fat in childhood is associated with a greater chance of high levels of adiposity in adulthood, and significant health and economic consequences for both the individual and wider society.[77–79] However, management of overweight and obesity can be a significant challenge at any age, particularly for individuals who have been over-fat for an extended period and/or experienced multiple failures in weight management. Furthermore, despite increased research attention, the evidence base for managing excess weight in children is somewhat limited. Therefore it is not surprising that progress to date in tackling childhood obesity has been slow and inconsistent.[80] In addition, studies have also been criticized for not providing a detailed methodology.[81] The key to the prevention and management of obesity in children and adolescents is modification of body composition through the promotion of regular PA and sound nutritional practices.[82–90] Severe dietary restriction should be avoided.

Individual assessment is highly recommended as this provides both child and family with an overview of health status and a basis for the incorporation of necessary lifestyle changes. Parental guilt and blame for childhood obesity is commonplace and thorough individual assessment can also help modulate this.[53,91] It is overly simplistic to blame a single factor such as family circumstances for childhood obesity, and consideration should be given to the broader psychosocial context.[92]

Exercise, diet, and behavioural interventions

The cornerstones of obesity management are diet, exercise, and behaviour modification.[53] A multi-component approach to weight management should ideally be family based and include nutrition, PA, and psychosocial support for overweight and obese young people.[93] Techniques commonly used to improve obese children's eating and activity behaviours include self-monitoring, social reinforcement, modelling, and social skills.[94] Family-focused behavioural interventions can provide positive health outcomes for both prepubertal children and adolescents.[80,95,96] A major focus of obesity management in young people should be restoration of energy balance to improve health.[2,88] Weight loss in growing individuals may be counter-productive; a healthier and more efficacious approach is to improve body composition by reducing body fat and maintaining or enhancing fat-free mass (FFM).[97,98] Sadly, a mainstream belief is that a decrease in body mass is the only acceptable measure of success in weight management, irrespective of the consequences for body composition.[65]

In summary, severe dietary restriction is contraindicated in children as growth and development may be jeopardized.[83,87] Excess body fat in growing children and adolescents may be managed by focusing on maintenance of body weight rather than unrealistic attempts to reduce body weight. As overweight or obese young people have an increase in body height, the proportion of body fat will decrease if body mass is stable. Concurrently, greater attention should be paid to increasing PA and exercise,[65,87,90,99] including the development of motor skills to assist in an active engagement in sport and PA.[100] A logical argument contends that because PA and exercise are active, unrestricted, and positive, whereas dieting is passive, restrictive, and negative, it is healthier to promote the benefits of positive and rewarding activity.[101] Readers are referred to the many reviews of PA and exercise for the prevention, treatment, and management of childhood and adolescent obesity.[60,83,102–105]

Importantly, the role of PA in the maintenance of weight loss[98,106] cannot be overstated. Considerable health and motor-skill related benefits are possible when individuals change from being inactive or sedentary to being regularly engaged in PA.[88,100]

The treatment and management of obesity in young people is challenging for both clinicians and parents. General clinical guidelines for obesity management[107] are available from a number of sources but, the process must be individualized and personalized, with a strong commitment from the individual and family to improve eating and activity behaviours. Interventions for overweight and obese children that are driven or motivated by parents, without a commitment from the individual child, are unlikely to succeed. Waters *et al.*[96] contend that interventions to improve child eating and activity behaviours are most effective if they are comprehensive and involve caregivers and the wider community.

Outlined in Box 25.1 are examples of key questions to help clinicians formalize a treatment and management plan:

From treatment and management to prevention

Prevention and management of obesity in children should be the highest priority of primary care, family-based and school-based programmes and initiatives.[95,96,107–110] In overweight and obese adults, high levels of PA are associated with greater weight loss and ability to maintain weight loss.[60] For many young people, the opportunity to increase daily energy expenditure through greater participation in PA and exercise may be sufficient to prevent obesity.[83] If PA was habitual and a non-negotiable lifestyle component from birth, the prevalence of obesity would be significantly lower. A logical argument is that a change in PA status may be simpler for non-obese youngsters than to encourage older individuals to be physically active once they become obese.[83] Parents, teachers, coaches, and medical practitioners have a collective responsibility to provide every opportunity for young people to be physically active.[87–89,100,111]

All children, irrespective of age, size, and shape love to move. It is very unfortunate that an increasing number of young people are not provided sufficient opportunity and encouragement to be physically active, whether in the form of spontaneous play and incidental activity, or more structured activity such as in school physical education and sport.[62,100,112]

It is also reasonable to suggest that quality experiences during childhood and adolescence may help to set the scene for a more

Box 25.1 Examples of key questions to help clinicians formalize a treatment and management plan

- What is the nature of the family environment, including physical characteristics of parents and siblings?
- How long has the individual been overweight or obese?
- Has the individual been relatively inactive for an extended period?
- Is the individual's willingness to participate in physical activity limited by low self-confidence and/or self-esteem?
- Has the individual been subjected to teasing and ridicule by peers?
- Is the individual genuinely concerned about their physical size and shape?
- Is the individual self-motivated with respect to improving body composition status?
- Is the individual committed to improving eating and activity behaviours?
- What is the individual's current health status and estimated risk?

active adulthood.[100,113] Some of the more important contributing factors to the maintenance of activity behaviours from childhood through to adulthood are success, fun, and enjoyment in PA experienced during the younger years.[62,88,100,102] Physical activity should not be regarded as a chore, but should be relevant and personally challenging for each individual. In young children, participation in a range of different activities should be encouraged, and competition minimized.[113] Perhaps not surprisingly, the earlier work of Epstein *et al.*[114,115] reported that activity programmes using lifestyle activities were more effective than programmed aerobic exercise.

Another important factor with a potential bearing on weight management is the level of societal knowledge, understanding, and appreciation of individual differences, including variability in size, shape, and body composition. For example, it is well documented that obesity in childhood can contribute to behavioural and emotional difficulties, such as depression, plus potentially result in stigmatization, poor socialization, and impairment in learning.[116,117] In addition to the traditional health benefits of PA like increased cardiorespiratory and muscular fitness, reduced body fatness, and enhanced bone health, quality physical education and other forms of PA can challenge stigma and stereotypes, improve psychosocial outcomes, and reduce symptoms of depression.[118]

Despite the basic premises of the energy balance equation, some individuals are predisposed to gain weight more readily than others and also have more difficulty losing weight.[119,120] The nature of biological determination in weight management has been hotly discussed for decades and is yet to be resolved.[54,56,57,121–125] Individuals who may be more predisposed to overweight or obesity than others need to be more vigilant regarding eating and activity behaviours. In this regard, it is critical that medical and other health professionals are conscious of the constellation of factors governing behaviour, including the possibility of precipitating the development of eating and weight disorders associated with a fear of fatness.[110]

Many demands are placed on individual settings, including schools.[126] However, the school setting could be better utilized to foster active behaviours[53,126] with quality physical education programmes across all levels and better use of facilities and available professionals.[100,118,126–128] Quality physical education and related physical activities should cater for all individuals and not be restricted to the more physically capable and potentially elite sportspersons. Regular participation in PA, including quality physical education, also has the potential to improve attention span and cognitive control of children.[118] Creative approaches to PA engagement must be both sensitive to curricular needs and student choice.[129]

The family environment[130] should include positive parental and sibling influences,[131,132] which are invaluable in the treatment and management of childhood obesity,[133] despite some of the major risk factors being parental obesity[53,134] and exercise habits.[53] Parents may facilitate and contribute to the maintenance of sedentary lifestyle behaviours[135] or parental exercise may contribute to lower levels of fatness in children, irrespective of whether the parent exercises with the child. Unfortunately, the most common scenario is that many children do not have the opportunity to walk or cycle to and from school and are not supervised by adults at home before and after school. This provides an additional opportunity for young people to make poor food choices, engage in inactive behaviours such as television viewing, and reduces the potential time for active pursuits.[94]

Evidence suggests that children's food choices are likely to be less healthy than their parents' choices, if young people are left to their own resources.[136,137] Even when parents are at home, inactive pursuits such as passive television viewing or video game play may be chosen as a convenient child-minding tools. Not surprisingly, excess television viewing and video gaming have been identified as contributing factors to childhood obesity[138,139] and may also enhance the intake of snacks low in energy and nutritional value.[140–142] Furthermore, if the content of television advertising to children is not controlled, children may be exposed to less healthy food options[140,143] and the types of food that parents may wish to limit.[144]

A focus of earlier research included the effects of reinforcing obese children for being more active and less sedentary.[115,145,146] Well before the more recent interest in sedentary behaviour and weight management, Epstein *et al.*[146] found that reducing access to preferred sedentary behaviours was superior to reinforcing active behaviour choices for weight control and fitness improvement at 1 year. Similarly,[147] highly valued sedentary activities such as television viewing can help to reinforce PA participation. Making television viewing available to children only while they were physically active resulted in an increase in activity time from 5 min at baseline to greater than 20 min when the contingency was in effect. Enhancing parental capacity to better manage children's reduced consumption of energy-dense food and participation in PA also has empirical support if comprehensive rather than conservative interventions are undertaken.[95,96,148–150]

The active involvement of at least one parent in the weight-management process with a child helps to improve short- and long-term weight regulation[134,151] and should be non-negotiable. All family members can benefit from the encouragement and support provided to an overweight or obese child in the adoption of new eating and exercise behaviours. Recent systematic reviews also support the role of parents of young children in school- and community-based obesity prevention interventions, suggesting parental influence extends to contexts beyond the family home.[95,96,150,152] Parents should be active role models and encourage all family members to participate in PA, ideally as a family unit. Numerous options exist for increased activity such as walking or cycling to and from school, taking the dog and children for a walk rather than being inactive, minimizing the use of motor vehicles, taking the stairs rather than lifts or escalators, and so on.

There is an urgent need for greater community responsibility and engagement to involve a wide range of sectors in the encouragement and promotion of exercise and PA.[88,95,96,100,109,150] Increasing opportunities for safe and appropriate PA, both structured and unstructured, and in and out of school, will likely provide significant benefits for all children and adolescents. A logical example is the greater use of walking and cycling to and from school.[118]

Box 25.2 provides suggestions on how to better support obese children and adolescents.

Evidence-based PA recommendations for the health of children, adolescents, and adults are now widely available,[153] as well as for weight management in children and adolescents.[107] However, there are numerous challenges regarding exercise and weight control in young people, including the difficulty of assessing the association

Box 25.2 Ways of supporting obese children and adolescents

- educating and informing children and adolescents
- actively discouraging dieting as a method to promote weight loss
- re-educating to correct poor eating and exercise habits while encouraging an improvement in overall health and well-being
- increasing self-esteem and body image including a positive mental attitude
- encouraging a positive 'can do' mentality. Everyone, irrespective of size and shape has the ability to improve their health status
- encouraging an acceptance of individual variability in body size and shape
- focus on health status not on weight, per se
- fostering an enjoyment in regular physical activity, commencing with low- to moderate-intensity activity and increasing as the individual improves in fitness
- downplaying the 'shame and blame' mentality regarding weight and fatness
- eating well and following recommended dietary guidelines.

between adiposity and enhanced PA (training) due to the lack of a standardized approach to the assessment of adiposity, PA, and energy expenditure.[154] Consequently, it is difficult to recommend a dose-response or minimal dose of exercise to maintain a desirable body composition in children.[102] Nonetheless, governments and 'expert' bodies in most developed nations have developed PA and sedentary behaviour guidelines (for example see Australian, UK, German, Canadian, and US examples.[153,155–157]). Due to differential growth and maturation, intervention programmes for young people should account for age-related preferences in activity and changes in PA levels during the growing years.[83,87,89,90] If children are actively involved in making decisions related to their PA and sports participation, there is also likely to be greater participation rates and enjoyment.[129,158] Despite the lack of definitive data regarding the tracking of PA experiences from the growing years to adult life, there is consensus that the level of enjoyment of PA in early years may be a key determinant of continued participation.[100,159]

Body satisfaction during the growing years: implications for eating and weight disorders

Maturation and a range of external factors, including psychosocial status, heavily influence the physical growth and development of children.[87] However, the relationships between body size and shape and psychological health are relatively poorly understood. For example, we know there is a strong association between increased body fatness and body dissatisfaction. However, gender differences have been identified,[160] suggesting differential responses to psychosocial pressure exist between boys and girls. In addition, it is unclear when dissatisfaction commences and/or at what age indicators of body image, such as dissatisfaction with one's body, are important enough to influence the global construct of self-esteem. Children as young as 3–5 years of age show a preference for thinner 'ideal' body shapes;[161] 6- to 8-year-old girls with existing internalized thin ideals show higher body satisfaction following exposure to idealized animated video characters.[162] Additionally, despite a lack of between-group differences on body image preference, 6- to 10-year-old girls who played with thin dolls for 10 min ate less than girls who played with building blocks.[163] Future research focus includes discovering how the key psychological indicators of health are linked and if they track with physical growth changes. It is also worth investigating how important the pubertal barrier is in the development of particular traits in this area, and what the role of PA participation, motor skill level, and body composition status is in relation to various psychological constructs.

Despite the interest in the area, relatively few studies have considered the interrelationships between body composition per se and body satisfaction during childhood and adolescence.[17] Preoccupation with body weight and fatness is just as common in childhood and adolescence as it is for adults. However, the strength of the association between body satisfaction and weight-related behaviours is unclear. Children as young as 3 years of age view obesity negatively,[164] and the stereotypes of thinness as attractive and desirable, and fatness as neither, are well established by 9 years of age.[165–167] Overweight and obese 9-year-old girls had significantly lower self-esteem related to physical appearance and athletic competence than their normal weight peers, but body weight had no impact on girls' rated importance of self-esteem. Heavier girls were less likely to be peer nominated as pretty, but did not differ in their popularity.

One of the limiting factors in this area of research has been the nature of the methods employed. For example, in studies of body image and weight control practices of children and adolescents, many studies have utilized instruments designed for adults.[168] We have investigated the effect of adult versus adolescent body-figure silhouette scales on ratings of body image[169] in adolescents and found significant between-scale differences. Adolescents displayed consistently lower body-image ratings when viewing adult as opposed to adolescent scales. These results confirm the need for population-specific measurement scales and the use of standardized assessment procedures.

Additionally, there are differences in the measures used to assess body satisfaction, particularly with reference to the body composition of participants. Hills and Byrne[169] investigated the effect of body composition on the association among three indices of body satisfaction in a group of adolescents. For individuals with higher weight-for-height and also greater body fat levels, Pearson correlation coefficients for body satisfaction were stronger than those for normal weight individuals. Hills and Byrne[17] also assessed appearance and weight-control attitudes and behaviours in adolescents and, as for previous work with this population,[169–172] found that males were significantly more satisfied than females with their physical appearance in general, and with weight-related aspects in particular. Despite both genders being less satisfied with a fatter physique, males perceived themselves as too thin and wished to be more muscular, while females felt they were too fat and desired to be thinner. Recent research has replicated these findings.[160]

Smolak *et al.*[173] have documented an association between puberty and an increase in body dissatisfaction in females, and Koff *et al.*[158] have reported a higher relationship between body image and self-concept for females at this stage of development. Earlier work by an Australian group[165] found that between 9 and

10 years of age, males and females do not differ significantly in their level of body satisfaction. Hills and Byrne[17] support the contention that the onset of puberty can influence body satisfaction, but for both sexes. In this study, a significant gender difference was found at 12 years of age, where females displayed a marked level of body dissatisfaction while males were satisfied with their physical appearance. At 14 years of age, males displayed a level of dissatisfaction with their physical appearance, comparable with females 2 years younger; this change dovetailed with the average age of puberty for males. Gender differences resumed by 16 years of age—males as a group were more satisfied as they approximated their mature adult physique, but females remained dissatisfied with their appearance.

It appears that current body size and fatness influence body satisfaction to some extent. A higher weight-for-height ratio and higher adiposity levels were associated with lower body satisfaction in both male and female adolescents. Those with higher adiposity thought and felt they were larger than their less-obese peers. However, there were no gender differences in body and weight satisfaction in adolescent males and females with lower levels of adiposity; additionally, females were no more likely than males to perceive themselves as overweight. These results confirm that body weight and level of adiposity are fundamental elements of physical attractiveness standards for both sexes.

The influence of body composition on disordered eating tendencies of adolescents

Given the higher prevalence of childhood obesity and the relationship between being above-average weight and dieting in adolescence,[25] it may be hypothesized that an increasing number of adolescents will employ restrictive dietary practices. Most studies have reported that dieting is predominantly a female characteristic. However, to date more research has focused on girls than boys. In the UK, an estimated 40% of girls and 25% of boys begin dieting in adolescence.[174] Some researchers have claimed that female concerns about weight and physical appearance and associated dieting have become so pervasive that they may be considered normal behaviour.[29,30,175,176] Of particular concern is that some studies have suggested that a substantial proportion of adolescent girls have used extreme weight-loss behaviours at least occasionally. However, a major shortcoming of many studies of weight-control practices has been the failure to make any reference to the actual physical size of individuals studied.

Work by Hills and Byrne[17] assessed weight concerns and dieting practices in a group of adolescent boys and girls and, consistent with previous work with a similar population,[19,176,177] found that females were significantly more likely than males to diet and fast for weight control. Females also employed more pathogenic weight control practices and counted the energy content of foods they consumed, although it is very difficult to assess the normalcy of these results given the range of reported prevalence in adults and adolescents. The gender differences found by Hills and Byrne[17] may again relate to the greater number of females who perceived themselves as overweight. Streigel-Moore *et al.*[178] have proposed that the body weight concerns of adolescent females are due to them equating 'normal' weight with 'underweight'. Another explanation[30] may be that females are aware of appropriate weight norms. However, females may deliberately try to violate them, reflecting dissatisfaction with body weight.

In summary, both relative weight-for-height (body mass index, BMI) and body-fat levels influenced body satisfaction and drive-for-thinness in males and females. Those who were bigger and fatter according to these measures were more dissatisfied with their physique, and displayed a greater concern with dieting, preoccupation with weight, and pursuit of thinness. These results suggest that body composition influences the prevalence of restrictive dietary practices. However, gender differences were still evident within each body composition categorization.

Exercise motivations of adolescents

In order to minimize distorted attitudes about body size and weight control it is important to determine the genesis of these attitudes, how they evolve over time, and which individuals are most vulnerable.[168,176] Hills and Byrne[169] investigated gender differences in exercise motivations in adolescents in relation to body composition status. Males displayed significantly greater body satisfaction than females, while females reported a greater concern for and preoccupation with weight and thinness. A similar proportion of males and females were overweight; however, nearly twice as many females perceived themselves as being overweight and more females reported exercising for weight control and to improve body tone. Those who were motivated to exercise for fitness, health, and enjoyment reported fewer disturbances in body image and body dissatisfaction, compared to those motivated to exercise for weight control, tone and attractiveness; this was a finding consistent with other studies.[177,179] However, once body composition was accounted for, there were no significant gender differences in exercise motivation at higher body-fat levels. In short, despite the evidence of gender differences being evident by adolescence, as seen in studies of adults, differences in exercise motivation may be attributed to both level of body dissatisfaction and body composition. McDonald and Thompson[177] have referenced the need to be concerned for individuals, particularly females, whose motivation for exercise is primarily cosmetic. Available evidence is particularly concerning and suggestive of an association between body composition, weight control behaviours, and health status from an early age. All health professionals and responsible adults must help to promote exercise as a means of achieving health and wellness, rather than helping to perpetuate the restrictive approach of using exercise merely as an avenue for weight control.[159]

Anorexia nervosa, bulimia nervosa, and binge eating disorder

Compared to anorexia, bulimia nervosa and binge eating disorder are more commonly described as beginning in young adults.[180] However, there are large numbers of adolescents with these conditions.[181] In each condition, the individual's self-evaluation is over-influenced by body weight and shape. Those individuals who do not meet the full DSM-5 criteria may be classified as having Avoidant/Restrictive Food Intake Disorder, Other Specified Feeding or Eating Disorder, or Unspecified Feeding or Eating Disorder. Both anorexia and bulimia nervosa are complex, closely related alterations in eating behaviour. Crisp[182] has suggested that both are pubertally-driven disorders with the common element being an underlying 'dyslipophobia' (or distressing 'fear of fatness'). Anorexia nervosa is characterized by weight loss, disturbed body image, an intense fear of weight gain and obesity, and particularly in girls a fear of the 'fatness' of the normal mature female body which is instigated at puberty.[182,183] Excessive PA also figures prominently as a symptom in both bulimia and the restricting subtype of anorexia nervosa.[184–188]

Mainstream bulimia nervosa, by contrast, occurs at or above normal adult body weight.[174] The condition is also characterized by an intense fear of fatness and the belief that other people consider this as a loss of control.[182] Bulimia is characterized by eating large quantities of food at one time (bingeing), which is purged from the body by vomiting, using laxatives or diuretics, fasting, and/or excessive exercise.[189] Bulimia is also frequently related to weight-reduction diets,[190] and may occur in younger people who are of normal or lower-than-average weight, where as binge eating is accompanied by strict dieting, self-induced vomiting, and low body weight.[191] Obese girls who diet obsessively may be at particular risk of developing an eating disorder.

Although, numerous diagnostic criteria have been employed to define each condition, those in Box 25.3 are adapted from the DSM-5.[180]

Box 25.3 Diagnostic criteria for anorexia nervosa, bulimia nervosa, and binge eating disorder

Diagnostic criteria for anorexia nervosa

A. Restriction of energy intake relative to requirements, leading to a significantly low body weight in the context of age, sex, developmental trajectory, and physical health. Significantly low weight is defined as a weight that is less than minimally normal or, for children and adolescents, less than that minimally expected.

B. Intense fear of gaining weight or of becoming fat, or persistent behaviour that interferes with weight gain, even though at a significantly low weight.

C. Disturbance in the way in which one's body weight or shape is experienced, undue influence of body weight or shape on self-evaluation, or persistent lack of recognition of the seriousness of the current low body weight.

Diagnostic criteria for bulimia nervosa

A. Recurrent episodes of binge eating. An episode of binge eating is characterized by both of the following:

1. Eating, in a discrete period of time (e.g. within any two-hour period), an amount of food that is definitely larger than what most individuals would eat in a similar period of time under similar circumstances.
2. A sense of lack of control over eating during the episode (e.g. a feeling that one cannot stop eating or control what or how much one is eating).

B. Recurrent inappropriate compensatory behaviours in order to prevent weight gain, such as self-induced vomiting, misuse of laxatives, diuretics, or other medications, fasting, or excessive exercise.

C. The binge eating and inappropriate compensatory behaviours both occur, on average, at least once a week for 3 months.

D. Self-evaluation is unduly influenced by body shape and weight.

E. The disturbance does not occur exclusively during episodes of anorexia nervosa.

Diagnostic criteria for binge eating disorder

A. Recurrent episodes of binge eating. An episode of binge eating is characterized by both of the following:

1. Eating, in a discrete period of time (e.g. within any 2-hour period), an amount of food that is definitely larger than what most people would eat in a similar period of time under similar circumstances.
2. A sense of lack of control over eating during the episode (e.g. a feeling that one cannot stop eating or control what or how much one is eating).

B. The binge-eating episodes are associated with three (or more) of the following:

1. Eating much more rapidly than normal.
2. Eating until feeling uncomfortably full.
3. Eating large amounts of food when not feeling physically hungry.
4. Eating alone because of feeling embarrassed by how much one is eating.
5. Feeling disgusted with oneself, depressed, or very guilty afterward.

C. Marked distress regarding binge eating is present.

D. The binge eating occurs, on average, at least once a week for 3 months.

E. The binge eating is not associated with the recurrent use of inappropriate compensatory behaviour as in bulimia nervosa and does not occur exclusively during the course of bulimia nervosa or anorexia nervosa.

Aetiology of anorexia and bulimia nervosa

Despite the lack of understanding of the specific aetiology of the eating disorders and the normal development of eating behaviour there is evidence that certain critical elements may be responsible. Risk factors identified to date include familial influences and genetic predisposition,[192,193] biological mechanisms such as a serotonin deficiency,[194,195] and personality and individual psychopathology.[196–198] More recently it has been proposed that the psychopathology sequelae associated with anorexia and bulimia nervosa are simply epiphenomena that follow after a sustained period of disordered eating.[33] Rather than psychopathology leading to anorexia or bulimia, disordered eating in this framework is the result of instrumental factors; neural reward centres become activated in response to dietary restraint and increased PA leading to chronic under-eating which manifests as an eating disorder. However, the authors do not discuss precipitants for dietary restraint and increased PA.

Casper[199] has outlined two categories of precipitating events in relation to the onset of anorexia nervosa—psychological or physical. Examples of psychological events include extreme disappointment in relation to an important relationship, the birth of a sibling, moving house, the loss of a friend, or a death in the family. Physical events may include early physical maturation and anxiety about puberty.

A number of researchers[16,200] have stated that participation in sport increases the risk for eating and weight problems as the biological risk for eating disorders relates to the common trend in many athletes to restrict energy intake. The dietary restraint needed to control intake may influence attitudes such as a preoccupation with eating and weight, and behaviours such as binge eating.[16]

The transition from childhood to adolescence is a time of substantial biological change and in females body fat stores increase as girls change from a child to a mature young woman. As organized sport and competition in the PA setting are commonplace, many individuals are faced with a dilemma; a biological change in physical characteristics and a desire to control eating and weight for both appearance and performance reasons.

Crisp[182] has indicated that anorexia has physical, social, and psychological handicaps, many of which the anorectic recognizes. At the same time, the individual denies the presence of illness and weight concerns, and will often be secretive and manipulative in an attempt to defend her bio-psychological avoidant stance. The individual with bulimia nervosa may also be secretive, commonly experiencing guilt, low self-esteem, and anger because of her incapacity to control food intake.[182]

The dieting and eating disorder continuum

Numerous studies acknowledge a continuum of risks for eating disorders,[23,201] ranging from normative concerns about body weight and shape, to rigid dieting, to subclinical, and subsequently, diagnosable eating disorders.[178,202–205] Similarly, Nylander[206] proposed that dieting behaviour lies on a continuum with no dieting behaviour and eating disorders at the extremes, and increasing levels of dieting severity between.

Clearly, not all individuals who diet develop eating disorders. However, dieting has been recognized as a prelude to anorexia and bulimia nervosa.[19,174,178,193,206] Smolak *et al.*[173] suggested that dieting should be viewed as problematic behaviour as it has the potential to lead to health-threatening weight cycling and binge eating. Dieting during adolescence is of particular concern as the highest incidence of anorexia nervosa occurs at the beginning of adolescence, and bulimia nervosa at the end.[174,175,207]

Prevalence of eating disorders

A number of issues need to be addressed when discussing the prevalence of disordered eating behaviours. For example, Brownell *et al.*[161] noted that to deal only with the 'clinical' entities of anorexia and bulimia nervosa would miss many 'subclinical' problems, such as preoccupation with food, obsessive thinking about weight, and disturbed body image. While the prevalence of anorexia nervosa in the general population is very low at approximately 1%, and bulimia estimated to be between one and 3%,[208] the number of people who suffer with eating and weight problems but do not meet strict diagnostic criteria is much greater.[208–210] Despite the relatively small number of adolescent girls who suffer from clinically diagnosable eating disorders[197] (3–5%), a sizeable portion of adolescent girls (40%) and boys (25%) report dieting behaviour.[174]

As many individuals have 'unusual' eating patterns but do not meet established diagnostic criteria for an eating disorder,[211] it is important that the terminology for clinically disordered eating practices is only used where appropriate. The misuse of the term 'eating disorder', or more specifically the terms anorexia or bulimia nervosa, may be another reason for the diversity in the reported figures regarding the prevalence of eating disorders.

Binge eating disorder

With the publication of the DSM-5 in 2013, binge eating disorder (BED), which was listed as a criterion for further study, is now included as psychological condition in an updated chapter named Feeding and Eating Disorders, along with anorexia nervosa, bulimia nervosa, and several other conditions.[212] Essential features under the new classification include recurrent episodes of three or more of the following at least once per week for a 3-month period:

i) Eating more rapidly than normal
ii) Eating until feeling uncomfortably full
iii) Eating large amounts of food when not feeling physically hungry
iv) Eating alone because of feeling embarrassed by how much one is eating
v) Feeling disgusted with oneself, depressed, or very guilty afterward.

Four levels of severity also apply from Mild (one to three binge-eating episodes per week) to Extreme (14 or more binges per week). The lifetime prevalence of BED is 1.6% and 0.8% for females and males respectively.[213] A recognized subpopulation of obese individuals, estimated to approximate 25% to almost 75% of those seeking treatment for the condition[49,214,215] undertake periodic bouts of binge eating. Obese binge-eaters are characterized as having experienced multiple weight loss failures followed by an abandonment of dietary restraint.[48] Interestingly, Wilson *et al.*[210] have reported that obese binge-eaters are more dissatisfied with their weight and have a higher preoccupation with their weight and food than other obese individuals.

Binge eating is often precipitated by negative emotions and individuals report feeling out of control.[214,216] When binge-eaters experience guilt, binges can be followed by increased dietary restraint which perpetuates an unbalanced relationship with food.

Prevention, treatment, and management

Treatment for each condition is largely experiential and behavioural.[182] Goals for the anorexic individual include weight gain[217] while weight maintenance may be more important for the bulimic or obese individual with binge-eating disorder. Robin *et al.*[211] have stressed the differential expression of anorexia and bulimia nervosa in children and adolescents compared to adults and suggested that multidisciplinary treatments should be tailored to the unique developmental, medical, nutritional, and psychological needs of young people. It is also important to acknowledge that the psychological profile in early onset (<16 years) anorexia differs from that in later onset.[218]

Recommendations for treatment and management by health professionals may include the elements of successful treatment as outlined by Comerci,[219] which include recognizing the disorder and restoring physiologic stability as soon as possible, establishing a trusting and therapeutic partnership with the young person, involving the family in treatment, and using a multi-disciplinary team approach.[220]

Box 25.4 Useful and practical points to emphasize when engaging with the young eating-disordered individual

i) The young person did not choose to develop an eating disorder, but they can choose to get better.
ii) Commonly, eating disorders reflect a means of coping with developmental issues e.g. the need to gain a sense of control, efficacy or identity.
iii) The individual may become angry and frustrated with treatment requirements, including the necessity for weight gain to improve health status.
iv) It is pointless to assign blame or guilt for the cause of the problem.
v) Professional help should focus on restoration of health (not merely weight gain).

Some of the useful and more practical aspects of engagement with the young eating disordered individual are to emphasize the points shown in Box 25.4 to parents and the individual.

Youngsters often have unresolved intrapersonal (self-esteem, self-efficacy) and interpersonal (school, home, or peers) conflicts, which generally relate to the common psychosocial adjustments during adolescence. Weight-control practices initiated to manage these issues tend to be reinforced by feedback. Examples may include compliments regarding appearance or the perception of mastery over what is eaten (or not eaten), and attempts to manage situations of overeating through exercise, vomiting, or the taking of laxatives. Negative feedback may also be commonplace, usually from family members and good friends, although this can commonly result in the opposite—further positive reinforcement.

The use of exercise in the treatment and management of these conditions appears to have considerable merit. For example, anorexic adolescents who are constantly looking for opportunities to participate in aerobic-based activities may benefit from individualized resistance training sessions to help preserve and strengthen skeletal muscle tissue.

The interested reader is referred to a number of other excellent sources for comprehensive details of prevention, treatment and management.[12,13,14,15,39,53,108]

Conclusions

Identification, treatment, and management of youth at all points along the weight spectrum from eating disordered behaviour to those with obesity continue to pose a challenge for clinicians and health care policy-makers. The challenges are exacerbated by a proliferation in developed and increasingly in developing nations undergoing nutritional transition to a more Western diet and lifestyle, which evidence suggests is associated with a preference for a lean physical appearance that paradoxically co-exists with increasing rates of obesity. This paradox remains poorly understood, yet it appears to be a pivotal element of chronic health problems related to body composition at both ends of the spectrum; lipophobia in the case of frank anorexia and bulimia nervosa, overweight, and obesity that in some cases is associated with binge-eating disorder, and associated morbidities across the spectrum. Early clinical identification, appropriate treatment, referral and follow up, and on-going management commencing with a general medical practitioner may be the most effective approach to mitigating this increasingly complex problem. However, models of care that begin in a medical setting and include clinical expertise in appropriate exercise and dietary prescriptions are relatively poorly defined and understudied. Further work is needed to develop effective interventions across this spectrum with a focus on clearly defined, healthy body composition outcomes.

Summary

- Obesity is an increasingly visible yet largely unaddressed problem
- Obesity is at one end of a spectrum of eating and weight-related disorders that includes frank anorexia and bulimia nervosa
- Identification of youth at each end of the spectrum, and those with maladaptive eating and exercise behaviours, is a serious challenge for clinicians and health policy makers
- Developmental factors are important considerations when identifying, treating, and managing body composition-related problems in youth
- Greater research focus on models of care that reflect the complexity of the problem are needed.

References

1. Batch JA, Baur LA. Management and prevention of obesity and its complications in children and adolescents. *Med J Aust*. 2005; 182: 130–135.
2. WHO. *Global strategy on diet physical activity and health*. Geneva: World Health Organization; 2004.
3. WHO. *Global status report on noncommunicable diseases* 2010. Geneva: World Health Organization; 2011.
4. WHO. *Diet, nutrition and the prevention of chronic diseases*. World Health Organ Tech Rep Ser. NO. 916 (TRS 916). Geneva: World Health Organization; 2003.
5. Caballero B. A Nutrition Paradox—Underweight and Obesity in Developing Countries. *N Engl J Med*. 2005; 352: 1514–1516.
6. Asfaw A. The effects of obesity on doctor-diagnosed chronic diseases in Africa: empirical results from Senegal and South Africa. *J Pub Health Policy*. 2006; 27: 250–264.
7. Monteiro CA, Hawkes C, Caballero B. The underweight/overweight paradox in developing societies: Causes and policy implications. In: Dubé L, Bechara A, Dagher A, *et al*. (eds.) *Obesity prevention: The role of brain and society on individual behavior*. Amsterdam: Academic Press; 2010. p. 463–469.
8. Black RE, Victora CG, Walker SP, *et al*. Maternal and child undernutrition and overweight in low-income and middle-income countries. *Lancet*. 2013; 382(9890): 427–451.
9. de Onis M, Blossner M, Borghi E. Global prevalence and trends of overweight and obesity among preschool children. *Am J Clin Nutr*. 2010; 92: 1257–1264.
10. Ng M, Fleming T, Robinson M, *et al*. Global, regional, and national prevalence of overweight and obesity in children and adults during 1980–2013: a systematic analysis for the Global Burden of Disease Study 2013. *Lancet*. 2014; 384(9945): 766–781.
11. Haby MM, Markwick A, Peeters A, Shaw J, Vos T. Future predictions of body mass index and overweight prevalence in Australia, 2005–2025. *Health Prom Int*. 2012; 27: 250–260.
12. Bratland-Sanda S, Sundgot-Borgen J. Eating disorders in athletes: overview of prevalence, risk factors and recommendations for prevention and treatment. *Eur J Sport Sci*. 2013; 13: 499–508.

13. Sundgot-Borgen J, Meyer NL, Lohman TG, *et al.* How to minimise the health risks to athletes who compete in weight-sensitive sports. Review and position statement on behalf of the Ad Hoc Research Working Group on Body Composition, Health and Performance, under the auspices of the IOC Medical Commission. *Br J Sports Med.* 2013; 47: 1012–1022.
14. Sundgot-Borgen J, Torstveit M. Aspects of disordered eating continuum in elite high-intensity sports. *Scand J Med Sci Sports.* 2010; 20: 112–121.
15. Werner A, Thiel A, Schneider S, Mayer J, Giel KE, Zipfel S. Weight-control behaviour and weight-concerns in young elite athletes—A systematic review. *J Eat Disord.* 2013; 1: 18.
16. Brownell KD, Rodin J, Wilmore JH. Eating, body weight and performance in athletes: an introduction. In: Brownell KD, Wilmore J (eds.) *Eating, body weight and performance.* Philadelphia: Lea and Febiger; 1992. p. 3–16.
17. Hills AP, Byrne NM. Body composition, body satisfaction, eating and exercise behaviour of Australian adolescents. In: Parizkova J, Hills AP (eds.) *Physical fitness and nutrition during growth.* Basel: Karger; 1998. p. 44–53.
18. McKinley NM. Resisting body dissatisfaction: fat women who endorse fat acceptance. *Body Image.* 2004; 1: 213–219.
19. Emmons L. Dieting and purging behaviour in black and white high school students. *J Am Diet Assoc.* 1992; 92: 306–312.
20. Boutelle K, Neumark-Sztainer D, Story M, Resnick M. Weight-control behaviors among obese, overweight, and nonoverweight adolescents. *J Pediatr Psychol.* 2002; 27: 531–540.
21. Committee on Sports Medicine and Fitness. Promotion of healthy weight-control practices in young athletes. *Pediatrics.* 2005; 116: 1557–1564.
22. Javed A, Tebben PJ, Fischer PR, Lteif AN. Female athlete triad and its components: toward improved screening and management. *Mayo Clinic Proc.* 2013: 996–1009.
23. Beals KA, Houtkooper L. Disordered eating in athletes. In: Burke L (ed.) *Clinical sports nutrition.* Sydney: McGraw-Hill; 2006. p. 201–223.
24. Brownell KD. Dieting and the search for the perfect body: Where physiology and culture collide. *Behav Ther.* 1991; 22: 1–12.
25. Paxton SJ, Wertheim EH, Gibbons K, Szmukler GI. Body image satisfaction, dieting beliefs, and weight loss behaviors in adolescent girls and boys. *J Youth Adol.* 1991; 20: 361–379.
26. Wertheim EH, Paxton SJ, Maude D, Szmukler GI. Psychosocial predictors of weight loss behaviors and binge eating in adolescent girls and boys. *Int J Eat Dis.* 1992; 12: 151–160.
27. Maude D, Wertheim EH, Paxton S, Gibbons K. Body dissatisfaction, weight loss behaviours, and bulimic tendencies in Australian adolescents with an estimate of female data representativeness. *Aust Psychol.* 1993; 28: 128–132.
28. Nowak M, Speare R, Crawford D. Gender differences in adolescent weight and shape related beliefs and behaviours. *J Paediatr Child Health.* 1996; 32: 148–152.
29. Mellin LM, Irwin CE, Scully S. Prevalence of disordered eating in girls: a survey of middle-class children. *J Am Diet Assoc.* 1992; 92: 851–853.
30. Koff E, Rierdan J. Perceptions of weight and attitudes toward eating in early adolescent girls. *J Adolesc Health.* 1991; 12: 307–312.
31. Patton GC, Selzer R, Coffey C, Carlin JB, Wolfe R. Onset of adolescent eating disorders: population based cohort study over 3 years. *BMJ.* 1999; 318(7186): 765–768.
32. Greenfeld D, Quinlan D, Harding M, Glass E, Bliss A. Eating behaviour in an adolescent population. *Int J Eat Dis.* 1987; 6: 99–111.
33. Zandian M, Ioakimidis I, Bergh C, Sodrsten P. Cause and treatment of anorexia nervosa. *Physiol Behav.* 2007; 92: 283–290.
34. Raevuori A, Keski-Rahkonen A, Hoek HW. A review of eating disorders in males. *Curr Opin Psychiatry.* 2014; 27: 426–430.
35. Spring B, Pingitore R, Bruckner E, Penava S. Obesity: idealized or stigmatized? Socio-cultural influences on the meaning and prevalence of obesity. In: Hills AP, Walqvist ML (eds.) *Exercise and obesity.* London: Smith-Gordon; 1994. p. 49–60.
36. Sikorski C, Luppa M, Luck T, Riedel-Heller SG. Weight stigma 'gets under the skin'-evidence for an adapted psychological mediation framework: a systematic review. *Obesity.* 2015; 23: 266–276.
37. Polivy J, Herman P. Dieting and bingeing: a causal analysis. *Am Psychol.* 1985; 40: 193–197.
38. Stice E, Presnell K, Shaw H, Rohde P. Psychological and behavioral risk factors for obesity onset in adolescent girls: a prospective study. *J Consult Clin Psychol.* 2005; 73: 195–202.
39. Hill A. Obesity and eating disorders. *Obes Rev.* 2007; 8(Suppl): 151–155.
40. Flynn M. Fear of fatness and adolescent girls: implications for obesity prevention. *Proc Nutr Soc.* 1997; 56: 305–317.
41. Wadden TA, Foster GD, Stunkard AJ, Linowitz JR. Dissatisfaction with weight and figure in obese girls: discontent but not depression. *Int J Obes.* 1988; 13: 89–97.
42. Hill A, Draper E, Stack J. A weight on children's minds: body shape dissatisfactions at 9 years old. *Int J Obes Relat Metab Disord.* 1994; 18: 383–389.
43. Wadden T, Foster G, Stunkard A, Linowitz J. Dissatisfaction with weight and figure in obese girls: discontent but not depression. *Int J Obes.* 1989; 13: 89–97.
44. Whitaker A, Davies M, Shaffer D, *et al.* The struggle to be thin: a survey of anorexic and bulimic symptoms in a non-referred adolescent population. *Psychol Med.* 1989; 19: 143–163.
45. Hill AJ. Pre-adolescent dieting: Implications for eating disorders. *Int Rev Psychiatry.* 1993; 5: 87–99.
46. Hill A. Causes and consequences of dieting and anorexia. *Proc Nutr Soc.* 1993; 52: 211–218.
47. Rodin J, Silberstein L, Striegel-Moore R. Women and weight: a normative discontent. In: Sonderegger TB (ed.) *Psychology and gender.* Lincoln: University of Nebraska Press; 1985. p. 267–307
48. Jebb S, Prentice A. Is obesity an eating disorder? *Proc Nutr Soc.* 1995; 54: 721–728.
49. de Zwaan M. Binge eating disorder and obesity. *Int J Obes Relat Metab Disord.* 2001; 25(Suppl 1): S51–S55.
50. Hay PJ, Mond J, Buttner P, Darby A. Eating disorder behaviors are increasing: Findings from two sequential community surveys in South Australia. *PLOS One.* 2008; 3(2).
51. Garfinkel P, Dorian B. Factors that may influence future approaches to the eating disorders. *Eat Weight Disord.* 1997; 2: 1–16.
52. Manore MM. *Weight management in the performance athlete.* Basel: Karger/Nestle Nutrition Institute; 2013.
53. Court JM. Strategies for management of obesity in children and adolescents. In: Hills AP, Wahlqvist ML (eds.) *Exercise and obesity.* London: Smith-Gordon; 1994. p. 181–194
54. Dietz WH. Childhood obesity. In: Cheung LWY, Richmond JB (eds.) *Child health, nutrition, and physical activity.* Champaign, IL: Human Kinetics; 1995. p. 155–170.
55. Gortmaker SL, Must A, Perrin JM, Sobol AM, Dietz WH. Social and economic consequences of overweight in adolescence and young adulthood. *N Engl J Med.* 1993; 329: 1008–1012.
56. Millward DJ. Energy balance and obesity: a UK perspective on the gluttony v. sloth debate. *Nutr Res Rev.* 2013; 26: 89–109.
57. Schutz Y, Byrne NM, Dulloo A, Hills AP. Energy gap in the aetiology of body weight gain and obesity: a challenging concept with a complex evaluation and pitfalls. *Obes Facts.* 2014; 7: 15–25.
58. Church TS, Thomas DM, Tudor-Locke C, *et al.* Trends over 5 decades in US occupation-related physical activity and their associations with obesity. *PLOS One.* 2011; 6: doi: 10.1371/journal.pone.0019657
59. Wadden TA, Butryn ML, Byrne KJ. Efficacy of lifestyle modification for long-term weight control. *Obesity Res.* 2004; 12(Suppl 3): 151S–162S.
60. Hill JO, Wyatt HR. Role of physical activity in preventing and treating obesity. *J Appl Physiol.* 2005; 99: 765–770.
61. Epstein LH. Exercise in the treatment of childhood obesity. *Int J Obes Relat Metab Disord.* 1995; 19(Suppl 4): S117–S121.
62. WHO. *Global recommendations on physical activity for health.* Geneva: World Health Organization; 2010.

63. Hills AP. Locomotor characteristics of obese children. In: Hills AP, Walqvist ML (eds.) *Exercise and obesity*. London: Smith-Gordon; 1994. p. 141–150.
64. Milligan R, Thompson C, Vandongen R, Beilin L, Burke V. Clustering of cardiovascular risk factors in Australian adolescents: association with dietary excesses and deficiencies. *J Cardiovasc Risk*. 1995; 2: 515–523.
65. Hills A, Byrne N. Exercise prescription for weight management. *Proc Nutr Soc*. 1998; 57: 93–103.
66. Labib M. The investigation and management of obesity. *J Clin Pathol*. 2003; 56: 17–25.
67. Lobstein T, Jackson-Leach R. Estimated burden of paediatric obesity and co-morbidities in Europe. Part 2. Numbers of children with indicators of obesity-related disease. *Int J Pediatr Obes*. 2006; 1: 33–41.
68. Shultz SP, Anner J, Hills AP. Paediatric obesity, physical activity and the musculoskeletal system. *Obes Rev*. 2009; 10: 576–582.
69. Shultz SP, Byrne NM, Hills AP. Musculoskeletal function and obesity: implications for physical activity. *Curr Obes Rep*. 2014; 3: 355–360.
70. Tsiros M, Coates A, Howe P, *et al*. Adiposity is related to decrements in cardiorespiratory fitness in obese and normal-weight children. *Pediatr Obes*. 2015; 11: 144–150.
71. Tsiros MD, Buckley JD, Howe PRC, Walkley J, Hills AP, Coates AM. Musculoskeletal pain in obese compared with healthy-weight children. *Clin J Pain*. 2014; 30: 583–588.
72. Haines L, Wan KC, Lynn R, Barrett TG, Shield JPH. Rising incidence of type 2 diabetes in children in the UK. *Diabetes Care*. 2007; 30: 1097–1101.
73. Goran MI, Ball GDC, Cruz ML. Obesity and risk of type 2 diabetes and cardiovascular disease in children and adolescents. *J Clin Endocrinol Metab*. 2003; 88: 1417–1427.
74. Sorof J, Daniels S. Obesity hypertension in children: A problem of epidemic proportions. *Hypertension*. 2002; 40: 441–447.
75. Groner JA, Joshi M, Bauer JA. Pediatric precursors of adult cardiovascular disease: noninvasive assessment of early vascular changes in children and adolescents. *Pediatrics*. 2006; 118: 1683–1691.
76. Gielen S, Hambrecht R. The childhood obesity epidemic: Impact on endothelial function. *Circulation*. 2004; 109: 1911–1913.
77. Freedman DS, Khan LK, Serdula MK, Dietz WH, Srinivasan SR, Berenson GS. The relation of childhood BMI to adult adiposity: The Bogalusa Heart Study. *Pediatrics*. 2005; 115: 22–27.
78. Litwin SE. Childhood obesity and adulthood cardiovascular disease. Quantifying the lifetime cumulative burden of cardiovascular risk factors. *J Am Coll Cardiol*. 2014; 64: 1588–1590.
79. Nader PR, O'Brien M, Houts R, *et al*. Identifying risk for obesity in early childhood. *Pediatrics*. 2006; 118: E594–E601.
80. Roberto CA, Swinburn B, Hawkes C, *et al*. Patchy progress on obesity prevention: emerging examples, entrenched barriers, and new thinking. *Lancet*. 2015; 385(9985): 2400–2409.
81. Collins CE, Warren J, Neve M, McCoy P, Stokes BJ. Measuring effectiveness of dietetic interventions in child obesity: A systematic review of randomized trials. *Arch Pediatr Adolesc Med*. 2006; 160: 906–922.
82. Ritchie L, Welk G, Styne D, Gerstein D, Crawford P. Family environment and pediatric overweight: what is a parent to do? *J Am Diet Assoc*. 2005; 105(Suppl 1): S70–S79.
83. Epstein L, Coleman K, Myers M. Exercise in treating obesity in children and adolescents. *Med Sci Sports Exerc*. 1996; 28: 428–435.
84. Must A. Morbidity and mortality associated with elevated body weight in children and adolescents. *Am. J. Clin Nutr*. 1996; 63: 445S–447S.
85. Barlow SE, Dietz WH. Obesity evaluation and treatment: Expert committee recommendations. *Pediatrics*. 1998; 102: e29.
86. Council on Sports Medicine and Fitness and Council on School Health. Active healthy living: Prevention of childhood obesity through increased physical activity. *Pediatrics*. 2006; 117: 1834–1842.
87. Hills AP, Byrne NM, Lindstrom R, Hill JO. 'Small changes' to diet and physical activity behaviors for weight management. *Obes Facts*. 2013; 6: 228–238.
88. Hills AP, Okely AD, Baur LA. Addressing childhood obesity through increased physical activity. *Nature Rev Endocrinol*. 2010; 6: 543–549.
89. Street S, Wells J, Hills A. Windows of opportunity for physical activity in the prevention of obesity. *Obes Rev*. 2015; 16: 857–870.
90. Todd AS, Street SJ, Ziviani J, Byrne NM, Hills AP. Overweight and obese adolescent girls: The importance of promoting sensible eating and activity behaviors from the start of the adolescent period. *Int J Environ Res Public Health*. 2015; 12: 2306–2329.
91. Schwartz M, Puhl R. Childhood obesity: a societal problem to solve. *Obes Rev*. 2003; 4: 57–71.
92. Covic T, Roufeil L, Dziurawiec S. Community beliefs about childhood obesity: its causes, consequences and potential solutions. *J. Public Health Med*. 2007; 29: 123–131.
93. Magarey AM, Perry RA, Baur LA, *et al*. A parent-led family-focused treatment program for overweight children aged 5 to 9 years: the PEACH RCT. *Pediatrics*. 2011; 127: 214–222.
94. Epstein LH, Saelens BE, O'Brien JG. Effects of reinforcing increases in active behavior versus decreases in sedentary behavior for obese children. *Int J Behav Med*. 1995; 2: 41–50.
95. Oude Luttikhuis H, Baur L, Jansen H, *et al*. Interventions for treating obesity in children. *Cochrane Data Syst Rev*. 2009; 1: doi: 10.1002/14651858.CD001872.pub2.
96. Waters E, de Silva-Sanigorski A, Hall BJ, *et al*. Interventions for preventing obesity in children. *Cochrane Data Syst Rev*. 2011; 12: doi: 10.1002/14651858.CD001871.pub3
97. Stiegler P, Cunliffe A. The role of diet and exercise for the maintenance of fat-free mass and resting metabolic rate during weight loss. *Sports Med*. 2006; 36: 239–262.
98. Catenacci V, Wyatt H. The role of physical activity in producing and maintaining weight loss. *Nat Clin Pract Endocrinol Metab*. 2007; 3: 518–529.
99. Schiffman S. Biological and psychological benefits of exercise in obesity. In: Hills AP, Walqvist ML (eds.) *Exercise and obesity*. London: Smith-Gordon; 1994. p. 103–114.
100. Hills AP, Dengel DR, Lubans DR. Supporting public health priorities: recommendations for physical education and physical activity promotion in schools. *Prog Cardiovasc Dis*. 2015; 57: 368–374.
101. Moore KA, Burrows GD. Behavioural management of obesity in an exercise context. In: Hills AP, Walqvist ML (eds.) *Exercise and obesity*. London: Smith-Gordon; 1994. p. 207–216.
102. Bar-Or O, Baranowski T. Physical activity, adiposity, and obesity among adolescents. *Pediatr Exerc Sci*. 1994; 6: 348–360.
103. Foreyt JP, Goodrick GK. Living without dieting: motivating the obese to exercise and to eat prudently. *Quest*. 1997; 47: 264–273.
104. Epstein LH. Exercise and obesity in children. *J Appl Sport Psych*. 1992; 4: 20–33.
105. Epstein L. Exercise in the treatment of childhood obesity. *Int J Obes Relat Metab Disord*. 1995; 19(Suppl 4): S117–S121.
106. Saris WHM, van Baak MA. Consequences of exercise on energy expenditure. In: Hills AP, Walqvist ML (eds.) *Exercise and obesity*. London: Smith-Gordon; 1994. p. 85–102.
107. National Health Medical Research Council. *Clinical practice guidelines for the management of overweight and obesity in adults, adolescents and children in Australia*. Melbourne: National Health and Medical Research Council; 2013.
108. Wilmore J. Weight gain, weight loss, and weight control: what is the role of physical activity? *Nutrition*. 1997; 13: 820–822.
109. Gill TP. Key issues in the prevention of obesity. *Br Med Bull*. 1997; 53: 359–388.
110. World Health Organization. *Obesity: Preventing and managing the global epidemic*. Geneva: World Health Organization; 2000.

111. Booth F, Hawley J. The erosion of physical activity in Western societies: an economic death march. *Diabetologia*. 2015; 58: 1730–1734.
112. Tremblay MS, Gray CE, Akinroye KK, Harrington DM, Katzmarzyk PT, Lambert EV, *et al*. Physical activity of children: a global matrix of grades comparing 15 countries. *J Phys Act Health*. 2014; 11(Supp 1): 113–125.
113. Allender S, Cowburn G, Foster C. Understanding participation in sport and physical activity among children and adults: a review of qualitative studies. *Health Educ Res*. 2006; 21: 826–835.
114. Epstein LH. A comparison of lifestyle change and programmed aerobic exercise on weight and fitness changes in obese children. *Behav Ther*. 1982; 13: 651–665.
115. Epstein LH, Wing RR, Koeske R, Valoski A. A comparison of lifestyle exercise, aerobic exercise, and calisthenics on weight loss in obese children. *Behav Ther*. 1985; 16: 345–356.
116. Miller AL, Lee HJ, Lumeng JC. Obesity-associated biomarkers and executive function in children. *Pediatr Res*. 2014; 77: 143–147.
117. Pizzi MA, Vroman K. Childhood obesity: effects on children's participation, mental health, and psychosocial development. *Occup Ther Health Care*. 2013; 27: 99–112.
118. McLennan N, Thompson J. Quality physical education (QPE): Guidelines for policy makers. Paris: UNESCO Publishing; 2015.
119. Speakman JR. Obesity: The integrated roles of environment and genetics. *J Nutr*. 2004; 134: 2090S–20105S.
120. Yang W, Kelly T, He J. Genetic epidemiology of obesity. *Epidemiol Rev*. 2007; 29: 49–61.
121. Bouchard C, Tremblay A, Despres J, *et al*. The response to long-term overfeeding in identical twins. *N Engl J Med*. 1990; 322: 1477–1482.
122. Stunkard A, Harris J, Pedersen N, McClearn G. The body-mass index of twins who have been reared apart. *N Engl J Med*. 1990; 322: 1483–1487.
123. Byrne NM, Hills AP. Biology or behavior: which is the strongest contributor to weight gain? *Curr Obes Rep*. 2013; 2: 65–76.
124. Byrne NM, Wood RE, Schutz Y, Hills AP. Does metabolic compensation explain the majority of less-than-expected weight loss in obese adults during a short-term severe diet and exercise intervention. *Int J Obes*. 2012; 36: 1472–1478.
125. Dhurandhar N, Schoeller D, Brown A, *et al*. Energy balance measurement: when something is not better than nothing. *Int J Obes*. 2015; 39: 1109–1113.
126. Booth M, Okely A. Promoting physical activity among children and adolescents: the strengths and limitations of school-based approaches. *Health Promot J Austr*. 2005; 16: 52–54.
127. Ward D, Bar-Or O. Role of the physician and physical education teacher in the treatment of obesity at school. *Pediatrician*. 1986; 13: 44–51.
128. Sallis JF, Chen AH, Castro CM. School-based interventions for childhood obesity. In: Cheung LWY, Richmond JB (eds.) *Child health, nutrition, and physical activity*. Champaign, IL: Human Kinetics; 1995. p. 179–204.
129. Smith A, Green K, Thurston M. 'Activity choice' and physical education in England and Wales. *Sport Educ Soc*. 2009; 14: 203–222.
130. Boonpleng W, Park CG, Gallo AM, Corte C, McCreary L, Bergren MD. Ecological influences of early childhood obesity: A multilevel analysis. *West J Nurs Res*. 2013; 35: 742–759.
131. Connell LE, Francis LA. Positive parenting mitigates the effects of poor self-regulation on body mass index trajectories from ages 4–15 years. *Health Psych*. 2014; 33: 757–764.
132. Stein RI, Epstein LH, Raynor HA, Kilanowski CK, Paluch RA. The influence of parenting change on pediatric weight control. *Obes Res*. 2005; 13: 1749–1755.
133. Golan M. Parents as agents of change in childhood obesity—from research to practice. *Int J Pediatr Obes*. 2006; 1: 66–76.
134. Epstein L. Family-based behavioural intervention for obese children. *Int J Obes Relat Metab Disord*. 1996; 20(Suppl 1): S14–S21.
135. Dietz W. The role of lifestyle in health: the epidemiology and consequences of inactivity. *Proc Nutr Soc*. 1996; 55: 829–840.
136. Klesges R, Stein R, Eck L, Isbell T, Klesges L. Parental influence on food selection in young children and its relationships to childhood obesity [published erratum appears in] *Am J Clin Nutr*. 1991; 53: 859–864.
137. Brown JE, Broom DH, Nicholson JM, Bittman M. Do working mothers raise couch potato kids? Maternal employment and children's lifestyle behaviours and weight in early childhood. *Soc Sci Med*. 2010; 70: 1816–1824.
138. Gortmaker SL, Must A, Sobol AM, Peterson K, Colditz GA, Dietz WH. Television viewing as a cause of increasing obesity among children in the United States, 1986–1990. *Arch Pediatr Adolesc Med*. 1996; 150: 356–362.
139. Farajian P, Panagiotakos DB, Risvas G, Malisova O, Zampelas A. Hierarchical analysis of dietary, lifestyle and family environment risk factors for childhood obesity: the GRECO study. *Eur J Clin Nutr*. 2014; 68: 1107–1112.
140. Dietz WH, Jr, Gortmaker SL. Do we fatten our children at the television set? Obesity and television viewing in children and adolescents. *Pediatrics*. 1985; 75: 807–812.
141. Salmon J, Campbell K, Crawford D. Television viewing habits associated with obesity risk factors: a survey of Melbourne schoolchildren. *Med J Aust*. 2006; 184: 64–67.
142. Borgogna N, Lockhart G, Grenard JL, Barrett T, Shiffman S, Reynolds KD. Ecological momentary assessment of urban adolescents' technology use and cravings for unhealthy snacks and drinks: Differences by ethnicity and sex. *J Acad Nutr Diet*. 2015; 115: 759–766.
143. Neville L, Thomas M, Bauman A. Food advertising on Australian television: the extent of children's exposure. *Health Promot Int*. 2005; 20: 105–112.
144. Wardle J. Parental influences on children's diets. *Proc Nutr Soc*. 1995; 54: 747–758.
145. Epstein L, Wing R, Penner B, Kress M. Effect of diet and controlled exercise on weight loss in obese children. *J Pediatr*. 1985; 107: 358–361.
146. Epstein LH, Saelens BE, Myers MD, Vito D. Effects of decreasing sedentary behaviors on activity choice in obese children. *Health Psych*. 1997; 16: 107–113.
147. Saelens B, Epstein L. Behavioral engineering of activity choice in obese children. *Int J Obes Relat Metab Disord*. 1998; 22: 275–277.
148. Janicke DM, Steele RG, Gayes LA, *et al*. Systematic review and meta-analysis of comprehensive behavioral family lifestyle interventions addressing pediatric obesity. *J Pediatr Psych*. 2014; 39: 809–825.
149. Muhlig Y, Wabitsch M, Moss A, Hebebrand J. Weight loss in children and adolescents. A systematic review and evaluation of conservative, non-pharmacological obesity treatment programs. *Deutsches Arzteblatt Int*. 2014; 111: 818–824.
150. WHO. *Population-based approaches to childhood obesity prevention*. Geneva: World Health Organization: 2012.
151. Wrotniak BH, Epstein LH, Paluch RA, Roemmich JN. Parent weight change as a predictor of child weight change in family-based behavioral obesity treatment. *Arch Pediatr Adolesc Med*. 2004; 158: 342–347.
152. Sobol-Goldberg S, Rabinowitz J, Gross R. School-based obesity prevention programs: A meta-analysis of randomized controlled trials. *Obesity*. 2013; 21: 2422–2428.
153. Department of Health and Aging. *Australia's physical activity and sedentary behaviour guidelines*. Canberra: Australian Federal Government; 2014.
154. Hills AP, Mokhtar N, Byrne NM. Assessment of physical activity and energy expenditure: an overview of objective measures. *Front Nutr*. 2014; 1(5): doi: 10.3389/fnut.2014.00005
155. American Heart Association. *Promoting Physical Activity in Children and Youth*. Available from: http://circ.ahajournals.org/content/114/11/1214.full. [Accessed October 2007].

156. Graf C, Beneke R, Bloch W, *et al.* Recommendations for promoting physical activity for children and adolescents in Germany. A consensus statement. *Obes Facts.* 2014; 7: 178–190.
157. Canadian Society for Exercise Physiology. *Canadian physical activity and sedentary behaviour guidelines handbook, 2012.* Ontario: Canadian Society for Exercise Physiology; 2012.
158. Koff E, Rierdan J, Stubbs ML. Gender, body image, and self-concept in early adolescence. *J Early Adolesc.* 1990; 10: 56–68.
159. Hills AP, Byrne NM. Relationships between body dissatisfaction, disordered eating and exercise motivations. *Int J Obes.* 1994; 18(Suppl 2): S31.
160. Pich J, Bibiloni Mdel M, Pons A, Tur JA. Weight self-regulation process in adolescence: The relationship between control weight attitudes, behaviors, and body weight status. *Front Nutr.* 2015; 2: 14.
161. Spiel EC, Paxton SJ, Yager Z. Weight attitudes in 3- to 5-year-old children: Age differences and cross-sectional predictors. *Body Image.* 2012; 9: 524–527.
162. Anschutz DJ, Engels R, Van Strien T. Increased body satisfaction after exposure to thin ideal children's television in young girls showing thin ideal internalisation. *Psych Health.* 2012; 27: 603–617.
163. Anschutz DJ, Engels R. The effects of playing with thin dolls on body image and food intake in young girls. *Sex Roles.* 2010; 63: 621–630.
164. Musher-Eizenman DR, Holub SC, Miller AB, Goldstein SE, Edwards-Leeper L. Body size stigmatization in preschool children: The role of control attributions. *J. Pediatr Psychol.* 2004; 29: 613–620.
165. Tiggerman M, Pennington B. The development of gender differences in body-size satisfaction. *Aust Psych.* 1990; 41: 246–263.
166. Clark L, Tiggemann M. Appearance culture in nine- to 12-year-old girls: Media and peer influences on body dissatisfaction. *Soc Dev.* 2006; 15: 628–643.
167. Slater A, Tiggemann M. Body image and disordered eating in adolescent girls and boys: A test of objectification theory. *Sex Roles.* 2010; 63: 42–49.
168. Byrne N, Hills A. Should body-image scales designed for adults be used with adolescents? *Percept Mot Skills.* 1996; 82: 747–753.
169. Hills AP, Byrne NM. Body composition, body satisfaction, and exercise motivation of girls and boys. *Med Sci Sports Exerc.* 1998; 30: S120.
170. Hills AP, Byrne NM. Body composition and body image: implications for weight-control practices in adolescents. *Int J Obes.* 1997; 21(Suppl 2): S115.
171. Hill A, Silver E. Fat, friendless and unhealthy: 9-year old children's perception of body shape stereotypes. *Int J Obes Relat Metab Disord.* 1995; 19: 423–430.
172. Phillips R, Hill A. Fat, plain, but not friendless: self-esteem and peer acceptance of obese pre-adolescent girls. *Int J Obes Relat Metab Disord.* 1998; 22: 287–293.
173. Smolak L, Levine MP, Gralen S. The impact of puberty and dating on eating problems among middle school girls. *J Youth Adolesc.* 1993; 22: 355–368.
174. Nicholls D, Viner R. Eating disorders and weight problems. *BMJ.* 2005; 330(7497): 950–953.
175. Krowchuk DP, Kreiter SR, Woods CR, Sinal SH, Du Rant RH. Problem dieting behaviours among young adolescents. *Arch Pediatr Adolesc Med.* 1998; 152: 884–888.
176. Killen J, Taylor C, Hammer L, *et al.* An attempt to modify unhealthful eating attitudes and weight regulation practices of young adolescent girls. *Int J Eat Disord.* 1993; 13: 369–84.
177. McDonald K, Thompson JK. Eating disturbance, body image dissatisfaction, and reasons for exercising: Gender differences and correlational findings. *Int J Eat Disord.* 1992; 11: 289–292.
178. Striegel-Moore RH, Silberstein LR, Rodin J. Toward an understanding of risk factors for bulimia. *Am Psych.* 1986; 41: 246–263.
179. Silberstein L, Striegel-Moore R, Timko C, Rodin J. Behavioural and psychological implications of body dissatisfaction: do men and women differ? *Sex Roles.* 1988; 19: 219–232.
180. American Psychiatric Association. *Diagnostic and statistical manual of mental disorders: DSM-5.* Washington, DC: American Psychiatric Association: 2013.
181. Schneider M. Bulimia nervosa and binge-eating disorder in adolescents. *Adolesc Med.* 2003; 14: 119–131.
182. Crisp A. The dyslipophobias: a view of the psychopathologies involved and the hazards of construing anorexia nervosa and bulimia nervosa as 'eating disorders'. *Proc Nutr Soc.* 1995; 54: 701–709.
183. Herzog D, Copeland P. Eating disorders. *N Engl J Med.* 1985; 313: 295–303.
184. Davis C. Eating disorders and hyperactivity: A psychobiological perspective. *Can J Psychiatry.* 1997; 42: 168–175.
185. Beumont P, Arthur B, Russell J, Touyz S. Excessive physical activity in dieting disorder patients: proposals for a supervised exercise program. *Int J Eat Disord.* 1994; 15: 21–36.
186. Davis C, Blackmore E, Katzman D, Fox J. Female adolescents with anorexia nervosa and their parents: a case-control study of exercise attitudes and behaviours. *Psychol Med.* 2005; 35: 377–386.
187. Kostrzewa E, Eijkemans MJC, Kas MJ. The expression of excessive exercise co-segregates with the risk of developing an eating disorder in women. *Psychiatry Res.* 2013; 210: 1123–1128.
188. Dalle Grave R, Calugi S, Marchesini G. Compulsive exercise to control shape or weight in eating disorders: prevalence, associated features, and treatment outcome. *Comprehen Psychiatry.* 2008; 49: 346–352.
189. Hilbert A, Pike KM, Goldschmidt AB, *et al.* Risk factors across the eating disorders. *Psychiatry Res.* 2014; 220: 500–506.
190. Westerterp KR, Saris WHM. Limits of energy turnover in relation to physical performance, achievement of energy balance on a daily basis. In: Williams C, Devlin JT (eds.) *Food, nutrition and performance.* London: E & FN Spon; 1992. p. 1–16.
191. Russell G. Bulimia nervosa: An ominous variant of anorexia nervosa. *Psych Med.* 1979; 9: 429–448.
192. Fichter MM, Noegel R. Concordance for bulimia nervosa in twins. *Int J Eat Disord.* 1990; 9: 255–263.
193. Hsu LKG, Chesler BE, Santhouse R. Bulimia nervosa in eleven sets of twins: A clinical report. *Int J Eat Disord.* 1990; 9: 275–282.
194. Goodwin GM, Fairburn CG, Cowen PJ. Dieting changes serotonergic function in women, not men: Implications for the aetiology of anorexia nervosa? *Psych Med.* 1987; 17: 839–842.
195. Kaye WH, Ballenger JC, Lydiard RB, *et al.* CSF monoamine levels in normal-weight bulimia: evidence for abnormal noradrenergic activity. *Am J Psychiat.* 1990; 147: 225–229.
196. Laberg JC, Wilson GT, Eldredge K, Nordby H. Effects of mood on heart rate reactivity in bulimia nervosa. *Int J Eat Disord.* 1991; 10: 169–178.
197. Laessle RG, Wittchen HU, Fichter MM, Pirke KM. The significance of subgroups of bulimia and anorexia nervosa: Lifetime frequency of psychiatric disorders. *Int J Eat Disord.* 1989; 8: 569–574.
198. Garner DM, Olmsted MP, Davis R, Rockert W, Goldbloom D, Eagle M. The association between bulimic symptoms and reported psychopathology. *Int J Eat Disord.* 1990; 9: 1–15.
199. Casper RC. Fear of fatness and anorexia nervosa in children. In: Cheung LWY, Richmond JB (eds.) *Child health, nutrition and physical activity.* Champaign, IL: Human Kinetics; 1995. p. 211–234.
200. Davis C, Kennedy SH, Ravelski E, Dionne M. The role of physical activity in the development and maintenance of eating disorders. *Psychol Med.* 1994; 24: 957–967.
201. Garfinkel P, Kennedy SH, Kaplan A. Views on classification and diagnosis of eating disorders. *Can J Psychiatry.* 1995; 40: 445–456.
202. Chamay-Weber C, Narring F, Michaud P. Partial eating disorders among adolescents: a review. *J Adolesc Health.* 2005; 37: 417–427.
203. Wilson G, Eldredge I. Pathology and development of eating disorders: implications for athletes. In: Brownell K, Rodin J, Wilmore JH (eds.) *Eating, body weight, and performance in athletes.* Philadelphia: Lea and Febiger; 1992. p. 128–145.
204. Patton G, Carlin J, Shao Q, *et al.* Adolescent dieting: healthy weight control or borderline eating disorder? *J Child Psychol Psychiatry.* 1997; 38: 299–306.
205. Favaro A, Ferrara S, Santonastaso P. The spectrum of eating disorders in young women: A prevalence study in a general population sample. *Psychosom Med.* 2003; 65: 701–708.

206. Nylander I. The feeling of being fat and dieting in a school population. Epidemiological interview investigation. *Acta Sociomed Scand.* 1971; 1: 17–26.
207. Brownell K, Fairburn C. *Eating disorders and obesity.* New York: Guilford Press; 1995.
208. Bunnell DW, Shenker IR, Nussbaum MP, Jacobson MS, Cooper P. Subclinical versus formal eating disorders: Differentiating psychological features. *Int J Eat Disord.* 1990; 9: 357–362.
209. Wilmore J. Eating and weight disorders in the female athlete. *Int J Sport Nutr.* 1991; 1: 104–117.
210. Wilson GT, Nonas CA, Rosenblum GD. Assessment of binge eating in obese patients. *Int J Eat Disord.* 1993; 13: 25–33.
211. Robin A, Gilroy M, Dennis A. Treatment of eating disorders in children and adolescents. *Clin Psych Rev.* 1998; 18: 421–446.
212. American Psychiatric Association. *Diagnostic and statistical manual of mental disorders: DSM-IV.* Washington, DC: American Psychiatric Association; 1994.
213. Hudson JI, Lalonde JK, Coit CE, *et al.* Longitudinal study of the diagnosis of components of the metabolic syndrome in individuals with binge-eating disorder. *Am J Clin Nutr.* 2010; 91: 1568–1573.
214. Spitzer RL, Devlin M, Walsh BT, *et al.* Binge eating disorder: A multisite field trial of the diagnostic criteria. *Int J Eat Disord.* 1992; 11: 191–203.
215. Higgins DM, Dorflinger L, MacGregor KL, Heapy AA, Goulet JL, Ruser C. Binge eating behavior among a national sample of overweight and obese veterans. *Obes.* 2013; 21: 900–903.
216. Stein R, Kenardy J, Wiseman C, Dounchis J, Arnow B, Wilfley D. What's driving the binge in binge eating disorder? A prospective examination of precursors and consequences. *Int J Eat Disord.* 2007; 40: 195–203.
217. Patel DR, Pratt HD, Greydanus DE. Treatment of Adolescents with Anorexia Nervosa. *J Adolesc Res.* 2003; 18: 244–260.
218. Abbate-Daga G, Piero A, Rigardetto R, Gandione M, Gramaglia C, Fassino S. Clinical, psychological and personality features related to age of onset of anorexia nervosa. *Psychopath.* 2007; 40: 261–268.
219. Comerci GD. Eating disorders in adolescents. *Pediatr Rev.* 1988; 10: 37–47.
220. Hay P, Chinn D, Forbes D, *et al.* Royal Australian and New Zealand College of Psychiatrists clinical practice guidelines for the treatment of eating disorders. *Aust N Zeal J Psychiatry.* 2014; 48: 1–62.

CHAPTER 26

Exercise, physical activity, and cerebral palsy

Annet J Dallmeijer, Astrid CJ Balemans, and Olaf Verschuren

Introduction

Cerebral palsy

Children with cerebral palsy (CP) experience difficulties in performing activities in daily living, including sports and exercise activities. As a result, most individuals with CP lead an inactive and sedentary lifestyle. Individuals with CP remained inactive because intensive exercise was assumed to increase spasticity and lead to detrimental effects on functional abilities. As a consequence, there was little information available about physical fitness levels and abilities to perform physical activity (PA). In the last decade, scientific interest in the potential benefits of exercise and PA for improving physical fitness, health, and daily physical activities has increased for children with CP, resulting in a growing number of publications addressing the importance of an active lifestyle.[1–3] This chapter describes the state of knowledge about fitness, exercise testing, training, and PA in children with CP. Practical advice in training and PA guidelines is also provided.

Cerebral palsy is the most common neurological disorder causing physical disability in childhood, with a prevalence in Europe of around two to three cases per 1000 live births.[4] The condition is attributed to non-progressive disturbances that occurred in the developing infant or foetal brain. The most important physical symptoms are mobility limitations caused by motor impairments, such as spasticity, muscle weakness, and impaired motor control. The condition is often accompanied by sensory, behavioural, and cognitive disturbances.[5] Limitations in mobility limit exercise performance, fitness, and PA levels.[3]

Classification

Individuals with CP typically present a variety of consequences, depending on the degree and location of brain damage. Over the years, classification has evolved that categorizes CP according to anatomical, neuromotor, and functional perspectives.[5] The anatomical classification distinguishes uni- or bilateral involvement. In the neuromotor classification three types of CP can be distinguished: spastic, dyskinetic, or ataxic. But mixed forms are common. Spastic CP is the most common subtype, affecting 85% of the total population of individuals with CP.

The Gross Motor Function Classification System (GMFCS) is a five-level functional classification system that has become the standard for classifying gross motor ability in children with CP.[6] Distinction between the five classification levels is based on their self-initiated movement, use of assistive mobility devices, use of wheeled mobility, and to a lesser extent, the quality of movement. Children classified as GMFCS level I walk indoors and outdoors and climb stairs without restriction, but have limitations in more advanced motor skills like running. Those with GMFCS level II walk indoors and outdoors without assistive devices, but experience limitations walking outdoors on uneven surfaces and inclines. Children in GMFCS level III walk indoors or outdoors with an assistive mobility device. Children in GMFCS level IV walk short distances with a device, but rely more on wheeled mobility at home and in the community. Children classified as GMFCS level V have no means of independent mobility.[6]

Exercise testing and physical fitness

Exercise testing

The assessment of exercise capacity in children with CP may be complicated by motor impairments, such as spasticity, limited range of motion, impaired selective motor control, and increased level of co-activation. Despite these difficulties both laboratory and field tests with acceptable validity and reliability have been developed to assess the fitness components in children with CP.[7] These tests include aerobic and anaerobic fitness tests and muscle strength tests. While most tests focus on ambulant children, tests for wheelchair-dependent children have also been recently described. Laboratory tests are characterized by high standardization of measurement, and are indicated when precise fitness measures are required for diagnostic purposes, or for training evaluation. Field tests can be used as a feasible alternative when no equipment is available or when the focus is on functional ability and more test specificity is required. Field tests generally reveal different outcomes that are more closely related to activities of daily life.

When conducting exercise tests in children with CP, the following points are important. Firstly, each test should be valid for the objective of the test. Secondly, the specificity of testing is important: the modality of the testing tool needs to be similar to the type of physical activity or exercise of interest. Next, the test should not require too much technical competence on the part of the child. Lastly, and importantly, care should be taken to make sure that the child understands exactly what is requested of him/her. For children with CP there is a core set of clinically feasible exercise tests, with an established level of evidence of the clinimetric properties for each outcome measure.[7–9] (see Table 26.1)

Table 26.1 Exercise tests for children with cerebral palsy

	Mode of testing	Target population	Test description	Clinimetric properties
Laboratory tests				
Aerobic exercise test				
Graded treadmill test[12,27]	Walking	GMFCS I-II	Walking with increments in speed each 1 or 2 min until exhaustion	Not available
Graded cycle ergometry test[13,19]	Cycling	GMFCS I-III	Cycling at constant speed with load increments each 1 or 2 min until exhaustion	*Test-retest reliability:* *Peak* $\dot{V}O_2$ ICC: 0.94, SEM: 5.4%[13] *Peak power output* Spearman's Rho = 0.92[19]
Graded arm ergometry exercise test[31]	Arm cranking	GMFCS III-IV	Arm cranking at constant speed with load increments each 1 or 2 min until exhaustion	Not available
Anaerobic exercise test				
20/30 s Wingate cycle test[19,20]	Cycling	GMFCS I-III	Cycling as fast as possible against constant load for 20 or 30 s	*Test-retest reliability:* *Mean power* Spearman's Rho = 0.95 (30s Wingate)[19] *Mean power* ICC: 0.96–0.99, SEM: 5.4–6.1% (20s Wingate)[20]
30 s Wingate arm cranking test[22]	Arm cranking	GMFCS III-IV	Arm cranking as fast as possible against constant load for 30 s	*Test-retest reliability: mean power* ICC: 0.99, LoA: −11.3–10.7 *Construct validity: mean power with muscle power sprint arm test:* ***r*** *= 0.88, p < 0.05*
Field tests				
Aerobic exercise test				
10 m Shuttle Run Test SRT-I (GMFCS I) and SRT-II (GMFCS II)[27,34]	Walking	GMFCS I-II	Crossing 10 m with increasing speed each min until exhaustion Speed: 5 km·h^{-1} (SRT-I) and 2 km·h^{-1} (SRT-II) with increment of 0.25 km·h^{-1} each minute	*Test-retest reliability:* *Number of shuttles (GMFCS I)* ICC: 0.97, SEM: 0.25, LoA: 1.01[27] *Number of shuttles (II)* ICC: 0.99, SEM: 0.42, LoA: 0.86[27] *Criterion validity:* *Peak* $\dot{V}O_2$ *on SRT I-II with* $\dot{V}O_2$ *peak on treadmill:* ***r*** = 0.96, LoA: 0.28–0.37[27] *Number of shuttles with peak* $\dot{V}O_2$ *on cycle ergometer:* ***r*** = 0.62 (I); ***r*** = 0.14 (II)[34]
7.5 m Shuttle Run Test (SRT-III protocol)[30]	Walking	GMFCS III	Crossing 7.5 m with increasing speed each min until exhaustion	*Test-retest reliability: Number of shuttles:* ICC: 0.98, SEM: 0.48
10 m Shuttle Ride Test (SRiT)[31]	Propelling a wheelchair	GMFCS III-IV	Crossing 10 m with increasing speed each min until exhaustion	*Test retest reliability: Number of shuttles* ICC: 0.99, SEM: 0.5 *Criterion validity:* peak $\dot{V}O_2$ *with armcrank* ***r*** = 0.84, p < 0.01
Anaerobic exercise test				
Muscle Power Sprint Test (MPST)[28,29]	Walking	GMFCS I-II	30 s: 6 all-out sprints at max speed (15 m)	*Test-retest reliability: mean power* ICC: 0.99; SEM: 9.0 LoA: 20[28] *Inter-observer reliability: mean power* ICC: 0.98 LoA: 24[28] *Criterion validity: MPST with Wingate cycle test* ***r*** = 0.90, p < 0.001[29] *Construct validity: difference mean power GMFCS I and II*, p = 0.006[28]
Muscle Power Sprint Test (wheelchair)[22]	Propelling a wheelchair	GMFCS III-IV	30 s: 6 all-out sprints at max speed (15 m)	*Test-retest reliability: mean power* ICC: 0.99 LoA:−7.1 to 6.4 *Construct validity: P20 mean with Wingate arm crank* ***r*** = 0.88, p < 0.05

GMFCS: Gross Motor Function Classification System; $\dot{V}O_2$ peak: peak oxygen uptake; ICC; Intraclass correlation coefficient; SEM: standard error of measurement; LoA: Limits of Agreement.

Aerobic fitness

Cardiorespiratory fitness is important for health in every individual.[10] It is an important determinant for cardiovascular health and life expectancy. It is therefore not surprising that this fitness component has been assessed over the years in children and adolescents with CP. Cardiopulmonary exercise testing with incremental loads is considered the 'gold standard' for the assessment of aerobic (i.e. cardiorespiratory) fitness. It enables determination of peak oxygen uptake ($\dot{V}O_2$) through measurements of ventilation, gas exchange, and heart rate for a direct assessment of aerobic fitness.[11] This laboratory-based test allows a standardized approach in terms of testing conditions and protocol and an objective determination of maximal exercise criteria. The objective criteria that should be achieved to indicate a maximal effort are: i) a heart rate (HR) > 180 beats·min^{-1} and ii) a respiratory exchange ratio ($\dot{V}CO_2/\dot{V}O_2$; R) > 1.00, and these should be accompanied by signs of subjective exhaustion in order to ensure a cardiorespiratory maximum.[7] (Interested readers are referred to Chapter 12 for a discussion of peak $\dot{V}O_2$ in healthy children).

The testing modality can be chosen based on the physical activities of the child in daily life, the type of exercise that should be evaluated, and on the feasibility of the modality for the particular child. Running on a treadmill[12] and cycling[13] are feasible methods when they are used to these modalities. Walking or running on a treadmill requires sufficient balance control, which is generally present in children with GMFCS I and II, while cycling is less dependent on balance control, allowing testing of children with GMFCS III, and sometimes GMFCS IV. This testing mode is, however, a less specific modality when walking is of interest. An arm-cranking test can be performed when mobility in daily life is mainly by wheelchair. All tests have a progressive character: exercise intensity (expressed in W) is incremented in the cycle and arm crank ergometer tests, and speed is increased in the treadmill test. Ideal test duration for determination of aerobic fitness is 8–12 min and the test terminates when the participant reaches exhaustion.

Peak $\dot{V}O_2$ is a direct measure of cardiorespiratory fitness. Aerobic performance measured with laboratory-based tests is sometimes expressed as power output (in cycling and arm cranking) or time (treadmill). However, these outcomes strongly depend on movement efficiency, which in turn varies with the level of motor involvement.[14] Table 26.1 shows the clinimetric properties of aerobic fitness tests for children with CP. The level of evidence is strong for good reliability of the aerobic cycle ergometer test for peak $\dot{V}O_2$ and limited for good reliability on peak power output, but there is no evidence of reliability of treadmill and arm crank ergometer tests.[7]

Although the primary deficit in CP occurs as a lesion in the brain, the impaired muscle function associated with CP in combination with reduced daily PA affects aerobic fitness. Peak $\dot{V}O_2$ measured on a cycle ergometer was 14–29% lower in children with CP than in typically developing children (Figure 26.1),[15] and 17% lower measured with a treadmill test.[12] As expected, peak power output measured on a cycle ergometer was 20–55% lower in children and was much more dependent on the severity of CP than peak $\dot{V}O_2$.[15] A reduced selective motor control, spasticity and co-contraction that are generally greater with higher motor involvement, may explain the lower power output with higher GMFCS levels (Figure 26.1). Peak $\dot{V}O_2$ was related to daily activity performance in children with a bilateral involvement,[16] suggesting that their aerobic fitness is influenced by physical inactivity leading to deconditioning.

Anaerobic fitness

Anaerobic fitness determines the ability to perform short bouts of high-intensity exercise. Anaerobic fitness is assumed to be a relevant fitness outcome in children, because most activities of daily living of children are characterized by intermittent short bursts of intensive exercise.[17] This activity pattern mainly relies on the anaerobic system.

As there is no direct non-invasive method available to measure the anaerobic energy turnover, the mean and peak power output

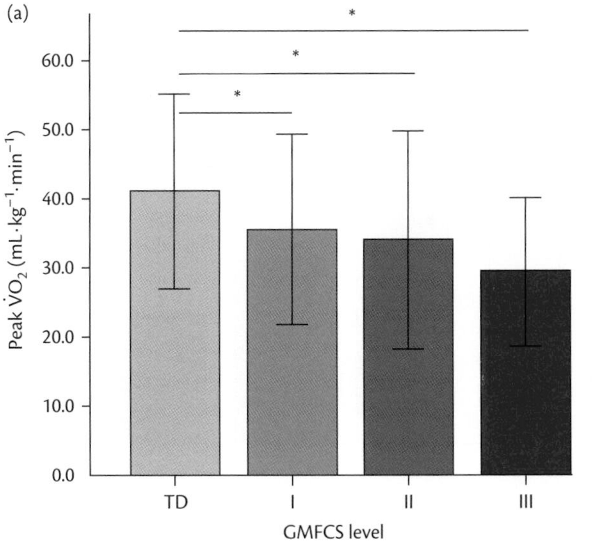

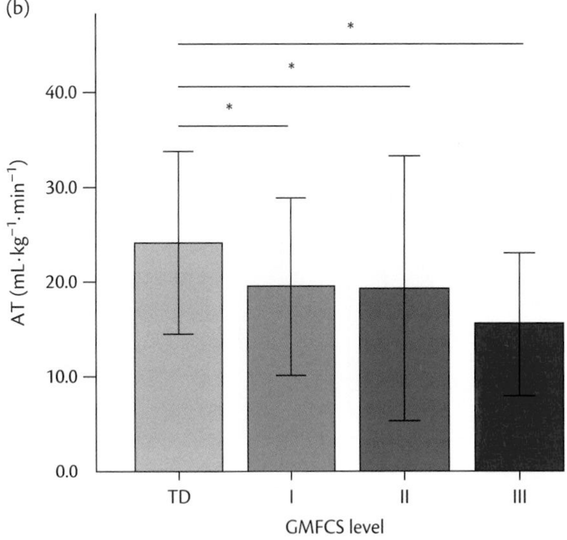

Figure 26.1 Peak oxygen uptake and anaerobic threshold in children with cerebral palsy and typically developing children.

Peak $\dot{V}O_2$ (a) = peak oxygen uptake, AT (b) = anaerobic threshold, CP = cerebral palsy, TD = typically developing children.

Balemans AC, Van Wely L, de Heer SJ, *et al*. Maximal aerobic and anaerobic exercise responses in children with cerebral palsy. Med Sci Sports Exerc. 2013; 45: 561–568.

that can be generated in a short period of intensive exercise are generally used to estimate anaerobic fitness. The Wingate anaerobic test (WAnT) is a laboratory-based cycle test that has been used to measure anaerobic fitness in children with CP.[15,18,19] The test consists of a full-out 30-s sprint test on a (child-adapted) cycle ergometer against a constant load. To allow optimal performance, the feet are strapped to the pedal using shoe fixation boxes, and the load is adapted to the ability of the child to avoid exercise limitations due to too high or too low speeds. (Interested readers are referred to Chapter 8 for a discussion of the use of the WAnT and other tests of high-intensity exercise with healthy children). The test showed acceptable reliability in children with CP.[19] A 20 s version of the WAnT that has been developed for children with CP also showed excellent reliability (Table 26.1).[20] Advantages of this shorter version include higher feasibility (test completion) and a smaller contribution of aerobic metabolism.[21]

The Wingate arm-cranking test was developed for children who mainly depend on their upper extremities for mobility. Children were instructed to crank the handles as fast as possible over a 30 s period. The load was set at 0.26 × body weight in Nm. This test also showed excellent reliability and construct validity (see Table 26.1).[22]

Using the 30 s WAnT, earlier studies found that peak and mean power output values are three to four standard deviations below the mean values for healthy controls, in children with moderate and severe CP.[18] Also a 50% lower mean power output was found in school-aged children with CP.[19] A more recent study showed that mean anaerobic power, measured with a 20 s WAnT, was 39–72% lower in children with GMFCS I-III compared to typically developing (TD) peers, and decreased with increasing GMFCS level (see Figure 26.2).[15]

Possible explanations for the lower anaerobic power include decreased muscle volumes and concomitant strength levels,[23] a reduction in fast type II muscle fibres,[24] and coordination problems like deficient synchronization between the agonist and antagonist muscle groups (co-activation).[25] The latter leads to lower effective force application and mechanical efficiency, which reduces the generated power output. It was also shown that children with CP have an impaired rapid force generation ability,[26] leading to difficulties in exerting explosive power. This can explain the lower overall power and larger variability (lower reliability) for peak power output.[20]

Aerobic and anaerobic field tests

Although the 'gold standard' assessment of exercise tolerance in children can be measured in a laboratory using a treadmill or cycle ergometer, the necessary equipment is expensive and may not be readily accessible. Moreover, highly skilled and devoted personnel are important.

Available field tests of aerobic and anaerobic capacity provide valid and reliable outcome measurements without the burden of expensive equipment in a sophisticated laboratory setting. The indications for field exercise testing in the group of children with CP are broad and have, as a general goal, the evaluation of exercise performance.

Field exercise tests are available for children classified at different GMFCS levels.[8] Most children classified as GMFCS levels I and II are able to walk and run without walking aids. For these children running-based field tests are available: the 10 m Shuttle Run Test (SRT)[27] and Muscle Power Sprint Test (MPST)[28,29] measure aerobic and anaerobic performance respectively. Children classified as GMFCS level III are able to walk with walking aids only and sometimes propel a manual wheelchair for short or long distances. Therefore, for this subgroup field exercise tests are related to walking[30] or propelling a wheelchair.[31] For children classified as GMFCS level IV, the field tests are related to propelling a wheelchair. CP-specific norm values are available for two field exercise tests: the 10 m SRT[32] and the MPST.[33] Clinimetric properties for all available field exercise tests are described in Table 26.1. The level of evidence is strong for good reliability for both aerobic and anaerobic field tests and for validity of the anaerobic field tests.[7] Interestingly, the peak $\dot{V}O_2$ achieved in a SRT has a good correspondence with the peak $\dot{V}O_2$ achieved on a treadmill, while the number of shuttles does not show an association with peak $\dot{V}O_2$ on the treadmill.[34] The number of shuttles is probably more a performance-related measure that takes running ability better into account.

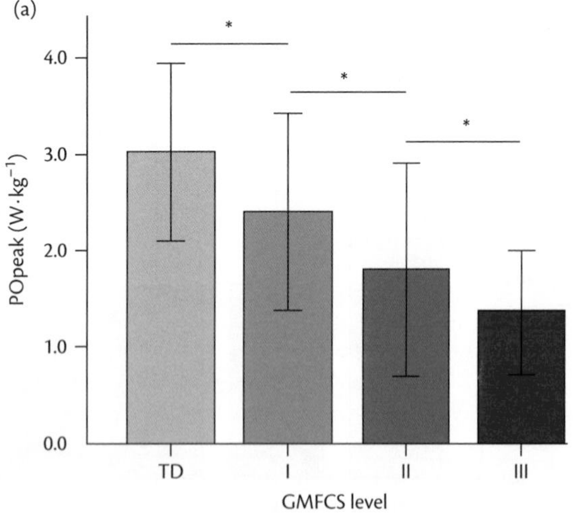

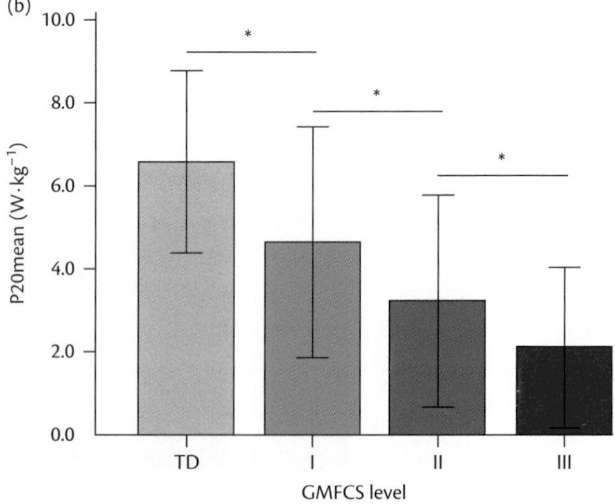

Figure 26.2 Peak aerobic power output and mean anaerobic power output in children with cerebral palsy and typically developing children.

POpeak (a) = peak aerobic power output, P20mean (b) = anaerobic power output.

CP = cerebral palsy, TD = typically developing children.

Balemans AC, Van Wely L, de Heer SJ, *et al.* Maximal aerobic and anaerobic exercise responses in children with cerebral palsy. Med Sci Sports Exerc. 2013; 45: 561–568.

Children classified at GMFCS level I and II have impaired anaerobic performance (measured with the MPST), as it is lower than that of their typically developing peers. This deficit increases with body height, especially in children classified at GMFCS level II.[35]

Muscle strength

Impairments of muscle function are prevalent characteristics in children with CP. As a result of the early damage to the motor pathways, primary impairments are spasticity, impaired motor control, and reduced muscle volume and force generating capacity. While the brain lesion is static, muscle impairments may increase over time, leading to further deterioration of muscle quality (i.e. decreased muscle volume, increased stiffness and intramuscular fat and collagen tissue).[24,36] Muscle strength is also limited by a reduced excitatory drive resulting in the inability to fully recruit all available motor units during maximal voluntary contractions.[37]

Strength testing in individuals with CP is limited by motor control problems. Increased co-activation reduces the net external joint torque, which is usually measured as a resultant of the force generation capacity of a specific muscle group. The increased activity of the antagonist muscle limits the effectiveness of the force application and thus the net joint torque, which may lead to an underestimation of the force generating capacity of the muscle itself.[38] Additionally, impaired selective motor control, i.e. the inability to execute single joint movements selectively, limits their capacity to generate effective joint torques. As these impairments increase with higher GMFCS levels (i.e. more severe disability) it is highly complicated, or even impossible, to evaluate muscle strength in children with GMFCS IV and V. As a consequence, little information is available about actual muscle strength levels of this group.

In children with GMFCS I-III isometric maximal muscle strength is most frequently measured using hand-held dynamometry. It has been shown that reliability of these tests is generally moderate to poor, depending on standardization of the testing procedure and experience of the assessor.[39] Reliability also varies between muscle groups and level of impairment.[40] Taking these limitations into account, valuable information regarding muscle strength can be obtained when multiple measurements are done (to reduce measurement error) or when results are interpreted on group level.[39]

Isokinetic dynamometers have been used to assess maximal dynamic strength and muscle endurance of merely the knee flexors and extensors over the whole range of motion. These laboratory tests showed also good reliability in children with CP (GMFCS I and II).[19]

There is ample evidence that muscle strength is reduced in walking children with CP when compared to age and gender-matched controls and strength levels decrease with larger motor involvement.[41–43] Isometric knee extensor strength of children GMFCS level I-III was reduced to 56–68% of age and gender-matched values in TD children. Knee flexor strength was reduced to 36–68%, hip abductors to 47–76%, hip flexors to 63–82%, and ankle plantar flexors to 37–57%.[41] In general, muscle weakness is reported to be more pronounced in the more distally located muscle groups, particularly the plantar flexors. Similar strength reductions were reported for maximal isokinetic muscle strength of the knee flexors and extensors (53% and 48% compared to controls respectively).[19] (The assessment and interpretation of muscle strength in healthy children is discussed in Chapter 7).

Walking economy

One of the consequences of the motor impairments and resulting gait deviations of children with CP is an increased energy demand of walking compared to TD children.[14,25] This reveals a low walking economy, or high energy cost, when expressing energy demands by covered distance (normalizing for speed). Although walking economy is not a fitness component, the combination of an increased energy expenditure during walking and a decreased aerobic fitness (i.e. peak $\dot{V}O_2$) leads to high physical strain levels during walking and daily life activities.[44] The high physical strain is suggested to be a cause of early fatigability in performing activities, which may limit their mobility and daily PA.[45] Fatigue in daily activities and reduced walking distance and duration are often reported complaints in this population.

Energy cost of walking can be determined reliably by measuring $\dot{V}O_2$ while children walk for 5–6 min at self-selected speed.[46] As expected, the energy cost of walking increases with more severe motor involvement in children with CP,[14,47]; energy cost can be up to three times higher in children with GMFCS level II or III when compared to TD children. Co-contraction accounted for up to 50% of the variability in $\dot{V}O_2$, suggesting that co-contraction is a major factor responsible for the higher energy cost of walking in children with CP. Also crouch gait, the flexed knee gait pattern that is often seen in CP, is suggested to be associated with increased energy cost.[48]

The physical strain, defined as the $\dot{V}O_2$ during walking expressed as a percentage of the maximal aerobic capacity (peak $\dot{V}O_2$), has been shown to be high in children with CP with GMFCS I (55%), II (62%), and III (78%), compared to 36% in TD children.[49] This leaves a smaller metabolic reserve, which is suggested to affect daily-life functioning and PA.[44] A significant relationship between the energy cost of walking and PA in 11 children with mild CP suggests that the high energy cost limits activity in daily life.[45] Consequently, the higher levels of physical strain while walking do not necessarily result in higher fitness levels, but, in contrast, may lead to physical inactivity and a concomitant deterioration in fitness level. The practical implementation of these findings is that health professionals should not only focus on treatments to improve walking economy, but should also consider training interventions to improve the maximal aerobic capacity.

Training effects

Aerobic training

Several training interventions have been developed to improve fitness in children with CP. Given the importance of cardiorespiratory fitness for health, the adaptive-response of this fitness component for children, adolescents, and adults with CP has been assessed over the years. Studies that evaluated the effects of aerobic and anaerobic training programmes on fitness outcomes are listed in Table 26.2. Exercise participation can be undertaken with a high level of safety by most people, including individuals with CP. Based on the safety issues for five randomized controlled trials that evaluated aerobic training in children with CP and reported no adverse events; there is a low risk of injury in children and adolescents with CP during

Table 26.2 Overview of randomized controlled studies evaluating aerobic and anaerobic training effects in children with cerebral palsy

	Participants	Frequency/duration	Intensity	Type	Outcome	Results
Aerobic training						
Van den Berg-Emons.[53]	N = 20 Age 7–13 years GMFCS I to IV (study predates GMFCS use)	2–4 times a week 9 months 45 min	70% HRR	–Cycling –Propelling wheelchair –Running –Swimming –Mat exercises	LAB: Peak power output during arm or cycle ergometer test Mean and peak power output of 30 s Wingate test	26% increase in peak power output No change on 30 s Wingate test
Unnithan *et al.*[51]	N = 13 Age 14–18 years GMFCS level II/III	Thrice weekly 12 weeks 20–22 min	65–75% HRmax	–Walking –Uphill walking	LAB: Peak $\dot{V}O_2$ during arm-ergometer test with gas analysis	18% increase in cardiorespiratory endurance (peak $\dot{V}O_2$)
Verschuren *et al.*[54]	N = 68 Age 7–20 years GMFCS level I/II	Twice a week 8 months 45 min	60–80% HRmax	Functional exercises: Running, steps-up and down, stepping over, bending, turning, getting up from the floor	FIELD: 10 m shuttle run test Mean power on Muscle Power Sprint Test (MPST)	41% increase on shuttle run test 27% increase on MPST
Nsenga *et al.*[50]	N = 20 Age 10–16 years GMFCS level I/II	Thrice weekly 8 weeks 40 min	50–65% peak $\dot{V}O_2$	–Cycling	LAB: Peak $\dot{V}O_2$ during cycle ergometer test with gas analysis	23% increase cardiorespiratory endurance (peak $\dot{V}O_2$)
Slaman *et al.*[52]	N = 42 Age 16–24 years GMFCS level I–IV	Twice a week 12 weeks 60 min	40–80% HRR	–Treadmill –Cycling –Arm cranking	LAB: Peak $\dot{V}O_2$ during cycle or arm-ergometer test with gas analysis	9% increase in cardiorespiratory endurance (peak $\dot{V}O_2$)
Anaerobic training						
Van Wely *et al.*[55]	N = 49 Age 7–12 years GMFCS level I/II/III	Once to twice a week 16 weeks 60 min	Maximal (no HR registered)	–Running –Slaloms	LAB: Peak $\dot{V}O_2$ during cycle-ergometer test with gas analysis Mean power output on 20 s Wingate Cycle test	No increase in cardiorespiratory endurance (peak $\dot{V}O_2$) and mean power output on the Wingate test
Verschuren *et al.*[54]	N = 68 Age 7–20 GMFCS level I/II	Twice a week 4 months 45 min	Maximal (no HR registered)	Functional exercises: Running, steps-up & down, stepping over, bending, turning, getting up from the floor	FIELD: 10 m shuttle run test Mean power on Muscle Power Sprint Test (MPST)	12% increase in aerobic performance 12% increase on MSPT

GMFCS: Gross Motor Function Classification System, HRR: heart rate reserve, HRmax: maximal heart rate.

aerobic training. The effectiveness of aerobic training was evaluated in these five studies, in which participants received exercise training versus placebo, or no intervention aimed at increasing aerobic fitness (see Table 26.2 for details).[50–54]

Three studies reported outcomes in peak $\dot{V}O_2$.[50–52] The other studies reported outcomes related to aerobic performance; power output measured with an arm cranking or cycle test,[53] and number of shuttles on the shuttle run test.[54] The reported increases in peak $\dot{V}O_2$ were 23% for an 8-week intervention with ambulant young people with CP (10–16 years),[50] 18% for a 3-month intervention with adolescents in GMFCS II and III (14–18 years)[51] and 9% for a 3-month intervention with adolescents/young adults (16–24 years) classified at GMFCS I-IV[52]. Performance measures increased with 41% on the SRT for an 8-month intervention with ambulant children (7–20 years)[54] and 26% on power output for a 9-month intervention in a mixed group of ambulant and wheelchair-using children (7–13 years).[53] Thus, according to these studies, one can conclude that cardiorespiratory training can effectively increase cardiorespiratory fitness and aerobic performance in children and young adults with CP. In these studies the participants exercised at least two to four times per week for a minimum of 20 min, and at a moderate intensity of about

60–75% of maximum HR, 40–80% of HR reserve, or 50–65% peak $\dot{V}O_2$.

Taken together, these results suggest that greater gains in cardiorespiratory fitness may occur with training programmes of longer duration and for children and adults with CP that have greater mobility and can engage in greater doses of training. (Interested readers are referred to Chapter 34 where the aerobic trainability of healthy young people is discussed).

Anaerobic training

An 8-month combined aerobic and anaerobic training programme in 68 ambulant children and adolescents with CP showed that the anaerobic power, evaluated with the MPST, was significantly increased by 12% during the second 4 months.[54] During these months the main focus of the training was on anaerobic performance, with functional exercises like sprinting, stepping, and turning. These findings suggest that anaerobic performance, measured as sprinting ability, is trainable in ambulant children/adolescents with CP.

Whether anaerobic power, measured with the WAnT, can be trained in children with CP is equivocal. There were no improvements found after a combined anaerobic-strength training focused on walking activities in 6- to 12-year-old children with CP.[55] A 9 month aerobic cycle training programme in 6- to 12-year-old children with spastic CP showed also no improvements in anaerobic power.[53] Lack of training effects in these studies could be explained by the non-specific test mode (walking vs. cycling) of the WAnT, the focus on aerobic[53] or strength training,[56] and low training frequency.[55] It is not determined yet whether the improvements in anaerobic performance on the MPST relate to increased anaerobic fitness or improved running skills.

Strength training

Previously, neurological treatment methods discouraged strength training because of a hypothesized aggravating effect on spasticity. However, over the last decades a number of studies showed that muscle strength can be improved by systematic strength training in children and adolescents with CP without any adverse effects such as increased spasticity.[57,58] Results of randomized-controlled studies are listed in Table 26.3. Data show that muscle strength can be improved in ambulant children, with effects ranging from 11–27%, varying among muscle groups and populations.[56,58–60] A home-based strength training programme in 21 children and adolescents with CP (8–18 years) reported significant improvement in combined measures of plantar flexor and knee extensor strength of 15%, but no effects on individual muscle groups.[58] A larger study of 51 children (6–13 years) showed improvements in knee extensors and hip abductors, and total strength ranging from 11–14%.[56]

Table 26.3 Overview of randomized control trials studying strength training effects in children with cerebral palsy

	Participants	Frequency/ duration	Intensity	Type	Outcome	Results
Dodd *et al.*[58]	N = 21 Age 8–18 GMFCS I/II/III	Thrice weekly 6 weeks	Three sets of 8–12 repetitions to fatigue	Multi-joint exercises (heel raises, half squats and step-ups)	Muscle strength: HHD ankle plantar flexors, knee extensors, hip extensors Other: mobility capacity	Significant increase combined strength of knee extensors and plantar flexors (15%)
Liao *et al.*[59]	N = 20 Age 5–12 GMFCS I/II	Thrice weekly 6 weeks	One set of ten repetitions at 20% 1RM One set of repetitions until fatigue at 50% 1RM One set of ten repetitions at 20% 1RM	Multi-joint exercises (sit-to-stand) loaded (using weight vest)	Muscle strength: HHD knee extensors, 1RM sit-to-stand Other: mobility capacity, gait speed	No effect on HHD, significant increase in 1RM sit-to-stand Sign increase in mobility capacity, no effect on gait speed
Scholtes *et al.*[56]	N = 51 Age 6–13 years GMFCS level I/II/III	Thrice weekly 12 weeks	Three sets of eight RM	Multi-joint exercises (leg press) and loaded functional exercises (using a weight vest)	Muscle strength: HHD multiple leg muscle groups, 6RM leg press Other: mobility capacity, gait	Significant increase in knee extensors (12%), hip abductors (11%), total HHD strength (8%), 6RM leg press (14%) No effects on mobility capacity and gait
Taylor *et al.*[60]	N = 48 Age 14–22 GMFCS level II/III	Twice a week 12 weeks	Three sets of 10–12 repetitions	Weight machines	Muscle strength HHD multiple leg muscle groups Other: mobility capacity, gait	Significant increase in strength (27%) of targeted muscle groups No effects on mobility capacity and gait

GMFCS = Gross Motor Function Classification System; HHD: hand-held dynamometry; PRE = Progressive Resistance Exercise; RM = repetition maximum.

Greater strength gains were reported in targeted muscles (27%) in 48 adolescents with CP (14–22 years) who received an individualized training programme to improve gait.[60] A recent meta-analysis combined data from both randomized and non-randomized studies.[61] They concluded that the effect sizes of most individual muscles were large, though insignificant for plantar flexors and hip muscles, and moderate to large for activities and gait variables. Despite these improvements in muscle strength, most programmes have proven less effective than expected, or sometimes not effective at all, for improving functional outcomes such as walking ability and other daily activities.[56,58,60] (Interested readers are referred to Chapter 35 for a discussion of resistance training with healthy children).

Physical activity

Physical activity in cerebral palsy

For all individuals, regular participation in PA and exercise benefits fitness, health, and participation in daily activities with peers. In children and adolescents with CP, fitness is lower than in TD peers and they are less active over the day.[62,63] Physical activity studies in CP showed that ambulant children with CP (GMFCS I-III) spend 73–82% of their waking hours being sedentary. They were engaged in light activities for 12–20%, and only 4–10% in moderate-to-vigorous activities (MVPA)[63–66], compared to 39% (sedentary time), 38% (light activities), and 29% (MVPA) in TD children.[63] Non-ambulant children spent as much as 97–99% of their waking hours sedentary, while they spent no time at MVPA.[64] The health effects in the long term are not yet completely understood, but the first results show detrimental effects on chronic conditions, such as cardiovascular conditions, diabetes, and arthritis in adults with CP.[67] The PA pattern across the whole activity continuum is therefore extremely important for youth with CP.

Describing the amount of activities needed to maintain and foster health is complicated. The dose-response relationship between volume of moderate- and vigorous-intensity aerobic activities and all-cause mortality is non-linear, with the most rapid reduction in risk occurring at the smallest increment of activity volume among the most sedentary individuals. Thus, for people who participate in high volumes of sedentary behaviour and who are also completely inactive (e.g. most people with CP), even small increases in the volume of PA may lead to profound health gains.

In general, youth with CP should strive to meet the public health recommendations for daily participation in MVPA, it should be developmentally appropriate and enjoyable, and it should involve a variety of activities (Table 26.4). However, for a subset of the CP population with excessive frailty, deconditioning, and/or mobility restriction, it is virtually impossible to meet the optimal recommendations of 60 min of daily MVPA.

Table 26.4 Recommendations for daily physical activity

Daily physical activity	Recommendations
Physical activity (moderate to vigorous)	
Frequency	≥ 5 days · week^{-1}
Intensity	Moderate-to-vigorous physical activity
Time	60 min
Type	A variety of activities
Physical activity (sedentary)	
Frequency	7 days · week^{-1}
Intensity	Sedentary (<1.5 METs)
Time	<2 h day or break up sitting for 2 min every 30–60 min
Type	Non-occupational, leisure-time sedentary activities such as watching television, using a computer, and/or playing video games

Sedentary behaviour

Although it is well established that PA is important for health, emerging evidence suggests that this is only part of the story. More recently, studies have shown that a large amount of sedentary behaviour, defined as any waking behaviour characterized by an energy expenditure ≤ 1.5 METs while in a sitting or reclining posture, is distinct from a lack of MVPA.[68] Sedentary behaviour is also associated with an increased risk of coronary heart disease, hypertension, diabetes, obesity, mortality, and some cancers in persons with a typical development.[69,70] Combining the findings from recent studies that have looked objectively at the PA level of children and adolescents with CP[63–66] show us that children and adults with CP spend 73–99% of their waking hours sedentary. Not only the total amount, but maybe even more problematic are prolonged periods of sedentary time with few breaks.[66,71] One study shows increased health risks which associate with sedentary behaviour in adults with CP,[72] but the emerging evidence in TD people indicates a need for interventions breaking up sedentary time. This is a promising intervention strategy as this may be more feasible for persons with mobility limitations.

Emphasizing increases in MVPA *and* replacing sedentary behaviour with light PA may therefore be beneficial for health in children and adolescents with CP. Focusing on the non-exercise segment of the activity continuum involves interventions to promote breaks in sedentary time, and replacement with light-intensity activities. A recent study[73] showed that by transitioning from seated to a standing position may contribute to the accumulation of light activity and reduce sedentary behaviour among children with CP.

Too much time spent in sedentary behaviour, especially when accrued in long, continuous bouts, is detrimental to cardiometabolic health.[69,71] Thus, specific interventions aimed at reducing sedentary behaviour in people with CP should be considered as a promising initial target to prevent cardiovascular complications. Indeed, evidence in the general population suggests that frequently interrupting sedentary time may have beneficial effects on metabolic health and haemostasis,[71] indicating that both the amount and patterns of sedentary behaviour contribute to changes in health. Encouraging people with CP to replace sedentary time with baseline activities is sensible, and although this is likely applicable for all children with CP, it is especially relevant for children classified in GMFCS levels IV and V, as reducing sedentary behaviour might be the only viable intervention.

Training recommendations

Aerobic training

To be able to develop universally accepted exercise prescription guidelines for children and adults with CP, a well-accepted framework of prescription nomenclature to operationalize the exercise variables from published randomized controlled studies in this population was used, including i) frequency, ii) intensity, iii) time, and iv) type (see Table 26.2). The extent to which recent training intervention studies were consistent with current recommendations related to cardiorespiratory (aerobic) exercise as provided by the American College of Sports Medicine (ACSM) has been evaluated.[10] Briefly, these guidelines recommend a frequency of 5 days $\cdot$ week^{-1} of moderate intensity exercise or 3 days $\cdot$ week^{-1} of vigorous intensity exercise. For deconditioned persons, the recommendation is to include light- to moderate-intensity exercise, and moderate- and vigorous-intensity exercise. The recommendation is 30–60 min $\cdot$ day^{-1} of purposeful moderate exercise, or 20–60 min $\cdot$ day^{-1} of vigorous intensity exercise, with regular, purposeful exercises that involve major muscle groups and is continuous and rhythmic in nature.

Frequency

All five studies on aerobic training[50–54] incorporated a training frequency of two to four sessions per week. From previous studies pertaining to CP, only two of the studies[50,51] were aligned with the ACSM guidelines for typically developing individuals that recommend at least three to five sessions per week. Interestingly, for the remaining studies in which frequency did not meet minimal recommendations, results demonstrated that training was still effective in increasing the cardiorespiratory fitness.[52–54] This may suggest that for persons with CP who are very deconditioned, it is possible and advisable to start with one to two sessions per week and progress gradually thereafter, as adaptations occur.

Intensity

Intensity refers to the effort of training (i.e. relative to maximal capacity), and is frequently prescribed relative to predicted maximal HR, heart rate reserve (HRR) (i.e. the difference between a person's measured or predicted maximum HR and resting HR), and/or peak $\dot{V}O_2$ (i.e. peak rate of $\dot{V}O_2$ as measured during incremental exercise). Although many factors need to be considered when evaluating these studies and respective findings (e.g. functional capacity of the participants), it is important to point out that intensity of training in each of these five studies was aligned with current ACSM guidelines. This suggests that many individuals with CP are capable to train at these intensities and benefit in fitness improvement of engaging in progressively intense aerobic exercise, similar to the extent recommended for TD peers.

Time

All training session had a duration of at least 20 min, which is aligned with the ACSM guidelines.

Type

For cardiorespiratory fitness, the ACSM recommends regular, purposeful exercise that involves major muscle groups and is continuous and rhythmic in nature. The types of activities provided in the five studies included running, step-ups, negotiating stairs, cycling, arm ergometry exercise, propelling a wheelchair, and swimming, and all were tailored to the specific condition of the included participants.

According to the existing intervention studies, exercise prescription focusing on aerobic capacity for children with CP should include: i) a minimum frequency of two to three times per week; ii) an intensity between 60–95% of peak HR, or between 40–80% of the HRR, or between 50–65% of peak $\dot{V}O_2$, and iii) a minimum time of 20 min per session, for at least eight consecutive weeks, when training three times a week, or for 16 consecutive weeks when training two times a week. Moreover, a pre-workout warm-up and cool-down could be added to reduce musculoskeletal injury and complications.

Anaerobic training

A fitness training programme predominantly anaerobic in nature is able to improve the anaerobic performance, measured with the MPST, in children with CP (see Table 26.2).[54]

Frequency

Prescription of anaerobic training for children with CP should include a 'familiarization' period, in which very low dosage training (i.e. minimal volume and intensity) occurs twice a week for at least 2 weeks.

Intensity

Training intensity for anaerobic training is at maximal intensity.

Time

Most children with CP are not used to strenuous exercise and they may need time to adapt to this maximal level of activity. Therefore, a few weeks of anaerobic training familiarization simply to reach the recommended training intensity is recommended. Longer interventions (e.g. 12–16 weeks) may be needed to experience significant or meaningful improvements in anaerobic performance. The duration of the anaerobic exercises are 20–30 s, with an activity to rest ratio of 1:3 to 1:5.

Type

The type of exercises need to be simple and require a minimal amount of motor skill, since this will interfere with the maximal intensity needed for a successful training intensity.

According to the existing intervention studies, exercise prescription focusing on anaerobic performance for children with CP should include: i) a minimum frequency of two times per week; ii) training at maximal intensity, and iii) a minimum time of 20 min per session, for at least 12 consecutive weeks.

Muscle strength training

The health benefits of enhancing muscular fitness have become well established in the general population. Higher levels of muscular strength are associated with significantly better cardiometabolic risk factor profiles,[74] lower risk of all-cause mortality, fewer cardiovascular disease events,[75] and lower risk of developing functional limitations. As CP results from an injury to motor regions of the developing brain, muscle weakness is a primary impairment, and there is strong evidence that children with CP are significantly weaker than typically developing children.[41–43]

Frequency

As is generally accepted for any novice trainee, prescription of resistance exercise for persons with CP should include a 'familiarization' period, in which very low dosage training (i.e. minimal volume and intensity) occurs twice a week for at least 2–4 weeks.

Intensity

One to four sets of 6–15 repetitions and gradual progression to meet the demands of improved muscular fitness are recommended.

Training intensity may be modified based on a targeted number of repetitions, or by increasing loading within a prescribed repetition-maximum range (e.g. 8–12 repetition maximum [RM]).[10] Because it is often challenging or unsafe to ascertain a true 1RM among individuals with CP, using the latter RM method to assign intensity is the most feasible, safe, and effective strategy.

Time

Most people with CP are not used to strenuous exercise and they may need time to adapt to this level of activity. Therefore, a few weeks of strength training familiarization simply to reach the recommended training volumes and intensities are recommended. Longer interventions with progressive intensities (e.g. 12–16 weeks) may be needed to experience significant or meaningful improvements in strength. Importantly, and as with cardiorespiratory endurance, greater doses of resistance exercise are required to improve muscle strength than is needed to maintain these improvements.[10]

Type of exercises

All three randomized controlled studies in children with CP[56,58,59] used multi-joint exercises (e.g. lateral step-ups, squatting) rather than single joint exercises (e.g. knee extension). However, single-joint resistance training may be more effective for very weak individuals, particularly at the beginning phases of training, as well as for children who tend to compensate when performing bilateral, multi-joint exercises.

According to the existing evidence exercise prescription focusing on muscle strength for children with CP should include: i) a minimum frequency of two times per week on non-consecutive days; ii) one to three sets of 6–15 repetitions, and gradually progress to meet the demands of improved muscular fitness, and; iii) a programme that lasts sufficiently long. Assuming a minimum of 8 weeks to experience changes in strength with simple activities, it is suggested that the duration of a programme is at least 12–16 weeks in order to maximize the likelihood of a training effect in people with CP.[76]

Conclusions

The low aerobic and anaerobic fitness levels of children with CP, as well as their extended muscle weakness, warrants specialized testing and training programmes for this vulnerable population. To maintain health and functional ability, comprehensive training and activity programmes are needed that are of sufficient frequency, intensity, and duration and focus on reducing sedentary behaviour, increasing PA and maintaining the balance between capacity and strain in daily activities.

Summary

- Children with cerebral palsy (CP) have major motor impairments that lead to reduced fitness and physical activity (PA) levels.
- Exercise tests need to be selected based on the physical ability of the child with CP and the goal of the assessment.
- Adapted laboratory and field tests to assess fitness with acceptable reliability and validity have been described for both ambulant and wheelchair-using children.
- Aerobic fitness is reduced when compared to typically developing children and is modifiable by (an)aerobic training.
- Anaerobic fitness is strongly reduced, depending on the level of the motor impairment, and anaerobic training can improve anaerobic (sprinting) performance.
- As CP results from an injury to the motor pathways, muscle weakness is an important impairment that can be improved by targeted strength training.
- Increased energy cost of walking in combination with reduced aerobic fitness induces high levels of physical strain that can lead to fatigue complaints and limited PA.
- Physical activity is low in children with CP and depends largely on the level of motor impairment.
- Low PA levels are believed to exaggerate deconditioning and muscle weakness that are present due the primary motor impairments.
- Sedentary time is higher in children with CP, especially in those using a wheelchair, emphasizing the need for reducing sedentary time.
- Reducing sedentary time and increasing PA are important to counteract the increased risk for health problems in adulthood in this population.
- Fitness training of sufficient frequency, intensity, and duration is recommended, or even required, to maintain and optimize health and functional ability in children with CP.

References

1. Damiano DL. Activity, activity, activity: rethinking our physical therapy approach to cerebral palsy. *Phys Ther.* 2006; 86: 1534–1540.
2. Fowler EG, Kolobe TH, Damiano DL, *et al.* Promotion of physical fitness and prevention of secondary conditions for children with cerebral palsy: section on pediatrics research summit proceedings. *Phys Ther.* 2007; 87: 1495–1510.
3. Maltais DB, Wiart L, Fowler E, Verschuren O, Damiano DL. Health-related physical fitness for children with cerebral palsy. *J Child Neurol.* 2014; 29: 1091–1100.
4. Oskoui M, Coutinho F, Dykeman J, Jette N, Pringsheim T. An update on the prevalence of cerebral palsy: a systematic review and meta-analysis. *Dev Med Child Neurol.* 2013; 55: 509–519.
5. Bax M, Goldstein M, Rosenbaum P, *et al.* Proposed definition and classification of cerebral palsy. *Dev Med Child Neurol.* 2005; 47: 571–576.
6. Palisano R, Rosenbaum P, Walter S, Russell D, Wood E, Galuppi B. Development and reliability of a system to classify gross motor function in children with cerebral palsy. *Dev Med Child Neurol.* 1997; 39: 214–223.
7. Balemans AC, Fragala-Pinkham MA, Lennon N, *et al.* Systematic review of the clinimetric properties of laboratory- and field-based aerobic and anaerobic fitness measures in children with cerebral palsy. *Arch Phys Med Rehab.* 2013; 94: 287–301.
8. Verschuren O, Balemans ACJ. Update of the core set of exercise tests for children and adolescents with cerebral palsy. *Pediatr Phys Ther.* 2015; 27: 187–189.
9. Verschuren O, Ketelaar M, Keefer D, *et al.* Identification of a core set of exercise tests for children and adolescents with cerebral palsy: a Delphi survey of researchers and clinicians. *Dev Med Child Neurol.* 2011; 53: 449–456.
10. Garber CE, Blissmer B, Deschenes MR, *et al.* American College of Sports Medicine position stand. Quantity and quality of exercise for developing and maintaining cardiorespiratory, musculoskeletal,

and neuromotor fitness in apparently healthy adults: guidance for prescribing exercise. *Med Sci Sports Exerc*. 2011; 43: 1334–1359.
11. Wasserman K, Hansen JE, Sue DY, Stringer WW, Whipp BJ. *Measurements during integrative cardiopulmonary exercise testing: Principles of exercise testing and interpretation,* 4th ed. Philadelphia: Lippincott Williams & Wilkins; 2005.
12. Verschuren O, Takken T. Aerobic capacity in children and adolescents with cerebral palsy. *Res Dev Disabil*. 2010; 31: 1352–1357.
13. Brehm MA, Balemans AC, Becher JG, Dallmeijer AJ. Reliability of a progressive maximal cycle ergometer test to assess peak oxygen uptake in children with mild to moderate cerebral palsy. *Phys Ther*. 2014; 94: 121–128.
14. Kamp FA, Lennon N, Holmes L, Dallmeijer AJ, Henley J, Miller F. Energy cost of walking in children with spastic cerebral palsy: relationship with age, body composition and mobility capacity. *Gait Posture*. 2014; 40: 209–214.
15. Balemans AC, Van Wely L, de Heer SJ, *et al*. Maximal aerobic and anaerobic exercise responses in children with cerebral palsy. *Med Sci Sports Exerc*. 2013; 45: 561–568.
16. Balemans AC, Van Wely L, Becher JG, Dallmeijer AJ. Longitudinal relationship among physical fitness, walking-related physical aactivity, and fatigue in children with cerebral palsy. *Phys Ther*. 2015; 95: 996–1005.
17. Bar-Or O. Role of exercise in the assessment and management of neuromuscular disease in children. *Med Sci Sports Exerc*. 1996; 28: 421–427.
18. Parker DF, Carriere L, Hebestreit H, Bar-Or O. Anaerobic endurance and peak muscle power in children with spastic cerebral palsy. *Am J Dis Child*. 1992; 146: 1069–1073.
19. van den Berg-Emons RJ, van Baak MA, de Barbanson DC, Speth L, Saris WH. Reliability of tests to determine peak aerobic power, anaerobic power and isokinetic muscle strength in children with spastic cerebral palsy. *Dev Med Child Neurol*. 1996; 38: 1117–1125.
20. Dallmeijer AJ, Scholtes VA, Brehm MA, Becher JG. Test-retest reliability of the 20-sec Wingate test to assess anaerobic power in children with cerebral palsy. *Am J Phys Med Rehabil*. 2013; 92: 762–767.
21. Chia M, Armstrong N, Childs D. The assessment of children's anaerobic performance using modifications of the Wingate Anaerobic test. *Pediatr Exerc Sci*. 1997; 9: 80–89.
22. Verschuren O, Zwinkels M, Obeid J, Kerkhof N, Ketelaar M, Takken T. Reliability and validity of short-term performance tests for wheelchair-using children and adolescents with cerebral palsy. *Dev Med Child Neurol*. 2013; 55: 1129–1135.
23. Noble J, Fry N, Lewis A, Keevil S, Gough M, Shortland A. Lower limb muscle volumes in bilateral spastic cerebral palsy. *Brain Dev*. 2014; 36: 294–300.
24. Mathewson MA, Lieber RL. Pathophysiology of muscle contractures in cerebral palsy. *Phys Med Rehabil Clin N Am*. 2015; 26: 57–67.
25. Unnithan VB, Dowling JJ, Frost G, Bar-Or O. Role of cocontraction in the O_2 cost of walking in children with cerebral palsy. *Med Sci Sports Exerc*. 1996; 28: 1498–1504.
26. Moreau NG, Falvo MJ, Damiano DL. Rapid force generation is impaired in cerebral palsy and is related to decreased muscle size and functional mobility. *Gait Posture*. 2012; 35: 154–158.
27. Verschuren O, Takken T, Ketelaar M, Gorter JW, Helders PJ. Reliability and validity of data for 2 newly developed shuttle run tests in children with cerebral palsy. *Phys Ther*. 2006; 86: 1107–1117.
28. Verschuren O, Takken T, Ketelaar M, Gorter JW, Helders PJ. Reliability for running tests for measuring agility and anaerobic muscle power in children and adolescents with cerebral palsy. *Pediatr Phys Ther*. 2007; 19: 108–115.
29. Verschuren O, Bongers BC, Obeid J, Ruyten T, Takken T. Validity of the muscle power sprint test in ambulatory youth with cerebral palsy. *Pediatr Phys Ther*. 2013; 25: 25–28.
30. Verschuren O, Bosma L, Takken T. Reliability of a shuttle run test for children with cerebral palsy who are classified at Gross Motor Function Classification System level III. *Dev Med Child Neurol*. 2011; 53: 470–472.
31. Verschuren O, Zwinkels M, Ketelaar M, Reijnder-van Son F, Takken T. Reproducibility and validity of the 10-meter shuttle ride test in wheelchair-bound children and adolescents with cerebral palsy. *Phys Ther*. 2013; 93: 967–974.
32. Verschuren O, Bloemen M, Kruitwagen C, Takken T. Reference values for aerobic fitness in children, adolescents, and young adults who have cerebral palsy and are ambulatory. *Phys Ther*. 2010; 90: 1148–1156.
33. Verschuren O, Bloemen M, Kruitwagen CAS, Takken T. Reference values for anaerobic performance and agility in ambulatory children and adolescents with cerebral palsy. *Dev Med Child Neurol*. 2010; 52: e222–e228.
34. Balemans ACJ, Van Wely L, Blonk J, Becher JG, Dallmeijer AJ. Comparing maximal cardiopulmonary exercise test and shuttle run test outcomes in children with cerebral palsy. *Dev Med Child Neurol*. 2015; 57(Suppl 5): 26–27.
35. Verschuren O, Maltais DB, Douma-van RD, Kruitwagen C, Ketelaar M. Anaerobic performance in children with cerebral palsy compared to children with typical development. *Pediatr Phys Ther*. 2013; 25: 409–413.
36. Barrett RS, Lichtwark GA. Gross muscle morphology and structure in spastic cerebral palsy: a systematic review. *Dev Med Child Neurol*. 2010; 52: 794–804.
37. Stackhouse SK, Binder-Macleod SA, Lee SC. Voluntary muscle activation, contractile properties, and fatigability in children with and without cerebral palsy. *Muscle Nerve*. 2005; 31: 594–601.
38. Hussain AW, Onambele GL, Williams AG, Morse CI. Muscle size, activation, and coactivation in adults with cerebral palsy. *Muscle Nerve*. 2014; 49: 76–83.
39. Willemse L, Brehm MA, Scholtes VA, Jansen L, Woudenberg-Vos H, Dallmeijer AJ. Reliability of isometric lower-extremity muscle strength measurements in children with cerebral palsy: implications for measurement design. *Phys Ther*. 2013; 93: 935–941.
40. Mulder-Brouwer AN, Rameckers EA, Bastiaenen CH. Lower extremity handheld dynamometry strength measurement in children with cerebral palsy. *Pediatr Phys Ther*. 2016; 28: 136–53.
41. Dallmeijer AJ, Rameckers EA, Houdijk H, de Groot S, Scholtes VA, Becher JG. Isometric muscle strength and mobility capacity in children with cerebral palsy. *Disabil Rehabil*. 2017; 39: 135–142.
42. Wiley ME, Damiano DL. Lower-extremity strength profiles in spastic cerebral palsy. *Dev Med Child Neurol*. 1998; 40: 100–107.
43. Eek MN, Tranberg R, Beckung E. Muscle strength and kinetic gait pattern in children with bilateral spastic CP. *Gait Posture*. 2011; 33: 333–337.
44. Dallmeijer AJ, Brehm MA. Physical strain of comfortable walking in children with mild cerebral palsy. *Disabil Rehabil*. 2011; 33: 1351–1357.
45. Maltais DB, Pierrynowski MR, Galea VA, Bar-Or O. Physical activity level is associated with the O_2 cost of walking in cerebral palsy. *Med Sci Sports Exerc*. 2005; 37: 347–353.
46. Brehm MA, Becher J, Harlaar J. Reproducibility evaluation of gross and net walking efficiency in children with cerebral palsy. *Dev Med Child Neurol*. 2007; 49: 45–48.
47. Johnston TE, Moore SE, Quinn LT, Smith BT. Energy cost of walking in children with cerebral palsy: relation to the Gross Motor Function Classification System. *Dev Med Child Neurol*. 2004; 46: 34–38.
48. Unnithan VB, Clifford C, Bar-Or O. Evaluation by exercise testing of the child with cerebral palsy. *Sports Med*. 1998; 26: 239–251.
49. Balemans ACJ, Bolster E, Bakels J, Blauw R, Becher JG, Dallmeijer AJ. Physical strain of walking in cerebral palsy. *Dev Med Child Neurol*. 2015; 57(Suppl 5): 65–66.
50. Nsenga AL, Shephard RJ, Ahmaidi S. Aerobic training in children with cerebral palsy. *Int J Sports Med*. 2013; 34: 533–537.
51. Unnithan VB, Katsimanis G, Evangelinou C, Kosmas C, Kandrali I, Kellis E. Effect of strength and aerobic training in children with cerebral palsy. *Med Sci Sports Exerc*. 2007; 39: 1902–1909.
52. Slaman J, Roebroeck M, Dallmeijer A, Twisk J, Stam H, van den Berg-Emons R. Can a lifestyle intervention programme improve physical behaviour

among adolescents and young adults with spastic cerebral palsy? A randomized controlled trial. *Dev Med Child Neurol.* 2015; 57: 159–166.
53. van den Berg-Emons RJ, van Baak MA, Speth L, Saris WH. Physical training of school children with spastic cerebral palsy: effects on daily activity, fat mass and fitness. *Int J Rehabil Res.* 1998; 21: 179–194.
54. Verschuren O, Ketelaar M, Gorter JW, Helders PJ, Uiterwaal CS, Takken T. Exercise training program in children and adolescents with cerebral palsy: a randomized controlled trial. *Arch Pediatr Adolesc Med.* 2007; 161: 1075–1081.
55. Van Wely L, Balemans AC, Becher JG, Dallmeijer AJ. Physical activity stimulation program for children with cerebral palsy did not improve physical activity: a randomised trial. *J Physiother.* 2014; 60: 40–49.
56. Scholtes VA, Becher JG, Comuth A, Dekkers H, Van Dijk L, Dallmeijer AJ. Effectiveness of functional progressive resistance exercise strength training on muscle strength and mobility in children with cerebral palsy: a randomized controlled trial. *Dev Med Child Neurol.* 2010; 52: e107–e113.
57. Damiano DL, Vaughan CL, Abel MF. Muscle response to heavy resistance exercise in children with spastic cerebral palsy. *Dev Med Child Neurol.* 1995; 37: 731–739.
58. Dodd KJ, Taylor NF, Graham HK. A randomized clinical trial of strength training in young people with cerebral palsy. *Dev Med Child Neurol.* 2003; 45: 652–657.
59. Liao HF, Liu YC, Liu WY, Lin YT. Effectiveness of loaded sit-to-stand resistance exercise for children with mild spastic diplegia: a randomized clinical trial. *Arch Phys Med Rehabil.* 2007; 88: 25–31.
60. Taylor NF, Dodd KJ, Baker RJ, Willoughby K, Thomason P, Graham HK. Progressive resistance training and mobility-related function in young people with cerebral palsy: a randomized controlled trial. *Dev Med Child Neurol.* 2013; 55: 806–812.
61. Park EY, Kim WH. Meta-analysis of the effect of strengthening interventions in individuals with cerebral palsy. *Res Dev Disabil.* 2014; 35: 239–249.
62. Van Wely L, Dallmeijer AJ, Balemans AC, Zhou C, Becher JG, Bjornson KF. Walking activity of children with cerebral palsy and children developing typically: a comparison between the Netherlands and the United States. *Disabil Rehabil.* 2014; 36: 2136–2142.
63. Balemans ACJ, Van Wely L, Middelweerd A, van den Noort JC, Becher JG, Dallmeijer AJ. Daily stride rate activity and heart rate response in children with cerebral palsy. *J Rehabil Med.* 2014; 46: 45–50.
64. Shkedy Rabani A, Harries N, Namoora I, Al-Jarrah M, Karniel A, Bar-Haim S. Duration and patterns of habitual physical activity in adolescents and young adults with cerebral palsy. *Dev Med Child Neurol.* 2014; 56: 673–680.
65. Nooijen C, Slaman J, Stam H, Roebroeck M, van den Berg-Emons R. Inactive and sedentary lifestyles amongst ambulatory adolescents and young adults with cerebral palsy. *J Neuroeng Rehabil.* 2014; 11: 49.
66. Obeid J, Balemans A, Noorduyn S, Gorter J, Timmons B. Objectively measured sedentary time in youth with cerebral palsy compared with age-, sex-, and season-matched youth who are developing typically: An explorative. *Phys Ther.* 2014; 94: 1163–1167.
67. Peterson MD, Ryan JM, Hurvitz EA, Mahmoudi E. Chronic conditions in adults with cerebral palsy. *JAMA.* 2015; 314: 2303–2305.
68. Gibbs BB, Hergenroeder AL, Katzmarzyk PT, Lee IM, Jakicic JM. Definition, measurement, and health risks associated with sedentary behavior. *Med Sci Sports Exerc.* 2015; 47: 1295–1300.
69. Katzmarzyk PT, Church TS, Craig CL, Bouchard C. Sitting time and mortality from all causes, cardiovascular disease, and cancer. *Med Sci Sports Exerc.* 2009; 41: 998–1005.
70. van der Ploeg HP, Chey T, Korda RJ, Banks E, Bauman A. Sitting time and all-cause mortality risk in 222 497 Australian adults. *Arch Intern Med.* 2012; 172: 494–500.
71. Healy GN, Dunstan DW, Salmon J, *et al.* Breaks in sedentary time: beneficial associations with metabolic risk. *Diabetes Care.* 2008; 31: 661–666.
72. Ryan JM, Hensey O, McLoughlin B, Lyons A, Gormley J. Reduced moderate-to-vigorous physical activity and increased sedentary behavior is associated with elevated blood pressure values in children with cerebral palsy. *Phys Ther.* 2014; 94: 1144–1153.
73. Verschuren O, Peterson MD, Leferink S, Darrah J. Muscle activation and energy-requirements for varying postures in children and adolescents with cerebral palsy. *J Pediatr.* 2014; 165: 1011–1016.
74. Jurca R, Lamonte MJ, Barlow CE, Kampert JB, Church TS, Blair SN. Association of muscular strength with incidence of metabolic syndrome in men. *Med Sci Sports Exerc.* 2005; 37: 1849–1855.
75. Gale CR, Martyn CN, Cooper C, Sayer AA. Grip strength, body composition, and mortality. *Int J Epidemiol.* 2007; 36: 228–235.
76. Verschuren O, Peterson MD, Balemans ACJ, Hurvitz EA. Exercise and physical activity recommendations for people with cerebral palsy. *Dev Med Child Neurol.* 2016; 58: 798–808.

CHAPTER 27

Exercise, physical activity, and cystic fibrosis

Susi Kriemler, Thomas Radtke, and Helge Hebestreit

Introduction

Cystic fibrosis (CF) is the most common genetic autosomal recessive disease of the Caucasian race, generally leading to death in early to mid-adulthood.[1] However, overall survival has markedly improved over the last decades for all individuals with CF, including those with poor lung function.[2] The frequency of the gene carrier (heterozygote) is 1:20–25 in Caucasian populations, 1:2000 in African-Americans, and very rare in Asian populations. The disease occurs in about 1 in every 2500 live births of the white population. The genetic defect causes a pathological electrolyte transport through the cell membranes by a defective chloride channel membrane transport protein (Cystic Fibrosis Transmembrane Conductance Regulator, or CFTR).[3] Functionally, this affects mainly the exocrine glands of secretory cells, sinuses, lungs, pancreas, liver, and the reproductive tract of the human body, leading to an impaired transepithelial fluid transport and resulting in impairments in the transport of secretions, ultimately leading to inflammation and destruction of affected organs. Transepithelial chloride transport may further be relevant for calcium release from sarcoplasmic reticulum in muscles that may alter muscle function.[4–6] The main symptoms of CF include chronic inflammatory pulmonary disease with a progressive loss of lung function, exocrine and sometimes endocrine pancreas insufficiency, and an excessive salt loss through the sweat glands.[1] A summary of the signs and symptoms of CF will be given with a special emphasis on the effect of exercise capacity and physical activity (PA).

Cystic fibrosis-related pathologies and exercise tolerance

General

Exercise tolerance in the child and adolescent with CF shows a wide variation. Some individuals with CF perform marathons or triathlons and others are hardly able to walk for a few minutes. Peak oxygen uptake ($\dot{V}O_2$) is usually reduced in children with CF even in those with mild pulmonary involvement.[7–12] The limitations in exercise performance aggravate with progression of the disease, for which some potential factors can be responsible. They are summarized in Figure 27.1.

In CF aerobic exercise capacity correlates significantly with resting pulmonary function.[13–16] As there are several confounders to this plausible relationship, the predictability of aerobic fitness based on resting pulmonary function for an individual is much lower due to other factors, such as nutrition,[13,17,18] peripheral muscle function,[19–21] cardiac function,[22–24] as well as daily PA.[25–27] Nevertheless, an increase in lung function parameters normally results in an improved exercise capacity.[28,29] In a healthy population, and also in mild CF lung disease,[30] maximal exercise is limited by muscle fatigue when the muscles become hypoxic and accumulate lactic acid. Those individuals with moderate to advanced pulmonary disease present an exaggerated ventilatory response during incremental exercise to exhaustion[8] and become more and more ventilatory limited. The limitation is normally correlated to the severity of the underlying lung disease. The rest of this section discusses possible limitations of exercise performance according to relevant organ system.

Respiratory system

The defect of the CFTR protein complex results in an impairment of mucociliary clearance, with the consequence of bronchial obstruction and recurrent or chronic infections in the lungs. Mechanisms include mucosal oedema secondary to chronic infection/inflammation, mechanical obstruction by abnormal viscous secretions, stimulation of autonomic nerve fibres caused by damage to respiratory epithelium, airway smooth muscle contraction by inflammatory mediators, or loss of CFTR function in sarcoplasmic reticulum of smooth muscles, and dynamic collapse of airways with partly destructed walls.[6,31] The recurrent inflammation/infection leads to a progressive destruction of the bronchial wall with bronchiectasis and to a progressive bronchial lability with a tendency of bronchial collapse, which further provokes mucostasis and inflammation.[3] The development of atelectatic, emphysematic, and fibrotic areas implies a progressive decline of functional lung tissue, the so-called cystic-fibrotic degeneration of the lung. The disease severity varies tremendously among patients, ranging from severe obstructive pulmonary disease in the infant up to a mild cough with normal pulmonary function in a 40-year-old patient. About 3–4% of adolescent or adult CF patients develop a spontaneous pneumothorax, mainly presenting as sharp thoracic pain and consequent tachypnoea or dyspnoea.[32] Respiratory insufficiency with hypercapnia, chronic hypoxaemia, and an exhaustion of the respiratory muscles is the cause of death in 70–80% of all CF patients.[33]

In mild disease, patients present with a normal lung function, despite the fact that ventilatory inhomogeneity may already be present. Newer techniques, such as multiple breath washout, are able

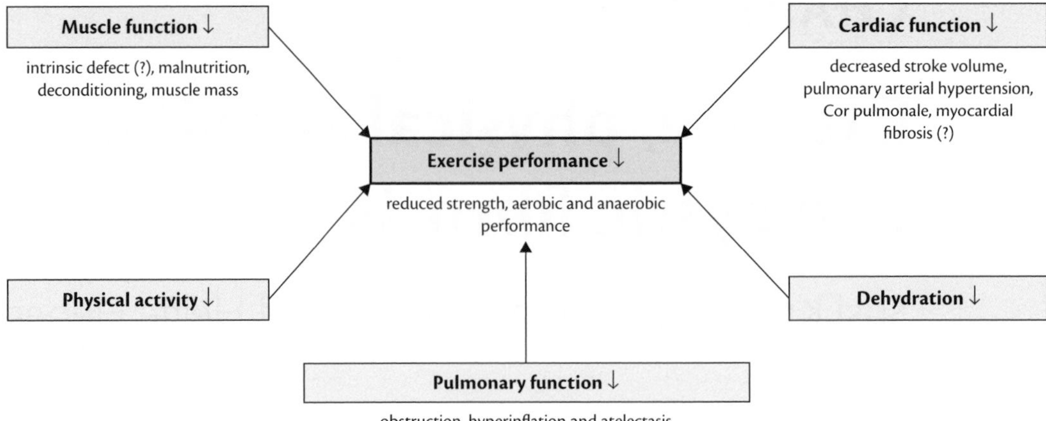

Figure 27.1 Potential factors responsible for exercise limitations in patients with cystic fibrosis.

to measure ventilatory inhomogeneity long before forced expiratory flow in one second (FEV_1) becomes abnormal. At a next stage of disease progression, patients normally present with an obstruction in their resting pulmonary function, including a decreased forced vital capacity (FVC), FEV_1, forced expiratory flow between 25 and 75% of vital capacity, peak expiratory flow, and an increased residual volume to total lung capacity.[34–36] In other words, there is bronchial obstruction and hyperinflation. A first consequence is the increase of dead space ventilation. which results in higher ventilation at any given workload and peak work capacity that becomes limited.[37,38] While a healthy child uses only about 70% of the maximal voluntary ventilation during maximal exercise, the patient with progressed CF uses a higher percentage, finally reaching 100% or even more.[39,40] Healthy people show a dead space to tidal volume ratio of about 30% at rest and a lower percentage at exercise. In patients with moderate or severe CF, the dead space to tidal volume ratio is increased at rest, and even more so at exercise. This is due to a limited tidal volume and a poor matching of ventilation and perfusion of the lungs.[41] Likewise, the relative ventilation for a given work load is increased, resulting in a higher oxygen cost of ventilation[42] and early fatigue of inspiratory muscle function. The oxygen cost of breathing in a healthy individual is in the range of 10% of peak $\dot{V}O_2$. However, it can reach 30–40% in those patients with severe respiratory limitations.[43] If peripheral oxygen demands cannot be met, desaturation occurs which further impairs respiratory muscle function. Furthermore, retention of airway secretions and destruction of lung tissue lead to ventilation of poorly perfused areas of the lung and thus progressive ventilation-perfusion mismatch. In consequence, an increased arterio-alveolar oxygen gradient and oxygen desaturation occur first during exercise and finally also at rest.[44]

Forced vital capacity decreases with progressive airway obstruction and hyperinflation, which limits an increase of tidal volume at increasing work loads.[45] Individuals with CF typically show lower increases in tidal volume that is partially compensated by a faster respiratory rate, without reaching the minute ventilations of healthy controls. However, this adaptive strategy of rapid shallow breathing has the disadvantage of increasing energy cost of breathing by inefficient dead space ventilation and by altered ribcage mechanics, beside increased airways resistance and decreased lung compliance, which contributes to early fatigue of the inspiratory muscles.[46] Furthermore, time to expire a given air volume is prolonged in obstructive airway disease. When combined with high breathing frequencies air trapping occurs and hyperinflation is aggravated. Inspiratory muscles are shortened and the diaphragm flattened, leading to a compromise of inspiratory muscle function.

High dead space ventilation can also jeopardize carbon dioxide (CO_2) elimination[45] and CO_2 retention occurs due to a lower increase in the ventilation due to low tidal volumes[47–49] and changes in the chemoreceptor set point for partial pressure of CO_2.[50] In CF, CO_2 retention during exercise has even been described as an early predictor of mortality[51] or as a predictor of a faster decline in FEV_1.[49] Whether CO_2 retention also contributes to limitations in maximal performance by increasing subjective dyspnoea sensation is not clear.

In general, patients with a FVC or a FEV_1/FVC ratio of >50% predicted are unlikely to show desaturation, even at high-intensity exercise, when desaturation is defined as a fall of oxygen saturation (SaO_2) <90%.[30,52] However, this is not true for all people with CF, and desaturation with exercise can neither be predicted nor excluded from pulmonary function testing alone.[53] In early reports, it was speculated that exercise performance in CF might be limited by oxygen availability, as indicated by a positive relationship between SaO_2 at peak exercise and peak $\dot{V}O_2$.[54] In a study by Nixon *et al.*[55] peak workload during exercise testing was not increased, despite oxygen supplementation in hypoxaemic CF patients. This led them to conclude that maximal exercise was not oxygen limited. Another elegant study, however, suggests that arterial hypoxaemia is indeed responsible for the exercise limitation.[56] A group of adult CF patients with moderate to severe disease and desaturation at maximal exercise underwent maximal exercise testing with and without added dead space. The condition with added dead space was tested under normoxia, as well as under hyperoxia. The addition of dead space caused reduced $\dot{V}O_2$ max with equal peak ventilation and desaturation than without added dead space, while $\dot{V}O_2$ max increased when oxygen was added to the additional dead space. The authors concluded that oxygen supplementation might help to improve maximal exercise performance by lowering minute ventilation and as such conserving energy of the respiratory muscles. Likewise, oxygen supplementation lowers heart rate and pulmonary arterial hypertension with the consequence of an improved ventilation-perfusion time.[55] It also seems to improve aerobic metabolism in the peripheral muscles as shown in calf muscles of patients with chronic obstructive pulmonary disease,[57] or it might reduce the sensation of dyspnoea at the end of exercise.[56]

Some patients experience a severe cough while exercising. It is important to mention to the patient, family, and teacher that this is not dangerous. In general, coughing is helpful as it facilitates the clearance of mucus from the bronchial system.[58] Usually, a short break during exercise is sufficient to stop the spells. In some patients, however, the cough or shortness of breath is a sign of exercise-induced bronchoconstriction.[31,59,60] The diagnosis of asthma in CF is problematic and it is difficult to determine which patients have a combination of CF and asthma and which have asthma-like symptoms, caused by the CF lung itself. The North American and European CF databases report that 17–32% of patients with CF have asthma and higher incidences were found when patients were tested several times, instead of a single test over a year.[61–63] The reported proportions of reactive airways range from as high as 65%[64] down to 2%,[65] but the average is around 40%.[59,60,66] The therapy is the same as for exercise-induced bronchoconstriction in the non-CF population, but some CF patients do not respond to bronchodilators as well as people with asthma, and should be tested repeatedly. Furthermore, 10% to 20% of CF patients treated with bronchodilators even demonstrate an acute decline in spirometric values.[67,68] Moreover, bronchodilators do not improve maximal exercise performance in CF, despite causing significant acute bronchodilation.[67,69] This lack of benefit occurred in all patients with ventilatory limitation during exercise and irrespective of a positive bronchoprovocation test.[69] Note that some authors also found bronchodilation with exercise, even without treatment.[65,66,69,70] An exercise-induced increase in mucus clearance or the re-opening of collapsed bronchi is thought to be responsible for the improvement in lung function. It is also possible that bronchoconstriction occurs due to airway instability by loss of bronchomotor tone leading to increased dead space ventilation, which could explain the lack of improvement in exercise performance.[69]

Cardiac system

Initially, the cardiovascular response to exercise appears to be relatively normal in CF and heart rates (HR) and cardiac output ($\dot{Q}$) are adequate for a given workload.[18,38] Cardiac output is often normal due to a more rapid rise of HR during exercise, thus compensating for a reduced stroke volume (SV), which seems to occur even in the absence of severe lung disease.[71] With disease progression, patients with CF often show a significant Cor pulmonale as a consequence of pulmonary artery hypertension.[72] The pathophysiology of Cor pulmonale and pulmonary arterial hypertension is explained by a progressive destruction of the lung parenchyma and pulmonary vasculature and to pulmonary vasoconstriction secondary to hypoxaemia. While some authors found right and left vetricular functional deficits during exercise others[13,38] basically found no abnormalities. Perrault *et al.*[23] measured the $\dot{Q}$ response during progressive upright and supine exercise in patients with CF of different disease severity. Cardiac output increased with exercise intensity in both positions, except in those patients with severe disease (FEV_1 40%). Despite a normal $\dot{Q}$ response all CF patients, irrespective of disease severity, failed to increase SV in response to the change from upright to the supine position. The authors concluded that this could reflect a limitation in end-diastolic ventricular filling by an alteration of ventricular diastolic function. In another study[14] several patients with CF showed a decrease in SV despite a normal $\dot{Q}$. Stroke volume correlated with hypoxaemia, but not with pulmonary function. This constellation is compatible with impaired left ventricular filling as a consequence of hypoxia induced pulmonary hypertension. In contrast, another study[24] found a more striking relationship between stroke volume (% predicted) and FEV_1 than with hypoxaemia, with an improvement of the SV response to exercise with improvement in ventilatory mechanics in some patients who were measured twice. In summary, cardiovascular limitations with decreases of SVs occur, but are often compensated by a higher HR, leading to a normal $\dot{Q}$. However, it needs to be determined whether or not the reduced SV is due i) to hypoxaemia causing pulmonary hypertension, ii) the consequence of an impaired left ventricular filling, iii) a decreased right ventricular performance as a consequence of increased pulmonary pressure and lung volumes, iv) poor nutrition, v) low PA, or vi) a combination of these factors. The decreased left ventricular filling has been linked to an inadequate coupling between the arterial and cardiac system, resulting in increased myocardial afterload.[74] A further reason could be multifocal myocardial fibrosis, which has been described in autopsies of patients with CF.[75]

Irrespective of all these cardiac alterations, arrhythmias in form of single ventricular extrasystoles and hypoxaemia during exercise have been described in about 25% of patients.[53,76] As SaO_2 and FEV_1 at rest were the strongest predictors of desaturation at maximal exercise a prediction formula was developed:

$$\begin{aligned} SaO_2 \text{ at peak exercise (in \%)} = {} & 1.1825 * SaO_2 \text{ at rest (in \%)} \\ & - 309.1474 / FEV_1 \text{ at rest (\% predicted)} \\ & - 16.4875 \end{aligned}$$

Although none of the patients had any symptoms and did not show any cardiac events and complications during 2–5 years of follow-up, the authors recommended performing routine exercise testing and to consider the option of additional oxygen under exercise.[53]

Habitual physical activity

Since some long-term exercise intervention studies[77,78] have been effective in slowing down pulmonary function decline and in increasing exercise performance, habitual PA might have an important impact on these parameters, which are documented predictors of mortality.[51,79,80] The relationship between habitual PA and lung function has been recently reported in 212 children and adolescents with CF over a 9-year period.[81] In this study, a greater increase in habitual PA was associated with a slower rate of decline in FEV_1, after adjustment for relevant confounders. In another longitudinal study[82] 7- to 17-year-old girls in the two lowest PA quartiles had a more rapid rate of decline in FEV_1 than girls in the two highest PA quartiles, while in boys PA was not related to FEV_1 decline. The authors concluded that a physically inactive lifestyle may partially explain the poorer survival of female patients with CF.[83] Children and adults with CF have been reported to have lower,[25] similar,[84] or even higher[7] levels of daily PA, compared to healthy children. In the latter study, children with CF performed more total and light intensity PA, but spent less time in moderate- to vigorous-intensity PA (MVPA) and vigorous-intensity PA (VPA) on both weekdays and weekend days.[7] This study showed weak to moderate correlations between MVPA or VPA and peak $\dot{V}O_2$ ($r = 0.39$–0.46).

In another study, Selvadurai *et al.*[26] documented an equal PA level in prepubertal boys and girls with CF, compared to controls. After onset of puberty, PA was higher in boys than girls with CF. It was even higher than in controls when lung disease was mild, but lower for those with moderate to severe lung disease. The best correlates of PA were nutritional status, aerobic capacity, anaerobic power, and quality of life, but not lung function. Surprisingly, there are few data in the literature on whether a relationship between PA and peak $\dot{V}O_2$ exists in CF and whether it reflects a direct effect or is mediated by confounding factors, such as pulmonary or muscle function. A cross-sectional study in 12–40-year-old patients with a broad range of disease severity found that PA beside body height, sex, FEV_1, and muscle power were identified as independent predictors of $\dot{V}O_2$ max.[27]

Despite the known benefits of a high PA level in CF, it is a major challenge for clinicians, physiotherapists, nurses, and exercise scientists to motivate children and their parents to follow a physically active lifestyle. Strategies to promote PA in CF are very limited. A recent Cochrane review on interventions for promoting PA including four studies and 199 participants with CF concluded that there is very limited evidence that exercise counselling and advice results in improvements in PA levels in this population.[85]

Nutrition, muscle mass, and muscle function

Exocrine pancreatic insufficiency with maldigestion and failure to thrive is a hallmark of CF, occurring in 85–90% of the CF population.[86] The impairment of the intraluminal digestion varies widely from the life-threatening event of a meconium ileus in the newborn, to a subclinical digestive residual function in the adult patient, and the severity of the disease seems to be in part related to the genetic defect.[87,88] It is nowadays well accepted that external factors like enzyme therapy or nutrition influence the progression and severity of the disease.[89–94] Undernutrition is often seen in patients with CF as a result of malabsorption, reduced energy intake, increased energy expenditure, and as a consequence of chronic pulmonary infection.

Cystic fibrosis disease increases energy demands, malabsorption causes energy loss, and external factors decrease energy intake. Consequently, there often is a net energy deficit, which is believed to impair respiratory and peripheral muscle function, leading to a progressive destruction of the pulmonary parenchyma and decrease immune regulation. This causes a worsening of the pulmonary function and increases the likelihood of pulmonary infections. The infections then provoke a further decrease of the lung function and may even cause anorexia and vomiting, which closes the vicious circle.[95]

It has to be considered that total daily energy expenditure in a resting stage,[96] as well as during exercise,[97–99] is increased in persons with CF, especially in the advanced stage with severe lung disease. It is therefore important that the energy intake is adjusted to the disease severity and the PA level.

In order to be able to calculate proper energy requirements, a first step is to assess the nutritional status and body composition. The body mass index (BMI) is widely used to assess nutritional status, but BMI does not inform about body composition. In patients with CF, there might be a normal BMI, although skeletal muscles might be wasted. This was indeed found in a group of young adults with CF, in whom a loss of fat-free mass, but a normal fat mass, measured by dual-energy X-ray absorptiometry (DEXA), was found in the presence of a normal BMI.[100] The loss of fat-free mass is often related to the severity of lung disease and the level of PA, suggesting that this pattern preferentially occurs in advanced lung disease and with frequent pulmonary exacerbations.[101] Whether the loss of fat-free mass leads to physical inactivity, or whether the loss of fat-free mass is rather a consequence of inappropriate use, remains a matter of debate. A low fat-free mass in adults with CF has also been found in other studies[102] and was related to more severe lung disease.[103]

There are several methods that have been used in studies reporting body composition in CF, including DEXA,[102–104] bioelectrical impedance,[104–106] and measurements of skinfold thickness.[104,105] Dual-energy X-ray absorptiometry is the preferred method, since it has been shown to be a useful and reliable method for body composition assessment and it also provides information about bone mass, which is often reduced in patients with CF. Studies in children and adults with CF found that skinfold thickness and bioelectrical impedance incorrectly estimate fat-free mass and fat mass in many patients compared with DEXA measurements.[104,105] Although results obtained using the three methods were highly correlated for the group, values for individual subjects varied widely and showed large differences with under- and overestimation.[107] So far, there are no CF-specific equations for skinfolds or bioelectrical impedance to assess body composition in CF that are reliable and valid enough on the individual level.

A better nutritional status is associated with higher aerobic[16,17] and anaerobic[108–110] exercise capacity in CF. Likewise, a poor nutritional status is considered as a risk factor for limited exercise capacity.[13,18] An increase in body weight through an adequate nutrition has been shown to improve exercise capacity[111] and muscle strength.[112] If the increase in energy intake is combined with exercise training, an improved exercise capacity and lean tissue gain are attained in some,[113] but not all studies.[112,114] In CF chronic airway obstruction leads to a catabolic metabolism, leading to secondary pulmonary infection and inflammation; a process which may induce protein breakdown and inhibit muscle development.[115,116] Yet, it is not clear whether impaired exercise performance is caused by a decrease in muscle mass or whether there is an intrinsic muscle defect. Moser *et al.*[19] tested the association between peak $\dot{V}O_2$ and muscle size in 7- to 18-year-old children and adolescents with CF and found that the reduced peak $\dot{V}O_2$ in CF was not solely explained by a reduction in muscle size, but that the reduction in peak $\dot{V}O_2$ was observed even when normalized to muscle cross-sectional area, which was only slightly lower in CF than in controls. This study is unique, since it directly assessed muscle mass by magnetic resonance imaging rather than relying on indirect estimates of muscle mass. Interestingly, Moser *et al.*[19] found that not only peak $\dot{V}O_2$ was reduced in CF, but also the $\Delta\dot{V}O_2/\Delta$work rate slope, describing reduced oxygen demands of exercise in CF at any intensity level. Whether this was caused by an increased work efficiency, by slowed oxygen kinetics,[117] or by a higher reliance on anaerobic pathways like in certain patients with congenital heart disease in which oxygen transport to muscle is reduced[118] was not clear. The authors also suggested that a change in adenosine triphosphate (ATP) metabolism as shown in patients with chronic disease[119] or an altered intrinsic muscle function[21] could have played a role. The latter hypothesis was based on a study that performed a magnetic resonance spectroscopy assessment of forearm and calf muscles of 12- to 17-year-old adolescents with CF during isometric exercise. This group found a higher intracellular pH, with less oxidative ATP turnover than in the healthy controls, suggesting an intrinsic defect in skeletal muscle function. In line with this hypothesis is the fact that, although peak $\dot{V}O_2$ was lower for muscle cross-sectional area in CF subjects, the abnormality causing this did not progressively worsen in older subjects. Whether the muscle function deficit is caused by the malnutrition, by the genetic defect[4,5] itself, or a combination of both is, however, not yet clear, and is still under debate.

Diabetes

Cystic fibrosis-related insulin-dependent diabetes mellitus (CFRDM) is a common complication of CF.[120,121] Cystic fibrosis-related insulin-dependent diabetes mellitus affects 9% of people with CF aged 5–9 years, 26% aged 10–20 years, and up to 50% by the age of 30 years.[122] Most of the patients are treated as in type I diabetes. The presence of CFRDM is associated with an accelerated decline in pulmonary function, poorer growth and nutritional status, and increased mortality.[121] CFRDM can be associated with exercise intolerance,[123] is almost always non-ketotic and has a slow, insidious onset. Physical activity should specially be promoted, because it may improve glucose tolerance,[124] is able to smooth the glucose peaks in the blood and prevents positive energy balance that is particularly prevalent among CFRDM patients.[121] As in type I diabetes the physically active child should be motivated to eat and drink before and during PA in order to avoid hypoglycaemia, especially when the activity is prolonged and intense. Based on the markedly improved long-term prognosis in CF it is more important than ever to provide a good management of the diabetes in order to prevent pulmonary function decline,[125] and micro- and macro-angiopathy. Regular PA should be firmly incorporated in the management of CF patients with CFRDM, due to the multiple recognized beneficial health effects, such as, but not limited to, cardiovascular disease prevention and better glucose homeostasis.[124,126–128] The improvement in glucose homeostasis could be explained by different mechanisms. These include the activation of the adenosine monophosphate kinase system, which enhances sensitivity of muscle glucose transport to insulin[129] by stimulation of glucose uptake by increased translocation of the glucose transporter GLUT4 to the plasma membrane,[130] or by circumventing upstream defects in insulin signal transduction via increased mitochondrial energy metabolism.[131] The major barrier to achieving perfect blood glucose control and minimizing secondary complications is still the risk of hypoglycaemia. Cystic fibrosis patients have normal hypoglycaemia awareness, but especially those with longer duration of CFRDM may be at increased risk because glucagon, as the body's defence hormone against insulin-induced hypoglycaemia, is impaired.[132] The incidence of exercise-induced hypoglycaemia is unknown in CF, but appears to be quite low.[133] It generally develops as a result of exercise without adequate reduction in insulin dose or increase in carbohydrate intake.

Osteopenia/osteoporosis

Children as well as adults with CF demonstrate low bone mass by reduced bone mineral density assessed by DEXA or quantitative peripheral computed tomography.[134–137] This may lead to osteoporosis with the potential of atraumatic bone fractures. Higher fracture incidences, in particular vertebral fractures, have been documented in adolescent and adult patients with CF.[134,138–141] In general, patients with advanced lung disease and those with the lowest muscle mass consistently show the lowest bone mass.[136,142,143] The severity of lung disease, rather than age per se, and cumulative use of steroids have been shown to explain half of the variance of bone mineral density. Irrespective of these two factors, muscle or fat-free mass is one of the most important predictors of bone mass, irrespective of disease state[144] and maintenance of bone mass, in large part, depends on skeletal muscle-derived mechanical loading.[145] It is possible that the severity of lung disease may be largely a surrogate marker of reduced muscle mass. Pathophysiologically, there is a decrease in bone formation and an increase in bone resorption.[136,146–148] Whether this is due to a direct genetic defect in bone where CFTR has been shown to be expressed in human osteoblasts, osteocytes, and osteoclasts,[149] or whether a secondary mechanism involving potential factors increasing bone resorption such as underlying inflammation, chronic respiratory acidosis, hyperglycaemia, and reduced PA play a critical role, is unknown. Cystic fibrosis-related insulin-dependent diabetes mellitus knockout mice show an abnormal skeletal phenotype with striking osteopenia, reduced cortical width and thinning of the trabeculae.[150] Although there is not yet proof, CFTR is expressed in bone cells and might have a physiological role in bone metabolism.

As in a healthy population, risk factors such as poor nutrition, low muscle mass, physical inactivity, delayed puberty, and steroid therapy are major causes of osteopenia. These factors often occur together in patients with CF and in concert increase the risk for low bone mass. There is a consistent correlation between body mass and bone density, with underweight patients showing the lowest bone mass,[134,135,137,151] compatible with the tight association between muscle and bone mass in general. There are scarce data on the effect of PA on bone mass in CF. Maximal $\dot{V}O_2$ and BMI have been found to be significant predictors of bone mass in CF[152] and the level of PA was associated with bone mineral density in children and adults with CF[153,154], suggesting that bone mass might indeed be influenced by impact loading not only in the general population but also in CF.

Dehydration

Patients with CF have a low tolerance to climatic heat stress which has been shown to increase morbidity and mortality among CF patients.[155,156] Dehydration might also decrease strength[157] and aerobic exercise performance.[158] The thermoregulatory ability among children with CF, who exercised 1.5–3 h in a hot climate, nevertheless seemed to be normal.[159] However, unlike healthy people who usually increase their extracellular osmolality as a result of sweating, CF patients had a decline in serum sodium chloride (NaCl) and osmolality compared to healthy controls during exposures to the heat,[159,160] resulting from the much higher loss of NaCl in the sweat of exercising CF patients.[159] In addition to hypovolaemia, an increase in extracellular osmolality triggers thirst by stimulating hypothalamic osmoreceptors.[161–163] It is thus possible that patients with CF, whose sweating does not induce a normal increase in extracellular osmolality, would be deprived of this trigger for thirst. Indeed, children with CF, when allowed to drink water *ad libitum* during exposure to a hot climate, drank half as much and dehydrate almost three times as much as healthy controls.[159] Despite the fact that this feature has not been shown in adults;[161] all patients with CF must therefore be encouraged to drink above and beyond thirst, especially when they exercise in warm or humid climates and during recovery from dehydration-inducing exercise. In addition, they should be encouraged to ingest electrolyte solutions with a high NaCl content (preferably 50 $mmol \cdot L^{-1}$ or more) which has been shown to prevent dehydration, rather than water alone.[164] It is possible that improvement in palatability of a high-sodium beverage would induce an even greater voluntary fluid intake.

Beneficial effects of exercise and physical activity

Many studies have been conducted over the last 30 years which suggest that exercise can improve aerobic fitness,[165,166] lessen the decrease of pulmonary function or even stop it,[167] and improve health-related quality of life (HRQoL).[40] A recent Cochrane review[168] including 13 randomized controlled short- and long-term studies with low to moderate risk of bias showed limited evidence that aerobic or anaerobic exercise, or a combination of both training modalities, has a beneficial effect on exercise capacity, pulmonary function, and HRQoL in individuals with CF. The authors highlighted that there is a clear need for high-quality randomized controlled studies with sufficient numbers of study participants and well-chosen, objectively measurable, reproducible, clinically relevant, and patient-orientated outcome measures.

Orenstein added an important reflection in his update on the role of exercise in CF[169] and pointed out that based on the expected decline in pulmonary function in patients with CF of 2% to 3% per year, an exercise intervention study shorter than 12 months may be unable to detect a difference in pulmonary function between control and exercise intervention participants. If one applies this statement to the existing randomized controlled studies, there are only four of the thirteen studies[29,77,78,167] that fulfil the suggested criterion regarding the 'appropriate' duration of a training intervention. These particular studies were able to show some beneficial effects of training including a lower rate of annual decline in FVC,[29,77,167] FEV1,[78] and an increase in exercise performance.[29,77,78]

Another recent Cochrane review[170] assessed the effect of inspiratory muscle training on lung function and exercise capacity in CF, including eight studies with a wide variation in quality. The review came to the conclusion that there is no evidence that this type of training is either beneficial or harmful.[170]

The reason why regular PA and exercise might be effective in decreasing the loss of pulmonary function over time is not well understood and still a matter of debate. It is possible that mechanical vibrations of the body and increased ventilation facilitate mechanical cleaning of the airways.[171,172] Aerobic exercise further inhibits the Amiloride-sensitive sodium channel in respiratory epithelium.[173] As such, the inhibition of luminal sodium conductance could increase fluid secretion into the airways during exercise and therefore facilitate mucus expectoration. Exercise has also been shown to stimulate anabolic mediators such as growth hormone and insulin-like growth factor-I in CF[116] and might further act—as in the healthy population—through improvement of insulin resistance, immune function,[174] induction of tissue growth factors, or through altered neuroendocrine control of metabolism, as suggested by Cooper *et al.*[175] All these factors may, at least in part, explain the beneficial effects of exercise in patients with CF.

In general, the majority of exercise training studies of CF have to be interpreted with caution. Factors such as small sample sizes, the lack of an adequate control group, merely no follow-up assessments, or short intervention periods of less than 2 months are some of the possible limitations to be considered. More studies are needed to test long-term effects, optimal training mode (aerobic vs anaerobic vs strength training) and context (supervised vs unsupervised, hospital vs home-based) to determine which approach is most beneficial and also most attractive to individuals with CF so that adherence to physical exercise training and PA stays high in the long term.

Harmful effects of exercise and physical activity

The risks of exercise and PA in patients with CF are consequences of the pathophysiological processes we have previously described. Risks are important to consider, but fortunately their occurrence is rare. A recent survey including 78 of 107 CF German facilities caring for 4208 patients responded to a caregiver's survey and 256 patients answered a web-based survey.[133] No serious adverse reactions (SARs) were reported for 713 exercise tests. With in-hospital training, the yearly incidence of exercise-related SARs such as pneumothorax, cardiac arrhythmia, injury, or hypoglycaemia was <1% each, the respective lifetime incidence reported by the patients was 0.8–6.3%. Sixty-seven per cent of the patients reported no SAR with exercise ever. Therefore, exercise testing when conducted under controlled conditions by trained personnel is safe in patients with CF, and SARs for in-hospital exercise training as well as during daily life are low. Nevertheless, it is wise to have potential SARs and risk constellations in mind (Table 27.1).

Table 27.1 Harmful effects of exercise in patients with cystic fibrosis.

Symptom	Comment
Hypoxaemia	Especially with $FEV_1 < 50\%$ predicted or resting $SaO_2 < 94\%$ at high altitude[199]
Exercise-induced bronchoconstriction	Repeated therapeutic control is recommended
Decreased body weight	Very rare, when increased demands are not compensated
Dehydration	Especially with long exercise in warm environment
Hypoglycaemia	Especially without adequate reduction in insulin dose or increase in carbohydrate intake under exercise
Fractures	With osteoporosis
Pneumothorax	More risk in contact sports, while diving or potentially with weight training (?)
Trauma to liver, spleen, oesophageal varices	With contact sports, bungee jumping, sky diving
Arrhythmias	Only detectable with standardized exercise testing including measurement of heart rhythm by electrocardiogram

For most sports there is no contraindication. There are several specific sports, however, which should be discouraged in CF, especially in an advanced stage of disease. One is scuba diving, and another is sports at high altitude. In both types of activities detrimental situations can occur in which oxygen becomes limited and severe desaturation can occur over longer periods. Furthermore, contact sports can cause trauma to an enlarged liver or spleen, and bungee jumping or sky diving increase the risk for pneumothorax and variceal bleeding.

Exercise testing and recommendations

Since $\dot{V}O_2$ max has become one of the strongest predictors of mortality in CF[51,79] and exercise has been proven to be helpful in improving health[29,167] and quality of life in CF[40,167] a regular exercise test is recommended for each child and adolescent for assessment of prognosis and individual patient counselling.[176] Recently, a statement on exercise testing in CF has been published with expert consensus recommendations on exercise testing protocols, outcome parameters, and interpretation of exercise tests.[176] Despite these recommendations, exercise testing is not performed on a regular base in most CF centres.[177,178] In addition to the determination of potential risk factors for exercise, exercise testing is useful to define training recommendations, to document training effects, and it may be a good means for motivation. If exercise testing is not done routinely, it is highly recommended in:

- those who experience some sort of symptoms at exercise, such as cough, dyspnoea, cyanosis, or fatigue
- those with a $FEV_1 < 50\%$ and/or $FVC < 70\%$ predicted
- those who fear to have any harmful effect from any type of PA
- those who want to start an exercise training programme
- those who want to document their training progress.

Most studies evaluating exercise capacity have used a progressive cycle or treadmill test, or field tests such as walking tests or step tests. The Godfrey cycle protocol[179] (Table 27.2) has been used most frequently in CF exercise research. It is preferably done with the measurement of ventilatory gas exchange and transcutaneous SaO_2. Alternatively, a treadmill protocol can be used, or the tests can be performed without gas measurements as long as SaO_2 is assessed.[176,180]

In general, the Godfrey cycle protocol yields acceptable reproducibility data for peak power output in 6- to 11-year-old children with CF, when the tests are performed 1 week apart.[181] Although the Godfrey protocol is often used, there is no single optimal testing protocol for children and adolescents with CF lung disease and several different exercise testing protocols have been tested in in different laboratories.[8,182]

Table 27.2 Godfrey exercise to assess aerobic exercise capacity.

Load (Watt)	Increment (Watt)	Height (cm)	Stage duration (min)
10	10	<120	1
15	15	120–150	1
20	20	>150	1

Werkman MS, Hulzebos EH, Helders PJ, Arets BG, Takken T. Estimating peak oxygen uptake in adolescents with cystic fibrosis. Arch Dis Child. 2014; 99: 21–25.

In the statement of exercise testing paper by Hebestreit *et al.*,[176] a rationale for the interpretation of a cardiopulmonary exercise test is provided and illustrated in (Figure 27.2).

If equipment for cardiopulmonary exercise testing (CPET) is not available, simple walking tests, shuttle run tests, or step tests can be used to assess a patient's functional exercise capacity. Field exercise tests are most commonly performed in paediatric lung transplant candidates with CF.[183] In the 6 min walking test children walk in a hospital corridor back and forth, while the walking distance (m) over a 6 min period is measured.[184–186] Incremental cycle ergometry,[187] the 6 min walking test,[184] and shuttle run[188] have been shown to be reliable and valid for children with CF. Limited reproducibility and validity data exist for the 3 min step test[189] as the test has a submaximal character and is unable to detect oxygen desaturation (fall in $SaO_2 > 4\%$), compared to CPET in children with CF.[190] For those who are unable or unwilling to perform a maximal exercise test or to document the change in functional exercise status, submaximal testing has been proposed.[191] Unfortunately, measurement properties such as responsiveness (to change) and the minimally important clinical difference have been poorly investigated for both cardiopulmonary and field exercise test outcomes in CF.

In order to find a level of exercise that is beneficial in patients with CF, the ventilatory threshold, which is defined as the point during incremental exercise when ventilation increases out of proportion to $\dot{V}O_2$, can be measured.[192] McLoughlin *et al.*,[193] however, showed that the ventilatory threshold significantly overestimates the lactate threshold in individuals with CF, because of impaired CO_2 excretion. This group suggested using the gas exchange threshold instead, which is the point during an incremental exercise where VCO_2 increases out of proportion to $\dot{V}O_2$. The gas exchange threshold has been shown to be reliable and valid in children[194] and adults with CF.[195]

There are two important test outcome parameters, i.e. the intensity of exercise where SaO_2 falls below 90% and the HR at which training should be performed. Whatever test is performed, it should identify those whose oxygen levels fall during exercise. It is recommended that individuals with CF should exercise at an intensity level where the SaO_2 is above 90%. Note that front head oximetry is the preferred method to assess oxygen saturation, since finger oximetry has been shown to be less accurate due to motion artefacts and altered digital perfusion that can even be more altered in CF than in a healthy population.[196] The HR at which oxygen saturation falls below 90% can be noted and the patient can make sure that his/her exercise intensity does not exceed this level. Today, small portable finger monitors are available that enable monitoring SaO_2 and HR during exercise or exercise breaks. If desaturation occurs at a very low intensity level, oxygen supplementation during exercise can be discussed.

Another aim of the test is to evaluate each individual's own maximal HR or ventilatory threshold, to be able to prescribe a training intensity. Generally, 70–80% of each maximal HR or 60–80% of peak $\dot{V}O_2$ is considered to be beneficial for efficient aerobic training in health and disease.

A change in body composition should always be considered when individual data are followed longitudinally. We recommend that the performance parameters of interest (e.g. peak $\dot{V}O_2$, peak workload) should at least be related to body weight, but better to fat-free mass or related to percent predicted values. Each training recommendation should include information about the frequency, intensity, and

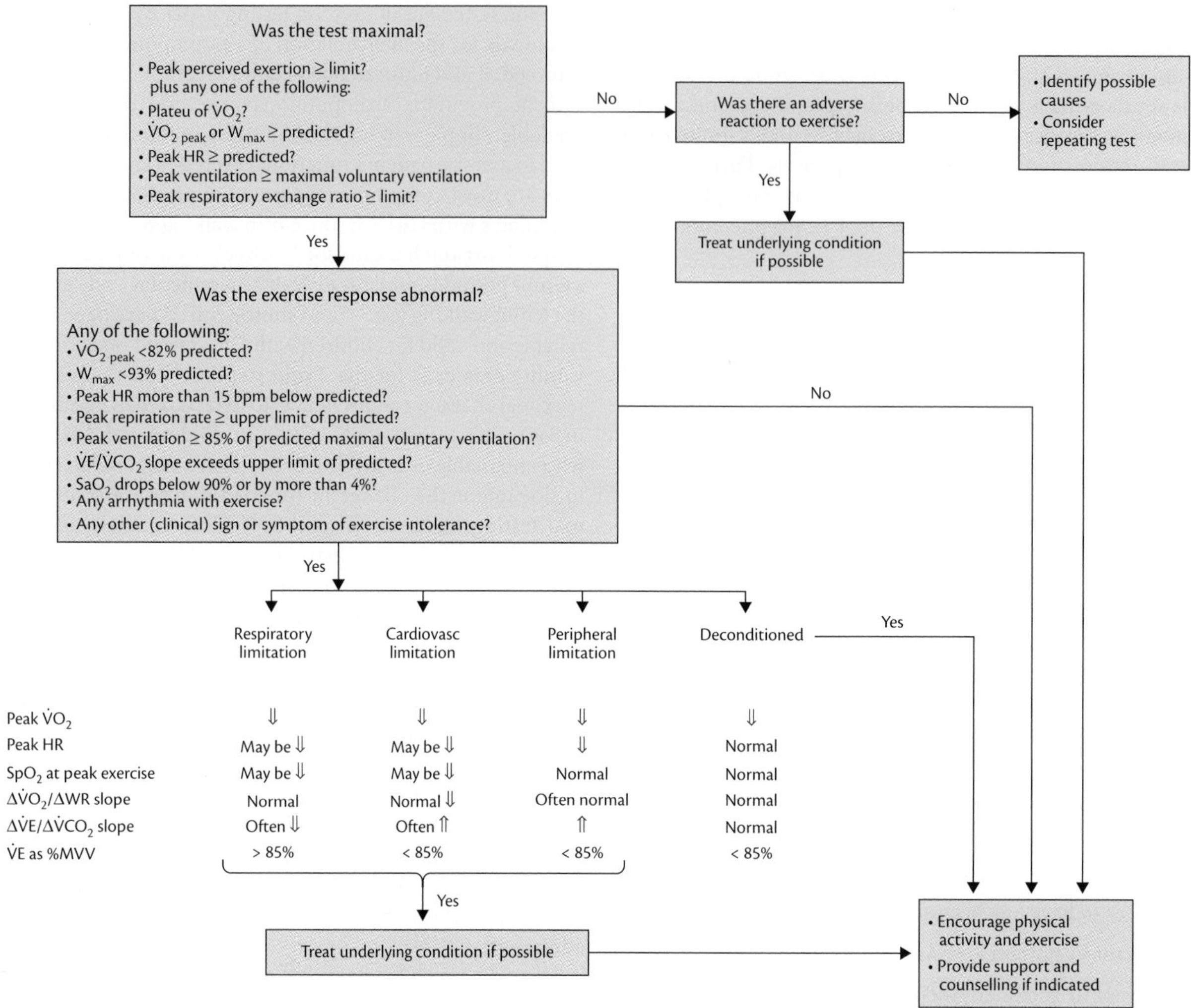

Figure 27.2 Approach for the interpretation of a cardiopulmonary exercise test.
Hebestreit H, Arets Hubertus GM, Aurora P, *et al*. Statement on Exercise Testing in Cystic Fibrosis. Respiration (2015), reprinted with permission of Karger Publishers.

duration or time of the exercise training programme. As in healthy persons, the training for those with CF should be performed at least three times per week, although five times per week is optimal, at an intensity level of 70–80% of maximal capacity, or at 85% of anaerobic threshold and for the duration of 30 min. Most beginners are not capable of performing such a programme initially and should be allowed to reach this level within 2–3 months. A good guide is a 10% increase per week, either in intensity or duration. Very often, intermittent training with a lot of breaks helps to start, or can be used for those unable to tolerate constant intensity exercise.[197] In this case, exercise bouts may last 0.5 to 2 min, interspersed with 1 min breaks. The exercise intensity can be set as for the constant intensity exercise, but might even be more intense due to the allowed recovery periods. Based on data from training programmes with CF patients, youngsters should be informed that a clear training effect is not expected before 2–3 months. Strength training can be applied as in the healthy population.

Selection of the type of sport and training

There is no single training method that can be considered to be most beneficial in terms of cardiorespiratory and muscular adaptions. Whatever type, intensity, and fragmentation is chosen, the most important factor to consider is long-term adherence. Modalities may include moderate constant load regimens[198] or high-intensity interval training[9,11,196] (interested readers are referred to Chapter 35 for a discussion of high-intensity interval training). The latter may be ideal for patients with advanced disease who use additional oxygen, but can be used for everybody.

We always recommend the young CF patient participates in various intense activities or sports. Team sports are extremely important for the self-esteem and social integration of any child with a chronic disease. It is helpful to inform the team and coach about the child's disease and to allow him/her to take breaks or run slower whenever needed. An individual sport has the advantage that it can be performed at an individual pace without interfering with anybody else. This is especially important when the disease becomes advanced in order to keep the young person active, but without constantly showing him/her the progression of the disease. In those progressed stages it can be very helpful to search for sports where skills like reactivity, coordination, and flexibility are more important than aerobic capacity or strength. Being a goalkeeper, playing tennis or table tennis, rock climbing, or dancing are some activities that might be appropriate. In general, the child should be allowed to perform any sport beside these exceptions. As long as the motivation and fun aspect is apparent, the best possible adherence and compliance is achieved. Again, the explanation to the coach and team members regarding the child's health condition seems to be the best way to allow an optimal tolerance and integration of the young patient with CF into the sports world.

Conclusions

Cystic fibrosis is a genetic disease resulting in an impaired mucociliary clearance, chronic bacterial airway infection, and inflammation that leads to progressive destruction of the lungs, which is the main cause for morbidity and premature death. Yet, diverse other organ systems such as heart, muscles, and bones, gastrointestinal tract, and sweat glands are often also affected, which can also interfere with exercise capacity. Exercise capacity is reduced when disease progresses mainly due to reduced functioning of the muscles, heart, and/or lungs. As there is growing evidence of positive effects of exercise training in CF on exercise capacity, decline of pulmonary function, and health-related quality of life, exercise should be implemented in all patients' care. More research is needed to understand pathophysiological mechanisms of exercise limitations and to find optimal exercise modalities to slow down disease progression, predict long-term adherence, and improve health-related quality of life.

Summary

- Exercise capacity in cystic fibrosis (CF) is reduced when disease becomes moderate to severe due to a reduced function of the muscles, heart and/or lungs. Whether these organ functions are impaired due to the inherited genetic defect of the cystic fibrosis transmembrane conductance regulator (CFTR) mutation itself, whether it is a consequence of progressive chronic disease, or whether it is rather physical inactivity related secondary to chronic progressive disease, is not fully understood.
- Although there is still limited evidence of positive effects of exercise training in CF on exercise capacity, decline of pulmonary function, and health-related quality of life, the observed effects are encouraging and there is no reason why exercise should not be implemented in all patients' care. Possible harmful effects of exercise such as hypoxaemia, hypoglycaemia, or bleeding from altered organs are rare, but have to be considered, especially with progression of the disease.
- Different gaps in our current knowledge need to be filled:
  - i. Search on pathophysiological mechanisms of exercise limitations to discover if they can be targeted (or not) by therapeutic strategies, and;
  - ii. More high-quality randomized controlled exercise trials are needed to find the best exercise modalities to slow down disease progression, to keep the compliance of the patients high, and to reach a maximum of health-related quality of life.

References

1. Ratjen F, Doring G. Cystic fibrosis. *Lancet*. 2003; 361: 681–689.
2. George PM, Banya W, Pareek N, *et al*. Improved survival at low lung function in cystic fibrosis: cohort study from 1990 to 2007. *BMJ*. 2011; 342: d1008.
3. Stoltz DA, Meyerholz DK, Welsh MJ. Origins of cystic fibrosis lung disease. *N Engl J Med*. 2015; 372: 1574–1575.
4. Lamhonwah AM, Bear CE, Huan LJ, *et al*. Cystic fibrosis transmembrane conductance regulator in human muscle: Dysfunction causes abnormal metabolic recovery in exercise. *Ann Neurol*. 2010; 67: 802–808.
5. Divangahi M, Balghi H, Danialou G, *et al*. Lack of CFTR in skeletal muscle predisposes to muscle wasting and diaphragm muscle pump failure in cystic fibrosis mice. *PLOS Genet*. 2009; 5: e1000586.
6. Cook DP, Rector MV, Bouzek DC, *et al*. Cystic Fibrosis Transmembrane Conductance Regulator in sarcoplasmic reticulum of airway smooth muscle: implications for airway contractility. *Am J Respir Crit Care Med*. 2015; 193: 417–426.
7. Aznar S, Gallardo C, Fiuza-Luces C, *et al*. Levels of moderate—vigorous physical activity are low in Spanish children with cystic fibrosis: a comparison with healthy controls. *J Cyst Fibros*. 2014; 13: 335–340.
8. Bongers BC, Werkman MS, Takken T, Hulzebos EH. Ventilatory response to exercise in adolescents with cystic fibrosis and mild-to-moderate airway obstruction. *Springerplus*. 2014; 3: 696.
9. Nguyen T, Obeid J, Ploeger HE, *et al*. Inflammatory and growth factor response to continuous and intermittent exercise in youth with cystic fibrosis. *J Cyst Fibros*. 2012; 11: 108–118.
10. Saynor ZL, Barker AR, Oades PJ, Williams CA. Impaired aerobic function in patients with cystic fibrosis during ramp exercise. *Med Sci Sports Exerc*. 2014; 46: 2271–2278.
11. Stevens D, Oades PJ, Williams CA. Airflow limitation following cardiopulmonary exercise testing and heavy-intensity intermittent exercise in children with cystic fibrosis. *Eur J Pediatr*. 2015; 174: 251–257.
12. de Meer K, Gulmans VA, van Der Laag J. Peripheral muscle weakness and exercise capacity in children with cystic fibrosis. *Am J Respir Crit Care Med*. 1999; 159: 748–754.
13. Marcotte JE, Canny GJ, Grisdale R. Effects of nutritional status on exercise performance in advanced cystic fibrosis. *Chest*. 1986; 90: 375–379.
14. Marcotte JE, Grisdale RK, Levison H, Coates AL, Canny GJ. Multiple factors limit exercise in cystic fibrosis. *Pediatr Pulmonol*. 1986; 2: 274–281.
15. Klijn PH, Terheggen-Lagro SW, Van Der Ent CK, *et al*. Anaerobic exercise in pediatric cystic fibrosis. *Pediatr Pulmonol*. 2003; 36: 223–229.
16. Klijn PH, van der Net J, Kimpen JL, Helders PJ, van der Ent CK. Longitudinal determinants of peak aerobic performance in children with cystic fibrosis. *Chest*. 2003; 124: 2215–2219.
17. Coates AL, Boyce P, Muller D, Mearns M, Godfrey S. The role of nutritional status, airway obstruction, hypoxia, and abnormalities in serum lipid composition in limiting exercise tolerance in children with cystic fibrosis. *Acta Paediatr Scand*. 1980; 69: 353–358.
18. Lands LC, Heigenhauser GJ, Jones NL. Analysis of factors limiting maximal exercise performance in cystic fibrosis. *Clin Sci (Lond)*. 1992; 83: 391–397.
19. Moser C, Tirakitsoontorn P, Nussbaum E, Newcomb R, Cooper DM. Muscle size and cardiorespiratory response to exercise in cystic fibrosis. *Am J Respir Crit Care Med*. 2000; 162: 1823–1827.
20. Selvadurai HC, Allen J, Sachinwalla T, *et al*. Muscle function and resting energy expenditure in female athletes with cystic fibrosis. *Am J Respir Crit Care Med*. 2003; 168: 1476–1480.
21. de Meer K, Jeneson JA, Gulmans VA, van der Laag J, Berger R. Efficiency of oxidative work performance of skeletal muscle in patients with cystic fibrosis. *Thorax*. 1995; 50: 980–983.
22. Benson LN, Newth CJ, Desouza M, *et al*. Radionuclide assessment of right and left ventricular function during bicycle exercise in young patients with cystic fibrosis. *Am Rev Respir Dis*. 1984; 130: 987–992.
23. Perrault H, Coughlan M, Marcotte JE, Drblik SP, Lamarre A. Comparison of cardiac output determinants in response to upright and supine exercise in patients with cystic fibrosis. *Chest*. 1992; 101: 42–51.

24. Hortop J, Desmond KJ, Coates AL. The mechanical effects of expiratory airflow limitation on cardiac performance in cystic fibrosis. *Am Rev Respir Dis*. 1988; 137: 132–137.
25. Nixon PA, Orenstein DM, Kelsey SF. Habitual physical activity in children and adolescents with cystic fibrosis. *Med Sci Sports* Exerc. 2001; 33: 30–35.
26. Selvadurai HC, Blimkie CJ, Cooper PJ, Mellis CM, Van Asperen PP. Gender differences in habitual activity in children with cystic fibrosis. *Arch Dis Child*. 2004; 89: 928–933.
27. Hebestreit H, Kieser S, Rudiger S, *et al*. Physical activity is independently related to aerobic capacity in cystic fibrosis. *Eur Respir J*. 2006; 28: 734–739.
28. Cerny FJ, Pullano T, Cropp GJA. Adaptation to exercise in children with cystic fibrosis. In: Nagle FJ, Montoye HJ (eds.) *Exercise in health and disease*. Springfield, IL: Thomas; 1982. p. 36–42.
29. Moorcroft AJ, Dodd ME, Morris J, Webb AK. Individualised unsupervised exercise training in adults with cystic fibrosis: a 1-year randomised controlled trial. *Thorax*. 2004; 59: 1074–1080.
30. Moorcroft AJ, Dodd ME, Morris J, Webb AK. Symptoms, lactate and exercise limitation at peak cycle ergometry in adults with cystic fibrosis. *Eur Respir J*. 2005; 25: 1050–1056.
31. Balfour-Lynn IM, Elborn JS. 'CF asthma': what is it and what do we do about it? *Thorax*. 2002; 57: 742–748.
32. Flume PA. Pneumothorax in cystic fibrosis. *Curr Opin Pulm Med*. 2011; 17: 220–225.
33. O'Sullivan BP, Freedman SD. Cystic fibrosis. *Lancet*. 2009; 373: 1891–1904.
34. Landau LI, Phelan PD. The spectrum of cystic fibrosis. *Am Rev Respir Dis*. 1973; 108: 593–602.
35. Zapletal A, Motoyama EK, Gibson LE, Bouhuys A. Pulmonary mechanics in asthma and cystic fibrosis. *Pediatrics*. 1971; 48: 64–72.
36. Corey M, McLaughlin FJ, Wiliams M, Levison H. A comparison of survival, growth, and pulmonary function in patients with cystic fibrosis in Boston and Toronto. *J Clin Epidemiol*. 1988; 41: 583–591.
37. Keochkerian D, Chlif M, Delanaud S, *et al*. Timing and driving components of the breathing strategy in children with cystic fibrosis during exercise. *Pediatr Pulmonol*. 2005; 40: 449–456.
38. Godfrey S, Mearns M. Pulmonary function and responses to exercise in cystic fibrosis. *Arch Dis Child*. 1971; 46: 144–151.
39. Lands LC, Heigenhauser GJF, Jones NL. Analysis of factors limiting maximal exercise performance in cystic fibrosis. *Clin Sci*. 1992; 83: 391–397.
40. Orenstein DM, Franklin BA, Doershuk CF, *et al*. Exercise conditioning and cardiopulmonary fitness in cystic fibrosis. The effects of a three-month supervised running program. *Chest*. 1981; 80: 392–398.
41. Webb AK, Dodd ME, Moorcroft J. Exercise in cystic fibrosis. *J Roy Soc Med*. 1995; 88 (Suppl): 30–36.
42. Mador MJ. Respiratory muscle fatigue and breathing pattern. *Chest*. 1991; 100: 1430–1435.
43. Levison H, Cherniack RM. Ventilatory cost of exercise in chronic obstructive pulmonary disease. *J Appl Physiol*. 1968; 25: 21–27.
44. Marcus CL, Bader D, Stabile MW, *et al*. Supplemental oxygen and exercise performance in patients with cystic fibrosis with severe pulmonary disease. *Chest*. 1992; 101: 52–57.
45. Keochkerian D, Chlif M, Delanaud S, *et al*. Breathing Pattern Adopted by Children with Cystic Fibrosis with Mild to Moderate Pulmonary Impairment during Exercise. *Respiration*. 2008; 75: 170–177.
46. Leroy S, Perez T, Neviere R, Aguilaniu B, Wallaert B. Determinants of dyspnea and alveolar hypoventilation during exercise in cystic fibrosis: impact of inspiratory muscle endurance. *J Cyst Fibros*. 2011; 10: 159–165.
47. Coates AL, Canny G, Zinman R, *et al*. The effects of chronic airflow limitation, increased dead space, and the pattern of ventilation on gas exchange during maximal exercise in advanced cystic fibrosis. *Am Rev Resp Dis*.1988; 138: 1524–1531.
48. Cerny FJ, Pullano T, Cropp GJA. Cardiorespiratory adaptations to exercise in cystic fibrosis. *Am Rev Respir Dis*. 1982; 126: 217–220.
49. Javadpour SM, Selvadurai H, Wilkes DL, Schneiderman-Walker J, Coates AL. Does carbon dioxide retention during exercise predict a more rapid decline in FEV1 in cystic fibrosis? *Arch Dis Child*. 2005; 90: 792–795.
50. Pianosi P, Wolstein R. Carbon dioxide chemosensitivity and exercise ventilation in healthy children and in children with cystic fibrosis. *Pediatr Res*. 1996; 40: 508–513.
51. Nixon PA, Orenstein DM, Kelsey SF, Doershuk CF. The prognostic value of exercise testing in patients with cystic fibrosis. *New Engl J Med*. 1992; 327: 1785–1788.
52. Henke KG, Orenstein DM. Oxygen saturation during exercise in cystic fibrosis. *Am Rev Respir Dis*. 1984; 129: 708–711.
53. Ruf K, Hebestreit H. Exercise-induced hypoxemia and cardiac arrhythmia in cystic fibrosis. *J Cyst Fibros*. 2009; 8: 83–90.
54. Cropp GJA, Pullano TP, Cerny FJ, Nathanson IT. Exercise tolerance and cardiorespiratory adjustments at peak work capacity in cystic fibrosis. *Am Rev Respir Dis*. 1982; 126: 211–216.
55. Nixon PA, Orenstein DM, Curtis SE, Ross EA. Oxygen supplementation during exercise in cystic fibrosis. *Am Rev Respir Dis*. 1990; 142: 807–811.
56. McKone EF, Barry SC, Fitzgerald MX, Gallagher CG. Role of arterial hypoxemia and pulmonary mechanics in exercise limitation in adults with cystic fibrosis. *J Appl Physiol*. 2005; 99: 1012–1018.
57. Payen JF, Wuyam B, Levy P. Muscular metabolism during oxygen supplementation in patients with chronic hypoxemia. *Am Rev Respir Dis*. 1993; 147: 592–598.
58. King M, Brock G, Lundell C. Clearance of mucus by simulated cough. *J Appl Physiol*. 1985; 58: 1776–1782.
59. Holzer FJ, Olinsky A, Phelan PD. Variability of airways hyperreactivity and allergy in cystic fibrosis. *Arch Dis Child*. 1981; 56: 455–459.
60. Silverman M, Hobbs FD, Gordon IR. Cystic fibrosis, atopy and airways lability. *Arch Dis Child*. 1978; 53: 873–878.
61. Morgan WJ, Butler SM, Johnson CA, *et al*. Epidemiologic study of cystic fibrosis: design and implementation of a prospective, multicenter, observational study of patients with cystic fibrosis in the US and Canada. *Pediatr Pulmonol*. 1999; 28: 231–241.
62. Koch C, McKenzie SG, Kaplowitz H, *et al*. International practice patterns by age and severity of lung disease in cystic fibrosis: data from the Epidemiologic Registry of Cystic Fibrosis (ERCF). *Pediatr Pulmonol*. 1997; 24: 147–154; discussion 159–161.
63. Konstan MW, Butler SM, Schidlow DV, *et al*. Patterns of medical practice in cystic fibrosis: part II. Use of therapies. Investigators and Coordinators of the Epidemiologic Study of Cystic Fibrosis. *Pediatr Pulmonol*. 1999; 28: 248–254.
64. Day G, Mearn HB. Bronchial lability in cystic fibrosis. *Arch Dis Child*. 1973; 48: 355–359.
65. Skorecki K, Levison H, Crozier DN. Bronchial lability in cystic fibrosis. *Acta Pediatr Scand*. 1976; 65: 39–42.
66. Price JF, Weller PH, Harper SA, Metthew DJ. Response to bronchial provocation and exercise in children with cystic fibrosis. *Clin Allergy*. 1979; 9: 563–570.
67. Dodd JD, Barry SC, Daly LE, Gallagher CG. Inhaled beta-agonists improve lung function but not maximal exercise capacity in cystic fibrosis. *J Cyst Fibros*. 2005; 4: 101–105.
68. Brand PL. Bronchodilators in cystic fibrosis. *J Roy Soc Med*. 2000; 93(Suppl 38): 37–39.
69. Serisier DJ, Coates AD, Bowler SD. Effect of albuterol on maximal exercise capacity in cystic fibrosis. *Chest*. 2007; 131: 1181–1187.
70. Kusenbach G, Friedrichs F, Skopnik H, Heimann G. Increased physiological dead space during exercise after bronchodilation in cystic fibrosis. *Pediatr Pulmonol*. 1993; 15: 273–278.
71. Pianosi P, Pelech A. Stroke volume during exercise in cystic fibrosis. *Am J Respir Crit Care Med*. 1996; 153: 1105–1109.
72. Hayes DJr, Tobias JD, Mansour HM, *et al*. Pulmonary hypertension in cystic fibrosis with advanced lung disease. *Am J Respir Crit Care Med*. 2014; 190: 898–905.
73. Chipps BE, Alderson PO, Roland JMA, *et al*. Non-invasive evaluation of ventricular function in cystic fibrosis. *J Pediatr*. 1979; 95: 379–384.

74. Hull JH, Ansley L, Bolton CE, *et al.* The effect of exercise on large artery haemodynamics in cystic fibrosis. *J Cyst Fibros.* 2011; 10: 121–127.
75. Nezelof C, Bouvier R, Dijoud F. Multifocal myocardial necrosis: a distinctive cardiac lesion in cystic fibrosis, lipomatous pancreatic atrophy, and Keshan disease. *Pediatr Pathol Mol Med.* 2002; 21: 343–352.
76. Lebecque P, Lapierre JG, Lamarre A, Coates AL. Diffusion capacity and oxygen desaturation effects on exercise in patients with cystic fibrosis. *Chest.* 1987; 91: 693–697.
77. Hebestreit H, Kieser S, Junge S, *et al.* Long-term effects of a partially supervised conditioning programme in cystic fibrosis. *Eur Respir J.* 2010; 35: 578–583.
78. Kriemler S, Kieser S, Junge S, *et al.* Effect of supervised training on FEV1 in cystic fibrosis: A randomised controlled trial. *J Cyst Fibros.* 2013; 12: 714–720.
79. Pianosi P, Leblanc J, Almudevar A. Peak oxygen uptake and mortality in children with cystic fibrosis. *Thorax.* 2005; 60: 50–54.
80. Kerem E, Reisman J, Corey M, Canny GJ, Levison H. Prediction of mortality in patients with cystic fibrosis. *New Engl J Med.* 1992; 326: 1187–1191.
81. Schneiderman JE, Wilkes DL, Atenafu EG, *et al.* Longitudinal relationship between physical activity and lung health in patients with cystic fibrosis. *Eur Respir J.* 2014; 43: 817–823.
82. Schneiderman-Walker J, Wilkes DL, Strug L, *et al.* Sex differences in habitual physical activity and lung function decline in children with cystic fibrosis. *J Pediatr.* 2005; 147: 321–326.
83. McIntyre K. Gender and survival in cystic fibrosis. *Curr Opin Pulm Med.* 2013; 19: 692–697.
84. Boucher GP, Lands LC, Hay JA, Hornby L. Activity levels and the relationship to lung function and nutritional status in children with cystic fibrosis. *Amer J Phys Med Rehab.* 1997; 76: 311–315.
85. Cox NS, Alison JA, Holland AE. Interventions for promoting physical activity in people with cystic fibrosis. *Cochrane Database Syst Rev.* 2013; 12: CD009448.
86. Ledder O, Haller W, Couper RT, Lewindon P, Oliver M. Cystic fibrosis: an update for clinicians. Part 2: hepatobiliary and pancreatic manifestations. *J Gastroenterol Hepatol.* 2014; 29: 1954–1962.
87. Borgo G, Astella G, Gasparini P, *et al.* Pancreatic function and gene deletion F508 in cystic fibrosis. *J Med Genet.* 1990; 27: 665–669.
88. Kerem E, Corey M, Kerem BS, *et al.* The relation between genotype and phenotype in cystic fibrosis. *New Engl J Med.* 1990; 323: 1517–1522.
89. Schoni MH, Casaulta-Aebischer C. Nutrition and lung function in cystic fibrosis patients: review. *Clin Nutr.* 2000; 19: 79–85.
90. Kraemer R, Rudeberg A, Hadorn B, Rossi E. Relative underweight in cystic fibrosis and its prognostic value. *Acta Paediatr Scand.* 1978; 67: 33–37.
91. Levy LD, Durie PR, Pencharz PB, Corey ML. Effects of long-term nutritional rehabilitation on body composition and clinical status in malnourished children and adolescents with cystic fibrosis. *J Pediatr.* 1985; 107: 225–230.
92. Shepherd RW, Holt TL, Thomas BJ. Nutritional rehabilitation in cystic fibrosis: controlled studies of effects on nutritional growth retardation, body protein turnover, and course of pulmonary disease. *J Pediatr.* 1986; 109: 788–794.
93. Liou TG, Adler FR, Fitzsimmons SC, *et al.* Predictive 5-year survivorship model of cystic fibrosis. *Am J Epidemiol.* 2001; 153: 345–352.
94. Shale DJ. Predicting survival in cystic fibrosis. *Thorax.* 1997; 52: 309.
95. Durie PR, Forstner GG. Pathophysiology of the exocrine pancreas in cystic fibrosis. *J R Soc Med.* 1989; 16: 1–20.
96. Allen JR, McCauley JC, Selby AM, *et al.* Differences in resting energy expenditure between male and female children with cystic fibrosis. *J Pediatr.* 2003; 142: 15–19.
97. Vaisman N, Penchanrz PB, Corey M, Canny GJ. Energy expenditure of patients with cystic fibrosis. *J Pediatr.* 1987; 111: 496–500.
98. Fried MD. The cystic fibrosis gene and resting energy expenditure. *J Pediatr.* 1991; 119: 913–916.
99. Richards ML, Davies PS, Bell SC. Energy cost of physical activity in cystic fibrosis. *Eur J Clin Nutr.* 2001; 55: 690–697.
100. Bolton CE, Ionescu AA, Evans WD, Pettit RJ, Shale DJ. Altered tissue distribution in adults with cystic fibrosis. *Thorax.* 2003; 58: 885–889.
101. Alicandro G, Bisogno A, Battezzati A, *et al.* Recurrent pulmonary exacerbations are associated with low fat free mass and low bone mineral density in young adults with cystic fibrosis. *J Cyst Fibros.* 2014; 13: 328–334.
102. Ionescu AA, Nixon LS, Evans WD, *et al.* Bone density, body composition, and inflammatory status in cystic fibrosis. *Am J Respir Crit Care Med.* 2000; 162: 789–794.
103. Ionescu AA, Nixon LS, Luzio S, *et al.* Pulmonary function, body composition, and protein catabolism in adults with cystic fibrosis. *Am J Respir Crit Care Med.* 2002; 165: 495–500.
104. Lands LC, Gordon C, Bar-Or O, *et al.* Comparison of three techniques for body composition analysis in cystic fibrosis. *J Appl Physiol.* 1993; 75: 162–166.
105. King S, Wilson J, Kotsimbos T, Bailey M, Nyulasi I. Body composition assessment in adults with cystic fibrosis: comparison of dual-energy X-ray absorptiometry with skinfolds and bioelectrical impedance analysis. *Nutrition.* 2005; 21: 1087–1094.
106. Quirk PC, Ward LC, Thomas BJ, *et al.* Evaluation of bioelectrical impedance for prospective nutritional assessment in cystic fibrosis. *Nutrition.* 1997; 13: 412–416.
107. Alicandro G, Battezzati A, Bianchi ML, *et al.* Estimating body composition from skinfold thicknesses and bioelectrical impedance analysis in cystic fibrosis patients. *J Cyst Fibros.* 2015; 14: 784–791.
108. Shah AR, Gozal D, Keens TG. Determinants of aerobic and anaerobic exercise performance in cystic fibrosis. *Am J Respir Crit Care Med.* 1998; 157: 1145–1150.
109. Cabrera ME, Lough MD, Doershuk CF, DeRivera GA. Anaerobic performance—assessed by the Wingate Test—in patients with cystic fibrosis. *Pediatr Exerc Sci.* 1993; 5: 78–87.
110. Boas SR, Joswiak ML, Nixon APA, Fulton JA, Orenstien DM. Factors limiting anaerobic performance in adolescent males with cystic fibrosis. *Med Sci Sports Exerc.* 1996; 28: 291–298.
111. Skeie B, Askanazi J, Rothkopf MM, *et al.* Improved exercise tolerance with long-term parenteral nutrition in cystic fibrosis. *Crit Care Med.* 1987; 15: 960–962.
112. Hanning RM, Blimkie CJR, Bar-Or O, *et al.* Relationships among nutritional status and skeletal and respiratory muscle function in cystic fibrosis: does early dietary supplementation make a difference? *Amer J Clin Nutr.* 1993; 57: 580–587.
113. Heijerman HGM, Bakker W, Sterk PJ, Dijkman JH. Long-term effects of exercise training and hyperalimentation in adult cystic fibrosis patients with severe pulmonary dysfunction. *Int J Rehab Res.* 1992; 15: 252–257.
114. Bertrand JM, Morin CL, Lasalle R, Ptrick J, Coates AL. Short-term clinical, nutritional, and functional effects of continuous elemental enteral alimentation in children with cystic fibrosis. *J Pediatr.* 1984; 104: 41–46.
115. Lands LC, Grey V, Smountas AA, Kramer VG, McKenna D. Lymphocyte glutathione levels in children with cystic fibrosis. *Chest.* 1999; 116: 201–205.
116. Tirakitsoontorn P, Nussbaum E, Moser C, Hill M, Cooper DM. Fitness, acute exercise, and anabolic and catabolic mediators in cystic fibrosis. *Am J Respir Crit Care Med.* 2001; 164: 1432–1437.
117. Hebestreit H, Hebestreit A, Trusen A, Hughson RL. Oxygen uptake kinetics are slowed in cystic fibrosis. *Med Sci Sports Exerc.* 2005; 37: 10–17.
118. Troutman WB, Barstow TJ, Galindo AJ, Cooper DM. Abnormal dynamic cardiorespiratory responses to exercise in pediatric patients after Fontan procedure. *J Am Coll Cardiol.* 1998; 31: 668–673.
119. American Thoracic Society and European Respiratory Society. Skeletal muscle dysfunction in chronic obstructive pulmonary disease: a statement. *Am J Respir Crit Care Med.* 1999; 159: S1–S40.
120. Kelly A, Moran A. Update on cystic fibrosis-related diabetes. *J Cyst Fibros.* 2013; 12: 318–331.

121. Brennan AL, Beynon J. Clinical updates in cystic fibrosis-related diabetes. *Seminars in Respir Crit Care Med.* 2015; 36: 236–250.
122. Moran A, Dunitz J, Nathan B, *et al.* Cystic fibrosis-related diabetes: current trends in prevalence, incidence, and mortality. *Diabetes Care.* 2009; 32: 1626–1631.
123. Ziegler B, Oliveira CL, Rovedder PM, *et al.* Glucose intolerance in patients with cystic fibrosis: sex-based differences in clinical score, pulmonary function, radiograph score, and 6-minute walk test. *Respir Care.* 2011; 56: 290–297.
124. Beaudoin N, Bouvet, GF, Rabasa-Lhoret R, Berthiaume Y. Effects of a partially supervised combined exercise program on glycemic control in cystic fibrosis: pilot study. (Abstract). *Pediatr Pulmonol.* 2015; 50(S41): 367.
125. Milla CE, Warwick WJ, Moran A. Trends in pulmonary function in patients with cystic fibrosis correlate with the degree of glucose intolerance at baseline. *Am J Respir Crit Care Med.* 2000; 162: 891–895.
126. Galassetti P, Riddell MC. Exercise and type 1 diabetes (T1DM). *Comp Physiol.* 2013; 3: 1309–1336.
127. Huttunen NP, Kaar ML, Knip M, *et al.* Physical fitness of children and adolescents with insulin-dependent diabetes mellitus. *Ann Clin Res.* 1984; 16: 1–5.
128. Sackey AH, Jefferson IG. Physical activity and glycaemic control in children with diabetes mellitus. *Diabet Med.* 1996; 13: 789–793.
129. Fisher JS, Gao J, Han DH, Holloszy JO, Nolte LA. Activation of AMP kinase enhances sensitivity of muscle glucose transport to insulin. *Am J Physiol Endocrinol Metab.* 2002; 282: E18–E23.
130. Towler MC, Hardie DG. AMP-activated protein kinase in metabolic control and insulin signaling. *Circ Res.* 2007; 100: 328–341.
131. Thyfault JP, Cree MG, Zheng D, *et al.* Contraction of insulin-resistant muscle normalizes insulin action in association with increased mitochondrial activity and fatty acid catabolism. *Am J Physiol Cell Physiol.* 2007; 292: C729–C739.
132. Moran A, Diem P, Klein DJ, Levitt MD, Robertson RP. Pancreatic endocrine function in cystic fibrosis. *J Pediatr.* 1991; 118: 715–723.
133. Ruf K, Winkler B, Hebestreit A, Gruber W, Hebestreit H. Risks associated with exercise testing and sports participation in cystic fibrosis. *J Cyst Fibros.* 2010; 9: 339–345.
134. Henderson RC, Madsen CD. Bone density in children and adolescents with cystic fibrosis. *J Pediatr.* 1996; 128: 28–34.
135. Bhudhikanok GS, Lim J, Marcus R, *et al.* Correlates of osteopenia in patients with cystic fibrosis. *Pediatrics.* 1996; 97: 103–111.
136. Bhudhikanok GS, Wang M-C, Marcus R, *et al.* Bone acquisition and loss in children and adults with cystic fibrosis: a longitudinal study. *J Pediatr.* 1998; 133: 18–27.
137. Gibbens DT, Gilsanz V, Boechat MI, *et al.* Osteoporosis in cystic fibrosis. *J Pediatr.* 1988; 113: 295–300.
138. Elkin SL, Fairney A, Burnett S, *et al.* Vertebral deformities and low bone mineral density in adults with cystic fibrosis: a cross-sectional study. *Osteoporosis Int.* 2001; 12: 366–372.
139. Aris RM, Renner JB, Winders AD, *et al.* Increased rate of fractures and severe kyphosis: sequelae of living into adulthood with cystic fibrosis. *Ann Int Med.* 1998; 128: 186–193.
140. Rossini M, Del Marco A, Dal Santo F, *et al.* Prevalence and correlates of vertebral fractures in adults with cystic fibrosis. *Bone.* 2004; 35: 771–776.
141. Ujhelyi R, Treszl A, Vasarhelyi B, *et al.* Bone mineral density and bone acquisition in children and young adults with cystic fibrosis: a follow-up study. *J Pediatr Gastroenterol Nutr.* 2004; 38: 401–406.
142. Haworth CS, Selby PL, Horrocks AW, *et al.* A prospective study of change in bone mineral density over one year in adults with cystic fibrosis. *Thorax.* 2002; 57: 719–723.
143. Gronowitz E, Mellstrom D, Strandvik B. Normal annual increase of bone mineral density during two years in patients with cystic fibrosis. *Pediatrics.* 2004; 114: 435–442.
144. Goodman CA, Hornberger TA, Robling AG. Bone and skeletal muscle: Key players in mechanotransduction and potential overlapping mechanisms. *Bone.* 2015; 80: 24–36.
145. Burr DB. Muscle strength, bone mass, and age-related bone loss. *J Bone Min Res.* 1997; 12: 1547–1551.
146. Baroncelli GI, De Luca F, Magazzu G, *et al.* Bone demineralization in cystic fibrosis: evidence of imbalance between bone formation and degradation. *Pediatr Res.* 1997; 41: 397–403.
147. Greer RM, Buntain HM, Potter JM, *et al.* Abnormalities of the PTH-vitamin D axis and bone turnover markers in children, adolescents and adults with cystic fibrosis: comparison with healthy controls. *Osteoporosis Int.* 2003; 14: 404–411.
148. Putman MS, Baker JF, Uluer A, *et al.* Trends in bone mineral density in young adults with cystic fibrosis over a 15-year period. *J Cyst Fibros.* 2015; 14: 526–532.
149. Shead EF, Haworth CS, Condliffe AM, *et al.* Cystic fibrosis transmembrane conductance regulator (CFTR) is expressed in human bone. *Thorax.* 2007; 62: 650–651.
150. Dif F, Marty C, Baudoin C, de Vernejoul MC, Levi G. Severe osteopenia in CFTR-null mice. *Bone.* 2004; 35: 595–603.
151. Grey AB, Ames RW, Matthews RD, Reid IR. Bone mineral density and body composition in adult patients with cystic fibrosis. *Thorax.* 1993; 48: 589–593.
152. Frangolias DD, Pare PD, Kendler DL, *et al.* Role of exercise and nutrition status on bone mineral density in cystic fibrosis. *J Cyst Fibros.* 2003; 2: 163–170.
153. Conway SP, Morton AM, Oldroyd B, *et al.* Osteoporosis and osteopenia in adults and adolescents with cystic fibrosis: prevalence and associated factors. *Thorax.* 2000; 55: 798–804.
154. Buntain HM, Greer RM, Schluter PJ, *et al.* Bone mineral density in Australian children, adolescents and adults with cystic fibrosis: a controlled cross sectional study. *Thorax.* 2004; 59: 149–155.
155. Kessler WR, Andersen DH. Heat prostration in fibrocystic disease of the pancreas and other conditions. *Pediatrics.* 1951; 8: 648–656.
156. Williams AJ, McKiernan J, Harris F. Heat prostration in children with cystic fibrosis. *BMJ.* 1976; 2: 297.
157. Bosco JS, Terjung RL, Greenleaf JE. Effects of progressive hypohydration on maximal isometric musclular strength. *J Sports Med Phys Fitness.* 1968; 8: 81–86.
158. Saltin B. Aerobic and anaerobic work capacity after dehydration. *J Appl Physiol.* 1964; 19: 1114–1118.
159. Bar-Or O, Blimkie CJ, Hay JD, *et al.* Voluntary dehydration and heat intolerance in cystic fibrosis. *Lancet.* 1992; 339: 696–699.
160. Orenstein DM, Henke KG, Costill DL, *et al.* Exercise and heat stress in cystic fibrosis patients. *Pediatr Res.* 1983; 17: 267–269.
161. Morimoto T, Slabochova Z, Naman RK, Sargent F, 2nd. Sex differences in physiological reactions to thermal stress. *J Appl Physiol.* 1967; 22: 526–532.
162. Nose H, Yawata T, Morimoto T. Osmotic factors in restitution from thermal dehydration in rats. *Am J Physiol.* 1985; 249: R166–R171.
163. Nose H, Mack GW, Shi X, Nadel ER. The role of plasma osmolality and plasma volume during rehydration in humans. *J Appl Physiol.* 1988; 65: 1–7.
164. Kriemler S, Wilk B, Schurer W, Wilson WM, Bar-Or O. Preventing dehydration in children with cystic fibrosis who exercise in the heat. *Med Sci Sports Exerc.* 1999; 31: 774–779.
165. Klijn PH, Oudshoorn A, van der Ent CK, *et al.* Effects of anaerobic training in children with cystic fibrosis: a randomized controlled study. *Chest.* 2004; 125: 1299–1305.
166. Selvadurai HC, Blimkie CJ, Meyers N, *et al.* Randomized controlled study of in-hospital exercise training programs in children with cystic fibrosis. *Pediatr Pulmonol.* 2002; 33: 194–200.
167. Schneiderman-Walker J, Pollock SL, Corey M, *et al.* A randomized controlled trial of a 3-year home exercise program in cystic fibrosis. *J Pediatr.* 2000; 136: 304–310.
168. Radtke T, Nolan SJ, Hebestreit H, Kriemler S. Physical exercise training for cystic fibrosis. *Cochrane Database Syst Rev.* 2015; 6: CD002768.
169. Orenstein DM, Higgins LW. Update on the role of exercise in cystic fibrosis. *Curr Op Pulmon Med.* 2005; 11: 519–523.

170. Houston BW, Mills N, Solis-Moya A. Inspiratory muscle training for cystic fibrosis. *Cochrane Database Syst Rev.* 2008: CD006112.
171. McIlwaine M. Chest physical therapy, breathing techniques and exercise in children with CF. *Paediatr Respir Rev.* 2007; 8: 8–16.
172. Orenstein DM, Henke KG, Cerny FJ. Exercise and cystic fibrosis. *Phys Sports Med.* 1983; 11: 57–63.
173. Hebestreit A, Kersting U, Basler B, Jeschke R, Hebestreit H. Exercise inhibits epithelial sodium channels in patients with cystic fibrosis. *Am J Respir Crit Care Med.* 2001; 164: 443–446.
174. Timmons BW, Tarnopolsky MA, Snider DP, Bar-Or O. Immunological changes in response to exercise: influence of age, puberty, and gender. *Med Sci Sports Exerc.* 2006; 38: 293–304.
175. Cooper DM. Exercise and cystic fibrosis: the search for a therapeutic optimum. *Pediatr Pulmonol.* 1998; 25: 143–144.
176. Hebestreit H, Arets HG, Aurora P, *et al.* Statement on Exercise Testing in Cystic Fibrosis. *Respiration.* 2015; 90: 332–351.
177. Barker M, Hebestreit A, Gruber W, Hebestreit H. Exercise testing and training in German CF centers. *Pediatr Pulmonol.* 2004; 37: 351–355.
178. Kaplan TA, ZeBranek JD, McKey RM, Jr. Use of exercise in the management of cystic fibrosis: short communication about a survey of cystic fibrosis referral centers. *Pediatr Pulmonol.* 1991; 10: 205–207.
179. Godfrey S, Davies CT, Wozniak E, Barnes CA. Cardio-respiratory response to exercise in normal children. *Clin Sci.* 1971; 40: 419–431.
180. Werkman MS, Hulzebos EH, Helders PJ, Arets BG, Takken T. Estimating peak oxygen uptake in adolescents with cystic fibrosis. *Arch Dis Child.* 2014; 99: 21–25.
181. Kent L, O'Neill B, Davison G, *et al.* Cycle ergometer tests in children with cystic fibrosis: reliability and feasibility. *Pediatr Pulmonol.* 2012; 47: 1226–1234.
182. Saynor ZL, Barker AR, Oades PJ, Williams CA. A protocol to determine valid $\dot{V}O_2$ max in young cystic fibrosis patients. *J Sci Med Sport.* 2013; 16: 539–544.
183. Radtke T, Faro A, Wong J, Boehler A, Benden C. Exercise testing in pediatric lung transplant candidates with cystic fibrosis. *Pediatr Transplant.* 2011; 15: 294–299.
184. Gulmans VA, van Veldhoven NH, de Meer K, Helders PJ. The six-minute walking test in children with cystic fibrosis. *Pediatr Pulmonol.* 1996; 22: 85–89.
185. Upton CJ, Tyrrell JC, Hillser EJ. Two minute walking distance in cystic fibrosis. *Arch Dis Child.* 1988; 63: 1444–1448.
186. Nixon PA, Joswiak ML, Fricker FJ. A six-minute walking test for assessing exercise tolerance in severely ill children. *J Pediatr.* 1996; 129: 362–366.
187. McKone EF, Barry SC, FitzGerald MX, Gallagher CG. Reproducibility of maximal exercise ergometer testing in patients with cystic fibrosis. *Chest.* 1999; 116: 363–368.
188. Selvadurai HC, Cooper PJ, Meyers N, *et al.* Validation of shuttle tests in children with cystic fibrosis. *Pediatr Pulmonol.* 2003; 35: 133–138.
189. Balfour-Lynn IM, Prasad SA, Laverty A, Whitehead BF, Dinwiddie R. A step in the right direction: assessing exercise tolerance in cystic fibrosis. *Pediatr Pulmonol.* 1998; 25: 278–284.
190. Narang I, Pike S, Rosenthal M, Balfour-Lynn IM, Bush A. Three-minute step test to assess exercise capacity in children with cystic fibrosis with mild lung disease. *Pediatr Pulmonol.* 2003; 35: 108–113.
191. Barry SC, Gallagher CG. The repeatability of submaximal endurance exercise testing in cystic fibrosis. *Pediatr Pulmonol.* 2007; 42: 75–82.
192. Wasserman K. The anaerobic threshold measurement to evaluate exercise performance. *Amer Rev Resp Dis.* 1984; 129: S35–S40.
193. McLoughlin P, McKeogh D, Byrne P, *et al.* Assessment of fitness in patients with cystic fibrosis and mild lung disease. *Thorax.* 1997; 52: 425–430.
194. Saynor ZL, Barker AR, Oades PJ, Williams CA. Reproducibility of maximal cardiopulmonary exercise testing for young cystic fibrosis patients. *J Cyst Fibros.* 2013; 12: 644–650.
195. Thin AG, Linnane SJ, McKone EF, *et al.* Use of the gas exchange threshold to noninvasively determine the lactate threshold in patients with cystic fibrosis. *Chest.* 2002; 121: 1761–1770.
196. Yamaya Y, Bogaard HJ, Wagner PD, Niizeki K, Hopkins SR. Validity of pulse oximetry during maximal exercise in normoxia, hypoxia, and hyperoxia. *J Appl Physiol.* 2002; 92: 162–168.
197. Gruber W, Orenstein DM, Braumann KM, Beneke R. Interval exercise training in cystic fibrosis—effects on exercise capacity in severely affected adults. *J Cyst Fibros.* 2014; 13: 86–91.
198. Wheatley CM, Baker SE, Morgan MA, *et al.* Effects of exercise intensity compared to albuterol in individuals with cystic fibrosis. *Respir Med.* 2015; 109: 463–474.
199. Schoene RB. Lung disease at high altitude. *Adv Exp Med Biol.* 1999; 474: 47–56.

CHAPTER 28

Exercise, physical activity, and children with physical or intellectual disabilities

Merrilee Zetaruk and Shareef F Mustapha

Riley has always played at the highest tier possible in our ice hockey association now playing Atom tier 3. He has always adapted to his weakness of being an amputee by playing a smarter game, naturally having better footwork than other kids by being forced to use his feet to compensate for his limited mobility in tight areas. Riley's shot compares to the best in the league now. He practices a lot on it, as it was always a weaker spot in his game. He is second in scoring on the team, averaging 1.5 points per game. He is the only amputee player that we know of in southern Alberta. We have had parents not even notice that he was missing an arm till months into the season, refs asking where his other glove is, and getting quite the reaction when he shows them his prosthetic. (Father of 10-year-old amputee athlete)

Introduction

Children with disabilities, whether mental or physical, have a right to the same respect and dignity afforded to able-bodied children. While many physical and psychological benefits of exercise and sport participation exist for children with disabilities, there is a number of challenges these children face. The incidence of sport-significant abnormalities detected on preparticipation screening in able-bodied individuals with typical development is relatively low (1–3%). In contrast, the rate may be as high as 40% in some disabled populations.[1] As such, it is important to understand the injuries to which children with disabilities are predisposed and the general strategies for prevention. Some adaptations via adjustments in rules and use of specialized equipment and prosthetic devices allow participation in a more diverse range of athletic activity for this population. Many opportunities exist for children with disabilities to participate in sports, from a local or recreational level all the way to the elite level in the Paralympic Games and Special Olympic World Games. Given the utility of physical activity (PA) for all and the increasing number of athletes with disabilities, it is important that health professionals become familiar with the unique challenges faced by these individuals.

A brief historical note

The first Paralympic games were held in Rome, Italy in 1960 and the first Paralympic Winter games were held in Ornskoldsvik, Sweden in 1976. The Paralympic games are the second-largest sporting event in the world. Today, there are many national and international organizations representing a variety of athletes with disabilities and elite level competitions have been established. Spectators watch in awe as these athletes reach new heights, at times rivalling their able-bodied counterparts.

Many athletes with disabilities have demonstrated great achievements beyond the competitive field. Two athletes who deserve special mention are Terry Fox and Rick Hansen. Terry Fox lost his right leg to cancer in 1977. Three years later, with the aid of a lower-limb prosthesis, he began a run across Canada to raise money for cancer research. Although his journey was terminated early due to a recurrence of the disease, he was able to raise $24 million for his cause. He received the prestigious Order of Canada award in 1980, 1 year before his death. Rick Hansen became paraplegic following a motor vehicle accident in 1973 and went on to become a celebrated Paralympic athlete. In order to raise money and awareness for accessibility and the potential of people with disabilities, he began a world tour that took him to 34 different countries over a 2-year period. He completed over 40 000 km by wheelchair and raised millions of dollars to help remove barriers for people with disabilities. These men have served not only as role models for young athletes with disabilities, but have become national heroes (see Figure 28.1).

Benefits of exercise and sport participation for children with physical or intellectual disabilities

Physical activity and sport participation are associated with a myriad of both physical and psychological health benefits. Health benefits of PA for children with physical or intellectual disabilities include decreased obesity, lower lifetime risk of cardiovascular disease, improved motor skills, improved functional ability, maintenance or improvement in range of motion of joints, and increased independence.[2] Through PA, children with disabilities can attempt to maintain their functional status, which is jeopardized by reduced mobility and to improve quality of life.[3,4] The psychosocial benefits[5] and improvements in overall well-being are immense.[3,4] Sport fosters healthy attitudes towards competition and fair play.[6] Children with disabilities may feel isolated from peers due to their disabilities. Participation of these children in sport and physical activities promotes inclusion.[3] Through sports, children develop

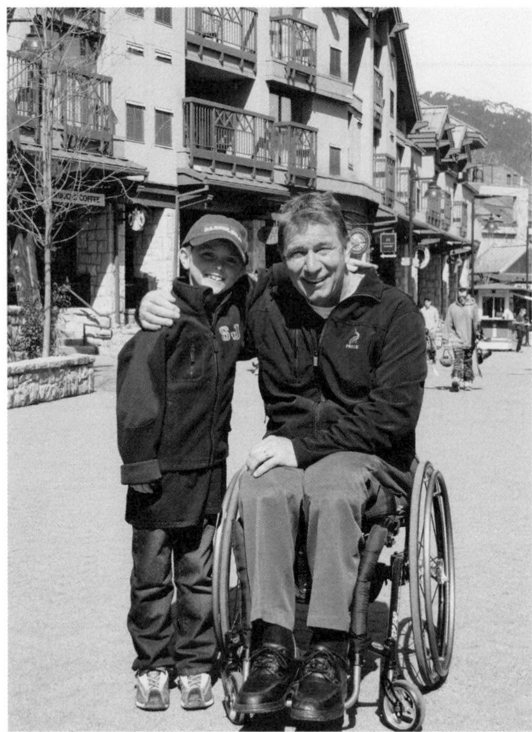

Figure 28.1 Rick Hansen with a young fan.

confidence in themselves and learn important social skills as they work together with their peers. At the same time, able-bodied children observe that despite an apparent 'handicap', children with disabilities can excel in many sports, a fact that is inspiring to both children and adults.

Childhood obesity is associated with hypertension, type 2 diabetes mellitus, fatty liver disease, coronary artery disease in adulthood, and musculoskeletal conditions such as slipped capital femoral epiphysis.[7,8] Of particular concern is that childhood obesity is a predictor of obesity in adult life. The prevalence of obesity among children and adolescents with disabilities was almost double that of the general population in a large retrospective study in the United States conducted in 2011.[9] Perhaps by encouraging children with intellectual disability to participate in sports or other physical activities, as adults they may be more active with a lower risk of obesity and all its health implications.

Cardiovascular disease is the most common medical problem in adults with intellectual disability.[10] Maximal oxygen uptake ($\dot{V}O_2$ max) as a measurement of cardiovascular fitness appears to be similar among children with and without intellectual disability.[11] As adolescents, those with intellectual disability have a substantially lower $\dot{V}O_2$ max than their unaffected peers.[11] This trend continues into adulthood and is particularly true for adults with Down syndrome (DS).[11] It appears that training can improve cardiovascular fitness in individuals with intellectual disability.[11] In order to reduce the risk of premature death due to coronary artery disease, individuals with intellectual disability should be encouraged to participate in activities that improve cardiovascular fitness.

Muscular strength and endurance appear to be lower in individuals of all ages with intellectual disability, compared to those with normal cognitive function.[11] As in the case of obesity, this difference is thought to be primarily due to lifestyle. Through training programmes aimed at increasing muscular endurance, this problem can largely be rectified.[11] Improved muscular strength improves work performance and level of independence.

Any individual with a visible disability may be at particularly high risk for psychological and social adjustment problems. Prejudices toward visible physical disabilities such as amputations can be greater than those toward functional ones. These children may be subject to bullying, marginalization, and eventual isolation by peers and society. Self-esteem can be adversely affected by these attitudes. Fortunately, sport participation and athletic competence in these individuals has been shown to correlate with higher self-esteem and improved body image.[12,13] Elite athletes with cerebral palsy (CP) report an improvement in overall health, quality of family life, and quality of social life.[4] Many forms of CP are accompanied by intellectual impairments or emotional disorders that often cause social difficulties among peers. For children with borderline or high-functioning intellectual disability, the social stigma attached to the impairment can be more handicapping than the condition itself. Sport participation can provide a means of social interaction for children with intellectual disability, while improving their fitness and self-concept.[14,15] Exercise and PA in this population may delay the need for institutionalization as well.[11]

Children with CP show deficits in strength compared with able-bodied peers.[3] A carefully designed and monitored programme of strength and flexibility training will improve flexibility, range of motion, and strength in these children.[16,17] Early PA helps maximize compensatory mechanisms of the central nervous system in order to decrease abnormal patterns of movement or posture among children with CP.[17,18] Participation in sports can help keep children and adolescents with CP engaged and motivated to continue exercising when prolonged physiotherapy is abandoned due to boredom or expense.[19]

The physiologic changes that take place during regular PA are similar in children with disabilities and in non-disabled children. The benefits of regular PA should also be similar in these two populations. In a systematic review of outcomes of cardiovascular exercise programmes for people with DS, improvement in peak oxygen consumption, peak minute ventilation, maximum work load, and increased time to exhaustion were demonstrated.[20] Participation in wheelchair sports improves $\dot{V}O_2$ max by an average of 20%, reduces risk of cardiovascular disease and respiratory infection, and improves self-image.[21] Exercise fosters good physical health through improvement of strength and endurance of the musculoskeletal system, as well as through improvements to nervous, cardiovascular, and endocrine systems. It nurtures positive mental attitudes and good overall psychological health.[1] Despite proven benefits, individuals with intellectual or physical disabilities still tend to have inadequate fitness levels. Sedentary individuals with paraplegia are at a threefold increased risk of hospitalizations compared with paraplegic athletes.[21]

There are many aspects of exercise and sport participation that are of particular benefit to visually impaired children. Physical activity helps develop a sense of orientation in space and improved mobility through enhancement of sense of touch, proprioception, balance, posture, and body control.[22,23] Through encouragement by parents and physicians, as well as the added motivation that is provided by participation in local blind sport association programmes or through organizations such as the Special Olympics, the overall health of individuals with disabilities will most certainly benefit.

Children with sensory impairments

The deaf child

Permanent, moderate to severe bilateral sensorineural hearing loss affects 0.5–1 per 1000 live births.[24] Such hearing loss can also occur at any time during childhood, resulting in a prevalence of 1.5–2 per 1000 children under 6 years of age.[24] Speech and language development can be impaired by hearing loss at a very young age, as can social and emotional development, behaviour, attention, and academic achievement.[24]

Deaf children became involved in organized sports in the United States in the 1870s when the Ohio School for the Deaf began to offer baseball and rugby for its students.[25,26] Soon after, football and basketball were introduced in a number of schools for the deaf. There were often no neuromuscular deficits in this population, so deaf athletes frequently played against hearing athletes. Today, we see many deaf children who are successful in both the deaf and hearing worlds of sport.

Hearing loss, per se, does not predispose children to any specific patterns of injury. Hearing-impaired children are at risk for balance deficits due to co-existing dysfunction of the vestibular apparatus.[27,28] Physical activities that require balance are more challenging in this setting. Activities that require climbing to heights, jumping on a trampoline, or diving into a pool should only be permitted if adequate safeguards are in place to prevent injury if the athlete loses balance and falls. Tumbling activities which require rotation should be attempted only if close supervision and spotting are available.[23] In the absence of concomitant vestibular dysfunction, the performance of deaf children compares favourably with that of hearing children in sport since their muscle function, strength, sensation, and coordination do not differ significantly.[29,30] The greatest problem for the hard-of-hearing or deaf athlete is communication with others, making participation in team sports more difficult.[31] Deaf children often participate in sports with hearing children, but are unable to hear verbal instructions or auditory cues from coaches and other players. Hearing aids may be helpful for some children. Co-existing speech impairments make communication even more difficult; however, many deaf children facilitate communication through sign language, lip reading, and other methods of visual cueing.[32,33] These skills, along with maximizing powers of observation and peripheral vision, allow children with hearing loss to participate in almost any sport; however, individual activities which require minimal communication (e.g. running or skiing) allow for the greatest success.

The World Games for the Deaf take place every 4 years. Winter events include Alpine and Nordic skiing, ice hockey, and speed skating. Summer events include badminton, basketball, cycling, men's wrestling, shooting, soccer, swimming, table tennis, team handball, tennis, track and field, volleyball, and water polo. The rules are essentially the same as those used in hearing competitions, with minor modifications such as visual cues to replace or supplement auditory cues.

The blind child

Visual impairment in children presents a challenge for sport participation. Approximately three in every thousand people are blind; as a result, a number of programmes have been developed in order to allow blind athletes to participate in various sports. According to the International Blind Sports Association (IBSA), any person with less than 10% of useful vision is eligible to compete as a blind athlete. The IBSA uses the logMAR visual acuity test to classify athletes from B1 to B3, based on testing of the better, corrected eye.[34] LogMAR (Logarithm of the Minimal Angle of Resolution) replaces the Snellen visual acuity test "(in parentheses below)". The finer grading scale allows for greater accuracy and reliability.

B1: Visual acuity poorer than LogMAR 2.6 (20/8000)

B2: Visual acuity ranging from LogMAR 1.5 (20/600) to 2.6 (20/8000) (inclusive) and/or visual field constricted to a diameter of less than 10°

B3: Visual acuity ranging from LogMAR 1.4 (20/500) to 1.0 (20/200) (inclusive) and/or visual field constricted to a diameter of less than 40°

Although visual impairment itself does not affect neuromuscular function, a fear of falling or colliding with objects results in a different pattern of movement than is observed in sighted children. Blind children often have postural problems such as rounded shoulders, stiffer posture, shorter stride, slower pace, and a shuffling gait. There is often hyperlordosis with a protruding abdomen.[22,33] Because of their restricted free movement in space, without early intervention through PA, blind children are apt to lead a sedentary lifestyle. Sedentary children become sedentary adults; therefore, it is important to encourage PA in all children, especially those with visual impairments. Auditory and tactile cues can be substituted for visual cues in a number of sports, thereby facilitating participation of blind children.[31] Through voice and touch, a guide can communicate with blind individuals to teach downhill skiing. The ski bra, invented in 1974, can be used initially to help with balance. This is a rigid device that keeps the ski tips about 7.5–10 cm apart, preventing crossing of the skis. Blind skiers, instructors, and guides wear a distinctive jacket or bib to allow easy identification by sighted skiers on the slopes.[35]

In addition to skiing, blind children compete in many different sports in which athletes without visual impairment participate, including competitive swimming, skating, baseball, track and field, and judo. Goal ball is a game uniquely designed for blind athletes. The ball has a bell inside it, allowing players to identify the trajectory of the ball and prevent it from crossing their goal line or entering the net. Like hearing loss, visual impairment alone does not affect the general fitness of individuals;[22] therefore, with modifications of rules and equipment, children with visual impairment can not only become physically active, but can attain a high level of performance in many sports.

Children with physical impairments

Children who have a disability that impairs their mobility often require the use of a wheelchair for PA or sport participation. Wheelchair sports include individuals with cerebral palsy, myelomeningocoeles, spinal cord injuries, or lower-extremity amputations. Not all children with these conditions require wheelchairs;

therefore, this section will include discussion of a range of disabilities from ambulatory to wheelchair athletes.

Children with cerebral palsy

Cerebral palsy (CP) is a non-progressive disorder of posture and movement resulting from a defect or lesion of the developing brain. Cerebral palsy is discussed in depth in Chapter 26. Here a brief summary is provided.

Cerebral palsy affects 3.6 per 1000 live births, with an estimated prevalence of two to three per 1000 in the general population.[36,37] Injuries to the cerebral cortex result in spasticity in one or more of the extremities, whereas injuries to the cerebellum or basal ganglia produce ataxia or athetosis, respectively. The most common patterns of spasticity as well as physiological parameters of exercise in CP are:

i) Monoplegia: one extremity involved, usually a lower extremity;
ii) Hemiplegia: involvement of the extremities on one side of the body; associated seizure disorder in one-third of affected children and cognitive impairments in one-quarter;
iii) Paraplegia: spasticity of both lower extremities;
iv) Diplegia: spasticity noted in all four extremities, with the upper extremities involved to a much lesser extent; likely to have normal intellectual development with a low incidence of seizure disorders;
v) Triplegia: three extremities involved, with sparing of one upper extremity;
vi) Quadriplegia: involvement of all four limbs; high rate of mental retardation and seizures.

Athetoid CP is the least common form of this disorder. It is characterized by hypotonia, athetoid movements, and slurring of speech. Seizures and intellectual impairment are uncommon in this group.

Although risk factors for injury are not unique to the child with CP, many risk factors are magnified in this population. Richter *et al.*[38] found an injury rate of 60% among athletes with CP at the 1988 Paralympic Games in South Korea. Imbalances in strength between agonist and antagonist muscle groups are risk factors for injury in typically-developing children.[39] These imbalances are even greater in CP due to the predilection of spasticity to affect primarily agonist muscle groups.[31] As a result of their spasticity, reduced range of motion, and dyscoordination, children with CP are at greater risk of soft tissue injuries during physical activities than other individuals with disabilities.[40] A good example of the effect of spasticity on muscle balance can be observed in the ankles. Spasticity of the gastrocnemius and soleus muscles results in tight heel cords and excessive plantar flexion of the foot.[31,36] Children with CP tend to be less active than their able-bodied peers, leaving them little opportunity to stretch their muscles on a regular basis without active encouragement and assistance from caregivers.[31] Joint contractures occur frequently in this population, adding to imbalances about the joints. Regular exercise programmes that incorporate stretching have been shown to improve flexibility in children with CP.[17]

Patellofemoral dysfunction occurs with increased frequency as growth and spasticity lead to tightening of the quadriceps and hamstring muscles. Gait disturbances predispose children with CP to joint malalignments. The result is increased stress across the patellofemoral joint, which leads to overuse injuries of the extensor mechanism.[31] Patellofemoral syndrome, while similar to that seen in able-bodied children, tends to be more severe in the CP population. In addition, there is increased risk of fragmentation of the distal patellar pole, such as is seen in Sinding-Larsen-Johansson syndrome. Children with this condition will present with pain and tenderness of the lower pole of the patella.

Spasticity not only causes an imbalance of muscles of the hip, but also can result in abnormal development of the hip joint itself. These abnormalities range from acetabular dysplasia and progressive arthritis to frank dislocation of the joint. These children present clinically with increasing hip pain associated with physical activity such as running. Marked adductor spasticity (scissor gait) contributes to the malalignments observed in the lower extremities.[18,41]

Children with athetoid CP exhibit slow, writhing, involuntary movements of the extremities, head, and neck. Activities that require accuracy, such as kicking a soccer ball, may be difficult in the more severely affected children. Sports that require balance will pose the greatest challenge, and perhaps the greatest risk, to children with the ataxic or atonic forms of CP. Their unsteady gait and lack of coordination make basic skills such as running and jumping quite difficult, and may lead to injury from falls.

The diverse presentations and range of severity of CP have necessitated the development of a functional classification system for athletic competition. The International Paralympic Committee (IPC) classification code used in the Paralympic Games takes into account trunk control, gross motor control, and strength of the extremities, as well as balance and fine motor control, with or without assistive devices. Classifications are specific for each sport because each sport requires a different set of abilities. Such a classification system is designed to permit more equitable competition among CP athletes with a wide range of disabilities.[42,43] Athletes with CP compete in many different sports, including cycling, power lifting, shooting, track, archery, bowling, table-tennis, snooker, football, basketball, volleyball, and swimming. The latter is a very good sport for children with CP, as swimming improves coordination and may relax spasticity.[18] Due to the high prevalence of epilepsy in CP, drowning is a real risk in this group; therefore, very close observation must be provided for all athletes with a seizure disorder. A history of a seizure disorder is not a contraindication to sport participation, if the seizures are well controlled. Athletes who have had a seizure within 6 months of sport participation or who have uncontrolled seizures should be carefully assessed prior to clearance.[44] Regardless of the sport, children with CP can benefit from PA and experience success in the competitive arena.

Children with myelomeningocoeles

Myelomeningocoele is the most common congenital anomaly of the nervous system. It results from a failure of the neural tube to close and affects approximately three to four per 10 000 live births.[45–47] Three-quarters of myelomeningocoeles occur in the lumbosacral region.[47] Myelomeningocoeles produce motor and sensory deficits as well as impairments in bowel and bladder function. Lesions in the lower sacral region have sparing of motor function. Eighty per cent of affected children have an associated hydrocephalus that can affect cognitive function and can further impair motor function. Furthermore, there is a high incidence of obesity in children with myelomeningocoele, making physical activity especially important.[48]

Children with myelomeningocoeles are classified according to their functional level, which corresponds to the most caudal functioning nerve root. Lower lesions may simply require bracing of the foot and ankle to permit sport participation, while athletes with higher lesions may perform best in a wheelchair. Swimming is a popular sport for many children with myelomeningocoeles since the upper extremities are often unaffected (see Figure 28.2). Sport participation depends not only on the functional level, but also on the presence of intellectual disability and degree of spasticity that results from associated hydrocephalus. These factors make this group extremely heterogeneous in abilities.

Type II Chiari defect, usually associated with myelomeningocoele, involves extension of cerebellar and brain stem tissue into the foramen magnum. Hydrocephalus, in association with a type II Chiari defect, develops in at least 80% of children with myelomeningocoele and often requires ventriculoperitoneal shunting.[47] Children with the associated Chiari malformation should be restricted from activities that have a significant risk of injury to the cervical spine such as diving, water skiing, and football.[5] In general, children with shunts should wear helmets for protection when participating in physical activities.[5]

Skin, bone, and muscle-tendon units are all at increased risk of injury in children with myelomeningocoeles. The lack of sensation below the level of the lesion leads to bruising, pressure sores, and skin breakdown from braces or wheelchair seats. Ensuring proper fit of adaptive equipment is paramount in the prevention of injuries, as is the use of appropriate cushioning and water absorptive clothing.[49] The risk of skin breakdown can be minimized by teaching children and their parents to inspect the skin regularly and to shift weight frequently. Lifting off the seat for 10–20 s intermittently throughout the day can be beneficial.[49] Racing wheelchair athletes may be at particularly high risk of pressure sores over the sacrum and ischium resulting from positioning of the knees higher than the hips for prolonged periods in these highly-specialized wheelchairs. Children who use braces should ensure that they are correctly positioned after each fall to reduce the likelihood of skin irritation from the brace.

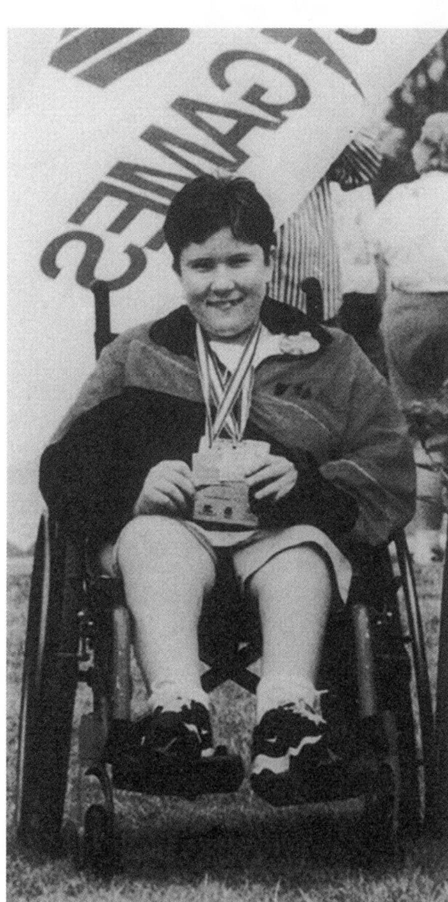

Figure 28.2 Young competitive swimmer proudly displays medals.

Limited weight-bearing results in osteopenia and increased risk of fractures. Fractures are particularly problematic in this group because of the sensory deficits that often result in delayed diagnosis. The incidence of fractures can be reduced by encouraging weight-bearing where possible and by limiting the period of immobilization following fracture.

Soft-tissue injuries such as muscle strains occur with greater frequency in this population. This is due to muscle weaknesses just above the level of the lesion and muscle imbalances resulting from spasticity. These children frequently have joint contractures that can significantly limit their range of motion. Special emphasis should be placed on range of motion and flexibility in the affected limbs, particularly if joint contractures are present.

Latex allergies are another concern in individuals with myelomeningocoeles. The reported prevalence of such allergies in this population ranges from 25–65%; therefore, it is important to ask for this pertinent past medical history and to avoid exposure in latex-allergic individuals.[50]

Children with spinal cord injuries

Evaluation of the epidemiology of spinal cord injuries in the United States over a 30-year period (1973 to 2003) revealed that 3.7% of cases occurred in patients under the age of 15 years and 51.6% occurred in people between the ages of 15 and 30 years.[51] Such injuries result in variable degrees of paralysis and sensory loss, along with dysfunction in other areas such as thermoregulation, circulation, and bowel and bladder control. The extent of the disability depends on the level of the spinal cord lesion and whether or not it is complete. Incomplete injuries allow some communication with areas distal to the injured cord. This results in some residual motor or sensory function below the level of the injury. Neurologic classification of spinal cord injury is based upon the lowest level of intact motor and sensory function.[52] In contrast, the functional classification system used in the Paralympic Games categorizes athletes according to their functional abilities.[32]

The most common injuries reported in young wheelchair athletes are blisters, wheel burns, bruises, and abrasions. These injuries result from contact with the wheelchair seat back, brakes, push rims, and wheels.[21] Lacerations can occur from collisions with other wheelchairs. Due to sensory and motor deficits, spinal cord-injured children experience many of the same problems as those with myelomeningocoeles. Contractures and muscle imbalances place these children at increased risk, with the shoulder being the most common site of injury to muscle-tendon units. The anterior shoulder is prone to excessive tightness due to poor posture and wheelchair pushing.[53] The latter can also result in muscle imbalances, with the shoulder flexor muscles being stronger than the extensors. Wheelchair athletes are at increased risk of shoulder injuries such as impingement syndromes and rotator cuff tendinitis. Proper pushing biomechanics can help prevent injuries to the shoulder.[54] The elbow and wrist are also frequent sites of overuse injuries, with medial and lateral epicondylitis as well as de Quervain's tenosynovitis being among the more common injuries at these sites.[21] Those who present with shoulder pain often have a relative weakness of the adductor muscles. Careful attention to stretching and to achieving balanced strength can reduce the likelihood of overuse injuries in the upper extremities. Skin breakdown and osteopenia also occur in the spinal cord-injured individual. The principles of management are the same as for those with myelomeningocoeles.

Nerve entrapment syndromes in the upper extremities are a problem for many wheelchair athletes. The numbness and weakness associated with carpal tunnel syndrome result from repetitive pressure of the heel of the hand on the push rim. Compression of the median or ulnar nerves can occur at the elbow as well. Radial tunnel syndrome should be considered in the differential diagnosis of lateral epicondylitis.[21]

Thermoregulation

Of particular concern for children with spinal cord injuries is impairment of thermoregulation. Able-bodied children are less efficient than adults at compensating for changes in ambient temperature. Children with lesions above T8 cannot maintain normal body temperature in the face of extreme environmental stresses.[31] Autonomic dysfunction impedes heat production mechanisms such as shivering, as well as heat dissipation mechanisms such as sweating, below the level of the spinal cord injury. While this problem also occurs in children with myelomeningocoeles, as mentioned previously, most of these neural tube defects occur in the lumbosacral region. The higher the lesion, the greater the impairment of thermoregulation; therefore, spinal cord-injured children with thoracic lesions are at greatest risk. Careful observation of both groups during events that take place in either high or low ambient temperatures will prevent hyperthermia or hypothermia respectively. Physicians who provide medical coverage at wheelchair athletic events must be prepared to deal with either outcome.

Autonomic dysreflexia

Autonomic dysreflexia occurs most frequently in quadriplegics and paraplegics with lesions above T6.[49] Noxious stimuli such as a full bladder or a fracture below the lesion cause mass activation of the sympathetic nervous system. Blood pressure rises dramatically as peripheral and splanchnic blood vessels vasoconstrict.[55,56] Due to sympathetic activation distal to the lesion, skin will be pale, cool, and clammy below the injury. Above the lesion, parasympathetic activation from the stimulation of carotid and aortic baroreceptors leads to marked vasodilation as well as facial flushing, sweating, nasal stuffiness, and bradycardia. This condition has been considered a medical emergency for years because of the potential for stroke. It also appears to enhance performance in wheelchair racing, which has prompted athletes to intentionally induce the condition by drinking excessively prior to a race or by clamping urinary catheters. This practice is extremely dangerous and is to be condemned. In the event that a wheelchair athlete presents with signs of autonomic dysreflexia, the urinary catheter should be inspected for a clamp or kink, and tight clothing or strapping of the lower extremities should be loosened. As it is difficult to place controls on the intentional induction of autonomic dysreflexia, athlete education may be the best defence against the potentially catastrophic outcome of this condition.

Amputees

Amputation refers to a partial or complete loss of one or more limbs and may be either congenital or acquired. Since the number of limbs affected and the level of the amputation vary considerably among amputees, classification systems based on these variables have been established for competition. The classification systems take into account whether the amputation is confined to a single arm or leg, or whether there are multiple amputations present. Athletes with amputations above the knee are distinguished from those with below-knee amputations. Similarly, athletes with above-elbow amputations compete in separate categories from those with below-elbow deficiencies. These systems provide a more equitable playing field for those whose disabilities vary greatly.[42]

Many amputees participate in physical activities with the use of prostheses (see Figures 28.3a and 28.3b) The prosthetic device is designed to compensate for any loss of function associated with the

(a)

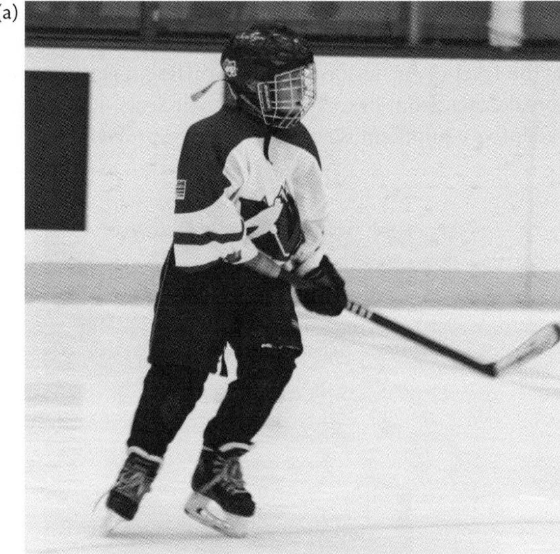

(b)

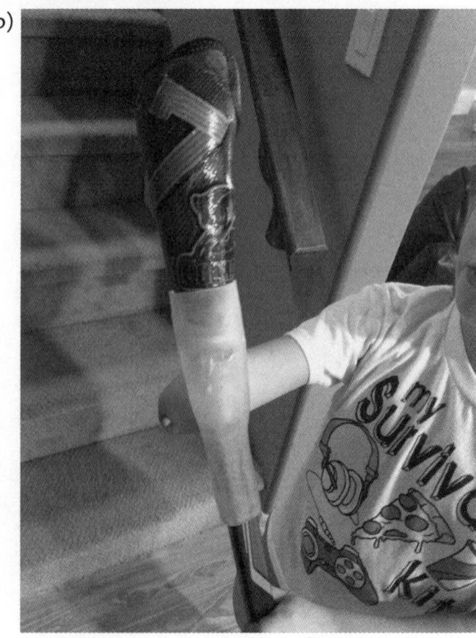

Figure 28.3 10-year-old amputee playing tier 3 hockey.

specific amputation. In the case of acquired amputations, early use of the prosthetic device facilitates its incorporation into the child's normal body actions.[57] It is very important that the prosthesis fit the child well; any discomfort may result in posture or gait disturbances. A good prosthesis alone is not enough to replace the deficient limb. The amputee must learn how to use the prosthesis, with some devices requiring more extensive training. Higher leg amputations may necessitate training with canes and crutches to master use of the prosthetic device.[57,58]

Children with amputations may have a decreased range of motion due to tight musculature or contractures. For example, a below-knee amputee who spends more time sitting than ambulating may develop tight hip and knee flexors. These children need to emphasize range of motion exercises in their training in order to reduce the risk of injuries to the muscle-tendon units. Balance is also adversely affected in amputees. For those with lower-limb amputations, this is due to the loss of proprioceptive feedback from the extremity. For those with acquired upper-limb amputations, the change in weight across the shoulder girdle affects balance. This is particularly hazardous in a sport such as figure skating, where balance is critical in preventing serious injuries from falls.[58]

In children, stump overgrowth is a frequent problem.[31] The bone begins to grow through the soft tissue left at the end of the stump, resulting in skin breakdown during physical activities. Children should be instructed to inspect the stump for erythema or skin breakdown, particularly if the stump begins to lose the cushioned feeling of the soft tissues. Surgical revision of the stump to prevent severe overgrowth may be required every 2–3 years and will facilitate continued pain-free participation in sports.[31] For those who wear a prosthesis during skiing, padding of the stump end can help prevent pressure sores and keep the stump warm.

An additional concern is for the integrity of the prosthesis. The stresses on the prosthesis during PA can be substantial, resulting in minor or major breakdowns of the device. Amputees should be instructed to inspect the prosthetic device regularly in order to detect problems before they develop into major breakdowns.

Specialized equipment and prosthetic devices for sport

In the evolution of any sport, technological advances in equipment may play a role in performance. Just as there have been advances in equipment for able-bodied individuals in sport, so have there been for athletes with physical disabilities. Highly specialized wheelchairs provide opportunities for non-ambulatory individuals with spinal cord injuries or myelomeningocoeles to participate in sports, such as wheelchair rugby, wheelchair basketball, and marathon racing.

Special mention should be made of snow skiing for amputees. In the early 1940s, Franz Wendel of Germany became the first person with a physical disability to compete as a skier after sustaining a leg injury that required amputation. Short ski tips were attached to the bottoms of crutches to aid in balance while skiing.[35] Since that time, significant improvements have been made to equipment design. Three-track skiing is used by those with a single leg amputation with or without one upper-extremity prosthesis. One full-length ski is attached to the sound leg, while two short outrigger skis on forearm crutches are manoeuvred by the upper extremities. Children tend to ski without their lower limb prostheses for improved balance and agility, while those with below-knee amputations who begin to ski during late adolescence tend to ski with the prosthesis, primarily for cosmetic reasons. Competitive athletes with above-knee amputations usually ski without their prosthesis.

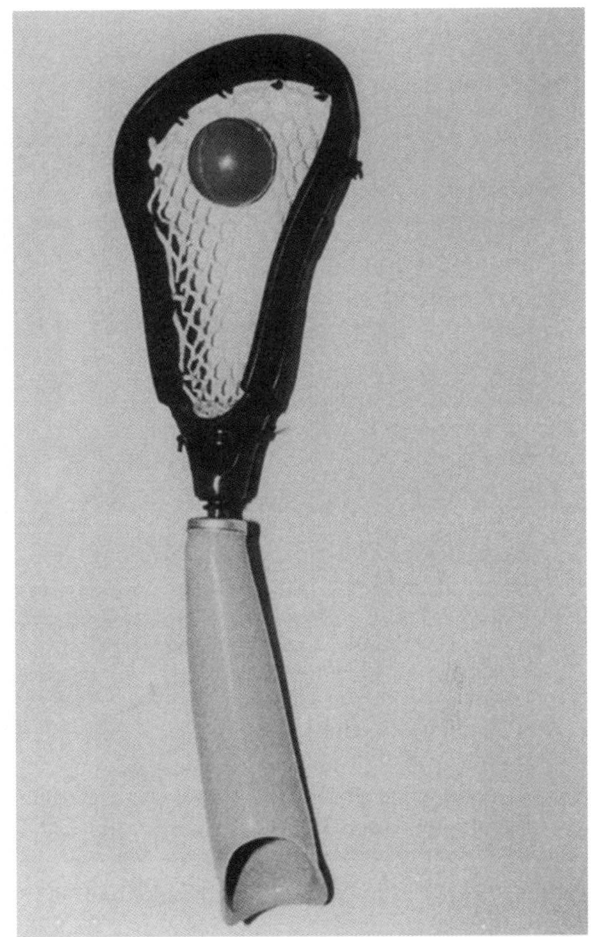

Figure 28.4 Terminal prosthesis to facilitate participation in baseball by children with upper limb amputations.

A number of highly specialized terminal prosthetic devices have been developed in order to allow children with amputations to participate in a wide variety of activities. Upper-limb prostheses have been used very successfully for a variety of physical activities including swimming, baseball (Figure 28.4), golf, basketball, skiing, dirt biking (Figure 28.5), cycling, and ice hockey. With the aid of a

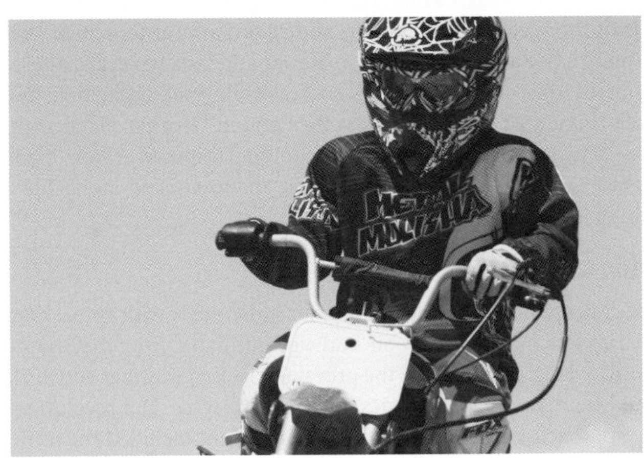

Figure 28.5 Specialized prosthesis for cycling and dirt biking.

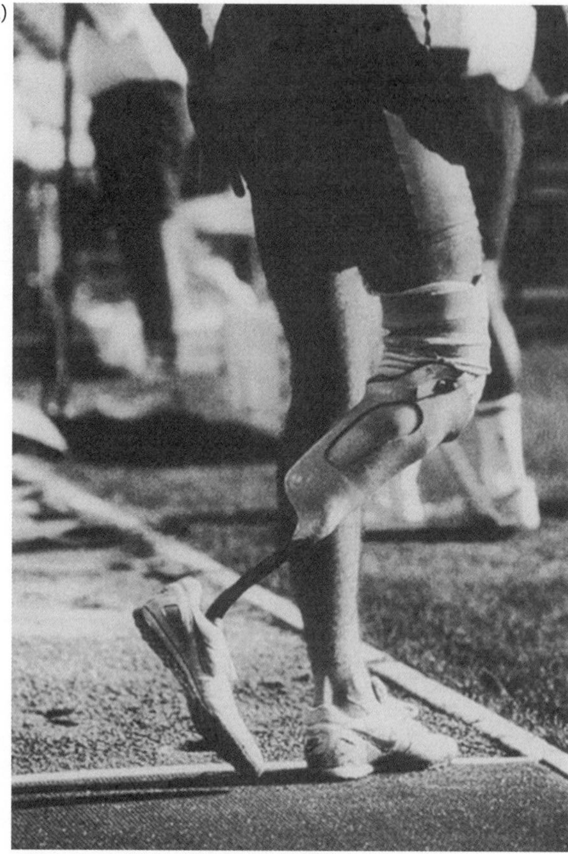

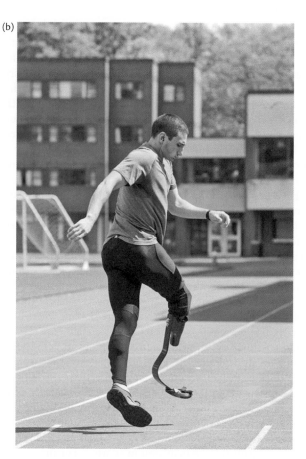

Figure 28.6 (a) Specialized prosthesis worn by an athlete at the Paralympic Games in Barcelona, 1992; (b) new carbon-fibre running prosthesis with blade positioned toward the rear of the socket.
Note the absence of a prosthetic heel.

hockey prosthesis, many young amputees are able to participate in hockey on a level equal to their able-bodied peers up to Bantam division (age 14 years).[95] Refinements in prosthetic design are ongoing, allowing improved performance in many different sports.

While performance has improved in both Olympic and Paralympic sports over the past couple of decades, none more so than in athletes with lower-limb amputations.[59,60] New lower-limb prosthetic devices provide amputees with near normal foot function. These carbon graphite prostheses store and release energy, which allows for an active push-off during running or jumping.[61] Design changes such as the repositioning of the blade toward the rear of the socket (Figures 28.6a and 28.6b) appear to benefit performance.[60] Such advances in material and design of prostheses facilitate involvement in sports such as volleyball, basketball, and track (Figure 28.7). Spectators at the London Olympic Games witnessed history in the making as a double amputee athlete using highly specialized running prosthetic devices raced alongside a field of able-bodied Olympians.

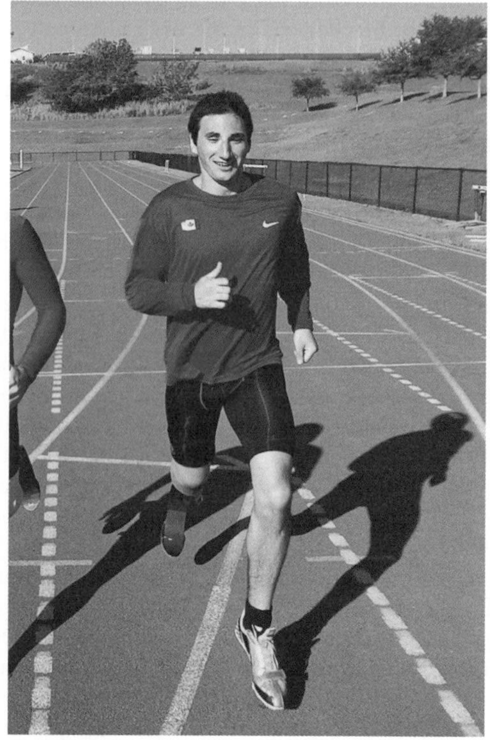

Figure 28.7 Elite Paralympic athlete training with carbon-fibre running prosthesis.

Wheelchair sports

The concept of sport participation for individuals with spinal cord injuries was introduced by Sir Ludwig Guttman during the Second World War, at a time when the prevailing feeling was that very little could be done for paraplegics and quadriplegics. His revolutionary approach to the spinal cord-injured patient included the introduction of the first competitive team sport for paraplegics, namely wheelchair polo. Soon after, wheelchair basketball and badminton were added to the list of sports for patients with spinal cord injuries, followed by archery and table tennis. On 28 July 1948, the Stoke Mandeville Games for the Paralysed were founded. They are held annually in Ayelsbury, England, except every fourth year, when they are held in the country hosting the Olympic Games. The first city to host the International Stoke Mandeville Games outside of England was Rome in 1960, when 400 athletes from 23 countries competed in the Olympic Stadium following the Olympic Games.[60] These Games became known as the Paraplegic Olympic Games, or Paralympics, and have grown dramatically since their inception. In 1992, more than one million spectators attended the Paralympics in Barcelona. Twenty years later, over 4200 athletes from 164 countries participated in the 2012 London Paralympics, with 2.7 million spectators in attendance.[62]

Popular wheelchair sports include tennis, volleyball, archery, bowling, track and field, marathon road racing, quad rugby, and basketball. Sport-specific modifications to wheelchairs optimize athletic performance. Wheelchair basketball was the first organized sport for paraplegics in the United States, with athletes achieving high skill levels. Modifications to rules have been made to facilitate wheelchair sports. For example, in basketball, a traveling violation occurs when an athlete performs three or more pushes of the wheelchair without bouncing the ball. Thanks to the initiative of Sir Ludwig Guttman and others around the world, spinal cord-injured individuals who were thought of as 'hopeless cripples'.[63] 50 years ago now participate in sports at an elite level and achieve things unimaginable to many able-bodied athletes.

Children with intellectual disability

Intellectual disability, which affects approximately 3% of the population, is characterized by impairments in measured intelligence and adaptive functioning.[64,65] The severity of intellectual disability is based on both clinical assessment of function and standardized testing of intelligence (IQ). Intellectual disability is considered to be approximately two standard deviations or more below the population mean, which equals an IQ score of 70 or below. Severity is based on an assessment of function across three domains; conceptual, social, and practical.[64] The conceptual domain includes skills in language, reading, writing, maths, reasoning, knowledge, and memory. The social domain refers to empathy, social judgment, interpersonal communication skills, the ability to make and retain friendships, and similar capacities. The practical domain centres on self-management in areas such as personal care, job responsibilities, money management, recreation, and organizing school and work tasks.[64,65]

The aetiology of intellectual disability can be categorized into prenatal, perinatal, and postnatal causes. Prenatal causes include genetic conditions (e.g. Down syndrome, fragile X syndrome, tuberous sclerosis, and inborn errors of metabolism), in-utero infections (e.g. cytomegalovirus, toxoplasmosis, and rubella) and toxin exposure (e.g. alcohol and lead).[65,66] Important perinatal causes of intellectual disability include infections (e.g. herpes simplex virus and meningitis), perinatal asphyxia, hyperbilirubinemia, and prematurity.[65] Postnatally, environmental and psychosocial factors can have a profound influence on developmental outcomes, including intellectual ability.[65,66] The effect that intellectual impairment has on function is as varied as the underlying causes. The most common genetic cause of intellectual disability is Down syndrome (DS). Children with DS must face many issues related to PA and sport participation that their 'normal' peers do not.

Down syndrome

Down syndrome, or Trisomy-21, is the most frequent human chromosomal syndrome, occurring in approximately one in 800 live births.[67] It occurs when an extra chromosome 21 is present through nondisjunction or translocation. If nondisjunction occurs after the first cell division following conception, only some of the cell lines will have trisomy 21, while others will have a normal chromosomal complement. Children affected by this mosaicism tend to have a milder phenotype.[67] The craniofacial features, including oblique palpebral fissures, epicanthic folds, brushfield spots, protruding tongue, prominent malformed ears, flat nasal bridge, and flat occiput, make DS the best recognized of the chromosomal syndromes. Of particular relevance to the sport medicine physician are the musculoskeletal and cardiovascular anomalies, as well as the cognitive impairment associated with this syndrome. Through proper screening prior to physical activity or sport participation, many children with DS can become active in a wide variety of sports and leisure activities.

Most of the musculoskeletal abnormalities observed in DS result from a defect in collagen synthesis that leads to ligamentous laxity and contributes to generalized hypotonia. As a result, children with DS are at increased risk of problems associated with hyperflexibility including atlantoaxial instability (AAI), patellofemoral syndrome, hip joint instability, and pes planus. The development of bunions is another common complaint that is often associated with the presence of pes planus and hyperpronation of the foot and is usually managed with shoe modifications.[68] Slipped capital femoral epiphysis is seen with slightly increased incidence in children with DS, and is likely due to the increased incidence of obesity and thyroid dysfunction in this population.[68,69] Many osseous abnormalities have been associated with patients with DS, including hypoplastic atlas/odontoid, congenitally abnormal C2, os odontoideum, ossicum terminale, bifid odontoid process, third condyle, bifid C1, scoliosis, multiple fused vertebrae, ovoid dens, and occipitalization of the atlas.[70]

Atlantoaxial instability

Atlantoaxial instability, which can lead to subsequent dislocation and spinal cord compression, is potentially the most serious musculoskeletal problem associated with DS.[71] It is also the most controversial area in the management of these children. The incidence of AAI in children with DS under 21 years of age is approximately 15%[72] and one to 2% of individuals with DS have symptomatic AAI.[73] The subluxation is due to laxity of the annular ligament of C1 as well as the generalized hypotonia seen in DS. Nearly all people with AAI who have suffered a catastrophic injury to the spinal cord have had preceding neurologic symptoms, which highlights the importance of a careful history and physical examination and an awareness of this association.

Because of the potential for permanent neurologic disability resulting from AAI, the Special Olympics issued a bulletin in 1983 restricting athletes with DS from participating in any activities that might cause injury to the neck and upper spine until they had been examined for AAI. Individuals who were found to have asymptomatic AAI were permanently restricted from participation in certain Special Olympics activities that placed them at increased risk of injury. These activities included gymnastics, diving, pentathlon, butterfly stroke in swimming, diving starts in swimming, high jump, and warm-up activities that placed undue stress on the head and neck muscles.[74,1] The following year, the American Academy of Pediatrics (AAP) issued a policy statement recommending that all children with DS who wished to participate in sports that involve possible trauma to the head and neck have lateral cervical spine radiographs in neutral, flexion, and extension prior to beginning training or competition.[75] This recommendation applied only to those who had not previously had normal radiologic findings. The AAP recommended restriction from high-risk sports when the distance between the odontoid process of the axis and the anterior arch of the atlas exceeded 4.5 mm or the odontoid was abnormal. Children with atlantoaxial subluxation and neurologic signs or symptoms were restricted from all strenuous activities and operative stabilization of the cervical spine was considered. Those with DS who did not have evidence of AAI could participate in all sports with no further follow-up unless neurologic signs or symptoms developed.[75]

The AAP retired the 1984 policy statement following a subject review in 1995.[72] The AAP reviewed the data on which their earlier recommendation was made and decided that there was uncertainty regarding the value of cervical spine radiographs in screening for possible catastrophic neck injury in individuals with DS and that radiologic screening for AAI failed to meet the criteria of Sackett *et al.*[76] Specifically, the radiologic test for AAI had poor reproducibility and there was limited evidence that screening programmes were effective in preventing symptomatic disease.

Assessing children with DS for neurologic signs and symptoms can be extremely challenging.[77] Their ability to verbalize regarding neuromotor difficulties or neck discomfort can be limited and they may not be cooperative during physical examinations.[78] Nevertheless, a careful neurological evaluation for signs and symptoms consistent with spinal cord compromise is the best clinical predictor of atlantoaxial instability. This screening should be done at least annually.[72,79] Health professionals and parents of children with DS should be aware of the importance of protecting the cervical spine during any anaesthetic, surgical, or radiographic procedure that requires extremes of head position. Parents should be advised that participation in some sports, including contact sports and gymnastics, places all children, but particularly those with DS, at increased risk of spinal cord injury. Potential dangers of trampolines should also be discussed with families, as children with DS may be at even greater risk of serious cervical spine injury than those without DS.[80,81] Importantly, parents of children with DS should receive counselling on the early signs of AAI. Any change in use of upper or lower extremities, change in gait, weakness, loss of bowel or bladder control, neck pain, radicular pain, stiff neck, torticollis, or change in general function should prompt an evaluation by a physician. Plain cervical spine radiography in the neutral position should be performed as part of the initial evaluation, keeping in mind that the child must be a minimum of 3 years of age to have adequate vertebral mineralization and epiphyseal development for accurate radiographic evaluation.[81] Children with signs or symptoms concerning for spinal cord compromise should have their cervical spine immobilized. Magnetic resonance imaging should be performed to evaluate the extent of spinal cord compression and they should be referred urgently to a surgical specialist for definitive treatment.

Although current evidence does not support the use of routine screening radiographs in asymptomatic children, it is important to note that Special Olympics still requires screening lateral radiographs of the cervical spine in children with DS prior to participation. Hankinson and Anderson[82] note that there have been no reports of cervical spinal cord injury during Special Olympics events, despite over 40 such cases reported in the literature. They suggest that screening may have played a role in prevention of injury in some cases.[82] O'Connor *et al.*[83] suggest that a single lateral radiograph with the neck in active flexion could be used to assess the atlanto-dens interval (ADI), rather than flexion, neutral, and extension views, since the ADI is widest in this position. This would minimize the exposure to radiation in situations where screening for AAI is still required for sport participation.

Cervical spine abnormalities occur in 40% of DS individuals.[84] Although AAI is by far the most common, other cervical spine abnormalities exist, such as abnormal vertebral bodies (especially C-2), multiple vertebral fusions, hypoplastic posterior arch of C-1, odontoid abnormalities, and spondylolysis and spondylolisthesis of the midcervical vertebrae.[85] The presence of an os odontoideum, seen in association with DS, can contribute to a greater risk of atlantoaxial instability requiring surgical stabilization.[70] In one series, 10 out of 12 cases of symptomatic AAI had an os odontoideum present.[71] If screening lateral radiographs are required by sport organizations prior to sport participation, not only should AAI be evaluated, but other craniocervical abnormalities should be ruled out.

Instability may also occur between the atlas and the occiput, increasing the risk of neurologic injury particularly if the neck is extended. Although radiographic evaluation and normative values for DS have not been well defined for the atlantooccipital region,[86] instability may be detected on lateral radiographs.[73,74] Atlantooccipital instability (AOI) has been shown to occur in about 18% of DS patients; however, neurologic symptoms relating to AOI are rare.[87] The utility of radiologic screening for AOI has not been established.

Other musculoskeletal issues

Patellofemoral instability is a concern for many children with DS. In 32% of individuals with DS, the patella subluxes or dislocates, resulting in significant impairment in sports and activities of daily living.[88] This instability results from ligamentous laxity in conjunction with anatomic abnormalities such as genu valgus, patella alta, or hypoplastic medial femoral condyle. Pes planus, also due to severe, generalized ligamentous laxity, is seen frequently in children with DS; therefore, use of orthotics may be necessary both in the management of patellofemoral symptoms and in the treatment of foot pain. Excessive joint laxity may affect the hips and often presents as a loud clunking or popping sound. This condition causes gradual degeneration of the hip joint, the extent of which is not certain. These individuals have poor gait and limited ambulation.[88] Prevention of hip damage is difficult but may be attempted using casting or abduction bracing. Even with surgical correction, hip instability may recur.

Medical conditions associated with Down syndrome

In addition to the various musculoskeletal problems that may afflict young individuals with DS, there are several medical problems that need to be followed carefully throughout infancy, childhood, and into adulthood. Children with DS have a higher prevalence of congenital heart anomalies and are at increased risk of thyroid disease, obesity, type 2 diabetes mellitus, obstructive sleep apnoea, gastrointestinal problems (intestinal atresias, Hirschprung's disease), seizures, and autoimmune conditions (coeliac disease, rheumatoid arthritis, type 1 diabetes mellitus, alopecia areata, autoimmune thyroiditis).[89] In addition, there may be psychological issues such as depression, behavioural problems, and varying degrees of intellectual disability that can impact participation in physical activities.[89]

Fifty percent of children with DS have congenital heart anomalies such as atrioventricular canal defects (endocardial cushion defects), ventricular septal defects, atrial septal defects, patent ductus arteriosus, and tetralogy of Fallot. As such, a cardiology consultation and echocardiogram are recommended in the neonatal period. Valvular disease, such as mitral valve prolapse, mitral regurgitation, and aortic regurgitation, is found more commonly in DS than in the general population and typically presents in early adulthood.[90] Prior to sport participation, children with DS should have a thorough history and physical examination with particular attention to the cardiovascular system. With respect to the gastrointestinal system, intestinal atresias occur at a higher frequency in DS than in the general population and typically present in the newborn period. Hirschsprung's disease typically presents in the newborn period in DS, but may present in childhood as chronic constipation.

Up to 75% of children with DS have some degree of hearing impairment; therefore, hearing should be tested every 6 months until normal hearing levels are established, then annually thereafter.[81] Ophthalmologic screening should be performed annually to 5 years of age, every 2 years from 5 to 13 years of age, and every 3 years thereafter, since 15% of patients develop cataracts and 50% of patients have severe refractive errors.[81]

It is estimated that half of all people with intellectual disability are overweight.[91] With obesity comes a multitude of potential medical complications, including hypertension, hypertriglyceridemia, and type 2 diabetes mellitus. Screening should be done at least yearly in the presence of obesity. Obesity is also associated with obstructive sleep apnoea (OSA). Symptoms of OSA such as snoring, brief periods of apnoea when sleeping, restless sleep, or excessive daytime sleepiness, should be screened for history and patients referred to a specialist as indicated. Obstructive sleep apnoea unabated can lead to sleep deprivation, symptoms of inattention and hyperactivity, and can adversely impact growth and overall development. Long term, it can have harmful effects on the cardiovascular system.[92]

Wound management in children with DS can be a challenge. Poorly controlled diabetes is associated with delayed wound healing;[91] therefore, emphasis on good glycaemic control and prevention of skin breakdown is vital. Proper fitting footwear and orthoses are essential.

Special Olympics

Special Olympics International began serving children and adults with intellectual disability in 1968. Participation in Special Olympics helps develop better socialization and physical skills in this population. It increases the individual's self-confidence and independence. Today, over 150 countries around the world offer this programme for children and adults with intellectual disabilities. Athletes, who are grouped according to age and ability, compete in summer sports such as track and field, swimming, powerlifting, rhythmic gymnastics, soccer, softball, and bowling. Official winter sports include Alpine and Nordic skiing, figure skating, speed skating, snowshoeing, and floor hockey. Over 30 000 athletes participate in the programme in Canada, and many more are involved throughout the world.[93] Athletes begin with local level competitions and, like their peers without intellectual disability, can progress to international competitions which are held every 4 years and are analogous to the Olympic Games.[93] The spirit of Special Olympics is encompassed in the Special Olympics athlete oath: 'Let me win but if I cannot win, let me be brave in the attempt'.

Conclusions

The twentieth century has witnessed a dramatic change in the public's perception of individuals with disabilities. New opportunities have allowed these children to experience the many benefits of sport participation once reserved exclusively for the able-bodied child. With this new participation, the field of sport medicine has had to expand in order to allow a greater understanding of the issues unique to each child with a disability. From the late 1800s, when baseball was first introduced at the Ohio School for the Deaf to the world-class Paralympic Games of today, athletes with disabilities have reached heights many of us will never achieve.

> You are the living demonstration of the marvels of the virtue of energy. You have given a great example, which we would like to emphasize, it can be a lead to all: you have shown what an energetic soul can achieve, in spite of apparently insurmountable obstacles imposed by the body. (Pope John XXIII, at the International Stoke Mandeville Games in Rome, 1960.[94])

Summary

- Children with disabilities experience many benefits from physical activity and sport participation, including increased confidence and self-esteem, improved physical fitness, and opportunities for social development.
- Deaf athletes often play and compete with hearing athletes, but have additional challenges related to communication with team members.
- Modifications of rules and equipment facilitate physical activity in children with visual impairment.
- Advances in equipment and prosthetic devices facilitate participation and optimize performance in many different sports by amputees and wheelchair athletes.
- Spasticity and joint contractures in children with cerebral palsy increase the risks of injury.
- Lack of sensation below the lesion in myelomeningocoeles or spinal cord injuries predisposes the child to pressure-related injuries; therefore, proper fit of adaptive devices and use of appropriate cushioning may prevent skin breakdown, bruising, and pressure sores.
- Osteopenia secondary to limited weight-bearing in wheelchair athletes increases the risk of fracture, which may be masked by sensory deficits.
- Latex allergies are common in individuals with myelomeningocoeles.

- Children with spinal cord lesions above T8 are particularly susceptible to heat-related illness due to impairment of heat production and dissipation mechanisms.
- Autonomic dysreflexia should be suspected in the wheelchair athlete with pale, cool, clammy skin below the lesion and facial flushing, nasal stuffiness, and sweating above the lesion. Hypertension and bradycardia are also present.
- If autonomic dysreflexia is suspected, urinary catheters should be inspected for clamps or kinks, and tight clothing or strapping of lower extremities should be loosened.
- The change in weight across the shoulder girdle in acquired upper-limb amputations affects balance and poses a greater risk for falls in some sports.
- Children with amputations should inspect their stumps regularly for skin breakdown and additional padding can help prevent pressure sores in some sports.
- Although evidence does not support the routine use of radiographs to screen for atlantoaxial instability in asymptomatic children with Down syndrome, such investigations are still required by Special Olympics prior to sport participation.
- A single lateral radiograph of the cervical spine in flexion may be adequate to assess the atlanto-dens interval where screening is still required by Special Olympics.
- A history of associated medical conditions should be sought in any athlete with a disability.

References

1. Birrer RB. The special olympics athlete: Evaluation and clearance for participation. *Clin Pediatr (Phila)*. 2004; 43: 777–782.
2. Rimmer JH, Braddock D, Fujiura G. Prevalence of obesity in adults with mental retardation: implications for health promotion and disease prevention. *Ment Retard*. 1993; 31: 105–110.
3. Murphy NA, Carbone PS. American Academy of Pediatrics council on children with disabilities: promoting the participation of children with disabilities in sports, recreation, and physical activities. *Pediatrics*. 2008; 121: 1057–1061.
4. Groff DG, Lundberg NR, Zabriskie RB. Influence of adapted sport on quality of life: perceptions of athletes with cerebral palsy. *Disabil Rehabil*. 2009; 31: 318–326.
5. Patel DR, Greydanus DE. Sport participation by physically and cognitively challenged young athletes. *Pediatr Clin North Am*. 2010; 57: 795–817.
6. Hyndman JC. The Growing Athlete. In Harries M, Williams C, Stanish WD, Micheli LJ (eds.) *Oxford textbook of sports medicine*, 2nd ed. Oxford: Oxford University Press; 1998. p. 727–741.
7. Haslam DW, James WPT. Obesity. *Lancet*. 2005; 366: 1197–1209.
8. Wang Y, Beydoun MA. The obesity epidemic in the United States gender, age, socioeconomic, racial/ethnic, and geographic characteristics: a systematic review and meta-regression analysis. *Epidemiol Rev*. 2007; 29: 6–28.
9. Segal M, Misha E, Phillips S, Bandini L, *et al*. Intellectual disability is associated with increased risk for obesity in a nationally representative sample of US children. *Disabil Health J*. 2016; 9: 392–398.
10. Pitetti KH, Campbell KD. Mentally retarded individuals—a population at risk? *Med Sci Sports Exerc*. 1991; 23: 586–593.
11. Fernhall B. Physical fitness and exercise training of individuals with mental retardation. *Med Sci Sports Exerc*. 1993; 25: 442–450.
12. Varni JW, Setoguchi Y. Correlates of perceived physical appearance in children with congenital/acquired limb deficiencies. *J Dev Behav Pediatr*. 1991; 12: 171–176.
13. Wetterhahn KA, Hanson C, Levy CE. Effect of participation in physical activity on body image of amputees. *Am J Phys Med Rehabil*. 2002; 81: 194–201.
14. Weiss J, Diamond T, Demark J, *et al*. Involvement in Special Olympics and its relations to self-concept and actual competency in participants with developmental disabilities. *Res Dev Disabil*. 2003; 24: 281–305.
15. Crawford C, Burns J, Fernie BA. Psychosocial impact of involvement in the Special Olympics. *Res Dev Disabil*. 2015; 45–46: 93–102.
16. Schindl MR, Forstner C, Kern H, *et al*. Treadmill training with partial body weight support in nonambulatory patients with cerebral palsy. *Arch Phys Med Rehabil*. 2000; 81: 301–306.
17. Fragala-Pinkham MA, Haley SM, Goodgold S. Evaluation of a community-based group fitness program for children with disabilities. *Pediatr Phys Ther*. 2006; 18: 159–167.
18. Guttman L. Sports for sufferers from cerebral palsy. In: Guttman L (ed.) *Textbook of sport for the disabled*. Aylesbury: HM+ M Publishers Ltd; 1976. p. 162–169.
19. Carroll KL, Leiser J, Paisley TS. Cerebral palsy: physical activity and sport. *Curr Sports Med Rep*. 2006; 5: 319–322.
20. Dodd KJ, Shields N. A systematic review of the outcomes of cardiovascular exercise programs for people with Down syndrome. *Arch Phys Med Rehabil*. 2005; 86: 2051–2058.
21. Schutz LK. The wheelchair athlete. In: Buschbacher RM, Braddom RL (eds.) *Sports medicine and rehabilitation: a sport-specific approach*. Philadelphia: Hanley & Belfus, Inc; 1994. p. 267–274.
22. Guttman L. Sports for the blind and partially sighted. In: Guttman L (ed.) *Textbook of sport for the disabled*. Aylesbury: HM+ M Publishers Ltd; 1976. p. 150–161.
23. Craft DH. Visual impairments and hearing losses. In: Winnick JP (ed.) *Adapted physical education and sport*. Windsor, ON: Human Kinetics; 1995. p. 143–166.
24. Haddad J. The Ear. In: Nelson WE (ed.) *Nelson textbook of paediatrics*, 17th ed. Philadelphia: Saunders Company; 2004. p. 2127–2150.
25. Winnick JP. Introduction to adapted physical education and sport. In: Winnick JP (ed.) *Adapted Physical Education and Sport*, 5th ed. Windsor, ON: Human Kinetics; 2011. p. 3–20.
26. Ohio School for the Deaf. Available from: www.ohioschoolforthedeaf.org/en-us/aboutus/ourhistory.aspx [Accessed 31 Jan 2016].
27. Hartman E, Houwen S, Visscher C. Motor skill performance and sports participation in deaf elementary school children. *Adapt Phys Activ Q*. 2011; 28: 132–145.
28. De Kegel A, Maes L, Baetens T, *et al*. The Influence of a vestibular dysfunction in the motor development of hearing-impaired children. *Laryngoscope*. 2012; 122: 2837–2843.
29. Guttman, L. Sports for the deaf. In: Guttman L (ed.) *Textbook of sport for the disabled*. Aylesbury: HM+ M Publishers Ltd; 1976. p. 170–173.
30. Palmer T, Weber KM. The deaf athlete. *Curr Sports Med Rep*. 2006; 5: 323–326.
31. Chang FM. Physically disabled athletes. In: Anderson SJ, Harris SS (eds.) *Care of the young athlete*, 2nd ed. Elk Grove Village, IL: American Academy of Pediatrics; 2010. p. 153–168.
32. Booth DW, Grogono BJ. Athletes with a disability. In: Harries M, Williams C, Stanish WD, Micheli LJ (eds.) *Oxford textbook of sports medicine*, 2nd ed. Oxford: Oxford University Press; 1998. p. 815–831.
33. Lieberman LJ. Hard of hearing, deaf, or deafblind. In: Winnick JP (ed.) *Adapted physical education and sport*, 5th ed. Windsor, ON: Human Kinetics; 2011. p. 251–267.
34. International Blind Sports Federation. Available from: www.ibsasport.org/classification. [Accessed 31 Jan 2016].
35. Laskowski ER. Snow skiing for the physically disabled. *Mayo Clin Proc*. 1991; 66: 160–172.
36. Spiegel DA. Cerebral Palsy. In: Dormans JP (ed.) *Pediatric orthopaedics and sports medicine—The requisites in paediatrics*. St. Louis, MS: Mosby; 2004. p. 373–415.

37. Johnston MV. Encephalopathies. In: Kliegman RM, Stanton BF, St Geme JW, Schor NF (eds.) *Nelson textbook of pediatrics*, 20th ed. Philadelphia, PA: Elsevier; 2016. p. 2896–2910.
38. Richter KE, Hyman SC, Mushett-Adams CA. Injuries in world-class cerebral palsy athletes at the 1988 South Korea Paralympics. *J Osteopath Sports Med.* 1991; 5: 15–18.
39. Soprano JV. Musculoskeletal injuries in the pediatric and adolescent athlete. *Curr Sports Med Rep.* 2005; 4: 329–334.
40. Patatoukas D, Farmakides A, Aggeli V, *et al.* Disability-related injuries in athletes with disabilities. *Folia Med.* 2011: 53: 40–46.
41. Poretta DL. Cerebral palsy, traumatic brain injury, and stroke. In: Winnick JP (ed.) *Adapted physical education and sport*, 5th ed. Windsor, ON: Human Kinetics; 2011. p. 269–289.
42. Tweedy SM, Vanlandewijck YC. International Paralympic Committee position stand—background and scientific principles of classification in Paralympic sport. *Br J Sports Med.* 2011; 45: 259–269
43. Simon LM, Ward DC. Preparing for events for physically challenged athletes. *Curr Sports Med Rep.* 2014; 13: 163–168.
44. Metzl JD. Preparticipation Examination of the Adolescent Athlete: Part 1. *Pediatr Rev.* 2001; 22: 199–204.
45. Parker SE, Mai CT, Canfield MA, *et al.* Updated National Birth Prevalence estimates for selected birth defects in the United States, 2004–2006. *Birth Defects Res A Clin Mol Teratol.* 2010; 88: 1008–1016.
46. Atta CAM, Fiest KM, Frolkis AD, *et al.* Global birth prevalence of spina bifida by folic acid fortification status: A systematic review and meta-analysis. *Am J Public Health.* 2016; 106: e24–e34.
47. Kinsman SL, Johnston MV. Congenital anomalies of the central nervous system. In: Kliegman RM, Stanton BF, St Geme JW, Schor NF (eds.) *Nelson textbook of pediatrics*, 20th ed. Philadelphia, PA: Elsevier; 2016. p. 2802–2819.e1.
48. van den Berg-Emons HJK, Bussmann JBJ, Meyerink HJ, *et al.* Body fat, fitness and level of everyday physical activity in adolescents and young adults with meningomyelocele. *J Rehabil Med.* 2003; 35: 271–275.
49. Dec K. The physically challenged athlete. In: Madden CC, Putukian M, Young CC, McCarty EC (eds.) *Netter's sports medicine.* Philadephia: Saunders; 2010. p. 101–109.
50. Randolph C. Latex allergy in pediatrics. *Curr Probl Pediatr.* 2001; 31: 135–153.
51. Jackson AB, Dijkers M, DeVivo MJ, *et al.* A demographic profile of new traumatic spinal cord injuries: change and stability over 30 years. *Arch Phys Med Rehabil.* 2004; 85: 1740–1748.
52. Kirshblum SC, Burns SP, Biering-Sorensen F, *et al.* International standards for neurological classification of spinal cord injury (Revised 2011). *J Spinal Cord Med.* 2011; 34: 535–546.
53. Aytar A, Zeybek A, Pekyavas NO, *et al.* Scapular resting position, shoulder pain and function in disabled athletes. *Prosthet Orthot Int.* 2015; 39: 390–396.
54. Churton E, Keogh JW. Constraints influencing sports wheelchair propulsion performance and injury risk. *BMC Sports Sci Med Rehabil.* 2013; 5: 3.
55. Blackmer J. Rehabilitation Medicine: 1. Autonomic Dysreflexia. *CMAJ.* 2003; 169: 931–935.
56. Perrouin-Verbe B. Autonomic dysreflexia (AD): What is it? Pathophysiology and criteria of diagnosis. *Ann Phys Rehabil Med.* 2014; 57: e226.
57. Poretta DL. Amputations, dwarfism, and les autres. In: Winnick JP (ed.) *Adapted physical education and sport*, 5th ed. Windsor, ON: Human Kinetics; 2011. p. 291–310.
58. Guttman, L. Sports for amputees. In: Guttman L (ed.) *Textbook of sport for the disabled.* Aylesbury: HM + M Publishers Ltd; 1976. p. 119–149.
59. Burkett B. Paralympic sports medicine—current evidence in winter sport: considerations in the development of equipment standards for paralympic athletes. *Clin J Sport Med.* 2012; 22: 46–50.
60. Grobler L, Ferreira S, Terblanche E. Paralympic sprint performance between 1992 and 2012. *Int J Sports Physiol Perform.* 2015; 10: 1052–1054.
61. Nolan L. Carbon fibre prostheses and running in amputees: a review. *Foot Ankle Surg.* 2008; 14:125–129.
62. International Paralympic Committee. Available from: www.paralympic.org/london-2012. [Accessed 31 Jan 2016].
63. Guttman, L. Wheelchair sports for spinal para- and tetraplegics. In: Guttman L (ed.) *Textbook of sport for the disabled.* Aylesbury: HM+ M Publishers Ltd; 1976. p. 21–46.
64. American Psychiatric Association. *Diagnostic and statistical manual of mental disorders*, 5th ed. Arlington, VA: American Psychiatric Publishing; 2013.
65. Shapiro BK, Batshaw ML. Intellectual Disability. In: Kliegman RM, Stanton BF, St Geme JW, Schor NF (eds.) *Nelson textbook of pediatrics*, 20th ed. Philadelphia, PA: Elsevier; 2016. p. 216–222.
66. Shevell M. Global developmental delay and mental retardation or intellectual disability: Conceptualization, evaluation, and etiology. *Pediatr Clin North Am.* 2008; 55: 1071–1084.
67. Bacino CA, Lee B. Cytogenetics. In: Kliegman RM, Stanton BF, St Geme JW, Schor NF (eds.) *Nelson textbook of pediatrics*, 20th ed. Philadelphia, PA: Elsevier; 2016. p. 604–627.
68. Pizzutillo PD, Herman MJ. Musculoskeletal concerns in the young athlete with down syndrome. *Oper Tech Sports Med.* 2006; 14: 135–140.
69. Bosch P, Johnston CE, Karol L. Slipped capital femoral epiphysis in patients with Down syndrome. *J Pediatr Orthop.* 2004; 24: 271–277.
70. Hwang SW, Jea A. A review of the neurological and neurosurgical implications of Down syndrome in children. *Clin Pediatr (Phila).* 2013; 52: 845–856.
71. Nader-Sepahi A, Casey AT, Hayward R, *et al.* Symptomatic atlantoaxial instability in Down syndrome. *J Neurosurg.* 2005; 103(3 Suppl): 231–237.
72. American Academy of Pediatrics. Atlantoaxial instability in Down syndrome: subject review. *Pediatrics.* 1995; 96: 151–154.
73. Pueschel SM. Should children with Down syndrome be screened for atlantoaxial instability? *Arch Pediatr Adolesc Med.* 1998; 152: 123–125.
74. Cohen WI. Atlantoaxial instability: what's next? *Arch Pediatr Adolesc Med.* 1998; 152: 119–122.
75. Committee on Sports Medicine. Atlantoaxial instability in Down syndrome. *Pediatrics.* 1984; 74: 152–154.
76. Sackett DL, Haynes RB, Guyatt GH, *et al.* *Clinical epidemiology: a basic science for clinical medicine*, 2nd ed. Boston, MA: Little, Brown, and Co; 1991.
77. Msall ME, Reese ME, DiGaudio K, *et al.* Symptomatic atlantoaxial instability associated with medical and rehabilitative procedures in children with Down syndrome. *Pediatrics.* 1990; 85: 447–449.
78. Pueschel SM, Scola FH, Pezzullo JC. A longitudinal study of atlanto-dens relationships in asymptomatic individuals with Down syndrome. *Pediatrics.* 1992; 89: 1194–1198.
79. Adam HM. In Brief—Atlantoaxial dislocation. *Pediatr Rev.* 2003; 24: 106–107.
80. Maranich AM, Hamele M, Fairchok MP. Atlanto-axial subluxation: a newly reported trampolining injury. *Clin Pediatr (Phila).* 2006; 45: 468–470.
81. Bull MJ, Committee on Genetics. Health supervision for children with Down syndrome. *Pediatrics.* 2011; 128: 393–406.
82. Hankinson TC, Anderson RCE. Craniovertebral junction abnormalities in Down syndrome. *Neurosurg.* 2010; 66: A32–A38.
83. O'Connor JF, Cranley WR, McCarten KM, *et al.* Commentary: atlantoaxial instability in Down syndrome: reassessment by the committee on sports medicine and fitness of the American Academy of Pediatrics. *Pediatr Radiol.* 1996; 26: 748–749.
84. Cope R, Olson S. Abnormalities of the cervical spine in Down's syndrome: diagnosis, risks, and review of the literature, with particular reference to the special olympics. *South Med J.* 1987; 80: 33–36.
85. Goldberg MJ. Spine instability and the Special Olympics. *Clin Sports Med.* 1993; 12: 507–515.
86. Chang FM. The disabled athlete. In: Stanitski CL, DeLee JC, Drez D (eds.) *Pediatric and adolescent sports medicine—Vol. 3.* Philadelphia: W.B. Saunders Company; 1994. p. 48–76.

87. El-Khoury M, Mourao MA, Tobo A, *et al*. Prevalence of atlanto-occipital and atlantoaxial instability in adults with Down syndrome. *World Neurosurg*. 2014; 82: 215–218.
88. Diamond LS, Lynne D, Sigman B. Orthopedic disorders in patients with Down's syndrome. *Orthop Clin North Am*. 1981; 12: 57–71.
89. Cooley WC. Down Syndrome. In: Osborn LM, DeWitt TG, First LR, Zenel JA (eds.) *Pediatrics*. Philadelphia: Mosby Inc; 2005. p. 1060–1064.
90. Hamada T, Gejyo F, Koshino Y, *et al*. Echocardiographic evaluation of cardiac valvular abnormalities in adults with Down's syndrome. *Tohoku J Exp Med*. 1998; 185: 31–35.
91. Platt, LS. Medical and orthopaedic conditions in Special Olympics athletes. *J Athl Train*. 2001; 36: 74–80.
92. Dincer HE, O'Neill W. Deleterious effects of sleep-disordered breathing on the heart and vascular system. *Respiration*. 2006; 73: 124–130.
93. Special Olympics Canada. Available from: www.specialolympics.ca [Accessed 31 Jan 2016].
94. L Guttman (ed.) *Textbook of sport for the disabled*. Aylesbury: HM+ M Publishers Ltd; 1976.
95. Paulsen, Doug. Rehabilitation Centre for Children, Winnipeg, Canada. Personal communication to author.

CHAPTER 29

Exercise, physical activity, and congenital heart disease

Roselien Buys, Tony Reybrouck, and Marc Gewillig

Introduction

Exercise testing in adult cardiac patients has mainly focused on ischaemic heart disease. The results of exercise testing with ECG monitoring are often helpful in diagnosing the presence of significant coronary artery disease. In children with heart disease, the type of pathology is different. Ischaemic heart disease is very rare. The majority of patients will present with congenital heart defects that will affect exercise capacity. In patients with congenital heart disease, exercise tests are frequently performed to measure exercise function or to assess abnormalities of cardiac rhythm. The risk of exercise testing is very low in the paediatric age group.[1] Findings from exercise testing show a reduced exercise capacity in many children with congenital heart disease and exercise responses differ between patients with different underlying heart defects. Results from exercise testing can provide insight into the clinical condition of the child and help decision making regarding patient management. However, exercise testing not only provides information about the heart, but also about the level of daily physical activity (PA). In general, PA has been found to be reduced in children with congenital heart disease, and below recommended guidelines. This has resulted in a shift in research attention from evaluating exercise responses of children with congenital heart disease towards investigating means to improve PA and exercise capacity for health.

Commonly used parameters to assess exercise performance and aerobic exercise function in children with cardiac disease

In exercise physiology, aerobic exercise performance is traditionally assessed by determination of the *maximal oxygen uptake* ($\dot{V}O_2$ max). This reflects the highest level of oxygen which does not further increase, despite an increase in exercise intensity. In paediatric exercise testing the $\dot{V}O_2$ max is frequently assessed by means of an incremental exercise test until voluntary exhaustion. However, although the measurement of $\dot{V}O_2$ max is useful, since it gives information about maximal exercise tolerance, the physiological definition of $\dot{V}O_2$ max is not always met in children. Only about 50% of children are able to reach such a plateau after repeated exercise tests.[2] Many children are not motivated to exercise to that point of exhaustion.[2] Therefore, other criteria should be used to confirm a maximal exercise effort such as i) a respiratory gas exchange ratio ($\dot{V}CO/\dot{V}O_2$) > 1.10, ii) a peak heart rate (HR) which is close to 200 beats$\cdot$min^{-1} and, iii) the subjective appearance of exhaustion. When one or more of these criteria are met, it is assumed that the peak $\dot{V}O_2$ is a maximal value. (Interested readers are referred to Chapter 12 for further discussion of peak $\dot{V}O_2$ and $\dot{V}O_2$ max during paediatric exercise testing). As shown in Figure 29.1a, peak $\dot{V}O_2$ is often reduced in children with congenital heart disease.

Additionally, the evaluation of the HR max provides important information. Some patients with congenital heart disease present with chronotropic limitation or are unable to raise their HR as expected according to the increase in workload.[3] Because of that, the HR max cannot always be used as a criterion for evaluating the maximal character of an exercise test in congenital heart disease.[2] Figure 29.1b shows average peak HR values for children with various congenital heart defects.

The *oxygen pulse* equals stroke volume (SV) times arteriovenous oxygen difference and is calculated by dividing $\dot{V}O_2$ by HR. In healthy subjects, the oxygen pulse continuously increases during submaximal exercise. Furthermore, the oxygen pulse has been used as a surrogate for SV during exercise and has been shown to correlate with SV during submaximal exercise.[4–7] The response of the oxygen pulse to exercise in children can be assumed to be somewhat different from the response in adults, but also in children, this parameter has been proposed as an indirect measure of SV.[8] Due to the child's smaller heart and total blood volume, SV is lower both at rest and during exercise.[9] A child can compensate for this by a higher HR response to submaximal exercise in comparison with adults. Oxygen uptake is further increased by a higher increase in arterial-mixed venous oxygen difference during submaximal exercise in children compared to adults. When the oxygen pulse is used as an indicative parameter for the evaluation of SV during graded exercise, the arterial-mixed venous oxygen difference is considered to remain fairly constant. Therefore, in children with congenital heart defects, the course of the oxygen pulse during an incremental exercise test gives an idea of the changes in SV in response to the increased workload and can provide interesting information regarding the patients' actual clinical condition.

In healthy children and adults, the blood remains fully oxygenated, even during maximal exercise. However, in congenital heart disease, the evaluation of *oxygen saturation during exercise* can provide clinicians with important information. When patients desaturate, this happens in a steady, progressive manner with the lowest numbers observed in the first minute after the load is removed.

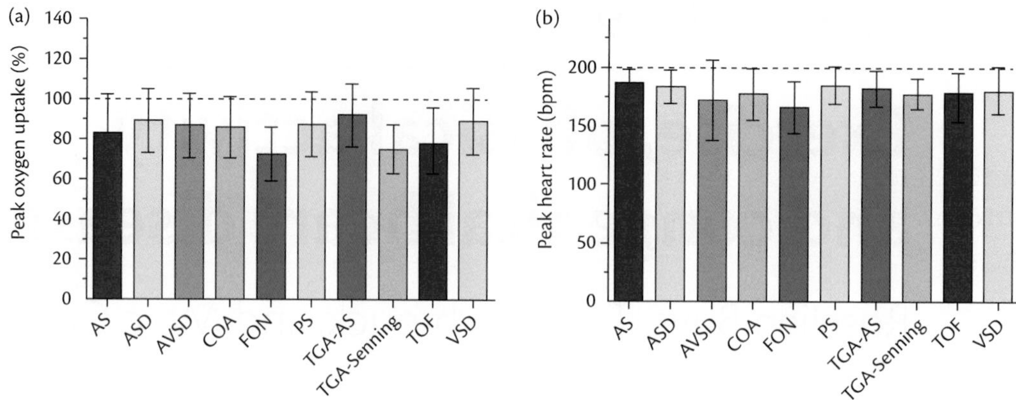

Figure 29.1 Peak oxygen uptake (a) and peak heart rate (b) in children with various congenital heart diseases.
AS, invasively treated aortic valve stenosis; ASD, surgically treated atrial septal defect; AVSD, surgically treated atrioventricular septal defect; COA, surgically treated aortic coarctation; FON, univentricular heart repaired with Fontan operation; PS, invasively treated pulmonary valve stenosis; TGA-AS, transposition of the great arteries surgically treated with the arterial switch operation; TGA-Senning, transposition of the great arteries surgically treated with the senning operation; TOF, surgically corrected tetralogy of Fallot; VSD, surgically treated ventricular septal defect. Dotted line represents peak values of healthy children.

Because maximal exercise tests may have several drawbacks in the paediatric population, clinical investigators have tried to define exercise parameters that are independent from reaching maximal effort. In the past, *heart rate response to exercise* has frequently been used to assess cardiovascular exercise performance.[10,11] However, in patients with congenital heart disease several drawbacks exist, as many patients may show a relative bradycardia during exercise, which is not associated with a high value for $\dot{V}O_2$ max, as should theoretically be expected. Therefore, the use of the HR response to exercise in the assessment of cardiovascular exercise performance can be misleading in patients with congenital heart disease, and cannot be considered to be a valid determinant of aerobic fitness.[12]

A more sensitive assessment of aerobic exercise function can be obtained by analysis of gas exchange. Therefore, considerable attention has been focused on the determination of the *ventilatory anaerobic threshold* in children, which is a very useful and reproducible indicator of aerobic exercise function in the paediatric age group.[13,14] This parameter reflects the highest exercise intensity at which a disproportionate increase in CO_2 elimination ($\dot{V}CO_2$) is found relative to $\dot{V}O_2$.[14,15] (Interested readers are referred to Chapter 10 and Chapter 12 for more detailed discussions of anaerobic and ventilation thresholds).

More recently, newer concepts have been developed to assess dynamic changes of respiratory gas exchange during exercise in patients with congenital heart disease.

The study of the steepness of the slope of $\dot{V}CO_2$ *versus* $\dot{V}O_2$ *above the ventilatory anaerobic threshold*, has been found to be a very sensitive and reproducible index for the assessment of cardiovascular exercise function in patients with congenital heart disease.[15]

Another objective and effort-independent parameter is the *oxygen uptake efficiency slope* (OUES), which was introduced as a measure of exercise capacity by Baba *et al.*[16] The OUES represents the slope of the semilog plot of minute ventilation (V_E) versus $\dot{V}O_2$ (see Figure 29.2). Thus OUES provides an estimation of the efficiency of V_E with respect to $\dot{V}O_2$, steeper slopes indicate a larger exercise capacity. The OUES has been shown to correlate highly with peak $\dot{V}O_2$ and to linearly increase with age during childhood and into adolescence.[17]

Also the $\dot{V}_E$ / $\dot{V}CO_2$-*slope* is supposed to be independent of achieving maximal exertion. This measure represents the slope of the regression line between $\dot{V}_E$ and CO_2 production. It provides information regarding ventilatory efficiency during exercise. A high $\dot{V}_E/\dot{V}CO_2$ slope observed in patients with repaired, non-cyanotic congenital heart disease can often indicate hypoperfusion due to an impaired cardiac output response to incremental exercise.[18] An inefficient ventilatory response to carbon dioxide will limit the exercise performance, as it indicates wasted ventilation. This ventilatory inefficiency has been related to worsening of the clinical condition of cardiac patients, as well as of mortality.[19,20]

The $\dot{V}O_2$ *versus exercise intensity* slope is a valid measurement of oxygen flow to the exercising tissues. Calculation of this slope can document limited oxygen flow to working muscles in congenital heart disease. As such a reduced slope of oxygen uptake versus exercise intensity constitutes another factor limiting exercise capacity as it reflects impaired oxygen delivery to the exercising tissues.[21]

In order to be able to answer important questions concerning the normality of exercise responses in patients, the results can be compared with normal reference values. It is recommended that each laboratory carefully chooses the normal values to which they compare the exercise tolerance, because geographical differences may

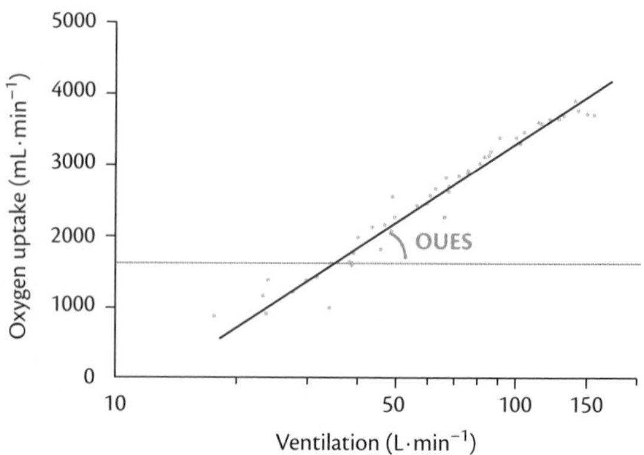

Figure 29.2 The oxygen uptake efficiency slope.
OUES, oxygen uptake efficiency slope.

influence the results of aerobic exercise performance. Reference values may also change over time and should be regularly updated and validated.

Cardiorespiratory response to exercise in specific congenital heart defects

Left-to-right shunts

Atrial septal defect

Children with atrial septal defect (ASD) usually have a normal or near normal exercise capacity. These children can attain normal or near normal values for $\dot{V}O_2$ max.[1,22] A number of haemodynamic abnormalities to exercise have been documented. The increase of cardiac output during exercise may be smaller than normal. Maximal HR response has been found to be lower than normal. In those who underwent surgical closure of the ASD, the age at surgery has been shown to influence exercise performance. In a consecutive series of 50 patients with ASD or ventricular septum defect evaluated in our laboratory, the ventilatory anaerobic threshold (as an estimate of aerobic exercise performance) was at the lower limit of normal (89 ± 14.4% of normal).[23] When studying the exercise response in children who underwent surgical closure of an ASD, a normal value was found in children who underwent surgery before 5 years of age, whereas a significantly lower value was found in children operated on after that age.[24]

In general, abnormalities detected in children either with unoperated or surgically closed ASD are usually minor and do not result in major limitations in exercise performance. Unless arrhythmia is a complication, these children should be encouraged to perform physical exercise and to participate in all sports at all levels. Exercise testing is generally indicated if symptoms of arrhythmia or dyspnoea on exercise are reported.

Ventricular septal defect

A small ventricular septal defect (VSD) will transmit only a small amount of blood from the left to the right side of the heart. Also during exercise, the shunt will remain small. Haemodynamic studies in this patient group showed that during graded exercise, patients with a VSD had a higher pulmonary circulation than systemic circulation, as could be expected. However, the relative shunt fraction decreased with increasing exercise intensity.[25] Subnormal values for cardiac output were found in this patient group. Studies during submaximal exercise testing, using gas exchange measurements, showed suboptimal values for ventilatory anaerobic threshold in a consecutive series of 43 patients with an unoperated VSD, evaluated in our laboratory. This value averaged 90 ± 15.3% of normal and was below the lower limit of the 95% confidence interval.[23] In this patient group, the decreased level of exercise capacity was correlated with decreased habitual PA. Finally, in a group of 18 patients who underwent surgical closure of a large VSD with pulmonary hypertension before age 1 year, the value for aerobic exercise performance was at the lower limit of normal (92 ± 17% of normal).[26] In a retrospective study about quality of life, Meijboom *et al.* [27] reported a normal exercise capacity in 84% of the patient group who underwent surgical closure of a VSD (n = 109). Also Binkhorst *et al.*[28] reported that children with patent or surgically closed VSDs have a normal exercise capacity, despite a mild chronotropic limitation in the latter. This shows that surgical correction of a congenital heart defect early in life can normalize the child's exercise performance.

Patent ductus arteriosus

Similarly, in patients with patent ductus arteriosus, results of exercise testing will generally be normal if the size of the shunt is moderate or small. These subjects will ordinarily be asymptomatic. In most conditions, these defects will be closed surgically or percutaneously, at an age when exercise testing is not feasible. Exercise testing will add little to the routine clinical evaluation of these patients.[1]

Valvular heart lesions

Aortic stenosis

Exercise testing in patients with aortic stenosis may show ST segment changes on the ECG, reflecting ischaemia, a drop in blood pressure, or an inadequate rise in blood pressure with increasing exercise intensity and eventually arrhythmia during exercise testing. The major haemodynamic determinant of ST segment changes during exercise is the inadequate oxygen delivery to the left ventricle. After relief of the gradient by surgery or balloon dilation, improvement of ST segment changes on the ECG during exercise has been reported.[29] A critical aortic stenosis can be identified by clinical findings and confirmed by echo-Doppler examination and eventually by cardiac catheterization.

During exercise testing, most of the patients show a reduced aerobic exercise performance which may be improved after surgery.[29] This may be related both to the inability of the cardiac output to increase adequately during exercise and also due to the effect of a medically imposed restriction of heavy PA and competitive sports. Sudden cardiac death (SCD) during exercise has been reported and has been ascribed to malignant arrhythmias. Fortunately, this is unlikely to happen in asymptomatic patients who present with mild to moderate stenosis.[22] In our experience, SCD has never occurred in follow up in over 200 patients with mild to moderate aortic stenosis (Doppler gradient < 60 mmHg). It allows them to perform up to moderate exercise, including recreational sports.

Pulmonary valve stenosis

Similarly to aortic stenosis, pulmonary valve stenosis results in a right ventricular overload. This may lead to a diminished pulmonary flow. In mild cases (gradients < 30 mmHg) normal or near normal values for ventilatory threshold have been found.[30]

During exercise the transvalvular pressure gradient in pulmonary stenosis may increase during graded exercise testing.[1] In mild cases (gradients < 30 mmHg), values for ventilatory anaerobic threshold have been found to be at the lower limit of normal.[30] In cases with moderate to severe pulmonary stenosis, right ventricular pressures may rise considerably during exercise, which may limit exercise capacity.[31] In patients with mild to moderate pulmonary stenosis (Doppler > 50 mmHg), relief of the stenosis results in an improvement of exercise tolerance. However, exercise performance may be limited in cases with severe pulmonary incompetence.

Cyanotic heart disease

Tetralogy of Fallot

Children who have undergone surgical repair of Tetralogy of Fallot (ToF), and who are felt postoperatively to have good results (no residual VSD and a pressure gradient between right ventricle and pulmonary artery below 20 mmHg), are generally asymptomatic at rest. However, a variety of abnormalities may be brought out by intensive exercise.[32] These include a high right ventricular pressure with values as high as 100 mmHg during maximal exercise, caused by a pressure gradient between right ventricle and pulmonary artery, a blunted increase in SV and HR, and the appearance of ventricular arrhythmias.

Despite these abnormalities, children who underwent total surgical repair for ToF are usually well during daily life. However, formal exercise testing has repeatedly shown subnormal values for $\dot{V}O_2$ max and also for ventilatory anaerobic threshold in this patient group.[15,33,34] Moreover, some individuals may reach normal values. Furthermore, after training, patients with this type of pathology can significantly increase maximal exercise capacity.[35] When the adequacy of the oxygen transport during exercise in patients with ToF repair was assessed by calculation of the slope of $\dot{V}O_2$ vs exercise intensity, reduced values have been found in patients after repair of ToF.[21] This was associated with increased values for the physiological dead space ventilation during exercise or the slope of V_E vs $\dot{V}CO_2$.[36] This is mostly attributed to significant residual haemodynamic abnormalities, such as severe pulmonary regurgitation and right ventricular dysfunction.

Postoperative ToF patients may have ventricular ectopy during exercise (exercise-induced arrhythmia). Exercise-induced ventricular arrhythmias are mainly seen in patients with late repair and poor right ventricular function.[37] Patients with important residual haemodynamic abnormalities such as those previously mentioned are at risk for cardiovascular events.[20]

Transposition of the great arteries

In simple transposition of the great arteries (TGA), the aorta arises from the right ventricle, while the pulmonary artery originates from the left ventricle. This results in severe cyanosis, as desaturated systemic venous blood is pumped in the systemic circulation, while the pulmonary venous return is pumped via left atrium and left ventricle in the lungs. Since this blood is already fully oxygenated, no more oxygen will be added to the blood.

The surgical approach to TGA from the late 1960s to early 1980s involved baffling or rerouting the systemic venous return (from the superior and inferior vena cava) to the mitral valve and left ventricle (atrial switch procedures, also referred to as Mustard or Senning procedure). Exercise testing following the atrial switch procedures has shown a variety of abnormalities even in patients who were asymptomatic at rest.[15,29,38] Also a variety of arrhythmias have been documented during exercise testing (junctional rhythm, premature atrial contractions, premature ventricular contractions).

Currently the arterial switch operation is the preferred surgical technique for transposition of the great arteries. Normal or near-normal values for exercise performance and normal ST on ECG have been reported in this patient group.[39,40] With earlier techniques coronary problems early and late after surgery were common. Improved surgical techniques appear to have resolved these problems.

Fontan circulation

In tricuspid atresia, there is a congenital absence of the tricuspid valve. In a Fontan circulation the caval veins are currently connected directly on the pulmonary arteries, bypassing the right heart. This means that there is no effective right heart pump. Although the survival and also exercise performance of these patients improve dramatically, most of these subjects still have a limited exercise tolerance.[41–43] The circulatory output after Fontan is primordially regulated by the pulmonary vasculature, which limits ventricular preload. The ventricle usually 'will pump whatever it gets'. Therefore, in the healthy Fontan patient, it may be the absence of a sub-pulmonary pump that limits normal increases in pulmonary pressures, trans-pulmonary flow requirements, and cardiac output that are required during exercise.[44]

The HR response is usually blunted in patients with Fontan circulation, and due to this, the term chronotropic incompetence is frequently incorrectly used. Using this definition depends on the comparison between patients and normal subjects regarding chronotropic incompetence: as a proportion of maximal exercise capacity, or in absolute values. Fontan patients have the reputation of having chronotropic impairment when HR is expressed relative to maximal normal value, but in absolute values they are even faster than controls. The term 'incompetence' suggests that increasing the HR would improve exercise tolerance; not only is this incorrect, but it is also dangerous. Heart rate response to exercise is indeed impaired in Fontan patients in comparison to healthy controls, but it is appropriate for the level of ventricular preload. A very fast HR with a limited preload would result in a decreased SV with hypotension, syncope, and eventually death. The lower oxygen saturation in the arterial blood sometimes seen in Fontan patients during exercise rather may be due to residual venous or atrial shunting.[45]

Fontan patients have a decline of exercise tolerance with increasing pulmonary vascular resistance and increasing ventricular end diastolic pressure; this downward slope may be slowed by regular exercise and may be very important for prolonging the favourable haemodynamic result in these patients. This is especially so as the pulmonary circulation in current Fontan circuits is characterized by absent pulsatility and limited increase in regular flow and pressure; this may result in increasing pulmonary vascular resistance.

Rhythm disturbances and conduction defects

Congenital complete atrioventricular block

In congenital complete atrioventricular block, the atrial rate increases normally during exercise, but ventricular rate does not accelerate adequately. In some cases, these patients may develop dizziness and syncope. Exercise testing in these patients shows subnormal values for peak $\dot{V}O_2$ or ventilatory anaerobic threshold and even for the increase of $\dot{V}O_2$ versus exercise intensity.[46] This results from the lack of acceleration of HR during exercise, one of the major components in increasing cardiac output and therefore oxygen delivery to the exercising tissues. In some cases with severe bradycardia and syncope, a pacemaker is inserted. These children should avoid competitive sports and physical activities where there is a danger of body collision as the wiring system that connects the pacemaker with the heart is easily damaged.

In the paediatric population, the frequency and significance of arrhythmia differs from adults.[46] As a general rule, the assessment of cardiac arrhythmia during exercise is useful in the management of these patients. If arrhythmia disappears with increasing exercise intensity, the prognosis of this type of arrhythmia is usually benign.

Congenital complete atrioventricular block after surgery

The anatomic structure of the sinus node is vulnerable to damage following cardiac surgery. Damage of the sinus node has been observed after surgical procedures that require extensive manipulations and sutures in the atria. Specific defects include D-transposition of the great arteries, repaired by atrial baffling procedures.[47] Fortunately, surgically acquired complete atrioventricular block is relatively uncommon, even with extensive surgery in the atria (e.g. D-transposition of the great arteries). In surgically acquired atrioventricular block there is usually no escape rhythm. Safety pacing is recommended.[48]

Habitual physical activity in children with congenital heart disease

Different methods have been applied in assessing the daily level of PA in paediatric patients. Physical activity can be assessed by self-report or objective measures. However, PA is difficult to assess and interpret, because no method is completely accurate.[49] (Interested readers are referred to Chapter 21 where PA assessment is extensively reviewed). However, despite their shortcomings, PA assessments are of value in children and adolescents with congenital heart disease. They can provide complementary information to exercise testing, which is useful in the interpretation of the exercise test results and in the formulation of PA advice to the patient.

It has been reported that children with congenital heart disease have reduced levels of PA when compared to healthy children and have PA levels below what is recommended.[50–52] However, results are conflicting in relation to PA.[53] Low levels of PA may be lifestyle-related in part, because patients with congenital heart disease have a potential to improve their physical fitness by PA similar to that of their healthy peers. Indeed, a relation between PA and exercise capacity also exists in children with congenital heart disease.[54]

Natural evolution of aerobic exercise performance and daily level of physical activity in children with congenital heart disease

It is a normal evolution to see the exercise capacity change during life. However, data regarding the progression of exercise intolerance with age in patients with congenital heart disease are scarce. Nevertheless, it is possible that the first signs of an impaired heart function are demonstrated by an exercise capacity that decreases faster than normal.[55]

To study the natural evolution of aerobic exercise performance during medium-term follow-up in patients with congenital heart disease, exercise performance tests were compared in patients who underwent exercise testing at least twice with a time interval of about 3 years. In our laboratory, serial exercise testing documented that cardiovascular exercise performance declines progressively in children with medically imposed restriction of intensive PA, such as aortic stenosis and in children with residual hemodynamic lesions. In the other patient groups we investigated, which were unoperated ventricular septal defect, pulmonary stenosis, and surgically closed ventricular septal defect, exercise performance remained stable during medium-term follow-up.[30] Moreover, the results of this study showed that at the initial evaluation all patients were in class I of the New York Heart Association (NYHA). At reassessment, about 3 years later, all patients remained in NYHA class I, except for two patients with a Fontan circulation, who belonged to class II and III at re-evaluation.[30] The daily level of PA, assessed by a standardized questionnaire, was significantly lower both at the first and second evaluation in patients with aortic stenosis, surgical repair of Tetralogy of Fallot, and Fontan repair, compared to the other patient groups. These subnormal values for the daily PA level were associated with a significant decrease of aerobic exercise function at re-assessment.[30]

We also performed a first longitudinal study in children and adolescents with atrial switch operation and concluded that in the overall group, the exercise performance remained stable during a follow-up of 3.5 ± 2 years, but that in individual patients, a decreasing exercise capacity was correlated with the development of haemodynamic lesions.[56] In a later study only investigating patients with Senning repair for complete transposition of the great arteries, we demonstrated that peak $\dot{V}O_2$ and peak oxygen pulse decreased faster with age than in healthy controls. This decline is most obvious during childhood and adolescence, and in female patients, when compared to young adults. In Figure 29.3, the decline in peak $\dot{V}O_2$ as a percentage of predicted values is plotted for children and adolescents with various congenital heart defects. The fact that the progressive decline is most obvious during childhood and adolescence suggests the impossibility to increase SV to the same extent as healthy peers during growth.[57] Moreover, a faster decline in peak oxygen pulse was related to a decrease in right ventricular contractility in this patient group.[57]

Fernandes *et al.*[58] found similar results in patients with a Fontan circulation in which a decline was particularly present in patients younger than 18 years; in adults this decline of exercise capacity tended to be similar to that of a normal population. Also Giardini *et al.*[59] showed a faster decline in exercise capacity compared to healthy controls in patients with a Fontan circulation, and this decline was stronger in patients with a morphologic right ventricle.

These data show the combined effect of the heart defect, the residual haemodynamic lesions, and hypoactivity on the evolution of aerobic exercise performance in these groups of patients. In children and adolescents with aortic stenosis, significantly lower values

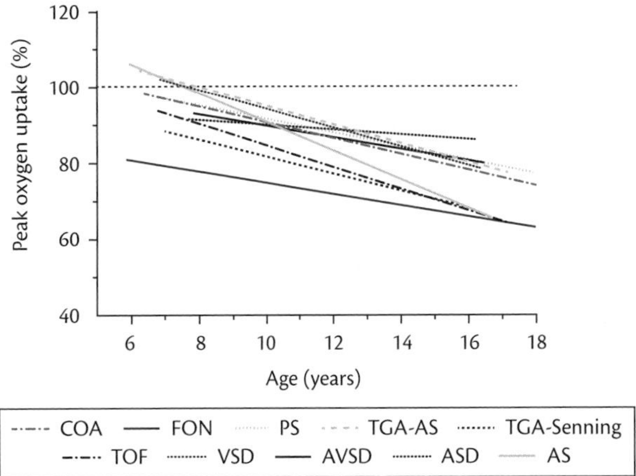

Figure 29.3 Changes in peak oxygen uptake with age.

AS, invasively treated aortic valve stenosis; ASD, surgically treated atrial septal defect; AVSD, surgically treated atrioventricular septal defect; COA, surgically treated aortic coarctation; FON, univentricular heart repaired with Fontan operation; PS, invasively treated pulmonary valve stenosis; TGA-AS, transposition of the great arteries surgivally treated with the arterial switch operation; TGA-Senning, transposition of the great arteries surgically treated with the senning operation; TOF, surgically corrected tetralogy of Fallot; VSD, surgically treated ventricular septal defect. Dotted line represents peak $\dot{V}O_2$ of healthy children.

for aerobic exercise performance were found both at first and second assessment. Similar data have been reported by Driscoll *et al.*[60]

The results of these studies show that the suboptimal aerobic exercise performance in children and adolescents with congenital heart disease are to some extent attributable to residual haemodynamic lesions after corrective surgery of the defect, and also to some degree of hypoactivity resulting from overprotection of the parents and the environment. However, in some patients there may also be an increase of the severity of the disease, which may prevent the individual from performing the same amount of physical exercise as their healthy peers. Therefore, except for some cases with severe disease progression and/or medically imposed restriction of intensive dynamic or static physical exercise, children and adolescents with congenital heart disease and their parents should be strongly encouraged to be more active, and to prevent the deleterious effect of physical deconditioning.

Exercise recommendations and rehabilitation of children with congenital heart disease

Nowadays most children with congenital heart disease are encouraged to be fully active and to participate in all recreational sport activities, even after corrective surgery. These recommendations are based on clinical findings that have shown that physical exercise in children with congenital heart disease has beneficial effects on physical, psychological, and social levels of both children and their parents/carers. In the majority of cases these children do not need to participate in a formal rehabilitation programme, but they should be encouraged to participate in recreational physical activities in leisure time and at school. Even after corrective surgery, a formal rehabilitation programme is mostly restricted to the hospitalization period and consists mainly of chest physiotherapy (breathing exercises) and early mobilization. As soon as the children are discharged from the hospital, they are encouraged to resume their normal physical activities at home. Unfortunately, despite this encouragement, many of these children are often (inappropriately) considered to be very fragile, resulting in overprotective behaviour from parents, and greater restriction from sports activities than is necessary. Unfortunately, greater inactivity and consequent deconditioning usually follow. With this in mind, performing regular physical exercise may be challenging for children with congenital heart disease, and encouraging an active lifestyle is paramount.[52,61,62]

A more formal paediatric cardiac rehabilitation programme might partially reverse the effects of physical inactivity and deconditioning, thereby improving exercise function. Controlled and clinical exercise studies in patients with congenital heart disease have shown that maximal exercise capacity can be improved following a period of physical training.[35] However, $\dot{V}O_2$ max did not improve in all studied subjects. The improvement of maximal exercise performance (assessed during cycle ergometry) without an increase in peak $\dot{V}O_2$ represents an improved mechanical efficiency during exercise. This may be beneficial for the patients, since the same level of exercise will be perceived as easier to perform and will induce less dyspnoea.[35]

Next to the benefit of an increased exercise and functional capacity, an exercise programme might also induce favourable benefits on the social level. It allows children with congenital heart disease to initiate exercise in a safe environment. An exercise programme might thus increase both parents' and children's level of confidence with regard to exercise; quite often there is also a positive effect regarding social interaction behaviours and well-being of the children. Indeed, playing or being active together with healthy peers may also help reduce children's feelings of being 'different'.

In the majority of cases of congenital heart disease there are only a few contraindications for physical exercise for both operated and non-operated cardiac defects.[37] Cumulative medical experience has shown that the potential risk of physical exercise in patients with congenital heart disease is very low.[35] In fact, only a few heart defects have been associated with sudden cardiac death during sports participation, which are mainly hypertrophic cardiomyopathy, severe aortic stenosis, congenital anomalies of the coronary arteries, Marfan's syndrome, and myocarditis. Fortunately, these anomalies represent only a small percentage of the total number of congenital heart defects in which sport participation is allowed. Since children, especially those who perform competitive sports, may be exposed to high levels of physiological stress, specific and detailed recommendations have been formulated for children with congenital heart disease.[22,37,63] These recommendations can be used for counselling children and adolescents with congenital heart disease.

Table 29.1 provides an overview of conditions requiring restrictions of heavy physical exercise and competitive sports, including moderate to severe aortic stenosis, left to right shunts with pulmonary hypertension, hypertrophic cardiomyopathy, pulmonary hypertension, and arrhythmia that worsens during exercise.[22,37,63,64] However, the final decision to allow the child with congenital heart disease to participate in physical exercise should always be based on a full cardiological examination. Regardless, as a general rule, cardiopulmonary exercise testing is advised in children with congenital heart defects before participation in sports activities is allowed.

Table 29.1 Exercise restrictions for the most common types of congenital heart disease.

No restrictions	Avoid high-intensity static sports	Avoid high-intensity static and dynamic sports
Mild AS	COA	Moderate–severe AS
ASD		FON
VSD		PS 30–50 mmHg gradient
AVSD		TGA-AS
PS < 30 mmHg gradient		PAH-CHD
TOF		HCMP
		Exercise induced arrhythmia

AS, aortic valve stenosis; ASD, atrial septal defect; AVSD, atrio-ventricular septal defect; COA, aortic coarctation; FON, univentricular heart repaired with Fontan operation; PS, pulmonary valve stenosis; TGA-AS, transposition of the great arteries surgivally treated with the arterial switch operation; TOF, Tetralogy of Fallot; VSD, ventricular septal defect, PAH, pulmonary arterial hypertension associated with congenital heart disease; HCMP, hypertrophic cardiomyopathy.

Conclusions

As a large proportion of patients with congenital heart disease are in the care of paediatric specialists, exercise testing equipment and exercise protocols have to be adapted for children. Functional performance should be assessed by performing exercise testing with measurement of gas exchange. In some groups of patients with congenital heart disease, suboptimal values have been found for aerobic exercise capacity. These values can be ascribed to haemodynamic dysfunction or residual haemodynamic lesions after surgery (e.g. in transposition of the great arteries, Tetralogy of Fallot, Fontan repair for univentricular heart). In other types of pathologies, medically imposed restriction of intensive physical exercise or competitive sports may determine to some extent a subnormal value of exercise performance. Finally, in some other types of congenital heart disease without overt haemodynamic dysfunction (e.g. ventricular septal defect or atrial septal defect, with normal pressures in the pulmonary circulation) a suboptimal value for aerobic exercise capacity is often related to reduced levels of PA in daily life. Exercise interventions to increase PA have been shown to generally be safe and beneficial in increasing exercise capacity in children with congenital heart disease, although further research in this area is necessary. Therefore, except for some cases with medically imposed restriction of intensive physical exercise, most patients are encouraged to be fully active during leisure time and to participate in all types of physical exercise at school.

Summary

- In children with congenital heart disease, maximal exercise testing is frequently performed to measure cardiorespiratory function and to assess abnormalities of cardiac rhythm.
- Both maximal and submaximal exercise parameters need to be taken into account in order to evaluate the child's clinical and physical condition.
- A reduced exercise capacity is common in children with congenital heart disease. This relates not only to the cardiac condition, but often also to a low level of physical activity in daily life.
- Serial exercise testing is particularly useful in children with congenital heart disease as it is possible that the first signs of an impaired heart function are demonstrated by an exercise capacity that decreases faster than normal.
- Exercise training interventions to increase physical activity have been shown to generally be safe and beneficial in increasing exercise capacity in children with congenital heart disease.
- Except for some cases with medically imposed restriction of intensive physical exercise, most patients are encouraged to be fully active during leisure time and to participate in all types of physical exercise at school.
- The final decision to allow the child with congenital heart disease to participate in physical exercise should always be based on a full cardiological examination along with cardiopulmonary exercise testing.

References

1. Gibbons RJ, Balady GJ, Bricker JT, *et al.* ACC/AHA 2002 guideline update for exercise testing: summary article. A report of the American College of Cardiology/American Heart Association Task Force on Practice Guidelines (Committee to Update the 1997 Exercise Testing Guidelines). *J Am Coll Cardiol.* 2002; 16; 408: 1531–1540.
2. Rowland TW. Aerobic exercise testing protocols. In: Rowland TW (ed.) *Pediatric laboratory exercise testing. Clinical guidelines.* Champaign, IL: Human Kinetics; 1993: 19–41.
3. Reybrouck T, Vangesselen S, Gewillig M. Impaired chronotropic response to exercise in children with repaired cyanotic congenital heart disease. *Acta Cardiol.* 2009; 646: 723–727.
4. Whipp BJ, Higgenbotham MB, Cobb FC. Estimating exercise stroke volume from asymptotic oxygen pulse in humans. *J Appl Physiol.* 1996; 816: 2674–2679.
5. Jones S, Elliott PM, Sharma S, McKenna WJ, Whipp BJ. Cardiopulmonary responses to exercise in patients with hypertrophic cardiomyopathy. *Heart.* 1998; 801: 60–67.
6. Hsi WL, Wong PL, Lai JS. Submaximal oxygen pulse divided by body weight during incremental exercise test. *Am J Phys Med Rehabil.* 1997; 764: 297–303.
7. Klainman E, Fink G, Lebzelter J, Krelbaumm T, Kramer MR. The relationship between left ventricular function assessed by multigated radionuclide test and cardiopulmonary exercise test in patients with ischemic heart disease. *Chest.* 2002; 1213: 841–845.
8. Bar-Or O, Rowland TW. Cardiovascular heart diseases. In: Robertson LD (ed.) *Pediatric exercise medicine: from physiological principles to health care application.* Leeds: Human Kinetics; 2004. p. 177–213.
9. Wilmore JH, Costill DL. *Children and adolescents in sport and exercise. Physiology of sport and exercise.* Leeds: Human Kinetics; 2004.
10. Adams FH, Linde LM. Physical working capacity: an index of cardiac fitness. *Chest.* 1961; 39: 577–578.
11. Adams FH, Duffie ERJr. Physical working capacity of children with heart disease. *Lancet.* 1961; 81: 493–496.
12. Washington RL, Bricker JT, Alpert BS, *et al.* Guidelines for exercise testing in the pediatric age group. From the Committee on Atherosclerosis and Hypertension in Children, Council on Cardiovascular Disease in the Young, the American Heart Association. *Circulation.* 1994; 904: 2166–2179.
13. Reybrouck T, Weymans M, Stijns H, Knops J, Van der Hauwaert L. Ventilatory anaerobic threshold in healthy children. Age and sex differences. *Eur J Appl Physiol Occup Physiol.* 1985; 543: 278–284.
14. Wasserman K. The anaerobic threshold measurement to evaluate exercise performance. *Am Rev Respir Dis.* 1984; 129(2 Pt 2): S35–S40.
15. Reybrouck T, Mertens L, Kalis N, *et al.* Dynamics of respiratory gas exchange during exercise after correction of congenital heart disease. *J Appl Physiol.* 1996; 802: 458–463.
16. Baba R, Nagashima M, Goto M, *et al.* Oxygen uptake efficiency slope: a new index of cardiorespiratory functional reserve derived from the relation between oxygen uptake and minute ventilation during incremental exercise. *J Am Coll Cardiol.* 1996; 15; 286: 1567–1572.
17. Akkerman M, van Brussel M, Bongers BC, Hulzebos EH, Helders PJ, Takken T. Oxygen uptake efficiency slope in healthy children. *Pediatr Exerc Sci.* 2010; 223: 431–441.
18. Mezzani A, Giordano A, Moussa NB, *et al.* Hemodynamic, not ventilatory, inefficiency is associated with high VE/VCO2 slope in repaired, noncyanotic congenital heart disease. *Int J Cardiol.* 2015; 191: 132–137.
19. Rausch CM, Taylor AL, Ross H, Sillau S, Ivy DD. Ventilatory efficiency slope correlates with functional capacity, outcomes, and disease severity in pediatric patients with pulmonary hypertension. *Int J Cardiol.* 2013; 1696: 445–448.
20. Muller J, Hager A, Diller GP, *et al.* Peak oxygen uptake, ventilatory efficiency and QRS-duration predict event free survival in patients late after surgical repair of tetralogy of Fallot. *Int J Cardiol.* 2015; 196: 158–164.
21. Reybrouck T, Mertens L, Brusselle S, *et al.* Oxygen uptake versus exercise intensity: a new concept in assessing cardiovascular exercise function in patients with congenital heart disease. *Heart.* 2000; 841: 46–52.

22. Hirth A, Reybrouck T, Bjarnason-Wehrens B, Lawrenz W, Hoffmann A. Recommendations for participation in competitive and leisure sports in patients with congenital heart disease: a consensus document. *Eur J Cardiovasc Prev Rehabil.* 2006; 133: 293–299.
23. Reybrouck T, Weymans M, Stijns H, Van der Hauwaert LG. Ventilatory anaerobic threshold for evaluating exercise performance in children with congenital left-to-right intracardiac shunt. *Pediatr Cardiol.* 1986; 71: 19–24.
24. Reybrouck T, Bisschop A, Dumoulin M, Van der Hauwaert LG. Cardiorespiratory exercise capacity after surgical closure of atrial septal defect is influenced by the age at surgery. *Am Heart J.* 1991; 122(4 Pt 1): 1073–1078.
25. Bendien C, Bossina KK, Buurma AE, *et al.* Hemodynamic effects of dynamic exercise in children and adolescents with moderate-to-small ventricular septal defects. *Circulation.* 1984; 706: 929–934.
26. Reybrouck T, Mertens L, Schulze-Neick I, *et al.* Ventilatory inefficiency for carbon dioxide during exercise in patients with pulmonary hypertension. *Clin Physiol.* 1998; 184: 337–344.
27. Meijboom F, Szatmari A, Utens E, *et al.* Long-term follow-up after surgical closure of ventricular septal defect in infancy and childhood. *J Am Coll Cardiol.* 1994; 245: 1358–1364.
28. Binkhorst M, van de Belt T, de Hoog M, van Dijk A, Schokking M, Hopman M. Exercise capacity and participation of children with a ventricular septal defect. *Am J Cardiol.* 2008; 1028: 1079–1084.
29. Pianosi PT, Driscoll DJ. Exercise testing. In: Allen HE, Driscoll D, Shaddy RE, Feltes TF (eds.) *Moss' heart disease in infants, children and adolescents.* Philadelphia: Wolters Kluwer—Lippincott Wiliams & Wilkins; 2008. p. 81–94.
30. Reybrouck T, Rogers R, Weymans M, *et al.* Serial cardiorespiratory exercise testing in patients with congenital heart disease. *Eur J Pediatr.* 1995;154: 801–806.
31. Rowland TW. Congenital obstructive and valvular heart disease. In: Goldberg B (ed.) *Sports and exercise for children with chronic health conditions.* Leeds: Human Kinetics; 1995. p. 183–207.
32. Fahey JT. Congenital Heart Disease—Shunt lesions and cyanotic heart disease. In: Goldberg B (ed.) *Sports and exercise in children with chronic health conditions.* Leeds: Human Kinetics; 1995. p. 208–224.
33. Reybrouck T, Weymans M, Stijns H, Van der Hauwaert LG. Exercise testing after correction of tetralogy of Fallot: the fallacy of a reduced heart rate response. *Am Heart J.* 1986; 1125: 998–1003.
34. Luijnenburg SE, De Koning WB, Romeih S, *et al.* Exercise capacity and ventricular function in patients treated for isolated pulmonary valve stenosis or tetralogy of Fallot. *Int J Cardiol.* 2012; 1583: 359–363.
35. Duppen N, Takken T, Hopman MT, *et al.* Systematic review of the effects of physical exercise training programmes in children and young adults with congenital heart disease. *Int J Cardiol.* 2013; 1683: 1779–1787.
36. Reybrouck T, Boshoff D, Vanhees L, Defoor J, Gewillig M. Ventilatory response to exercise in patients after correction of cyanotic congenital heart disease: relation with clinical outcome after surgery. *Heart.* 2004; 902: 215–216.
37. Takken T, Giardini A, Reybrouck T, *et al.* Recommendations for physical activity, recreation sport, and exercise training in paediatric patients with congenital heart disease: a report from the Exercise, Basic and Translational Research Section of the European Association of Cardiovascular Prevention and Rehabilitation, the European Congenital Heart and Lung Exercise Group, and the Association for European Paediatric Cardiology. *Eur J Prev Cardiol.* 2012; 195: 1034–1065.
38. Reybrouck T, Gewillig M, Dumoulin M, Van der Hauwaert LG. Cardiorespiratory exercise performance after Senning operation for transposition of the great arteries. *Br Heart J.* 1993; 702: 175–179.
39. Reybrouck T, Eyskens B, Mertens L, Defoor J, Daenen W, Gewillig M. Cardiorespiratory exercise function after the arterial switch operation for transposition of the great arteries. *Eur Heart J.* 2001; 2212: 1052–1059.
40. Muller J, Hess J, Horer J, Hager A. Persistent superior exercise performance and quality of life long-term after arterial switch operation compared to that after atrial redirection. *Int J Cardiol.* 2013; 1662: 381–384.
41. Gewillig M. The Fontan circulation. *Heart.* 2005; 916: 839–846.
42. Gewillig MH, Lundstrom UR, Bull C, Wyse RK, Deanfield JE. Exercise responses in patients with congenital heart disease after Fontan repair: patterns and determinants of performance. *J Am Coll Cardiol.* 1990; 156: 1424–1432.
43. Diller GP, Dimopoulos K, Okonko D, *et al.* Exercise intolerance in adult congenital heart disease: comparative severity, correlates, and prognostic implication. *Circulation.* 2005; 1126: 828–835.
44. La Gerche A, Gewillig M. What limits cardiac performance during exercise in normal subjects and in healthy fontan patients? *Int J Pediatr.* 2010; 10: 1–8.
45. Gewillig MH, Lundstrom UR, Bull C, Wyse RK, Deanfield JE. Exercise responses in patients with congenital heart disease after Fontan repair: patterns and determinants of performance. *J Am Coll Cardiol.* 1990; 156: 1424–1432.
46. Reybrouck T, Vanden Eynde B, Dumoulin M, Van der Hauwaert LG. Cardiorespiratory response to exercise in congenital complete atrioventricular block. *Am J Cardiol.* 1989; 6414: 896–899.
47. Paul MH, Wessel HU. Exercise studies in patients with transposition of the great arteries after atrial repair operations (Mustard/Senning): a review. *Pediatr Cardiol.* 1999; 201: 49–55.
48. Eliasson H, Sonesson SE, Salomonsson S, Skog A, Wahren-Herlenius M, Gadler F. Outcome in young patients with isolated complete atrioventricular block and permanent pacemaker treatment: A nationwide study of 127 patients. *Heart Rhythm.* 2015; 1211: 2278–2284.
49. Warren JM, Ekelund U, Besson H, Mezzani A, Geladas N, Vanhees L. Assessment of physical activity—a review of methodologies with reference to epidemiological research: a report of the exercise physiology section of the European Association of Cardiovascular Prevention and Rehabilitation. *Eur J Cardiovasc Prev Rehabil.* 2010; 172: 127–139.
50. Arvidsson D, Slinde F, Hulthen L, Sunnegardh J. Physical activity, sports participation and aerobic fitness in children who have undergone surgery for congenital heart defects. *Acta Paediatr.* 2009; 989: 1475–1482.
51. De Bleser L, Budts W, Sluysmans T, *et al.* Self-reported physical activities in patients after the Mustard or Senning operation: comparison with healthy control subjects. *Eur J Cardiovasc Nurs.* 2007; 63: 247–251.
52. Massin MM, Hovels-Gurich HH, Gerard P, Seghaye MC. Physical activity patterns of children after neonatal arterial switch operation. *Ann Thorac Surg.* 2006; 812: 665–670.
53. Ewalt LA, Danduran MJ, Strath SJ, Moerchen V, Swartz AM. Objectively assessed physical activity and sedentary behaviour does not differ between children and adolescents with and without a congenital heart defect: a pilot examination. *Cardiol Young.* 2012; 221: 34–41.
54. Weymans M, Reybrouck T. Habitual level of physical activity and cardiorespiratory endurance capacity in children. *Eur J Appl Physiol Occup Physiol.* 1989; 588: 803–807.
55. Fredriksen PM, Veldtman G, Hechter S, *et al.* Aerobic capacity in adults with various congenital heart diseases. *Am J Cardiol.* 2001; 873: 310–314.
56. Reybrouck T, Mertens L, Brown S, Eyskens B, Daenen W, Gewillig M. Long-term assessment and serial evaluation of cardiorespiratory exercise performance and cardiac function in patients with atrial switch operation for complete transposition. *Cardiol Young.* 2001; 111: 17–24.
57. Buys R, Budts W, Reybrouck T, Gewillig M, Vanhees L. Serial exercise testing in children, adolescents and young adults with Senning repair for transposition of the great arteries. *BMC Cardiovasc Disord.* 2012; 12: 88.
58. Fernandes SM, McElhinney DB, Khairy P, Graham DA, Landzberg MJ, Rhodes J. Serial cardiopulmonary exercise testing in patients with previous Fontan surgery. *Pediatr Cardiol.* 2010; 312: 175–180.

59. Giardini A, Hager A, Pace NC, Picchio FM. Natural history of exercise capacity after the Fontan operation: a longitudinal study. *Ann Thorac Surg*. 2008; 853: 818–821.
60. Driscoll DJ, Wolfe RR, Gersony WM, *et al*. Cardiorespiratory responses to exercise of patients with aortic stenosis, pulmonary stenosis, and ventricular septal defect. *Circulation*. 1993; 87(2 Suppl): I102–I113.
61. Longmuir PE, Brothers JA, de Ferranti SD, *et al*. Promotion of physical activity for children and adults with congenital heart disease: a scientific statement from the American Heart Association. *Circulation*. 2013; 12721: 2147–2159.
62. Muller J, Hess J, Hager A. Daily physical activity in adults with congenital heart disease is positively correlated with exercise capacity but not with quality of life. *Clin Res Cardiol*. 2012; 1011: 55–61.
63. Graham TP, Jr., Bricker JT, James FW, Strong WB. 26th Bethesda conference: recommendations for determining eligibility for competition in athletes with cardiovascular abnormalities. Task Force 1: congenital heart disease. *Med Sci Sports Exerc*. 1994; 26(Suppl): S246–S253.
64. Pelliccia A, Fagard R, Bjornstad HH, *et al*. Recommendations for competitive sports participation in athletes with cardiovascular disease: a consensus document from the Study Group of Sports Cardiology of the Working Group of Cardiac Rehabilitation and Exercise Physiology and the Working Group of Myocardial and Pericardial Diseases of the European Society of Cardiology. *Eur Heart J*. 2005; 2614: 1422–1445.

PART 3

Sport science

CHAPTER 30

Development of the young athlete

Neil Armstrong and Alison M McManus

Introduction

Millions of young people enjoy sport and it is estimated that in England ~80% of youth participate in competitive sport each year.[1] Youth sport is, however, performed at several levels which can be simplistically illustrated in a performance pyramid with mass participation at the foundation and elite youth sport at the pinnacle. At each level of the pyramid competition becomes more intense and inevitably young people will voluntarily withdraw (drop-out) or be systematically excluded (cut) for lack of attainment in a more competitive environment (Figure 30.1). This chapter discusses young athletes who have committed to club membership, are regularly competing at regional, national, or international level, and have reached or aspire towards reaching the peak of the performance pyramid.

Youth sport takes place within a matrix of biocultural factors but success in most youth sports is founded on physical and physiological variables which function in accord with individual biological clocks. An analysis of the development and trainability of physical and physiological variables in youth and their impact on sport performance is the principal focus of the chapter.

It has been estimated that the conversion rate from youth sport participation to professional sport is ~0.01%. Even among young athletes who are identified as talented and selected from an early age for inclusion in training programmes that are specifically designed for elite performance, very few (range ~0.02–0.46% depending on sport) become elite adult athletes.[2] Young athletes are cut or drop-out of sport for a plethora of reasons, including physical injuries, stress, adverse personal experiences, excessive external pressure, and inappropriate or abusive behaviour by peers or dominant adults. Exploration of these challenges to young athletes' personal development, health, and well-being is a complementary objective of the chapter.

The chapter is structured not only to provide a free-standing analysis of the physical and physiological factors underpinning sport performance and a discussion of potential risks to the health and well-being of young athletes, but also to serve as an introduction to the sections on Sport Science and Sport Medicine. Where appropriate, interested readers are referred to other chapters where issues are addressed in detail and with a more specific brief.

Genetics

Sport performance depends on both genetic and environmental (e.g. training) factors and the extent to which they affect performance or other sport-related traits that vary according to the trait. The genetic influence on physical and physiological variables is acknowledged with, for example, the heritability of stature, muscle strength, peak oxygen uptake (peak $\dot{V}O_2$), and anaerobic power estimated to be ~80%, ~15–90%, ~50%, and ~46–84%, respectively with the genetic influence on trainability of peak $\dot{V}O_2$ estimated at ~50%.[3] Recent advances in molecular exercise physiology and their potential application to youth sport performance are beyond the scope of this chapter, but are insightfully addressed in Chapter 31.

Chronological age, biological maturity, and the young athlete

Successful performance in youth sport is underpinned by a range of physical and physiological variables, including body size, body shape, body composition, muscle strength, muscle metabolism, aerobic fitness, and anaerobic fitness, which operate in a sport-specific, asynchronous, and non-linear manner. The influence of these variables on sport performance varies with sex and on an individual basis in accord with chronological aging and biological maturation. Throughout this chapter 'age' will refer to chronological age.

Biological maturation

All young people experience a similar pattern of biological maturation but there are wide individual variations in its timing and tempo. Boys successful in youth sports tend to be advanced or, at least, on time in biological maturation. With the notable exceptions of artistic gymnasts and divers, few later-maturing boys are successful in sport during early- and mid-puberty. However, some later-maturing boys, if they retain interest in sport, reach elite status in age-group sports by 16–18 years, facilitated by catch-up growth and the reduced effect of maturity-associated variation in body size on performances at this time. The biological maturation-related changes in physical and physiological characteristics associated with success in youth sport are less prominent in girls than boys. Earlier-maturing girls are advantaged in some sports but other sports favour the physical characteristics of later-maturing girls.[4]

There is no compelling evidence to suggest that intensive training affects the timing or tempo of biological maturation,[5] but selection and retention in many youth sports are related to biological maturity. Data indicate that in a range of team and individual sports boys in the age group 10–12 years have skeletal ages which span the spectrum from delayed to advanced biological maturation. However, in older age-group sports, the numbers of earlier

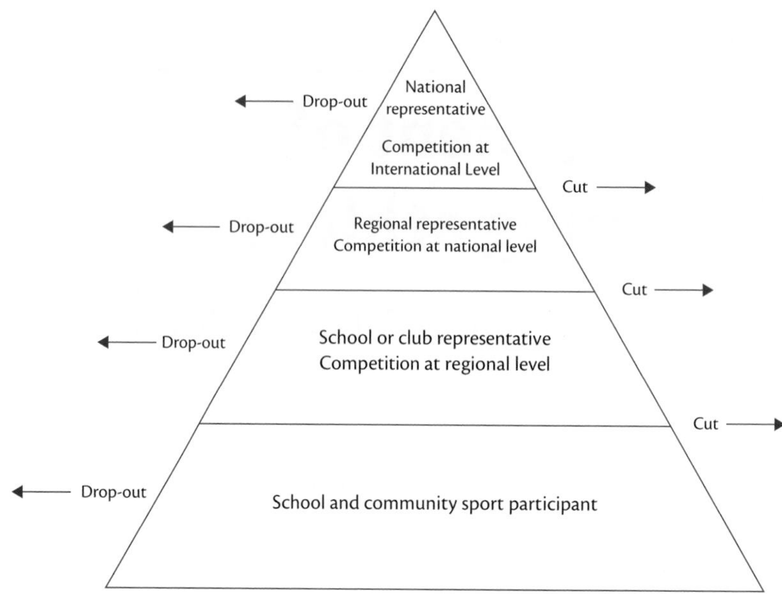

Figure 30.1 Young athlete performance pyramid.
Participation and levels of competition showing the reduction in number of participants as young athletes either dropout or are cut from the squad.

maturing and skeletally mature athletes increase with a corresponding decline in the number of later maturing boys. Similarly, with few exceptions (e.g. artistic gymnastics) ages at peak height velocity (PHV) are consistent with earlier biological maturation of young male athletes.[6]

Data from girls are largely limited to swimming, athletics, and artistic gymnastics. Among 13- to16-year-old track and field athletes, skeletal ages are advanced in jumpers and throwers but generally lag chronological age in runners. Swimmers under 14 years span the maturity spectrum but tend to be early or on time in skeletal age. Swimmers still competing at 14–15 years are primarily on time or advanced in skeletal age, with most swimmers aged 16–17 years skeletally mature. In contrast, among 5- to 10-year-old artistic gymnasts, late and early maturing girls are equally represented but subsequently skeletal ages lag behind chronological ages with the difference more marked in later adolescence. Sparse data from young athletes indicate ages at PHV close to the general population, except for artistic gymnasts who are delayed. Athlete ages at menarche also approximate the general population except for artistic gymnasts and divers who, on average, tend to be later, although still within the normal range of variability.[6]

Body size and shape

In developed countries the onset of girls' growth spurt normally occurs between 8.2 and 10.3 years with PHV reached between 11.3 and 12.2 years. Boys, on average, lag ~2 years behind girls. There is, however, marked variation among individual children in both the timing of the initiation of the spurt and the timing and magnitude of PHV. Early maturing boys might reach PHV at ~12.0 years having started their spurt at ~10.5 years, while late maturing boys might begin their spurt at ~14.5 years, and not reach PHV until ~16.0 years. Corresponding variation occurs in girls. The rate of growth in stature slows from PHV but growth continues to ~16–18 years in girls and ~18–20 years in boys, although it might persist into the early twenties. The maturity-associated variation in body size is particularly marked from 9 to 14 years when sport participation is at its zenith, but it is also noticeable from ~15–17 years with the catch-up of later maturing individuals.[7] (Interested readers are referred to Chapter 2 where growth and maturation are discussed in detail).

As well as changes in body size, young people experience changes in body proportions and shape which markedly influence sport performance. The growth spurt in leg length precedes that of the trunk, and hands and feet grow out of phase with leg, arm, and trunk growth. This might lead to a young athlete temporarily having to cope with a change in centre of mass and deterioration in some motor skills presenting what has been called 'adolescent awkwardness'. Earlier-maturing boys, however, enjoy changes in body size and body shape that are advantageous in most sports.[8]

Earlier-maturing girls have advantages over later-maturing girls in sports that are reliant on large body size, but their wider hips, relatively shorter legs, and greater body fatness are characteristics which can be disadvantageous in some sports. Later-maturing girls present more linear physiques, less body fat, relatively longer legs, lower hip-to-shoulder ratios, and often higher strength-to-mass ratios than earlier-maturing girls, and these characteristics are more suitable for success in several sports.[9]

There is no convincing evidence to suggest that intensive training compromises adult stature or the growth of body segments and data from both sexes must be considered in the context of the selection and retention criteria applied to various youth sports.[5] Young athletes in many sports (e.g. rowing, swimming, tennis, and volleyball) have statures that equal or exceed the 50th percentile, although in some sports there is variation by playing position (e.g. basketball, soccer, and rugby). In contrast, artistic gymnastics and diving are sports which consistently present a profile of below-average stature.[10] (Interested readers are referred to Chapter 32 for more detailed analysis).

Body mass

Body mass follows a similar but, due to energy balance issues, less stable pattern to stature with a marked increase in infancy and early childhood, a steady increase during mid-childhood, a rapid increase during puberty, and a slower increase into adulthood. The growth spurt in body mass is similar in shape to that of stature but occurs ~0.2–0.4 years later in boys and ~0.3–0.9 years later in girls. Young athletes' body mass is normally at or above the 50th percentile, but distance runners, artistic gymnasts, and divers consistently present with body masses below the average of less-athletic youth.[10]

Body composition

Body fatness

Small sex differences in fat mass and % body fat are evident from mid-childhood, but girls' body fat increases substantially in puberty, reaching ~26–31% of body mass. Increases in boys' body mass in puberty are primarily due to gains in skeletal tissue and muscle mass, with % fat mass declining from ~16% to ~12–14%.

Intensive training is associated with a reduction in body fatness in both sexes, but the difference between athletes and non-athletes is greater in females. Young female athletes are generally leaner than their non-athletic peers, but body fatness varies with sports. Values as low as ~14% body fat have been recorded in female gymnasts, with distance runners and cross-country skiers reported to present ~21–25% body fat, and swimmers, track and field athletes, lacrosse, soccer, softball, and volleyball players noted to have body-fat percentages of ~27%.[9]

Bone

Bone mass progressively increases from birth through childhood and puberty into early adulthood. Bone mineral density (BMD) adapts to the mechanical strain placed upon it by skeletal loading and changes are localized to the induced strain. Intermittent loading high in both magnitude and rate produces an osteogenic effect. Therefore, resistance exercise and short bursts of explosive exercise are effective for bone development.[11] (Interested readers are referred to Chapter 18 for a review of physical activity and bone health).

The effect of intensive training on BMD is sport specific. Racquet sport athletes and little league baseball players have been observed to have ~20% higher BMD in their dominant arm than non-athletes, and soccer players, weight lifters, and gymnasts have been reported to have higher BMD than age-matched peers.[9] In contrast, intensive training associated with altered menstrual function has been associated with demineralization of bones in some very active female athletes. It has been suggested that a point may exist up to which intensive training has a beneficial effect on bone mineralization, and beyond which it has an opposite effect in sexually mature young people.[7]

Skeletal muscle

Skeletal muscle mass increases progressively with age in boys before exhibiting a marked pubertal growth spurt. Peak muscle mass velocity (PMV) is a relatively late event in puberty occurring several months after PHV, but by ~17 years boys' muscle mass comprises ~54% of body mass. Girls do not experience a similar spurt in muscle mass to boys and from 5 to 13 years their % muscle mass increases from ~40–45% before, in relative terms, declining due to increased fat accumulation.

Muscle strength

The relationship between muscle mass development and expression of muscle strength during growth and maturation is complex. The maximal force that can be generated by skeletal muscle is a function of muscle size. But, in addition to muscle size, increases in the expression of strength are dependent on the maturation of the central nervous system, including increases in neural myelination, enhanced motor unit recruitment, synchronization, and firing frequency. Changes in muscle pennation angle, skeletal lever ratios, and moment arm lengths during growth also influence the expression of muscle strength, especially in adolescence.[12]

Muscle strength refers to the ability of the skeletal muscles to exert force for the purpose of resisting or moving external loads or to propel objects against gravity. Muscle strength increases in a near-linear manner with age from early childhood until ~13–15 years of age when there is marked surge in boys' strength followed by a slower increase into the early, mid-, or even late twenties. The spurt in muscle strength lags behind PMV and although substantial sport-related benefits do not become apparent until late puberty, earlier-maturing boys enjoy significant advantages over similarly aged but later-maturing peers. There is no compelling evidence of girls experiencing an adolescent strength spurt and their muscle strength begins to plateau in late adolescence.[13]

Differences in the muscle strength of boys and girls are small prior to puberty and there is an overlap of male and female scores on strength assessments. The prepubertal strength difference is greatly magnified during puberty, and by late puberty very few girls can compete with age-matched boys on strength measures. The age at which sex differences become noticeable is both muscle group- and muscle action-specific and confounded by the individual timing and tempo of biological maturation. Sex-related strength differences in the arms and upper body are more evident and appear earlier than those in the legs. By age ~17 years boys are ~50% stronger than girls in the quadriceps, but have biceps strength that is almost double that of girls.[14] (Interested readers are referred to Chapter 7 for a detailed review of muscle strength).

Superior muscle strength and the rate at which it is applied (power) are important determinants of success in many youth sports, and in boys they often differentiate the elite young athlete from the less successful performer. High relative strength also confers advantages to female athletes who tend to be stronger than age-matched peers. One study reported that elite girl gymnasts, swimmers, and tennis players expressed ~20% greater quadriceps and biceps strength than less athletic school girls, but no difference between sports was revealed when muscle strength was co-varied for body mass.[15]

Muscle strength can be enhanced with training and there is no minimum age requirement for beginning a resistance exercise training programme. Children of 5 to 6 years of age have made noticeable improvements in muscle strength following exposure to appropriate resistance exercise, but it is age 7–8 years before most children are ready for structured resistance training.[16,17] Several learned societies have published guidelines and recommendations for resistance exercise training with young people after concluding that it is a safe form of exercise when closely monitored and consistent with participants' technical competency, age, and biological maturity.[16–18]

The response of young people to resistance training is dependent on the age, biological maturity, and sex of the individual, as well as the exercise intensity, duration, and frequency of the training programme. A meta-analysis revealed that training-induced strength gains reported in the literature range from 10 to 90%.[19] A more focused position statement concluded that, following a well-designed, 8- to 20-week training programme, expected strength gains in untrained youth are typically ~30–40%, but on cessation of the training programme strength gains rapidly decay.[16]

Training-induced strength gains in prepubertal children are principally due to neural adaptations. In adolescence, facilitating alterations in neural mechanisms are sustained, but the effects of resistance training, particularly in late-adolescent boys, are primarily a function of substantial increases in lean body mass and muscle cross-sectional area.[11] The trainability of muscle strength increases with age and biological maturity, but there is no discernible spurt in the ability to enhance muscle strength through training in puberty.[19] There is a minor sex-associated effect on absolute and relative strength gains following training among prepubertal children.[20] However, in adolescence, sex-associated differences in trainability emerge with boys generally showing significantly greater training-induced strength gains than girls.[21] (Interested readers are referred to Chapter 36 for a review of resistance training).

Muscle metabolism

Synthesis of data from a range of invasive and non-invasive methodologies strongly supports an age effect on muscle metabolism during exercise. (Interested readers are referred to Chapter 6 where research in muscle metabolism is reviewed). Data are consistent with age-related differences in estimates of muscle energy stores, oxidative and glycolytic enzymes activity, substrate utilization, anaerobic and anaerobic respiration, % of type I muscle fibres, patterns of recruitment of higher threshold (type II) motor units, and rate of recovery from high-intensity exercise. There is interplay of anaerobic and aerobic metabolism in which children present a relatively higher oxidative capacity than adolescents or adults. Anaerobic glycolytic flux increases with age at least into adolescence, and possibly into young adulthood. Independent effects of biological maturity remain to be empirically proven. Muscle metabolism is influenced by sex, but data from girls are relatively sparse and further work is required to tease out evidence-based explanations of sex differences in relation to age and biological maturity.[22]

Young athletes therefore appear well-equipped for long-duration, moderate-intensity exercise. With increasing age (and perhaps biological maturity), the enhanced ability to utilize anaerobic metabolism to support exercise is reflected by marked improvements in performance in sports reliant on short-duration, high-intensity exercise, particularly in boys.[23]

Stable isotope tracer studies have demonstrated that the oxidation rate of ingested ^{13}C-labelled enriched carbohydrate drinks (CHOexo) during exercise is higher in boys than in men and related to biological maturity. The enhanced oxidation rate of CHOexo has been showed to not only spare endogenous CHO and fat, but also to enhance endurance performance. Exogenous CHO spares endogenous substrate utilization in girls in an age-related manner, but the magnitude of CHOexo oxidation does not appear to be different in female children and adolescents. The optimal CHOexo feeding regime during exercise to sustain endurance performance in youth is unknown, but is evidently related to biological maturity in boys.[24–28]

Investigations of the effects of training on muscle energy stores and enzymes activity are sparse and require confirmation. Data mainly emanate from muscle biopsy studies involving a small number of male participants with no comparator groups and inadequately described exercise training regimens. Nevertheless, muscle biopsy data are consistent and indicate that training induces increases in resting stores of adenosine triphosphate (ATP), phosphocreatine (PCr), and glycogen and in both aerobic and anaerobic enzymes activity.[29–31] In contrast, a cross-sectional study of trained and untrained 12- to 15-year-old boys, using magnetic resonance spectroscopy, reported no significant differences in 'anaerobic metabolic ability'.[32] However, even substantial training-induced % changes in muscle metabolism during exercise are unlikely to result in similar % changes in sport performance.[31]

Aerobic fitness

Aerobic fitness may be defined as the ability to deliver oxygen to the muscles and to utilize it to generate energy to support muscle activity during exercise. Peak $\dot{V}O_2$ limits the rate at which oxygen can be provided during exercise and a high peak $\dot{V}O_2$ is a pre-requisite of elite performance in many sports, but it does not describe all aspects of aerobic fitness. In several sports and in everyday life intermittent exercise and the ability to engage in rapid changes in exercise intensity are at least as important as peak $\dot{V}O_2$. Under these conditions it is the transient kinetics of $p\dot{V}O_2$ which best describe the relevant component of aerobic fitness. Furthermore, during sustained exercise, lactate accumulates within the muscle and diffuses into the blood to provide an estimate of the relative aerobic and anaerobic contribution to the exercise. Blood lactate accumulation therefore provides a useful indicator of aerobic fitness with reference to the ability to sustain submaximal exercise.

As components of aerobic fitness are comprehensively discussed in Chapter 12 and Chapter 13, and aerobic trainability is reviewed in Chapter 34, only salient points will be addressed herein.

Peak oxygen uptake

Boys' peak $\dot{V}O_2$ increases in a near-linear manner by ~150% from 8 to 16 years. Girls' peak $\dot{V}O_2$ increases by ~80% over the same age range, but data are less consistent with some indications of it levelling off at ~14 years of age. The sex difference increases from ~10% at 8 years to ~35% at 16 years of age. Boys' greater increase in muscle mass in puberty accounts for much of the sex difference in peak $\dot{V}O_2$, but supplementary factors include boys' greater cardiac index, higher blood haemoglobin concentration, and, possibly, better matching of muscle oxygen delivery to muscle oxygen utilization. In both sexes biological maturity has a positive effect on peak $\dot{V}O_2$ independent of age and changes in body size, body mass, and body composition.[33]

When peak $\dot{V}O_2$ is expressed in ratio with body mass ($mL \cdot kg^{-1} \cdot min^{-1}$) a different picture emerges, with boys' values remaining unchanged or declining slightly with age, whereas girls' values steadily decline from 8 to 18 years. Although ratio scaling of body mass is informative for young athletes who carry their body mass,[34] it has clouded understanding of peak $\dot{V}O_2$ during growth and maturation. In puberty body mass often increases at a greater rate than peak $\dot{V}O_2$ and comparative studies of ratio scaled aerobic fitness favour individuals with low body mass.[35] It is therefore futile to compare prepubertal and adolescent youth or to compare and contrast the aerobic fitness of young athletes from different sports using ratio scaling (e.g. artistic gymnasts vs rugby players). When body mass is appropriately controlled using allometry or multi-level modelling, boys' peak $\dot{V}O_2$ progressively increases from childhood into young adulthood, and girls' values increase from childhood into mid-teens and then show no observable decline into young adulthood.[36]

Trained young athletes of both sexes are generally reported to have a higher peak $\dot{V}O_2$ than their untrained peers, but data are often confounded by the use of ratio scaling. In addition as comparisons of young athletes with untrained youth report cross-sectional data, differences in peak $\dot{V}O_2$ might be due to initial selection for sport rather than subsequent training programmes.[37] To address the issue, the International Olympic Committee (IOC) convened an 'expert conference' on training the elite young athlete.[38] The resulting consensus statement was underpinned by a systematic review of the paediatric literature on aerobic training.[39] The review acknowledged the genetic variability in aerobic trainability and noted the wide range of training-induced changes in peak $\dot{V}O_2$ reported in several studies. However, it concluded that current evidence supports the view that a 12-week, constant-intensity exercise training (CIET) programme, with heart rate maintained in the range ~85–90% of maximum, for 20 min, three times·week^{-1}, will induce, on average, an 8–9% increase in peak $\dot{V}O_2$. No well-controlled, long-term studies of young athletes satisfied the stringent criteria for inclusion in the systematic review but it was noted that a 52-week observational study of prepubertal, girl swimmers reported a 38% increase in peak $\dot{V}O_2$ (in L·min^{-1}) compared with a 13% increase in peak $\dot{V}O_2$ in a matched control group over the same time period.[40] The effect of CIET on peak $\dot{V}O_2$ was revealed to be independent of sex, age, and biological maturity. No persuasive evidence to suggest training-induced changes in either maximal heart rate or maximal arteriovenous oxygen difference during youth was present, and the review concluded that increases in peak $\dot{V}O_2$ are primarily a function of enhanced stroke volume.[39]

The IOC sponsored systematic review refuted Katch's[41] well-cited hypothesis of a 'trigger point' or 'maturation threshold' below which the effects of training are minimal or non-existent. It also not only failed to identify 'critical periods'[42] during which responses to training have been postulated to be augmented, but also observed that studies which have directly investigated the responses of children and adults to the same relative CIET have not reported significantly different training-induced changes in peak $\dot{V}O_2$.[39] A subsequent series of focused studies further addressed the concept of a potential maturation threshold below which responses to training are blunted, and provided empirical evidence that age and biological maturity do not influence the magnitude of responses to cardiopulmonary training in youth.[43,44] (The evidence supporting and refuting a maturation threshold is analysed in Chapter 34).

High-intensity interval training (HIIT), which consists of repeated sessions of brief, intense bouts of exercise interspersed by short periods of rest or low-intensity exercise, has been shown to be an effective and time-efficient approach to training in adults.[45] As children recover more rapidly from intermittent bouts of high-intensity exercise than do adults, it is therefore surprising that HIIT protocols have not been prioritized in paediatric training studies.[46] It was demonstrated over 20 years ago that prepubertal girls could improve their peak $\dot{V}O_2$ through either CIET or HIIT,[47] but it is only recently that research has focused on HIIT as a means of enhancing the aerobic fitness of young athletes.[48–50] Further investigations with well-defined participant groups of young athletes, using CIET, HIIT, and combined CIET and HIIT protocols are required to tease out the relative efficacy of CIET and HIIT in increasing the aerobic fitness of young athletes.[46] (Interested readers are referred to Chapter 35 for a review of HIIT).

Pulmonary oxygen uptake kinetics

Pulmonary $\dot{V}O_2$ kinetic responses at the onset of exercise can be analysed across four exercise domains and three phases as illustrated in Figure 12.3. In all exercise domains the initial rise in $p\dot{V}O_2$ (phase I) is dissociated from $\dot{V}O_2$ at the muscles due to the almost instantaneous increase in cardiac output, which is initiated by vagal withdrawal and the mechanical pumping action of the contracting muscles. Little is known about age- biological maturity-, and sex-related differences in the duration of phase I across exercise domains as investigations have been constrained by methodological challenges.[52]

Children are characterized by a greater oxygen cost and a shorter primary (phase II) time constant (τ) at the onset of moderate-intensity exercise and heavy-intensity exercise compared with adults. Boys present a shorter primary τ than men at the onset of very heavy-intensity exercise, but there are no comparative data on females. Secure data from the onset of severe-intensity exercise are sparse. Despite significant differences in peak $\dot{V}O_2$ there is no sexual dimorphism in the primary τ at the onset of exercise below the lactate threshold (T_{LAC}), but during the transition from rest to heavy-intensity exercise boys present a significantly shorter primary τ than girls. Longitudinal studies have noted that at the onset of heavy-intensity exercise the primary τ increases with age in both children and adolescents. Independent effects of biological maturation on the primary τ remain to be proven.[53]

In the moderate-exercise domain a steady state in $p\dot{V}O_2$ (phase III) is reached within ~2 min but during exercise above T_{LAC}, phase III is characterized by the oxygen cost increasing over time as a slow component of $p\dot{V}O_2$ is superimposed. In the heavy-exercise domain, prepubertal children present a $p\dot{V}O_2$ slow component which contributes ~10% of the end-exercise $p\dot{V}O_2$ after 10 min of exercise, and increases in size with age. Girls present a significantly larger $p\dot{V}O_2$ slow component than boys from prepuberty through adolescence. There is a phase III $p\dot{V}O_2$ slow component in both children and adolescents during very heavy-intensity exercise which increases with age, at least in boys. Data from females are absent and sexual dimorphism has not been addressed in this exercise domain. In the severe-intensity exercise domain a $p\dot{V}O_2$ slow component is not discernible from the primary component.[51]

Children's higher oxygen cost of exercise and shorter τ during the primary component indicate an age-related enhanced oxidative function. The increase in amplitude of the $p\dot{V}O_2$ slow component with age is probably a function of preferential recruitment of type I muscle fibres by children. As boys appear to have a greater % of type I muscle fibres than girls this is consistent with their $p\dot{V}O_2$ kinetics responses.[51]

Training interventions that either speed the primary τ (reducing the oxygen deficit) or attenuate the $p\dot{V}O_2$ slow component (reducing the total oxygen cost of the exercise) will improve exercise tolerance. No prospective data on the trainability of the $p\dot{V}O_2$ kinetics of young athletes are available, and current understanding is founded on four cross-sectional studies which have reported a shorter τ in trained swimmers[54,55] and footballers[56,57] than their untrained peers. In adults the primary τ and the $p\dot{V}O_2$ slow component have been shown to respond positively and rapidly to both

CIET and HIIT, but the optimal training programme for young athletes remains to be determined.

Blood lactate accumulation

In youth, a positive relationship between age and blood lactate accumulation during and following submaximal and maximal exercise is generally observed, but there is no convincing evidence of sex differences in blood lactate accumulation. A convincing theoretical argument can be made for a biological maturity effect on muscle lactate production and subsequent blood lactate accumulation during exercise, but empirical studies have consistently failed to provide compelling supportive evidence.[58–60]

The T_{LAC} expressed as % peak $\dot{V}O_2$ has been reported as negatively correlated with age.[58] Young athletes accumulate less blood lactate than untrained youth at the same relative exercise intensity and in trained youth the T_{LAC} occurs at a higher % of peak $\dot{V}O_2$[23] (see Figure 39.3). No study has specifically investigated the mechanisms underpinning the training-induced reduction in blood lactate accumulation in youth, but data from adults suggest that the primary mechanism is likely to be an increase in the oxidative capacity of the exercising muscles.[63]

Anaerobic fitness

Anaerobic fitness can be described as the ability to support metabolism by non-oxidative pathways.[62] High anaerobic fitness is essential for elite performance in many sports, but the complexity of measuring physiological variables during non-steady-state exercise has limited understanding of the mechanisms underpinning anaerobic performance.[63] Unlike aerobic fitness, there is no gold standard laboratory technique for the assessment of anaerobic fitness, and few data are available from sport-specific tests of young athletes.[64]

Anaerobic fitness is routinely described in terms of peak power output (PP) and mean power output (MP) assessed using variants of the Wingate anaerobic test.[65] Peak power is normally determined over a 1 s or 5 s period and MP over a 30 s test period. Mean power is a complex variable as, although primarily supported by anaerobic energy sources, it includes an unquantified contribution from aerobic metabolism, which has been estimated to vary from 10 to 44% and is higher during youth, an unquantified proportion of which can be attributed to faster $p\dot{V}O_2$ kinetics.[66]

There is a near-linear increase in PP from 7 to 12 years with girls often outscoring boys of similar age due to their more advanced biological maturation. From ~13 years boys experience a marked spurt in PP through to young adulthood, and often beyond.[71] From 7 to 17 years, boys' values have been reported to increase by ~375% compared to a ~295% increase in girls' PP, resulting in a ~50% sex difference by age ~17 years.[67] Biological maturity has been shown to be positively related to both boys' and girls' PP independent of age and body mass.[68] Earlier maturers therefore have a clear advantage over later maturers of similar age in sporting activities primarily supported by anaerobic metabolism.

In contrast to aerobic fitness, anaerobic fitness increases at a greater rate than body mass from the onset of puberty.[69] The determinants of enhanced anaerobic fitness during biological maturation include changes in muscle fibre size, % muscle fibre type, and muscle metabolism. Neuromuscular factors, particularly the ability in late puberty to better recruit and more fully use higher threshold motor units than prepubescents, play a crucial role in improving anaerobic performance.[70] (Interested readers are referred to Chapter 8 where maximal intensity exercise is discussed in detail).

Anaerobic and aerobic performances are enhanced by both age and biological maturity, but they increase at different magnitudes and rates, which impacts on the tempo of changes in various sport performances during youth. Longitudinal data on the same young people show that from 12–17 years PP and MP increase by ~120% and ~113% respectively in boys and by ~65% and ~60% in girls. Increases in peak $\dot{V}O_2$ over the same age range are somewhat smaller at ~70% and ~25% for boys and girls, respectively.[33,69]

There is compelling evidence that young people can increase their anaerobic fitness with training, but well-structured training studies are sparse compared with those investigating aerobic fitness. Outcome data on the magnitude of training-induced improvements in anaerobic fitness are less clear than with other physiological variables, and gains from short-term training programmes have been estimated to fall within a range of 5 to 12%, with PP improving more than MP.[71]

Although comparative studies are confounded by the influence of selection and retention in sports, higher than normal anaerobic power values have been consistently reported in elite young swimmers, gymnasts, tennis players, and handball players.[71] Data from well-controlled and meticulously executed training intervention studies with young athletes are sparse. One study, however, compared trained prepubertal, pubertal, and postpubertal female swimmers with untrained girls in similar stages of biological maturation and noted that no interaction was evident between training status and biological maturity, with similar magnitudes of difference between trained and untrained swimmers at all three stages of biological maturity.[72] These data are similar to those from aerobic fitness and resistance training, and reinforce the view that young athletes' responses to exercise training are not influenced by critical periods, trigger points, or maturation thresholds.[73]

Resistance to fatigue

Young people have consistently been reported to recover more quickly than adults from repeated bouts of high-intensity exercise. This facility advantages the young athlete and has been attributed to maturational changes in both aerobic and anaerobic metabolism.[74] However, comparing recovery rates of children, adolescents, and adults is complex, and it has been argued that as they generate lower power outputs, young people's faster recovery from maximal exercise or repeated bouts of high-intensity exercise is not directly comparable to adults as they have less to recover from.[75] Nevertheless, the consensus from numerous studies is that the ability to recover quickly during intermittent bouts of high-intensity exercise undergoes a progressive decline from childhood to adulthood in males, whereas in females an adult profile is established by 14–15 years of age.[76–78] The age-related resistance to fatigue impacts on the appropriate design of HIIT programmes for young athletes. (Interested readers are referred to Chapter 9 for further discussion of fatigue and recovery).

Speed

For the present purpose speed is considered as rate of over ground running which is influenced by adaptations in a plethora of physical and physiological variables. Contributory factors to speed increases in youth include enlargement of muscle cross-sectional area and length, morphological alterations to muscle and tendon, growth of limb length, changes in muscle exercise metabolism, neural development, and enhanced biomechanical and motor coordination.[79] Speed is included herein as an example of how a vital component of sport performance is reliant on a complex amalgam of physical and physiological factors influenced by age and biological maturity.[80] (Interested readers are referred to Chapter 37 for a more detailed analysis).

As would be expected on the basis of the complexity of the timing and tempo of the development of the underlying characteristics, speed increases in youth follow a non-linear pathway which is difficult to predict. Specific periods for accelerated advances in speed have been hypothesized from 5–9 years in both sexes, from 11–14 years in girls, and from 12–16 years in boys,[42] but the postulates lack both precision and convincing empirical evidence.

Prepubescent boys and girls show similar progression in sprint speed with age, which probably reflects the development of the central nervous system, motor skills, and biomechanical coordination.[81] (Interested readers are referred to Chapter 3 and Chapter 4 for detailed discussion). From ~12 years speed development in girls is diminished compared with boys, with the disparity likely due to differential changes in muscle metabolism, muscle strength, muscle power, body shape, body size, and body composition in accord with biological maturation, as described herein.[80]

Rigorously designed and executed studies investigating the trainability of speed in youth are remarkably sparse, but data are consistent in supporting the efficacy of training. As with other aspects of performance during youth, there is no compelling evidence to support the existence of a maturation threshold below which training is ineffective. Training-induced increases in speed can be made throughout childhood and adolescence although the mechanisms involved probably differ with biological maturity.[80] A recent review of the extant literature concluded that prepubertal and postpubertal boys experience training-induced changes in speed of similar magnitude (~1.1–3.5%) but the response in midpuberty is attenuated.[82] There are few data on the trainability of girls' speed.

Further research is required to evaluate the mechanisms underlying the normal development and potential trainability of speed in youth, but in relation to age it has a significant but non-linear impact on sport performance.

Chronological age, biological maturity, and performance in youth sport

Biological clocks run at different rates and earlier-maturing boys are generally taller, heavier, broader shouldered, longer limbed, and more muscular than later-maturing boys of the same age. Even small increases in shoulder breadth can result in large increases in upper trunk muscle. When this is combined with the greater leverage of longer arms, the advantages in rowing, throwing, and racquet sports become readily apparent. Earlier-maturing boys experience a marked increase in muscle strength in advance of similarly aged but later-maturing boys. The muscle enzyme profile needed to promote the anaerobic generation of energy is augmented as boys move through puberty into young adulthood and this is reflected by an increase in speed and a surge in performance reliant on anaerobic metabolism. Aerobic fitness is enhanced with aging- and biological maturation-related increases in stroke volume, blood haemoglobin concentration, and muscle mass. As youth sport is organized on the basis of age, earlier-maturing boys are strongly advantaged in a wide range of sports[8].

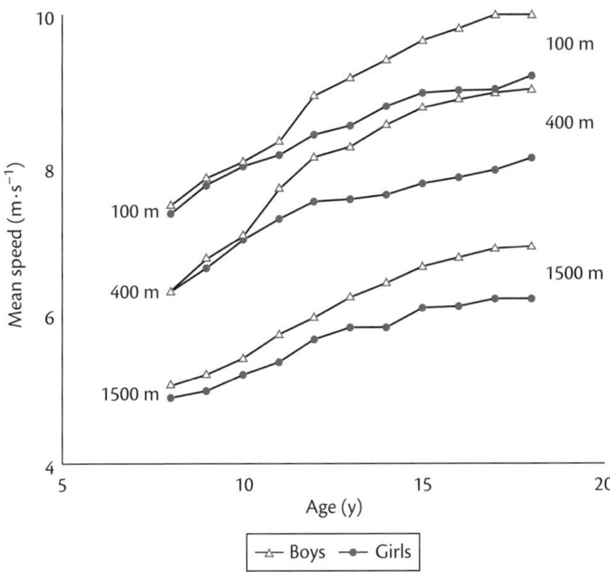

Figure 30.2 World best performances in 100 m, 400 m, and 1500 m in relation to chronological age and sex.

The 100 m is primarily supported by the catabolism of phosphocreatine and anaerobic glycolysis with ~10% of the energy provided by aerobic metabolism. The 400 m is ~60–70% supported by anaerobic metabolism, predominantly glycolysis, with minor support from aerobic sources. The 1500 m is a ~80% aerobic event although increases in pace (e.g. final sprint) have high anaerobic components.

Earlier-maturing girls benefit from increases in muscle strength, anaerobic fitness, and aerobic fitness, which can all promote sport performance, but differences in physical and physiological characteristics associated with biological maturation are less pronounced in girls than in boys. The linear physiques, with less mass for stature, lower % of body fat, relatively longer legs, lower hip-to-shoulder ratios, greater strength-to-mass ratios, and higher resistance to fatigue of later-maturing girls are more suitable for success in many sports. Earlier-maturing girls do not therefore dominate female youth sport.[9]

Selection and retention in age-group sports are often driven by biological maturity but there are no persuasive data to suggest that intensive exercise training influences the timing or tempo of biological maturation. Both prepubertal and pubertal athletes benefit from appropriate exercise training and generally present superior muscle strength, aerobic fitness, anaerobic fitness, and speed than their untrained peers. There is, however, no convincing evidence of a maturation threshold or trigger point below which appropriate training is ineffective. Several popular long-term athlete development models are founded on hypotheses of 'windows of opportunity' or 'critical periods' for optimal development or effects of training, but there is a paucity of empirical evidence to support their existence.[89]

The non-linear and asynchronous progression of performance in different sporting events is clearly illustrated in Figure 30.2 which shows world's best performances in relation to age and sex in track events primarily sustained by different energy systems.

Early specialization in youth sport

It is not unusual to see 2-year-olds in gymnastics initiation programmes and involvement in organized sport often begins as young as 5 years of age, when children are still developing basic movement patterns. Professional soccer clubs are reputed to recruit talented

5-year-olds to their development programmes to prevent rival clubs securing their signature. A 5-year-old prodigy in the Ajax soccer academy was described as 'well worth this investment of time and attention, because 1 day he might be sold to Chelsea or Real Madrid or Juventus for millions'.[83(p369)] The early recruitment to soccer schools of excellence or Premier League academies with the potential of huge financial rewards can focus the minds of children (and their parents), persuade them to concentrate on soccer, and dissuade them from experiencing other sports.

The belief that early specialization leads to enhanced sport performance in adulthood is largely founded on an unsound concept, which is popularly known as the '10 000 hour rule'. This postulate is based on the retrospective data of Ericsson *et al.*[84] which describe the *average* number of hours of solitary practice undertaken by expert violinists during their development. The data were misconstrued in a popular book[85] into an assertion that an individual requires 10 000 h of deliberate practice (i.e. ~3 $h \cdot day^{-1}$ for 10 years) to attain mastery in a sport or activity. Numerous subsequent scientific studies[3] and popular books[86] have shown the '10 000 hour rule' to be fatally flawed, with genetics being at least as important as the environment for elite sporting performance. In a recent editorial Ericsson[87] himself argued that his data were misinterpreted to support a '10 000 hour rule', a term which he had never used in his own papers. He emphasized the huge *variance* in hours of practice reported by expert musicians during their development, stated that 'There is nothing magical about exactly 10 000 h', and acknowledged that 'it is possible to reach international level in much less time'. [87(p534)]

It is clearly evident from the physical and physiological variables described herein that sport performance in youth changes in an asynchronous, non-linear, and sport-specific manner with age and in accord with individual biological clocks. It is therefore not surprising that early specialization in a single sport often turns out to be inappropriate for the young athlete's late adolescent or post-pubertal physiology, body size, body shape, or body composition. Very few young athletes earmarked and groomed for future success in a single sport from an early age achieve their aspirations. Survey data from Eastern Europe illustrate the low success rate of early selection, recruitment, and enrolment in specialist sport schools. For example, of ~20 000 10- to 13-year-olds selected for youth sport schools in the German Democratic Republic (GDR), 25% were relegated after the first year in a promotion programme. Of ~35 000 young Russian athletes enrolled in youth sports schools, only 0.14% were subsequently successful in senior international competition.[88]

A growing body of research suggests that diverse activity experiences and sport sampling, and not early sport specialization, promote both personal and athletic development.[89] The developmental model of sport participation, proposed by Côté,[90,91] provides a powerful and flexible framework that emphasizes the transitions from play to practice and from diversity to intensity in accord with the young athlete's development, including growth and biological maturation. Côté and Erikson[2] argue persuasively that the incorporation of diversification and deliberate play into the early stages of sport development facilitates the progress of elite performance, but at a much lower social cost than early sport specialization.

Chronological age-group sport

In youth, participation in competitive sport is regulated by age groups (e.g. under 15, under 16, under 17, and under 18) and many young people with potential to succeed are denied access to and retention in youth sport through selection policies influenced by date of birth in relation to the selection year or age-deception practises.

The relative age effect

In addition to earlier biological maturation, age relative to the selection year influences chances of being selected for and retained in age-group sports teams. Birth date discrimination, referred to as the relative age effect (RAE), creates a marked advantage for those, particularly boys, who are eldest in their age-group and therefore more likely to be bigger and more biologically mature than those youngest in the age group. Youth born early in the selection year are more likely to be identified as talented by professional clubs and to eventually become involved with the sport as a professional. Young people born late in the selection year are more likely to drop out of competitive sport, often as early as 12 years of age.[92]

A recent review incorporating a meta-analysis revealed that participants from the youngest birth quartile within age groups were less likely to be selected from 14 years of age, even less likely to be a member of representative teams from 15–18 years, and very unlikely to become elite adult athletes. In addition, the presence of a linear profile with the RAE increasing with the number of months away from the referent group was identified.[93]

The existence of the RAE has been verified in numerous sports, with soccer probably the most documented. In a comprehensive study, the birth date distributions in relation to selection year (1st January to 31st December) of male under 15, under 16, under 17, and under 18 national soccer teams of ten European countries, and female under-18 participants in an international tournament were analysed. Both by country and across Europe statistically significant differences by birth quartile were demonstrated with 43% of male players born in the first quarter and 9% born in the last quarter of the selection year (see Figure 30.3). Data on girls were limited to one relatively old age group, but the RAE was much less pronounced in elite female under-18 soccer players with 31% born in the first quarter and 17% born in the final quarter of the selection year. The authors suggested that approaching 18 years of age, most female players are fully mature physically and that the technical aspect of the game might be of more importance than the physical component in the women's game.[92]

As successful youth players receive more specialist coaching, devote more time to honing their skills and understanding of the game, become known to selectors of representative teams and club scouts, and are less likely to drop out of the sport than their unselected peers, it is not surprising that the RAE persists into the adult game.[94]

Chronological age deception

The influence of date of birth on sport performance in age-group sport in itself creates a challenge for fair competition, but the problem is compounded further by cheating the system through the use of age-deception techniques, such as altering passports and registrations for personal gain or national prestige. To combat cheating, international sport organizations have made strenuous attempts to develop objective methods to accurately determine age,[95] but there is currently no fool-proof method of age verification.[96]

Instances of cheating are well-documented with parents, young athletes, and even National Governing Bodies (NGBs) of sport participating in age-deception practices. In sports where strength,

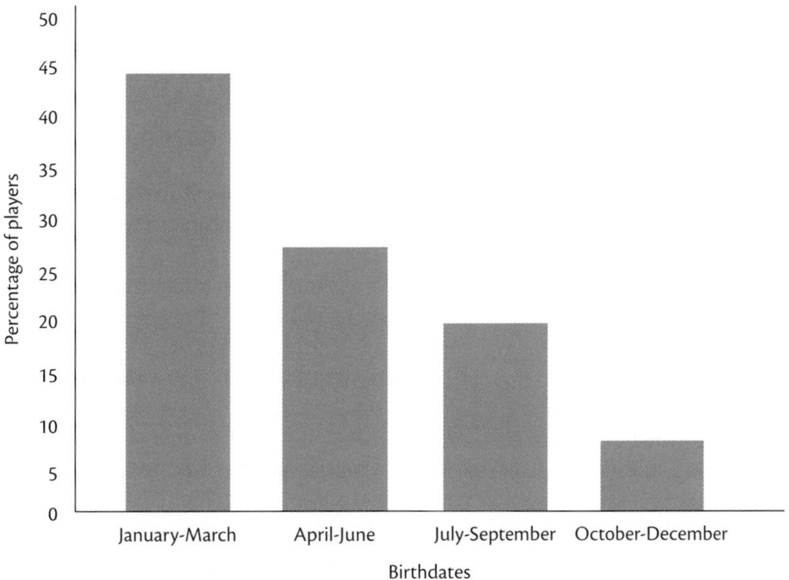

Figure 30.3 The relative age effect.

Birthdates of the under 15, under 16, under 17, and under 18 national soccer teams from ten European countries showing the imbalance in birthdates in the selection year which begins on 1st January and ends on 31st December. Figure drawn from data in Helsen *et al.*[102] reprinted from Armstrong N. Sport and children. In: Whyte GP, Loosemore M, Williams C, (eds.) ABC of sport and exercise medicine, 4th ed. Chichester: Wiley; 2015: 97–101, with permission.

power, and speed provide a competitive advantage (e.g. soccer) registrations have been falsified to allow older players to compete. The head of the Chilean Football Federation altered the licences of 16 juniors out of a squad of 18 so that older players could participate in junior World Cup qualification games.[97]

In sports which favour pre- and early-pubertal athletes (e.g. artistic gymnastics) legal documents have been altered to allow participation by athletes below the prescribed age limit. When a Romanian Olympic gold medallist finally admitted that she had been given a false date of birth to allow her to compete in the Olympics, the President of the Romanian Gymnastic Federation responded without apparent remorse that, 'Falsifying the age of gymnasts is a worldwide practice. We copied what the others were doing'.[97(p50)]

Risks to young athletes' health and well-being

Participation in sport provides a positive environment for the promotion of personal development, physical fitness, health, and well-being during youth.[98] However, risks to young athletes' health and well-being have also been identified and extensively documented. Evidence is accumulating that youth sport, particularly in the upper echelons of the performance pyramid, offers substantial challenges to all stakeholders including parents, coaches, medical staff, sport scientists, administrators, sport governing bodies, and young athletes themselves.[89]

Physical, psychological, and sexual abuse

In a sporting environment where discipline and obedience are often important elements, young athletes find it difficult to question adults who are not only entrusted with their care, but on whom they might be heavily dependent for their future careers in the sport.[97] Numerous studies have indicated that, in several sports, young athletes who are legally minors, have been socialized into accepting that abuse, intimidation, and threat (or actual use) of physical violence is part of the culture and practice of their sport.[99]

A retrospective study of 1430 youth athletes in the UK revealed that 26% of male and 23% of female respondents reported experiencing behaviour categorized as causing psychological or physical harm, such as being hit, shaken, or forced to train when injured or exhausted.[100] Professional soccer provides several pertinent case studies. One study of professional soccer academies in England and Wales reported that psychological (public verbal) abuse of young players (aged 16–18 years) was a common technique used by coaches with little regard for the welfare of the young person.[99] The verbal abuse and derogatory language to which young players are often subject to in soccer academies appears to be seen as part of the steep learning curve they are obliged to undertake while preparing for a career in professional soccer.[101] The use of physical violence by dominant adults against young players is not unknown. Kelly and Waddington[102] documented the response of the manager of an English Premier League soccer club who, on noticing the changing room to be untidy, lined up his youth team and smacked them all on the head with a cricket bat.

Data on the health and well-being of young soccer players who do not make the cut into the major professional leagues are sparse. However, a recent newspaper article[103] revealed that 55% of ~100 15- to 18-year-olds surveyed suffered from mental illnesses such as depression and anxiety, or engaged in drug use that contributed to impaired functioning within 1 month of being released from their clubs without a professional contract. The same source reported that the charity XPRO supported ~60 players under 20 years of age who had depression and a further 250 players who were currently in young offenders institutions having been released by their clubs without a contract.

Sexual abuse and harassment occurs at all ages, and not just in sport, but there is a high risk of abuse in sports where there is early specialization or where talent identification occurs around the age of puberty. The risk of sexual abuse is also high when the athlete is on the verge of success with an increased dependency on the perpetrator. The abuser may be a coach, a parent, a doctor, an administrator, or other athletes preying on a vulnerable teammate or squad member.[104]

Interest in protecting young athletes from psychological, physical, and sexual abuse in sport and concern for their future health and well-being is recognized by the IOC and other sport governing bodies. These concerns have stimulated consensus statements,[105] powerful recommendations for sports organizations,[106] and the development of a comprehensive 'safeguarding children in sport' framework, which is discussed in Chapter 50.

Coach and parental pressure

By their early teens some young athletes are training for ~30–40 $h \cdot week^{-1}$,[5] with, in certain sports (e.g. artistic gymnastics), ~30% of elite participants reported to having already experienced the adverse effects of overtraining.[107] The question arises of whether this heavy commitment to training is made freely by the young athlete. Ethically, for consent to participate in intensive sport training and competition to be provided voluntarily, there must be an absence of implied pressure. With the power differentials between coaches or parents and young athletes there is always the possibility of coercion of the young person to over-commit to an exhaustive and time-consuming regimen of training and competition. Inappropriate and unrealistic demands and expectations on young athletes can lead to disempowerment, lack of autonomy, a unidimensional identity, depression, and numerous other psychological stresses, often referred to generically as 'burnout'.[108] (Interested readers are referred to Chapter 38 for further discussion of the overtraining syndrome).

The excessive time committed to training and competition by some young athletes has been associated with child abuse and, if classified as child labour, the amount of time devoted to training would certainly be illegal in several countries.[109]

The fervour of parents for their child to succeed is epitomized by the father of one teenage tennis prodigy who, according to David,[97] screamed, 'Kill the bitch'! when his daughter, later a major international star, was competing against another child. The determination of coaches and parents to win at all costs is reflected further in several studies of parent, coach, and young athlete behaviour. For example, in a study of 11- to 14-year-old athletes' moral behaviour, it was noted that 9% acknowledged cheating and 13% admitted attempts to injure an opponent; however, it was also reported that 7% received encouragement from their coaches to cheat and 8% were encouraged by their coaches to injure opponents.[110] In another study, 60% of youth tennis players claimed that their parents had embarrassed them, 30% indicated that their parents had yelled or screamed at them, and, remarkably, 13% reported that their parents had hit them after a match.[111]

It is well documented that a problem with self-report surveys of behaviour is the tendency for respondents to represent themselves in a positive light. Thus, there are often discrepancies between parents' and young athletes' reports of the same incidences. But, as Holt and Knight[112] discuss, young athletes' perceptions of parental behaviours may be more important than the behaviours per se.

Financial exploitation

Elite young athletes can earn huge sums of money, e.g. Jennifer Capriati had won US$1 000 000 in tennis prize money alone by the time she was 16 years of age. Driven by the pursuit of professional contracts there is a plethora of evidence of economic exploitation and abuse of trust by adults engaging with young athletes, who are minors in the eyes of the law. In many countries legislation protects the earnings of minors in the entertainment industry, but young athletes are not covered by these laws. There are cases recorded where parents (or legal guardians) have spent their children's earnings from sport without consulting them, leaving young athletes to 'retire' without the financial security they had earned and expected.[97]

Financial investment in young athletes is a risk; there is no guarantee of future success and very few young athletes become elite adult athletes. Yet, sport management groups search the world to identify future sport stars at an early age and widely publicise success stories. For example, tennis player Anna Kournikova was contracted to agents at 10 years of age with the stipulation that she and her mother move from Moscow to live in Florida. Formula One racing team McLaren contracted 15-year-old Lewis Hamilton, a talented go-kart driver, for US$2 000 000 before he had a driving licence. The number of talented young athletes who do not fulfil their aspirations can, however, only be vaguely estimated.

A recent development in youth sport is the activity of unscrupulous agents in the trafficking and sale of talented young athletes, particularly from Africa and South Asia to Europe and the US. Few reliable data are available, but an inquiry carried out by the Italian Senate Commission for Children revealed that 5282 licensed soccer players less than 16 years of age came from countries outside the European Union, mainly from Africa. Only 23 had their contract properly registered and most had been trafficked to Italy illegally. Only a small minority of these players eventually obtained professional contracts and in many cases as adults they became illegal migrants.[97]

Performance-enhancing drugs

Modern state organized use of performance-enhancing drugs (PEDs) by young athletes dates back to GDR State Plan 14.25 initiated in the 1960s. Highly selected and talented youngsters were enrolled, often without their knowledge, on systematic programmes of anabolic androgenic steroid use administered and monitored by sport medicine doctors.[113] Not only did this criminal abuse lead to premature deaths and severe adverse health effects in the young athletes themselves, but also to the inheritance of serious health problems by their offspring.[114]

Many young athletes compete in elite senior competitions and although there might no longer be state plans that focus on the introduction of PEDs to talented children and adolescents, there are currently persuasive allegations of state-sponsored PED programmes and positive test cover-ups for potential Olympians, with both national (e.g. Russia) and international (e.g. International Association of Athletic Federations, IAAF) governing bodies implicated.

Thirty-three athletes aged less than 15 years competed in the 2012 Olympic Games; the youngest competitor was aged 13 years and the youngest gold medallist was 15 years old. In most countries, potential Olympians are subject to sophisticated year-round testing for PEDs in advance of the Games. But, the ethics and legality of NGBs insisting on regular, non-therapeutic blood sampling of 12-year-old children in the year prior to the Games on the basis that they *might* be selected for the Olympic Games are dubious. Moreover, the interpretation of data collected from young athletes experiencing growth and biological maturation at individual rates is challenging.

Recent evidence of young athletes being victims of external pressure to use banned substances lies in the obsessive obligation to 'make weight at all costs' for competition in sports organized in body-weight categories. In the 2010 and 2014 Youth Olympics (for athletes aged 14–18 years), anti-doping rule violations for the use of diuretics were reported in wrestling and Taekwondo. In the 2014 Commonwealth Games, a 16-year-old weightlifting gold medallist had her medal rescinded after testing positive for a banned diuretic.

Significant numbers of young athletes have admitted to the use of PEDs[115] with 13–68% admitting anabolic androgenic steroid use in a sporting context.[89] The results of a survey of ~6000 16-year-olds who practised sport on average 10 h·week^{-1}, with 22% participating at either national or international level, indicate possible sources of PEDs. It was reported that ~4% of young athletes claimed to have been enticed into using PEDs, but the most remarkable revelation was that the PEDs were mostly supplied by friends, parents, and family doctors.[116] In an attempt to protect young athletes from inducements by members of their entourage to take PEDs, the World Anti-Doping Agency introduced in 2015 a Prohibited Association clause to their Code. This clause, as discussed in Chapter 49, 'prohibits association by an athlete, in a professional or sport-related capacity, with any support person who is serving a period of doping-related ineligibility or who has been criminally or professionally found guilty of an offence within the past 6 years for conduct that would have constituted an anti-drug rule violation'.

Dietary supplementation, disordered eating, and eating disorders

Body mass and composition are crucial performance characteristics in some sports (e.g. rugby and artistic gymnastics) and there are concerns over subtle, or even overt, pressure by coaches to enhance performance through manipulation of body mass by dietary supplementation or the maintenance of an energy deficit. In extreme cases, this behaviour is clearly child abuse.

The most frequently used supplements among young athletes are vitamins and minerals taken for perceived health reasons,[117] but dietary supplementation for enhanced performance is common, especially among young male athletes.[118] (Interested readers are referred to Chapter 48 where the benefits and risks of dietary supplements are reviewed). Using rugby union as an example, it has been reported that ~50% of schoolboy rugby players under 16 years in South Africa 'bulk up' through dietary supplements.[119] In 2013 the England under-18 rugby union squad mean body weight was greater than the 2003 senior World Cup-winning squad. Vague definitions and the resistance of some national associations to keeping transparent records make accurate cataloguing of the prevalence of rugby union injuries difficult but, coinciding with the marked increase in body mass, injuries in youth rugby union appear to have doubled.[120] At least one public health expert has questioned whether schoolboys playing competitive rugby (and their parents or guardians) are sufficiently cognizant of the risks of serious injury to be able to give informed consent to participate in the game.[121]

In sports where body size and mass are crucial for optimum performance, self-imposed or external demands promote the prevalence of Relative Energy Deficiency in Sport (RED-S),[122] the combined outcome of low-energy intake and high levels of energy expenditure. The concept of RED-S originates from the Female Athlete Triad, a syndrome of three inter-related conditions, namely menstrual dysfunction, disordered eating, and premature osteoporosis caused by low energy availability in female athletes. Evidence now shows that low energy availability results in a far greater range of health risks from menstrual dysregulation to cardiovascular impairment than previously recognized.[122] Additionally, although this is primarily an issue for young female athletes, low energy availability has also been reported in male athletes in sports where low body mass is an expectation.[123] As the level of RED-S risk increases, so does the likelihood of the young athlete developing a disturbed body image and clinical eating disorder. The incidence of eating disorders also increases at the commencement of sport specialization and escalates further during periods of intensive competition.[124] The diagnosis of RED-S and disordered eating is complex, but the risks for health and well-being accentuate the importance of coach and parent vigilance. To reduce the risk of RED-S, early detection through health screening of young athletes, particularly those in endurance and weight category sports, is necessary. However, in the longer term, athlete, parent, and coach education is essential.[125] (Interested readers are referred to Chapter 47 where the evidence is presented and the issue discussed).

Sport injuries

Sport is the leading cause of injury in youth accounting for ~35% of all injuries in this population. Sport injuries are, however, comprehensively covered in other chapters in this book, and will only be highlighted herein with interested readers referred to appropriate chapters.

Early specialization, intensive training, inadequate recovery, and frequent participation in sport competitions are associated with a rising prevalence of overuse injuries[126] (see Chapter 40). The prevalence of injuries in both contact (see Chapter 42) and non-contact (see Chapter 43) sport is escalating, with lower extremity injuries the most common (see Chapter 45). The highest injury rates for girls are in gymnastics, basketball, soccer, ice hockey, field hockey, running, and handball. For boys, injuries predominantly occur in rugby, soccer, ice hockey, basketball, American football, wrestling, and running.[127]

There is increased recognition of the seriousness of continuing to compete when injured. Non-life threatening cases of medical mismanagement of injuries, in particular the excessive use of analgesic medication by team doctors in youth soccer, are regularly reported[128] (see Chapter 50). But, it took the death of a 14-year-old rugby player, who was treated three times for blows to the head and sent back onto the field on each occasion, before collapsing and dying from 'second impact syndrome' to stimulate a serious debate on the management of concussion in youth rugby (see Chapter 42 and Chapter 46).

The largest prospective study to date revealed an 11.4% risk of a youth rugby union player sustaining a concussion over a season, equivalent to one or two players in every season, in every school or club youth rugby team of 15 players.[129] The conclusion of a systematic review of the likelihood of sustaining a concussion in youth rugby went as far as to recommend that rugby should not be a compulsory component of school physical education.[130] (Injuries in physical education classes are discussed in Chapter 41). As youth are more vulnerable to concussion and its effects than adults, concerns are also being expressed in other contact sports. Following a class-action lawsuit in California, the United States Soccer Federation banned players under 10 years of age from heading the ball and limited the amount of 'headers' in practise by 11–13-year-olds. Clearly, more research into youth sport-related concussions and other head injuries is urgently required.

Conclusions

The physiological bases of paediatric sport science are well documented. Coaches and young athlete support teams not only need to be cognizant of the influence of aging, biological maturation, and training on current and future sport performance, but also need to implement development programmes which are evidence-based.

The vast majority of participants gain great pleasure from youth sport, some aspire to elite status, and a select few achieve international success. However, talented young athletes drop-out of sport, often through lack of mentoring and inappropriate behaviour by dominant adults in their entourage or team members. Other youth are denied opportunities in age-group sport through selection and retention policies which are related to biological maturity and the arbitrary timing of the selection year.

The optimum development of the young athlete, not the optimum development of the sport, should be the focus of attention. Key issues include fostering participation in a range of sports, nurturing talent regardless of the ticking of individual biological clocks, and educating and supporting young athletes to effectively and enjoyably manage their health, well-being, and sport-life balance.

Summary

- Success in youth sport is strongly influenced by physical and physiological variables which operate in a chronological age-, biological maturity-, and sex-related manner.
- Earlier-maturing boys are generally taller, heavier, broader shouldered, longer limbed, and more muscular than later-maturing boys of the same chronological age. They also benefit from biological maturity-related increases in muscle strength, anaerobic fitness, and aerobic fitness.
- Competitive youth sport is organized by chronological age group and in many sports earlier-maturing boys are strongly advantaged when competing against less mature boys with similar chronological ages.
- Boys who are oldest in their age group gain an advantage from the relative age effect which persists into elite adult sport.
- Earlier-maturing girls benefit from increases in muscle strength, anaerobic fitness, and aerobic fitness, but the differences in physiological variables associated with biological maturity are less marked in girls.
- Later-maturing girls' more linear physiques, with less mass for stature, lower % of body fat, relatively longer legs, lower hip-to-shoulder ratios, higher resistance to fatigue, and greater strength-to-mass ratios are more suitable for success in some sports.
- Earlier-maturing girls do not dominate all female youth sport. The relative age effect persists but is less pronounced in girls.
- There is no compelling evidence to suggest that intensive exercise or training affects the timing or tempo of biological maturation, growth of body segments, or adult stature.
- Muscle strength, anaerobic fitness, speed, and aerobic fitness are enhanced by appropriate training, but data do not support the existence of 'windows of opportunity' 'critical periods', or 'maturation thresholds'.
- Parents, coaches, and scientific support teams involved in youth sport should focus on nurturing talent regardless of the speed of biological clocks.
- Participation in youth and community sport provides a positive environment for the promotion of young people's enjoyment, personal development, health, and well-being, but participation in elite youth sport also presents inherent challenges to young athletes and their entourage.
- Cases of psychological, physical, and sexual abuse of young athletes are well documented.
- Power differentials between coaches or parents and young athletes can lead to coercion of the young person to over-commit to exhaustive regimens of training and competition.
- Disordered eating patterns are common in some sports. Evidence is accumulating that both legal and illegal ergogenic aids are used to enhance performance in youth sport.
- Early specialization, intensive training, inadequate recovery, and frequent participation in sport competitions are associated with a rising prevalence of overuse injuries.
- Parents, coaches, and the scientific and medical entourage should prioritize the optimal development of the young athlete, who should be actively supported to effectively and enjoyably manage their health, well-being, and sport-life balance.

References

1. The Health and Social Care Information Centre. *Statistics on obesity, physical activity and diet—England 2013.* London: National Health Service; 2013.
2. Côté J, Erikson K. Diversification and deliberate play during the sampling years. In: Baker J, Farrow D (eds.) *Routledge handbook of sport expertise.* London: Routledge; 2015. p. 305–316.
3. Tucker R. Collins M. What makes champions? A review of the relative contribution of genes and training to sporting success. *Br J Sports Med.* 2014; 46: 555–561.
4. Armstrong N, McManus AM. (eds.) *The elite young athlete.* Basel: Karger; 2011.
5. Malina RM. Baxter-Jones ADG, Armstrong N, *et al.* The role of intensive training in the growth and maturation of artistic gymnasts. *Sports Med.* 2013; 43: 783–802.
6. Malina RM, Rogol AD, Cumming SP, Coelha e Silva MJ, Figueiredo AJ. Biological maturation of youth athletes: assessment and implications. *Br J Sports Med.* 2015; 49: 852–859.
7. Malina RM, Bouchard C, Bar-Or O. *Growth, maturation and physical activity*, 2nd ed. Champaign, IL: Human Kinetics; 2004.
8. Armstrong N, McManus AM. Physiology of elite young male athletes. *Med Sport Sci.* 2011; 56: 1–22.
9. McManus AM, Armstrong N. Physiology of elite young female athletes. *Med Sport Sci.* 2011; 56: 23–46.
10. Malina RM. Physical growth and biological maturation of young athletes. *Exerc Sport Sci Rev.* 1994; 22: 389–434.
11. Lloyd RS, Faigenbaum AD, Stone MH, *et al.* Position statement on youth resistance training: the 2014 International Consensus. *Br J Sports Med.* 2014; 48: 498–505.
12. Blimkie CJR. Age- and sex-associated variation in strength during childhood: Anthropometric, morphologic, neurologic, biomechanical,

endocrinologic, genetic, and physical activity correlates. In: Gisolfi CV, Lamb DR (eds.) *Youth, exercise, and sport*. Carmel, CA: Benchmark Press; 1989. p. 99–161.
13. Jones DA, Round JM. Muscle development during childhood and adolescence. In: Hebestreit H, Bar-Or O (eds.) *The young athlete*. Oxford: Blackwell; 2008. p. 18–26.
14. Round JM, Jones DA, Honour JW, Nevill AM. Hormonal factors in the development of differences in strength between boys and girls during adolescence: A longitudinal study. *Ann Hum Biol*. 1999; 26: 49–62.
15. Maffuli N, King JB, Helms P. Training in elite young athletes (the training of young athletes [TOYA] study): injuries, flexibility, and isometric strength. *Br J Sports Med*. 1994; 28: 123–136.
16. Faigenbaum AD, Kraemer WJ, Blimkie CJR, *et al*. Youth resistance training: Updated position statement paper from the National Strength and Conditioning Association. *J Strength Cond Res*. 2009; 23: S60–S79.
17. Lloyd R, Faigenbaum A, Stone M, *et al*. Position statement on youth resistance training: the 2014 International Consensus. *Br J Sports Med*. 2014; 48: 498–505.
18. Stratton G, Jones M, Fox KR, *et al*. BASES position statement on guidelines for resistance exercise in young people. *J Sport Sci*. 2004: 22: 383–390.
19. Behringer M, vom Heede A, Yue Z, Mester J. Effects of resistance training in children and adolescents: A meta-analysis. *Pediatrics*. 2010; 126: e1199–e1210.
20. Falk B, Tenenbaum G. The effectiveness of resistance training in children: a meta-analysis. *Sports Med*. 1996; 22: 176–186.
21. Lillegard WA, Brown EW, Wilson DJ, *et al*. Efficacy of strength training in prepubescent to early postpubescent males and females: effects of gender and maturity. *Pediatr Rehabil*. 1997; 1: 147–157.
22. Armstrong N, Barker AR. New insights in paediatric exercise metabolism. *J Sport Health Sci*. 2012; 1: 18–26.
23. Armstrong N, Barker AR, McManus AM. Muscle metabolism changes with age and maturation: How do they relate to youth sport performance? *Br J Sports Med*. 2015; 49: 860–864.
24. Timmons BW, Bar-Or O, Riddell MC. Oxidation rate of exogenous carbohydrate during exercise is higher in boys than in men. *J Appl Physiol*. 2003; 94: 278–284.
25. Timmons BW, Bar-Or O, Riddell MC. Influence of age and pubertal status on substrate utilization during exercise with and without carbohydrate intake in healthy boys. *Appl Physiol Nutr Metab*. 2007; 32: 416–425.
26. Timmons BW, Bar-Or O, Riddell MC. Energy substrate utilization during prolonged exercise with and without carbohydrate intake in preadolescent and adolescent girls. *J Appl Physiol*. 2007; 103: 995–1000.
27. Riddell MC, Bar-Or O, Wilk B, Parolin ML, Heigenhauser GJF. Substrate utilization during exercise with glucose plus fructose ingestion in boys ages 10–14 yr. *J Appl Physiol*. 2001; 90: 903–911.
28. Timmons BW, Bar-Or O. RPE during prolonged cycling with and without carbohydrate ingestion in boys and men. *Med Sci Sports Exerc*. 2003; 35: 1901–1907.
29. Eriksson BO, Gollnick PD, Saltin B. The effect of physical training on muscle enzyme activities and fiber composition in 11-year-old boys. *Acta Paediatr Belg*. 1974; 28: 245–252.
30. Fournier M, Ricci J, Taylor AW, Ferguson RJ, Montpetit RR, Chaitman BR. Skeletal muscle adaptation in adolescent boys: sprint and endurance training and detraining. *Med Sci Sports Exerc*. 1982; 14: 453–456.
31. Cadefau J, Casdemont J, Grau JM, *et al*. Biochemical and histochemical adaptation to sprint training in young athletes. *Acta Physiol Scand*. 1990; 140: 341–351.
32. Kuno SY, Takahashi H, Fujimoto K, *et al*. Muscle metabolism during exercise using P-31 nuclear magnetic resonance spectroscopy in adolescents. *Eur J Appl Physiol*. 1995; 70: 301–304.
33. Armstrong N, Welsman JR. Peak oxygen uptake in relation to growth and maturation in 11–17-year-old humans. *Eur J Appl Physiol*. 2001; 85: 546–551.
34. Nevill A, Rowland TW, Goff D, Martell L, Ferrone L. Scaling or normalizing maximum oxygen uptake to predict 1-mile run time in boys. *Eur J Appl Physiol*. 2004; 92: 285–288.
35. Welsman JR, Armstrong N. Scaling for size: Relevance to understanding effects of growth on performance. In: Hebestreit, H, Bar-Or O (eds.) *The young athlete*. Oxford: Blackwell; 2008. p. 50–62.
36. Welsman JR, Armstrong N, Kirby BJ, Nevill AM, Winter EM. Scaling peak $\dot{V}O_2$ for differences in body size. *Med Sci Sports Exerc*. 1996; 28: 259–265.
37. Armstrong N, Tomkinson GR, Ekelund U. Aerobic fitness and its relationship to sport, exercise training and habitual physical activity during youth. *Brit J Sports Med*. 2011; 45: 849–858.
38. Mountjoy M, Armstrong N, Bizzini L, *et al*. IOC consensus statement: Training the elite child athlete. *Br J Sports Med*. 2008; 42: 163–164.
39. Armstrong N, Barker AR. Endurance training and elite young athletes. *Med Sport Sci*. 2011; 56: 59–83.
40. Obert P, Courteix D, Lecoq AM, Guenon P. Effect of long-term intense swimming training on the upper body peak oxygen uptake of prepubertal girls. *Eur J Appl Physiol*. 1996; 73: 136–143.
41. Katch VL. Physical conditioning of children. *J Adolesc Health Care*. 1983; 3: 241–246.
42. Viru A, Loko J, Harro M, Volver A, Laaneots L, Viru M. Critical periods in the development of performance capacity during childhood and adolescence. *Eur J Phys Educ*. 1999; 4: 75–119.
43. McNarry MA, Welsman JR, Jones AM. Influence of training and maturity status on the cardiopulmonary responses to ramp incremental cycle and upper body exercise in girls. *J Appl Physiol*. 2011; 119: 375–381.
44. McNarry MA, Mackintosh KA, Stoedefalke K. Longitudinal investigation of training status and cardiopulmonary responses in pre- and post-pubertal children. *Eur J Appl Physiol*. 2014; 114: 1573–1580.
45. Gist NH, Fedewa MV, Dishman RK, Cureton KJ. Sprint interval training effects on aerobic capacity: A systematic review and meta-analysis. *Sports Med*. 2014; 44: 269–279.
46. Armstrong N, McNarry MA, Aerobic fitness and trainability in healthy youth: Gaps in our knowledge. *Pediatr Exerc Sci*. 2016; 28: 171–177.
47. McManus AM, Armstrong N, Williams CA. Effect of training on the aerobic power and anaerobic performance of prepubertal girls. *Acta Paediatr*. 1997; 86: 456–459.
48. Armstrong N. Aerobic fitness and training in children and adolescents. *Pediatr Exerc Sci*. 2016; 28: 7–10.
49. Costigan SA, Eather N, Plotnikoff RC, Taaffe DR, Lubans DR. High-intensity interval training for improving health-related fitness in adolescents: A systematic review and meta-analysis. *Br J Sports Med*. 2015; 49: 1253–1261.
50. Harrison CB, Gill ND, Kinugasa T, Kilding AE. Development of aerobic fitness in young team sport athletes. *Sports Med*. 2015; 45: 969–983.
51. Armstrong N, Barker AR. Oxygen uptake kinetics in children and adolescents. A review. *Pediatr Exerc Sci*. 2009; 21: 130–147.
52. Fawkner SG, Armstrong N. Oxygen uptake kinetic response to exercise in children. *Sports Med*. 2003; 33: 651–669.
53. Fawkner SG, Armstrong N. Can we confidently study $\dot{V}O_2$ kinetics in young people? *J Sport Sci Med*. 2007; 6: 277–285.
54. McNarry NA, Welsman JR, Jones AM. Influence of training status and exercise modality on pulmonary O_2 uptake kinetics in pubertal girls. *Eur J Appl Physiol*. 2011; 111: 621–631.
55. Winlove MA, Jones AM, Welsman JR. Influence of training status and exercise modality on pulmonary O_2 uptake kinetics in pre-pubertal girls. *Eur J Appl Physiol*. 2010; 108: 1169–1179.
56. Marwood S, Roche D, Rowland TW, Garrard M, Unnithan VB. Faster pulmonary oxygen uptake kinetics in trained versus untrained male adolescents. *Med Sci Sports Exerc*. 2010; 42: 127–134.
57. Unnithan VB, Roche DM, Garrard M. Oxygen uptake kinetics in trained and untrained adolescent females. *Eur J Appl Physiol*. 2015; 115: 213–220.
58. Pfitzinger P, Freedson P. Blood lactate responses to exercise in children: Part 2. Lactate threshold. *Pediatr Exerc Sci*. 1997; 9: 299–307.
59. Williams JR, Armstrong N. The influence of age and sexual maturation on children's blood lactate responses to exercise. *Pediatr Exerc Sci*. 1991; 3: 111–120.

60. Welsman JR, Armstrong N. Assessing post-exercise blood lactates in children and adolescents. In: Van Praagh E (ed.) *Pediatric anaerobic performance*. Champaign, IL: Human Kinetics; 1998. p. 137–153.
61. Holloszy JO. Biochemical adaptations in muscle-effects of exercise on mitochondrial on oxygen uptake and respiratory enzyme activity in skeletal muscle. *J Biol Chem*. 1967; 242: 2278–2282.
62. McNarry MA, Jones AM. The influence of training status on the aerobic and anaerobic responses to exercise in children. A review. *Eur J Sport Sci*. 2014; 14(Suppl): S57–S68.
63. Van Praagh E, Dore E. Short-term muscle power during growth and maturation. *Sports Med*. 2002; 32: 701–728.
64. Barker AR, Armstrong N. Exercise testing elite young athletes. *Med Sport Sci*. 2011; 56: 106–125.
65. Inbar O, Bar-Or O, Skinner JS. *The Wingate anaerobic test*. Champaign, IL: Human Kinetics; 1996.
66. Chia M, Armstrong N, Childs D. The assessment of children's performance using modifications of the Wingate test. *Pediatr Exerc Sci*. 1997; 9: 80–89.
67. Martin RJ, Dore E, Twisk J, Van Praagh E, Hautier CA, Bedu M. Longitudinal changes of maximal short-term peak power in girls and boys during growth. *Med Sci Sports Exerc*. 2004; 36: 498–503.
68. Armstrong N, Welsman JR, Kirby BJ. Performance on the Wingate anaerobic test and maturation. *Pediatr Exerc Sci*. 1997; 9: 253–261.
69. Armstrong N, Welsman JR, Chia MYA. Short-term power output in relation to growth and maturation. *Br J Sports Med*. 2001; 35: 118–124.
70. Inbar O, Chia M. Development of maximal anaerobic performance: An old issue revisited. In: Hebestreit H, Bar-Or O (eds.) *The young athlete*. Oxford: Blackwell; 2008. p. 27–38.
71. Ratel S. High intensity and resistance training and elite young athletes. *Med Sport Sci*. 2011; 56: 84–96.
72. McNarry MA, Welsman JR, Jones AM. Influence of training and maturity status on girls' responses to short-term, high-intensity upper- and lower- body exercise. *Appl Physiol Nutr Metab*. 2011; 36: 344–352.
73. McNarry MA, Barker AR, Lloyd RS, Buchheit M, Williams CA, Oliver JL. BASES expert statement on trainability during childhood and adolescence. *Sport Exerc Sci*. 2014; 41: 22–23.
74. Ratel S, Kluka V, Vicencio SG, *et al*. Insights into the mechanisms of neuromuscular fatigue in boys and men. *Med Sci Sports Exerc*. 2015; 47: 2319–2328.
75. Falk B, Dotan R. Child-adult differences in the recovery from high-intensity exercise. *Exerc Sport Sci Rev*. 2006; 34: 107–112.
76. Ratel S, Martin V. Is there a progressive withdrawal of physiological protections against high-intensity induced fatigue during puberty? *Sports*. 2015; 3: 346–357.
77. Dipla K, Tsirini T, Zafeiridis A, *et al*. Fatigue resistance during high-intensity intermittent exercise from childhood to adulthood in males and females. *Eur J Appl Physiol*. 2009; 106: 645–653.
78. Ratel S, Duche P, Williams CA. Muscle fatigue during high-intensity exercise in children. *Sports Med*. 2006; 36: 1031–1065.
79. Ford P, De Ste Croix M, Lloyd R, *et al*. The long-term athlete development model: physiological evidence and application. *J Sport Sci*. 2010; 29: 389–402.
80. Oliver JL, Rumpf MC. Speed development in youth. In: Lloyd RS, Oliver JL (eds.) *Strength and conditioning for young athletes: Science and application*. London: Routledge; 2014. p. 80–93.
81. Haywood KM, Getchell N. *Life span motor development*. 6th ed, Champaign, IL: Human Kinetics; 2014.
82. Rumpf MC, Cronin JB, Oliver JL, Hughes MG. Effect of different training methods on running sprint times in male youth. *Pediatr Exerc Sci*. 2012; 24: 170–186.
83. Malina RM. Early sport specialization: Roots, effectiveness, risks. *Curr Sports Med Rep*. 2010; 6: 364–371.
84. Ericsson, KA, Krampe RT, Tesch-Romer C. The role of deliberate practice in the acquisition of expert performance. *Psychol Rev*. 1993; 100: 343–406.
85. Gladwell M. *Outliers: The story of success*. New York: Little Brown; 2008.
86. Epstein D. *The sports gene*. London: Yellow Jersey Press; 2013.
87. Ericsson KA. Training history, deliberate practice and elite sports performance: an analysis in response to Tucker and Collins review-what makes champions? *Br J Sports Med*. 2013; 47: 533–535.
88. Vaeyens R, Gullich A, Warr CR, Philippaerts R. Talent identification and promotion of Olympic athletes. *J Sports Sci*. 2009; 27: 1367–1380.
89. Bergeron MF, Mountjoy M, Armstrong N, *et al*. International Olympic Committee consensus statement on youth athletic development. *Br J Sports Med*. 2015; 49: 843–851.
90. Côté J. The influence of the family in the development of talent in sport. *Sport Psychol*. 1999; 13: 395–417.
91. Côté J, Abernethy B. A developmental approach to sport expertise. In: Murphy S (ed.) *The Oxford handbook of sport and performance psychology*. Oxford: Oxford University Press; 2012. p. 435–437.
92. Helsen WF, Van Winckel J, Williams M. The relative age effect in youth soccer across Europe. *J Sports Sci*. 2005; 23: 629–636.
93. Cobley S, Baker J, Wattie N, McKenna J. Annual age-grouping and athlete development: A meta-analytical review of relative age effects in sport. *Sports Med*. 2009; 39: 235–256.
94. Brewer J, Balsom P, Davis J. Seasonal birth distribution amongst European soccer players. *Sports Exerc Injury*. 1995; 1: 154–157.
95. Engebretsen L, Steffen K, Bahr R, *et al*. International Olympic Committee Consensus Statement on age determination in high-level young athletes. *Br J Sports Med*. 2010; 44: 476–484.
96. Malina RM. Skeletal age and age verification in youth sport. *Sports Med*. 2011; 41: 926–947.
97. David P. *Human rights in youth sport*. London: Routledge; 2005.
98. Mountjoy M, Andersen LB, Armstrong N, *et al*. International Olympic Committee consensus statement on the health and fitness of young people through physical activity and sport. *Br J Sports Med*. 2011; 45: 839–848.
99. Platts C, Smith A. Health, well-being and the 'logic' of elite youth sports work. In: Green K, Smith A (eds.) *Routledge handbook of youth sport*. Oxford: Routledge; 2016. p. 492–504.
100. Alexander K, Stafford A, Lewis R. *The experiences of children participating in organized sport in the UK*. Edinburgh: University of Edinburgh Press; 2011.
101. Roderick M. *The work of professional football. A labour of love?* London: Routledge; 2006.
102. Kelly S, Waddington J. Abuse, intimidation and violence as aspects of managerial control in professional soccer in Britain and Ireland. *Int Rev Soc Sport*. 2006; 41: 147–164.
103. Ducker J. From superstars to scrapheap: meet the game's lost generation. *The Times*. 2015 15 January: 68–69.
104. Mountjoy M. Doubt. *Curr Sports Med Rep*. 2015; 14: 77–79.
105. Brackenridge C, Fasting K. International Olympic Committee Consensus Statement on sexual harassment and abuse in sport. *Int J Sport Exerc Psych*. 2008: 6: 442–449.
106. Mountjoy M, Rhind DJA, Tiivas A, Leglise M. Safeguarding the child athlete in sport; a review, a framework and recommendations for the IOC youth athlete development model. *Br J Sports Med*. 2015; 49: 883–886.
107. Matos NF, Winsley RJ, Williams CA. Prevalence of overreaching/overtraining in young English athletes. *Med Sci Sports Exerc*. 2011; 43: 1287–1294.
108. Winsley RJ, Matos N. Overtraining and elite young athletes. *Med Sport Sci*. 2011; 56: 97–105.
109. Rowland TW. On the ethics of elite-level sports participation by children. *Pediatr Exerc Sci*. 2000; 12: 1–5.
110. Shields D, Bredemeir BL, La Voi N, Power FC. The sport behavior of youth, parents, and coaches: the good, the bad, and the ugly. *J Res Character Educ*. 2005; 3: 43–59.
111. DeFrancesco C, Johnson P. Athlete and parent perceptions in junior tennis. *J Sport Behav*. 1997; 22: 29–36.
112. Holt NL, Knight CJ. *Parenting in youth sport*. London: Routledge; 2015.
113. Frahke WW, Berendonk B. Hormonal doping and androgenization of athletes: a secret program of the German Democratic Republic government. *Clin Chem*. 1997; 43: 1262–1279.

114. Ungerleider S. *Faust's gold. Inside the East German doping machine.* New York: Dunne; 2001.
115. Harmer PA. Anabolic-androgenic steroid use among young male and female athletes: is the game to blame? *Br J Sports Med.* 2010; 44: 26–31.
116. Laure P, Binsinger C. Adolescent athletes and the demand and supply of drugs to improve their performance. *J Sports Sci Med.* 2005; 4: 272–277.
117. McDowall JH. Supplement use by young athletes. *J Sports Sci Med.* 2007; 6: 337–342.
118. Diehl K, Thiel A, Zipfel S, Mayer J, Schnell A, Schneider S. Elite adolescent athletes' use of dietary supplements: characteristics, opinions and sources of supply and information. *Int J Sport Nutr Exerc Metab.* 2012; 22: 165–174.
119. Duvenage KM, Meltzer ST, Chantler SA. Initial investigation of nutrition and supplement use, knowledge and attitudes of under-16 rugby players in South Africa. *S Africa J Sports Med.* 2015; 27: 67–71.
120. Freitag A, Kirkwood G, Scharer S, Ofori-Asenso R, Pollock AM. Systematic review of rugby injuries in children and adolescents under 21 years. *Br J Sports Med.* 2015; 49: 511–519.
121. Pollock AM. *Tackling rugby.* London: Verso; 2014.
122. Mountjoy M, Sundgot-Borgen J, Burke L, *et al.* The IOC consensus statement: beyond the Female Athlete Triad—Relative Energy Deficiency in Sport (RED-S). *Br J Sports Med.* 2014; 48: 491–497.
123. Sundgot-Borgen J, Garthe I. Elite athletes in aesthetic and Olympic weight-class sports and the challenge of body weight and body compositions. *J Sports Sci.* 2011; 29: S101–S114.
124. Campbell K, Peebles R. Eating disorders in children and adolescents: state of the art review. *Pediatrics.* 2014; 134: 582–592.
125. Sundgot-Borgen J, Meyer NL, Lohman TG, *et al.* How to minimise health risks to athletes who compete in weight-sensitive sports review and position statement on behalf of the Ad Hoc Research Working Group on Body Composition, Health and Performance, under the auspices of the IOC Medical Commission. *Br J Sports Med.* 2013; 47: 1012–1022.
126. American Academy of Pediatrics Council on Sports Medicine and Physical Fitness. Overuse injuries, overtraining, and burnout in child and adolescent athletes. *Pediatrics.* 2007; 119: 1242–1245.
127. Emory CA, Thierry-Olivier R, Whittaker JL, Nettel-Aguirre A, van Mechelen W. Neuromuscular training injury prevention strategies in youth sport: a systematic review and meta-analysis. *Br J Sports Med.* 2015; 49: 865–870.
128. Tscholl P, Feddermann N, Junge A, Dvorak J. The use and abuse of painkillers in international soccer: data from 6 FIFA tournaments for female and youth players. *Am J Sports Med.* 2009; 37: 260–265.
129. McIntosh As, McCrory P, Finch CF, *et al.* Head, face and neck injury in youth rugby: incidence and risk factors. *Br J Sport Med.* 2010; 44: 188–193.
130. Kirkwood G, Parekh N, Ofori-Asenso R, Pollock AM. Concussion in youth rugby union and rugby league: a systematic review. *Br J Sports Med.* 2015; 49: 506–510.

CHAPTER 31

Molecular exercise physiology

Henning Wackerhage, Jonathon Smith, and Darren Wisniewski

Introduction

Definition of and introduction to molecular exercise physiology

Molecular exercise physiology is the study of exercise physiology using molecular biology methods.[1] Molecular biology methods were introduced to exercise physiology by pioneers like the exercise physiologist Frank W Booth and the sport and exercise geneticist Claude Bouchard, to elucidate the mechanisms of adaptation to exercise and to understand how differences in our deoxyribonucleic acid (DNA) sequence affect sport and exercise-related traits, respectively. Also, transgenic mice have revealed genes whose mutation increases or decreases exercise performance or affects sport- and exercise-related traits. Additionally, molecular biology has been a key tool for developmental biologists, as it has allowed us to test whether the increased or decreased function of a gene affects pre- or postnatal development.

Overall there are strong links between molecular biology, adaptation to exercise, the genetics of sport- and exercise-related traits, and the development of the exercising human being. There are a plethora of questions in this area:

- By what mechanisms does the exercise of a child promote or hinder the development of muscles, joints, tendons, the cardiovascular system, the nervous system, and overall growth?
- Do the exercise and diet habits of mothers and fathers affect their children? If so, what are the underlying mechanisms?
- What are the mechanisms that explain variations in trainability with different developmental stages?
- Can we use genetic tests to predict the talent of a child for sport? If so, what are the ethical considerations?

We do not have satisfactory answers for all these questions. This chapter introduces molecular exercise physiology to those that work in paediatric exercise physiology in a way that is not overly technical. It first discusses signal transduction and introduces the development of skeletal muscle (myogenesis), tendon, and bone (osteogenesis) as examples for the development of key exercise organs. It then discusses some questions related to development, nutrition, and exercise. Afterwards it introduces the modern signal transduction hypothesis of adaptation in relation to resistance and endurance exercise. It covers molecular genetics and highlights that athletic talent is all about DNA sequence variations. Finally, it reviews how our genome has evolved and given us unique exercise capabilities, the genetics of maturation and body height, strength, and endurance-related traits, and asks whether genetic performance tests make any sense.

Development of key exercise organs

Using examples, this first section discusses how development is regulated on a cellular and molecular level, and specifically reviews the development of muscle, bones, and tendons. It then provides examples of how exercise and nutrition affect development.

On a cellular level, while cells become more and more specialized during development and thereby reduce their potency. The fertilized oocyte is a totipotent stem cell, as it is able to differentiate into all the cells of the body. With ongoing development, pluripotent and multipotent cells emerge that can differentiate into several, but not all, cell types (pluripotent cells can differentiate into more cell types than multipotent cells). Fully differentiated cells have reached their final point in development and, under normal circumstances, are not able to differentiate into other cell types. However, in adult tissues, adult stem cells, such as satellite cells in skeletal muscle, exist. These regenerate organs, for example, after sports injuries and support postnatal growth.

On a molecular level, transcription factors regulate the differentiation and identity of cells. Transcription factors are proteins that bind specific, short regulatory DNA motifs to switch on or off the expression of genes, or to open up or close down specific parts of the genome, such as the muscle or brain parts. Generally, half of all transcription factors are expressed in any one cell type[2] and while some regulate the gene expression response to signals like exercise, other factors, termed core or pioneer factors, are capable of regulating the identity of a cell. In other words, their expression determines whether a cell is a stem cell, muscle cell, or a neuron.

The ability of so-called core or pioneer transcription factors to regulate the cell type is perhaps best demonstrated by seminal experiments by the group of the Nobel Prize recipient Shinya Yamanaka. They expressed the transcription factors Oct3/4, Sox2, c-Myc, and Klf4 in mouse[3] and human fibroblasts[4] and found that this changed the identity of the cells from fibroblasts to induced pluripotent stem cells (iPSC). These experiments both confirmed that transcription factors can determine the identity of a cell, which was already known, and that transcription factors could be used to turn a fully differentiated cell into a pluripotent stem cell. This represented a major breakthrough in life sciences research, as induced pluripotent stem cells could potentially be used to regenerate diseased organs.

In other research, MyoD (gene symbol *MyoD1*) was identified as a muscle-making transcription factor.[5,6] In this study, the authors used the DNA altering agent 5-azacytidine on fibroblasts, which allowed new genes to be switched on. In rare cases the fibroblasts turned into muscle cells, termed myoblasts, suggesting that some of the newly expressed proteins had muscle-making properties. The authors then carried out further molecular analyses to identify the muscle-making protein that was expressed after 5-azacytine treatment. They found a protein, which they named MyoD, and confirmed that it can indeed turn fibroblasts into muscle cells. Subsequent experiments showed that the forced expression of MyoD could turn all sorts of cells into muscle cells, or at least switch on the expression of muscle genes.[7] Taken together, especially core or pioneer transcription factors regulate the differentiation of cells from the totipotent, fertilized oocyte to the various fully differentiated cell types in the adult body. The sets of transcription factors that are critical for certain cell types are increasingly identified.[8]

The development of muscle: myogenesis

This next section discusses the development of specific tissues. The development of skeletal muscle (myogenesis), tendon, and bone (osteogenesis) are examples of the development of key exercise organs.

After fertilization, the cells in the oocyte divide and form the primary germ layers of the embryo which will then go on to differentiate into organs in a process termed organogenesis. The germ layers are:[9]

i) Ectoderm (outer layer): these cells will develop into the epidermis of the skin, brain, and nervous system.

ii) Endoderm (inner layer): these cells will develop into the epithelium of the digestive tube and its organs, including the lungs.

iii) Mesoderm (middle layer): these cells will form blood, heart, kidney, gonads, bones, muscles, and connective tissues.

Skeletal muscle is the key exercise organ as it converts the chemical energy in nutrients into force, movement, and heat. Muscle development (see Figure 31.1) begins when cells form somites, which are blocks of mesodermal cells that form to the left and right of the head-to-tail axis of the embryo.[10,11] Myogenesis is then initiated by the expression of *Myf5, Mrf4,* and *MyoD*, which are closely related myogenic regulatory factors.[10] The expression of these genes is essential for myogenesis because if *Myf5, Mrf4,* and *MyoD* are knocked out then muscle does not form in mouse embryos.[12,13] *Myf5, Mrf4,* and *MyoD*-expressing muscle cells are cells with one nucleus, termed myoblasts. Later, such myoblasts fuse to form multi-nucleated myotubes, which further mature into muscle fibres. The fusion of myoblasts is regulated by myogenin, another myogenic regulatory factor.[10,14,15] Adult muscle fibres of long human muscles, such as the sartorius and gracilis, can be up to 20 cm long[16] and may contain tens of thousands of nuclei.[1] Human skeletal muscles are often comprised of hundreds of thousands of muscle fibres, but their numbers differ greatly between individuals. For example, the vastus lateralis muscles of males around 20 years of age contain between 393 000 and 903 000 muscle fibres.[17] Also, there are slow type I, intermediate type IIa, and fast type IIx muscle fibres in humans,[18] and there is great inter-individual variation between their relative percentages, with sprinters having more type II and endurance runners having more type I muscle fibres.[19,20] The number of muscle fibres per

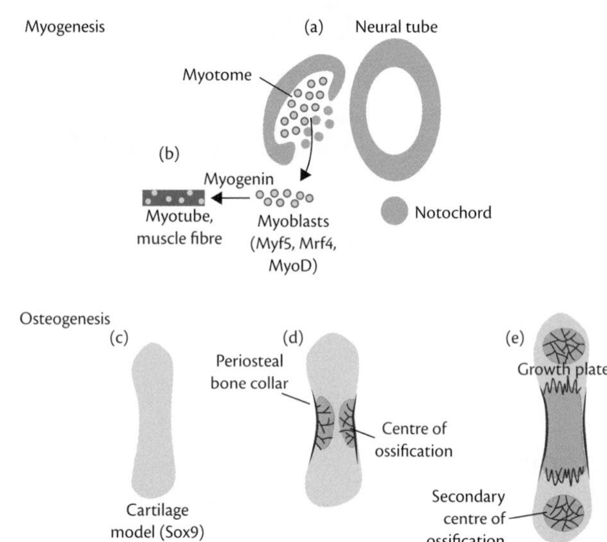

Figure 31.1 Schematic depicting key events during myogenesis and osteogenesis. Myogenensis.
(a) Somites form left and right of the head-to-tail axis of the embryo. From somatic cells the myotome develops which comprises myoblasts that express. (b) Myf5, Mrf4 or Myod as muscle-making transcription factors. Especially myogenin regulates then the fusion of myoblasts into myotubes that further mature into muscle fibres. Osteogenesis through endochondral ossification.[32] (c) A cartilage model of the future bone forms. (d) Ossification starts and a so-called periosteal bone collar forms. The primary centre of ossification expands towards the ends of the cartilage model. (e) Secondary centres of ossification form at each end of the bone to the outside of the growth plate or epiphyseal plate. When growth ends, the growth plate cartilage is replaced by bone tissue. At this stage, cartilage only exists at the ends of the bone, as the articular cartilage of joints.

muscle and the fibre type proportions are likely dependent mainly on differences in the DNA sequence of individuals, as environmental factors such as training have little effect.

Muscle fibres cannot regenerate themselves, as the nuclei in muscle fibres do not divide anymore. This task is instead carried out by the resident stem cells of skeletal muscle, termed satellite cells, which were discovered by electron microscopy.[21] Satellite cells express the transcription factor Pax7 and the knockout of Pax7 results in the loss of almost all satellite cells, and thus impaired skeletal muscle growth.[22] The function and importance of satellite cells is controversial in the literature, but mouse models have allowed researchers to deplete satellite cells in mouse muscle and provide a suitable experimental model to finally address key questions of satellite cell biology. As expected, satellite cells are essential for the regeneration of skeletal muscle.[23–25] However, and perhaps surprisingly, the depletion of satellite cells does not prevent the initial overload-induced hypertrophy,[26] although the hypertrophied muscle cannot be maintained over longer periods if it lacks satellite cells.[27] Thus, satellite cells are key for the regeneration of muscle, but not for an initial muscle hypertrophy in response to overload, as this mainly depends on the protein accretion of muscle fibres.

The development of tendons

Tendons are mechanically tough connective tissues that connect muscles to bone. Cells that commit to the tendon lineage express a transcription factor termed scleraxis (gene symbol *Scx*).[28] Scleraxis is not only a marker of tendons and tendon progenitors, but it also contributes to their development, as *Scx* knockout mice have severe tendon defects.[29] This suggests that *Scx* is only one of several transcription factors that are necessary for normal tendon development. In the actual tendons, fibroblasts that are also called tenocytes then synthesize the stringy protein collagen I and these collagen I fibres align parallel to the tendon axis. Tendons then connect to muscle via the myotendinous junction, and to bone via the enthesis.[30] Muscle is required for tendon formation because the loss of almost all muscle in MyoD and Myf5 double-knockout mice also leads to the loss of *Scx* expression.[31]

The formation of bone: chondrogenesis and osteogenesis

Bones form the skeleton, and their longitudinal growth determines the overall growth of a child and adolescent. Bone forms through one of two processes, depending on the type of bone:[9,13]

- *Intramembranous ossification*: the process that leads to the formation of the flat bones, for example, the skull. During this process embryonic mesenchymal cells differentiate directly into bone.
- *Endochondral ossification*: (see Figure 31.1) the process that forms the long bones of the arms and legs, in addition to most other bones. During this process, embryonic mesenchymal cells first form a cartilage model of a bone as an intermediate, which then turns into bone in a second step, termed ossification. The longitudinal growth of such bones takes place at the growth plate (also known as physis or epiphyseal plate) until adult height is reached, at which point the growth plate also turns into bone.

A plethora of molecular signalling processes governs the differentiation of the initial mesenchymal cells into chondrocytes, the proliferation, and further differentiation of chondrocytes before endochondral ossification, which is the actual formation of bones through mineralization.[32] In chondrocytes, the expression of the transcription factor Sox9 is key; a knockout of Sox9 blocks the formation of cartilage and bone.[33] This suggests that Sox9 is essential for chondrogenesis. Moreover, if Sox9 is artificially expressed in hypertrophic chondrocytes (i.e. chondrocytes that are about to turn into bone) then bone does not form, suggesting that chondrocytes need to switch off Sox9 to ossify.[34] Together this implies that Sox9 is essential for the formation of chondrocytes prior to endochondral ossification. At the same time, Sox9 prevents the last step of osteogenesis by suppressing ossification, vascularization, and bone marrow formation. After the formation of chondrocytes, the key transcription factor Runx2 (also known as Cbf1a) is required for ossification. The best evidence for this is in mice where Runx2 is knocked out; these mice do not form bone due to the blocking of endochondral and intramembranous ossification.[35] Further research shows that Runx2 is required for chondrocyte maturation and for the formation of osteoblasts.[32]

Mechanical signals and cell differentiation

After discussing the development of muscle, tendon, and bone we will now discuss how mechanical signals resulting from muscle contraction, or the mechanical properties of a cell, regulate differentiation. Mechanical signals influence development and cellular behaviour, and also cause muscle, tendon, and bone adaptations in children and adults. To investigate the effect of mechanical signals on development, researchers have pharmacologically paralysed the muscles in chick limbs or used MyoD and Myf5 double knockout mice, that form little or no muscle.[36] These animal models generally show that the paralysis or absence of muscle results in impaired joint and bone development. For example, MyoD and Myf5 double knockout mice have altered long bones with less mineralization. Additionally, these mice have more bone-degrading osteoclasts in newly formed bone, suggesting that muscle and the resultant mechanical loading are already important for normal bone mineralization during early development.[37] Thus, even prenatal 'exercise' of the embryo will influence the development of its body.

However, mechanical signals not only regulate the gene expression, development, and size of organs, but they can also affect the cell type into which stem cells differentiate. If mesenchymal stem cells are cultured on substrates with different stiffness, then this affects the differentiation of these cells. When grown on soft substrate (0.1–1 kPa elasticity) the mesenchymal cells express neurogenic markers, such as *GDNF*, *TUBB4/1*, and *NCAM1*, and turn into neurons. When grown on medium substrate (8–17 kPa elasticity) then the cells express myogenic regulators, such as *MYOG*, *PAX7*, and *MEF2C*, and turn into myoblasts. Finally, when grown on hard substrate (25–40 kPa elasticity) then the cells express bone markers, such as *SMAD*s and *RUNX2* (CBF1), and turn into osteoblasts.[38] In another study, the signalling events that regulate cell behaviour in relation to stiffness were investigated. The authors found that a stiff substrate led to the expression of genes that are typically regulated by the so-called Hippo pathway.[39] Together, the stiffness of the cell niche plus mechanical loading affect the lineage into which mesenchymal cells differentiate; the adaptations of cells of the skeleton to loading and the Hippo pathway are key regulators of such responses. It is unknown whether mechanical stimuli in utero affect development of organs through these mechanisms.

Epigenetic regulation of development: does maternal nutrition and exercise affect the offspring?

Epigenetics refers to the study of long term changes in gene expression that occur in the absence of changes to the DNA sequence.[40] This section reviews histone acetylation, DNA methylation, and microRNAs, which are the much-studied epigenetic changes in relation to exercise. Histone acetylation refers to the addition of an acetyl group by a histone acetyltransferase (HAT). This typically promotes gene transcription by unravelling DNA and exposing sites for the transcriptional machinery. Conversely, histone deacetylases (HDACs) remove acetyl groups. Such deacetylation changes the conformational layout of chromatin to a more condensed state, essentially wrapping DNA more tightly around the histone molecules, making sites inaccessible to transcriptional machinery. Thus, histone deacetylation is associated with transcriptional repression.[41] Deoxyribonucleic acid methylation involves the addition of a methyl group at CpG and non-CpG sites throughout the genome (where C = a cystosine nucleobase, G = a guanine nucleobase and p = the phosphate in-between) by the DNA methyltransferase family of enzymes (DNMTs).[42] The effect this modification elicits on gene expression depends on its location, i.e. DNA methylation at promoter or enhancer regions of genes is associated with transcriptional repression,[43] whereas DNA methylation within the gene body is associated with active transcription.[44] Lastly, microRNAs are non-coding ribonucleic acids (RNAs) that have the ability to bind and decrease the stability of messenger RNA (mRNA). This can lead to degradation of the mRNA or repress its translation into a fully functioning protein.[45] Additionally, the binding of microRNAs to mRNA can directly up- or down-regulate its translation into protein.[46,47] Together, these nuclear changes and posttranscriptional modifications govern tissue and cell specific gene expression, and, thus, overall organismal phenotype.

So why is the study of epigenetics relevant for paediatric exercise physiologists? Firstly, it is becoming increasingly apparent that epigenetic traits as a consequence of nutrition or exercise may be inherited over generations[48] (and that atypical epigenomes are associated with numerous diseases).[45,49] As such, an individual's epigenome may not only increase their own susceptibility to certain diseases, but also the susceptibility of their offspring. Of particular importance is the epigenetic influence of perinatal nutrition, as a link between foetal malnutrition in the womb and development of disease in later life. This was first proposed by David J P Barker who showed that a lower birth weight, which is partially dependent on foetal nutrition (the genetics of birth weight will be discussed later), was significantly correlated with an increased risk of developing insulin resistance, type 2 diabetes, and other pathologies in later life.[50] This phenomenon has been termed the 'Barker' or 'thrifty phenotype' hypothesis and is supported by retrospective studies on pregnant women and their offspring during the Dutch Winter Famine (1944–1945), the Leningrad Siege (1941–1944), and the Chinese Famine (1959–1961). It has been hypothesized that, in such conditions, under-nutrition is sensed by the foetus and that this leads to long-term epigenetic adaptations that enable the greatest chance of survival by preparing the individual for a life of malnourishment.[51] It may not just be the nutrition of the mother that influences the epigenome of offspring, either, as a recent study has added to the body of evidence suggesting that paternal prenatal health may also play a role. In a recent report, epigenetic differences between the sperm of lean and obese men in areas of the genome implicated in obesity and appetite regulation were discovered.[52] Although the nature of the study means that a causal link between paternal and offspring obesity cannot be confirmed, it further suggests that environmental factors can have a profound epigenetic impact on germ cells. This could potentially influence embryo development and the resulting phenotype of the child.

Secondly, given that exercise has a profound effect on epigenetic markers, especially for mitochondria, it is intuitive to suggest that the maternal and paternal pre- and perinatal exercise may impact the expression of genes that have a lasting influence on the athletic prowess of their offspring. In support of this, maternal exercise during gestation reduces PGC-1α hypermethylation and ameliorates age-related metabolic dysfunction in C57BL/6 mice at 9 months of age.[53] Furthermore, comparing the molecular and phenotypic evidence suggests that moderate maternal exercise during early pregnancy can enhance foetal growth[54] whereas high volumes of maternal exercise during the later stages of pregnancy can reduce foetal growth.[55] In relation to this, Chalk and Brown[56] propose a dose-dependent, hypothetical model for the effects of maternal exercise on the foetal epigenome, which tentatively suggests that maternal exercise is beneficial at low to moderate doses but potentially detrimental at high doses. Together this suggests that pre- and postnatal development is not solely driven by a genetic programme that proceeds without regard for nutrition or exercise signals. Instead, nutrition and exercise especially influence the epigenome of the embryo, which may have consequence for its health and, potentially, also exercise abilities later in life.

The signal transduction model of adaptation

This section discusses the mechanism that results in the adaptation to exercise in children, adolescents, and adults. Training scientists had listed 'principles of training', such as overload, but these often trivial principles are not mechanisms of adaptation and are of little practical use. Others had generalized the supercompensation or overcompensation time course of glycogen (i.e. the increase of glycogen values above resting values after exhausting exercise, recovery, and feeding) as a pseudo-mechanism that explains adaptation to exercise.[57] While such a time course may seem intuitive as a training mechanism and has been experimentally demonstrated,[58] there are few other systems that follow such a time course. Also, according to the supercompensation hypothesis, post-exercise rest periods would be essential for adaptation. However, for key exercise organs this is not true. The heart never rests and adapts to exercise. Similarly, chronic, low-frequency electrical stimulation of skeletal muscle for weeks without rest leads to extreme endurance exercise-like adaptations.[59,60] Together this demonstrates that the supercompensation hypothesis is not a mechanism that describes the general adaptation to exercise.

So, what are the actual mechanisms that mediate adaptation to exercise? Research by molecular exercise physiologists into the mechanisms of adaptation to exercise training has unequivocally demonstrated that signal transduction proteins mediate the adaptation to exercise. Firstly, sensor proteins (SE in Figure 31.2) sense exercise-induced signals such as tension, adenosine monophosphate (AMP), glycogen, calcium (Ca^{2+}), oxygen (O_2), and hormones. In the second step, signal transduction proteins (SP in Figure 31.2), which are organized as pathways and networks, convey, amplify, and compute this information. In the third step, signal transduction proteins regulate effector proteins (EP in Figure 31.2) that then control processes, such as gene expression, protein synthesis, protein breakdown, and other processes such as proliferation or cell death. In their sum, these are the adaptation to exercise training. This experimentally well-supported, generalized theory is schematically illustrated in Figure 31.2.

An important point regarding adaptation is that the magnitude of adaptations differs between individuals, as the $\dot{V}O_2$ max adaptation to endurance exercise,[61] strength and muscle hypertrophy adaptations to resistance training,[62] and health adaptations to endurance training[63] all vary greatly in the human population. The trainability of key exercise variables not only differs between individuals, but there is also an ongoing debate as to how trainability changes in children and adolescents, and whether there are 'windows of [enhanced] trainability'.[64] Genetic studies have started to identify DNA sequence variations that partially explain the trainability of individuals.

Genetics

Introduction to genetics and exercise

The athletic development of a child depends on its unique genome, i.e. its DNA sequence, and on environmental factors of which training, nutrition, and a pro-sports environment are probably the most important. David Epstein has illustrated this in his popular science book 'The Sports Gene' in which he eloquently debunks the '10 000 h of practice is all it takes' hypothesis. Instead he demonstrates to the wider readership that DNA sequence variations are roughly as important as the environment for elite sporting performance.[65] But while everyone can potentially train hard and eat a performance-promoting diet it is impossible to alter athletic talent, which is essentially determined by an individual's DNA sequence variations that encode sporting ability. Generally, DNA sequence variations

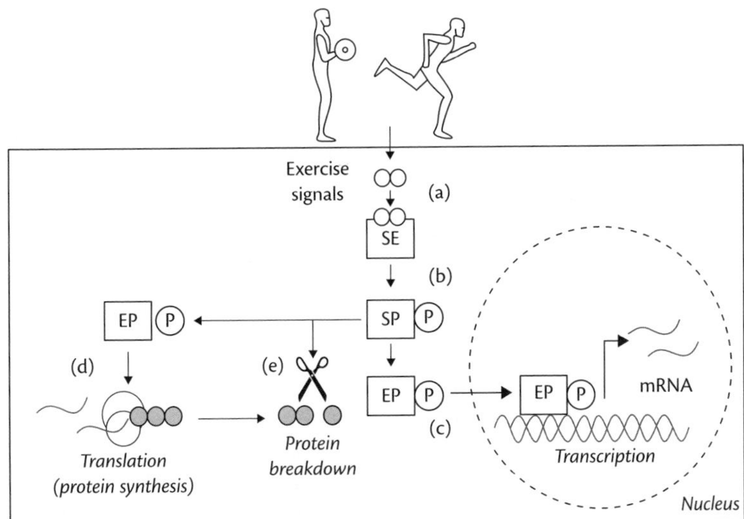

Figure 31.2 Schematic drawing of the signal transduction theory of adaptation to exercise.
(a) Resistance and endurance exercise each induce a specific set of signals in skeletal muscle (shown here) and other organs. These signals include changes in the concentration of small molecules such as Ca^{2+} or O_2, mechanical signals or hormones. All of these signals are sensed by sensor proteins (SE). (b) Active sensor proteins then regulate the activity, binding, modification, and localization of signal transduction proteins (SP). Such signal transduction proteins are organised as pathways and networks, which convey, amplify and compute this information. A common form of signalling is reversible protein phosphorylation (the circled 'P' indicates a phosphate group). (c) Active signal transduction proteins regulate effector proteins (EP) that then mediate cellular processes. Together, these are the adaptation to exercise. A key group of effector proteins are transcription factors, which bind specific, short DNA motifs to regulate gene expression. (d) A second class of effector proteins is the translational regulators, which regulate the translation of RNA into protein by ribosomes and, thus, cell hypertrophy. (e) Finally, protein breakdown and other cellular processes are also regulated by active effector proteins.

strongly influence the baseline values of sport and exercise-related traits, such as maximal oxygen uptake ($\dot{V}O_2$ max), strength, or body height, as well as the trainability of traits that can be improved.[1] Having favourable DNA sequence variations for most of these traits and the right environment in a highly motivated girl or boy gives a high chance that she or he will develop into an elite athlete later in life, if the training regime is effective and if injuries do not stop athletic development.

How does the unique DNA sequence of an embryo, child, adolescent, or adult encode athletic talent? The DNA in the human genome encodes roughly 3.3 billion DNA base pairs (Gb) for a haploid genome, where only one of each chromosome pair is counted, and 6.6 Gb for the whole diploid genome, where both copies of the 22 autosomes and two sex chromosomes are counted. A particular version of DNA on one chromosome is termed an allele and, as chromosomes come in pairs (the sex chromosomes in men being an exception), we generally carry two alleles for each bit of DNA. Our genome encodes just over 20 000 protein-coding genes and 8500 RNA genes, which are not translated into protein but are still important. For example, ribosomes, the protein synthesis machines of our cells, are mainly made out of ribosomal RNA and, in addition, there are many regulatory RNAs, some of which we have partially discussed. The DNA of humans, and also the DNA of most of the cells within our own body, differ because errors occur when cells divide and double up their DNA, in a reaction termed replication. This is a nearly, but not fully, error-proof process and so, despite faithful replication and effective repair mechanisms, it has been estimated that errors occur in roughly 1 per 100 000 bases.[66] Even though nearly 80% of the genome has a function, at least in some cells,[67] most mutations have probably no or hardly any effect, as they do not change the sequence of a protein or they lie in DNA that has no or only minor regulatory functions. Mutations that change amino acids in a protein or convert them to premature stop codons or mutations that change regulatory DNA are likely to change the function of the affected cells and of the whole organism.

Mutations will result in DNA sequence variations that can either be variations of one base (e.g. from CAG to CTG), termed single nucleotide polymorphism (SNP, pronounced 'snip'), or can be more complex changes of the DNA which are typically insertions or deletions (abbreviated as Indels). Insertions and deletions can occur when mitosis or DNA repair malfunctions.

Deoxyribonucleic acid sequence variations can be common (the minor allele or variant is >5%) or rare (the minor allele or variant is <5%). Somewhat confusing polymorphisms are DNA sequence variations that occur at least in 1% of the population. The 1000 Genomes Project has quantified the DNA sequence variation in the human genome. They estimate that each individual carries 30 000–150 000 rare (<0.5% frequency), 120 000–680 000 low-frequency (0.5–5% frequency) and 3.6–3.9 million common (>5%) DNA sequence variations.[68] Generally, common DNA sequence variations, especially SNPs, have a small effect size; in other words they affect traits such as the $\dot{V}O_2$ max, height, or fasting blood glucose only a tiny bit. This is because if a DNA sequence variation has a large positive or negative effect on a phenotype that affects fitness, then it will either become fixed in the population (i.e. after several generations the whole species will carry the fitness-increasing variant and then it is not a variant anymore) or it will not or rarely be passed on because it reduces the chance of having offspring. This is the case for many Mendelian diseases that are caused by one detrimental mutation. Only DNA sequence variations with no or small effect sizes can remain variations in the population over long periods, as there is minimal selection for or against the DNA sequence variation. Thus, in summary, common DNA sequence variations generally have a small effect size whereas some rare DNA sequence variations can have a large positive or negative effect size.

Sequence variations: large and small effects

So do exceptional athletes carry the favourable alleles of thousands of common DNA sequence variations, or is it rare DNA sequence variations that play an important role? This question is not yet answered, but there are examples for rare DNA sequence variations with a large effect size on sport and exercise-related traits. Deoxyribonucleic acid sequence loss-of-function variations in myostatin (gene symbol *Gdf8*)[69] have a large effect on muscle size in several species, including humans.[70] It is likely that such mutations not only increase mass but also muscle function, as whippet dogs that are heterozygous (i.e. only one of the two copies is affected) for a premature stop codon in the myostatin gene have a greater muscle mass and are significantly faster than wildtype dogs.[71] Nonetheless, such myostatin loss-of-function mutations are rare because the large muscle mass presumably requires a large food intake and will reduce endurance capacity, which might have been detrimental in ancient times. Similarly, DNA sequence gain-of-function variations in the Epo receptor (gene symbol *EPOR*) have a large effect size on the haematocrit.[72] One carrier of this mutation, Eero Mäntyranta, had a haematocrit of over 60% and won three gold, two silver and two bronze medals in cross-country skiing during Olympic games. Intriguingly, no homozygous individuals appear to be born.[72] This perhaps suggests that high doses of the *EPOR* mutant are lethal, which might explain why this DNA sequence variation has remained rare. Several mutations of *EPOR* or of genes that are involved in the sensing of oxygen have been reported and result in a similar phenotype.[73]

In contrast, many common diseases and most sport- and exercise-related traits are complex traits characterized by a normal, rather than on/off, distribution. For example, although type 2 diabetes is diagnosed in an 'on/off' fashion, the diagnostic criterion of fasting blood glucose concentration varies greatly in human populations. Similarly, body height, maximal running speed, or $\dot{V}O_2$ max are not 'on/off' or 'high/low' traits, but follow a normal distribution. Such continuous or quantitative traits are typically influenced by many common DNA sequence variations with generally small effect sizes. However, this does not exclude the possibility of rare genotypes that only occur in a few cases, where they have a large effect size on traits otherwise shaped by many common DNA sequence variations with small effect sizes. Examples are DNA sequence variations of genes such as *HNF4α, GCK, HNF1α, PDX1*, or *HNF1β* that, on their own, are sufficient to cause maturity-onset diabetes of the young (MODY).[74] Similarly, while body height is a continuous, polygenic trait, mutations that change an arginine to a stop codon in the *AIP* gene are sufficient to cause gigantism, as they result in benign pituitary adenomas that secrete excess hormone.[75] Conversely, activating mutations of the *FGFR3* gene are sufficient to cause a form of dwarfism, termed achondroplasia, as active FGFR3 inhibits the proliferation of chondrocytes and, thus, longitudinal bone growth at the growth plate.[76] In summary, many common diseases and sport- and exercise-related traits are polygenic and are generally dependent on hundreds to thousands of common DNA sequence variations with small affect sizes. This does not exclude that, in some rare cases, mutations of single genes can be sufficient to cause a large effect size, as in the case of the double-muscled myostatin boy[70] or individuals with a high haematocrit due to *EPOR* mutations.[72] It is unknown whether many of the truly exceptional athletes carry rare DNA sequence variants that greatly affect a trait that is key for their performance.

Genotypic and phenotypic associations

So how are associations between genes and phenotypes discovered? Mendelian gene-phenotype associations, where individual genes have a large effect (e.g. *DMD* mutations in muscular dystrophy, *CTGF* mutations in cystic fibrosis), were typically discovered by linkage analyses using affected families or by studying candidate genes in individuals with striking phenotypes, as was the case in the double-muscled myostatin boy.[70] For the discovery of more common alleles, with smaller effect sizes, genome-wide association studies (GWAS) have been developed. In such studies, microchips are used to detect alleles of hundreds of thousands of SNPs in thousands or tens of thousands of individuals, where inherited traits, such as body height, have been determined. Importantly, GWAS analyses not only indicate whether the measured SNPs themselves influence the trait, but significant SNPs also indicate heritability in the vicinity of the SNP.[77] Another breakthrough in genetic analysis has been the development of next generation (DNA) sequencing, which has scaled up DNA sequencing so that many laboratories can now sequence a whole human genome in just several days.[78] This has shifted the problem from DNA sequencing to the bioinformatical analysis of the results to identify the genetic needles in the genome haystack that are responsible for the trait. Thus, sequencing the genomes of truly exceptional athletes is the easy bit; identifying the DNA sequence variations that make these athletes exceptional is the difficult part!

The genetics of development, maturation, and body height

Deoxyribonucleic acid sequence variations affect pre- and postnatal development, infancy, childhood, the onset of puberty, growth, and the body height that a girl or boy eventually reaches. Here, a much-studied factor is birth weight, which is associated with many exercise and health-related variables, including positive associations with adult grip strength (i.e. larger babies are stronger later in life[79]) being overweight,[80] cancer,[81] and negative associations with the risk of developing type 2 diabetes mellitus (i.e. lighter babies are more likely to develop diabetes[82]), cardiovascular mortality,[83] and all-cause mortality.[83] Birth weight depends on many factors that influence the growth of the embryo in the uterus, including DNA sequence variations in the embryo and mother.

A GWAS meta-analysis and other analyses, involving up to 70 000 individuals, have identified seven loci confirming *CCNL1* and *ADCY5*, which were already known, and newly identifying *HMGA2, LCORL, ADRB1, CDKAL1*, and a locus on chromosome 5 as loci associated with birth weight.[84] So what do the genes in these loci do? The birth weight-lowering alleles of *ADCY5* and *CDKAL1* were previously linked to a greater risk of type 2 diabetes, and the authors propose that these alleles lower foetal insulin and, thus, lower growth, which also increases the risk of type 2 diabetes.[84] Additionally, the birth weight-lowering alleles of *HMGA2* and *LCORL* were also associated with lower adult height and may slow growth.[84] This study shows that some DNA sequence variations partially determine our birth weight, carbohydrate metabolism, and growth.

After birth there is fast infant growth, slowing mild-childhood growth, and a pubertal growth spurt, before the growth plate ossifies and individuals reach their adult height. The timing and extent of growth varies greatly and is important for the sporting performance of children and adolescents at a given age ((interested readers are referred to Chapter 30 where this is dicussed further). To identify DNA sequence variations that determine when and by how much children and adolescents grow, researchers measured prepubertal height in females and males at 10 and 12 years, height change between age 8 and >18 years as total pubertal growth, and height change between age 14 and >18 years as late pubertal growth. The authors then performed a GWAS analysis to identify genes and loci that significantly affected these variables.[85] The authors identified nine loci that affected the variables investigated, of which *LIN28B* was previously known to influence pubertal growth. *LIN28B* is an interesting hit, as it regulates the timing of development in lower organisms, such as the worm, and regulates the proliferation and differentiation of stem cells.[86] Another hit was *MAPK3* gene, which encodes the ERK1 protein, whose deactivation has previously been linked to increased bone growth in mice. In addition to *LIN28B* and *MAPK3*, other significant loci and genes are *GNA12, ZBTB38, CABLES1, ADAMTS3, EFEMP1, ADCY3-POMC*, and *VGLL3*.[85]

The final result of pre- and postnatal growth is adult body height, a variable that is roughly 80% inherited and that can be measured cheaply, quickly, and reliably. Because of that, body height has been measured as a variable in many GWAS studies, making height the darling of variables for GWAS researchers. In the latest GWAS meta-analysis, the GWAS data of 253 288 individuals of European ancestry were incorporated to identify genomic loci that affect human body height.[87] The analyses show that 21%, 24%, and 29% of the variance in human height can be explained by the best 2000, 3700, and 9500 SNPs. This suggests that DNA sequence variations in thousands of genes and loci determine human height.[87] The authors then performed analyses to identify expression patterns and processes that are common to the genes that affect human height and found that the genes are highly expressed in tissues related to chondrocytes and osteoblasts, and other musculoskeletal, cardiovascular, and endocrine tissues. Also, the genes were involved in processes such as ossification, embryonic skeletal system development, and limb development.[87] Together this suggests that, while there are rare Mendelian disorders of body height such as dwarfism caused e.g. by *FGFR3* mutations,[76] or acromegaly as a consequence of mutations of the *AIP* gene,[75] generally body height is affected by DNA variations of thousands of genes that regulate growth pre- and postnatally.

Genetics of endurance and strength-related traits

Twin and family studies have been used to roughly estimate the inheritance of endurance and strength. For $\dot{V}O_2$ max, as a measure of aerobic fitness, the estimates range between 40% and 93%.[88,89] Recent estimates suggest that the heritability of $\dot{V}O_2$ max is 50%[90] and the trainability of $\dot{V}O_2$ max (i.e. the $\dot{V}O_2$ max change after a given amount of endurance training) is 47%.[91] For strength-related variables, the heritability estimates range from 14–90%.[92] As a very rough estimate, a heritability of 50% or more for strength should not be too far off, which is supported by a heritability of 50–60% for grip strength in the largest study of its kind.[93]

So what are the DNA sequence variations that explain the genetic variation of strength and endurance? We start to answer this question by reviewing human evolution, which is also the story of the occurrence and selection of DNA sequence variation that has shaped the exercise capabilities of modern day humans. Hominins have evolved from roughly 7 to 4 million years ago in the Savannah, in the rain shadow of the East African rift.[94] Around 1.9–1.8 million years ago, key events in human evolution happened: hominin brain size increased dramatically,[94] the shoulder morphology changed to allow the high-speed throwing of projectiles through utilization of elastically stored energy,[95] and hominins evolved endurance running capabilities.[96] In contrast, the great apes that evolved in the Western rain forests are characterized by smaller brains and have comparatively low endurance but high power, as judged by their extreme jumping ability.[97] Thus, at that point in time, DNA sequence variations that are now fixed in our current genomes entered the human gene pool, were selected, and now encode the typical intellectual and exercise abilities of modern day humans.

While hominin species did migrate at other times, the key migration event was when modern *Homo sapiens* left Africa, roughly 50 000–100 000 years ago, and populated the whole planet—from the arctic to the equator, from maritime areas to deserts, and from lowlands to mountainous areas of over 3000 m. There is evidence that modern-day humans have adapted genetically to their different habitats, with skin colour being the most obvious genetic adaptation to a specific environment. But there are other examples. For example, researchers compared Greenlandic Inuit with European controls using a Metabochip for SNPs associated with cardiometabolic phenotypes. The strongest signal came from loci of fatty acid desaturase genes, suggesting genetic adaptation to the unique high-meat and high-fat diet of the Inuit.[98] Similarly a genome-wide allelic differentiation scan of high altitude Tibetans and lowland Han Chinese,[99] and the sequencing of the exomes of 50 Tibetians,[100] led to the discovery of unique DNA sequence variations of the *EPAS1* gene in the Tibetans. *EPAS1* encodes the HIF2α transcription factor that mediates adaptation to hypoxia. Intriguingly, the Tibetans carried DNA sequence variations that promote a lower haematocrit, which prevents excessive haematocrit levels and resultant detrimental effects while living and exercising at high altitude. We have already discussed the example of Finnish families where some members have activating mutations in the *EPOR* receptor gene, which results in a very high haematocrit.[72] Interestingly, carriers appear to be heterozygous for the mutation and there are no homozygous individuals, presumably because the haematocrit is then lethal, which might explain why this genotype has not become enriched in the wider population.

The aforementioned Greenlanding Inuit, Tibetean, *EPOR*, and myostatin genotypes are examples for DNA-sequence variations with a large effect size that are otherwise rare in the global population. This poses the question whether unique DNA sequence variations with a large effect size can be found in populations with a high proportion of elite athletes. Examples of such populations are Kenian Kalenjin, Ethiopian Oromo, and Ugandan Sebei populations, with many elite endurance runners, and sprinters from West Africa or of West African descent, as well as Sherpa high-altitude mountaineers from Nepal.[65] Comparing populations that harbour a high frequency of athletes with close control populations, using methods such as genome-wide allelic differentiation scans or next-generation sequencing, should be a suitable strategy of identifying the genetic causes of the unique exercise capacity of some individuals in these populations, especially in pure endurance, power, strength, or high altitude sports.

What about the normal variation of strength and endurance-related traits in the normal population? In relation to this, molecular genetics started with the measurements of common DNA sequence variations that were first discovered and studied in a disease context. Much studied examples are the *ACE* I/D (reviewed by Puthucheary *et al.*[101]) and *ACTN3* R577X DNA sequence variants (reviewed by Eynon *et al.*[102]). However, while such DNA sequence variations may influence strength or endurance, their effect size is small and perhaps comparable to the variation caused by a difference of 1–2°C in the ambient temperature during a $\dot{V}O_2$ max test. This has recently been highlighted by Claude Bouchard, the perpetual pioneer of sport and exercise genetics, who has urged a shift to the unbiased exploration of the genome, with an emphasis on large subject numbers.[103]

Some GWAS studies have been performed in relation to sport- and exercise-related traits. In a key study, 473 sedentary adults, which is a low number for a GWAS study, performed a 20-week endurance exercise programme to determine the trainability of $\dot{V}O_2$ max. The researchers also obtained the DNA of the individuals and performed a GWAS analysis by measuring 324 611 SNPs.[104] The researchers found 39 SNPs that were significantly associated with the gain of $\dot{V}O_2$ max, with $P < 1.5 \times 10^{-4}$. A SNP score based on 21 alleles showed that individuals who carried nine or fewer favourable alleles improved their $\dot{V}O_2$ max by 221 $mL \cdot min^{-1}$ and those who carried ≥19 favourable alleles improved their $\dot{V}O_2$ max by 604 $mL \cdot min^{-1}$,[104] potentially making this a genetic test for cardiovascular fitness trainability, if it can be validated. In a follow-up study, the authors sought to determine the biological significance of their findings by performing additional analyses that incorporated biological knowledge and connections between genes in the analyses.[105] The fatty CoA synthetase long-chain family member 1 *(ACSL1)* was a key SNP that can potentially be related to changes in $\dot{V}O_2$ max. The analyses performed revealed other genes and pathways as candidates for $\dot{V}O_2$ max adaptation to exercise. Future studies will show whether the predictions resulting from these analyses are real, and if they indeed mediate the magnitude of the adaptive response.

In the Hunter community (n = 2088) and the Sydney Memory and Ageing (n = 541) GWAS studies, the genetic variants that determine grip strength in elderly men and women were investigated. The authors found no results of genome-wide significance and the results of the Hunter study were not replicated in the smaller Sydney study.[106] Gene-based analyses in the Hunter study identified *ZNF295* and *C2CD2* as significant genes. This study confirmed that very large datasets from, ideally, homogenous populations are needed for GWAS studies to have a chance of detecting common DNA sequence variations.

Another source of information regarding genes whose mutations affect endurance and strength are transgenic mouse models. Given that all genes are affected by DNA sequence variations in the human genome, transgenic mouse studies can allow researchers to identify candidate genes where DNA sequence variations change strength, endurance or other sport and exercise-related traits. For example, the identification of DNA sequence variations in the double-muscled myostatin boy[70] was informed by the prior discovery that the knockout of myostatin (gene symbol *Gdf8*) in mice results in double muscled mice.[69] Currently the International Mouse Phenotyping Consortium performs the extensive phenotyping of transgenic mouse models for 20 000 mouse genes.[107] The limitation for exercise physiologists is that grip strength is the only muscle strength-related phenotype that is measured. There is already a plethora of transgenic mouse models with exercise-related phenotypes. This includes a transgenic mouse that overexpresses the enzyme Pepck (gene symbol *Pck1*) in skeletal muscle.[108] These mice have a greatly enhanced endurance running performance when compared to wildtype mice. So, another approach for the discovery of rare DNA sequence variations, with larger effect sizes, could be to sequence candidate genes in individuals with unusual sport and exercise-related traits.

Genetic testing

Given that many sport- and exercise-related traits are significantly and typically 50% inherited, genetic tests could potentially be used to predict athletic talent or other related variables, such as adult body height or the susceptibility to injury. The possibility of such tests poses two key questions that we aim to answer. Firstly, are such genetic performance tests meaningful in a sense that they predict reliably whether an individual has athletic talent? Secondly, are such tests ethical?

If a genetic test for a sport- and exercise-related trait is to be meaningful, then the result must predict a large proportion of the trait. Thus, if just a single DNA sequence variation is measured, then this should have a Mendelian 'talent versus no talent' effect size for the test to be meaningful. This is true for the very rare human myostatin[70] and *EPOR*[72] genotypes but not for common genotypes such as the *ACE* I/D[101] or *ACTN3* R577X[102] polymorphisms, which have a small effect size that only explains a small fraction of athletic talent. Most sport- and exercise-related traits are probably highly polygenic, similar to body height,[87] which itself contributes to talent in many sports. For example, to determine the talent for National Basketball Association basketball in a child through a genetic test, one would need to measure thousands of DNA sequence variations for height alone,[87] in addition to DNA sequence variation that influence traits including speed and power, aerobic and anaerobic endurance, motor skill learning, visual perception, and resistance to injury. The only way to detect common and rare DNA sequence variations that determine the talent for basketball would be to sequence the whole genome of the individual, which is possible now,[78] followed by extensive bioinformatical analyses to detect hundreds or thousands of causative alleles. Frankly, classical talent identification, which is an indirect genetic test, is much more effective! In line with this, researchers have highlighted issues with direct-to-consumer marketing of genetic tests aimed at identifying a child's athletic talent. The researchers agree that genetic tests have currently no role in talent identification or individualized training prescription.[109]

The second, and potentially more important, issue is whether genetic tests are ethical. For example, is it ethical to take a DNA sample from an embryo, child, or adolescent to predict athletic talent? This has been discussed in a review related to a British Association of Sport and Exercise Sciences (BASES) position stand on the issue,[110] and in a recent review.[109] Key arguments in this debate are:

- *Testing of embryos*: As the DNA sequence of an individual does not change, the predictive power of a genetic test is the same no matter if it is performed using the DNA of embryos, children, adolescents, or adults. This is very different to most classical performance tests, as their predictive power depends on the age at which they are performed. For example, $\dot{V}O_2$ max or one repetition maximum tests in toddlers are almost meaningless but might accurately predict adult aerobic performance when performed in adolescents. Thus there is a danger that genetic performance tests could be performed in embryos and the findings used to decide whether to carry out an abortion.

- *Unknown disease implications:* Some DNA sequence variations may later turn out to be associated with major disease. For example, a polymorphism in the human bradykinin *B2BKR* receptor is associated not only with exercise-induced cardiac hypertrophy[111] and mechanical efficiency,[112] but also with increased cardiac disease risk.[113] It seems plausible that some growth-related alleles also predispose for cancer and this would potentially be devastating news for the carrier.

In summary, the current best forms of genetic testing are the classical performance tests, as they comprehensively assess the genetic basis of athletic talent, even if in an indirect way. Current molecular genetic tests focused on single or few polymorphisms are not meaningful, as SNPs typically have small effect sizes and so yield minimal information about the genetic basis of athletic talent.[103,109] However, the combination of next generation sequencing[78] and powerful bioinformatics may potentially uncover rare and common DNA sequence variations that explain a great fraction of athletic talent. Such tests might be meaningful but, here, professional genetic counselling,[109] data protection, the prohibition of the testing of embryos or minors, and a way to deal with alleles that predict major disease, are important.

Conclusions

Molecular exercise physiology in the context of paediatric exercise physiology is a large field where developmental physiology, molecular biology, and classical exercise physiology converge. Studying the pre- and postnatal development of key exercise organs will reveal how they develop and may help to explain differences between individuals. Of particular interest are maternal influences such as maternal nutrition and exercise. Adaptation to exercise is mediated by signal transduction networks in three steps: i) The sensing of exercise-induced signals e.g. by tension, AMP, glycogen, Ca^{2+}, O_2, and hormone-sensing proteins; ii) The transduction and computation of such signals by signal transduction proteins; iii) The regulation of adaptations such as mitochondrial biogenesis, protein synthesis, or apoptosis by effector proteins. Sport and exercise genetics currently experience a change of direction as researchers realize that the study of common DNA sequence variants with generally small effect sizes in <100 individuals yields little useful information. Studies on traits such as body height reveal that such traits depend on hundreds, if not thousands, of common DNA sequence variations and, in rare cases, on rare DNA sequence variants with a large effect size. Thus, a change in approach and methodology is needed. Animal studies have revealed genes where mutations have a large effect size on performance and it will be key to determine whether the talent of elite athletes is based on rare DNA sequence variations or whether it is the cumulative effect of many favourable common DNA sequence variations.

Summary

- Molecular exercise physiology is the study of exercise physiology using molecular biology methods.
- The development of organs, including key exercise organs, depends on transcription factors that determine the identity of cells. MyoD is an example for a muscle-making transcription factor and Sox9 for a chondrocyte-making factor. Chondrocytes can further develop into bone.
- Maternal nutrition and exercise can regulate foetal development especially through epigenetic mechanisms.
- Adaptation to exercise occurs in three steps: i) sensor proteins sense exercise-induced signals such as tension, AMP, glycogen, Ca^{2+}, O_2, and hormones; ii) signal transduction proteins, which are organized as pathways and networks, convey, amplify, and compute this information; iii) effector proteins regulate things like gene expression, protein synthesis, protein breakdown, and other processes such as proliferation or cell death.
- 'Athletic talent' is a term that describes the DNA sequence variants that determine the potential for being an athlete.
- Common DNA sequence variations generally have a small effect size. In contrast, rare DNA sequence variations can have a large effect size. Examples for the latter are loss-of-function mutations of the myostatin (gene symbol *GDF8*) gene that are associated with increased muscle size, and gain-of-function mutations of the *EPOR* gene that are increased with a high haematocrit.
- Human body height depends on hundreds if not thousands of common DNA sequence variations. In rare cases mutations of the *FGFR3* gene and *AIP* gene have a large effect size as they cause dwarfism or acromegaly, respectively.
- Current genetic performance tests based on common DNA sequence variations yield little useful information and they are therefore discouraged. Additionally, there are ethical considerations in that genetic testing can potentially be performed on embryos and that some sport and exercise-related genotypes may later be identified as disease-associated genotypes.

References

1. Wackerhage H. *Molecular exercise physiology. An introduction*. Oxford: Routledge; 2014.
2. Vaquerizas JM, Kummerfeld SK, Teichmann SA, Luscombe NM. A census of human transcription factors: function, expression and evolution. *Nature Rev Genet*. 2009; 10: 252–263.
3. Takahashi K, Yamanaka S. Induction of pluripotent stem cells from mouse embryonic and adult fibroblast cultures by defined factors. *Cell*. 2006; 126: 663–676.
4. Takahashi K, Tanabe K, Ohnuki M, *et al*. Induction of pluripotent stem cells from adult human fibroblasts by defined factors. *Cell*. 2007; 131: 861–872.
5. Lassar AB, Paterson BM, Weintraub H. Transfection of a DNA locus that mediates the conversion of 10T1/2 fibroblasts to myoblasts. *Cell*. 1986; 47: 649–656.
6. Davis RL, Weintraub H, Lassar AB. Expression of a single transfected cDNA converts fibroblasts to myoblasts. *Cell*. 1987; 51: 987–1000.
7. Weintraub H, Tapscott SJ, Davis RL, *et al*. Activation of muscle-specific genes in pigment, nerve, fat, liver, and fibroblast cell lines by forced expression of MyoD. *Proc Nat Acad Sci*. 1989; 86: 5434–5438.
8. D'Alessio AC, Fan ZP, Wert KJ, *et al*. A systematic approach to identify candidate transcription factors that control cell identity. *Stem Cell Rep*. 2015; 5: 763–775.
9. Gilbert SF. *Developmental biology*, 10th ed. Sunderland, MA: Sinauer; 2014.

10. Buckingham M, Rigby PW. Gene regulatory networks and transcriptional mechanisms that control myogenesis. *Dev Cell.* 2014; 28: 225–238.
11. Buckingham M, Bajard L, Chang T, *et al.* The formation of skeletal muscle: from somite to limb. *J Anat.* 2003; 202: 59–68.
12. Rudnicki MA, Schnegelsberg PN, Stead RH, Braun T, Arnold HH, Jaenisch R. MyoD or Myf-5 is required for the formation of skeletal muscle. *Cell.* 1993; 75: 1351–1359.
13. Kassar-Duchossoy L, Gayraud-Morel B, Gomes D, *et al.* Mrf4 determines skeletal muscle identity in Myf5:Myod double-mutant mice. *Nature.* 2004; 431: 466–471.
14. Neuhaus P, Braun T. Transcription factors in skeletal myogenesis of vertebrates. *Results Probl Cell Differ.* 2002; 38: 109–126.
15. Buckingham M, Vincent SD. Distinct and dynamic myogenic populations in the vertebrate embryo. *Curr Opin Genet Dev.* 2009; 19: 444–453.
16. Heron MI, Richmond FJ. In-series fiber architecture in long human muscles. *J Morphol.* 1993; 216: 35–45.
17. Lexell J, Taylor CC, Sjostrom M. What is the cause of the ageing atrophy? Total number, size and proportion of different fiber types studied in whole vastus lateralis muscle from 15- to 83-year-old men. *J Neurol Sci.* 1988; 84: 275–294.
18. Schiaffino S. Fibre types in skeletal muscle: a personal account. *Acta Physiol.* 2010; 199: 451–463.
19. Costill DL, Fink WJ, Pollock ML. Muscle fiber composition and enzyme activities of elite distance runners. *Med Sci Sports.* 1976; 8: 96–100.
20. Costill DL, Daniels J, Evans W, Fink W, Krahenbuhl G, Saltin B. Skeletal muscle enzymes and fiber composition in male and female track athletes. *J Appl Physiol.* 1976; 40: 149–154.
21. Mauro A. Satellite cell of skeletal muscle fibers. *J Biophys Biochem Cytol.* 1961; 9: 493–495.
22. Seale P, Sabourin LA, Girgis-Gabardo A, Mansouri A, Gruss P, Rudnicki MA. Pax7 is required for the specification of myogenic satellite cells. *Cell.* 2000; 102: 777–786.
23. Murphy MM, Lawson JA, Mathew SJ, Hutcheson DA, Kardon G. Satellite cells, connective tissue fibroblasts and their interactions are crucial for muscle regeneration. *Development.* 2011; 138: 3625–3637.
24. Lepper C, Partridge TA, Fan CM. An absolute requirement for Pax7-positive satellite cells in acute injury-induced skeletal muscle regeneration. *Development.* 2011; 138: 3639–3646.
25. Sambasivan R, Yao R, Kissenpfennig A, *et al.* Pax7-expressing satellite cells are indispensable for adult skeletal muscle regeneration. *Development.* 2011; 138: 3647–3656.
26. McCarthy JJ, Mula J, Miyazaki M, *et al.* Effective fiber hypertrophy in satellite cell-depleted skeletal muscle. *Development.* 2011; 138: 3657–3666.
27. Fry CS, Lee JD, Jackson JR, *et al.* Regulation of the muscle fiber microenvironment by activated satellite cells during hypertrophy. *FASEB Journal.* 2014; 28: 1654–1665.
28. Schweitzer R, Chyung JH, Murtaugh LC, *et al.* Analysis of the tendon cell fate using Scleraxis, a specific marker for tendons and ligaments. *Development.* 2001; 128: 3855–3866.
29. Murchison ND, Price BA, Conner DA, *et al.* Regulation of tendon differentiation by scleraxis distinguishes force-transmitting tendons from muscle-anchoring tendons. *Development.* 2007; 134: 2697–2708.
30. Gaut L, Duprez D. Tendon development and diseases. *WIREs Dev Biol.* 2016; 5: 5–23.
31. Brent AE, Braun T, Tabin CJ. Genetic analysis of interactions between the somitic muscle, cartilage and tendon cell lineages during mouse development. *Development.* 2005; 132: 515–528.
32. Mackie EJ, Tatarczuch L, Mirams M. The skeleton: a multi-functional complex organ: the growth plate chondrocyte and endochondral ossification. *J Endocrinol.* 2011; 211: 109–121.
33. Akiyama H, Chaboissier MC, Martin JF, Schedl A, de Crombrugghe B. The transcription factor Sox9 has essential roles in successive steps of the chondrocyte differentiation pathway and is required for expression of Sox5 and Sox6. *Genes and Dev.* 2002; 16: 2813–2828.
34. Hattori T, Muller C, Gebhard S, *et al.* SOX9 is a major negative regulator of cartilage vascularization, bone marrow formation and endochondral ossification. *Development.* 2010; 137: 901–911.
35. Komori T, Yagi H, Nomura S, *et al.* Targeted disruption of Cbfa1 results in a complete lack of bone formation owing to maturational arrest of osteoblasts. *Cell.* 1997; 89: 755–764.
36. Nowlan NC, Sharpe J, Roddy KA, Prendergast PJ, Murphy P. Mechanobiology of embryonic skeletal development: Insights from animal models. *Birth Defects Res C Embryo Today.* 2010; 90: 203–213.
37. Gomez C, David V, Peet NM, *et al.* Absence of mechanical loading in utero influences bone mass and architecture but not innervation in Myod-Myf5-deficient mice. *J Anat.* 2007; 210: 259–271.
38. Engler AJ, Sen S, Sweeney HL, Discher DE. Matrix elasticity directs stem cell lineage specification. *Cell.* 2006; 126: 677–689.
39. Dupont S, Morsut L, Aragona M, *et al.* Role of YAP/TAZ in mechanotransduction. *Nature.* 2011; 474: 179–183.
40. Dolinoy DC. The agouti mouse model: an epigenetic biosensor for nutritional and environmental alterations on the fetal epigenome. *Nutr Rev.* 2008; 66(Suppl 1): S7–S11.
41. de Ruijter AJ, van Gennip AH, Caron HN, Kemp S, van Kuilenburg AB. Histone deacetylases (HDACs): characterization of the classical HDAC family. *Biochem J.* 2003; 370: 737–749.
42. Denis H, Ndlovu MN, Fuks F. Regulation of mammalian DNA methyltransferases: a route to new mechanisms. *EMBO Reports.* 2011; 12: 647–656.
43. Deaton AM, Bird A. CpG islands and the regulation of transcription. *Genes and Dev.* 2011; 25: 1010–1022.
44. Jones PA. Functions of DNA methylation: islands, start sites, gene bodies and beyond. *Nature Genetics.* 2012; 13: 484–492.
45. Heyn H, Esteller M. DNA methylation profiling in the clinic: applications and challenges. *Nature Genet.* 2012; 13: 679–692.
46. Da Sacco L, Masotti A. Recent insights and novel bioinformatics tools to understand the role of microRNAs binding to 5' untranslated region. *Int J Mol Sci.* 2012; 14: 480–495.
47. Vasudevan S. Posttranscriptional upregulation by microRNAs. *WIREs RNA.* 2012; 3: 311–330.
48. Carone BR, Fauquier L, Habib N, *et al.* Paternally induced transgenerational environmental reprogramming of metabolic gene expression in mammals. *Cell.* 2010; 143: 1084–1096.
49. Bartlett TE, Zaikin A, Olhede SC, West J, Teschendorff AE, Widschwendter M. Corruption of the intra-gene DNA methylation architecture is a hallmark of cancer. *PLOS One.* 2013; 8: e68285.
50. Barker DJ. Maternal nutrition, fetal nutrition, and disease in later life. *Nutrition.* 1997; 13: 807–813.
51. Gluckman PD, Hanson MA, Buklijas T, Low FM, Beedle AS. Epigenetic mechanisms that underpin metabolic and cardiovascular diseases. *Nat Rev Endocrinol.* 2009; 5: 401–408.
52. Donkin I, Versteyhe S, Ingerslev LR, *et al.* Obesity and bariatric surgery drive epigenetic variation of spermatozoa in humans. *Cell metabolism.* 2015; 23: 369–378.
53. Laker RC, Lillard TS, Okutsu M, *et al.* Exercise prevents maternal high-fat diet-induced hypermethylation of the Pgc-1alpha gene and age-dependent metabolic dysfunction in the offspring. *Diabetes.* 2014; 63: 1605–1611.
54. Clapp JF 3rd, Kim H, Burciu B, Schmidt S, Petry K, Lopez B. Continuing regular exercise during pregnancy: effect of exercise volume on fetoplacental growth. *Am J Obstet Gynecol.* 2002; 186: 142–147.
55. Clapp JF3rd, Kim H, Burciu B, Lopez B. Beginning regular exercise in early pregnancy: effect on fetoplacental growth. *Am J Obstet Gynecol.* 2000; 183: 1484–1488.
56. Chalk TE, Brown WM. Exercise epigenetics and the fetal origins of disease. *Epigenomics.* 2014; 6: 469–472.
57. Koutedakis Y, Metsios GS, Stavropoulos-Kalinoglou A. Periodization of exercise training in sport. In: MacLaren D (ed.) *The physiology of training.* Edinburgh: Elsevier; 2006. p. 1–21.
58. Bergstrom J, Hultman E. A study of the glycogen metabolism during exercise in man. *Scand J Clin Lab Invest.* 1967; 19: 218–228.

59. Henriksson J, Chi MM, Hintz CS, *et al.* Chronic stimulation of mammalian muscle: changes in enzymes of six metabolic pathways. *Am J Physiol.* 1986; 251: C614–C632.
60. Chi MM, Hintz CS, Henriksson J, *et al.* Chronic stimulation of mammalian muscle: enzyme changes in individual fibers. *Am J Physiol.* 1986; 251: C633–C642.
61. Bouchard C, An P, Rice T, *et al.* Familial aggregation of $\dot{V}O_2$ max response to exercise training: results from the HERITAGE Family Study. *J Appl Physiol.* 1999; 87: 1003–1008.
62. Hubal MJ, Gordish-Dressman H, Thompson PD, *et al.* Variability in muscle size and strength gain after unilateral resistance training. *Med Sci Sports Exerc.* 2005; 37: 964–972.
63. Bouchard C, Blair SN, Church TS, *et al.* Adverse metabolic response to regular exercise: is it a rare or common occurrence? *PLOS One.* 2012; 7: e37887.
64. McNarry MB, Barker A, Lloyd,RS, Buchheit M, Williams C, Oliver J. The BASES expert statement on trainability during childhood and adolescence. *Sport Exerc Sci.* 2014; 41: 22–23.
65. Epstein D. *The sports gene.* London: Yellow Jersey Press; 2013.
66. Pray LA. DNA replication and causes of mutation. *Nature Educ.* 2008; 1: 214.
67. Bernstein BE, Birney E, Dunham I, Green ED, Gunter C, Snyder M. An integrated encyclopedia of DNA elements in the human genome. *Nature.* 2012; 489: 57–74.
68. 1000 Genomes Project Consortium, Abecasis GR, Auton A, Brooks LD, DePristo MA, Durbin RM, *et al.* An integrated map of genetic variation from 1,092 human genomes. *Nature.* 2012; 491: 56–65.
69. McPherron AC, Lawler AM, Lee SJ. Regulation of skeletal muscle mass in mice by a new TGF-beta superfamily member. *Nature.* 1997; 387: 83–90.
70. Schuelke M, Wagner KR, Stolz LE, *et al.* Myostatin mutation associated with gross muscle hypertrophy in a child. *N Engl J Med.* 2004; 350: 2682–2688.
71. Mosher DS, Quignon P, Bustamante CD, *et al.* A mutation in the myostatin gene increases muscle mass and enhances racing performance in heterozygote dogs. *PLOS Genet.* 2007; 3: e79.
72. de la Chapelle A, Traskelin AL, Juvonen E. Truncated erythropoietin receptor causes dominantly inherited benign human erythrocytosis. *Proc Nat Acad Sci.* 1993; 90: 4495–4499.
73. Huang LJ, Shen YM, Bulut GB. Advances in understanding the pathogenesis of primary familial and congenital polycythaemia. *Brit J Haematol.* 2010; 148: 844–852.
74. Fajans SS, Bell GI. MODY: history, genetics, pathophysiology, and clinical decision making. *Diabetes Care.* 2011; 34: 1878–1884.
75. Chahal HS, Stals K, Unterlander M, *et al.* AIP mutation in pituitary adenomas in the 18th century and today. *N Engl J Med.* 2011; 364: 43–50.
76. Foldynova-Trantirkova S, Wilcox WR, Krejci P. Sixteen years and counting: the current understanding of fibroblast growth factor receptor 3 (FGFR3) signaling in skeletal dysplasias. *Hum Mutation.* 2012; 33: 29–41.
77. Visscher PM, Brown MA, McCarthy MI, Yang J. Five years of GWAS discovery. *Am J Hum Genet.* 2012; 90: 7–24.
78. Koboldt DC, Steinberg KM, Larson DE, Wilson RK, Mardis ER. The next-generation sequencing revolution and its impact on genomics. *Cell.* 2013; 155: 27–38.
79. Sayer AA, Syddall HE, Gilbody HJ, Dennison EM, Cooper C. Does sarcopenia originate in early life? Findings from the Hertfordshire cohort study. *J Gerontol Biol Sci Med Sci.* 2004; 59: M930–M934.
80. Schellong K, Schulz S, Harder T, Plagemann A. Birth weight and long-term overweight risk: systematic review and a meta-analysis including 643,902 persons from 66 studies and 26 countries globally. *PlOS One.* 2012; 7: e47776.
81. Risnes KR, Vatten LJ, Baker JL, *et al.* Birthweight and mortality in adulthood: a systematic review and meta-analysis. *Int J Epidemiol.* 2011; 40: 647–661.
82. Whincup PH, Kaye SJ, Owen CG, *et al.* Birth weight and risk of type 2 diabetes: a systematic review. *JAMA.* 2008; 300: 2886–2897.
83. Risnes KR, Vatten LJ, Baker JL, Jameson K, Sovio U, Kajantie E, *et al.* Birthweight and mortality in adulthood: a systematic review and meta-analysis. *Int J Epidemiol.* 2011; 40: 647–61.
84. Horikoshi M, Yaghootkar H, Mook-Kanamori DO, *et al.* New loci associated with birth weight identify genetic links between intrauterine growth and adult height and metabolism. *Nature Genet.* 2013; 45: 76–82.
85. Cousminer DL, Berry DJ, Timpson NJ, *et al.* Genome-wide association and longitudinal analyses reveal genetic loci linking pubertal height growth, pubertal timing and childhood adiposity. *Hum Mol Genet.* 2013; 22: 2735–2747.
86. Tsialikas J, Romer-Seibert J. LIN28: roles and regulation in development and beyond. *Development.* 2015; 142: 2397–2404.
87. Wood AR, Esko T, Yang J, *et al.* Defining the role of common variation in the genomic and biological architecture of adult human height. *Nature Genet.* 2014; 46: 1173–1186.
88. Bouchard C, Lesage R, Lortie G, *et al.* Aerobic performance in brothers, dizygotic and monozygotic twins. *Med Sci Sports Exerc.* 1986; 18: 639–646.
89. Klissouras V. Heritability of adaptive variation. *J Appl Physiol.* 1971; 31: 338–344.
90. Bouchard C, Daw EW, Rice T, *et al.* Familial resemblance for $\dot{V}O_2$ max in the sedentary state: the HERITAGE family study. *Med Sci Sports Exerc.* 1998; 30: 252–258.
91. Bouchard C, An P, Rice T, *et al.* Familial aggregation of $\dot{V}O_2$ max response to exercise training: results from the HERITAGE Family Study. *J Appl Physiol.* 1999; 87: 1003–1008.
92. Peeters MW, Thomis MA, Beunen GP, Malina RM. Genetics and sports: an overview of the pre-molecular biology era. *Med Sport Sci.* 2009; 54: 28–42.
93. Silventoinen K, Magnusson PK, Tynelius P, Kaprio J, Rasmussen F. Heritability of body size and muscle strength in young adulthood: a study of one million Swedish men. *Genet Epidemiol.* 2008; 32: 341–349.
94. Maslin MA, Shultz S, Trauth MH. A synthesis of the theories and concepts of early human evolution. *Philos Trans R Soc Lond B Biol Sci.* 2015; 370: 20140064.
95. Roach NT, Venkadesan M, Rainbow MJ, Lieberman DE. Elastic energy storage in the shoulder and the evolution of high-speed throwing in Homo. *Nature.* 2013; 498: 483–486.
96. Bramble DM, Lieberman DE. Endurance running and the evolution of homo. *Nature.* 2004; 432: 345–352.
97. Scholz MN, D'Aout K, Bobbert MF, Aerts P. Vertical jumping performance of bonobo (Pan paniscus) suggests superior muscle properties. *Proc Biol Sci.* 2006; 273: 2177–2184.
98. Fumagalli M, Moltke I, Grarup N, *et al.* Greenlandic Inuit show genetic signatures of diet and climate adaptation. *Science.* 2015; 349: 1343–1347.
99. Beall CM, Cavalleri GL, Deng L, *et al.* Natural selection on EPAS1 (HIF2alpha) associated with low hemoglobin concentration in Tibetan highlanders. *Proc Nat Acad Sci.* 2010; 107: 11459–11464.
100. Yi X, Liang Y, Huerta-Sanchez E, *et al.* Sequencing of 50 human exomes reveals adaptation to high altitude. *Science.* 2010; 329: 75–78.
101. Puthucheary ZA, Rawal J, McPhail M, *et al.* Acute skeletal muscle wasting in critical illness. *JAMA.* 2013; 310: 1591–1600.
102. Eynon N, Hanson ED, Lucia A, *et al.* Genes for elite power and sprint performance: ACTN3 leads the way. *Sports Med.* 2013; 43: 803–817.
103. Bouchard C. Exercise genomics-a paradigm shift is needed: a commentary. *Br J Sports Med.* 2015; 49: 1492–1496.
104. Bouchard C, Sarzynski MA, Rice TK, *et al.* Genomic predictors of the maximal O_2 uptake response to standardized exercise training programs. *J Appl Physiol.* 2011; 110: 1160–1170.
105. Ghosh S, Vivar JC, Sarzynski MA, *et al.* Integrative pathway analysis of a genome-wide association study of $\dot{V}O_2$ max response to exercise training. *J Appl Physiol.* 2013; 115: 1343–1359.
106. Chan JP, Thalamuthu A, Oldmeadow C, *et al.* Genetics of hand grip strength in mid- to late life. *Age.* 2015; 37: 9745.
107. Brown SD, Moore MW. The International Mouse Phenotyping Consortium: past and future perspectives on mouse phenotyping. *Mammalian Genome.* 2012; 23: 632–640.

108. Hakimi P, Yang J, Casadesus G, *et al.* Overexpression of the cytosolic form of phosphoenolpyruvate carboxykinase (GTP) in skeletal muscle repatterns energy metabolism in the mouse. *J Biol Chem.* 2007; 282: 32844–32855.
109. Webborn N, Williams A, McNamee M, *et al.* Direct-to-consumer genetic testing for predicting sports performance and talent identification: Consensus statement. *Br J Sports Med.* 2015; 49: 1486–1491.
110. Wackerhage H, Miah A, Harris RC, Montgomery HE, Williams AG. Genetic research and testing in sport and exercise science: A review of the issues. *J Sports Sci.* 2009; 27: 1–8.
111. Brull D, Dhamrait S, Myerson S, *et al.* Bradykinin B2BKR receptor polymorphism and left-ventricular growth response. *Lancet.* 2001; 358: 1155–1156.
112. Williams AG, Dhamrait SS, Wootton PT, *et al.* Bradykinin receptor gene variant and human physical performance. *J Appl Physiol.* 2004; 96: 938–942.
113. Dhamrait SS, Payne JR, Li P, *et al.* Variation in bradykinin receptor genes increases the cardiovascular risk associated with hypertension. *Eur Heart J.* 2003; 24: 1672–1680.

CHAPTER 32

The influence of physical activity and training on growth and maturation

Robert M Malina

Introduction

Studies spanning almost a century have noted potential benefits of regular physical activity (PA) on growth, and at the same time expressed concerns about the effects of competitive sports, specifically on boys.[1–4] The latter continues as a contemporary concern and is the focus of this chapter. The historical background of issues related to studies of PA and sport is initially considered. The potential effects of PA on indicators of growth and maturation in the general population of youth and of training for sport in youth athletes are then evaluated.

Historical background

Beneficial effects of PA on growth in height were suggested in early studies of largely late adolescent boys 14–22 years[5,6] and male gymnasts.[7,8] Others, however, were not convinced.[1,9] Sampling and lack of control for individual differences in maturity status were potential confounders,[6] although pubertal effects were noted.[8]

With the emergence of organized sport in the United States in the early part of the last century, especially high school sport, apprehension about the extension of interschool sport into lower grade levels was expressed by medical and educational authorities,[10–12] and also at the 1930 White House Conference on Child Health and Protection.[13] Moreover, two early studies suggested a negative effect of sport participation on growth in height. Smaller height gains over 2 years in interschool touch football sport participants than non-participants ~13–16 years implied a negative influence on growth, but sampling bias associated with earlier biological maturation of athletes was also noted.[14] Smaller estimated six monthly height gains were noted across the respective seasons in 7th–8th grade interschool football and basketball players leading to the conclusion that '… growth of the long bones of the body is influenced negatively by strenuous activity'.[15(p49)] Though limited in analysis, the two studies were often cited as evidence that sport participation may negatively influence growth in stature.[1,16,17]

The issue of maturity-related variation in studies of male athletes was noted by the Joint Committee on Athletic Competition for Children of Elementary and Junior High School age.[18] Reference was made to a comparison of 1028 male high school athletes and non-athletes; the former were advanced in skeletal age by about 2 years. Shortly thereafter, two studies reported that the majority of participants in the 1955 and 1957 Little League World Series (baseball) were advanced in pubertal development[19] and skeletal age.[20] The observations suggested selectivity along a maturity gradient which has been consistently noted in male participants in many sports.[21]

Discussions of the pros and cons of competitive sports for youth prompted the Oregon Association of District Superintendents to call for a '… study whether current practices were harmful to the physical and emotional welfare of the participants'. [22(p2)] Thus, the Medford Boys' Growth Study was initiated at the University of Oregon in 1955 '… to investigate problems pertaining to interschool competitive athletics among elementary school boys'.[22(p3)] The analyses compared athletes in four sports to non-athletes in upper elementary, junior high, and senior high school grades. Athletes in football, basketball, and track were, on average, taller and heavier, and advanced in skeletal age, especially between 12 and 15 years. At the other levels, differences in size and maturity between players and non-players were negligible. Baseball was not offered as a junior high sport.

Opportunities for organized sport among girls were quite limited in the first half of the last century, and discussions of high school sport focused exclusively on boys. One of the first reported studies of young females regularly involved in sport considered the growth, sexual maturation, and functional characteristics of 30 elite teenage swimmers.[23] The swimmers were taller and heavier than Swedish reference values at 7 years of age (before systematic training) and at 14 years, while mean age at menarche (12.9 ± 1.1 years) was somewhat earlier than that of the Swedish population.

Physical activity ≠ training

Moderate to vigorous PA and associated health and fitness-related benefits are the current focus of national discussions of youth.[24,25] Methods for quantifying PA include direct observations, questionnaires, videos, diaries, interviews, mechanical counters, and accelerometry. Each method has limitations and advantages.[26] Accelerometry is the preferred method at present; it provides estimates of time spent in activities of sedentary, light, moderate, and vigorous intensities. Specific contexts of PA are not ordinarily provided. (Interested readers are referred to Chapter 21 for an analysis of the assessment of PA).

Time has major limitations as an indicator of the intensity of activity. Children and youth are rarely continuously active, and activities of younger children are largely intermittent. Nevertheless, many studies classify youth as active and less active based on self-, teacher-, and/or parent-reported time in specific activities.

Sport is a major context of PA, but it is important to distinguish between participation in sport both informal and formal (organized), and systematic training for sport. Sport training and practice include major intervals of reduced activity—warm-up, stretching, instruction, rest intervals between repetitions or drills, recovery, etc. Intensity of activities also varies during competitions. Soccer and field hockey matches involve reasonably continuous activity of variable intensity. Baseball and American football games involve brief periods of activities of variable intensities among regular intervals of relative inactivity. Substitutions in basketball and ice hockey provide regular rest intervals throughout a match. Intermittent activities are characteristic of gymnastics, diving, racquet sports, and some field events in athletics, while bouts of continuous activity are common in swimming, running, rowing, and sports or sport disciplines with a major endurance component. Time in PA of different intensities in several local level[27–29] and elite[30–32] youth sports is quite variable. Care is essential in generalizing PA levels and intensities from reported time. Estimated energy expenditure (in METs) by intensity of effort in different sports has been summarized.[33, 34]

Indicators of growth and maturation

A major question in evaluating PA and/or training as a factor affecting growth and maturation is if the effects of PA or training can be partitioned from changes which occur with normal growth and maturation. Many factors, both genetic and environmental, influence these processes; they are beyond the scope of this overview.[26] Children will grow and mature whether or not they are physically active or participate/train in sport.

The subsequent discussion considers height, weight, and proportions (where relevant); maturity status—skeletal age (SA), pubertal status; maturing timing—chronological ages (CAs) at peak height velocity (PHV), menarche; and aspects of body composition. Methods are summarized in Chapter 1.

Physical activity, growth, and maturation in the general population

Height and weight

Longitudinal data for Dutch boys and girls 6–12 years,[35] Canadian boys 8–16 years[36] and Belgian boys 13–18 years[37] classified as active and less active showed no consistent differences in mean heights and weights, although data for weight were more variable. Several anthropometric dimensions also did not differ between active and less active Belgian boys. It is reasonable to conclude that elevated levels of habitual PA, though variably defined, did not influence growth in height and weight of children and adolescents.

Body composition

Given its close relationship with growth in height, fat-free mass (FFM) has received somewhat less attention than fat mass (FM, adiposity). Given advances in technology, estimates of lean tissue mass (LTM), bone mineral content (BMC), and bone mineral density (BMD) have received increased attention.

Fat-free mass

Multilevel modelling analysis, allowing for height, maturity timing (years from PHV), and PA (questionnaires) in a longitudinal series of Canadian youth shows an independent effect of PA on growth in LTM in both sexes;[38] the effect was greater in boys than in girls when height and years from PHV were controlled. The results also suggested relatively larger gains in LTM associated with PA prior to PHV in both sexes. Of potential relevance, peak velocity of growth in LTM occurred, on average, after PHV in this sample.[39] The results highlight the need to control for individual differences in height and maturation when evaluating changes in FFM associated with PA.

A 10-month programme (30 min $\cdot$ day^{-1}, 3 days $\cdot$ week^{-1}) of high-impact strength and aerobic activities among 9- and 10-year-old girls was associated with a larger mean increment in LTM compared to girls who followed their normal pattern of activity. The active girls also showed a smaller increase in FM.[40] There was considerable overlap between groups, and changes in height, weight, and pubertal status were not controlled in making comparisons.

Allowing for the preceding, available data relating regular activity to growth in FFM is limited and highlights the need to account for changes that accompany normal growth and maturation in children and especially adolescents.

Bone mineral

Evidence from a variety of cross-sectional and longitudinal comparisons of active and less active youth indicated a beneficial effect of regular PA on BMC and/or BMD.[24,25,41] Most data were based upon pre-and early-pubertal children of both sexes, girls more often than boys; observations among youth nearing maturity or already mature were more variable, though generally positive. Physical activity interventions aimed at augmenting BMC were consistent with the preceding.[24] Programmes generally met 2–3 times $\cdot$ week^{-1} for moderate- to high-intensity activities, weight-bearing activities of a longer duration (45–60 min), and/or high-impact activities over a shorter duration (10 min). More recent data (three-dimensional imaging) suggested changes in bone geometry indicative of a positive role of habitual PA in enhancing bone strength; short bouts of activity may have been as effective as sustained activity.[42]

In the longitudinal series of Canadian youth, youth of both sexes who were active during the interval of maximal growth accrued more BMC than less active youth,[43] suggesting an enhanced effect of PA on bone mineral during the period of rapid adolescent growth in both sexes. Peak velocity of growth in BMC in this sample occurred, on average, about one-half of a year after PHV.[39]

Adiposity

The literature addressing the influence of PA on indicators of adiposity is reasonably extensive. The longitudinal studies of Dutch boys and girls[35] and Belgian boys[37] indicated no differences in skinfolds between active and less active groups. Other studies with a longitudinal component were variable in design and largely short term.[24,44] Results generally indicated no or only small changes in adiposity with PA in normal-weight children and adolescents. Studies with an extended longitudinal component showed somewhat variable results. In a mixed-longitudinal study spanning

8–15 years, a higher level of PA (questionnaire) was associated with a lower accumulation of FM in boys, but not in girls after controlling for maturity (years from PHV) and FFM.[45] The results also suggested that PA prior to PHV may negatively influence the accumulation of FM in boys, consistent with the positive effect of PA prior to PHV on LTM.[38]

Among boys and girls aged 3–5 years at entry and followed to 11 years, high levels of PA (estimated from accelerometry) were associated with a later adiposity rebound.[46] Although the rebound implies a gain in fatness, evidence suggests that growth in LTM and not FM is characteristic of the rebound.[47]

Enhanced PA programmes spanning about 10–20 weeks appear to have a minimal effect on adiposity in normal weight youth.[44] Most programmes included relatively continuous PA, usually of the endurance type. Physical activity doses across programmes were difficult to ascertain, but results did not vary with programme duration. Several studies of longer duration showed mixed results. It is possible that normal weight youth require a greater PA volume to influence indicators of adiposity. In contrast, PA interventions with overweight and obese youth were associated with reductions in overall and visceral adiposity.[24,44] Persistence of PA-related changes in adiposity was not ordinarily considered.

Maturation

Information on the potential influence of PA on indicators of maturity status and timing are limited. Two longitudinal studies of boys aged 11–15 years[48] and 13–18 years of age[37] indicated similar progress in SA and CA in active and less active boys. Progress in SA also did not differ between beginning gymnasts and controls followed from 5 to 7 years of age (Lewis and Malina, unpublished). Other data for girls are lacking.

Data on pubertal status and progress are also lacking. Some epidemiological data suggested an association, albeit not strong, between habitual PA and later menarche[49,50] but other analyses did not.[51] There is a need to consider other factors associated with this pubertal event; these are considered in more detail in the Growth and maturity characteristics of young athletes section.

Estimated ages at PHV (timing) and estimated peak velocities of growth in height in four longitudinal studies did not differ between active and less active boys.[36,37,52–54] Data for girls are lacking.

Growth and maturity characteristics of young athletes

Youth athletes have been used to highlight potential benefits and risks of PA for growth and maturation. It is assumed that athletes have been regularly active in sport-specific training, and differences relative to non-athletes, both positive and negative, can be attributed to training-related activity.

Limitations of studies of young athletes

Studies of youth athletes have several limitations in the preceding context. First, definition and classification of youth as sport participants or as athletes are variable. Second, sport is characterized by differential persistence and dropout, either voluntary or forced, as in cutting. Third, sport is selective or exclusive; selection tends to follow a maturity-related gradient in many sports.[21,55] Fourth, successful young athletes of both sexes, especially the elite, tend to be different from non-athletes and also from dropouts in some sports in size, composition, and maturation.[56–58]

Allowing for the preceding, generalizations from athletes to the general population need caution, and vice versa. Two other issues need attention. As noted, time (hours, weeks, months, and years) has limited utility as an indicator of sport-specific training. Details of training activities are not ordinarily specified. Additionally, environments associated with training, specific clubs, or specific coaches (styles, demeanours, perceptions, etc.) are not considered. The environments comprise the 'culture' of specific sports or a particular programme, gymnasium, or club, and need more attention in addressing growth and maturation, as well as behavioural development of youth athletes.

In order to evaluate the potential influence of training for a specific sport on the growth and maturation of young athletes, it is essential to have a grasp of their growth and maturity status compared to the general population of youth.

Size attained

Youth athletes of both sexes in several team sports (basketball, soccer, handball, volleyball, ice hockey) and in several individual sports (swimming, tennis, alpine skiing, track and field disciplines except distance running) have, on average, statures and weights that approximate or exceed reference medians for the general population.[54,59,60] Extensive data on mean heights for youth male soccer players tend to fluctuate above and below the reference medians through childhood and adolescence, while mean weights tend to exceed the reference in late adolescence.[61] The adolescent trend suggests greater weight-for-height, which likely reflects physique differences. Less extensive data for youth ice hockey players suggest a similar trend. Data on youth female participants in the two sports are limited, though numbers of participants in both sports are increasing.

The pattern of growth in height and weight relative to reference values is more variable among athletes in several individual sports. Artistic gymnasts and figure skaters of both sexes present, on average, a profile of short stature and lighter body mass, but weight is appropriate for height. Heights of elite youth male and female divers tend to be slightly below the reference median, while weights tend to approximate the median. Means heights of male youth distance runners tend to cluster at or below reference medians in early adolescence, but are generally below reference medians in later adolescence. Mean heights of female distance runners tend to cluster about the reference medians through adolescence. In contrast, mean weights of distance runners of both sexes vary between the 10th percentiles and medians from late childhood through adolescence with few exceptions. The data suggest low weight-for-height of youth distance runners of both sexes.

The preceding observations suggest variation in weight-for-height of athletes in several individual sports. Proportionally low weight-for-height is often a concern among female athletes in some sports. Body mass indices of individual athletes in several sports were graded relative to international criteria for mild, moderate, and severe thinness.[62] Mild and moderate thinness occurred more often among elite female gymnasts; severe thinness was uncommon. Thinness of female athletes was related to later maturation. Information on menarcheal status of athletes 10–16 years was available for US Junior Olympic divers, US artistic gymnasts at a national training camp, US and Canadian figure skaters, and

Polish distance runners. Of 33 athletes in the four sports with mild or moderate thinness, 23 were premenarcheal (mild 21, moderate two). Among elite female artistic gymnasts 13–16 years (Rotterdam World Championship in 1987), 34 of 129 (26%) were mildly or moderately thin; 29 of the 34 were premenarcheal (Malina, unpublished). Less weight-for-height is related in part to linearity of physique which is characteristic of later maturation in both sexes.[26] Corresponding data for male athletes were limited to divers and distance runners. Mild thinness was somewhat more common among distance runners.[62]

Body composition

Attention has often focused on FM and % fat in young athletes given the generally negative influence of fatness on performances in which the body is moved or projected, and perhaps perceptions of coaches. Free-fat mass is highly correlated with and shows a growth pattern very similar to height.[26] As such, one would expect FFM in youth athletes to vary with heights of athletes. Bone is a component of FFM that has received considerable attention among young athletes. Higher BMC and BMD are generally noted in youth athletes of both sexes compared to the general population, but there are exceptions.[63] Effects of training on bone mineral in youth athletes are considered in the Bone mineral section.

Estimates of % fat are more available for youth athletes in individual in contrast to team sports. Earlier estimates were based largely on densitometry and total body water, while more recent estimates were increasingly based upon dual energy X-ray absorptiometry (DEXA) and bioelectrical impedance analysis (BIA). Allowing for variation in methodology, among samples and in sports/sport disciplines represented, several trends were apparent. Athletes have, on average, lower % fat than non-athletes of the same CA, more so in males than in females. Percentage fat tends to decline in male athletes during adolescence (as in the general population due to rapid growth of FFM),[26] while % fat changes relatively little in female athletes from late childhood into adolescence. Estimates of % fat vary among and within sports, allowing for variation in CA, growth, and maturity status, and with size-mass demands of specific disciplines (throwing events in athletics) and positions in team sports where mass is a factor (linemen in American football).

Estimates of % fat predicted from skinfolds complement the preceding and include athletes in several team sports. Technical errors in the measurement[63] and errors associated with equations for predicting % fat (3–5%)[65,66] should be noted. Trends across age and relative to reference values for non-athletes are generally similar to those discussed, except for greater variability among estimates.

Maturity status and timing

The subsequent discussion of maturity status and timing in youth athletes is based on several recent reviews.[21,55,59,61] Information on the maturity status of youth athletes is based largely on SA and stage of pubertal development. The data for both indicators are derived from samples of European ancestry, with several exceptions.

Skeletal maturation

Skeletal age data are largely limited to youth ≥10 years of age and are more available for male than for female youth athletes. Data for artistic gymnasts are an exception; SA data extend to 5 years and are more available for females. Female gymnasts have, on average, SAs that approximate CAs between 5 and 10 years; subsequently, SAs lag behind CAs so that average and later maturing athletes are more prevalent during adolescence. It is likely that significant numbers of gymnasts aged 15–18 years were skeletally mature, although this is not always reported. Less extensive data for male gymnasts suggest a similar trend, and many gymnasts aged 16–18 years are skeletally mature.

Late- and early-maturing boys are about equally represented in samples of male athletes in a variety of sports at 10–11 years. With increasing CA during adolescence, numbers of late-maturing male athletes decline and early-maturing and skeletally mature athletes increase. Late-maturing boys may attain success in some sports in later adolescence (16–18 years), e.g. track and basketball. This emphasizes catch-up in skeletal maturation (all youth eventually reach maturity) and the reduced significance of maturity-associated variation in body size in late adolescence. It also highlights variation in the make-up of samples of athletes in early, mid- and late adolescence.

After gymnastics, SA data for female athletes are most available for swimming and athletics. Swimmers under 14 years span the maturity spectrum from early through late maturation, though more tend to be average and early. Swimmers 14–15 years are primarily average or advanced in SA, while most swimmers 16–17 years are skeletally mature. Among track and field athletes 13–16 years, SAs tend to lag somewhat behind CAs in runners, but are advanced in jumpers and throwers.

Pubertal status

Commonly used indicators of pubertal status include stages of pubic hair (PH) and genital (G) development in males and stages of PH and breast (B) development in females (see Chapter 1). Distributions of stages within single-year CA groups are not ordinarily reported. Studies commonly include competitive age groups that span 2 years, or combine youth across several CAs, which limit the utility of the data.

Given the preceding limitations, data spanning late childhood through adolescence are not extensive for youth athletes of both sexes; an exception is youth male soccer players.[55,61] Stages PH1 through PH4 were represented in players 11 years old, and all five stages were represented among players 12 and 13 years old, thus spanning the spectrum from prepuberty to maturity. The majority of players who were 14, 15, and 16 years old were near maturity (PH 4) or mature (PH 5). The general maturity gradient was consistent with advanced SA and testicular volume in players 14–16 years of age.[21,67]

Age at peak height velocity

In contrast to SA and pubertal status, corresponding information on maturity timing is quite limited.[55] Twelve estimates of age at PHV are available for male athletes of European ancestry. Several are limited by the age span considered, i.e. studies likely began too late and ended too early, so that ages at PHV in earlier- and later-maturing boys could not be successfully modelled. Among 76 soccer players followed longitudinally 4–5 years, from 10 to 13 years, to 14–17 years, ages at PHV could be estimated for only 33 players; CA approximated SA at initial observation.[68] Peak height velocity could not be estimated for 43 players; 25 were advanced in SA and 18 were delayed in SA relative to CA at initial observation.

Allowing for the preceding and also differential persistence/dropout in sport, mean estimated ages at PHV for male athletes in cycling, rowing, athletics, and combined sports tend to be somewhat earlier than non-athletes, while those for athletes in soccer, ice hockey, and basketball tend to approximate estimates from several European longitudinal growth studies. The one estimate for male gymnasts is consistent with later maturation.

Only five estimates of age at PHV are available for female athletes of European ancestry.[55] Mean ages for participants in rowing, athletics, and combined sports approximate the averages for non-athletes, while mean ages for two samples of artistic gymnasts are later.

Estimated ages at PHV for Japanese and South Korean youth athletes are generally consistent with trends noted in European youth.[55] Except for a sample of elite male distance runners, males were non-select school athletes while females were select prefecture or school level athletes in team sports. Male soccer players were an exception (later PHV), which contrasted elite J League Academy players 13–15 years who were advanced in skeletal maturation.[69]

Age at menarche

Prospective data are based on actual ages at menarche for individual athletes followed longitudinally; samples are often small and select, and some data are short term. *Status quo* data provide a median age at menarche for a sample of athletes; samples commonly include athletes of different skill levels at younger ages and more select athletes at older ages. Selective persistence in a sport and exclusion/dropout are confounding factors with both methods.

Prospective data for youth athletes are limited to 12 samples: five of artistic gymnasts, three of swimmers, and one each for tennis, rowing, athletics, and combined sports. Status quo data are limited to 11 samples: three for athletics, two for swimming and gymnastics, and one each for figure skating, diving, soccer, and combined team sports.[55,57] The estimate for elite gymnasts at the 1987 World Championship (15.6 ± 2.1 years) was based on athletes 13–21 years;[70] given the CA cut-off for competition, the sample included no younger gymnasts. Most mean/median ages at menarche for prospective and status quo samples of athletes are within the range of normal variation and tend to approximate those for the general population; artistic gymnasts, figure skaters, ballet dancers, and perhaps divers are exceptions.

Training for sport and the growth and maturation of young athletes

Longitudinal data are essential to evaluate potential effects of systematic training on the growth and maturation of young athletes. Given the exclusive nature of sport, such data are limited. Studies of athletes in several sports are initially considered, followed by separate discussions of training among youth artistic gymnasts and later ages at menarche in athletes.

Studies from Poland and the former Czechoslovakia

The growth, maturation, and performance of youth athletes in a variety of sports have been the focus of study in the former Eastern Bloc countries. Several are subsequently summarized.

Two prospective studies considered youth training in sport schools in Warsaw (Poland). Selection was based on body size (specifically stature), performance on a battery of motor proficiency tests, and a medical examination. Training protocols were elaborated by specialists in the respective sports and approved by the Ministry of Education.[71]

The first study included a mixed-longitudinal sample of 78 boys and 40 girls followed from 11–14 years.[54,72,73] Boys participated in athletics (n = 33, running, jumping events), wrestling (n = 26), basketball (n = 11) and sailing (n = 7); girls participated in athletics (n = 23) and rowing (n = 17). Programmes extended over 9 months·year^{-1}; training increased from 8 h·week^{-1} in the first year to 12 h·week^{-1} in the third year. Heights and weights of boys and girls in the sport school were taller than Polish reference data. Estimated height velocities of boys suggested earlier maturation, while those of girls suggested average maturation compared to Swiss reference values.[74] Estimated ages at entry into stages of PH and G in boys were consistent with earlier maturation, while estimated ages at entry into stages of PH and B in girls approximated the reference for non-athletes.

The second prospective study followed 52 boys and 49 girls longitudinally from ~11–18 years of age.[75–77] The samples included 21 boys (athletics n = 10, rowing n = 11) and 23 girls (athletics n = 13, rowing n = 9, swimming n = 1) who were training about 12 h·week^{-1} for 9 months of the year in sport schools or clubs. The remaining youth did not systematically participate in sport but had regular physical education. Youth athletes of both sexes were, on average, taller and heavier than non-active peers. The trends suggested less weight-for-height among athletes. Male athletes attained PHV earlier than non-athletes, while peak velocities of growth in height did not differ. Female athletes and non-athletes differed negligibly in age at PHV, peak velocity, age at menarche, and the interval between ages at PHV and at menarche. Estimated ages at attaining stages B3, B4, and B5 and stages PH3, PH4, and PH5, and intervals between adjacent stages also did not differ between female athletes and non-athletes.[75] Subsequent analyses noted an earlier age at PHV for boys in rowing compared to athletics, while girls training in rowing and athletics did not differ in ages at PHV and menarche.[55]

A third study of Polish youth active in sport was retrospective. Longitudinal records spanning 8–18 years for 25 boys and 13 girls active in sport during late childhood, adolescence, and young adulthood were extracted from the Wrocław Growth Study (WGS) and the Wrocław Longitudinal Twin Study.[54,78,79] In the case of twins, the more actively involved twin was selected; otherwise, one member was randomly selected.

Male athletes were taller and heavier than the WGS reference from 11–18 years; differences for weight increased from mid- to late adolescence in male athletes. Skeletal ages of male athletes were similar to CAs at 9 and 10 years, but then in advance so that by 14 and 15 years, the difference was, on average, 1 year. Consistent with the preceding, estimated ages at take-off and PHV, and ages at attaining PH2 and PH4 and G2 and G4 were earlier in athletes compared to WGS. The pattern of maturation of male athletes was that associated with early maturation.

Female athletes were also taller and heavier than the reference from 11–18 years. In contrast to males, SA and CA did not differ among athletes from 10 to 15 years; age at take-off also did not differ relative to WGS.[79,80] In contrast, ages at PHV and menarche, and ages at reaching stages PH2 and PH4 and B2 and B4 of athletes were slightly later than in WGS. The interval between ages at PHV and menarche in athletes was similar to athletes in Warsaw sport schools and non-athletes.[75] The pattern of maturation among female athletes approximated that of average maturing girls.

The growth and skeletal maturation of male athletes in Brno (former Czechoslovakia) were monitored longitudinally from 12–15 years.[81] Cyclists (n = 6), rowers (n = 11), ice hockey players (n = 16), and participants in various sports (n = 17, tennis, volleyball, handball, athletics, hockey goal keepers, rowing steersman, and others) were included. Samples of non-athletes (n = 34) and dropouts (n = 19) were also followed. Sport-specific training increased over time in cyclists, rowers, and ice hockey players. Training time among participants in several sports and dropouts was more variable.

Heights and weights of athletes were, on average, similar to the non-athletes, allowing for variation in skeletal maturity status. Cyclists were, on average, advanced in SA relative to CA by ~0.5 year over the four observations. Skeletal age and CA were similar in rowers over the first year, but SA was in advance of CA by ~0.5 year in the final two observations. In contrast, SA was delayed relative to CA by about ~0.5 year in ice hockey players. The trends suggested somewhat earlier maturation among cyclists and rowers, and somewhat later maturation among hockey players. Skeletal age-CA differences (<0.5 year) for the mixed-sports group, dropouts and non-athletes were generally consistent with the ice hockey players. Allowing for variation in status, progress in SA relative to CA between 12 and 15 years was similar among athletes, dropouts, and non-athletes; by inference, training across the pubertal years did not influence skeletal maturation.

Graphic interpolation of individual height curves (four points) was used to interpolate the CA at which the 'point of inflection' was attained (estimate of age at PHV). Estimated mean ages were consistent with earlier maturation among cyclists and rowers and average maturation among ice-hockey players compared to dropouts and non-athletes. The estimate for athletes participating in several sports was intermediate.[81]

Progress in SA was evaluated among elite Czechoslovak female adolescent athletes in four sports over the interval of their competitive years: artistic gymnasts (n = 24) and figure skaters (n = 16) at 12 and 16 years, and tennis (n = 14), soccer (n = 23), and volleyball (n = 12) players 12–18 years.[82] Chronological ages ranged from 12–15 years and from 16–18 years at the two observations. Mean SAs approximated mean CAs at both evaluations, except in figure skaters among whom SA lagged behind CA by ~0.5 year at initial observation. Skeletal ages of 17 athletes (19%) changed in maturity classification between observations, but there was no clear pattern: early to average, four; average to early, three; average to late, six; and late to average, four. Some athletes probably attained skeletal maturity at the second observation (not reported) which would influence maturity classifications. Allowing for this limitation, the process of skeletal maturation was not affected by intensive training and competition during adolescence.

Perhaps the most widely cited study from Czechoslovakia (Prague) focused on body composition and working capacity.[16,53,83–85] The project started in 1961 with ~140 boys 11 years of age[86]; 'boys with markedly accelerated or retarded somatic development were eliminated'. [16p(235)]

Longitudinal records for height, weight, and body composition (% fat via densitometry, FM, FFM) from 11–18 years were available for 39 boys. Potential for selective persistence and dropout should be noted. The boys comprised three activity groups: active (n = 8), intermediate activity (n = 18), and least active (n = 13), but descriptions of activity levels differed somewhat.[16,53,85] The composition of the active group is relevant to the present discussion; it included 6 or 7 basketball players and 2 or 1 in athletics (running).[53,85] It was likely that the most active boys were youth athletes training for sport, primarily basketball; they were taller than boys in the other groups throughout the study and heavier from 13–18 years.

The small groups differed only slightly in body composition at 11–12 years. Subsequently, the most active boys (athletes) gained more FFM and less FM than the moderately and least active boys. The latter differed slightly in FFM but the least active group had greater % fat. The greater gains in FFM among the most active boys were generally attributed to the stimulating effects of regular PA.

Variation in biological maturation was not considered in the analyses. Skeletal ages were monitored.[48] In an analysis of the groups between 11 and 15 years, active boys (n = 14, described as training regularly in basketball and athletics, in addition to other sports) were, on average, advanced in SA (SA minus CA) at each age compared to boys intermediate (n = 32) and lowest (n = 24) in activity; the differences were most marked at 14 and 15 years, suggesting earlier maturation. Although samples sizes were a bit different, data from the same research unit indicated advanced SA relative to CA in 12 active (labelled sportsmen, nine in basketball, three in light athletics) compared to 16 least-active boys at each age from 11 through 17 years, but especially from 14–17 years.[87] It is thus likely that growth of FFM during adolescence was influenced by advanced skeletal maturity in the most active boys. Moreover, progress in skeletal maturation was not affected by PA/training during adolescence.

A question of relevance is the timing of the adolescent spurt. An early report indicated no differences in age at PHV among groups,[16] but a subsequent report indicated an earlier age at PHV (graphic interpolation) in the active (14.1 ± 0.9 years) compared to moderately- (14.5 ± 1.0 years) and least-active (14.6 ± 1.2 years) boys.[53] Estimated peak velocities did not differ among groups. Application of the Preece-Baines model 1 to mean heights of the three samples[84] showed similar results, but earlier estimated ages at PHV: active 13.2 years, moderately-active 13.9 years, and least-active 13.9 years, and no differences in estimated peak velocities among groups, 7.9, 7.6, and 7.5 $cm \cdot year^{-1}$, respectively (Malina, unpublished). Estimates for the active group were consistent with data for adolescents active in sport, i.e. earlier maturation.[55] Overall, the greater heights and FFM in active boys were due in large part to subject selectivity/persistence and advanced maturation.

Training of Young Athletes study

The Training of Young Athletes (TOYA) study of youth athletes from the greater London area was mixed-longitudinal. Several cohorts in four sports were followed for 3 years spanning 9 to 18 years: gymnastics (81 girls, 38 boys), swimming (60 girls, 54 boys), tennis (81 girls, 74 boys), and soccer (65 boys).[88] Training was described as intensive; median weekly hours varied with sport and age: gymnastics, 10–15 h; swimming, 9–13 h; tennis, 5–10 h; soccer, 3–10 h.

On average, heights of male tennis players, swimmers, and soccer players overlapped during late childhood and adolescence, while gymnasts were consistently shorter. Late adolescent heights of swimmers and tennis players were greater than those of soccer players.[89] Stages G2, G3, and G4 were attained, on average, later among gymnasts compared to the other athletes. Testicular volume did not differ among athletes in the four sports between 9 and 13 years of age and was within the normal range for healthy boys. Testicular volume was less among gymnasts 14 through 17 years, but did not differ among athletes in the four sports by 19 years. The results highlighted variation among athletes in the four sports during puberty which reflected differential timing.

Among females, swimmers and tennis players did not differ in height across the age range, but were consistently taller than gymnasts. Mean late adolescent heights of swimmers and tennis players reached the 75th percentile of the reference, whereas mean heights of gymnasts reached the reference median.[90] Youth athletes in the three sports did not differ in ages at attaining stages B2, B3, and B4, and also PH2, PH3, and PH4, but gymnasts attained B5 and PH5 significantly later than swimmers and tennis players. Age at menarche was, on average, identical among tennis players and swimmers, 13.3 ± 1.4 years, and was later in gymnasts, 14.5 ± 1.5 years.[90,91] When ages at attaining the respective stages of puberty were aligned on time before and after menarche, there were no differences among athletes in the three sports.

Other studies

Consistent with observations on progress in SA in 14 female tennis players,[82] observations of small samples (n = 6 in each sex) of elite Japanese female and male tennis players indicated similar progress in SA and CA between 12 and 14 years.[92] A 2-year prospective study indicated no differences in progress in height and weight of male ice hockey players and a combined sample of female gymnasts, figure skaters, and runners compared to controls between 12 and 14 years.[93] Hockey players were, on average, taller and heavier than controls, but the samples did not differ in pubertal status at each observation. In contrast, the combined group of female athletes was, on average, shorter and lighter than controls, and also somewhat less mature in pubertal status at 13 and 14 years of age.

Short-term observations (12 and 22 months) of elite distance runners indicated no effect of run training on size attained and growth rate.[94] In a mixed-longitudinal sample of elite distance runners spanning adolescence, SAs of 11 female and 10 male runners were, on average, ~0.5 year behind CAs at initial observation. Subsequently, heights of both female and male runners did not differ, on average, from reference values, but weights were consistently lighter from 10 to 18 years. Estimated velocities of growth also did not differ from the reference. By inference, training for distance running during childhood and adolescence did not influence attained size and rate of growth in height and weight.[95] Application of Preece-Baines model 1 to mean heights of the runners suggested slightly later ages at PHV in the runners, 12.4 years in girls, and 14.3 years in boys, consistent with SA at initial observation.

Overview of longitudinal studies

Allowing for variation in sampling and sports represented, and in methodology among the longitudinal studies, results were consistent in showing no effect, positive or negative, of regular training for sport on size attained, growth rate in height, and several indicators of maturity status and timing. The pattern of growth and maturation observed in Polish and Czech athletes was generally consistent with early maturation in males, and average or on-time maturation in females. The trends were likewise similar with most cross-sectional data for youth athletes. Results of the TOYA study highlighted sport-related variation in pubertal timing, specifically between gymnasts and athletes in the other sports considered.

Two persistent questions

The preceding suggests that systematic training for sport does not negatively influence linear growth, maturity status, and maturity timing in youth athletes. Yet, two concerns are evident in the literature. First, the shorter stature and later maturation of gymnasts, specifically females, are the outcomes of intensive training beginning at relatively early ages. Second, intensive training before menarche is associated with later menarche.

Training and the growth and maturation of artistic gymnasts

A consensus committee convened by the Scientific Commission of the International Gymnastics Federation arrived at the following conclusions:

> 'Adult height or near adult height of female and male artistic gymnasts is not compromised by intensive gymnastics training at a young age or during the pubertal growth spurt. …
>
> Gymnastics training does not attenuate growth of upper (sitting height) or lower (legs) body segment lengths. …
>
> Gymnastics training does not appear to attenuate pubertal growth and maturation, including SA, secondary sex characteristics and age at menarche, and rate of growth and timing and tempo of the growth spurt.[58(p798)]

The subsequent discussion elaborates on several related issues. Gymnasts are shorter before the onset of training, i.e. in early childhood.[96,97] and tend to have, on average, shorter parents,[89,90,96,98–100] though some data are variable.[97]

Youth who persist and drop out of the sport differ in growth and maturation, highlighting selectivity of the sport. Among Polish gymnasts followed longitudinally from 10 to 12 years through adolescence,[98] those who persisted (5 females, 6 males) were, on average, shorter and lighter than those who dropped out (4 females, 8 males). Youth who persisted also attained PHV later than those who dropped out, but estimated peak velocities did not differ.[101] Among Swiss female gymnasts selected between 7 and 14 years, 12 subsequently dropped out. Girls who persisted were shorter and lighter at selection, delayed in skeletal maturation, and attained menarche later than girls who dropped out.[102] Height and weight at 16–18 years, however, did not differ significantly.

Differential persistence and dropout have implications for interpreting cross-sectional comparisons. Samples of gymnasts differ in composition with increasing CA. Mid- and late-adolescent samples are largely later maturing, reflecting in part the persistence and perhaps selection of late maturing youth in the sport.

Data addressing SA of youth gymnasts longitudinally are limited. Among advanced level American female gymnasts followed from 7–9 years of age, mean SA lagged slightly behind CA, but both CA and SA showed similar progress over three observations. Classification of maturity status (early, average, late) changed in only two girls, one from late to average and another from early to average (Lewis and Malina, unpublished). Skeletal age was delayed relative to CA in female and male gymnasts in the former East Germany between 12 and 14 years, but both CA and SA showed similar progress over the three observations.[100,103] In contrast, SA and CA did not differ among Czechoslovak female gymnasts at 12 and 16 years, and both made similar progress over the interval of 4 years.[82] Classification of maturity status changed between the two observations in seven gymnasts, but there was no clear pattern: early to average, one; average to early, two; average to late, three; and late to average, one. Overall, evidence from the four studies indicated no influence of training on progress in skeletal maturation of youth gymnasts of both sexes.

Several short-term studies of the sexual maturity status of gymnasts are limited by methods of reporting and sampling. For example, ratings of pubertal stages were combined into a single score or mean stage, athletes were grouped by pubertal status independent of CA, only mean CAs of youth at different stages were reported, and/or athletes of specific pubertal status were selected, e.g. pre- or early pubertal.[58] In the TOYA study, variation in pubertal maturation of female and male gymnasts relative to athletes in other sports reflected differential timing; gymnasts were later maturing, but progressed through puberty as expected.[89,90]

Given the shorter heights and later maturation of gymnasts of both sexes and the trend for gymnasts to have shorter parents, another relevant question is how gymnasts compare with other short adolescents. Estimated ages at PHV of gymnasts from two longitudinal samples of girls and one of boys, three short-term mixed-longitudinal samples of girls, and a mixed-longitudinal sample of boys were compared with estimates for three samples of short late-maturing youth: late-maturing youth with short parents, short normal late-maturing youth, and youth with idiopathic short stature.[58,101] Estimated ages at PHV and peak velocities among gymnasts and short late-maturing non-gymnasts of both sexes were generally similar, which suggested that gymnasts of both sexes have the characteristics of short, normal, late-maturing youth with short parents. The growth and maturity characteristics of gymnasts reflect primarily constitutional and/or familial factors interacting with the selective criteria of the sport and differential persistence and dropout.

The shorter heights of gymnasts of both sexes have been related to reduced leg length in the context of selection for shorter limbs[100,104] and/or stunted growth of the lower limbs with intensive training.[104,105] Observations from short-term studies are limited due to lack of control for variation associated with CA per se, and individual differences in maturation, especially during adolescence.[55] As in the general population, peak velocities of growth in leg length and sitting height occur, respectively, before and after PHV in gymnasts.[106] Among gymnasts of contrasting maturity status, differences in leg length and sitting height are negligible when data are aligned on estimated age at PHV.[107]

It has also been suggested that gymnasts have proportionally shorter legs for their heights, but maturity status was not considered.[108] However, mean sitting height/height ratios of female gymnasts 10 to 17 years were consistent with reference values for the general population.[55] Elite gymnasts advanced in maturity status do have proportionally shorter legs than less-mature gymnasts of the same CA,[109] but this contrast reflects variation in maturity status.[26]

Training and menarche

Most discussions of maturation among female athletes focus on menarche, which is a late-pubertal event. Menarche occurs, on average, a year or so after PHV in both non-athletes and athletes.[75]

Only the prospective and status quo methods deal with athletes who are in the process of maturing. The former is based on actual ages at menarche for individual athletes in longitudinal studies. The latter is based on the distributions of athletes by menarcheal status (pre- or post-) across ages spanning late childhood through adolescence, and provides an estimated median for the sample (see Chapter 1). Prospective and status quo estimates of age at menarche in youth athletes are limited in the number and in sports represented. Mean/median ages at menarche are within the range of normal variation and most tend to approximate mean/median ages for the general population; artistic gymnasts, figure skaters, ballet dancers, and divers are exceptions.[55,110]

In contrast, most data for athletes are retrospective, based on recalled ages at menarche in samples of late adolescent and adult athletes. Retrospective ages are influenced by memory, recall bias (the shorter the recall interval, the more accurate the recall, and vice versa), and by a tendency to report ages in whole years, typically age at the birthday before menarche.[26] Mean ages at menarche based on the retrospective method are within the range of normal variation, and tend to be later in athletes in many, but not all, sports.[26,57,59,110] Reported mean ages also vary within sports, among sports, and also between 'early' and 'late' entry sports.

Later mean ages at menarche were attributed to regular training before menarche with the conclusion that training 'delays' menarche.[111–113] The nature of the training stimulus was not specified except in general terms. The term 'delay' implies that training 'causes' menarche to occur later. Data dealing with the inferred relationship, however, are correlational and do not permit statements of causality.

The association between training before menarche and later menarche may be an artefact. For example, two girls begin 'training' at 8 years of age. One girl is genotypically an early maturer and attains menarche at 10 years, while another is genotypically a late maturer and attains menarche at 15 years. The early maturing girl has only 2 years of training before menarche, while the late maturing girl has 7 years of training.[114]

Issues that need to be addressed include discovering what, if anything, in the sport environment contributes to later menarche in some athletes or athletes in specific sports. Is it the physical and/or physiological act of training? Is it the psychological stress of training and competition? Is it the sport environment, including other athletes, coaches and the sport system? Is it the interactions among these factors and others? Additionally, there is also a need to consider athletes who begin sport training after menarche.

Factors that need consideration include the select, non-random nature of athlete samples, differential persistence and dropout in a sport, athletes who change sports, ethnic variation, and diet and nutritional status. These factors are rarely considered in studies of athletes.[57,110, 115]

Familial aggregation and environmental circumstances require consideration. Mothers of athletes tend to be later maturing, and mother-daughter and sister-sister correlations for age at menarche are of similar magnitude as those for non-athletes.[26,58,91,116] Family size is an additional factor; larger family size is associated with later menarche and some data indicate that athletes come from larger families.[117,118] The estimated sibling effect on age at menarche, controlling for birth order, ranged from 0.15–0.22 years and from 0.08–0.19 years per additional sibling in families of athletes and non-athletes, respectively.[118]

The home environments of young athletes also merit study. In the context of life history theory, high-quality, warm home environments during development are associated with later menarche, while socially adverse home environments during development are associated with earlier menarche.[119,120] It is proposed that ...

> '... quality of parental investment, as indexed by measures such as Parental Supportiveness, is the most important mechanism through

which young children receive information about levels of stress and support in their local environments, and that this information provides a basis for adaptively adjusting pubertal timing'.[120(p1814)]

This implies interactions between behavioural development and biological maturation.

Parents are primary socializing agents for participation in sport and major influences on psychosocial outcomes associated with sport.[121,122] Parental involvement in elite athletes (swimming, tennis) was similar to parental investment in talented individuals in the arts (concert pianists, sculptors) and sciences (research mathematicians, neurologists) who had attained international status at relatively young ages.[123] Given parental investments (social, emotional, economic) in the sport training and achievements of their offspring, does later menarche reflect familial correlation and a high-quality, warm home developmental environment? Indicators of a positive developmental environment, parental approval, greater family cohesiveness, frequency of positive interactions, and so on, merit further study. Unknown factors in the development of young athletes are coaches and sport systems, which may function to complement or to disrupt the lives of young athletes.

Like other aspects of growth and maturation, a variety of factors are related to the timing of menarche. If training for sport is a factor, it likely interacts with or is confounded by other factors, so that a specific effect may be difficult to extract. Two comprehensive discussions of the issue have concluded with two observations: first, menarche occurs, on average, later in athletes in some sports, and second, the relationship between later menarche and training for sport is not causal.[124,125]

Training and body composition

With few exceptions, body composition studies of youth athletes are short term, which makes it difficult to partition changes associated with training from those associated with growth and maturity maturation.

Fat-free mass and fat mass

Two studies of boys dating to the 1960s and 1970s illustrate the trends and related issues. The first study of Czech boys[16,84] was discussed in the Studies from Poland and the former Czechoslovakia section. Height, weight, and body composition of three groups followed from 11–18 years were compared: active (n = 8), moderately active (n = 18) and least active (n = 13). The groups differed slightly in body composition at 11–12 years. During the course of the study, the most active boys gained more FFM and less FM than the moderately- and least-active boys. The latter differed only slightly in FFM and the least-active group had greater % fat. The larger gains in FFM among the most active boys were generally attributed to the effects of regular PA. The active boys, however, were likely athletes training for sport, primarily basketball. They were taller than boys in the other groups throughout the study, heavier from 13–18 years, advanced in skeletal maturation, and also attained PHV earlier. It is reasonable that the greater heights and FFM in active boys were due in large part to subject selectivity/persistence and advanced maturation.

The second study evaluated the influence of a 4-month endurance training programme (1 $h \cdot day^{-1}$, 3 $days \cdot week^{-1}$ plus a 1-month more intensive training camp) on the body size and estimated body composition of nine Swedish boys, 11–13 years.[126] Height, weight and ^{40}K (proxy for FFM) were measured before and within 3 weeks after the programme, an interval of ~0.5–0.6 year. Ages ranged from 11.6 to 13.5 years at the second observation, when testicular volume was also measured. Estimated changes in body size and ^{40}K after training are summarized in Table 32.1.

Table 32.1 Age-adjusted changes in size and potassium-40 of boys after training.

	n	Height (cm)	Weight (kg)	^{40}K (g)
Total sample	9	3.9 ± 0.3	0.8 ± 0.8	12.3 ± 1.4
TV < 9 mL	6	2.7 ± 0.4	0.3 ± 1.1	11.2 ± 0.6
TV ≥ 9 mL	3	5.1 ± 0.7	1.1 ± 1.8	12.0 ± 0.9

(TV = testicular volume)

Source data from Von Döbeln W, Eriksson BO. Physical training, maximal oxygen uptake and dimensions of the oxygen transporting and metabolizing organs in boys 11–13 years of age. Acta Paediatr Scand. 1972; 61: 653–660.

Although limited, it appears that observed gains in height and ^{40}K were influenced by age per se, sexual maturation, and perhaps the adolescent spurt. Results of the two studies highlight the need to consider both growth and maturation in efforts to document effects of systematic training on growth of FFM in adolescent boys.

Other studies monitoring changes in FFM and FM with sport-specific training and competition among youth athletes are often focused on changes during a season. A study of nine adolescent wrestlers (15.4 ± 0.3 years) and seven non-athletes (15.0 ± 0.4 years) monitored body composition (densitometry) across a season.[127] Body mass and estimated FFM and % fat declined in wrestlers from pre- to late-season, which likely reflected concern for 'making weight'. The three variables then increased from pre- to post-season. Non-athletes also increased in body mass and FFM but did not change in % fat. The gain in FFM from pre- to post-season was the same in both wrestlers and non-athletes; increments in height and SA were also similar in the two groups. Overall, the changes were relatively small and should be viewed in the context of growth and maturation, and sport-specific emphasis on body weight during the season.

Similar trends were apparent in 15 late adolescent/young adult collegiate female swimmers (19.1 ± 1.3 years).[128] Densitometric estimates of body composition were made at three points during the season, October, December, and March. Body mass, FM, and % fat decreased while FFM increased from October to December. Weight training (high repetition, low resistance) typically preceded swim training early in the season. Changes in mass and body composition were generally maintained from December to March, as swimmers tapered in preparation for the national championship. Other studies of athletes are limited to two observations, pre- and post-season, and as such provide limited insights into variation in training emphases and competitions during a season.[63]

Bone mineral

Mixed-longitudinal observations spanning 4–10 years of age showed greater accretion of BMC among gymnasts compared to ex-gymnasts (dropouts) and non-gymnasts.[129] Short-term studies of prepubertal female gymnasts indicated greater BMC and BMD especially at weight-bearing sites compared to controls.[130,131] Short-term observations of pre- and peripubertal male gymnasts also indicated greater bone mineral compared to non-athlete controls.[31] Change in pubertal status during the studies was not indicated. Controlling for maturity status (breast stages, estimated time from PHV), female gymnasts accrued greater BMC and BMD across puberty compared to non-athletes.[132] Training-related gains in BMD during childhood and adolescence persisted into young adulthood in female gymnasts.[130,133]

The extreme unilateral activity associated with tennis training shows localized increases in bone mineral accretion in both sexes. Comparisons of 47 pre-, peri- (early) and postpubertal female tennis players 8–17 years indicated variation in bone areas and strength between the mid- and distal regions of the playing and non-playing humeri.[134] The effects of loading were specific to region and surface of the bone, and varied with stage of puberty. In addition to bone variables (BMC, total and cortical areas, bending strength), muscle areas were larger in the dominant compared to the non-dominant arms in this sample of female tennis players, but relative differences in bone variables and muscle area did not increase across maturity groups.[135] Differences in muscle areas between playing and non-playing arms explained relatively small percentages of the variance in BMC, cortical areas, and bending strength (12–16%). A comparison of upper arm and forearm muscle size and characteristics of the humeri, radii, and ulnae of the playing and non-playing arms of elite youth tennis players of both sexes (13.5 ± 1.9 years) also indicated marked differences.[136] As in the preceding study,[135] bone characteristics were related to corresponding muscle size differences, but a role for factors other than muscle size that influence training-related side-to-side differences in bone was indicated.

Both pre-/peri-pubertal (n = 13) and postmenarcheal (n = 32) tennis players 10 to 17 years of age experienced significantly greater changes in bone variables in the playing compared to the non-playing humeri over 1 year; relative gains were greater among younger pre/peripubertal players.[137] Consistent with studies of youth tennis players, the long-term positive influence of racquet sport training (tennis, squash) on BMC and bone strength was apparent in the dominant versus non-dominant arms of female players grouped by recalled ages at which formal training began.[138–140]

A systematic review of studies of youth swimmers (mean ages 8.7–16.1 years) indicated a BMD similar to sedentary controls (14 studies, seven of males, seven of females), but lower than athletes participating in 'osteogenic', weight-bearing impact sports (nine studies, seven in females, primarily gymnastics and soccer).[141] By inference, swim training does not influence bone mineral accrual.

Although distance running is a weight-bearing activity, observations on female high school endurance runners suggested reduced BMC accrual associated with training, menstrual function, reduced energy intake and/or disordered eating behaviour across the adolescent years.[142–144] Moreover, female runners with low BMC at baseline (~15 years) were more likely to have low BMC 3 years later.[145]

Long-term data for late adolescent athletes in different sports are limited, but what is available provides additional insights and raises questions. Bone mineral content and BMD were compared among adolescent cyclists <17 years (15.5 ± 0.9 years) and ≥17 years (18.4 ± 1.4 years) with 2–7 years of training in the sport, and age-matched controls involved in recreational sports.[146] Total body BMC and BMD was less in cyclists than controls in both age groups, but regional variation in BMC and BMD was substantial. Among cyclists <17 years, BMC of the legs was lower and that of the hip was significantly higher compared to age-matched controls, while among cyclists ≥17 years, BMC in the pelvis, femoral neck, and legs was lower compared to age-matched controls. Bone mineral density was also lower, on average, among both groups of cyclists than controls at most sites, though differences were significant only among older cyclists. Allowing for limited numbers, the results suggested that training in cycling '... may adversely affect bone mass during adolescence'.[146(p8)]

In a similar vein, total body BMD and spine and femoral neck BMD were compared in male ice hockey players and non-athlete controls at 16, 19, and 22 years.[147] Baseline bone density measures at 16 years were slightly greater among hockey players, while at 19 years, hockey players had significantly greater total body and femoral neck BMD compared to non-athletes. At 22 years of age, differences between active hockey players and non-athletes in total body, spine, and femoral neck BMD were marked, while corresponding measures for formerly active players were intermediate between active players and non-athletes. The evidence suggested that BMD advantages associated with active participation in sport may not persist with the cessation of regular participation and training in the sport; the trend was especially evident for the femoral neck.

Conclusions

Physical activity in the general population of youth and systematic training for sport among youth athletes have no effect on size attained and rate of growth in height and on maturity status and timing, but may influence body weight and indicators of body composition.

Summary

- Physical activity in the general population of youth and systematic training for sport among youth athletes has no effect on size attained and rate of growth in height and on maturity status and timing.
- Physical activity and training may influence body weight and composition. Both favourably influence bone mineral, but variable effects are noted in some sports. Physical activity has a minimal effect on fatness in normal-weight youth, but regular training generally has a positive influence on fatness in youth athletes. Data for fat-free/lean tissue mass are suggestive, but limited.
- Menarche occurs later in athletes in some but not all sports, but the relationship between later menarche and training is not causal. Data for adolescent athletes are limited.
- Constitutional factors play a central role in the selection and retention of young athletes in a sport. These factors and others, e.g. aesthetic criteria of specific sports, requisite skills, differential retention and dropout, and complexities of adult-controlled elite sport environments need careful consideration when evaluating potential effects of training on the growth and maturation of youth athletes.

References

1. Steinhaus AH. Chronic effects of exercise. *Physiol Rev*. 1933; 13: 103–147.
2. Rarick GL. Exercise and growth. In Johnson WR (ed.) *Science and medicine of exercise and sports*. New York: Harper and Brothers; 1960. p. 440–465.
3. Malina RM. Exercise as an influence upon growth: Review and critique of current concepts. *Clin Pediatr*. 1969; 8: 16–26.
4. Malina RM. The effects of exercise on specific tissues, dimensions and functions during growth. *Stud Phys Anthropol*. 1979; 5: 21–52.

5. Beyer HG. The influence of exercise on growth. *J Exp Med.* 1896; 1: 546–558.
6. Schwartz L, Britten RH, Thompson LR. *Studies in physical development and posture.* Public Health Bulletin No. 179. Washington, DC: Government Printing Office; 1928.
7. Matthias E. *Der Einfluss der Leibesübungen auf das Körperwachstum im Entwicklungsalter.* Zurich: Rascher and Company; 1916.
8. Godin P. *Growth during school age: Its application to education.* Boston: Gorham Press; 1920.
9. Crampton CW. *Boy's book of strength.* New York: McGraw Hill; 1936.
10. Savage WL. Effect of athletics upon growing boys. *Am Phys Educ Rev.* 1901; 6: 143–150.
11. Orr W. The place of athletics in the curriculum of secondary schools for girls and boys. *Am Phys Educ Rev.* 1907; 12: 49–59.
12. Maurer AH. Football in high school. *Educ Rev.* 1910; 40: 132–137.
13. White House Conference on Child Health and Protection. *Growth and development of the child. Part I. General considerations; Part IV. Appraisement of the child.* New York: Century Company; 1932.
14. Rowe FA. Growth comparison of athletes and non-athletes. *Res Q.* 1933; 4: 108–116.
15. Fait HF. *An analytical study of the effects of competitive athletics upon junior high school boys.* PhD [dissertation]. Iowa City, IA: Iowa State University; 1951. Available from: Michigan State University library, GV 345, microcard, East Lansing, MI.
16. Pařizkova J. Particularities of lean body mass and fat development in growing boys as related to their motor activity. *Acta Paediatr Belg.* 1974; 28(Suppl): 233–244.
17. Lopez R, Pruett DM. The child runner. *J Phys Educ Rec Dance.* 1982; 53: 78–81.
18. American Association for Health, Physical Education, and Recreation. *Desirable athletic competition for children: Joint committee report.* Washington, DC: American Association for Health, Physical Education, and Recreation; 1952.
19. Hale CJ. Physiological maturity of Little League baseball players. *Res Q.* 1956; 27: 276–284.
20. Krogman WM. Maturation age of 55 boys in the Little League World Series, 1957. *Res Q.* 1959; 30: 54–56.
21. Malina RM. Skeletal age and age verification in youth sport. *Sports Med.* 2011; 41: 925–947.
22. Clarke HH. *Physical and motor tests in the Medford Boy's Growth Study.* Englewood Cliffs, NJ: Prentice-Hall; 1971.
23. Åstrand PO, Engström L, Eriksson BO, *et al.* Girl swimmers. *Acta Paediatr.* 1963; 147(Suppl): 1–75.
24. Strong, WB, Malina RM, Blimkie CJR, *et al.* Evidence based physical activity for school youth. *J Pediatr.* 2005; 146: 732–737.
25. Physical Activity Guidelines Committee. *Physical activity guidelines advisory committee report 2008, Part G, Section 9: Youth.* Washington, DC: Department of Health and Human Services; 2008.
26. Malina RM, Bouchard C, Bar-Or O. *Growth, maturation, and physical activity*, 2nd ed. Champaign, IL: Human Kinetics; 2004.
27. Katzmarzyk PT, Walker P, Malina RM. A time-motion study of organized youth sports. *J Hum Move Stud.* 2001; 40: 325–334.
28. Leek D, Carlson JA, Cain KL, *et al.* Physical activity during youth sports participation. *Arch Pediatr Adol Med.* 2011; 154: 294–299.
29. Wickel EE, Eisenmann JC. Contribution of youth sport to total daily physical activity among 6- to 12-yr-old boys. *Med Sci Sports Exerc.* 2007; 39: 1493–1500.
30. Daly RM, Rich PA, Klein R. Hormonal responses to physical training in high-level peripubertal male gymnasts. *Eur J Appl Physiol.* 1998; 79: 74–81.
31. Daly RM, Rich PA, Klein R, Bass S. Effects of high-impact exercise on ultrasonic and biochemical indices of skeletal status: A prospective study in young male gymnasts. *J Bone Min Res.* 1999; 14: 1222–1230.
32. Rhea MR, Hunter RL, Hunter TJ. Competition modeling of American football: Observational data and implications for high school, collegiate, and professional player conditioning. *J Strength Cond Res.* 2006; 20: 58–61.
33. Ridley K, Olds TS. Assigning energy costs to activities in children: A review and synthesis. *Med Sci Sports Exerc.* 2008; 40: 1439–1446.
34. Ridley K, Ainsworth BE, Olds S. Development of a compendium of energy expenditures for youth. *Int J Beh Nutr Phys Act.* 2008; 5: 45–52.
35. Saris WHM, Elvers JWH, van't Hof MA, Binkhorst RA. Changes in physical activity of children aged 6 to 12 years. In Rutenfranz J, Mocellin R, Klimt F (eds.) *Children and exercise XII.* Champaign, IL: Human Kinetics; 1986. p. 121–130.
36. Mirwald RL, Bailey DA. *Maximal aerobic power.* London, ON: Sports Dynamics; 1986.
37. Beunen GP, Malina RM, Renson R, Simons J, Ostyn M, Lefevre J. Physical activity and growth, maturation and performance: A longitudinal study. *Med Sci Sports Exerc.* 1992; 24: 576–585.
38. Baxter-Jones ADG, Eisenmann JC, Mirwald RL, Faulkner RA, Bailey DA. The influence of physical activity on lean mass accrual during adolescence: A longitudinal analysis. *J Appl Physiol.* 2008; 105: 734–741.
39. Iuliano-Burns S, Mirwald RL, Bailey DA. The timing and magnitude of peak height velocity and peak tissue velocities for early, average and late maturing boys and girls. *Am J Hum Biol.* 2001; 13: 1–8.
40. Morris FL, Naughton GA, Gibbs JL, Carlson JS, Wark JD. Prospective ten-month exercise intervention in premenarcheal girls: Positive effects on bone and lean mass. *J Bone Min Res.* 1997; 12: 1453–1462.
41. Baptista F, Janz KF. Habitual physical activity and bone growth and development in children and adolescents: A public health perspective. In Preedy VR (ed.) *Handbook of growth and growth monitoring in health and disease.* New York: Springer; 2012. p. 2395–2411.
42. MacDonald H, Kontulainenm S, Petit M, Janssen P, McKay H. Bone strength and its determinants in pre- and early pubertal boys and girls. *Bone.* 2006; 39: 598–608.
43. Bailey DA, McKay HA, Mirwald RL, Crocker PRE, Faulkner RA. A six-year longitudinal study of the relationship of physical activity to bone mineral accrual in growing children: The University of Saskatchewan Bone Mineral Accrual Study. *J Bone Min Res.* 1999; 14: 1672–1679.
44. Malina RM, Howley E, Gutin B. *Body mass and composition.* Report prepared for the Youth Health Subcommittee, Physical Activity Guidelines Advisory Committee; 2007.
45. Mundt CA, Baxter-Jones ADG, Whiting SJ, Bailey DA, Faulkner RA, Mirwald RL. Relationships of activity and sugar drink intake on fat mass development in youths. *Med Sci Sports Exerc.* 2006; 38: 1245–1254.
46. Moore LL, Gao D, Bradlee ML, *et al.* Does early physical activity predict body fat change throughout childhood? *Prev Med.* 2003; 37: 10–17.
47. Campbell MWC, Williams J, Carlin JB, Wake M. Is the adiposity rebound a rebound in adiposity? *Int J Pediatr Obes.* 2011; 6: e207–e215.
48. Černý L. The results of an evaluation of skeletal ages of boys 11–15 years old with different régime of physical activity. In Kral J, Novotny V (eds.) *Physical fitness and its laboratory assessment.* Prague: Charles University; 1970. p. 56–59.
49. Moisan J, Meyer F, Gingras S. Leisure physical activity and age at menarche. *Med Sci Sports Exerc.* 1991; 23: 1170–1175.
50. Merzenich, H, Boeing H, Wahrendorf J. Dietary fat and sports activity as determinants for age at menarche. *Am J Epidemiol.* 1993; 138: 217–224.
51. Moisan J, Meyer F, Gingras S. A nested case-control study of the correlates of early menarche. *Am J Epidemiol.* 1990; 132: 953–961.
52. Kobayashi K, Kitamura K, Miura M, *et al.* Aerobic power as related to body growth and training in Japanese boys: A longitudinal study. *J Appl Physiol.* 1978; 44: 666–672.
53. Šprynarova S. The influence of training on physical and functional growth before, during and after puberty. *Eur J Appl Physiol.* 1987; 56: 719–724.
54. Malina RM. Physical activity and training: Effects on stature and the adolescent growth spurt. *Med Sci Sports Exerc.* 1994; 26: 759–766.

55. Malina RM, Rogol AD, Cumming SP, Coelho e Silva MJ, Figueiredo AJ. Biological maturation of youth athletes: Assessment and implications. *Br J Sports Med.* 2015; 49: 852–859.
56. Malina RM. Physical growth and biological maturation of young athletes. *Exerc Sport Sci Rev.* 1994; 22: 389–433.
57. Malina RM. Growth and maturation of young athletes—Is training for sport a factor? In: Chan KM, Micheli LJ (eds.) *Sports and children.* Hong Kong: Williams and Wilkins; 1998. p. 133–161.
58. Malina RM, Baxter-Jones ADG, Armstrong N, *et al.* Role of intensive training in the growth and maturation of artistic gymnastics. *Sports Med.* 2013; 43: 783–802.
59. Malina RM. *Crescita e maturazione di bambini ed adolescenti praticanti atletica leggera—Growth and maturation of child and adolescent track and field athletes* (in both Italian and English). Rome: Centro Studi e Ricerche, Federazine Italiana di Atletica Leggera; 2006.
60. Beunen G, Malina RM. Growth and biologic maturation: relevance to athletic performance. In: Hebestreit H, Bar-Or O (eds.) *The young athlete.* Malden, MA: Blackwell; 2008. p. 3–17.
61. Malina RM, Coelho e Silva MJ, Figueiredo AJ. Growth and maturity status of youth players. In: Williams AM (ed.) *Science and soccer: Developing elite performers*, 3rd ed. Abingdon: Routledge; 2013. p. 307–332.
62. Malina RM, Rogol AD. Sport training and the growth and pubertal maturation of young athletes. *Pediatr Endoc Rev.* 2011; 9: 441–455.
63. Malina RM, Geithner CA. Body composition of young athletes. *Amer J Lifestyle Med.* 2011; 5: 262–278.
64. Malina RM. Anthropometry. In: Maud PJ, Foster C (eds.) *Physiological assessment of human fitness.* Champaign, IL: Human Kinetics; 1995. p. 205–219.
65. Lohman TG. Skinfolds and body density and their relationship to body fatness. *Hum Biol.* 1981; 53: 181–225.
66. Lohman TG. Applicability of body composition techniques and constants for children and youths. *Exerc Sport Sci Rev.* 1986; 14: 325–357.
67. Cacciari E, Mazzanti L, Tassinari D, *et al.* Effects of sport (football) on growth: Auxological, anthropometric and hormonal aspects. *Eur J Appl Physiol.* 1990; 61: 149–158.
68. Philippaerts RM, Vaeyens R, Janssens M, *et al.* The relationship between peak height velocity and physical performance in youth soccer players. *J Sports Sci.* 2006; 24: 221–230.
69. Hirose N. Relationships among birth-month distribution, skeletal age and anthropometric characteristics in adolescent elite soccer players. *J Sports Sci.* 2009; 27: 1159–1166.
70. Claessens AL, Malina RM, Lefevre J, *et al.* Growth and menarcheal status of elite female gymnasts. *Med Sci Sports Exerc.* 1992; 24: 755–763.
71. Woynarowska B, Wójcik M, Gorynski P. Wydolnośc fizyczna dzieci o róznym stopniu aktywności ruchowej. *Wychowanie Fizyczne i Sport.* 1974; 4: 81–87.
72. Malina RM, Eveld DJ, Woynarowska B. Growth and sexual maturation of active Polish children 11–14 years of age. *Hermes, Tijdschrift van het Intituut voor Lichamelijke Opleiding* (Journal of the Institute of Physical Education, Catholic University of Leuven, Belgium). 1990; 21: 341–353.
73. Malina RM, Beunen G, Lefevre J, Woynarowska B. Maturity-associated variation in peak oxygen uptake in active adolescent boys and girls. *Ann Hum Biol.* 1997; 24: 19–31.
74. Prader A, Largo RH, Molinari L, *et al.* Physical growth of Swiss children from birth to 20 years of age: First Zurich Longitudinal Study of Growth and Development. *Helvet Paediatr Acta.* 1989; 52(Suppl): 1–125.
75. Geithner CA, Woynarowska B, Malina RM. The adolescent spurt and sexual maturation in girls active and not active in sport. *Ann Hum Biol.* 1998; 25: 415–423.
76. Geithner CA, Satake T, Woynarowska B, Malina RM. Adolescent spurts in body dimensions: Average and modal sequences. *Amer J Hum Biol.* 1999; 11: 287–295.
77. Malina RM, Woynarowska B, Bielicki T, *et al.* Prospective and retrospective longitudinal studies of the growth, maturation, and fitness of Polish youth active in sport. *Int J Sports Med.* 1997; 18(Suppl 3): S179–S185.
78. Malina RM, Bielicki T. Growth and maturation of boys active in sports: Longitudinal observations form the Wrocław Growth Study. *Pediatr Exerc Sci.* 1992; 4: 68–77.
79. Malina RM, Bielicki T. Retrospective longitudinal growth study of boys and girls active in sport. *Acta Paediatr.* 1996; 85: 570–576.
80. Malina RM, Kozieł SM. Validation of maturity offset in a longitudinal sample of Polish girls. *J Sports Sci.* 2014; 32: 1374–1382.
81. Kotulan J, Řeznickova M, Placheta Z. Exercise and growth. In: Placheta Z (ed.) *Youth and physical activity.* Brno: JE Purkyne University Medical Faculty; 1980. p. 61–117.
82. Novotný V. Veränderungen des Knochenalters im Verlauf einer mehrjährigen sportlichen Belastung. *Med u Sport.* 1981; 21: 44–47.
83. Pařizkova J. Longitudinal study of the relationship between body composition and anthropometric characteristics in boys during growth and development. *Glasnik Antropoloskog Drustva Jugoslavije.* 1970; 7: 33–38.
84. Pařizkova J. Body fat and physical fitness. The Hague: Martinus Nijhoff; 1977.
85. Šprynarova S. Longitudinal study of the influence of different physical activity programs on functional capacity of the boys from 11 to 18 years. *Acta Paediatr Belg.* 1974; 28(Suppl): 204–213.
86. Pařizkova J. Growth and growth velocity of lean body mass and fat in adolescent boys. *Pediatr Res.* 1976; 10: 647–650.
87. Ulbrich J. Individual variants of physical fitness in boys from the age of 11 up to maturity and their selection for sports activities. *Medicina dello Sport.* 1971; 24: 118–136.
88. Baxter-Jones ADG, Helms PJ. Effects of training at a young age: A review of the Training of Young Athletes (TOYA) study. *Pediatr Exerc Sci.* 1996; 8: 310–327.
89. Baxter-Jones ADG, Helms P, Maffulli N, Baines-Preece JC, Preece M. Growth and development of male gymnasts, swimmers, soccer and tennis players: A longitudinal study. *Ann Hum Biol.* 1995; 22: 381–394.
90. Erlandson MC, Sherar LB, Mirwald RL, Maffulli N, Baxter-Jones ADG. Growth and maturation of adolescent female gymnasts, swimmers, and tennis players. *Med Sci Sports Exerc.* 2008; 40: 34–42.
91. Baxter-Jones ADG, Helms P, Baines-Preece J, Preece M. Menarche in intensively trained gymnasts, swimmers and tennis players. *Ann Hum Biol.* 1994; 21: 407–415.
92. Kanehisa H, Kuno S, Katsuta S, Fukunaga T. A 2-year follow-up study on muscle size and dynamic strength in teenage tennis players. *Scand J Med Sci Sports.* 2006; 16: 93–101.
93. Fogelholm M, Rankinen R, Isokääntä M, Kujala U, Uusitupa M. Growth, dietary intake and trace element status in pubescent athletes and schoolchildren. *Med Sci Sports Exerc.* 2000; 32: 738–746.
94. Daniels J, Oldridge N. Changes in oxygen consumption of young boys during growth and running training. *Med Sci Sports.* 1971; 3: 161–165.
95. Eisenmann JC, Malina RM. Growth status and estimated growth rate of young distance runners. *Int J Sports Med.* 2002; 23: 168–173.
96. Peltenburg AL, Erich WBM, Zonderland ML, Bernink MJE, van den Brande JL, Huisveld IA. A retrospective growth study of female gymnasts and girl swimmers. *Int J Sports Med.* 1984; 5: 262–267.
97. Damsgaard R, Bencke J, Matthiesen G, Petersen JH, Müller J. Is prepubertal growth adversely affected by sport? *Med Sci Sports Exerc.* 2000; 32: 1698–1703.
98. Ziemilska A. *Wpływ intensywnego treningu gimnastycznego na rozwój somatyczny i dojrzewanie dzieci.* Warsaw: Akademia Wychowania Fizycznego; 1981.
99. Theintz GE, Howald H, Allemann Y, Sizanenko PC. Growth and pubertal development of young female gymnasts and swimmers: A correlation with parental data. *Int J Sports Med.* 1989; 10: 87–91.
100. Keller E, Fröhner G. Growth and development of boys with intensive training in gymnastics during puberty. In: Laron L, Rogol AD (eds.) *Hormones and sport.* New York: Raven Press; 1989. p. 11–20.

101. Malina RM. Growth and maturation of elite female gymnasts: Is training a factor? In: Johnston FE, Zemel B, Eveleth PB (eds.) *Human growth in context*. London: Smith-Gordon; 1999. p. 291–301.
102. Tönz O, Stronski SM, Gmeiner CYK. Wachstum und Pubertät bei 7- bis 16 jahrigen Kunstturneirinnen: eine prospektive Studie. *Schweiz med Wschr*. 1990; 120: 10–20.
103. Fröhner G, Keller E, Schmidt G. Wachstumsparameter von Sportlerinnen unter Bedingungen hoher Trainingsbelastungen. *Ärztl Jugend*. 1990; 81: 375–379.
104. Jahreis G, Kauf E, Fröhner G, Schmidt HE. Influence of intensive exercise on insulin-like growth factor-I, thyroid and steroid hormones in female gymnasts. *Growth Regulat*. 1991; 1: 95–99.
105. Theintz GE, Howald H, Weiss U, Sizonenko PC. Evidence for a reduction of growth potential in adolescent female gymnasts. *J Pediatr*. 1993; 122: 306–313.
106. Thomis M, Claessens AL, Lefevre J, Philippaerts R, Beunen GP, Malina RM. Adolescent growth spurts in female gymnasts. *J Pediatr*. 2005; 146: 239–244.
107. Baxter-Jones ADG, Maffulli N, Mirwald RL. Does elite competition inhibit growth and delay maturation in some gymnasts? Probably not. *Pediatr Exerc Sci*. 2003; 15: 373–382.
108. Buckler JMH, Brodie DA. Growth and maturity characteristics of schoolboy gymnasts. *Ann Hum Biol*. 1977; 4: 455–463.
109. Claessens AL, Lefevre J, Beunen GP, Malina RM. Maturity-associated variation in the body size and proportions of elite female gymnasts 14–17 years of age. *Eur J Pediatr*. 2006; 165: 186–192.
110. Malina RM. Menarche in athletes: A synthesis and hypothesis. *Ann Hum Biol*. 1983; 10: 1–24.
111. Märker K. Zur Menarche von Sportlerinnen nach mehrjährigem in Training in Kindesalter. *Medizin un Sport*. 1979; 19: 329–332.
112. Warren MP. The effect of exercise on pubertal progression and reproductive function in girls. *J Clin Endocrinol Metab*. 1980; 51: 1150–1157.
113. Frisch RE, Gotz-Welbergen AV, McArthur JW, *et al*. Delayed menarche and amenorrhea of college athletes in relation to age of onset of training. *JAMA*. 1981; 246: 1559–1563.
114. Stager JM, Wigglesworth JK, Hatler LK. Interpreting the relationship between age of menarche and prepubertal training. *Med Sci Sports Exerc*. 1990; 22: 54–58.
115. Malina RM. Growth and maturation: Interactions and sources of variation. In: Mascie-Taylor CGN, Yasukouchi A, Ulijaszek S (eds.) *Human variation from the laboratory to the field*. Boca Raton, FL: CRC Press/Taylor and Francis Group; 2010. p. 199–218.
116. Malina RM, Ryan RC, Bonci CM. Age at menarche in athletes and their mothers and sisters. *Ann Hum Biol*. 1994; 21: 417–422.
117. Malina RM, Bouchard C, Shoup RF, Lariviere G. Age, family size and birth order in Montreal Olympic athletes. In: Carter JEL (ed.) *Physical structure of Olympic athletes: Part I. The Montreal Olympic Games Anthropological Project*. Basel: Karger; 1982. p. 13–24.
118. Malina RM, Katzmarzyk PT, Bonci, CM, Ryan RC, Wellens RE. Family size and age at menarche in athletes. *Med Sci Sports Exerc*. 1997; 29: 99–106.
119. Ellis BJ. Timing of pubertal maturation in girls: An integrated life history approach. *Psychol Bull*. 2004; 130: 920–958.
120. Ellis BJ, Essex MJ. Family environments, adrenarche, and sexual maturation: A longitudinal test of a life history model. *Child Develop*. 2007; 78: 1799–1817.
121. Weiss MR. Social influences on children's psychosocial development in youth sports. In: Malina RM, Clark MA (eds.) *Youth sports: Perspectives in a new century*. Monterey, CA: Coaches Choice; 2003. p. 109–126.
122. Brustad RJ. Parental roles and involvement in youth sport: Psychosocial outcomes for children. In: Malina RM, Clark MA (eds.) *Youth sports: Perspectives in a new century*. Monterey, CA: Coaches Choice; 2003. p. 127–138.
123. Sloane KD. Home influences on talent development. In: Bloom BS (ed.) *Developing talent in youth*. New York: Ballantine Books; 1985. p. 439–476.
124. Loucks, AB, Vaitukaitis J, Cameron JL, *et al*. The reproductive system and exercise in women. *Med Sci Sports Exerc*. 1992; 24: S288–S293.
125. Clapp JF, Little KD. The interaction between regular exercise and selected aspects of women's health. *Am J Obstet Gynecol*. 1995; 173: 2–9.
126. Von Döbeln W, Eriksson BO. Physical training, maximal oxygen uptake and dimensions of the oxygen transporting and metabolizing organs in boys 11–13 years of age. *Acta Paediatr Scand*. 1972; 61: 653–660.
127. Roemmich JN, Sinning WE. Weight loss and wrestling training: effects on nutrition, growth, maturation, body composition, and strength. *J Appl Physiol*. 1997; 82: 1751–1759.
128. Meleski BW, Malina RM. Changes in body composition and physique of elite university-level swimmers during a competitive season. *J Sports Sci*. 1985; 3: 33–40.
129. Erlandson MC, Kontulainen SA, Chilibeck PD, Arnold CA, Baxter-Jones ADG. Bone mineral accrual in 4- to 10-year-old precompetitive, recreational gymnasts: A 4-year longitudinal study. *J Bone Min Res*. 2011; 26: 1313–1320.
130. Bass S, Pearce G, Bradney M, *et al*. Exercise before puberty may confer residual benefits in bone density in adulthood: studies in active prepubertal and retired female gymnasts. *J Bone Miner Res*. 1998; 13: 500–507.
131. Nickols-Richardson SM, O'Connor PJ, Shapses SA, Lewis RD. Longitudinal bone mineral density changes in female child artistic gymnasts. *J Bone Miner Res*. 1999; 14: 994–1002.
132. Nurmi-Lawton JA, Baxter-Jones AD, Mirwald RL, *et al*. Evidence of sustained skeletal benefits from impact-loading exercise in young females: a 3-year longitudinal study. *J Bone Miner Res*. 2004; 19: 314–322.
133. Ducher G, Hill BL, Angeli T, Bass SL, Eser P. Comparison of pQCT parameters between ulna and radius in retired elite gymnasts: The skeletal benefits associated with long-term gymnastics are bone- and site-specific. *J Musculoskel Neuronal Interact*. 2009; 9: 247–255.
134. Bass SL, Saxon L, Daly RM, *et al*. The effect of mechanical loading on the size and shape of bone in pre-, peri-, and post-pubertal girls: A study in tennis players. *J Bone Min Res*. 2002; 17: 2274–2280.
135. Daly RM, Saxon L, Turner CH, Robling AG, Bass SL. The relationship between muscle size and bone geometry during growth and in response to exercise. *Bone*. 2004; 34: 281–287.
136. Ireland A, Maden-Wilkinson T, McPhee J, *et al*. Upper limb muscle-bone asymmetries and bone adaptation in elite youth tennis players. *Med Sci Sports Exerc*. 2013; 45: 1749–1758.
137. Ducher G, Bass SL, Saxon L, Daly RM. Effects of repetitive loading on the growth-induced changes in bone mass and cortical bone geometry: A 12-month study in pre/peri- and postmenarcheal tennis players. *J Bone Mine Res*. 2011; 26: 1321–1329.
138. Kannus P, Haapasalo H, Sankelo M, *et al*. Effect of starting age of physical activity on bone mineral in the dominant arm of tennis and squash players. *Ann Intern Med*. 1995; 123: 27–31.
139. Kannus P, Sievanen H, Vuori I. Physical loading, exercise, and bone. *Bone*. 1996; 18: 1S–3S.
140. Kontulainen S, Kannus P, Haapasalo H, *et al*. Good maintenance of exercise-induced bone gain with decreased training of female tennis and squash players: a prospective 5-year follow-up study of young and old starters and controls. *J Bone Miner Res*. 2001; 17: 195–201.
141. Gomez-Bruton A, Montero-Marín J, Gonzalez-Agüero A, *et al*. The effect of swimming during childhood and adolescence on bone mineral density: A systematic review and meta-analysis. *Sports Med*. 2016; 46: 335–379.
142. Barrack MT, Rauh MJ, Nichols JF. Cross-sectional evidence of suppressed bone mineral accrual among female adolescent distance runners. *J Bone Min Res*. 2010; 25: 1850–1857.
143. Barrack MT, Rauh MJ, Barkai HS, Nichols JF. Dietary restraint and low bone mass in female adolescent endurance runners. *Amer J Clin Nutr*. 2008; 87: 36–43.

144. Barrack MT, Van Loan MD, Rauh MJ, Nichols JF. Physiologic and behavioral indicators of energy deficiency in female adolescent runners with elevated bone turnover. *Amer J Clin Nutr*. 2010; 92: 652–659.
145. Barrack MT, Van Loan MD, Rauh MJ, Nichols JG. Body mass, training, menses, and bone in adolescent runners: A 3-yr follow-up. *Med Sci Sports Exerc*. 2011; 43: 959–966.
146. Olmedillas H, Gonzälez-Agüero A, Moreno LA, Casajús JA, Vicente-Rodriguez G. Bone related health status in adolescent cyclists. *PLOS One*. 2011; 6: e24841.
147. Gustavsson A, Olsson T, Nordstrom P. Rapid loss of bone mineral density of the femoral neck after cessation of ice hockey training: A 6-year longitudinal study in males. *J Bone Min Res*. 2003; 18: 1964–1969.

CHAPTER 33

Hormones and training

Jaak Jürimäe

Introduction

There has been great interest in the influence of sport training on growth and maturation in children and adolescents during recent years. Regular physical exercise plays an important role in the developing child. It stimulates somatic growth, influences muscle development, strengthens bones, modulates adipose tissue, and contributes to the development of the cardiorespiratory system and sexual maturation.[1] These growth and maturation processes are regulated by the secretion and action of the endocrine system, including the growth hormone (GH)—insulin-like growth factor-1 (IGF-I) axis, the hypothalamic-pituitary-gonadal (HPG) axis, and thyroid hormone concentrations.[1,2] While prepubertal growth is almost exclusively dependent on GH, IGF-I, and thyroid hormones, the marked acceleration in growth velocity during puberty is dependent on the interaction of the GH-IGF-I and HPG axes with the continued permissive effect of thyroid hormone.[2] Somatic growth and sexual maturation processes are also influenced by the nutritional status.[2,3] Marked undernutrition combined with heavy training and competition can suppress growth and maturation and delay pubertal development,[3] while chronic overnutrition may result in early maturation and an increased growth velocity.[2] The influence of nutritional status on linear growth and pubertal timing is also demonstrated by the fact that a critical amount of body fat is known to be essential for onset of puberty,[4] while a marked delay in onset of oestrogen can permanently cause the skeleton to be undermineralized.[3] Accordingly, it appears that the growth and maturation of young athletes, especially in weight-controlled aesthetic sports face an additional burden of possible negative energy balance.[3]

Energy homeostasis is regulated by a complex neuroendocrine system including central and peripheral tissues.[5,6] Important to this regulatory system is the existence of several adipose and gut tissue hormones that communicate the status of body energy stores to the hypothalamus.[5,6] These include, but are not limited to, several highly active molecules such as leptin, adiponectin, ghrelin, and some more classical molecules such as interleukin (IL)-6 and tumour necrosis factor-α (TNF-α).[5,6] These inflammatory cytokines are related to obesity, and obesity may be considered as a low-grade systemic inflammatory disease in children.[7] In addition, their concentrations are often related to such factors as biological age and maturation.[5,8] The concentrations of inflammatory mediators may vary depending on specific physical activity[9] and physical performance[10] levels in children during linear growth and maturation.

It is well known that young athletes sometimes employ very high training loads and achieve international recognition at a very young age in some sport disciplines (e.g. gymnastics, figure skating). This may lead to delayed puberty and slowed growth rate due to increased energy expenditure coupled with limited nutritional intake.[5] In contrast, it is worth investigating whether chronic exposure to high training loads in the presence of adequate nutrition accelerates the rate of somatic growth and maturation[2] (interested readers are referred to Chapter 32 for further discussion).

Research on how these potential outcomes are related to different hormones during growth and maturation is limited. In addition, as training efficiency depends on the intensity, volume, duration, and frequency of training load and on the athlete's ability to tolerate it, imbalance between the training load and the athlete's tolerance may lead to under- or overtraining[11] (interested readers are referred to Chapter 38 for further discussion). The exposure of growing athletes to a high level of training stress is also indicated by the activation of the hypothalamic-pituitary-adrenal (HPA) axis, where circulating cortisol increases as a result of exercise-induced negative energy balance.[6,12] However, the behaviour of the catabolic hormone cortisol as a result of training stress is not studied enough in growing athletes.[1] Accordingly, there is a need to find specific blood hormonal markers that can objectively describe the balance between training load and the athlete's tolerance. As the endocrine system modulates anabolic and catabolic processes and plays an important role in the adaptation to training load,[6,11] different hormone levels could be used to describe the training status of a young athlete. At present, there is not enough information about the possible overtraining syndrome using different hormone parameters in young athletes.[6] There are several examples where some talented young athletes after long periods of intensive training end their career due to overtraining, while others may have dropped out of elite sport through the lack of success by the age of 16–17 years. Compared to adults, relatively few data are available on the role of the endocrine system and its influences on both athletic performance and hormone responses to frequent exercise-related stress in young athletes during growth and maturation.[11,13]

It should be taken into account that the effects of athletic training on growing children may not be similar to those on adults, especially when the hormone concentrations could be elevated due to the process of growth rather than a reflection on a specific training environment.[2] Therefore, the effect of exercise training on anabolic hormones and inflammatory mediators is particularly important during puberty, since there is a spontaneous increase in anabolic hormones that leads to a marked growth spurt during this period of growth.[11] According to Roemmich,[2] the main adaptive changes in the endocrine system that occur during intense training periods in children during growth include: i) altered basal and maximal exercise-induced hormone concentrations; ii) decreased

Table 33.1 Summary of reported main basal hormonal responses to pubertal maturation and sport training in growing athletes.

Hormone	Puberty	Prolonged training	Possible overreaching
Growth hormone-insulin-like growth factor-1 axis			
Growth hormone	↑	↑ or ↔	↓ or **?**
IGF-I	↑	↔ or ↑	↓
IGF-I/IGFBP-3 ratio	↑	↔ or ↑	↓
Hypothalamic-pituitary-gonadal axis			
Testosterone	↑	↔	**?**
Oestrogens	↑	↔	↓
Hypothalamic-pituitary-adrenal axis			
Cortisol	↔	↔ or ↑	**?**
Adipocytokines			
Leptin	↑	↔ or ↓	↓
Adiponectin	↓	↔ or ↑	**?**
Gastrointestinal hormones			
Ghrelin	↓	↑ or ↔	↑ or**?**

↑ increase; ↓ decrease; ↔ no change; **?** presently unknown.

magnitude of hormonal responses to acute training stimuli; and/or iii) altered number of circulating binding proteins that bind the specific hormone. This chapter focuses on the available information about the specific effects of prolonged exercise training on the hormones of the GH-IGF-I, HPG and HPA axes, and different inflammatory mediators in young sportsmen at different stages of linear growth and sexual maturation throughout childhood and adolescence (Table 33.1).

Sport training and the growth hormone-insulin-like growth factor-1 axis

The GH-IGF-I axis is a hormonal axis that is involved in GH release from the pituitary and IGF-I from the liver.[1] This axis controls somatic and tissue growth, and is also known to play a role in metabolic adaptation to exercise training.[11,14,15] Interestingly, exercise training is also associated with changes in inflammatory cytokines, and the balance between the anabolic hormones and inflammatory mediators is believed to determine the effects of training load.[11,16] It should be considered that while exercise training stimulates anabolic components of the GH-IGF-I axis, it may also increase catabolic pro-inflammatory cytokines such as IL-6 and TNF-α[11,16] Unfortunately, data on the balance between these anabolic and catabolic hormones during the whole training season in young athletes are scarce.[11] Eliakim and Nemet[11] have proposed that the assessment of changes in these antagonistic circulating growth mediators may assist in monitoring the effects of different types of prolonged exercise training in growing athletes.

Significant relationships of functional (i.e. cardiorespiratory fitness determined by peak oxygen consumption [peak $\dot{V}O_2$]) and structural (i.e. thigh muscle volume determined by magnetic resonance imaging) parameters of physical fitness with resting GH, GH binding protein (GHBP), and IGF-I secretion in prepubertal and adolescent children have been found.[11,17,18] The association between peak $\dot{V}O_2$ and mean overnight GH levels has probably resulted from an increase in peak GH amplitude.[11] Eliakim *et al.*[14] argued that the stimulation of the GH-IGF-I axis by repetitive training sessions contributes to an increase in muscle mass and improved cardiorespiratory responses to exercise (such as peak $\dot{V}O_2$). Increasing levels of physical activity stimulate GH pulsatility and consequently circulating IGF-I concentrations.[14] In agreement with this, mean and peak GH levels were significantly higher in elite young athletes compared to non-elite athletes and sedentary controls.[19] A strong correlation between GH levels and mean weekly training volume was also found in these elite athletes who trained at least 12 h·week^{-1}.[19] However, in spite of higher GH levels, no difference in circulating IGF-I levels was found between studied groups, nor were any correlations found between circulating GH and IGF-I levels.[19] There is speculation that the differences in IGF-I levels between these studies can be attributed to differences in age, maturation, and physical fitness levels. Taken together, these data suggest that physical fitness is associated with anabolic adaptations of the GH-IGF-I system already in prepubertal and adolescent years in young sport participants, even as spontaneous growth proceeds.[11]

Typically, there are no differences in basal IGF-I and IGF binding protein (IGFBP) concentrations in growing athletes when compared with untrained controls.[11,12,20–22] For example, Courteix *et al.*[20] reported no differences in IGF-I levels between adolescent rhythmic gymnasts and untrained controls, despite reduced adiposity and leptin levels in rhythmic gymnasts. It was argued that although IGF-I is regulated by energy balance, and reduced body fat is often related to decreased IGF-I levels, exercise preserved IGF-I concentrations in the rhythmic gymnasts.[20] In support of this, baseline or pulsatility values of IGF-I as well as IGFBP-I and IGFBP-3 appear to be unaffected by menstrual status (amenorrhea vs eumenorrhea) in young female athletes.[23] It has also been reported that IGF-I levels do not change as a result of prolonged training in young athletes.[12,24] Furthermore, Maimoun *et al.*[25] demonstrated that serum IGF-I and the IGF-I/IGFBP-3 ratio as an index of free IGF-I were increased with pubertal stages in rhythmic gymnasts, showing a similar pattern with untrained controls.[12] No differences in IGF-I, IGFBP-3, and the IGF-I/IGFBP-3 ratio were found between adolescent swimmers, rhythmic gymnasts, sprinters, and untrained controls.[21] In contrast, there are also studies that have found lower basal IGF-I values in adolescent athletes compared to untrained controls.[26,27] It has been suggested that energy status interferes with IGF-I secretion as negative energy balance has been related to reduced serum IGF-I levels in both young male and female athletes.[11,12] Furthermore, the discrepant findings in basal IGF-I levels could also be due to the time of sampling in relation to the young athletes' sport season.[12,28] It has been argued that while GH-IGF-I axis hormone concentrations may vary during training in prepubertal rhythmic gymnasts, these fluctuations have no reflection on linear growth over the next 4 years when entering into puberty, although a delay in pubertal progression was observed in the studied rhythmic gymnasts.[28]

The function of the GH-IGF-I axis may be suppressed in child athletes during strenuous training periods showing a catabolic hormonal environment, which may be attributed to an imbalance between energy intake and expenditure.[11,12] For example, a dietary restriction during the wrestling season in male adolescent wrestlers produced a partial GH-resistance in later parts of the season.[29,30] Roemmich and Sinning[29] proposed that the partial GH resistance may have been caused by a reduced negative hypothalamic feedback by IGF-I or a decrease in GHBP concentration. The growth effects of GH are enhanced by GHBP, and GH secretion would need to increase to account for the reduced GHBP concentration to ensure continuation of normal growth.[2] It has been suggested that the GH-IGF-I axis is regulated by energy balance through the GH receptor, and the effects of the training season are reversible on the reduction of the training load (i.e. energy expenditure) and increase in energy intake in male adolescent athletes.[29] Furthermore, it should be considered that, even when incremental growth rate in male adolescent wrestlers is suppressed during the season, an incremental (i.e. catch-up) growth during post-season occurs.[29,30]

Reduced IGF-I levels during heavy training periods are associated with a loss of body mass in child female gymnasts[31] and adolescent male wrestlers,[29,30] which provides clear evidence for a negative energy balance and catabolic state in these young athletes.[11] In another study, Nemet *et al.*[15] demonstrated that, although inadequate energy intake and negative energy balance are the major reasons for the training-induced decrease in IGF-I concentration, IGF-I level may fall even when energy balance and weight stability are maintained in late-adolescent male wrestlers. It has also been demonstrated that while circulating IGF-I decreases as a result of an intense training period, aerobic fitness may still improve in growing children.[32] Accordingly, changes in basal IGF-I appear to be good markers of general condition and energy balance of the young athlete, while they may not necessarily be good markers for functional performance of athletes.[11] Furthermore, while tapering of the training intensity has been associated with increased circulating IGF-I concentrations and improved performance in athletes, Eliakim and Nemet[11] have proposed that an inability to increase IGF-I levels before major competitions should be an alarming sign that the general condition is not optimal for an elite growing athlete. To avoid possible overtraining, basal IGF-I concentrations should be measured several times during the whole training season to detect possible training-related changes in this hormone level in elite young athletes.

Sport training and the hypothalamic-pituitary-gonadal axis

There is a positive association between GH, IGF-I, and reproductive hormones, and the interaction of the reproductive hormones with the GH-IGF-I axis is likely a major contributor to pubertal growth and maturation outcomes.[8] The reproductive hormones of the HPG axis are also highly sensitive to the physiological stress of sport training in growing athletes.[12] Accordingly, the high level of exercise training completed by young growing athletes and the possible risks associated with it has generated considerable interest in paediatric exercise science. In particular, alterations in the HPG axis during heavy training have been documented in male[29] and female[12] growing athletes. These negative reactions in the HPG axis may lead to reduced growth velocity[12] and delayed skeletal maturation[33] in both male and female child athletes, and delayed menarche in young female athletes[1] (Interested readers are referred to Chapter 32 for further discussion).

The impact of sport training on circulating testosterone levels in adults has been relatively well studied. Typically, testosterone concentrations in blood are lowered after prolonged endurance training[34] and increased after prolonged resistance training[35] periods in adult athletes. Similarly, testosterone concentrations were decreased after 43 weeks of swimming training in pubertal boys.[36] In another study, testosterone levels were followed over an entire competitive season in elite under 15 and under 17 male soccer players, and there was a significant decrease in testosterone concentration at the end of the competitive season as compared with the beginning of the season in both age groups.[37] In adolescent male wrestlers, reduced testosterone levels were found in the late season due to the dietary restrictions necessary to obtain and/or maintain the desired weight category.[29] However, testosterone concentrations were returned to normal levels after the season. These changes were unrelated to oestradiol, prolactin, or cortisol concentrations, which modulate the activity of the HPG axis.[29] It was concluded that the low testosterone concentrations were caused by a reduction in testosterone production during the season as hormone binding proteins remained in the normal range.[29] In contrast, there were no changes in testosterone concentration during a 2-month sport season in adolescent male runners.[38] Furthermore, no relationship between basal level of testosterone and training volume has been found in adolescent male runners[38] or gymnasts.[39] It appears that a short period of endurance training does not lower circulating testosterone levels in pubertal male athletes, while a longer training season accompanied with caloric deficit may negatively affect testosterone release, which returns back to normal after the season.[1] In contrast to adult athletes, it could be suggested that a chronic decrease in basal testosterone levels is not likely to occur over a prolonged training period in maturing young athletes due to: i) the possibility that observed lowered testosterone concentrations in young people may have been a function of an increase in receptor binding, which would be a positive effect[38,39] and ii) the reduction in circulating testosterone levels have only been observed in those adult athletes who have been endurance training for several years.[40]

A recent study by Zinner *et al.*[41] investigated the effect of a 2-week high-intensity interval training (HIIT) block microcycle on circulating testosterone concentrations in well-trained adolescent male triathletes. The training adaptations to a relatively short block periodization training programme included increases in circulating testosterone levels in addition to significant gains in peak power output and time trial performance in young triathletes.[41] Accordingly, greater testosterone levels indicate that even a short, 2-week HIIT programme causes a heightened anabolic state in junior triathletes. It was suggested that the positive effects of this training period might be explained by the ability of testosterone to stimulate erythropoiesis and lactate transport capacities in these adolescent triathletes.[41] These results show that a one block microcycle may have positive anabolic effects on endurance performance even in adolescent athletes. In addition, a positive association between basal testosterone level and peak $\dot{V}O_2$ has been observed in boys with different levels of maturation.[42] In another study, circulating testosterone was related to aerobic fitness as determined by a Yo-Yo intermittent endurance test in preadolescent soccer players.[43] While testosterone was associated with muscle power, as determined by a countermovement jump (CMJ) test, in preadolescent players,[43] testosterone was not related to CMJ scores in adolescent soccer players.[37] Furthermore, it was suggested that changes in testosterone and changes in muscle power were not related over a 1-year competitive season in elite under 15 and under 17 soccer players.[37] Differences in the testosterone results in these studies with young soccer players[37,43] could be explained by the differences in maturation and exercise stress.

Pubertal maturation increases testosterone levels in both boys[13,42] and girls[12,44] during linear growth. In adolescent girls, Kraemer *et al.*[44] found that a 7-week competitive season caused higher resting- and exercise-induced testosterone concentrations in runners. Therefore, it was argued that the increased testosterone response could be attributed to training and/or maturation in adolescent female athletes.[44] In another study, testosterone was increased after 3 days of heavy training in child female gymnasts,[31] while testosterone levels were relatively stable over a 1-year training period in elite adolescent female swimmers.[27] Overall, pubertal maturation and short-term exercise training affects baseline testosterone levels in female athletes.[1] In young male soccer players, the mean testosterone levels were associated with both chronological age and pubertal stages.[13] Sport training did not change resting testosterone concentration or affect the onset of puberty in male gymnasts.[39] This demonstrates that sport training does not result in advanced onset of puberty, and young athletes in team sports excel because of their early maturation[39,45] (interested readers are referred to Chapter 30 for further discussion). In contrast to athletes from team sports, young gymnasts train hard from an early age and have been found to be shorter than age-matched untrained controls.[39,46] This has led to the question whether short stature in pubertal gymnasts is the result of selection bias or a result of delayed puberty due to altered reproductive hormones during intense training.[39,46,47] However, no differences in circulating testosterone concentrations between high-level peripubertal[47] and adolescent[39] gymnasts with age-matched untrained controls have been found. Furthermore, Daly *et al.*[47] found no difference in resting testosterone levels between peripubertal gymnasts and control subjects over a 10-month study period. These results together show that high levels of prolonged sport training in growing athletes appear to have no effect on basal testosterone levels or pubertal maturation in young athletes (interested readers are referred to Chapter 32 for further discussion).

It is well established that intense training with inadequate energy intake during growth exerts an inhibitory effect on the HPG axis in female athletes.[12,33,48] For example, no significant rise in oestradiol concentrations was observed in pubertal female gymnasts, which is in contrast to age-matched untrained controls.[12,49] Adolescents competing in high-level sports are therefore at risk of developing the female athletic triad,[12] which is defined as the association of eating disorders, functional hypothalamic amenorrhea, and reduced bone mineral density.[2,48] It appears that exercise-induced menstrual dysfunction, which includes primary and secondary amenorrhea and oligomenorrhea, may occur in a wide range of adolescent female athletes and across a wide spectrum of sports disciplines.[12] The estimated prevalence of secondary amenorrhea among young athletes is 4–20 times higher than in the general population.[50] It appears to be higher mainly in younger female athletes who train intensively, resulting in low energy availability,[48] with the highest prevalence observed in sports emphasizing leanness and low body mass, such as gymnastics, figure skating, and running, although other sports with fewer nutritional constraints but high energy expenditure, such as swimming and skiing are also affected.[2,12] For example, gymnasts often present menarche delayed by 2–3 years, as well as oligomenorrhea or athletic amenorrhea.[12] Athletic amenorrhea is characterized by reduced oestrogen concentrations,[48] which are linked to the reduced gonadotropin-releasing hormone (GnRH) pulsatility.[12] The evidence indicates that energy deficiency is the major factor that alters reproductive hormone secretion in female athletes, rather than exercise stress or an increase in exercise energy expenditure.[12,51] There is an energy availability threshold of about 20–25 $\text{kcal} \cdot \text{kg}^{-1}$ (83.7–104.7 $\text{kJ} \cdot \text{kg}^{-1}$) lean body mass, and menstrual disturbance occurs when energy availability is below this threshold.[51] Consequently, athletic amenorrhea is mainly a nutritional problem and may be reversed by dietary modifications.[48] However, nutrient deficiency is extremely concerning in young female athletes, as the immature reproductive hormone axis could be less resilient to nutritional stress, which in turn may cause late menarche or primary amenorrhea,[52] and perhaps even lifelong alterations in reproductive function[2] (interested readers are referred to Chapter 47 for further discussion).

Elite young female athletes, e.g. gymnasts, who are training intensively with limited dietary intake year round may be at greater risk for limiting their growth velocity and pubertal maturation.[2] Accelerated or catch-up growth after retirement from competitive sport has been described in former young gymnasts,[53] which suggests reduced growth potential during training.[54] When the growth and maturation of female gymnasts and swimmers were compared, adolescent female gymnasts presented delayed age at menarche and lower growth velocity in addition to lower oestradiol and IGF-I concentrations.[54,55] However, it has to be taken into account that the adult height of female and male gymnasts is not compromised by intensive gymnastics training.[33] In contrast, the growth and maturation characteristics of gymnasts may be due to genetic factors, since elite young gymnasts are shorter than age-matched controls before intensive gymnastics training, and they generally have relatively short parents who also had later than average puberty.[55] At present, available data on the separate effect of intensive gymnastics training on growth, maturation, and the reproductive hormone system in young female and male gymnasts are still inadequate.[2,33] Further longitudinal studies are needed to better understand the issue of intensive gymnastics training and alterations within the whole endocrine system in growing and maturing young athletes.

Sport training and the hypothalamic-pituitary-adrenal axis

Sport disciplines like gymnastics, figure skating, and swimming, among others, require high performance levels during the growth period, and expose young athletes to high levels of physiological and psychological stress at a relatively early age.[12] The HPA axis plays a critical role in the ability of the growing athlete to respond to this stress.[56] However, unlike the HPG axis, the HPA axis does not undergo dramatic shifts in activity with age once the normal diurnal variation in cortisol concentrations is established in early life.[56] Accordingly, in young soccer players, no differences in basal cortisol levels were observed between different pubertal stages, and no relationship between cortisol and pubertal stages was found.[13] Furthermore, no difference in resting cortisol concentration at any time during a 10-month period was found in peripubertal male gymnasts and an untrained, control group of boys.[47] Similarly, Kraemer *et al.*[44] reported that a 7-week high-school track season did not affect resting cortisol levels in adolescent female distance runners, while cortisol concentrations remained relatively unchanged in adolescent wrestlers and their age-matched control subjects in pre-season, late season, and post-season.[29] These results indicate that basal cortisol concentrations are not affected by prolonged sport training during sexual maturation in young athletes. More studies are needed to clarify the chronic effect of sport training on the basal cortisol concentration in growing athletes to better understand its significance.[1]

The HPA axis has been reported to be activated by a negative energy balance[56] and as an adaptation to exercise stress.[12] Relatively high basal cortisol values have frequently been observed in adolescent and young adult female athletes and, to a greater degree, in amenorrheic athletes.[12,57] In addition, the cortisol response to intense exercise is reduced in amenorrheic athletes compared with eumenorrheic athletes because of their high basal cortisol values.[57] In another study, no difference in basal cortisol levels was found between elite young female sports gymnasts with normal menstruation and those with amenorrhea.[58] However, the diurnal variation in circulating cortisol levels was abolished in elite gymnasts, which probably reflects the adaptation to prolonged heavy training and chronic energy deficit.[58] Accordingly, a negative energy balance as a result of sport training is necessary for the increase in basal cortisol concentrations in growing athletes. While a significantly reduced basal cortisol level may already be an indicator of chronic overtraining syndrome in adult athletes,[34] it is still not possible to draw specific conclusions about the interaction between basal cortisol level and the specific amount of physical stress during prolonged sport training in elite growing athletes.

Sport training and the peripheral signals of energy homeostasis

The complex feedback mechanisms reporting peripheral fat and energy stores to the central nervous system consist of several appetite hormones, including adipose tissue and gastrointestinal hormones.[12,56] Accordingly, adipose tissue is not simply an energy storage organ, but also a secretory organ that synthesizes multiple adipocytokines and acts as an endocrine organ.[5] These adipocytokines include leptin, adiponectin, resistin, visfatin, IL-6, and TNF-α among others.[8] Among the gastrointestinal peptides secreted in response to changes in energy homeostasis are ghrelin and peptide YY.[12,56] While ghrelin remains unique as the only known circulating hormone that stimulates appetite,[56,59] peptide YY has received more attention from appetite supressing hormones among the gastrointestinal peptides.[60] In addition to the regulation of energy homeostasis, these appetite hormones promote appetite and satiety signals as well as an inflammatory response.[5,8,56] Various studies have examined the effects of exercise and sport training on alterations in different peripheral signals of energy homeostasis.[5,6,61] However, most of the research in this area has been conducted on leptin, adiponectin, and ghrelin.[61] Furthermore, the core feedback signals in the energy homeostatic mechanism for energy intake appear to be leptin and ghrelin,[56] while leptin, adiponectin, and ghrelin assist in somatic and pubertal growth in children in addition to regulating energy balance.[5]

Leptin

Leptin is the most investigated hormone in relation to energy homeostasis.[5,6] In the light of its role as a permissive signal for the normal functioning of the HPG axis,[62] leptin appears to be the molecular link among adequate energy stores, adipose tissue, and the onset of puberty in children.[63] It has been suggested that leptin stimulates the regulation of GnRH, thus allowing for the pituitary secretion of gonadotropins necessary for pubertal onset.[8] Elevations in leptin concentration contribute to the activation of the HPG axis and may also lead to the activation of the GH-IGF-I axis, which results in a positive feedback to the HPG axis.[8] This suggests that leptin may be a molecular signal linking nutritional status to the pubertal activation of the HPG axis.[64] It appears that circulating leptin is present at similar concentrations in both sexes over the prepubertal years, and the initiation of puberty has been linked to increased leptin concentrations.[63] After onset of puberty in which the maturation of the reproductive system is in progress,[8] a more dramatic increase in leptin concentration has been observed in girls compared with boys.[8,63] Leptin peaks at pubertal stage 2 in boys and, thereafter, leptin levels decline to reach a nadir at the end of puberty in boys.[8] There is a progressive increase in leptin through prepuberty into early puberty in girls, and then it peaks at the end of puberty, mostly likely because of the increase in adipose tissue stores that occurs during pubertal development in girls.[8,63] Consequently, leptin is related to various factors including energy status and body composition as well as pubertal onset and progression in children during linear growth.[5]

Leptin concentrations have been found to be lowered after prolonged high-volume training in adult athletes.[34] Similarly, low leptin levels have been reported in growing athletes in relation to their reduced body fat mass and as a direct result of chronic exercise training.[5,12] This is particularly observed in gymnastics, running, swimming, and aesthetic activities such as ballet dancing,[12,49,65–68] as well as in team sports like basketball and soccer.[12] For example, at least 2 years of strenuous training with relatively high energy expenditure caused lowered leptin levels in prepubertal rhythmic gymnasts with mean age of 8 years in comparison with age-matched healthy untrained controls.[69] Furthermore, Parm *et al.*[70] found that leptin was not changed as a result of a 12-month training period in prepubertal rhythmic gymnasts, while significant increases in leptin were observed in untrained controls over the same period. In highly trained rhythmic gymnasts, leptin levels were elevated in those athletes who were in pubertal stages 4

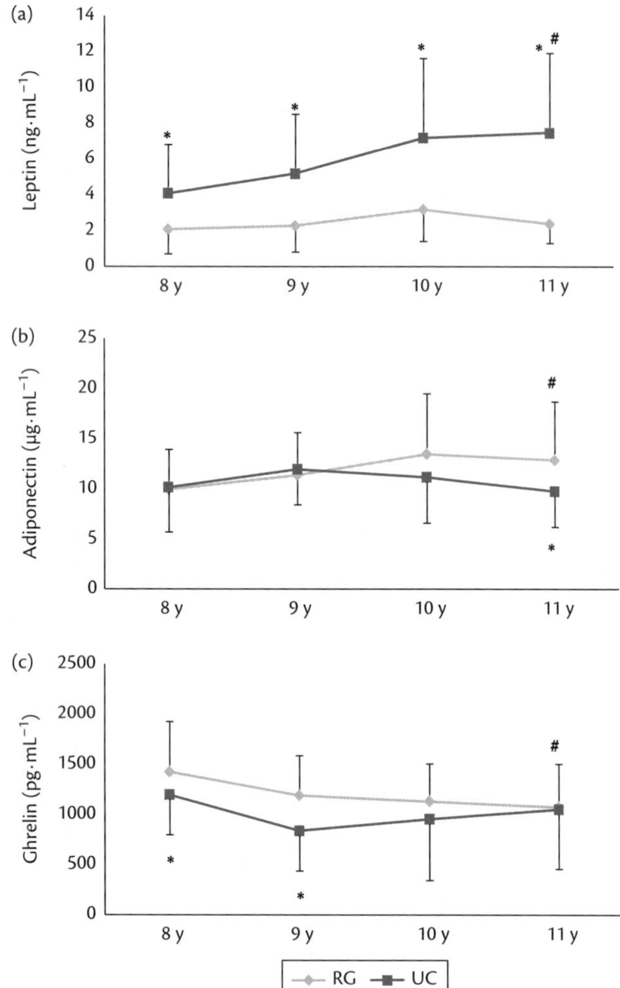

Figure 33.1 Leptin (a), adiponectin (b), and ghrelin (c) concentrations in rhythmic gymnasts and untrained controls entering into puberty.
RG = rhythmic gymnasts; UC = untrained controls.
* Significant difference between RG and UC; $p < 0.05$; # Significant difference from 8 year-old girls; $p < 0.05$.
Data from Võsoberg K, Tillmann V, Tamm AL, *et al.* Adipocytokine and ghrelin levels in relation to body composition in rhythmic gymnasts entering into puberty: a 3-year follow-up study. Pediatr Exerc Sci. 2014; 26: 477–484.

and 5 when compared with athletes in pubertal stages 1 and 2.[71] Therefore, it was argued that leptin levels rise in parallel with increases in body fat mass in highly trained rhythmic gymnasts despite the reduced amount of adipose tissue in young female athletes at different stages of maturation.[71] A longitudinal study[65] showed that leptin concentrations remained relatively unchanged in rhythmic gymnasts advancing from prepuberty to midpuberty (from pubertal stage 1 to pubertal stages 2 and 3), while significant increases in leptin levels were seen in age-matched, untrained controls over the same time period (Figure 33.1a). Furthermore, changes in body fat mass were related to changes in leptin concentrations over the 36-month study period in these young athletes.[65] It has been suggested that the specific, heavy-training volume seen in these rhythmic gymnasts during the prepubertal years may have counterbalanced the age-dependent increase in circulating leptin, and the increase in leptin levels could be sometimes seen in later stages of pubertal maturation in female athletes.[5]

Intense sport training can delay the normal pattern of pubertal development in athletes,[2,72] and basal leptin concentrations have been reported to be lower in these young athletes.[12,72] For example, Weimann[72] found that circulating leptin concentrations were lower in elite female and male sport gymnasts and remained unchanged at different maturational levels when compared with healthy untrained controls. In both genders, total energy consumption and nutritional intake were insufficient, although to a lesser extent in male gymnasts.[72] A long history of intense training (~7 years in girls, ~4 years in boys) with high volume (~22 $h \cdot week^{-1}$ in girls; ~16 $h \cdot week^{-1}$ in boys) during the sensitive phases of pubertal maturation led to lowered leptin concentrations in sport gymnasts of both sexes, although the lowered leptin levels were more pronounced in female athletes as they had a longer history of high-demand training sessions when compared to male athletes.[72] In addition, girls also displayed low oestrogen levels, reduced body fat mass, and retarded menarche, while the pubertal development in elite male gymnasts remained almost unaltered.[72] It was argued that high sport training load and consequently high energy expenditure impair the development of body fat mass appropriate for age, and the lack of body fat reserves, per se, leads to low leptin levels.[72] This effect was further aggravated by insufficient caloric intake due to current aesthetic standards in this sport discipline and accordingly leptin concentrations were substantially lower; this in turn may not allow the HPG axis to be activated properly to induce puberty in a timely manner.[72] The persistent low leptin levels in young athletes may influence the age of menarche by delaying it for 1–3 years.[12] These results demonstrate that training history may have an impact on basal leptin levels and pubertal development in elite adolescent athletes.

Also, no difference in basal leptin concentration was found in adolescent female swimmers with advancing age and pubertal stage after onset of puberty.[68] Therefore, leptin concentrations were relatively unchanged despite significant increases in IGF-I and oestradiol concentrations during this 24-month study period in female swimmers.[68] Leptin levels also remained unchanged in male swimmers advancing from prepuberty to puberty, while IGF-I and testosterone concentrations were increased according to pubertal maturation over the 24-month study period.[73] In addition, basal leptin concentrations were correlated with body fat mass in young female[68] and male[73] swimmers. These results suggest that reduced basal leptin concentrations could be used as a sign of increased training stress in adolescent sportsmen and lowered leptin levels depend on low body fat mass, while the hormones of the HPG axis are within normal range in both male and female adolescent athletes.[5] Reduced basal and acute exercise-induced leptin levels have been suggested to be indicative of a short-term overreaching state in adult athletes.[34] Clearly, further studies are needed to understand the exact role of circulating leptin in conditions of high training stress and inadequate recovery in maturing young athletes.

Adiponectin

Apart from the prominent role of leptin, another adipocytokine that has raised considerable interest as a mediator in energy homeostasis is adiponectin.[5,12] Unlike many other adipocytokines, adiponectin is exclusively secreted from adipose tissue, detected in high levels in blood, and involved in metabolism, reproductive function, insulin resistance, and inflammatory processes.[5,12] Circulating adiponectin is influenced by pubertal maturation, although these changes are sex specific.[5,8,74] Adiponectin levels may not change during puberty in girls, while the concentrations decrease during puberty in boys.[8,74] The decreased adiponectin levels in boys may likely reflect a direct inhibitory role of androgens on circulating adiponectin,[8] as adiponectin has negatively been correlated with testosterone in adolescent boys.[74] It appears that pubertal maturation that moderates changes in body composition is also related to adiponectin levels at least in boys.[5]

Well-trained adult athletes present relatively high baseline adiponectin concentrations.[6] However, it has been suggested that sport training increases adiponectin levels only when accompanied by body fat reduction and weight loss.[12] Given the relatively strict diets of elite adolescent athletes in aesthetic sports like rhythmic gymnastics and ice skating, adiponectin might be considered a starvation hormone, signalling low energy availability.[5,12] Roupas *et al.*[75] found that in elite rhythmic gymnasts participating in the World Championships, salivary adiponectin levels were associated with the amount of reported weekly training volume (40.8 $h \cdot week^{-1}$). Furthermore, when young athletes were divided according to the amount of weekly training load, elite rhythmic gymnasts with very heavy training loads (>41 $h \cdot week^{-1}$) showed significantly higher adiponectin levels in comparison with elite rhythmic gymnasts adopting less heavy training loads ($\leq$41 $h \cdot week^{-1}$). However, it was suggested that the association between adiponectin and training volume may reflect the deterioration of energy balance rather than exercise stress, per se, and support the role of adiponectin as a starvation hormone, signalling low energy availability.[75] In contrast, no association of adiponectin levels with reproductive function was documented in elite female rhythmic gymnasts.[75] In addition, higher levels of salivary adiponectin have been found in elite rhythmic gymnasts when compared with age-matched untrained controls.[76]

It has also been indicated that adiponectin levels may not be different between prepubertal and pubertal athletes in comparison with age-matched untrained controls.[5,67] For example, no differences in adiponectin concentrations have been observed between prepubertal and pubertal rhythmic gymnasts with untrained controls,[67,69] and between pubertal swimmers and untrained controls.[77] In another study, circulating adiponectin concentrations were similarly increased and were not different in 8-year-old prepubertal rhythmic gymnasts and age-matched, untrained controls over a 12-month study period.[70] However, in certain circumstances basal adiponectin levels could be higher in growing athletes as a result of heavily increased energy expenditure.[5,65] Adiponectin concentrations were increased in rhythmic gymnasts advancing from prepuberty to midpuberty (from pubertal stage 1 to pubertal stages 2 and 3), while no changes in adiponectin were seen in age-matched, untrained controls in the same time period (Figure 33.1b).[65] It was also found that a bigger increase in adiponectin level was associated with a lower increase in body mass index over the 36-month study period in the rhythmic gymnasts group.[65] These results together suggest that basal adiponectin concentrations could be increased as a result of increased training stress in young athletes after onset of puberty and adiponectin could be used as a marker of energy deprivation in elite female adolescent athletes.[5]

Ghrelin

Ghrelin is another peripheral signal which has been associated with the appetite-regulating responses at the hypothalamic and pituitary levels.[12] Specifically, ghrelin is an endogenous ligand of the GH secretogogue receptor, but its role in body mass regulation is more prominent than its role in GH secretion.[56] Ghrelin promotes positive energy balance by increasing appetite and food intake.[56,60] Ghrelin levels decrease after caloric intake and increase while fasting.[5] Furthermore, it has also been proposed that ghrelin could influence growth and physical development.[78] A negative correlation of circulating ghrelin concentration with age[78] and pubertal development[79] has been found. It has been hypothesized that ghrelin provides a link between energy homeostasis, body composition, and pubertal maturation through action on the hypothalamus,[80] where ghrelin stimulates the secretion of GnRH, which in turn stimulates the pituitary production and secretion of the gonadotropins required for pubertal onset.[8] The initiation of puberty substantially decreases circulating ghrelin concentrations in both sexes,[5,78] and a negative correlation between ghrelin and testosterone has been observed in boys entering puberty.[79] The increase in testosterone concentrations at the beginning of puberty stimulates the GH-IGF-I axis and thus via negative feedback may supress ghrelin secretion.[79] The decrease in ghrelin levels at the onset of puberty is apparent despite the fact that puberty is characterized by increased appetite and food intake,[78] and ghrelin is known to stimulate appetite.[60] Whatmore *et al.*[78] suggested that there could be an increased sensitivity for appetite stimulation by ghrelin throughout puberty to sustain linear growth. Thus, pubertal maturation is associated with ghrelin, concentrations of which decrease with advancing pubertal maturation.[5]

Long-term chronic exercise has been demonstrated to produce increases in circulating ghrelin concentrations in adult athletes,[6] and sport training also increases ghrelin levels in adolescents.[5,61] For example, a cross-sectional study investigated basal ghrelin concentrations in female adolescent swimmers and age-matched, physically inactive controls.[22] Accounting for age, body composition, and pubertal stage, it was found that young athletes have higher ghrelin levels in comparison with inactive controls.[22] In accordance, prepubertal rhythmic gymnasts had higher ghrelin levels when compared with untrained controls.[69] However, basal ghrelin concentrations decreased in both prepubertal rhythmic gymnasts and age-matched, untrained controls over the 12-month study period,[70] demonstrating that increasing age decreases ghrelin levels similarly in both groups despite large differences in daily energy expenditure.[5] Therefore, ghrelin concentrations were significantly higher in rhythmic gymnasts when compared with untrained controls in both measurement times during prepuberty.[70] It could be argued that regular sport training still causes higher ghrelin concentrations to stimulate appetite and food intake to cover higher energy homeostasis in these young athletes.[22] Ghrelin may act as a hormone signalling a need for energy conservation, and ghrelin secretion is triggered to counter a further deficit of energy storage to help to maintain normal body mass in growing athletes.[5,60] However, when rhythmic gymnasts and untrained controls reached puberty (from pubertal stage 1 to mostly pubertal stages 2 and 3), basal ghrelin levels were decreased in both groups and were no longer significantly different between groups with different energy expenditure levels (Figure 33.1c).[65]

In another longitudinal study monitoring male swimmers from prepuberty (pubertal stage 1) to midpuberty (pubertal stages 3 and 4), a significant decrease in circulating ghrelin was also seen after the evolution of puberty.[73] Basal ghrelin levels were not changed in adolescent female swimmers with advancing pubertal maturation over a 24-month period.[68] These results together indicate that ghrelin levels are higher in prepubertal children who participate in sport training in comparison with age-matched, untrained controls. However, ghrelin concentrations decrease after onset of puberty in young athletes even in the presence of chronically elevated energy expenditure.[5] It appears that pubertal maturation reduces basal ghrelin levels in growing athletes of both sexes, despite heavy athletic activity.[5]

In heavily exercising adolescent female athletes, menstrual disturbances have been linked to an energy deficiency, where caloric intake is inadequate for exercise energy expenditure,[81] and higher basal ghrelin levels have been observed in amenorrheic athletes than in normally menstruating exercise trainers.[12,61] There are data to suggest that young female athletes with varying severities of menstrual disturbances can be distinguished from each other based on their circulating ghrelin concentrations.[81–83] Therefore, increased ghrelin levels in young athletes with amenorrhea may have a role in a reproductive system.[5,12] An inverse correlation between acylated ghrelin and gonadal steroids was observed in adolescent athletes,[82] and acylated ghrelin levels may differentiate between adolescent athletes who will or will not develop functional hypothalamic amenorrhea during heavy training.[12,61] Accordingly, it is likely that high ghrelin levels contribute to functional hypothalamic amenorrhea by altering GnRH and luteinizing hormone pulsatility.[12,56,83] It appears that both ghrelin and leptin contribute independently to the variability in luteinizing hormone pulsatility and secretion.[83] In addition, body fat mass is an important negative determinant of basal ghrelin levels in amenorrheic athletes.[82,83] Therefore, an increase in energy intake in amenorrheic athletes induces a decrease in basal ghrelin levels, which is paralleled by increases in body mass and resumption of menses.[12] It appears that circulating ghrelin concentration is a biomarker of energy imbalance across the menstrual cycle in adolescent females.

Conclusions

Since more children worldwide practice sport, more research on the chronic exercise-related modification of the endocrine system appears to be essential in young athletes. The increased participation of growing children in competitive sport at a relatively early age in recent years, especially when associated with inadequate caloric intake, exposes young athletes to several health risks. Further longitudinal studies are warranted of the relationships between specific hormone responses to training stress during the prepubertal years and pubertal maturation in athletes. More specifically, an effort should be made to find objective hormonal parameters to quantify the balance between actual sport training and the tolerance of this specific training load by growing athletes. To date, there is no single hormonal marker that could describe a possible overtraining syndrome in growing and maturing athletes. It should be considered that in those sport disciplines where heavy training with large energy expenditure starts at a relatively young age, and in which a thin body is required, such as in gymnastics, there is a greater risk for developing the female athletic triad during the adolescent period.[5] Therefore, exercise-related reproductive dysfunction may have consequences for growth velocity and peak bone mass acquisition.[84] Recent findings also highlight the endocrine role of adipose tissue and energy balance in the regulation of energy homeostasis and reproductive function in young athletes.[12] Recently, in addition to adipose tissue, the endocrine role of bone tissue in energy homeostasis in rhythmic gymnasts was also demonstrated.[85] Specifically, Jürimäe *et al.*[85] suggested that sclerostin and preadipocyte factor-1 may be involved in energy homeostasis, at least in those prepubertal girls who have experienced significant alterations in daily energy expenditure such as rhythmic gymnasts. The number of peripheral factors revealed to participate in energy homeostasis is continuously increasing and further studies are required to find out which specific hormones can be used to better characterize training stress and maturation in growing athletes. In conclusion, young athletes should be monitored at short intervals to better understand the influence of a high training load on different hormonal markers that are responsible for overall growth and energy homeostasis.

Summary

- Physical performance is associated with anabolic adaptations of the GH-IGF-I system in prepubertal and adolescent athletes even as spontaneous growth proceeds.
- The function of the GH-IGF-I axis may be suppressed in growing athletes during strenuous training periods, which is attributed to a negative energy balance.
- Heavy training appears to have no effect on basal testosterone concentrations or pubertal maturation in male athletes.
- Energy deficiency is the major factor that alters reproductive hormone secretion in adolescent female athletes, rather than exercise stress or an increase in exercise energy expenditure.
- Basal cortisol concentrations are not affected by prolonged sport training during sexual maturation in athletes.
- Basal leptin levels may be reduced and remain unchanged advancing from prepuberty to pubertal maturation in athletes.
- Reduced basal leptin concentrations can be used as a sign of increased training stress in adolescent athletes.
- Basal adiponectin concentrations can be increased as a result of heavy training stress in athletes after onset of puberty, and adiponectin could be used as a marker of energy deprivation in elite female adolescent athletes.
- Basal ghrelin concentrations are elevated in growing athletes, while pubertal onset decreases ghrelin levels even in the presence of chronically elevated energy expenditure in athletes.
- Basal ghrelin levels can be used as an indicator of energy imbalance across the menstrual cycle in adolescent athletes.

References

1. Rubin DA, Tufano JJ, McMurray RG. Endocrine responses to acute and chronic exercise in the developing child. In: Constantini N, Hackney AC (eds.) *Endocrinology of physical activity and sport*. New York: Humana Press; 2013. p. 417–436.
2. Roemmich JN. Growth, maturation and hormonal changes during puberty: influence of sport training. In: Kraemer WJ, Rogol AD (eds.) *The endocrine system in sports and exercise. The encyclopedia of sports medicine*. Oxford: Blackwell; 2005. p. 512–524.
3. Hills AP, Byrne NM. An overview of physical growth and maturation. *Med Sport Sci*. 2010; 55: 1–13.

4. Weise M, Eisenhofer G, Merke DP. Pubertal and gender-related changes in the sympathoadrenal system in healthy children. *J Clin Endocrinol Metab*. 2002; 87: 5038–5043.
5. Jürimäe J. Adipocytokine and ghrelin responses to acute exercise and sport training in children during growth and maturation. *Pediatr Exerc Sci*. 2014; 26: 392–403.
6. Jürimäe J, Mäestu J, Jürimäe T, Mangus B, von Duvillard SP. Peripheral signals of energy homeostasis as possible markers of training stress in athletes: a review. *Metabolism*. 2011; 60: 335–350.
7. Utsal, L, Tillmann V, Zilmer M, *et al*. Elevated serum IL-6, IL-8, MCP-1, CRP, and IFN-γ levels in 10- to 11-year-old boys with increased BMI. *Horm Res Paediatr*. 2012; 78: 31–39.
8. Casazza K, Hanks LJ, Alvarez JA. Role of various cytokines and growth factors in pubertal development. *Med Sport Sci*. 2010; 55: 14–31.
9. Jimenez-Pavon D, Ortega FB, Artero EG, *et al*. Physical activity, fitness, and serum leptin concentrations in adolescents. *J Pediatr*. 2012; 160: 598–603.
10. Utsal L, Tillmann V, Zilmer M, *et al*. Negative correlation between serum IL-6 level and cardiorespiratory fitness in 10- to 11-year-old boys with increased BMI. *J Pediatr Endocrinol Metab*. 2013; 26: 503–508.
11. Eliakim A, Nemet D. Exercise training, physical fitness and the growth hormone-insulin-like growth factor-1 axis and cytokine balance. *Med Sport Sci*. 2010; 55: 128–140.
12. Maimoun L, Georgopoulos NA, Sultan C. Endocrine disorders in adolescent and young female athletes: impact on growth, menstrual cycles, and bone mass acquisition. *J Clin Endocrinol Metab*. 2014; 99: 4037–4050.
13. Di Luigi L, Baldari C, Gallotta MC, *et al*. Salivary steroids at rest and after a training load in young male athletes: relationships with chronological age and pubertal development. *Int J Sports Med*. 2006; 27: 709–717.
14. Eliakim A, Nemet D, Cooper DM. Exercise, training, and the GH-IGF-I axis. In: Kraemer WJ, Rogol AD (eds.) *The endocrine system in sports and exercise. The encyclopedia of sports medicine*. Oxford: Blackwell; 2005. p. 165–179.
15. Nemet D, Conolly PH, Pontello-Pescatello AM, *et al*. Negative energy balance plays a major role in the IGF-I response to exercise training. *J Appl Physiol*. 2004; 96: 276–282.
16. Eliakim A, Nemet D. Interval training and the GH-IGF-I axis—a new look into an old training regimen. *J Pediatr Endocrinol Metab*. 2012; 25: 815–821.
17. Eliakim A, Brasel JA, Mohan S, Barstow TJ, Berman N, Cooper DM. Physical fitness, endurance training, and the growth hormone-insulin-like growth factor-I system in adolescent females. *J Clin Endocrinol Metab*. 1996; 81: 3986–3992.
18. Eliakim A, Scheett TP, Newcomb R, Mohan S, Cooper DM. Fitness, training, and the growth hormone --> insulin-like growth factor I axis in prepubertal girls. *J Clin Endocrinol Metab*. 2001; 86: 2797–2802.
19. Ubertini G, Grossi A, Colobianchi D, *et al*. Young elite athletes of different sport disciplines present with an increase in pulsatile secretion of growth hormone compared with non-elite athletes and sedentary subjects. *J Endocrinol Invest*. 2008; 31: 138–145.
20. Courteix D, Rieth N, Thomas T, *et al*. Preserved bone health in adolescent elite rhythmic gymnasts despite hypoleptinemia. *Horm Res*. 2007; 68: 20–27.
21. Gruodyte R, Jürimäe J, Saar M, Jürimäe T. The relationship among bone health, insulin-like growth factor-1 and sex hormones in adolescent female athletes. *J Bone Miner Metab*. 2010; 28: 306–313.
22. Jürimäe J, Cicchella A, Jürimäe T, *et al*. Regular physical activity influences plasma ghrelin concentrations in adolescent girls. *Med Sci Sports Exerc*. 2007; 39: 1736–1741.
23. Waters DL, Qualls CR, Dorin R, Veldhuis JD, Baumgartner RN. Increased pulsatility, process irregularity, and nocturnal trough concentrations of growth hormone in amenorrheic compared to eumenorrheic athletes. *J Clin Endocrinol Metab*. 2001; 86: 1013–1019.
24. Daly RM, Rich PA, Klein R, Bass S. Effects of high-impact exercise on ultrasonic and biochemical indices of skeletal status: a prospective study in young male gymnasts. *J Bone Miner Res*. 1999; 14: 1222–1230.
25. Maimoun L, Coste O, Galtier F, *et al*. Bone mineral density acquisition in peripubertal female rhythmic gymnasts is directly associated with plasma IGF-1/IGF-binding protein-3 ratio. *Eur J Endocrinol*. 2010; 163: 157–164.
26. Zanker CL, Swaine IL. Bone turnover in amenorrheic and eumenorrheic women distance runners. *Scand J Med Sci Sports*. 1998; 8: 20–26.
27. Maimoun L, Coste O, Philibert P, *et al*. Testosterone secretion in elite adolescent swimmers does not modify bone mass acquisition: a 1-year follow-up study. *Fertil Steril*. 2013; 99: 270–278.
28. Adiyaman P, Ocal G, Berberoglu M, *et al*. Alterations in serum growth hormone (GH)/GH dependent ternary complex components (IGF-I, IGFBP-3, ALS, IGF-I/IGFBP-3 molar ratio) and the influence of these alterations on growth pattern in female rhythmic gymnasts. *J Pediatr Endocrinol Metab*. 2004; 17: 895–903.
29. Roemmich JN, Sinning WE. Weight loss and wrestling training: effects of growth-related hormones. *J Appl Physiol*. 1997; 82: 1760–1764.
30. Roemmich JN, Sinning WE. Sport-seasonal changes in body composition, growth, power and strength of adolescent wrestlers. *Int J Sports Med*. 1996; 17: 92–99.
31. Jahreis G, Kauf E, Fröhner G, Schmidt HE. Influence of intensive exercise on insulin-like growth factor-I, thyroid and steroid hormones in female gymnasts. *Growth Regul*. 1991; 1: 95–99.
32. Scheett TP, Nemet D, Stoppani J, Maresh CM, Newcomb R, Cooper DM. The effect of endurance-type exercise training on growth mediators and inflammatory cytokines in pre-pubertal and early pubertal males. *Pediatr Res*. 2002; 52: 491–497.
33. Malina RM, Baxter-Jones ADG, Armstrong N, *et al*. Role of intensive training in the growth and maturation of artistic gymnasts. *Sports Med*. 2013; 43: 783–802.
34. Mäestu J, Jürimäe J, Jürimäe T. Monitoring of performance and training in rowing. *Sports Med*. 2005; 35: 597–617.
35. Fry AC, Kraemer WJ, Ransany CT. Pituitary-adrenal-gonadal responses to high-intensity resistance exercise overtraining. *J Appl Physiol*. 1998; 85: 2352–2359.
36. Carli G, Martelli G, Viti A, Baldi L, Bonifazi M, Lupo di Prisco C. Modulation of hormone levels in male swimmers during training. In: Hollander AP, Huijing PA, de Groot D (eds.) *Biomechanics and medicine in swimming*. Champaign, IL: Human Kinetics; 1983. p. 33–40.
37. Arruda AF, Aoki MS, Freitas CG, Spigolon LM, Franciscon C, Moreira A. Testosterone concentration and lower limb power over an entire competitive season in elite young soccer players. *J Strength Cond Res*. 2015; 29: 3380–3385.
38. Rowland TW, Morris AH, Kelleher JF, Haag BL, Reiter EO. Serum testosterone response to training in adolescent runners. *Am J Dis Child*. 1987; 141: 881–883.
39. Gurd B, Klentrou P. Physical and pubertal development in young male gymnasts. *J Appl Physiol*. 2003; 95: 1011–1015.
40. Hackney AC. Endurance exercise training and reproductive endocrine dysfunction in men: alterations in the hypothalamic-pituitary-testicular axis. *Curr Pharm Design*. 2001; 7: 261–273.
41. Zinner C, Wahl P, Achtzehn S, Reed JL, Mester J. Acute hormonal responses before and after 2 weeks of HIT in well trained junior triathletes. *Int J Sports Med*. 2014; 35: 316–322.
42. Pomerants T, Tillmann V, Karelson K, Jürimäe J, Jürimäe T. Ghrelin response to acute aerobic exercise in boys at different stages of puberty. *Horm Metab Res*. 2006; 38: 752–757.
43. Moreira A, Mortatti A, Aoki M, Arruda A, Freitas C, Carling C. Role of free testosterone in interpreting physical performance in elite young Brazilian soccer players. *Pediatr Exerc Sci*. 2013; 25: 186–197.
44. Kraemer RR, Acevedo EO, Synovitz LB, Herbert EP, Gimpel T, Castracane VD. Leptin and steroid hormone responses to exercise in adolescent female runners over a 7-week season. *Eur J Appl Physiol*. 2001; 86: 85–91.
45. Cacciari F, Mazzanti L, Tassinari D, *et al*. Effect of sport (football) on growth: auxological, anthropometric and hormonal aspects. *Eur J Appl Physiol*. 1990; 61: 149–158.

46. Daly RM, Rich PA, Klein R, Bass SL. Short stature in competitive prepubertal and early pubertal male gymnasts: the result of selection bias or intense training? *J Pediatr.* 2000; 137: 510–516.
47. Daly RM, Rich PA, Klein R. Hormonal responses to physical training in high-level peripubertal male gymnasts. *Eur J Appl Physiol.* 1998; 79: 74–81.
48. Eliakim A, Beyth Y. Exercise training, menstrual irregularities and bone development in children and adolescents. *J Pediatr Adolesc Gynecol.* 2003; 16: 201–206.
49. Weimann E, Blum WF, Witzel C, Schwidergall S, Böhles HJ. Hypoleptinemia in female and male elite gymnasts. *Eur J Clin Invest.* 1999; 29: 853–860.
50. Loucks AB, Horvath SM. Athletic amenorrhea: a review. *Med Sci Sports Exerc.* 1985; 17: 56–72.
51. Loucks AB, Heath EM. Induction of low T_3 syndrome in exercising women occurs at a threshold of energy availability. *Am J Physiol.* 1994; 266: R817–R823.
52. Constantini NW. Clinical consequences of athletic amenorrhea. *Sports Med.* 1994; 17: 213–223.
53. Caine D, Lewis R, O´Connor P, Howe W, Bass S. Does gymnastics training inhibit growth of females? *Clin J Sports Med.* 2001; 11: 260–270.
54. Theintz GE, Howald H, Weiss U, Sizonenko PC. Evidence for a reduction of growth potential in adolescent female gymnasts. *J Pediatr.* 1993; 122: 306–312.
55. Theintz GE, Howald H, Allemann Y, Sizonenko PC. Growth and pubertal development of young female gymnasts and swimmers: a correlation with parental data. *Int J Sports Med.* 1989; 10: 87–91.
56. Fugua JS, Rogol AD. Neuroendocrine alterations in the exercising human: implications for energy homeostasis. *Metabolism.* 2013; 62: 911–921.
57. De Souza MJ, Maguire MS, Maresh CM, Kraemer WJ, Rubin KR, Loucks AB. Adrenal activation and the prolactin response to exercise in eumenorrheic and amenorrheic runners. *J Appl Physiol.* 1991; 70: 2378–2387.
58. Georgopoulos NA, Rottstein L, Tsekouras A, *et al.* Abolished circadian rhythm of salivary cortisol in elite artistic gymnasts. *Steroids.* 2011; 76: 353–357.
59. King JA, Wasse LK, Stensel DJ. The acute effects of swimming on appetite, food intake, and plasma acylated ghrelin. *J Obes.* 2011; 351628.
60. Jürimäe J, Jürimäe T. Ghrelin responses to acute exercise and training. In: Constantini N, Hackney AC (eds.) *Endocrinology of physical activity and sport.* New York: Humana Press; 2013. p. 207–220.
61. Kraemer RR, Castracane VD. Effect of acute and chronic exercise on ghrelin and adipocytokines during pubertal development. *Med Sport Sci.* 2010; 55: 156–173.
62. Barash JA, Cheung CC, Weigle DS, *et al.* Leptin is a metabolic signal to the reproductive system. *Endocrinology.* 1996; 137: 3144–3147.
63. Clayton PE, Gill MS, Hall CM, Tillmann V, Whatmore AJ, Price DA. Serum leptin through childhood and adolescence. *Clin Endocrinol.* 1997; 46: 727–733.
64. Rogol AD, Roemmich JN, Clark PA. Growth at puberty. *J Adolesc Health.* 2002; 31: 192–200.
65. Võsoberg K, Tillmann V, Tamm AL, *et al.* Adipocytokine and ghrelin levels in relation to body composition in rhythmic gymnasts entering into puberty: a three-year follow-up study. *Pediatr Exerc Sci.* 2014; 26: 477–484.
66. Munoz MT, de la Piedra C, Barrios V, Garrido G, Argente J. Changes in bone density and bone markers in rhythmic gymnasts and ballet dancers: implications for puberty and leptin levels. *Eur J Endocrinol.* 2004; 151: 491–496.
67. Gruodyte R, Jürimäe J, Cicchella A, Stefanelli C, Passariello C, Jürimäe T. Adipocytokines and bone mineral density in adolescent female athletes. *Acta Paediatr.* 2010; 99: 1879–1884.
68. Jürimäe J, Lätt E, Haljaste K, Purge P, Cicchella A, Jürimäe T. A longitudinal assessment of ghrelin and bone mineral density with advancing pubertal maturation in adolescent female athletes. *J Sports Med Phys Fitness.* 2010; 50: 343–349.
69. Parm AL, Jürimäe J, Saar M, *et al.* Plasma adipocytokine and ghrelin levels in relation to bone mineral density in prepubertal rhythmic gymnasts. *J Bone Miner Metab.* 2011; 29: 717–724.
70. Parm AL, Jürimäe J, Saar M, *et al.* Bone mineralization in rhythmic gymnasts before puberty: no longitudinal associations with adipocytokine and ghrelin levels. *Horm Res Paediatr.* 2012; 77: 369–375.
71. Maimoun L, Coste O, Jaussen A, Mariano-Goulart D, Sultan C, Paris F. Bone mass acquisition in female rhythmic gymnasts during puberty: no direct role for leptin. *Clin Endocrinol.* 2010; 72: 604–611.
72. Weimann E. Gender-related differences in elite gymnasts: the female athlete triad. *J Appl Physiol.* 2002; 92: 2146–2152.
73. Jürimäe J, Lätt E, Haljaste K, Purge P, Cicchella A, Jürimäe T. Influence of puberty on ghrelin and BMD in athletes. *Int J Sports Med.* 2009; 30: 403–407.
74. Böttner A, Kratzsch J, Müller G, *et al.* Gender differences of adiponectin levels develop during the progression of puberty and are related to serum androgen levels. *J Clin Endocrinol Metab.* 2004; 89: 4053–4061.
75. Roupas ND, Maimoun L, Mamali I, *et al.* Salivary adiponectin levels are associated with training intensity but not with bone mass or reproductive function in elite rhythmic gymnasts. *Peptides.* 2014; 51: 80–85.
76. Roupas ND, Mamali I, Armeni AK, *et al.* The influence of intensive physical training on salivary adipokine levels in elite rhythmic gymnasts. *Horm Metab Res.* 2012; 44: 980–986.
77. Ageloussi S, Theodorou AA, Paschalis V, *et al.* Adipocytokine levels in children: effects of fatness and training. *Pediatr Exerc Sci.* 2012; 24: 461–471.
78. Whatmore AC, Hall CM, Jones J, Westwood M, Clayton PE. Ghrelin concentrations in healthy children and adolescents. *Clin Endocrinol.* 2003; 59: 649–654.
79. Pomerants T, Tillmann V, Jürimäe J, Jürimäe T. Relationships between ghrelin and anthropometrical, body composition parameters and testosterone levels in boys at different stages of puberty. *J Endocrinol Invest.* 2006; 29: 962–967.
80. Budak E, Fernandez-Sanchez SM, Bellver J, Cervero A, Simon C, Pellicer A. Interactions of the hormones leptin, ghrelin, adiponectin, resistin, and PYY3-36 with the reproductive system. *Fertil Steril.* 2006; 85: 1563–1581.
81. Scheid JL, De Souza MJ. Menstrual irregularities and energy deficiency in physically active women: the role of ghrelin, peptide YY, and adipocytokines. *Med Sport Sci.* 2010; 55: 82–102.
82. Christo K, Cord J, Mendes N, *et al.* Acylated ghrelin and leptin in adolescent athletes with amenorrhea, eumenorrheic athletes and controls: a cross-sectional study. *Clin Endocrinol.* 2008; 69: 628–633.
83. Ackerman KE, Slusarz K, Guereca H, *et al.* Higher ghrelin and lower leptin secretion are associated with lower LH secretion in young amenorrheic athletes compared with eumenorrheic athletes and controls. *Am J Physiol Endocrinol Metab.* 2012; 302: E800–E806.
84. Maimoun L, Coste O, Mura T, *et al.* Specific bone mass acquisition in elite female athletes. *J Clin Endocrinol Metab.* 2013; 98: 2844–2853.
85. Jürimäe J, Tillmann V, Cicchella A, *et al.* Increased sclerostin and preadipocyte factor-1 levels in prepubertal rhythmic gymnasts: associations with bone mineral density, body composition, and adipocytokine values. *Osteoporos Int.* 2016; 27: 1239–1243.

CHAPTER 34

Aerobic trainability

Melitta A McNarry and Neil Armstrong

Introduction

Training occurs in many guises with a variety of intended outcomes, but the underlying concept is of a series of practices where the end result is to render a human or an animal, as quickly and completely as possible, fit for the performance of a given amount of work.[1] Although this definition was published more than 120 years ago, it is essentially unchanged in the current Oxford dictionary. Perhaps more surprising is that the list of unanswered questions regarding the influence of training in paediatric populations remains almost equally unchanged, notwithstanding an increasing body of research on the physiology of training of the adult population. The applicability of such research to paediatric populations is limited, however, as children are not mini-adults, and their responses are not simply scaled-down versions of adult responses.[2] Indeed, there is still debate on the most fundamental questions of whether children are physiologically trainable and, if so, how this trainability manifests itself.[3,4] Furthermore, as the majority of evidence is derived from cross-sectional data, it remains unclear whether training-induced changes in the aerobic fitness of young athletes are attributable to initial selection for sport, (including genetic predisposition), subsequent training programmes, or a combination thereof.[5]

The resolution of such questions is increasingly urgent given the rising levels of engagement of young people in sporting activities,[3,6] with concomitant increases in the duration, frequency, and intensity of the training, all of which are believed to lead to success at ever younger ages. These trends emphasize the importance of examining the interactions between training and physiological adaptations through normal growth and maturation. Understanding these interactions may provide insights into the dose-response relationship, thereby allowing training programmes to be structured and orientated to young athletes. Appropriate tailoring of training programmes to paediatric populations could avoid deleterious effects on long-term health and have significant implications for the motivation and continuing enjoyment of the participants.

Understanding of the development of aerobic fitness during growth and maturation is not only applicable in a sporting context, however, because it has important implications for the design of evidence-based strategies for tackling problems, such as obesity, throughout childhood and adolescence. Intensive training lies on one extreme of the physical activity (PA) spectrum, but a greater understanding of the dose-response relationship between PA and physiological and psychosocial health would be beneficial in improving current guidelines on health-related PA levels.

This chapter examines the influence of training or trained status on young people's responses to exercise. It examines the effects of training and its potential mechanistic basis on the four key parameters of aerobic fitness summarized in Figure 34.1; maximal (or peak) oxygen uptake ($\dot{V}O_2$), the lactate or gas exchange threshold, exercise economy, and the kinetics of pulmonary (p) $\dot{V}O_2$.[7] The controversy regarding the presence or otherwise of a 'maturation threshold', a concept suggesting that a 'trigger point' must be surpassed for training-induced adaptations to be manifest, is also discussed. Finally, it considers potential methodological issues which limit interpretation of the available evidence and identifies directions for future research.

In accord with Chapter 12, which complements the present chapter, the term 'prepubertal children' will be used when prepuberty is confirmed in the research cited; 'children' represents those 12 years and younger but without proof of pubertal status; 'adolescents' refers to 13- to 18 year olds; and 'youth' or 'young people' describes both children and adolescents.

Peak oxygen uptake

Maximal $\dot{V}O_2$ was first reported by Hill and Lupton[8] as the p$\dot{V}O_2$ that cannot be increased during exercise despite further increases in exercise intensity. However, in a single incremental exercise test to volitional exhaustion a plateau in p$\dot{V}O_2$ is only observed in a minority of children and the highest p$\dot{V}O_2$ achieved is referred to as peak $\dot{V}O_2$. This parameter is the most extensively measured variable in paediatric exercise science[9] and is generally considered to be the gold standard measure of youth aerobic fitness.[10,11] However, the measurement and interpretation of peak $\dot{V}O_2$ is problematic, not least being whether the peak $\dot{V}O_2$ achieved in an exercise test is representative of a true maximum effort,[12] as discussed in Chapter 12. A further limitation of peak $\dot{V}O_2$ is its restricted practical applicability, especially within training and performance environments, where it does not represent a strong predictor of future performance[13] and cannot readily be used to set optimal training intensities.[14,15] Thus, while recognizing that peak $\dot{V}O_2$ is an important measure of aerobic fitness, it should not be considered the sole indicator of aerobic fitness, as is frequently the case in paediatric studies. Indeed, such a reliance to date has largely confounded our interpretation of the wider aerobic adaptations associated with exercise training.

Influence of training on peak oxygen uptake

Early studies often concluded that training elicited minimal or no training-induced increases in children's peak $\dot{V}O_2$.[16–19] However, such findings must be interpreted with caution as they may largely be attributable to methodological limitations, such as a lack of commonality between the training and testing modalities, the implementation of low training volume programmes, and/or inconsistent

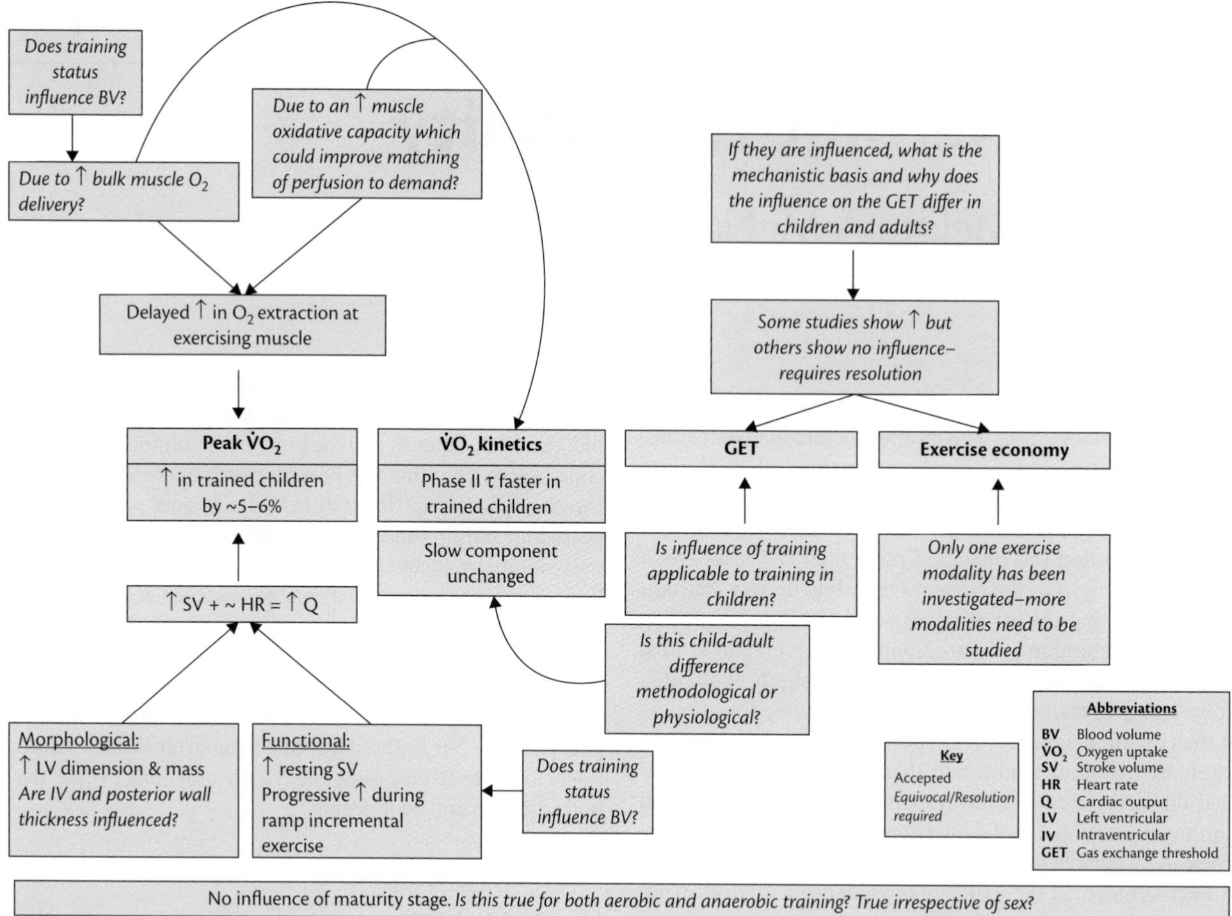

Figure 34.1 Summary of current understanding and controversies regarding the influence of training status on parameters of aerobic fitness.
Generally accepted findings are indicated in black whilet italics illustrate areas of controversy and debate. See text for further details and supporting references.
Reprinted from McNarry M, Jones A. The influence of training status on the aerobic and anaerobic responses to exercise in children: A review. Eur J Sport Sci. 2014; 14: S57–S68, with permission from Taylor and Francis.

data collection time points during longitudinal studies. In contrast, more recent studies report training-induced increases in peak $\dot{V}O_2$ from cross-sectional,[20–22] longitudinal,[16,23,24] and intervention-based studies.[25–29] Despite this growing consensus, the extent of the peak $\dot{V}O_2$ increase with training remains controversial. A meta-analysis suggested an increase of 5 to 6% following aerobic training to be typical in children and adolescents,[30] but there is large inter-participant variation, with studies reporting changes in peak $\dot{V}O_2$ ranging from −10% to + 25%. Much of the variance has been attributed to the pre-training peak $\dot{V}O_2$,[31] but other factors include differences in training volumes (frequency, duration, and, particularly, intensity), adherence to training programmes, the motivation of participants during peak $\dot{V}O_2$ tests, and familiarization with the testing protocol. The principal factor, however, may be the influence of genetics on the ability to respond to training, but data from young people are sparse (see the section on Maturation threshold and Chapter 31).

While the majority of training studies are based on sustained periods of constant intensity exercise training, (CIET) there is a growing body of research suggesting a similar efficacy of high-intensity interval training (HIIT) in eliciting training-induced adaptations.[32] High-intensity interval training consists of repeated bouts of short, high-intensity exercise interspersed by short periods of low-intensity exercise or passive rest. Given the similarity of such bouts of exercise to children's habitual PA patterns,[33] and their preference for, and rapid recovery from, such exercise modalities,[34] the paucity of studies in paediatric populations is surprising. (Children's rapid recovery from high-intensity exercise is discussed in detail in Chapter 9).

The positive influence of HIIT on the peak $\dot{V}O_2$ of prepubertal girls was first reported over 20 years ago,[35] but a concerted research effort has only recently emerged. High-intensity interval training is comprehensively reviewed in Chapter 35 but it is pertinent here to note the findings of a recent meta-analysis which concluded that HIIT is effective in increasing peak $\dot{V}O_2$ in pubertal youth.[36] Although there is currently insufficient evidence to draw such conclusions in prepubertal children, HIIT presents a promising alternative to traditional training methods for 'time poor' children and adolescents.[36]

Mechanistic bases of training adaptations on peak oxygen uptake

The higher peak $\dot{V}O_2$ demonstrated in trained children is generally accepted to be associated with an enhanced stroke volume (SV) and consequently increased cardiac output ($\dot{Q}$), as maximal heart rate (HR max) is unaffected by training.[20,21,37] Less clear, however, is the cause of this enhanced SV, and Figure 34.1 shows suggested morphological and/or functional adaptations of the myocardium which may be related.

Increased left ventricular dimension and mass are the most widely reported morphological adaptations in children.[21,38] Though an increased intraventricular and posterior wall thickness has also been suggested,[39] it remains controversial,[21,38,40] perhaps because there is an age-related progression in morphological training adaptations.[41] All of these morphological adaptations occur in adults following training.[41,42] A progression in children could be associated with the changes in testosterone levels which occur during puberty,[42,43] or represent an overload limitation due either to the inherently lower blood pressures in children during exercise[44] or to the shorter history of training in children.[38]

Functional adaptations have also been suggested by studies reporting an enhanced SV at rest[21,42,44] and an altered SV response pattern during exercise in trained, compared to untrained, children.[19,46] As illustrated in Figure 34.2, in contrast to the conventional plateau in SV at ~40–50% of peak $\dot{V}O_2$, SV increases progressively until exhaustion in trained children.[19,44,45] A similar progressive increase throughout incremental exercise has been suggested to be related to enhanced diastolic filling in trained adults,[45] but the applicability of this explanation to younger populations remains to be established. Specifically, in adults an enhanced diastolic filling is postulated to be related, at least in part, to a training-induced increase in blood volume.[47,48] There are no secure data on the influence of training on blood volume in children, probably because direct measurements are largely precluded by ethical constraints. However, limited indirect evidence derived from Doppler echocardiography supports earlier invasive studies in suggesting a potential influence of training on blood volume in children.[41,49–51]

In accord with the Fick equation, the training-induced increase in peak $\dot{V}O_2$ may alternatively, or additionally, be associated with an enhanced arteriovenous oxygen difference (a-vO_2 diff). The a-vO_2 diff is the amount of oxygen extracted from the arterial

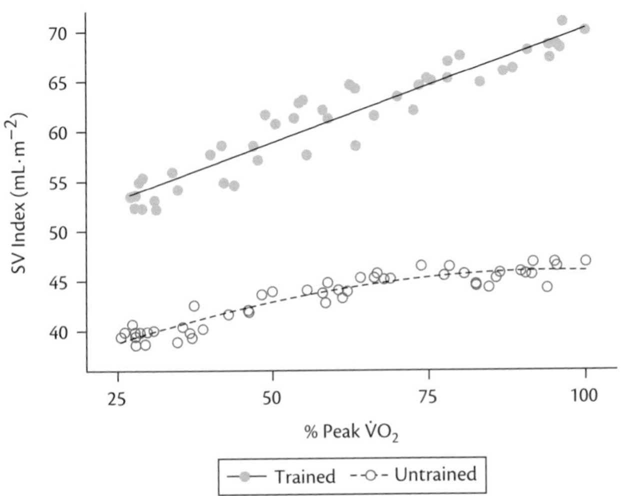

Figure 34.2 The stroke volume response pattern during incremental cycle ergometry.
Figure illustrates data from a representative trained and untrained girl.
Reproduced from McNarry MA, Welsman JR, Jones AM. Influence of training and maturity status on the cardiopulmonary responses to ramp incremental cycle and upper body exercise in girls. J Appl Physiol. 2011; 110: 375–381 with permission from The American Physiological Society.

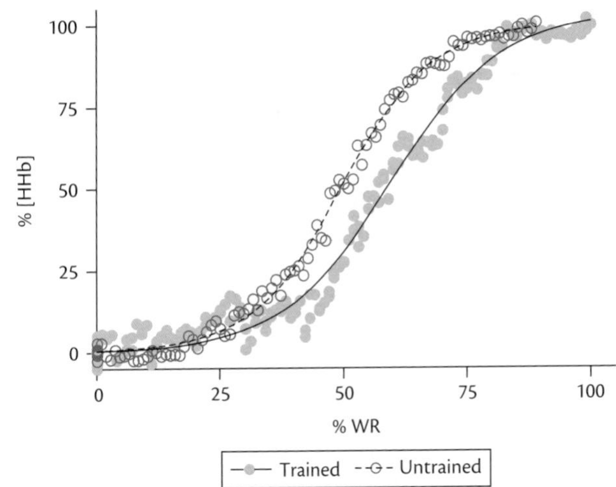

Figure 34.3 Deoxyhaemoglobin and myoglobin response as a function of relative work rate during incremental cycle ergometry.
[HHb] is deoxyhaemoglobin and myoglobin; WR is work rate. Figure illustrates data from a representative trained and untrained girl.
Reproduced from McNarry MA, Welsman JR, Jones AM. Influence of training and maturity status on the cardiopulmonary responses to ramp incremental cycle and upper body exercise in girls. J Appl Physiol. 2011; 110: 375–381 with permission from The American Physiological Society.

blood (i.e. fractional oxygen extraction), and reflects the balance between oxygen delivery and utilization. While assessment of the a-vO_2 diff was conventionally confounded by the necessity to calculate this parameter from the rearrangement of the Fick equation, technological advances now enable fractional oxygen extraction to be estimated using near-infrared spectroscopy (NIRS) to measure the concentrations of deoxygenated haemoglobin and myoglobin ([HHb]).[46–48]

The a-vO_2 diff does not appear to be influenced by training in children, either at rest or at maximal-exercise intensity.[41,43,48] However, there are suggestions that training status may influence the response pattern during incremental exercise, with a significant rightward shift in the sigmoidal oxygen extraction curve relative to % peak power in trained children.[20] The physiological basis for this rightward shift, shown in Figure 34.3, remains to be elucidated, but an elevated bulk muscle oxygen delivery and/or closer matching of local perfusion to metabolic rate within the muscle in trained children may delay the drive for increased oxygen extraction. Improved matching of perfusion to metabolic rate may be associated with the increased muscle oxidative capacity, which has been reported in trained children.[49,50]

Lactate and gas exchange thresholds

The lactate threshold (T_{LAC}), determined during an incremental exercise test, refers to the rate at which the blood lactate accumulation first begins to increase above baseline values. The concomitant bicarbonate buffering of lactic acidosis allows this threshold to be estimated non-invasively through respiratory gas analysis from the disproportionate increase in carbon dioxide output relative to $\dot{V}O_2$, known as the gas exchange threshold (GET) or ventilatory threshold (T_{VENT}). The GET typically occurs in between 45% and 70% of peak $\dot{V}O_2$ in children.[49,50] It has been suggested that the T_{LAC}/GET represents the optimal training intensity for improvements in aerobic fitness in adults,[51,52] providing a high-quality aerobic training stimulus without an accumulation of lactate that may compromise training duration.[53,54] However, a meta-analysis reported that training interventions with children must involve an exercise intensity >80% of peak HR for an influence of training on peak $\dot{V}O_2$ to be manifest,[30] a conclusion supported by a more recent systematic review.[55] As this intensity is significantly above the GET/T_{LAC}, the importance of these thresholds in setting training intensity probably lies in enhancing the ability to sustain submaximal exercise rather than increase peak $\dot{V}O_2$.[26,35]

Influence of training on lactate and gas exchange thresholds

Young athletes involved in aerobic sports generally accumulate less blood lactate than their untrained peers at the same submaximal exercise intensity.[55] Endurance training moves the blood lactate accumulation versus treadmill speed curve to the right and the T_{LAC} has been reported to occur at a higher percentage of peak $\dot{V}O_2$ following training,[2] as described in Chapter 39 (see Figure 39.3). The T_{LAC} therefore has the potential to provide a means of demonstrating improvements in muscle oxidative capacity with endurance training, often in the absence of changes in peak $\dot{V}O_2$. However, data from young people are sparse. Similarly, in adults, training has been observed to elicit a dissociation between the T_{LAC} and the GET/T_{VENT};[56] whether the same is true in children is presently unknown, not least due to a lack of research regarding the influence of training on the T_{LAC} during growth and maturation.

The present discussion focuses on the influence of training on the GET/T_{VENT} in children and adolescents, which remains largely unresolved with results seemingly dependent on the method of expressing the GET/T_{VENT}. Specifically, there is a significant increase in the treadmill speed at which the threshold occurs following training.[54,55] However, when considered relative to peak $\dot{V}O_2$, most,[20,57–61] but not all,[26,59–62] studies have failed to find a significant influence of training. The conflicting results are likely attributable to a number of experimental limitations, including small sample sizes, varied training programmes, and a failure to account and control for pubertal status. However, these limitations may also arise from differences in the assumptions used in data analysis. For example, Paterson and colleagues,[62] conducted a 5-year longitudinal study and reported the T_{VENT} as a fraction of peak $\dot{V}O_2$ to increase in a cohort of boys from 11–15 years. They attributed this increase to training, but as no control group was studied the influence of growth and maturation cannot be accounted for. Furthermore, these conclusions are based on evidence suggesting T_{VENT} as a fraction of peak $\dot{V}O_2$ decreases with age,[63–65] which is refuted by more recent studies.[66–68] In the debate surrounding the potential efficacy of HIIT at eliciting training-induced adaptations in the GET, it is pertinent to note the findings of McManus *et al.*,[27] who reported that only HIIT, and not CIET, significantly influence the GET. Interestingly, despite these conflicting data, the GET/T_{LAC} still appears to be a strong predictor of children's aerobic performance.[69–71]

Mechanistic bases of training adaptations on lactate and gas exchange thresholds

While the occurrence of the GET/T_{LAC} at a higher exercise intensity post-training is a clear indicator of an enhanced endurance capacity,[72] its mechanistic bases remain to be elucidated. Specifically, the limited evidence available, principally drawn from adult studies, suggests that a positive change in the GET/T_{LAC} may be related to a decreased rate of muscle lactate production.[73] Lactate production may be reduced because of a lower rate of muscle glycogen utilization[73–76] or due to faster $p\dot{V}O_2$ kinetics, which would reduce the initial reliance on non-oxidative glycogen utilization. Alternatively, the shift in the GET/T_{LAC} may reflect a training-induced improvement in the ability to eliminate lactate from the blood[77–80] by an increased uptake and oxidization of lactate in the liver and muscles[81], enabled by the increased oxidative enzyme capacity of trained participants[82]. The applicability of such findings to children and adolescents remains to be determined.

Exercise economy

Exercise economy can be defined as the steady-state $p\dot{V}O_2$ required at a given absolute exercise intensity, and therefore describes the relationship between oxygen consumption and, for example, running, cycling, or swimming speed or exercise intensity. An enhanced exercise economy (i.e. a lower $p\dot{V}O_2$ for a given absolute running speed or exercise intensity) is advantageous because it enables the energy demands of a given exercise intensity to be met by a lower % of peak $\dot{V}O_2$, thereby delaying the onset of fatigue and increasing exercise tolerance. Despite the relevance of such concepts to training and performance, little research has been conducted concerning the influence of training on the exercise economy of children and adolescents. Some evidence suggests that training does not significantly affect exercise economy, even when peak $\dot{V}O_2$ is increased,[26,83–86] although improvements in running economy and performance with no concomitant change in peak $\dot{V}O_2$ have also been reported.[83,87] It is difficult to draw more definite conclusions because of methodological limitations, such as the almost exclusive focus on a single exercise modality (running), the use of a potentially insufficient training duration, and the variety of speeds used for the determination of exercise economy. A further limitation of exercise economy as an indicator of aerobic fitness is that at exercise intensities above the GET/T_{VENT} the slow component of $p\dot{V}O_2$ confounds its determination.

Pulmonary oxygen uptake kinetics

Pulmonary $\dot{V}O_2$ kinetics describe the time-course of increase in $p\dot{V}O_2$ towards a new steady-state following a sudden increase in metabolic demand, and provide a useful assessment of the integrated capacity of an organism to transport and utilize oxygen to support the increased rate of energy turnover in the contracting myocytes.[88]

Below the GET, the $p\dot{V}O_2$ response is characterized by three phases: an initial cardiodynamic phase (phase I) which reflects the rapid elevation in $\dot{Q}$ and pulmonary blood flow, a second phase (phase II) during which $p\dot{V}O_2$ increases exponentially, reflecting the increasing muscle $\dot{V}O_2$,[89,90] and a final steady-state phase (phase III) which is typically achieved after ~2 min of constant-intensity exercise.[76,77] Above the GET the attainment of a steady-state is delayed, or even precluded, by the presence of a supplementary slow component of $p\dot{V}O_2$.[91–93] Early studies questioned the presence of a slow component in the response to heavy-intensity exercise in children,[94,95] but the general consensus from more recent studies is that it is present, albeit of a reduced magnitude compared to that in adults.[58,59,96–98] Pulmonary $\dot{V}O_2$ kinetics is discussed in more detail in Chapter 12 and Chapter 13.

Influence of training on pulmonary oxygen uptake kinetics

In contrast to the evidence in adults demonstrating that training represents a potent stimulus to the dynamic $p\dot{V}O_2$ response, the first studies of prepubertal children indicated that the trained state was not associated with either a reduced phase II time constant (τ)[96,99] or a reduced amplitude of the $p\dot{V}O_2$ slow component.[96] However, these conclusions may be a consequence of methodological limitations, such as the use of only a single exercise transition to characterize $p\dot{V}O_2$ kinetics, the prescription of exercise intensity as a fraction of the peak $\dot{V}O_2$, the use of mixed sex cohorts, and/or a lack of commonality between the training and testing modalities.[96,99] More recent studies that have avoided these pitfalls have reported a significant influence of trained status on $p\dot{V}O_2$ kinetics in both prepubertal[58,100] and pubertal athletes,[22,57,59] although these differences were restricted to a faster phase II τ. It is also pertinent to note the importance of exercise modality in revealing trained status-related differences in prepubertal children; significant influences of trained status were only evident during upper body ergometry in trained prepubertal swimmers,[58] a sport which predominately engages the upper body.[101] Figure 34.4 illustrates the influence of trained status and the importance of exercise modality on $p\dot{V}O_2$ kinetics.

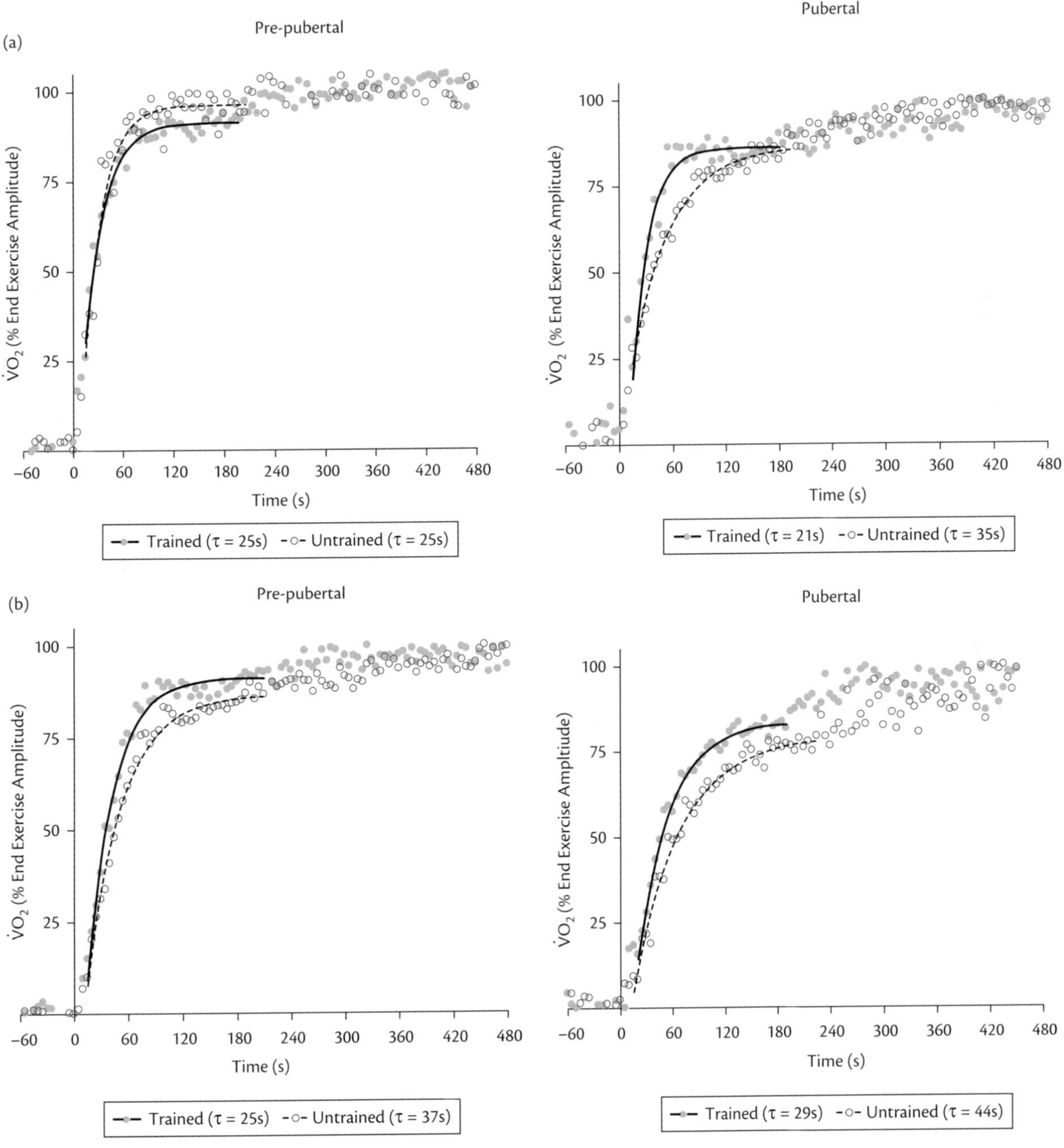

Figure 34.4 Pulmonary oxygen uptake response to a step increment in exercise intensity from an unloaded baseline to heavy intensity exercise.

Figures illustrate data from a representative trained and untrained girl during (a) cycle and (b) upper body exercise. In each case the increment in exercise intensity at the onset of exercise is to 40% of the difference between the gas exchange threshold and peak oxygen uptake.

Reproduced from Winlove MA, Jones AM, Welsman J. Influence of training status and exercise modality on pulmonary O_2 uptake kinetics in pre-pubertal girls. Eur J Appl Physiol. 2010; 108: 1169–1179 and McNarry MA, Welsman JR, Jones AM. Influence of training status and exercise modality on pulmonary O_2 uptake kinetics in pubertal girls. Eur J Appl Physiol. 2010; 111: 621–631 with permission from Springer.

Interestingly, a recent study investigating the influence of a short-term, high-intensity intervention in obese children has highlighted the potential utility of p$\dot{V}O_2$ kinetics, relative to traditional peak $\dot{V}O_2$ measures, in identifying the physiological impact of training. Specifically, while the peak $\dot{V}O_2$ of obese children was not influenced, the dynamic p$\dot{V}O_2$ response to heavy intensity exercise was 20% faster following just 6 weeks of training.[100] These findings are therefore in accord with studies in adults demonstrating the dynamic p$\dot{V}O_2$ response to be similarly influenced by HIIT and CIET modalities.[102]

Although research on young people's dynamic p$\dot{V}O_2$ response at the onset of exercise is sparse, p$\dot{V}O_2$ recovery kinetics, which closely reflect muscle phosphocreatine (PCr) kinetics,[103,104] have received even less attention. This is surprising because incomplete PCr recovery would be anticipated to have deleterious consequences for subsequent exercise performance.[105,106] Only 2 studies to date have sought to investigate the influence of training on the recovery p$\dot{V}O_2$ kinetics during youth, and have reported largely contradictory findings. McNarry *et al.*[107] found training to be associated with a significantly faster p$\dot{V}O_2$ phase II τ in both prepubertal and pubertal swimmers, but Marwood *et al.*[108] observed no influence of training on the responses of pubertal soccer players. This discrepancy may be related to the sex of the participants as sex influences the p$\dot{V}O_2$ on-kinetics of prepubertal children,[109] although the applicability of such findings either to adolescents, or to the recovery response, remains to be established. Alternatively, these discrepancies may be related to differences in the volume of training undertaken, disparities between training and testing modalities, or to the intensity of exercise utilized to investigate the p$\dot{V}O_2$ recovery responses. Further research is urgently required.

Mechanistic bases of training adaptations on pulmonary oxygen uptake kinetics

The mechanistic basis for training adaptations in the p$\dot{V}O_2$ kinetic response remains a contentious issue in both children and adults, and both muscle oxygen delivery and oxygen utilization have been postulated as rate-limiting determinants.[110] Ethical constraints have limited the measurement of the potential mediators in children, but technological advances, such as NIRS, are facilitating the non-invasive investigation of the determinants of p$\dot{V}O_2$ kinetics during childhood and adolescence.

Nevertheless, little information is presently available regarding the mechanistic basis of the faster p$\dot{V}O_2$ kinetics in trained children and adolescents, and a lack of standardization in the interpretation of changes in the [HHb] response further obfuscates the issue. Marwood *et al.*[57] found the [HHb] response to be unchanged in trained adolescents during moderate-intensity exercise, whereas McNarry *et al.*[59] observed trained adolescent swimmers to demonstrate significantly faster [HHb] kinetics during heavy-intensity exercise. Differences in trained status, exercise intensity, and sex may explain these discrepancies, but both studies were taken to indicate that training elicited central (bulk oxygen delivery) and peripheral (enhanced oxygen utilization) adaptations. Similar findings in trained adults[102] have been attributed to an enhanced muscle oxidative capacity consequent to an increased mitochondrial volume and oxidative enzyme activity.[111,112] Although a similarly increased muscle oxidative capacity has been reported in trained children,[113,114] there are insufficient data available on the effects of training on muscle fibre type and oxidative capacities in children and adolescents to establish the mechanisms responsible for the enhanced oxygen extraction kinetics. Several studies agree that training is associated with faster HR kinetics in pubertal children: if HR kinetics is accepted to reflect muscle blood flow kinetics then there may also be enhanced oxygen delivery to the muscle, in accord with studies in adults reporting faster conduit artery flow and vascular conductance following training.[115,116] However, it is important to note that increased bulk oxygen delivery in the trained state does not necessarily imply that oxygen availability was limiting in the untrained state. When considering the potential mechanistic basis for training-induced adaptations in the dynamic p$\dot{V}O_2$ response, it is interesting to note the dissociation between the phase II τ and peak $\dot{V}O_2$ in both children[58,109] and adults,[117] suggesting different mechanisms may be responsible for these adaptations. However, further conclusions regarding these discrepancies are presently precluded.

Therefore, while current evidence does not permit the complete elucidation of the factors limiting p$\dot{V}O_2$ kinetics in adolescents, the faster p$\dot{V}O_2$ kinetics following training are likely to be a function of both a faster oxygen delivery and greater oxygen extraction, as similarly concluded in adults.[110,118,119] With regards to this conclusion, it is pertinent to note the absence of comparable data in prepubertal children; although Winlove *et al.*[58] reported no influence of training on the dynamic HR response, no data are presently available regarding the influence of training on the [HHb] response in prepubertal children.

Parameters of aerobic fitness and sport performance

The relevance of various parameters of aerobic fitness to sporting performance remains unclear, especially within young populations. Indeed, the sparse data available are equivocal, although this could largely be a reflection of the sport-specific nature of performance prediction. For example, while improvements in running economy and performance have been reported in concert with no changes in peak $\dot{V}O_2$,[83,87] others have reported peak $\dot{V}O_2$ to be the principal physiological determinant of performance in children and adolescents.[120,121] Although there is currently no information regarding the relevance of training-induced enhancements in the dynamic p$\dot{V}O_2$ response of children and adolescents, evidence from adult studies indicates that performance improvements may not be related to faster p$\dot{V}O_2$ kinetics and/or a reduced slow component amplitude.[122–125] However, such findings should be interpreted in the context that faster p$\dot{V}O_2$ kinetics may nonetheless be important due to their role in reducing the oxygen deficit, which has been correlated with increased time to exhaustion in some,[125] but not all studies.[123] Further work is required to determine the applicability of such conclusions to young people.

Maturation threshold

The weight of current evidence indicates that children are trainable, with significant changes being manifest in the majority of parameters of aerobic fitness. The only studies that have directly compared the trainability of children and adults found comparable increases in peak $\dot{V}O_2$ irrespective of age.[126,127] Generally, however, the changes in children and adolescents are considerably smaller in magnitude than those in adults: following an 8- to 12-week training

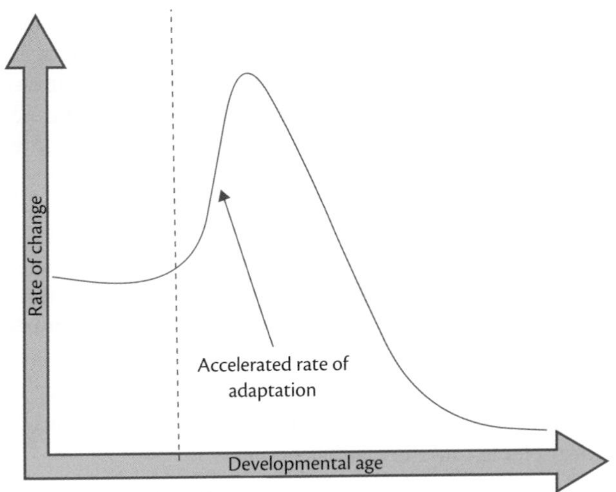

Figure 34.5 Schematic of the accelerated rate of change in aerobic performance parameters often suggested to be associated with puberty and referred to as 'windows of trainability'.
Dashed line indicates the onset of puberty.
Source data from McNarry MA, Barker A, Lloyd R, Buchheit M, Williams CA, Oliver J. The BASES expert statement on trainability during childhood and adolescence. The Sport and Exercise Scientist. 2014; 41: 22–23.

programme children typically demonstrate an 8–9% improvement in peak $\dot{V}O_2$,[30] compared to ~15–30% in adults.[128] Conventionally, this reduced magnitude has been attributed to the higher baseline fitness levels and/or higher habitual PA levels in children which limit the potential for improvements. There is certainly evidence of an inverse relationship between baseline fitness and training-induced adaptations,[29,30,106–108] but this relationship may explain less than 10% of the variation in peak $\dot{V}O_2$.[129]

In their narrative review, Pate and Ward[130] concluded that habitual PA levels may play an important role in aerobic fitness. However, although Rowland and Boyajian[131] provided support for this hypothesis by demonstrating an inverse relationship between habitual PA and the training-induced increase in peak $\dot{V}O_2$, this postulate has largely been discounted by more recent studies.[129,132] Indeed, such a notion appears untenable as data demonstrate that children rarely experience the volume or intensity of PA required to enhance peak $\dot{V}O_2$[133] and that their habitual PA is not related to peak $\dot{V}O_2$.[5,134] An alternative hypothesis to explain the child-adult disparity is that there is an optimal chronological age or maturation stage at which training will be most effective, or that there is a trigger point during maturation that must be surpassed for training-related adaptations to be realized.[40,112] This threshold, illustrated in Figure 34.5, was originally suggested to be related to the hormonal milieu, particularly the hormones that initiate puberty. Several subsequent studies purported to support the notion of a maturation threshold.[16,113–116]

In an early longitudinal study Kobayashi *et al.*[16] determined the peak $\dot{V}O_2$ of 7 boys annually from 9.7–15.8 years old, reporting that increases in peak $\dot{V}O_2$ were only significantly greater than those attributable to growth and maturation alone in the year before peak height velocity (PHV). However, interpretation of these findings is limited by the lack of a control group prior to PHV and failure to report the intensity of training undertaken. Indeed, the findings of several early studies may be a reflection of an inadequate training programme (insufficient duration, frequency, and intensity), a conclusion supported by numerous studies showing similar influences of training irrespective of stage of maturation.[20,24,83,126] Perhaps the strongest demonstrations of the absence of a maturation threshold are a recent longitudinal study which found no interaction between the influence of training and maturation stage,[24] and two studies investigating the influence of training on monozygotic twins.[61,135] Weber *et al.*[135] reported that 10 weeks of endurance training elicited significant increases in the peak $\dot{V}O_2$ of pre- and postpubertal, but not pubertal, twins, while Danis *et al.*[61] reported significant increases in the peak $\dot{V}O_2$ of prepubertal but not pubertal twins. Further evidence against a maturation threshold is provided by the results of a recent systematic review of the literature which found similar magnitude of increases in peak $\dot{V}O_2$ in both prepubertal (7.7%) and pubertal (8.6%) children.[55]

Despite this negative evidence, the concept of a maturation threshold or window of opportunity has been widely adopted. It is integral to various models of long-term athletic development and there is a widespread belief that training does not have significant effects on aerobic fitness before puberty. It is important to highlight, however, that it remains to be rigorously demonstrated that intensive training prior to puberty is associated with any greater benefit during adulthood than commencing intensive training at a later stage of maturation. Furthermore, potential benefit must be balanced against the increased chances of burnout or injury which are widely associated with intensive training at a young age.[136–140] (See Chapter 38 for a discussion of the overtraining syndrome).

Methodological issues

At several points in this chapter we have drawn attention to the methodological limitations of particular studies. This is such a common failing in this field that it justifies reiteration. Perhaps the most prominent limitation is the utilization of cross-sectional research designs which preclude the attribution of effects to training per se, as they may be a reflection of a participant's genetic phenotype which has been estimated to account for ~50–70% of the inter-individual variation in, for example, peak $\dot{V}O_2$.[61] (Interested readers are referred to Chapter 31 for further discussion of the genetic aspects of trainability). Nonetheless, cross-sectional designs do provide certain intrinsic advantages, such as the ability to study the influence of long-term, intensive training, and their results should by no means be discounted. Further confounding factors in the literature are the variety of training programmes implemented, which frequently involve insufficient training frequency, duration, and/or intensity to provide valid conclusions regarding trainability. Furthermore, few studies report adherence or attendance rates, although this information is vital to the evaluation of the efficacy of training interventions.

The demanding nature of training studies and of the assessment of parameters of aerobic fitness often engenders a self-selection bias within sample populations, thus limiting the generalizability of findings. This limitation is further compounded in studies employing only small numbers of participants (often only boys) and which frequently lack a control group with which to account for the concomitant influences of growth and maturation. Indeed, despite the widely debated modulatory role of maturation in determining the potential influence of training, few studies assess maturity, relying on chronological age to delineate participant groups and failing to assess the influence of training across the stages of maturation. Furthermore, the literature has a substantial male bias. Consequently, important questions regarding the potential sex-specificity of a maturation threshold, as might be expected given the considerably greater influence of androgens on performance parameters of adolescent boys, remain to be resolved. The resolution of such methodological issues should allow us to investigate whether the effect of maturation is associated with a discrete threshold, per se, or is perhaps a more refined continuum of effects.

Finally, a limitation inherent to the investigation of paediatric physiology with its attendant ethical issues is the reliance on non-invasive, and consequently indirect, methodologies. Techniques such as magnetic resonance imaging and spectroscopy have not been widely used, and these and other technological advances offer the prospect of more comprehensive measurements which may resolve many pertinent questions in paediatric physiology. In the meantime, we are heavily reliant on the results from a few early studies which used highly invasive methodologies.

Conclusions

This chapter reviews the evidence and concludes that children do not lack trainability, and significant influences of training status are evident across parameters of aerobic fitness reflecting both central and peripheral adaptations, as summarized in Figure 34.1. Most significantly, training increases peak $\dot{V}O_2$, associated with an enhanced SV and $\dot{Q}$; p$\dot{V}O_2$ kinetics is faster in trained children; and both SV and [HHb] response patterns are advantageously influenced by training. Further research is urgently required, but, at present, the weight of evidence strongly suggests that the effects of training on aerobic fitness are not reliant on a maturation threshold and are modulated by training volume and the commonality between training and testing modalities.

Many questions remain to be resolved regarding the influence of training on young people's responses to exercise and the mechanistic bases underpinning training adaptations. These include the mechanistic bases for the influence of training on the SV and [HHb] responses to incremental ramp exercise, as well as many aspects of the p$\dot{V}O_2$ kinetics responses, such as the faster phase II τ with training, the reduced slow component magnitude compared to adults, and the apparent lack of training influence on this parameter. When considering these mechanistic bases, it is pertinent to note the role of genetic predisposition in determining the magnitude of training-induced adaptations, resulting in a spectrum of non-to-high responders, as discussed in Chapter 31.

A number of applied questions also remain. Establishing whether training-induced enhancements during prepuberty predispose individuals to greater training benefits during adulthood will have considerable impact within sport performance environments. However, given the current trend for low PA levels[141] and increasing obesity, the development of our understanding of the dose-response relationship between exercise training and physiological adaptations across stages of maturation is perhaps more important. A central tenet to such an understanding is establishing which parameters of aerobic fitness provide the greatest predictive or prognostic value; peak $\dot{V}O_2$ may be the most researched parameter, but this should not be misconstrued as it being the most informative. It may be argued that the notion of a single gold standard predictor is simplistic and we should rather be seeking to consider all parameters of aerobic fitness, a conclusion supported by the present authors.

Gaps in our knowledge of aerobic fitness and its trainability need to be clearly identified in the context of the continuum from sickness to elite performance. Recently developed non-invasive techniques and technologies need to be harnessed and utilized to provide new insights into optimum aerobic training programmes for young people.[142]

Summary

- Despite early studies suggesting that children were not aerobically trainable, more recent studies demonstrate significant training-induced adaptations in aerobic fitness.
- Irrespective of stage of maturation, training-induced increases in peak $\dot{V}O_2$ are evident and have been attributed to an enhanced stroke volume, and thus cardiac output.
- A training-induced enhancement in stroke volume is suggested to be related to both functional and morphological myocardial adaptations.
- Increased peripheral oxygen utilization may contribute to the higher peak $\dot{V}O_2$ in trained children and adolescents.
- Trained children demonstrate faster p$\dot{V}O_2$ kinetics due to both central (enhanced bulk oxygen delivery) and peripheral (improved matching of perfusion to demand/increased oxidative capacity) adaptations.
- Training has not been demonstrated to influence the magnitude of the p$\dot{V}O_2$ slow component in children or adolescents.
- Trained children demonstrate a lactate threshold and, possibly, a gas exchange threshold which occurs at higher exercise intensity than in their untrained peers, although the underpinning mechanistic bases remain to be elucidated.
- The influence of training on exercise economy is presently unclear, with only limited information focusing primarily on running economy available.
- The majority of evidence refutes the notion of a maturation threshold, suggesting that children are trainable irrespective of stage of maturity.
- There is currently a lack of appropriate prospective data to fully elucidate the interaction between maturity and training on the parameters of aerobic fitness.
- Longitudinal studies across defined stages of maturity with sufficient power and an appropriate control group are required to further elucidate the influence of training on measures of aerobic fitness throughout childhood and adolescence.

References

1. Lagrange F. Training. *In: Physiology of bodily exercise*. London: Kegan Paul, Trench & Co; 1889. p. 210–223.
2. Armstrong N, Welsman J. *Young people and physical activity*. Oxford: Oxford University Press; 2002.
3. Baxter-Jones ADG, Mundt C. The young athlete. In: Armstrong N (ed.) *Pediatric exercise physiology*. Philadelphia: Churchill Livingstone Elsevier; 2007. p. 299–324.
4. Tolfrey K. Responses to training. In: Armstrong N (ed.) *Paediatric exercise physiology*. Philadelphia: Churchill Livingstone Elsevier; 2007. p. 213–234.

5. Armstrong N, Tomkinson G, Ekelund U. Aerobic fitness and its relationship to sport, exercise training and habitual physical activity during youth. *Br J Sports Med.* 2011; 45: 849–858.
6. American Academy of Pediatrics Committee on Sports Medicine and Fitness. Intensive training and sports specialization in young athletes. *Pediatrics.* 2000; 106: 154–157.
7. Whipp BJ, Davis JA, Torres F, Wasserman K. A test to determine parameters of aerobic function during exercise. *J Appl Physiol.* 1981; 50: 217–221.
8. Hill AV, Lupton H. Muscular exercise, lactic acid, and the supply and utilization of oxygen. *QJMed.* 1923; 16: 135–171.
9. Armstrong N, Welsman JR. Development of aerobic fitness during childhood and adolescence. Pediatr Exerc Sci. 2000; 12: 128–149.
10. Rowland TW. *Exercise and children's health.* Champaign, IL: Human Kinetics; 1990.
11. Tomkinson GR, Olds TS. Field tests of fitness. In: Armstrong N, van Mechelen W (eds.) *Paediatric exercise science and medicine*, 2nd ed. Oxford: Oxford University Press; 2008. p. 109–128.
12. Barker AR, Williams CA, Jones AM, Armstrong N. Establishing maximal oxygen uptake in young people during a ramp cycle test to exhaustion. *Br J Sports Med.* 2009; 45: 498–503.
13. Matos N, Winsley RJ. Trainability of young athletes and overtraining. *J Sport Sci Med.* 2007; 6: 353–367.
14. Bosch AN. Exercise science and coaching: Correcting common misunderstandings. *Sports Sci and Coach.* 2006; 1: 77–87.
15. Jones AM. The physiology of the world record holder for the women's marathon. *Int J Sports Sci Coach.* 2006; 1: 101–116.
16. Kobayashi K, Kitamura K, Miura M, Sodeyama H, Miyashita M, Matsui H. Aerobic power as related to body growth in Japanese boys: a longitudinal study. *J Appl Physiol.* 1978; 44: 666–672.
17. Mirwald RL, Bailey DA, Cameron N, Rasmussen RL. Longitudinal comparison of aerobic power in active and inactive boys aged 7.0 to 17.0 years. *Ann Hum Biol.* 1981; 8: 405–414.
18. Welsman J, Armstrong N, Withers S. Responses of young girls to two modes of aerobic training. *Br J Sports Med.* 1997; 31: 139–142.
19. Welsman J, Armstrong N, Chedzoy S, Withers S. Aerobic training in 10-year-old and adult females. (Abstract). *Med Sci Sports Exerc.* 1996; 28: 3.
20. McNarry MA, Welsman JR, Jones AM. Influence of training and maturity status on the cardiopulmonary responses to ramp incremental cycle and upper body exercise in girls. *J Appl Physiol.* 2011; 110: 375–381.
21. Rowland TW, Bougault V, Walther G, Nottin S, Vinett A, Obert P. Cardiac responses to swim bench exercise in age-group swimmers and non-athletic children. *J Sci Med Sport.* 2009; 12: 266–272.
22. Unnithan V, Roche D, Garrard M, Holloway K, Marwood S. Oxygen uptake kinetics in trained adolescent females. *Eur J Appl Physiol.* 2015; 115: 213–220.
23. Baxter-Jones A, Goldstein H, Helms P. The development of aerobic power in young athletes. *J Appl Physiol.* 1993; 75: 1160–1167.
24. McNarry MA, Mackintosh KA, Stoedefalke K. Longitudinal investigation of training status and cardiopulmonary responses in pre- and early-pubertal children. *Eur J Appl Physiol.* 2014; 114: 1573–1580.
25. Baquet G, Gamelin FX, Mucci P, Thevenet D, Van Praagh E, Berthoin S. Continuous vs. interval aerobic training in 8- to 11-year-old children. *J Strength Cond Res.* 2010; 24: 1381–1388.
26. Baquet G, Berthoin S, Dupont G, Blondel N, Fabre C, van Praagh E. Effects of high intensity intermittent training on peak $\dot{V}O_2$ in prepubertal children. *Int J Sports Med.* 2002; 23: 439–444.
27. McManus A, Cheng C, Leung M, Yung T, Macfarlane D. Improving aerobic power in primary school boys:A comparison of continuous and interval training. *Int J Sports Med.* 2005; 26: 781–786.
28. Barbeau P, Johnson MH, Howe CA, *et al.* Ten months of exercise improves general and visceral adiposity, bone, and fitness in black girls. *Obesity.* 2007; 15: 2077–2085.
29. Carrel AL, Clark R, Peterson SE, Nemeth BA, Sullivan J, Allen DB. Improvement of fitness, body composition, and insulin sensitivity in overweight children in a school-based exercise program: A randomized, controlled study. *Arch Pediatr Adolesc Med.* 2005; 159: 963–968.
30. Baquet G, Van Praagh E, Berthoin S. Endurance training and aerobic fitness in young people. *Sports Med.* 2003; 33: 1127–1143.
31. Mahon AD. Aerobic training. In: Armstrong N, van Mechelen W (eds.) *Paediatric exercise science and medicine*, 2nd ed. Oxford: Oxford University Press; 2008. p. 513–529.
32. Gist N, Fedewa M, Dishman R, Cureton K. Sprint interval training effects on aerobic capacity: A systematic review and meta-analysis. *Sports Med.* 2014; 44: 269–279.
33. Bailey RB, Olson J, Pepper SL, Porszasz J, Barstow TJ, Cooper DM. The level and tempo of children's physical activities: an observational study. *Med Sci Sport Exerc.* 1995; 27: 1033–1041.
34. Bond B, Williams C, Isic C, *et al.* Exercise intensity and postprandial health outcomes in adolescents. *Eur J Appl Physiol.* 2014; 115: 927–936.
35. McManus AM, Armstrong N, Williams CA. Effect of training on the aerobic power and anaerobic performance of prepubertal girls. *Acta Paediatr.* 1997; 86: 456–459.
36. Costigan SA, Eather N, Plotnikoff RC, Taaffe DR, Lubans DR. High-intensity interval training for improving health-related fitness in adolescents: a systematic review and meta-analysis. *Br J Sports Med.* 2015; 49: 1253–1261.
37. Rowland TW, Garrard M, Marwood S, Guerra E, Roche D, Unnithan VB. Myocardial performance during progressive exercise in athletic adolescent males. *Med Sci Sports Exerc.* 2009; 41: 1721–1728.
38. Nottin S, Nguyen LD, Terbah M, Obert P. Left ventricular function in endurance-trained children by tissue Doppler imaging. *Med Sci Sports Exerc.* 2004; 36: 1507–1513.
39. Ayabakan C, Akalin F, Mengutay S, Cotuk B, Odabas I, Ozuak A. Athlete's heart in prepubertal male swimmers. *Cardiol Young.* 2006; 16: 61–66.
40. Obert P, Nottin S, Baquet G, Thevenet D, Gamelin FX, Berthoin S. Two months of endurance training does not alter diastolic function evaluated by TDI in 9–11-year-old boys and girls. *Br J Sports Med.* 2009; 43: 132–135.
41. Katch VL. Physical conditioning of children. *J Adolesc Health.* 1983; 3: 241–246.
42. Obert P, Mandigouts S, Nottin S, Vinet A, N'Guyen LD, Lecoq AM. Cardiovascular responses to endurance training in children: effect of gender. *Eur J Clin Invest.* 2003; 33: 199–208.
43. Rowland TW, Unnithan VB, Macfarlane NG, Gibson NG, Paton JY. Clinical manifestations of the athletes heart in prepubertal male runners. *Int J Sports Med.* 1994; 15: 515–519.
44. Nottin S, Vinet A, Stecken F, *et al.* Central and peripheral cardiovascular adaptations to exercise in endurance-trained children. *Acta Physiol Scand.* 2002; 175: 85–92.
45. Rowland TW. Endurance athletes' stroke volume response to progressive exercise: A critical review. *Sports Med.* 2009; 39: 687–695.
46. DeLorey DS, Kowalchuk JM, Paterson DH. Relationship between pulmonary O_2 uptake kinetics and muscle deoxygenation during moderate-intensity exercise. *J Appl Physiol.* 2003; 95: 113–120.
47. Ferreira LF, Townsend DK, Lutjemeier BJ, Barstow TJ. Muscle capillary blood flow kinetics estimated from pulmonary O_2 uptake and near-infrared spectroscopy. *J Appl Physiol.* 2005; 98: 1820–1828.
48. Grassi B, Pogliaghi S, Rampichini S, *et al.* Muscle oxygenation and pulmonary gas exchange kinetics during cycling exercise on-transitions in humans. *J Appl Physiol.* 2003; 95: 149–158.
49. Fawkner S, Armstrong N. Assessment of critical power with children. *Pediatr Exerc Sci.* 2002; 14: 259–268.
50. Fawkner S, Armstrong N. Longitudinal changes in the kinetic response to heavy-intensity exercise in children. *J Appl Physiol.* 2004; 97: 460–466.
51. Mader A. Evaluation of the endurance performance of marathon runners and theoretical-analysis of test-results. *J Sports Med Phys Fit.* 1991; 31: 1–19.
52. Weltman A, Snead D, Seip R, *et al.* Percentages of maximal heart-rate, heart-rate reserve and $\dot{V}O_2$ max for determining endurance training intensity in male runners. *Int J Sports Med.* 1990; 11: 218–222.
53. Weltman A. The lactate threshold and endurance performance. *Adv Sports Med Fitness.* 1989; 2: 91–116.

54. Macdougall JD. The anaerobic threshold: its significance for the endurance athlete. *Can J Appl Physiol.* 1977; 2: 137–140.
55. Armstrong N, Barker AR. Endurance training and elite young athletes. *Med Sport Sci.* 2011; 56: 59–83.
56. Poole DC, Gaesser GA. Response of ventilatory and lactate thresholds to continuous and interval training. *J Appl Physiol.* 1985; 58: 1115–1121.
57. Marwood S, Roche D, Rowland TW, Garrard M, Unnithan V. Faster pulmonary oxygen uptake kinetics in trained versus untrained male adolescents. *Med Sci Sport Exerc.* 2010; 42: 127–134.
58. Winlove MA, Jones AM, Welsman J. Influence of training status and exercise modality on pulmonary O_2 uptake kinetics in pre-pubertal girls. *Eur J Appl Physiol.* 2010; 108: 1169–1179.
59. McNarry MA, Welsman JR, Jones AM. Influence of training status and exercise modality on pulmonary O_2 uptake kinetics in pubertal girls. *Eur J Appl Physiol.* 2010; 111: 621–631.
60. Rotstein A, Dotan R, Baror O, Tenenbaum G. Effect of training on anaerobic threshold, maximal aerobic power and anaerobic performance of preadolescent boys. *Int J Sports Med.* 1986; 7: 281–286.
61. Danis A, Kyriazis Y, Klissouras V. The effect of training in male prepubertal and pubertal monozygotic twins. *Eur J Appl Physiol.* 2003; 89: 309–318.
62. Paterson DH, McLellan TM, Stella RS, Cunningham DA. Longitudinal study of ventilation threshold and maximal oxygen uptake in athletic boys. *J Appl Physiol.* 1987; 62: 2051–2057.
63. Cooper DM, Weilerravell D, Whipp BJ, Wasserman K. Aerobic parameters of exercise as a function of body size during growth in children. *J Appl Physiol.* 1984; 56: 628–634.
64. Kanaley JA, Boileau RA. The onset of the anaerobic threshold at 3 stages of physical maturity. *J Sports Med Phys Fit.* 1988; 28: 367–374.
65. Gaisl G, Buchberger J. Changes in aerobic-anaerobic transition in boys after 3 years in special physical education. In: Ilmarinen J, Valimaki I (eds.) *Children and sport.* New York: Springer-Verlag; 1984. p. 156–161.
66. Rowland TW, Green GM. Physiological-responses to treadmill exercise in females—adult-child differences. *Med Sci Sports Exerc.* 1988; 20: 474–478.
67. Mahon AD, Duncan GE, Howe CA, DelCorral P. Blood lactate and perceived exertion relative to ventilatory threshold: boys versus men. *Med Sci Sports Exerc.* 1997; 29: 1332–1337.
68. Mahon AD, Gay JA, Stolen KQ. Differentiated ratings of perceived exertion at ventilatory threshold in children and adults. *Eur J Appl Physiol Occup Physiol.* 1998; 78: 115–120.
69. Fernhall B, Kohrt W, Burkett LN, Walters S. Relationship between the lactate threshold and cross-country run performance in high school male and female runners. *Pediatr Exerc Sci.* 1996; 8: 37–47.
70. Zanconato S, Baraldi E, Rigon F, Vido L, Da Dalt L, Zacchello F. Gas exchange during exercise in obese children. *Eur J Pediatr.* 1989; 148: 614–617.
71. Hebestreit H, Staschen B, Hebestreit A. Ventilatory threshold: a useful method to determine aerobic fitness in children? *Med Sci Sports Exerc.* 2000; 32: 1964–1969.
72. Jones AM, Carter H. The effect of endurance training on parameters of aerobic fitness. *Sports Med.* 2000; 29: 373–386.
73. Favier RJ, Constable SH, Chen M, Holloszy JO. Endurance exercise training reduces lactate production. *J Appl Physiol.* 1986; 61: 885–889.
74. Saltin B, Karlsson J. Muscle glycogen utilization during work of different intensties. In: Pernow B, Saltin B (eds.) *Muscle metabolism during exercise.* New York: Plenum; 1971. p. 289–299.
75. Fitts RH, Booth FW, Winder WW, Holloszy JO. Skeletal muscle respiratory capacity, endurance and glycogen utilisation. *Am J Physiol.* 1975; 228: 1029–1033.
76. Saltin B, Nazar DL, Costill DL, *et al.* The nature of the training response: peripheral and central adaptations in one legged exercise. *Acta Physiol Scand.* 1976; 96: 289–305.
77. Donovan CM, Pagliassotti MJ. Endurance training enhances lactate clearance during hyperlactatemia. *Am J Physiol.* 1989; 73: 782–789.
78. Freund H, Lonsdorfer J, Oyono-Enguelle S, Lonsdorfer A, Bogui P. Lactate exchange and removal abilities in sickle cell patients and in trained and untrained healthy humans. *J Appl Physiol.* 1992; 73: 2580–2587.
79. Bonen A, Baker SK, Hatta H. Lactate transport and lactate transporters in skeletal muscle. *Can J Appl Physiol.* 1997; 22: 531–552.
80. MacRae HSH, Dennis SC, Bosch AN, Noakes TD. Effects of training on lactate production and removal during progressive exercise in humans. *J Appl Physiol.* 1992; 72: 1649–1656.
81. Sumida KD, Urdiales JH, Donovan CM. Enhanced gluconeogenesis from lactate in perfused livers after endurance training. *J Appl Physiol.* 1993; 264: 156–160.
82. Stallknecht B, Vissing J, Galbo H. Lactate production and clearance in exercise. Effects of training. A mini-review. *Scan J Med Sci Sport.* 1998; 8: 127–131.
83. Daniels J, Oldridge N, Nagle FJ, White B. Differences and changes in $\dot{V}O_2$ among young runners 10 to 18 years of age. *Med Sci Sport Exer.* 1978; 10: 200–203.
84. Unnithan VB, Timmons JA, Brogan RT, Paton JY, Rowland TW. Submaximal running economy in run-trained pre-pubertal boys. *J Sports Med Phys Fit.* 1996; 36: 16–23.
85. Petray CK, Krahenbuhl GS. Running training, instructions on running technique and running economy in 10-year-old males. *Res Q Exerc Sport.* 1985; 56: 251–255.
86. Unnithan V, Holohan J, Fernhall B, Wylegala I, Rowland TW, Pendergast DR. Aerobic cost in elite female adolescent swimmers. *Int J Sports Med.* 2009; 30: 194–199.
87. Krahenbuhl GS, Morgan DW, Pangrazi RP. Longitudinal changes in distance-running performance of young males. *Int J Sports Med.* 1989; 10: 92–96.
88. Whipp BJ, Ward SA. Physiological determinants of pulmonary gas-exchange kinetics during exercise. *Med Sci Sport Exer.* 1990; 22: 62–71.
89. Grassi B, Poole DC, Richardson RS, Knight DR, Erickson BK, Wagner PD. Muscle O_2 uptake kinetics in humans: Implications for metabolic control. *J Appl Physiol.* 1996; 80: 988–998.
90. Krustrup P, Jones AM, Wilkerson DP, Calbet JAL, Bangsbo J. Muscular and pulmonary O_2 uptake kinetics during moderate- and high-intensity sub-maximal knee-extensor exercise in humans. *J Physiol.* 2009; 587: 1843–1856.
91. Barstow TJ, Mole PA. Linear and nonlinear characteristics of oxygen-uptake kinetics during heavy exercise. *J Appl Physiol.* 1991; 71: 2099–2106.
92. Jones AM, Grassi B, Christensen PM, Krustrup P, Bangsbo J, Poole DC. The slow component of $\dot{V}O_2$ kinetics: mechanistic bases and practical applications. *Med Sci Sport Exer.* 2011; 43: 2046–2062.
93. Whipp BJ, Wasserman K. Oxygen uptake kinetics for various intensities of constant-load work. *J Appl Physiol.* 1972; 33: 351–356.
94. Armon Y, Cooper DM, Flores R, Zanconato S, Barstow TJ. Oxygen-uptake dynamics during high-intensity exercise in children and adults. *J Appl Physiol.* 1991; 70: 841–848.
95. Williams CA, Carter H, Jones AM, Doust JH. Oxygen uptake kinetics during treadmill running in boys and men. *J Appl Physiol.* 2001; 90: 1700–1706.
96. Obert P, Cleuziou C, Candau R, Courteix D, Lecoq AM, Guenon P. The slow component of O_2 uptake kinetics during high-intensity exercise in trained and untrained prepubertal children. *Int J Sports Med.* 2000; 21: 31–36.
97. Fawkner S, Armstrong N. Oxygen uptake kinetic response to exercise in children. *Sports Med.* 2003; 33: 651–669.
98. Fawkner S, Armstrong N. Modelling the $\dot{V}O_2$ kinetic response to heavy intensity exercise in children. *Ergonomics.* 2004; 47: 1517–1527.
99. Cleuziou C, Lecoq AM, Candau R, Courteix D, Guenon P, Obert P. Kinetics of oxygen uptake at the onset of moderate and heavy exercise in trained and untrained prepubertal children. *Sci Sports.* 2002; 17: 291–296.
100. McNarry MA, Lambrick D, Westrupp N, Faulkner J. The influence of a six-week, high-intensity games intervention on the pulmonary

oxygen uptake kinetics in prepubertal obese and normal-weight children. *Appl Physiol Nutr Met.* 2015; 40: 1012–1018.
101. Ogita F, Hara M, Tabata I. Anaerobic capacity and maximal oxygen uptake during arm stroke, leg kicking and whole body swimming. *Acta Physiol Scand.* 1996; 157: 435–441.
102. Bailey SJ, Wilkerson DP, DiMenna FJ, Jones AM. Influence of repeated sprint training on pulmonary O_2 uptake and muscle deoxygenation kinetics in humans. *J Appl Physiol.* 2009; 106: 1875–1887.
103. Barker A, Welsman J, Fulford J, Welford D, Williams C, Armstrong N. Muscle phosphocreatine and pulmonary oxygen uptake kinetics in children at the onset and offset of moderate intensity exercise. *Eur J Appl Physiol.* 2008; 102: 727–738.
104. Rossiter HB, Ward SA, Howe FA, Kowalchuk JM, Griffiths JR, Whipp BJ. Dynamics of intramuscular ^{31}P-MRS Pi peak splitting and the slow components of PCr and O_2 uptake during exercise. *J Appl Physiol.* 2002; 93: 2059–2069.
105. Ferguson C, Rossiter HB, Whipp BJ, Cathcart AJ, Murgatroyd SR, Ward SA. Effect of recovery duration from prior exhaustive exercise on the parameters of the power-duration relationship. *J Appl Physiol.* 2010; 108: 866–874.
106. Vanhatalo A, Jones AM. Influence of prior sprint exercise on the parameters of the 'all-out critical power test' in men. *Exp Physiol.* 2009; 94: 255–263.
107. McNarry MA, Welsman JR, Jones AM. Influence of training status and maturity on pulmonary O_2 uptake recovery kinetics following cycle and upper body exercise in girls. *Pediatr Exerc Sci.* 2012; 24: 246–261.
108. Marwood S, Roche D, Garrard M, Unnithan V. Pulmonary oxygen uptake and muscle deoxygenation kinetics during recovery in trained and untrained male adolescents. *Eur J Appl Physiol.* 2011; 111: 2775–2784.
109. Fawkner S, Armstrong N. Sex differences in the oxygen uptake kinetic response to heavy-intensity exercise in prepubertal children. *Eur J Appl Physiol.* 2004; 93: 210–216.
110. Poole DC, Barstow TJ, McDonough P, Jones AM. Control of oxygen uptake during exercise. *Med Sci Sport Exer.* 2008; 40: 462–474.
111. Holloszy JO. Biochemical adaptations in muscle—effects of exercise on mitochondrial oxygen uptake and respiratory enzyme activity in skeletal muscle. *J Biol Chem.* 1967; 242: 2278–2282.
112. Mogensen M, Bagger M, Pedersen PK, Fernstrom M, Sahlin K. Cycling efficiency in humans is related to low UCP3 content and to type I fibres but not to mitochondrial efficiency. *J Physiol.* 2006; 571: 669–681.
113. Eriksson BO, Gollnick PD, Saltin B. Muscle metabolism and enzyme activities after training in boys 11–13 years old. *Acta Physiol Scand.* 1973; 87: 485–497.
114. Fournier M, Ricci J, Taylor AW, Ferguson RJ, Montpetit RR, Chaitman BR. Skeletal-muscle adaptation in adolescent boys—sprint and endurance training and detraining. *Med Sci Sport Exer.* 1982; 14: 453–456.
115. Krustrup P, Hellsten Y, Bangsbo J. Intense interval training enhances human skeletal muscle oxygen uptake in the initial phase of dynamic exercise at high but not at low intensities. *J Physiol.* 2004; 559: 335–345.
116. Shoemaker JK, Phillips SM, Green HJ, Hughson RL. Faster femoral artery blood velocity kinetics at the onset of exercise following short-term training. *Cardiovasc Res.* 1996; 31: 278–286.
117. Fawkner S, Armstrong N, Potter CR, Welsman J. Oxygen uptake kinetics in children and adults after the onset of moderate-intensity exercise. *J Sports Sci.* 2002; 20: 319–326.
118. Jones AM, Koppo K. Effect of training on VO_2 kinetics and performance. In: Jones AM, Poole DC (eds.) *Oxygen uptake kinetics in sport, exercise and medicine.* London: Routledge; 2005. p. 373–397.
119. McKay BR, Paterson DH, Kowalchuk JM. Effect of short-term high-intensity interval training vs. continuous training on O_2 uptake kinetics, muscle deoxygenation, and exercise performance. *J Appl Physiol.* 2009; 107: 128–138.
120. Duché P, Falgairette G, Bedu M, Lac G, Robert A, Coudert J. Analysis of performance of prepubertal swimmers assessed from anthropometric and bio-energetic characteristics. *Eur J Appl Physiol Occup Physiol.* 1993; 66: 467–471.
121. Jurimae J, Haljaste K, Cicchella A, *et al.* Analysis of swimming performance from physical, physiological, and biomechanical parameters in young swimmers. *Pediatr Exerc Sci.* 2007; 19: 70–81.
122. Billat VL, Richard R, Binsse VM, Koralsztein JP, Haouzi P. The VO_2 slow component for severe exercise depends on type of exercise and is not correlated with time to fatigue. *J Appl Physiol.* 1998; 85: 2118–2124.
123. Billat VL, Mille-Hamard L, Demarle A, Koralsztein JP. Effect of training in humans on off- and on-transient oxygen uptake kinetics after severe exhausting intensity runs. *Eur J Appl Physiol.* 2002; 87: 496–505.
124. Norris SR, Petersen SR. Effects of endurance training on transient oxygen uptake responses in cyclists. *J Sports Sci.* 1998; 16: 733–738.
125. Demarle AP, Slawinski JJ, Laffite LP, Bocquet VG, Koralsztein JP, Billat VL. Decrease of O_2 deficit is a potential factor in increased time to exhaustion after specific endurance training. *J Appl Physiol.* 2001; 90: 947–953.
126. Savage MP, Petratis MM, Thomson WH, Berg K, Smith JL, Sady SP. Exercise training effects on serum lipids in prepubescent boys and adult men. *Med Sci Sport Exerc.* 1986; 18: 197–204.
127. Eisenmann PA, Golding LA. Comparison of effects of training on VO_2 max in girls and young women. *Med Sci Sport Exerc.* 1975; 7: 136–138.
128. Rowell L. *Human cardiovascular control.* New York: Oxford University Press; 1993.
129. Tolfrey K, Campbell IG, Batterham AM. Aerobic trainability of prepubertal boys and girls. *Pediatr Exerc Sci.* 1998; 10: 248–263.
130. Pate RR, Ward DS. Endurance exercise trainability in children and youth. In: Grana WA, Lombardo JA, Sharkey BJ, Stone EJ (eds.) *Advances in sports medicine and fitness.* Chicago, IL: Year Book Medical Publishers; 1990. p. 37–55.
131. Rowland TW, Boyajian A. Aerobic response to endurance exercise training in children. *Pediatrics.* 1995; 96: 654–658.
132. Rowland TW. *Children's exercise physiology*, 2nd ed. Champaign, IL: Human Kinetics; 2005.
133. Armstrong N, Welsman J. The physical activity patterns of European youth with reference to methods of assessment. *Sports Med.* 2006; 36: 1067–1086.
134. Armstrong N, Fawkner SG. Aerobic fitness. In: Armstrong N (ed.) *Paediatric exercise physiology.* Edinburgh: Churchill-Livingstone; 2007. p. 161–187.
135. Weber G, Kartodihardjo W, Klissouras V. Growth and physical-training with reference to heredity. *J Appl Physiol.* 1976; 40: 211–215.
136. Hemery D. *Should a child specialize in just one sport? The pursuit of sporting excellence: A study of sport's highest achievers.* Champaign, IL: Human Kinetics; 1988.
137. Baxter-Jones ADG, Helms P. Effects of training at a young age: A review of the training of young athletes (TOYA) study. *Pediatr Exerc Sci.* 1996; 8: 310–327.
138. Starosta W. Selection of children in sport. In: Rogozkin V, Maughan RM (eds.) *Current research in sport sciences: An international perspective.* London: Plenum Press; 1996. p. 21–25.
139. Hollander EB, Meyers MC, LeUnes A. Psychological factors associated with overtraining: Implications for youth sport coaches. *J Sport Behav.* 1995; 18: 3–20.
140. Salguero A, Gonzalez-Boto R. Identification of dropout reasons in young competitive swimmers. *J Sports Med Phys Fit.* 2003; 43: 530–534.
141. Riddoch C, Mattocks C, Deere K, *et al.* Objective measurement of levels and patterns of physical activity. *Arch Dis Child.* 2007; 92: 963–969.
142. Armstrong N, McNarry MA. Aerobic fitness and trainability in youth: gaps in our knowledge. *Pediatr Exer Sci.* 2016; 28: 171–177.

CHAPTER 35

High-intensity interval training

Keith Tolfrey and James W Smallcombe

Introduction

High-intensity interval training (HIIT) describes exercise 'characterised by brief, intermittent bursts of vigorous activity, interspersed by periods of rest or low-intensity exercise'.[1(p1047)] The popularity of this type of training has increased recently as a time-efficient and potent alternative to 'traditional' moderate-intensity continuous training (MCT). With a global crisis in chronic, non-communicable diseases[2] providing an alarming backdrop, much of this attention has centred on the potential of HIIT to assist in the fight against lifestyle-related disease (e.g. cardiovascular disease and type 2 diabetes mellitus).

The popular discourse surrounding HIIT has been fuelled by renewed academic interest in this form of exercise,[3–6] and emerging evidence that supports the notion that HIIT may induce physiological adaptations comparable to those from higher volume MCT.[5] Perhaps the most alluring feature of HIIT is the priority afforded to intensity over duration, and thus, the purported time efficiency.[7] The remarkably low-volume of exercise performed typically during HIIT is also likely to be appealing to a modern society, which frequently cites a 'lack of time' as a major barrier to regular exercise participation.[8]

Although HIIT has only been aligned recently to public health promotion, the origins of this training method may be traced back to, at least, the early twentieth century.[9] The history of modern sport is littered with accounts of elite athletes and coaches using, and honing through anecdotal inquiry, various forms of HIIT to optimize sport performance. High-intensity interval training is by no means a new phenomenon, but instead a training concept long-appreciated by athletes. This training technique has, however, evolved recently from rudimentary origins into a contemporary exercise tool utilized by sport- and health-professionals alike. This chapter examines the scientific evidence supporting the efficacy of HIIT to confer benefit to both sports performance and health in children and adolescents (young people).

The use of HIIT by young people is particularly relevant for a number of reasons. Firstly, it seems that high-intensity exercise may be completed by children without substantial fatigue compared with adults.[10] (Interested readers are referred to Chapter 9 for a detailed discussion on fatigue resistance). Secondly, it has been suggested that HIIT may resemble the spontaneous, intermittent nature of habitual physical activity (PA) in young people.[11] Thirdly, it is possible that HIIT is less susceptible to the monotony that young people often associate with MCT[12] and is, consequently, more conducive to longer-term exercise adherence. However, considering that most young people fail to meet international PA guidelines,[13] perhaps the most compelling rationale for HIIT is that it could offer them a viable alternative to more traditional forms of exercise and encourage greater engagement during these formative years.[14] Of course, HIIT is not a panacea; indeed, numerous caveats come with HIIT training in young people; these caveats are addressed throughout the chapter.

When critically appraising any research findings, the contextual framework is very important. For example, training is defined as methods used to enhance or develop skills and/or knowledge with the intention of improving one or more predetermined outcomes. In this chapter, however, training refers specifically to PA or exercise, which is completed repeatedly over time, to enhance a physical, physiological, or sports performance outcome that can be quantified using recognized measurement techniques. Moreover, because training implies sustainable improvements are sought, we will make every effort to differentiate chronic training adaptations from acute exercise responses. We define 'high intensity' as exercise that can be sustained for up to 4 min (240 s) before a rest interval is required.

It is also critical to determine whether the emphasis on exercise training is for gains in sports performance or physical health. The literature includes some outcome measures that relate explicitly to one of these two paradigms and others apply to both (e.g. peak oxygen uptake [$\dot{V}O_2$]; a measure of cardiorespiratory fitness [CRF]). We review the literature from both perspectives and there may be some overlap.

Finally, there are many detailed reviews on the scientific basis and prescription of HIIT,[9,15–19] which are based on a multitude of laboratory and field studies with adults. Buchheit and Laursen[9] indicated recently that further research is required with youth; therefore, it is not our intention to indicate how HIIT should be prescribed for young people, but to critically appraise the current scientific literature to evaluate the efficacy of this form of exercise training with young people. Importantly, while most researchers use traditional null-hypothesis significance testing (NHST) methods to compare outcome measures over time and between groups or training conditions, we have used their published means and standard deviations to estimate pairwise effect sizes to determine whether the findings might be meaningful from a sport performance or health perspective. Thus, the descriptors suggested by Cohen[20] are used to describe the range of effect sizes, specifically: trivial <0.2, small 0.2 to <0.5, moderate 0.5 to <0.8 and large ≥0.8.

High-intensity interval training and the young performance athlete

Participation in organized youth sport is progressing constantly to new heights of competitiveness and sophistication. Indeed, optimizing the performance of young athletes has emerged as a burgeoning area of interest for sport scientists and coaches alike. The provision of highly-structured training now pervades the broad spectrum of youth sport. Although not comparable in number to those conducted with adults, various studies have examined the efficacy of HIIT to improve sport performance outcomes in young people, and we highlight the key findings, with specific focus on the physiological parameters associated with sporting success. At this point, it is important that the reader recognizes some of the difficulties faced when attempting to evaluate the effect of a training intervention on sporting performance, per se. The complex nature of sports performance—dependent on a number of intricately linked physiological, biomechanical, psychological, technical, and tactical factors—renders the laboratory-based assessment of sporting capability inherently difficult. Consequently, many researchers rely on the assessment of the components of fitness (e.g. speed, aerobic endurance, and strength) associated with successful sport performance. While tightly controlled laboratory measures can provide reliable, valid, and comparable data, it is much more challenging to interpret these data and establish whether training-induced changes in such parameters translate to meaningful improvements in sport performance under free-living, competitive conditions. There has, however, been some endeavour to bridge this gap in knowledge and an emerging body of research provides valuable insight into the role that HIIT might play in enhancing athletic performance.

An array of studies has examined the effect of HIIT on a wide range of performance outcomes in male and female athletes aged 8–18 years (Table 35.1). The characteristics of the training protocols vary considerably with the interventions spanning 11 days to 10 weeks and two or three training sessions per week. The repetitions range from 3 to 40 and last between 10 s and 4 min. In most studies, exercise intensity was fixed at 90–95% predicted maximum heart rate (HR max). Alternatively, high-intensity exercise was defined as all-out (maximum) intensities; >95% maximal aerobic speed (MAS); and/or >90% of personal best time.

Cardiorespiratory fitness

Cardiorespiratory fitness is recognized as an important determinant of athletic performance in sports requiring a high aerobic energy provision. Hence, its response to HIIT in the context of sports performance is examined here; the section High-intensity interval training for health approaches it from a health perspective. Peak $\dot{V}O_2$, measured during exhaustive exercise, is widely recognized as the criterion measure of CRF. Although a high level of CRF alone does not guarantee sporting success, it is often exhibited by elite athletes. It has been reported consistently that the performance of 14–30 HIIT sessions, over a period ranging from 11 days to 10 weeks, leads to significant increases in CRF in both trained and untrained young people (Table 35.1). These studies have demonstrated that HIIT is effective in increasing peak $\dot{V}O_2$ by 6–12%, typically. A number of studies have employed laboratory-based measures of gas exchange (e.g. indirect calorimetry) to quantify HIIT-induced changes in peak $\dot{V}O_2$, while others have used field-based fitness tests to estimate it; the former is prioritized for discussion in this section.

Baseline CRF is an important factor when assessing training-induced changes. As young athletes regularly engage in structured aerobic exercise training programmes, they will have an enhanced capacity for oxidative metabolism at baseline, compared with their untrained counterparts. Hence, gains may be more difficult to achieve through increased sub-maximal training load alone.[21,22,23] Consequently, it has been suggested that HIIT may be a particularly useful training tool to use with youth athletes. Impressive baseline fitness ≥63 $mL \cdot kg^{-1} \cdot min^{-1}$ was seen in two studies,[24,25] though the former was scaled using lean body mass. The 8.3% increase found by Chamari *et al.*[24] was in 14-year-old male footballers who completed 8 weeks of HIIT, comprised of 4 min intervals at 90–95% individual HR max. Similarly, it was reported that an 8-week HIIT programme resulted in a 10.1% increase in peak $\dot{V}O_2$ in late-adolescent male footballers.[25] Collectively, these studies support the efficacy of HIIT in already well-trained youth athletes, but the omission of a control group in both studies precludes the establishment of direct causality. Furthermore, as HIIT was performed alongside their regular technical and tactical sessions, it is not possible to attribute the change in CRF to HIIT exclusively.

Athletes and coaches may question how HIIT-induced changes in CRF compare to those conferred by high-volume MCT; some studies have compared the different regimes directly (Table 35.1). In a randomized, crossover study conducted in 9- to 11-year-old competitive swimmers, Sperlich and colleagues[31] compared changes in peak $\dot{V}O_2$ after 5 weeks of HIIT and, what was called high-volume training (HVT). The within measures research design eliminates between group variance common to all mixed design studies and the 8.5-week wash-out period should have countered a possible period effect. Significant, moderate, and small ($d = 0.57$ and 0.46) increases were observed after HIIT (10.2%) and HVT (8.5%), respectively. It was concluded that desirable, short-term changes in CRF could be achieved through HIIT despite a comparatively reduced training time (2 h less each week) and volume (5.5 vs 11.9 $km \cdot week^{-1}$). Importantly, the authors recognized the limitation of a cycle ergometer-based test in swimmers. Indeed, this was reflected in the modest baseline peak $\dot{V}O_2$ values (~40 $mL \cdot kg^{-1} \cdot min^{-1}$), which were considerably lower than might be expected in children accustomed to training at least four times $\cdot$ $week^{-1}$. However, the difficulties associated with the in-pool measurement of gaseous exchange with young children were highlighted and provided as justification for the surrogate use of cycle ergometry.

In a later study conducted with 14-year-old footballers using a between-measures experimental design, it was reported that peak $\dot{V}O_2$ increased significantly by ~7% following 5 weeks of HIIT yet was unchanged (non-significant, ~2% increase) following 5 weeks of high-volume training.[32] Although the boys continued to participate in regular football-specific training during the intervention period, this additional training load was similar in both groups. Other studies suggest that similar changes in CRF are induced by both HIIT and continuous cycle ergometer training in untrained prepubertal girls and boys.[34,35] Interestingly, in the latter of these studies, the interval training group exhibited pre- to post-increases in a number of physiological parameters, including ventilatory threshold, that were not observed in the continuous training group.[35] This limited body of research provides preliminary evidence that HIIT appears to be at least as efficacious as MCT in enhancing CRF in young athletes.

The time frame over which CRF may be enhanced through HIIT represents an interesting point for discussion. While the majority of studies with young athletes (Table 35.1) have examined the effect of 4–10 weeks of HIIT on peak $\dot{V}O_2$, mixed findings emerged from two studies that assessed the efficacy of a shorter 'shock microcycle'.[28,40] It was demonstrated, in a well-controlled study conducted

Table 35.1 Prospective high-intensity interval training studies with children and adolescents that assessed athletic performance outcomes

Citation	HIIT sample	Control sample	Sex	Sport	Age (years)	Length (wk)	Training programme	Performance (Δ%)		
Baquet *et al.*[26]	33	20[a]	M & F	N/A	8–11	7	F2, 30 min of short intermittent aerobic running (10 or 20 s) at 100 to 130% MAS	Peak $\dot{V}O_2$: MS:	+8*† +5*†	
Baquet *et al.*[27]	36	36[a]	M &F	N/A	8–11	7	F2, 30 min of high-intensity intermittent running (10 or 20 s) at 100 to 130% MAS	MS: SBJ:	+5*† +10*†	
Breil *et al.*[28]	13	8[b]	M & F	Alpine Skiing	16–17	11 days	Shock Micro-cycle of HIIT. 15 high-intensity aerobic interval sessions in 11 days. 4 × 4-min at 90–95% HRmax, 3-min recovery periods	Peak $\dot{V}O_2$ PPO: VT: Lac_{max}: Tlim: CMJ: SJ:	+6* +6* +10* +11* +5 −5* −4*	
Buchheit *et al.*[29]	**G1:**15 **G2:**17	N/A	M & F	Handball	15.5	10	**G1:** F2, HIIT, 12–24 × 15-s runs at 95% MAS, with 15-s passive recovery **G2:** F2, Small-sided handball games performed over similar time period	 V_{IFT}: T_{lim}: RSA: 10-m Sprint: CMJ:	**G1:** +6* +36* +3* +1 +3	**G2:** +7* +27* +5* +2 +3
Buchheit *et al.*[30]	**G1**: 7 **G2**: 8	N/A	M	Football	14.5	10	**G1**: F1, Repeated Sprint Training: 2–3 sets of 5–6 × 15 to 20 m repeated shuttle sprints with 14 s of passive or 23 s of active recovery **G2:** F1, Explosive Strength Training: 4–6 series of 4–6 explosive strength exercises	 10-m Sprint: 30-m Sprint: RSAmean: CMJ: Hop:	**G1:** +2 +2* +3* +7* +14*	**G2:** +33 +2* +1* +15*† +28*
Chamari *et al.*[24]	18	N/A	M	Football	14.0	8	F2, 1 session 4 × 4 min at 90–95% HRmax. 3 min active recovery One session 4 × 4 min small sided games (4 × 4 players) at 90–95% HRmax	Peak $\dot{V}O_2$: Peak $\dot{V}O_2$ (abs): RE: Hoff-Test:	+8 +15* +14* +10*	
Delextrat and Martinez[31]	**G1:** 9 **G2:** 9	N/A	M	Basketball	**G1:** 16.0 **G2:** 16.3	6	**G1**: F2, HIIT. Intermittent running at 95% maximal aerobic performance. 15 s exercise bouts interspersed with 15 s of active recovery for 8–13 min e.g. 2 × (8–13 min of 15 s—15 s) **G2:** F2, Small-sided games. 2 vs 2 small sided games. e.g. 2 × (2–3 × 3 min 45 s—4 min 15 s)	 V_{IFT}: Defence: Offence:	**G1:** +3* −3 +4*	**G2:** +4* +5 +7*
Faude *et al.*[32]	**G1 & G2:** 10 Crossover	N/A	M & F	Swimming	16.6	4	**G1**: F6, HIIT, 30.8% above individual anaerobic threshold. Various interval duration and repetitions **G2:** F6, High-volume Training, 23.3% above individual anaerobic threshold. Various interval duration and repetitions	 IAT: T_{100}: T_{400}:	**G1:** +* −1 0	**G2:** +* −1 0

(*continued*)

Table 35.1 Continued

Citation	HIIT sample	Control sample	Sex	Sport	Age (years)	Length (wk)	Training programme	Performance (Δ%)		
Impellizzeri *et al.*[33]	**G1:** 15 **G2:** 14	N/A	M	Football	17.2	4 & 8	**G1:**F2, Generic Interval Training. 4 × 4 min at 90–95% HRmax with 3 min active recovery **G2:** F2, Small-sided Football Games	 Peak $\dot{V}O_2$: $\dot{V}O_2$ at LT: V at LT: Eckblom: Distance run: HI running: LI running: Walking:	**G1:** +8* +13* +9* +14* +6* +23* +18* −9*	**G2:** +7* +11* +10* +16* +4* +26* +7* −8*
McManus *et al.*[34]	**G1**: 11 **G2**: 12	7[a]	F	N/A	9.6	8	**G1:** F3, Sprint Running. 3 × 10 s maximal speed sprints with 10 s rest followed by 3 × 30 s sprints with 90 s rest. Increased to four, five, and six sets after 2, 4 and 6 weeks, respectively **G2:** F3, Cycle Ergometer Exercise 20 min cycling at HR 160–170 $b \cdot min^{-1}$	 Peak $\dot{V}O_2$: PPO: MPO:	**G1:** +8* +10* +3	**G2:** +10* +20* −1
McManus *et al.*[35]	**G1**:10 **G2**:10	15[a]	M	N/A	10.3	8	**G1:** F3, Interval training. 7 × 30 s maximal speed sprint on cycle ergometer with 2 min 45 s active recovery **G2:** F3, Continuous training. 20 min steady state cycling at HR 160–170 $b \cdot min^{-1}$	 Peak $\dot{V}O_2$: PPO: $\dot{V}O_2$ at VT:	**G1:** +12* +33*† +22*†	**G2:** +6* +22 +3
McMillan *et al.*[25]	11	N/A	M	Football	16.9	10	F2, Football-specific running. 4 × 4 min at 90–95% HRmax separated by 3 min recovery at 70% HRmax	Peak $\dot{V}O_2$: RE: CMJ: SJ: 10-m Sprint:	+10* 0 +3* +7* 0	
Meckel *et al.*[36]	**G1**:11 **G2**:13	N/A	M	Football	14.3	7	**G1:** F3, Short-sprint repetition training. Four to six sets of 4 × 50 m reps of all-out sprints with 2 and 4 min rest between reps and sets, respectively **G2:** F3, Long-sprint repetition training. 4–6 200 m reps at 85% max 100 m speed with 5 min rest between reps	 Peak $\dot{V}O_2$: T_{250} 30-m Sprint $T_4 \times {}_{10}$ SBJ:	**G1:** +7* +4* +3* +3* +1	**G2:** +10* +3* +2* +1* +2
Rotstein *et al.*[37]	16	12[a]	M	N/A	10.8	9	F3, Interval Running. 1–2 sets of 3 × 600 m with 2.5 min rest, 5 × 400 m with 2 min rest and 6 × 150 m with 1.5 min rest. Varying intensity	Peak $\dot{V}O_2$: T_{1200} PPO MPO LAIV	+8* +10* +14* +10* +2*	

Sperlich *et al.*[38]	**G1 & G2:** 26 Crossover	N/A	M and F	Swimming	10.5	5	**G1:** F5, HIIT. 30 min, 50–300 m intervals. Intensity 92% personal best 100 m freestyle time **G2:** F5, High Volume Training. 60 min, 100–800 m intervals, Intensity 85% personal best for each distance		**G1:**	**G2:**
								Peak $\dot{V}O_2$:	+12*	+9*
								Lac_{max}	+26*	−24*
								LEN:	+17*	+6
								T_{2000}:	+3*	0
								T_{100}:	+2	+2
Sperlich *et al.*[39]	**G1**: 9 **G2**: 8	N/A	M	Football	13.5	5	**G1**: F3–4, HIIT. <30-min running session (4–15 × 30 s–4 min) at 90–95% HR max. Intervals separated by 1 to 3 min jogging at 50–60% HRmax **G2:** F3–4, High Volume Training. 45- to 60 min exercise session at 50–70% HRmax		**G1:**	**G2:**
								Peak $\dot{V}O_2$:	+7*	+2
								T_{1000}:	+4*	+2
								20-m Sprint:	+4*	+4*
								30-m Sprint:	+4*	+4*
								40-m Sprint:	+3*	+3*
								Drop Jump:	+15	+7
								CMJ:	+12	+26
								SJ:	+11	+14
Wahl *et al.*[40]	**G1:** 8 **G2:** 8	N/A	M & F	Triathlon	15.4	2	Shock Micro-cycle. 15 sessions within three, 3-day training blocks over 14 days. HIIT training at 90–95% HRmax. 40 s–4 min intervals. Variable sets and repetitions **G1:** Active recovery **G2:** Passive Recovery		**G1:**	**G2:**
								Peak $\dot{V}O_2$:	−1	+3
								TT_{PO} ($W{\cdot}kg^{-1}$)	+3	+14*
								$TT_{Lactate}$	+12	+23*
								Wingate PPO:	+2	−2
								Wingate MP:	+5*	−2

Peak $\dot{V}O_2$—peak oxygen uptake ($mL{\cdot}kg^{-1}{\cdot}min^{-1}$); **MS**—maximal speed (velocity) at the end of a graded field test; **SBJ**—standing broad jump; **PPO**—peak power output; **VT**—ventilatory threshold; **Lac_{max}**—maximal blood lactate concentration; **T_{lim}**—time to exhaustion at relative, pre-intervention exercise intensity; **CMJ**—counter movement jump; **SJ**—squat jumps; **V_{IFT}**—velocity reached at end of the $30–15_{IFT}$ test; **RSA (mean)**—mean sprint time during repeated sprint ability test; **10/20/30/40-m Sprint**—sprint time over 10/20/30/40 metres; **Hop**—mean height during hopping test; **Peak $\dot{V}O_2$ (abs)**—peak oxygen uptake ($L{\cdot}min^{-1}$); **RE**—running economy; **Hoff-Test**—football-specific circuit; **Defence**—defensive agility; **Offence**—offensive agility; **IAT**—individual anaerobic threshold; **T_{100}**—maximal 100-m swim time; **T_{400}**—maximal 400-m swim time; **$\dot{V}O_2$ at LT**—oxygen uptake at lactate threshold; **Vat LT**—velocity at lactate threshold; **Eckblom**—football-specific endurance test; **Distance run**—distanced run during competitive football match; **HI running**—time spent in high-intensity running during competitive football match; **LI running**—time spent in low-intensity running during competitive football match; **Walking**—time spent walking during competitive football match; **MPO**—mean power output; **$\dot{V}O_2$ at VT**—oxygen uptake at ventilatory threshold; **T_{250}**—250-m running time; **$T_{4\times10}$**—4 × 10-m shuttle running time; **T_{1200}**—1200-m running time; **LAIV**—lactate inflection point velocity; **LEN**—Ligue Européenne de Natation, the European governing body—international pointing system for competition performance; **T_{2000}**—maximal 2000-m swim time; **TT_{PO}**—time trial power output; **$TT_{Lactate}$**—time trial blood lactate concentration; **Wingate PPO**—peak power output during Wingate test; **Wingate MP**—mean power out during Wingate test.

* Significant difference pre- to post-intervention; † Significant difference between-groups. [a] Habitual Physical Activity; [b] Habitual Training.

in the off-season preparatory period, that 15 HIIT sessions performed over 11 days resulted in a 6% increase in peak $\dot{V}O_2$ in late-adolescent alpine skiers.[28] In contrast, a control group exhibited no change in cardiorespiratory fitness following maintenance of their habitual training patterns. The magnitude of change was relatively modest in comparison to those reported following HIIT regimes spanning a longer period of time with young athletes (Table 35.1). The authors suggested that the high frequency of HIIT may have compromised the efficiency of the training with regard to the maximal capacity for improvement in aerobic capacity. However, it is reasonable to conclude that a moderate 6% (d = 0.58) increase in peak $\dot{V}O_2$ represents a generous return from 11 days of training for skiers with good baseline fitness (53 $mL \cdot kg^{-1} \cdot min^{-1}$).

In contrast to these findings, Wahl and colleagues[40] reported no meaningful change (d = 0.02) in peak $\dot{V}O_2$ in 16 young triathletes following a similar microcycle of HIIT consisting of 15 sessions performed over 14 days. The authors speculated that a slight decrease in post-HIIT haemoglobin concentration [Hb], possibly the result of a loss of red blood cells due to the high impact of the HIIT regime, might explain the failure of the training microcycle to induce meaningful improvements. It is possible that these losses could not be fully compensated in the 7-day recovery period post-intervention. A particularly pertinent finding of this latter study was that significant decreases were observed in some dimensions of the Persons Perceived Physical State Scale (PEPS), including perceived physical energy, perceived physical flexibility, and readiness to train, highlighting the exhausting nature of this training intervention. This, of course, raises important questions surrounding the extent to which this form of high-frequency HIIT may be tolerated, as well as the possibility that such training, if not carefully managed, might lead to the manifestation of overtraining symptoms and the impairment of performance often associated with this condition. (Interested readers are referred to Chapter 38 for further discussion of overtraining). Future research is undoubtedly warranted to further elucidate the optimal combination of HIIT frequency, intensity, and recovery time for use with young athletes.

Similar increases in aerobic performance—estimated using field-based fitness tests—have also been reported.[27,29,31,32,36] Typically, such studies have employed incremental fitness tests, the assessment of intermittent exercise performance (e.g. shuttle run test [20MST], intermittent fitness test), and/or physiological parameters such as individual anaerobic threshold as surrogate measures of aerobic capacity. Of course, field-based estimates of endurance performance do not provide the quality of data associated with the sophisticated laboratory assessment of gas exchange. However, such field-based tests represent a convenient and inexpensive method of estimating endurance performance and represent a valuable tool to track changes over a period of training, especially with large groups of athletes. Ultimately, the emerging findings from these studies provide further, albeit weaker, evidence supporting the efficacy of HIIT to induce desirable improvements in endurance performance, which are likely to be underpinned by CRF in young people.

Explosive strength

The effect of HIIT on explosive strength (power), the ability to exert maximal muscular contraction in the shortest possible time, has been examined in several studies (Table 35.1) using a battery of jump tests. Typically, a selection of jump tests has been used to assess training-induced changes in the explosive strength of the lower limbs. These include counter movement jump (CMJ); drop jump (DJ); standing broad (long) jump (SBJ); squat jump (SJ); and vertical jump (VJ). Explosive strength is a component of physical fitness that may be particularly important to sports in which sprinting and/or jumping (vertical and/or horizontal) are integral to successful performance, with the obvious examples being the 100-m sprint and long jump. There are, however, many other sports in which explosive strength represents an essential, yet more subtle, determinant of sports performance and/or skill execution. Of course, sports performance outcomes are normally very complex and it is likely that the changes in the ability to produce explosive strength, as measured by the performance of simple jump tasks in isolation to other sport-related skills, represents an ill-defined fraction of these outcomes. Nonetheless, jumping ability remains a useful performance assessment tool and a number of noteworthy findings have emerged from HIIT studies in which explosive strength has been assessed by this method.

Changes in power are more heterogeneous than CRF following HIIT; untrained, prepubertal children, completing 7 weeks of high-intensity interval running (10 or 20 s at 100–130% MAS) experienced a significant, but moderate increase (d = 0.62; 9.6%) in SBJ distance.[27] The authors concluded that HIIT performed at velocities greater than MAS enhanced lower limb explosive strength and speculated that this likely resulted from a combination of both neurological adaptations and/or alterations in muscle fibre type characteristics; however, it was suggested that the former was likely to be the primary mechanism responsible for the observed improvement. It should be reiterated that this study was conducted in untrained boys and girls, which could magnify the increase. This suggestion is supported by trained, late-adolescent professional footballers who experienced only small gains in CMJ (d = 0.35; 2.7%) and SJ (d = 0.42; 6.9%) performance after 10 weeks of HIIT involving football-specific interval running at a fixed intensity of 90–95% of HR max.[25] As expected, these 'statistically significant', but small, effects in jump performance did not translate into a concomitant improvement in 10-m sprint time, which illustrates that jump-specific measures of explosive strength may not always translate to a holistic enhancement of power-related performance.

A number of studies have reported no meaningful improvement in explosive jump performance following HIIT. Buchheit and colleagues[29] demonstrated that 10 weeks of HIIT resulted in trivial changes in CMJ (d = 0.13) and 10-m sprint time (d = 0.13) in well-trained male and female handball players. Similarly, trivial and small increases in SBJ were exhibited amongst youth football players following a 7-week HIIT programme consisting of either all-out short-sprint repetitions (50 m; d = 0.19) or long-sprint repetitions (200 m; d = 0.32) performed at 85% of maximal 100 m time.[36] These findings were contrary to the authors' hypothesis that the short-sprint programme would yield improvements in jump ability and led to the conclusion that the technical aspects of jump performance may need to be practised during HIIT if meaningful improvements in performance are to be conferred. Finally, in a well-designed, but somewhat underpowered study, 5 weeks of HIIT resulted in only small increases in CMJ or SJ performance in adolescent football players.[39] Although these studies reported no meaningful improvement in jump performance following HIIT, it is equally noteworthy that the weekly performance of two to three sessions of high-intensity exercise over a period of 5–10 weeks resulted in no impairment of power-related performance. This is particularly encouraging given concerns about potential incompatibility of endurance training and maintenance of power-related performance. The evidence that has emerged from studies conducted with young people may reassure athletes and coaches that HIIT, if designed and supervised appropriately, can be utilized to enhance important components of fitness (e.g. CRF) without compromising explosive strength and power-related performance.

The importance of design and management of HIIT is, however, highlighted further by the findings of Breil *et al.*[28] Following an 11-day shock micro-cycle of HIIT consisting of 15 sessions, participants experienced a moderate reduction (d = –0.54; 4.8%) in CMJ performance. This performance decrement was observed despite an improvement in CRF. The authors speculated that the high-frequency training microcycle could have contributed to persistent muscle fatigue and subsequent impairment of performance. The authors[28] concluded that participants may have needed more than 7 days post-HIIT recovery to fully restore explosive strength capacity.

Overall, the weight of the available evidence suggests that HIIT, if carefully managed, is unlikely to result in an impairment of explosive strength and, in some cases, might lead to performance enhancement. It is important, however, for young athletes and their coaches to consider the frequency of HIIT sessions carefully as well as the recovery time provided between exercise bouts. Furthermore, particular attention should be paid to the recovery period following the completion of an intensive block of HIIT, especially in the lead-up to competition.

Sport-specific performance outcomes

A small number of studies have attempted to assess the effect of HIIT on competitive sporting performance and/or sport-specific capacities directly. Impellizzeri *et al.*[33] used a matched, randomized, parallel-group experimental model with young footballers. Employing increases in total running distance, number of sprints performed, and time spent performing at higher-exercise intensities, they concluded that competitive match performance had improved after HIIT. These improvements in sport-specific parameters were accompanied by an increase in peak $\dot{V}O_2$. Another interesting finding from this study was the observed improvement in performance during the football-specific Ekblom aerobic endurance field test, which comprises several activities typical of football, including changes in direction, jumps, and backwards running.[41] Similar changes in football performance and CRF were also observed in a parallel experimental group following small-sided game-based training.[33] The authors of this study concluded that HIIT and small-sided game training were equally effective modes of aerobic training for use with youth football players. Another important consideration is that the training interventions were completed in addition to the players' regular football training (technical and tactical sessions). Although the authors reported that this additional football-specific training was performed at low intensities, it is possible that it provided an additional training stimulus. It is, therefore, impossible to isolate the effect of HIIT and establish a causal and independent relationship between the training interventions and the changes in sport-specific outcome measures.

Faude and colleagues[32] found that 4 weeks of HIIT resulted in no improvement in 100 or 400 m swim times in competitive adolescent swimmers; however, they did report that seven out of nine swimmers swam personal best times (PBs) in the 3 months after the HIIT training cycle. Whether these PBs can be attributed to HIIT directly is questionable. In another swimming study by Sperlich *et al.*,[38] competitive performance was assessed before and after 5 weeks of HIIT and HVT. Significant changes in 2000 m swim time and scoring on the LEN (Ligue Européenne de Natation, the European Governing Body) international point system for competition performance were reported only after HIIT (not HVT); however, the magnitude of these effects was small (d ≤ 0.48). Moreover, the group reduction in 100 m swim times was trivial (d ≤ 0.18). Based on these differences between HIIT and HVT, Sperlich *et al.*[38] concluded that high training volumes provided no advantage compared to lower volumes of HIIT. They went on to suggest that the use of HIIT may enable a greater proportion of training time to be spent on technical development, while conferring similar benefit to physiological parameters.

The efficacy of a 2-week shock microcycle of HIIT to enhance cycling performance in young triathletes has been assessed using average power output (PO in Watts; W) during a 20 min time trial (TT) performance test,[40] which is deemed a valid and reliable simulation of a race event in adults.[42] Wahl *et al.*[40] also compared passive and active recovery by dividing the 16 girls and boys equally into two separate training groups. Time trial average PO increased significantly from 2.9 to 3.3 $W \cdot kg^{-1}$ in the passive group (d = 0.66; 12%), whereas the change in the active recovery group was only small (d = 0.24; ~3%) and within the reported coefficient of variation for this performance measure. The increase in 20 min TT performance was observed despite non-significant, trivial (d ≤ 0.19) changes in peak $\dot{V}O_2$ in both groups; interestingly, the total cycling distance achieved during the TT was not reported. This finding led the authors to recommend that when working with athletes, the measurement of performance should represent the main criterion for the efficacy of a training programme as physiological parameters may not be sensitive to change.

High-intensity interval training for health

Cardiorespiratory fitness

In line with the general paediatric exercise science and medicine literature, CRF is one of the most commonly measured outcome variables in studies that have that examined the efficacy of HIIT in young people (Tables 35.1 and 35.2). Although it is normally defined as peak $\dot{V}O_2$, some studies have included endurance performance measures (e.g. 20MST),[14,27,55] maximal endurance speed[56], running economy[26] or gas exchange threshold.[44] While it can be argued that most young people rarely exercise at intensities that would elicit peak $\dot{V}O_2$, it has a strong empirical relationship with cardiometabolic health; therefore, the results from health-focused HIIT studies including 20MST are included.

We are aware that numerous early studies employed interval training techniques, common to endurance athletes, with healthy young people; however, they were not designed specifically to examine the efficacy of HIIT. Consequently, their study design features often do not allow us to isolate the independent effect of the high-intensity elements of the research. Nevertheless, much can be learned from these pioneers. For example, Rotstein *et al.*[37] reported a large (d = 1.41; 8%) increase in peak $\dot{V}O_2$ in sixteen 10- to 11-year-old boys who completed a series of 150–600 m runs, three times $\cdot$ week^{-1} over 9 weeks, compared with an age and activity matched non-training control group (Table 35.2). The precise exercise intensity

Table 35.2 Peak oxygen consumption: prospective high-intensity interval training studies with children and adolescents that included a comparison with either an untrained control or at least two different training programmes.

Citation	Sample sizes[a]	Sex & body size[b]	Age (years)	Length (wk)	HIIT (min)[c]	HIIT training programme	Peak $\dot{V}O_2$ (Δ%)[d]
Baquet *et al.*[26]	33:20 (53)	M & F NW-OB	8–11	7	93	F2[e], 4 sets × 5–10 reps × 10–20 s @ 100–130% MAS run	8[§] vs −2
Baquet *et al.*[27]	22:22:19 (77)	M & F NW-OW	8–11	7	152	F3, 5 sets × 5–10 reps × 10–20 s @ 100–130% MAS run	5[§] vs 7[§] vs −2
Baquet *et al.*[43]	22:22:19 (77)	M & F NW-OW	8–11	7	152	F3, 5 sets × 5–10 reps × 10–20 s @ 100–130% MAS run	
Baquet *et al.*[56]	503:48	M & F NW-OW	10–16	10	35	F1[e], 2 sets × 10 reps × 10 s @ 100–120% MAS run	
Barker *et al.*[44]	10 (10)	M NW	15	2	16.5	F3, 1 set × 4–7 reps × 30 s 'all-out' cycling	5[§]
Bond *et al.*[45]	13 (16)	M & F NW-OW	13	2	54	F3, 1 set × 8–10 reps × 60 s @ 90% peak aerobic cycling power	3
Buchan *et al.*[14]	17:16:24	M & F NW-OW	16	7	54	F3, 1 set × 4–6 reps × 30 s 'all-out' running	
Buchan *et al.*[55]	42:47	M & F NW	16	7	54	F3, 1 set × 4–6 reps × 30 s 'all-out' running	
Corte de Araujo[46]	15:15 (39)	M & F OB	8–12	12	108	F2, 1 set × 3–6 reps × 60 s @ MAS run	15[§] vs 13[§]
Ingul *et al.*[47]	10:10 (20)	M & F OB	14	13	416	F2, 1 set × 4 reps × 240 s @ 90% HR_{max} run	9[§]
Koubaa *et al.*[48]	14:15	M OB	13	12	504	F3, 1 set × 7 reps × 120 s @ 80–90% MAS run	11[§] vs 5[§]
Lau *et al.*[62]	15:21:12 (48)	M & F OW	11	6	54	F3, 1 set × 12 reps × 15 s @ 120% MAS run	
Logan *et al.*[49]	5:5:6:5:5 (29)	M NW-OB	16	8	21 to 107	F2, 1–5 sets × 4 reps × 20 s 'all-out' various exercise modes	5 vs 7[§] vs 3 vs 9[§] vs 7[§]
McManus *et al.*[34]	11:12:7 (45)	F NW	9	8	72	F3, 3–6 × 10 s + 3–6 × 30 s 'all-out' running	8[§] vs 10[§] vs −2
McManus *et al.*[35]	10:10:15 (45)	F NW	10	8	84	F3, 3–6 × 10 s + 3–6 × 30 s 'all-out' cycling	11[§] vs 8[§] vs 2
Nourry *et al.*[50]	9:9 (24)	M & F NW	10	8	187	F2, 4 sets × 5–10 reps × 10–20 s @ 100–130 MAS run	16[§] vs −1
Racil *et al.*[51]	11:11:12 (36)	F OB	16	12	264	F3, 2 sets × 6–8 reps × 30 s @ 100–110 MAS run	8[§] vs 5[§] vs 1
Rosenkranz*[52]	8:8 (18)	M & F NW-OW	7–12	8	107	F2, 4 sets × 5–10 reps × 10–20 s @ 100–130 MAS run	25[§] vs −8
Rotstein *et al.*[37]	16:12 (28)	M NW	10–11	9	Not known	F3, 1–2 sets: 3 × 600-m + 5 × 400-m + 6 × 150 m, 'high' intensity running	8[§] vs 2
Tjønna† *et al.*[53]	22:20 (54)	M & F OW-OB	14	12	384	F2, 1 set × 4 reps × 240 s @ 90% HR_{max} run	9[§] vs 0 11[§] vs −1
Williams *et al.*[54]	12:13:14 (45)	M NW	10	8	72	F3, 3–6 × 10 s + 3–6 × 30 s 'all-out' running	−2 vs 5

[a] HIIT: Other training: Habitual control (starting total sample size).

[b] M—male, F—female; NW—normal weight, OW—overweight, OB—obese.

[c] Total HIIT time (does not include warm-up or cool down).

[d] Percentage changes for HIIT vs other training and/or habitual control.

[e] F—weekly training frequency (e.g., F3 = 3 sessions per week).

[§] Significant within HIIT group change.

* Low maximum heart rates suggest peak $\dot{V}O_2$ were invalid.

† Top row of results (n = 20) 3 months of HIIT; bottom row of results (n = 13) 12 months of HIIT.

was not provided, but described as being suitable to each participant's condition at baseline; it is also unclear how long it took the boys to complete the various intervals. Moreover, each training session lasted 45 min with a 15–20 min warm-up; therefore it does not fit the time-efficient model regularly characterized as HIIT. Despite these limitations, in the context of this chapter, this study was published when there was considerable doubt whether it was possible for children (i.e. preadolescents) to increase their CRF via exercise training,[57] and the mean baseline peak $\dot{V}O_2$ was an impressive 54 $mL \cdot kg^{-1} \cdot min^{-1}$. Before attempting to tease out potential moderators of HIIT effects on CRF, the focus now turns to a study[44] that adopted a very similar research design as Burgomaster *et al.*,[4] which stimulated the recent renewed interest in HIIT. In Barker *et al.*'s study[44], ten adolescent boys were exposed to only six maximal intensity cycling training sessions spanning 14 days (Table 35.2). The training progressed from 4 × 30 s 'all-out' sprints on the cycle ergometer (i.e. Wingate anaerobic tests) with 4 min active recovery in session one to seven × 30 s sprints in the final session. The change in peak $\dot{V}O_2$ was small (d = 0.30; 5%) whether expressed relative to body mass or not. Interestingly, the mean change of 2.7 $mL \cdot kg^{-1} \cdot min^{-1}$ is almost identical to that found in a recent meta-analysis of eight studies with adolescents[58] who completed between 13 and 36 HIIT sessions over 5–15 weeks. The authors[44] justified the exclusion of a control group by suggesting that growth or maturation changes would be minimal over just 2 weeks. They indicated any changes could be ascribed to HIIT because the participants agreed to suspend their habitual organized sports activities for the duration of the study; a similar argument has been posited by the same group in a different study measuring endothelial and autonomic function.[45]

Numerous potential moderators may influence the size of the HIIT-induced effect, the most obvious being the training programme components and participant characteristics or behaviours. Costigan *et al.*[58] included 20 HIIT studies with adolescents in a recent meta-analytic review, and from eight of these it was found that study duration, type of comparison group, and risk of bias were not significant moderators. The outcome of our review of studies with participants ranging from normal-weight to obese, suggests that obese participants are more likely to experience large gains in CRF following HIIT.[46–48,51,53] It was apparent that the obese participants in these studies were exposed to a greater dose (volume) of the high-intensity exercise stimulus—this was usually because the training programme extended over a longer period (minimum 12 weeks[46–48,51,53] vs. 2–9 weeks[34,35,37,44,50,55]) than in normal-weight young people coupled with a lower baseline level of fitness, which is more susceptible to change.[59] While changes in normal-weight prepubescent girls[34] and late-adolescent boys and girls[55] range from large to trivial respectively, closer scrutiny of both studies reveals that McManus *et al.*[34] only reported changes in absolute peak $\dot{V}O_2$, which may not account completely for subtle changes in body size over the 8-week training period. Buchan and colleagues[55] measured endurance performance via the 20MST rather than oxygen consumption; however, other publications by the same group, using the same training intervention, but with a heterogeneous mixed-sex sample that included healthy and overweight participants, found that changes in 20MST performance were small[14]. It should be noted that most effect sizes reported by Buchan *et al.*[14] appeared to be inflated compared with pairwise values derived from the means and standard deviations provided in their results (i.e. mean difference × $SD^{-1}_{(pooled)}$)—it is not clear how they calculated their effect sizes specifically.

A key question when examining so-called 'traditional' MCT has been whether biological maturation is an important moderator. Katch[57] hypothesized that training-induced changes in cardiovascular function could only be small before the onset of puberty because of a maturational 'trigger point', which had been proposed initially by Gilliam and Freedson[60] after scrutinizing the findings of their small mixed-sex, school-based training study. However, Shephard[61] cited early study design limitations, including inadequate sample sizes, missing control groups, poor training programme characteristics relative to baseline levels of fitness, and inadequate exposure to the training stimulus, when dismissing differences in the training response between children and adolescents. While there is now considerable evidence from MCT studies that a blunted adaptation is common in children, scrutiny of the small number of HIIT studies that have measured peak $\dot{V}O_2$ appear to be equivocal. There is considerable heterogeneity from the nine available studies with prepubertal children.[26,27,34,37,43,46,50,52,54] After randomly assigning 45 prepubertal boys equally to sprint interval training (SIT), continuous cycling training (CCT), and habitual control (CON) groups, Williams *et al.*[54] found that peak $\dot{V}O_2$ did not change meaningfully in SIT (n = 12; d = –0.11), whereas CCT experienced a small increase (n = 13; d = 0.35); as expected CON was virtually unchanged (n = 14; d = 0.04). It is possible that the relatively high baseline fitness (~55 $mL \cdot kg^{-1} \cdot min^{-1}$) of the boys contributed to this outcome; however, a direct comparison with the Rotstein study[37], where prepubertal, healthy weight boys also had a high baseline, but increased their peak VO_2 substantially, does not support this. The contrasting large (d = 1.00; ~15%) increase in peak VO_2 reported in a well-controlled study of Brazilian children by Corte de Araujo *et al.*[46] was most likely because the children were obese with very low baseline fitness (~26 $mL \cdot kg^{-1} \cdot min^{-1}$). Furthermore, the substantial inter-study difference in total HIIT times (108 min[46] vs. 72 min[54]) will have been a critical factor—the obese boys and girls also 'recovered' at 50% of their peak aerobic velocity between the high-intensity running bouts, whereas the boys in the Williams[54] study rested passively. When considering inter-study differences, the contribution of a warm-up, exercise recovery periods between repetitions, and an active cool-down should not be underestimated when they are incorporated into every training session.

The influence of participant sex on the training effect could be an important factor; however, it is very difficult to identify an independent sex effect that is not due to baseline differences in peak $\dot{V}O_2$ or maturation. The majority of HIIT studies we reviewed recruited mixed-sex samples (Tables 35.1 and 35.2) and often pooled the participants after failing to find a statistically significant sex by time interaction, which should not be interpreted as meaning the study was powered adequately from the outset. In the study with the largest sample,[55] there was an imbalance between the number of girls (n = 12) and boys (n = 30) who completed the HIIT; this is not meant as a criticism, as first-hand experience has shown that girls are more difficult to recruit than boys. The statistical analyses included power calculation details, but fell short of partitioning the sample into sub-groups to account for the independent sex effect. Only two studies were identified that included girls exclusively,[34,51] with both reporting large increases in peak $\dot{V}O_2$. Racil[51] studied obese, post-adolescent girls with a total HIIT time of 264 min, whereas McManus[34] recruited healthy-weight, prepubertal girls who accumulated 72 min of HIIT over 8 weeks; direct comparisons are obviously difficult. Hence, more research with girls is needed and their data should be analysed separately from boys' in studies designed specifically to address this intriguing question.

Total HIIT time calculated from the training characteristics included in Table 35.2 is a possible moderator. This should not be confused with volume, a composite of time and intensity, which was too complicated to estimate because of the intra- and inter-study variation in intensity. The HIIT time varied from 16.5[44]–416 min[47]—these equated to 2.75 and 16 min of exercise per training session, respectively. Despite the dichotomous training times, the effect sizes were small,[44] and small to moderate,[47] depending on the factor used to scale the peak $\dot{V}O_2$ data. This comparison is included specifically to highlight that there are a multitude of factors that determine to what extent young participants adapt when exposed to chronic exercise stimuli; the amount of training is only a single factor. About half of the studies that measured peak $\dot{V}O_2$ before and after HIIT reported a large effect[34,35,37,46,48,50,51,53], with the remaining being small to trivial (Table 35.2). A very recent study[49] was designed, using novel analytical techniques, to examine whether HIIT-training effects are dose-dependent; the final sample was twenty six 16-year-old boys assigned randomly to one of five training groups (n ≅ five per group). Each group completed 4 × 20 s near maximal effort bursts across a variety of exercise modes with the dose being titrated from one to five sets per session (i.e. 80–400 s HIIT per session), twice a week for 8 weeks. While the exercise fidelity was good, the quadratic trend used to identify the dose-adaptation explained >2% of the variance in the data. The authors highlighted the wide variation in individual responses across all five groups, despite group one doing only a fifth of the exercise volume compared with those in group five. This likely reflected large differences in baseline fitness ranging from 34–41 $mL \cdot kg^{-1} \cdot min^{-1}$. Finally, many studies rationalise HIIT training by claiming it may be more efficacious than MCT for increasing health via improvement in peak $\dot{V}O_2$; however, few include an MCT comparison group to examine this directly.[34,35,37,46,48,50,51,53] Notwithstanding difficulties in matching participant characteristics in independent groups, three studies[37,50,53] found HIIT (10.0%) was more efficacious than MCT (2.8%) and four[34,35,46,48] had similar effects HIIT (9.8%) ≅ MCT (9.5%); all of these studies were better than a habitual control group. Although Williams *et al.*[54] concluded that neither HIIT nor MCT changed peak $\dot{V}O_2$, the small MCT-induced increase (d = 0.35; 5.1%) was marginally better than HIIT (d = −0.11; −1.6%).

Body size and composition

Obesity is at the forefront of public consciousness because it is more overt than many other health problems and it has numerous disease co-morbidities.[63] It is, therefore, not surprising that measurement of various body size variables is as common in HIIT studies as CRF; in fact, researchers have questioned whether fitness or fatness may be more important from a public health perspective.[64] Most readers will be aware that changes in body size or composition, particularly adipose tissue, require longer-term exposure to an exercise-induced energy deficit; however, it is a critical adjunct to dietary intervention and lasting weight or fat loss. Most HIIT interventions in young people are between 2 and 13 weeks long, which is relatively short when considering meaningful changes in body composition; hence, of the 17 studies shown in Table 35.3, 13 found only trivial or small changes. Although some studies reported that the changes in body size were statistically significant,[49,46] the effect sizes suggest these are unlikely to be meaningful; however, it is possible that prolonged adherence to HIIT may result in changes that have long-term health implications if sustained. Ongoing growth and maturation can confound exercise interventions unless controlled adequately with well-matched comparison groups; although the HIIT group may not reduce body size or composition, it is possible that the exercise could delay changes relative to habitual controls,[55] but this has yet to be shown consistently and with adequate dietary control.

Of the studies that reported a moderate or large change in body size measures,[37,47,51,53,62] two used skinfolds[37,62] with healthy and overweight prepubertal participants, respectively. Neither controlled for habitual dietary or PA variations over the intervention period, but the relative changes (~12%) were very similar, and seemingly impressive, following only 9 and 6 weeks of HIIT. Using bioelectrical impedance analysis (BIA), 11 mixed-maturation, obese, 15-year-old girls reduced their body fat from 37% to 34% (~8%) over 12 weeks.[51] The total HIIT time (264 min) is one of the highest reported in this rare girls-only study; differences in maturation between the girls were accounted for statistically, and, although diet was measured at baseline, it was not clear if it or habitual PA changed over the 12 weeks. Racil *et al.*[51] concluded that HIIT may be a better approach to improving health in 'young women' than moderate-intensity training, but added that their study was only an important first step. The two studies from Wisløff's team, in Norway,[47,53] with obese adolescents are included here because of the large total HIIT time (~416 min) and the studies are well-designed and controlled. They are, however, considered to be proof of concept studies with small mixed-sex samples, which precludes widespread application of the results. The same HIIT protocol, consisting of 4 × 4 min bouts of uphill walking or running at 90–95% HR max per session, was completed twice a week for 3 months. In the Tjønna study[53], 13 of the 20 HIIT participants who completed the 3-month HIIT also trained at home or in a gym for a further 9 months twice a week (not included in HIIT time calculations shown in Table 35.3). Dual-energy X-ray absorptiometry (DEXA) derived measures showed that changes in body fat were small in both studies, regardless of training programme length (d ≤ −0.43; ~5%). However, a moderate effect (d = −0.67; ~7%) for waist circumference was evident after 12 months.[53] It is important to note that eight and a further seven participants were lost to follow-up after the 3-month and 12-month training periods, respectively; though, it was suggested the data did not differ from those who completed all measurements. Ingul *et al.*[47] have suggested that the objective of exercise interventions for obese adolescents should be weight stagnation rather than reduction, with subtle improvements in lean and adipose tissue; when allied with improved CRF it should be possible to 'decrease the risk of developing obesity-related comorbid conditions despite minimal weight loss'.[47(p858)]

Table 35.3 Body size, biochemical metabolites, and vascular health: prospective high-intensity interval training studies with children and adolescents that included a comparison with either an untrained control or at least two different training programmes (only high-intensity interval training group results displayed for biochemical metabolites).

Citation	Body size (Δ%)[a]	Biochemical metabolites (Δ%)[a]						Vascular health (Δ%)[a]		
		Glu[b]	Ins	TAG	HDL	LDL	TC	SBP	DBP	FMD
Baquet *et al.*[26]	%BF −4 vs −3									
Baquet *et al.*[27]	%BF 1 vs 1									
Baquet *et al.*[43]	BMI 1 vs 1 vs −2									
Baquet *et al.*[56]	%BF 9 vs 6									
Barker *et al.*[44]	BMI <1							1	3	
Bond *et al.*[45]		0	<1	−8	5	−5	−2	−2 & 0	−11 & −11	F 15§ & 15§ P 29§ & 17§
Buchan *et al.*[14]	%BF −3 vs −11§ vs 0	−9	112	65§	20	−24	3	−5 vs −4 vs −4	−3 vs 0 vs −6	
Buchan* *et al.*[55]	WC <1 vs 2	2	8	10	21	−44§	−16	−4§ vs −3	−1 vs −6	
Corte de Araujo[46]	%BF −3 vs −3	−3	−29§	−10	7	2	<1	−8§ vs 0	−6 vs −8	
Ingul *et al.*[47]	%BF −5§							−6§	−13§	
Koubaa *et al.*[48]	WC −2			−6§	4§	−2	−1	−2§ vs −2§	−3§ vs −2	
Lau *et al.*[62]	ΣSF −14§ vs −1 vs 8§									
Logan *et al.*[49]	−1 vs −4§ vs −6§ vs −2 vs −6§							−6§ to 5§	−13§ to 3	
Nourry *et al.*[50]	%BF −8 vs −3									
Racil* *et al.*[51]	%BF −8§ vs −5§ vs −1	−2	−27§	−7§	6§	−12§	−7§			
Rosenkranz[52]	%BF −10 vs −4	6	-	−17	22	−36§	−13§	−2 vs −2	−4 vs −2	
Tjønna† *et al.*[53]	%BF −12§ vs −3§	−6§	−29§	−11	10			−7§ vs −2§	−8§ vs −3	5§ vs 4
	%BF −3§ vs <1	−6§	−34§	−18	10			−6§ vs −4§	−7§ vs −1	6§ vs 1

Participant and training characteristics are displayed in Table 34.2.

[a] HIIT vs other training and/or habitual control.

[b] All fasting: Glu—glucose, Ins—insulin, TAG—triacylglycerol, HDL & LDL—high & low density lipoprotein cholesterol, TC—total cholesterol.

* Plasma metabolites presented to only one decimal place, which may have led to inflated %Δ estimations.

§ Significant within HIIT group change.

† Top row of results (n=20) 3 months of HIIT; bottom row of results (n=13) 12 months of HIIT.

Biochemical metabolites

We identified eight HIIT studies that included blood samples (Table 35.3); due to the wide array of metabolites measured in these studies, we attempt to identify study or participant characteristics that may have exerted a meaningful influence on the results. Racil *et al.*'s[51] study with obese adolescent girls stands out for its numerous adaptations indicative of improved physical health (see Tables 35.2 and 35.3). Large ($d \geq 0.80$), significant reductions in fasting concentrations of insulin ($d = -2.78$; 27%), triacylglycerol (TAG) ($d = -0.83$; 7%), low-density lipoprotein cholesterol (LDL-C) ($d = -1.29$; 12%), total cholesterol (TC) ($d = -1.17$; 7%) and homeostatic model assessment for insulin resistance (HOMA-IR) ($d = -2.28$; 30%) were found; whereas, high-density lipoprotein cholesterol (HDL-C) increased ($d = 1.20$; 6%) over the 12 weeks. In contrast, a small reduction in fasting glucose concentration was reported ($d = -0.23$), which is a common finding in the other HIIT studies reviewed.[14,45,49,55] The only exception was Tjønna *et al.*,[53] who reported meaningful reductions in obese adolescents after 3 and 12 months of training; this study measured both fasting glucose and after an oral glucose load test ($d = -0.58$ to -0.94). Meaningful reductions in fasting insulin[46,53] and HOMA-IR[46] were also reported in other studies with obese participants who completed HIIT programmes with total exercise times ranging from 108–416 min. This improvement in glucose control and insulin sensitivity is less likely to be experienced by participants who are relatively healthy at the start of short interventions.[14,45,55]

Changes in the lipid profile varied considerably across the studies, which will be a function of the large day-to-day variability[65] (particularly for triacylglycerol concentration), baseline concentrations, and total training time, but the small group of HIIT studies provide little empirical direction on moderators. Half (four) of the HIIT studies that estimated changes in LDL-C reported significant reductions, with effects ranging from small[49] to large.[51,52] Only the obese boys who completed the running programme by Koubaa *et al.*[48] had a moderate (d = 0.78; 4%) increase in HDL-C, which was similar in relative terms to Racil's[51] girls above. However, a lack of dietary control means it is not possible to be certain changes were exercise-induced in this Tunisian study.[48] Measurement of high-sensitivity C-reactive protein (hs-CRP), adiponectin, and interleukin 6 (IL-6) are still rare in HIIT studies with young people,[14,49,51,53,55] and the results are inconsistent. For example, effect sizes for adiponectin range from −1.41 (51% reduction)[14] to 2.43 (34% increase);[51] although an increase in this adipose tissue derived adipokine has been found in obese adults undergoing chronic exercise training, it has not been shown consistently.[66] Only Logan[49] reported a significant increase in IL-6 across their five small training groups, ranging from 5 to 62%, but the omnibus effect size (d = 0.45) probably underestimated within-group pairwise effects. Two separate studies by Buchan *et al.*[14,55] reported small reductions (d ≤ −0.35) in IL-6 after 54 min of HIIT spanning 7 weeks. Finally, only two studies[45,49] stated explicitly that their post-intervention measures were completed at least 48 h after the final training session to ensure the results reflected a chronic training adaptation rather than an acute, last exercise bout response. It is unfortunate that this important design feature is rarely built into the studies, which means it is difficult to differentiate acute responses from chronic adaptations.

Vascular health

In this final health-related sub-section, we examine HIIT-induced adaptations in blood pressure and endothelial function (flow mediated dilation; FMD). Although blood pressure is often measured in exercise studies with young people, endothelial function is still considered a 'novel' cardiovascular disease (CVD) risk factor that may precede changes in more 'traditional' risk factors in the atherosclerotic pathway[67] (interested readers are referred to Chapter 17 for further discussion of cardiovascular disease risk factors). Significant decreases in systolic blood pressure (SBP) are reported in the majority of HIIT studies (Table 35.3); the magnitude of effects are small,[55] moderate,[14,47,53] and large[46,48] (d = −0.36 to −1.00; 2 to 8%). Higher baseline SBP (≥125 mmHg) in obese young people who experienced the greatest total HIIT times (>100 min), or longest training programmes (>12 weeks), appear to be requisite characteristics for meaningful reductions in SBP. Although fewer studies found significant or meaningful reductions in diastolic blood pressure (DBP), there were those that managed to supervise their young obese or overweight charges through HIIT programmes lasting at least 12 weeks[47,48,53] (Table 35.3).

Tjønna *et al.*[53] used high-resolution vascular ultrasound to measure FMD with random, investigator-blinded analyses in their study of obese boys and girls. They reported improvements of 5.1% and 6.3% above baseline after 3 and 12 months of training, respectively; this compared well with the multidisciplinary training group (3.9% and return to baseline) who experienced standard clinical practice over the same period. The authors linked concomitant changes in HDL-C, blood glucose, and insulin with enhanced bioavailability of nitrous oxide (NO), the primary regulator of endothelial function, and large increases in the anti-inflammatory hormone adiponectin. Importantly, they hypothesized that exercise training improves endothelial function regardless of changes in body size providing CRF improved—this may be a very important strategy to consider when helping overweight or obese young people to choose to exercise regularly. Also from Norway, Ingul *et al.*[47] designed a HIIT study to see if it 'corrected' impaired measures of resting and exercise cardiac function in obese adolescents when compared with a lean group of age and sex-matched 13–16-year-olds. Interested readers are encouraged to refer to the publication directly to access the methods, which are too detailed to include here; the Dubois body surface area (m^2) formula[68] was used to scale cardiac dimensions for between group differences in body size. The 32 min of HIIT per week over 3 months increased most measures of systolic function and left ventricular (LV) volumes that were impaired originally so that pre-training obese vs. lean group differences were eradicated; these included large effects for stroke volume index (d = 1.13), global strain rate (d = 1.94), fractional shortening (d = 1.22), and peak systolic tissue velocity (S`; d = 1.00). In contrast, LV end-systolic volume and cardiac output were virtually unchanged. Similarly, significant HIIT-induced normalization of diastolic function in the obese group was seen, with large effects for deceleration time (DT; d = −1.33) and isovolumetric relaxation time (IVRT; d = −0.81). Echo with Tissue Doppler and Doppler flow velocities revealed pre-intervention impaired mitral annulus excursion (MAE; 24%), flow velocity time integral of the LV outflow tract (16%), global strain rate (32%), global strain (22%), and peak early tissue Doppler velocity (18%) in the obese versus lean at both rest and exercise. However, most of these impairments were resolved following HIIT with small to moderate, non-significant differences (d ≤ −0.62) between the obese and lean groups. Although the difference in global strain was more than halved, it was still large (d = −0.90) and in favour of the lean participants (~8.5%). In contrast, MAE improved to such an extent at rest that it was slightly higher in the obese group (d = 0.77). Despite these very promising changes in the exercise-trained obese adolescents, the authors[47] highlighted that they need to be replicated in a multicentre study with a representative sample and intent-to-treat research design.

The very low-volume HIIT used by Bond and colleagues[45] consisted of just six training sessions spread over 2 weeks, similar to previously published studies with sedentary[69] and type-2 diabetic adults.[70] The study was designed so that it was possible to separate the acute response from the last exercise session, and the chronic 2-week training adaptation by including pre-exercise, 1-day post-exercise, and 3-day post-exercise measurements; however, a non-exercise-matched control group was not included due to the brevity of the training period. Statistically significant changes ($P \leq 0.04$) in FMD, baseline arterial diameter, and heart rate variability (HRV) were found; effect sizes ranged from small to large (d = 0.39–0.97). The 1-day post-exercise effects were larger than those found 3 days after the last exercise training session (compared with the pre-exercise baseline). There were also some subtle, but noteworthy, differences between fasting and postprandial measures, which could mean post-meal measurements provide a more insightful window to metabolism than overnight fasting conditions. The postprandial reductions in FMD and HRV were expected given the test breakfast meal had a very high energy content of 7134 kJ (~1704 kcal) amounting to a large proportion (≥82%) of the samples' measured mean daily energy intakes. The authors highlighted the primary study outcomes as: i) a HIIT-induced improvement in endothelial function and HRV in boys and girls; ii) changes in novel and traditional CVD risk factors may occur independently; and iii) the changes (Δ) in endothelial function and HRV were transient (%Δ1-day > %Δ3-day), which suggest their findings may reflect an acute response from the last exercise training bout rather than a chronic physiological or metabolic adaptation.

Time efficiency and enjoyment of high-intensity interval training

Two commonly cited potential advantages of HIIT, compared with MCT, are the purported time-efficiency of the exercise modality and the enjoyment associated with this form of training. Although the amount of time spent exercising (i.e. actively engaged in power-producing activity) during HIIT is relatively small, it is questionable how much time may actually be 'saved' by this form of exercise, especially when one considers the time committed to an appropriate warm-up, active or passive recovery between interval repetitions and, finally, post-session recovery. The importance of exercise volume, per se, and the impact this may have on long-term exercise adherence, should not be dismissed; it may represent an interesting avenue for future research with young people.

Physical activity enjoyment has been identified as a consistent predictor of childhood PA levels.[71] Unfortunately, very little research exists that has quantified exercise enjoyment during HIIT with young people. Encouragingly, however, evidence derived from studies conducted with adults suggests that HIIT may be a more enjoyable form of exercise, compared with continuous, steady-state exercise of a lower intensity.[70,72,73,74] Furthermore, a recent study conducted with children indicates that the perceived enjoyment of steady-state exercise may be increased by the addition of intermittent all-out sprints, despite the latter exercise resulting in a greater total amount of work compared to steady-state exercise alone.[12] Although additional research is required to confirm this finding, it raises important questions surrounding the optimal manipulation of exercise intensity and duration to maximize enjoyment and adherence during childhood and adolescence. Longitudinal experimental studies are undoubtedly warranted to examine perceived enjoyment during HIIT as well as adherence to this form of exercise over a prolonged period of time. Such studies may also provide valuable insight into the extent to which this form of exercise training can be tolerated and sustained by young people. They may also help to further delineate the priority that should be afforded to this form of training.

Conclusions

It is clear from our comprehensive search and critical appraisal of the literature that research examining the efficacy of HIIT in young people is still in its infancy. Nevertheless, there are some promising findings for sports performance and health outcome measures. However, these are all based on training studies that are limited by their brevity and need to be followed up with longer studies involving both male and female children and adolescents in more representative samples. There is insufficient evidence to suggest that young people, even highly motivated athletes, can sustain such high-intensity exercise over longer than 3 consecutive months and retain their interest, motivation, and enjoyment while remaining free from exercise training-induced injury. These issues must be addressed systematically before we can be confident in prescribing this type of training for performance or health gains in young people.

Summary

- Inclusion of high-intensity interval training (HIIT) in programmes for young athletes may complement moderate continuous activity in light of widespread non-compliance with the current international recommendations for physical activity in young people.
- Despite recent growth in the number of scientific studies examining the efficacy of HIIT in young people, longitudinal studies are rare; these studies have focused on both sports performance and health outcomes with athletes and non-athletes. This dual focus reflects the continued interest in maximizing sports performance, but also the growing concern about perceived low levels of cardiometabolic fitness and the high proportion of young people who are overweight or obese, with related co-morbidities, in this segment of the population.
- Cardiorespiratory fitness, defined as peak $\dot{V}O_2$, has been the most popular outcome measure of sports performance and health-related studies with young people. High-intensity interval training can increase peak $\dot{V}O_2$ meaningfully, but whether it is better than alternative exercise regimes has yet to be confirmed reliably. Longer-term studies, which include comprehensive, valid measures of compliance, injuries, and enjoyment are required.
- Explosive strength (power) gains following HIIT in young athletes are small to moderate, but do not appear to be impaired. Recovery time, built into individual training sessions and cycles, should be considered carefully when leading into competitive performance.
- The effects of HIIT on direct measures of sports performance are limited to only a few studies and the results suggest that the gains are moderate at best. However, it should be recognized that even small gains in performance for young people who are already well-trained may be meaningful if maintained and applied consistently.
- Changes in body size and composition following HIIT have, typically, been trivial to small, which reflects study design more than the efficacy of the training, per se. This is because HIIT has only been prescribed typically from 2 to 13 weeks in the scientific literature.
- The few studies which take blood samples before and after HIIT make it difficult to identify any trends in the variety of biochemical metabolites investigated; reductions in fasting insulin and LDL-C are promising findings to date, particularly in obese girls and boys. However, these need to be verified in larger studies extended over longer periods.
- Finally, three HIIT studies have focused on vascular health; unsurprisingly, they are dependent on the baseline levels of the outcome variables like systolic blood pressure and cardiac function. Again, more well-controlled research is required to reach firmer conclusions.

References

1. Gibala MJ, Little JP, MacDonald MJ, Hawley JA. Physiological adaptations to low-volume, high-intensity interval training in health and disease. *J Physiol.* 2012; 590: 1077–1084.
2. Beaglehole R, Bonita R, Horton R, *et al.* Priority actions for the non-communicable disease crisis. *Lancet.* 2011; 377: 1438–1447.
3. Tabata I, Irisawa K, Kouzaki M, Nishimura K, Ogita F, Miyachi M. Metabolic profile of high intensity intermittent exercises. *Med Sci Sports Exerc.* 1997; 29: 390–395.
4. Burgomaster KA, Hughes SC, Heigenhauser GJF, Bradwell SN, Gibala MJ. Six sessions of sprint interval training increases muscle oxidative potential and cycle endurance capacity in humans. *J Appl Physiol.* 2005; 98: 1985–1990.
5. Gibala, MJ, Little JP, van Essen M, *et al.* Short-term sprint interval versus traditional endurance training: similar initial adaptations in human skeletal muscle and exercise performance. *J. Physiol.* 2006; 575: 901–911.
6. Babraj JA, Vollaard NB, Keast C, Guppy FM, Cottrell G, Timmons JA. Extremely short duration high intensity interval training substantially improves insulin action in young healthy males. *BMC Endocr Disord.* 2009; 9: 3
7. Gibala MJ. High-intensity interval training: a time-efficient strategy for health promotion? *Curr Sports Med Rep.* 2007: 6: 211–213.
8. Trost SG, Owen N, Bauman AE, Sallis JF, Brown W. Correlates of adults' participation in physical activity: review and update. *Med Sci Sports Exerc.* 2002; 34: 1996–2001.
9. Buchheit M, Laursen P. High-intensity interval training, solutions to the programming puzzle: Part 1: cardiopulmonary emphasis. *Sports Med.* 2013; 43: 313–338.
10. Hebestreit H, Mimura, K, Bar-Or O. Recovery of muscle power after high intensity short-term exercise: Comparing boys and men. *J Appl Physiol.* 1993; 74: 2875–2880.
11. Bailey RC, Olson J, Pepper SL, Porszasz J, Barstow TJ, Cooper DM. The level and tempo of children's physical activities: an observation study. *Med Sci Sports Exerc.* 1995; 27: 1033–1041.
12. Crisp NA, Fournier PA, Licari MK, Braham R, Guelfi KJ. Adding sprints to continuous exercise at the intensity that maximises fat oxidation: implications for acute energy balance and enjoyment. *Metabolism.* 2012; 61: 1280–1288.
13. Hallal PC, Andersen LB, Bull FC, Guthold R, Haskell W, Ekelund U. Global physical activity levels: surveillance progress, pitfalls, and prospects. *Lancet.* 2012; 380(9838): 247–257.
14. Buchan DS, Ollis S, Young JD, *et al.* The effects of time and intensity of exercise on novel and established markers of CVD in adolescent youth. *Am J Hum Biol.* 2011; 23: 517–26.
15. Billat LV. Interval training for performance: a scientific and empirical practice. Special recommendations for middle- and long-distance running. Part I: aerobic interval training. *Sports Med.* 2001; 31: 13–31.
16. Billat LV. Interval training for performance: a scientific and empirical practice. Special recommendations for middle- and long-distance running. Part II: anaerobic interval training. *Sports Med.* 2001; 31: 75–90.
17. Laursen PB, Jenkins DG. The scientific basis for high-intensity interval training: optimising training programmes and maximising performance in highly trained endurance athletes. *Sports Med.* 2002; 32: 53–73.
18. Bishop D, Girard O, Mendez-Villanueva A. Repeated sprint ability. Part II: recommendations for training. *Sports Med.* 2011; 41: 741–756.
19. Iaia FM, Bangsbo J. Speed endurance training is a powerful stimulus for physiological adaptations and performance improvements of athletes. *Scand J Med Sci Sports.* 2010; 20(Suppl 2): 11–23.
20. Cohen J. *Statistical power analysis for the behavioural sciences*, 2nd ed. Hillsdale, NJ: Lawrence Erlbaum Associates; 1988.
21. Londeree BR. Effect of training on lactate/ventilatory thresholds: a meta-analysis. *Med Sci Sports Exerc.* 1997; 29: 837–843.
22. Costill DL, Flynn MG, Kirman JP, *et al.* Effects of repeated days of intensified training on muscle glycogen and swimming performance. *Med Sci Sports Exerc.* 1988; 20: 249–254.
23. Lake MJ, Cavanagh PR. Six weeks of training does not change running mechanics or improve running economy. *Med Sci Sports Exerc.* 1996; 28: 860–869.
24. Chamari K, Hachana Y, Kaouech F, Jeddi R, Moussa-Chamari I, Wisløff U. Endurance training and testing with the ball in young elite soccer players. *Br J Sports Med.* 2005; 39: 24–28.
25. McMillan K, Helgerud J, Macdonald R, Hoff J, *et al.* Physiological adaptations to soccer specific endurance training in professional youth soccer players. *Br J Sports Med.* 2005; 39: 273–277.
26. Baquet G, Berthoin S, Dupont G, Blondel N, Fabre C, Van Praagh E. Effects of high intensity intermittent training on peak VO(2) in prepubertal children. *Int J Sports Med.* 2002; 23: 439–444.
27. Baquet G, Guinhouya C, Dupont G, Nourry C, Berthoin S. Effects of a short-term interval training program on physical fitness in prepubertal children. *J Strength Cond Res.* 2004; 18: 708–713.
28. Breil FA, Weber SN, Koller S, Hoppeler H, Vogt M. Block training periodization in alpine skiing: effects of 11-day HIT on $\dot{V}O_2$max and performance. *Eur J Appl Physiol.* 2010; 109: 1077–1086.
29. Buchheit M, Laursen PB, Kuhnle J, Ruch D, Renaud C, Ahmaidi S. Game-based training in young elite handball players. *Int J Sports Med.* 2009; 30: 251–258.
30. Buchheit M, Mendez-Villanueva A, Delhomel G, Brughelli M, Ahmaidi S. Improving repeated sprint ability in young elite soccer players: repeated sprints vs. explosive strength training. *J Strength Cond Res.* 2010; 24: 2715–2722.
31. Delextrat A, Martinez A. Small-sided game training improves aerobic capacity and technical skills in basketball players. *Int J Sports Med.* 2014; 35: 385–391.
32. Faude O, Meyer T, Scharhag J, Weins F, Urhausen A, Kindermann W. Volume vs. intensity in the training of competitive swimmers. *Int J Sports Med.* 2008; 29: 906–912.
33. Impellizzeri FM, Marcora SM, Castagna C, *et al.* Physiological and performance effects of generic versus specific aerobic training in soccer players. *Int J Sports Med.* 2006; 27: 483–492.
34. McManus AM, Armstrong N, Williams CA. Effect of training on the aerobic power and anaerobic performance of prepubertal girls. *Acta Paediatr.* 1997; 86: 456–459.
35. McManus AM, Cheng CH, Leung MP, Yung TC, Macfarlane DJ. Improving aerobic power in primary school boys: a comparison of continuous and interval training. *Int J Sports Med.* 2005; 26: 781–786.
36. Meckel Y, Gefen Y, Nemet D, Eliakim A. Influence of short versus long repetition sprint training on selected fitness components in young soccer players. *J Strength Cond Res.* 2012; 26: 1845–1851.
37. Rotstein A, Dotan R, Bar-Or O, Tenenbaum G. Effect of training on anaerobic threshold, maximal aerobic power and anaerobic performance of preadolescent boys. *Int J Sports Med.* 1986; 7: 281–286.
38. Sperlich B, Zinner C, Heilemann I, Kjendlie PL, Holmberg HC, Mester J. High-intensity interval training improves $\dot{V}O_2$ peak, maximal lactate accumulation, time trial and competition performance in 9–11-year-old swimmers. *Eur J Appl Physiol.* 2010; 110: 1029–1036.
39. Sperlich B, De Marées M, Koehler K, Linville J, Holmberg HC, Mester J. Effects of 5 weeks of high-intensity interval training vs. volume training in 14-year-old soccer players. *J Strength Cond Res.* 2011; 25: 1271–1278.
40. Wahl P, Zinner C, Grosskopf C, Rossmann R, Bloch W, Mester J. Passive recovery is superior to active recovery during a high-intensity shock microcycle. *J Strength Cond Res.* 2013; 27: 1384–1393.
41. Balsom P. Evaluation of physical performance. In: Ekblom B (ed.) *Football (soccer).* Oxford: Blackwell Scientific Publications; 1994. p. 102–123.
42. Currell K, Jeukendrup AE. Validity, reliability and sensitivity of measures of sporting performance. *Sports Med.* 2008; 38: 297–316.
43. Baquet G, Gamelin FX, Mucci P, Thévenet D, Van Praagh E, Berthoin S. Continuous vs. interval aerobic training in 8- to 11-year-old children. *J Strength Cond Res.* 2010; 24: 1381–1388.

44. Barker AR, Day J, Smith A, Bond B, Williams CA. The influence of 2 weeks of low-volume high-intensity interval training on health outcomes in adolescent boys. *J Sports Sci.* 2014; 32: 757–765.
45. Bond B, Cockcroft EJ, Williams CA, *et al.* Two weeks of high-intensity interval training improves novel but not traditional cardiovascular disease risk factors in adolescents. *Am J Physiol Heart Circ Physiol.* 2015; 309: H1039–H1047.
46. Corte de Araujo AC, Roschel H, Picanço AR, *et al.* Similar health benefits of endurance and high-intensity interval training in obese children. *PLOS One.* 2012; 7: e42747.
47. Ingul CB, Tjønna AE, Stolen TO, Stoylen A, Wisløff U. Impaired cardiac function among obese adolescents: effect of aerobic interval training. *Arch Pediatr Adolesc Med.* 2010; 164: 852–859.
48. Koubaa A, Trabelsi H, Masmoudi L, *et al.* Effect of intermittent and continuous training on body composition cardio-respiratory fitness and lipid profile in obese adolescents. *IOSR-JPBS.* 2013; 3: 31–37.
49. Logan GR, Harris N, Duncan S, Plank LD, Merien F, Schofield G. Low-active male adolescents: A dose response to high-intensity interval training. *Med Sci Sports Exerc.* 2016; 48: 481–490.
50. Nourry C, Deruelle F, Guinhouva C, *et al.* High-intensity intermittent running training improves pulmonary function and alters exercise breathing pattern in children. *Eur J Appl Physiol.* 2005; 94: 415–423.
51. Racil G, Ben Ounis O, Hammouda O, *et al.* Effects of high vs. moderate exercise intensity during interval training on lipids and adiponectin levels in obese young females. *Eur J Appl Physiol.* 2013; 113: 2531–2540.
52. Rosenkranz S K, Rosenkranz, RR, Hastmann TJ, Harms CA. High-intensity training improves airway responsiveness in inactive nonasthmatic children: Evidence from a randomized controlled trial. *J Appl Physiol.* 2012; 112: 1174–1183.
53. Tjønna AE, Stølen TO, Bye A, *et al.* Aerobic interval training reduces cardiovascular risk factors more than a multi-treatment approach in overweight adolescents. *Clin Sci (Lond).* 2009; 116: 317–326.
54. Williams CA, Armstrong N, Powell J. Aerobic responses of prepubertal boys to two modes of training. *Br J Sports Med.* 2000; 34: 168–173.
55. Buchan DS, Ollis S, Young JD, Cooper SM, Shield JP, Baker JS. High intensity interval running enhances measures of physical fitness but not metabolic measures of cardiovascular disease risk in healthy adolescents. *BMC Public Health.* 2013; 13: 498.
56. Baquet G, Berthoin S, Gerbeaux M, Van Praagh E. High-intensity aerobic training during a 10-week one-hour physical education cycle: effects on physical fitness of adolescents aged 11 to 16. *Int J Sports Med.* 2001; 22: 295–300.
57. Katch VL. Physical conditioning of children. *J Adolesc Health Care.* 1983; 3: 241–246.
58. Costigan SA, Eather N, Plotnikoff RC, Taaffe DR, Lubans DR. High-intensity interval training for improving health-related fitness in adolescents: a systematic review and meta-analysis. *Br J Sports Med.* 2015; 49: 1253–1261.
59. Tolfrey K. (2007). Responses to training. In: Armstrong N (ed.) *Paediatric exercise physiology*. London: Elsevier; 2007. p. 213–234.
60. Gilliam TB, Freedson PS. Effects of a 12-week school physical fitness program on peak $\dot{V}O_2$, body composition and blood lipids in 7 to 9 year old children. *J Sports Med.* 1980; 1: 73–78.
61. Shephard RJ. Effectiveness of training programmes for prepubescent children. *Sports Med.* 1992; 13: 194–213.
62. Lau PWC, Wong del P, Ngo JK, Liang Y, Kim CG, Kim HS. Effects of high-intensity intermittent running exercise in overweight children. *Eur J Sport Sci.* 2015; 15: 182–190.
63. Lobstein T, Jackson-Leach R. Estimated burden of paediatric obesity and co-morbidities in Europe. Part 2. Numbers of children with indicators of obesity-related disease. *Int J Pediatr Obes.* 2006; 1: 33–41.
64. Barry VW, Baruth M, Beets MW, Durstine JL, Liu J, Blair SN. Fitness vs fatness on all-cause mortality: a meta-analysis. *Prog Cardiovasc Dis.* 2014; 56: 382–391.
65. Tolfrey K, Campbell IG, Jones AM. Intra-individual variation of plasma lipids and lipoproteins in prepubescent children. *Eur J Appl Physiol.* 1999; 79: 449–456.
66. Lee S, Kwak HB. Effects of interventions on adiponectin and adiponectin receptors. *J Exerc Rehabil.* 2014; 10: 60–68.
67. Juonala M, Viikari JS, Laitinen T, *et al.* Interrelations between brachial endothelial function and carotid intima-media thickness in young adults: the Cardiovascular Risk in Young Finns study. *Circulation.* 2004; 110: 2918–2923.
68. DuBois D, DuBois EF. A formula to estimate the approximate surface area if height and weight be known. *Arch Intern Medicine.* 1916; 17: 863–871.
69. Hood MS, Little JP, Tarnopolsky MA, Myslik F, Gibala MJ. Low-volume interval training improves muscle oxidative capacity in sedentary adults. *Med Sci Sports Exerc.* 2011; 43: 1849–1856.
70. Little JP, Gillen JB, Percival ME, *et al.* Low-volume high intensity interval training reduces hyperglycemia and increases muscle mitochondrial capacity in patients with type 2 diabetes. *J Appl Physiol.* 2011; 111: 1554–1560.
71. DiLorenzo TM, Stucky-Ropp RC, Vander Wal JS, Gotham HJ. Determinants of exercise among children. II. A longitudinal analysis. *Prev Med.* 1998; 27: 470–477.
72. Boyd JC, Simpson CA, Jung ME, Gurd BJ. Reducing the intensity and volume of interval training diminishes cardiovascular adaptation but not mitochondrial biogenesis in overweight/obese men. *PLOS One.* 2013; 8: e68091.
73. Bartlett JD, Close GL, MacLaren DP, Gregson W, Drust B, Morton JP. High-intensity interval running is perceived to be more enjoyable than moderate intensity continuous exercise: implications for exercise adherence. *J Sports Sci.* 2011; 29: 547–553.
74. Jung ME, Little JP, Gillen J, Gibala MJ. It's not too hard! Perceived enjoyment for high-intensity interval training in type 2 diabetes. *Med Sci Sports Exerc.* 2011; 43(Suppl 1): 20.

CHAPTER 36

Resistance training

Avery D Faigenbaum and Rhodri S Lloyd

Introduction

Resistance training can be a safe and effective method of conditioning for children and adolescents, provided the programme is supervised by qualified professionals and consistent with the needs, interests, and abilities of youth. While much of what we understand about the stimulus of resistance exercise has been gained from research on adults, a compelling body of evidence indicates that regular participation in a developmentally appropriate resistance-training programme offers observable health and fitness benefits to children and adolescents.[1–3] Although some observers questioned the safety and efficacy of youth resistance training in the 1980s and 1990s, new perspectives for promoting resistance exercise as part of a long-term approach to youth physical development highlight the importance of integrating resistance training into youth fitness programmes.[1,4,7]

Youth who fail to enhance their muscular strength and motor skill proficiency early in life may not be prepared to achieve global recommendations of at least 60 min of daily moderate to vigorous physical activity (MVPA).[6,8] Youth with muscular weakness or low motor coordination tend to have less confidence and competence in their physical abilities, which in turn, limits participation in exercise, games, and sport activities.[9–12] Conversely, youth with higher levels of muscular fitness (i.e. muscular strength, muscular power, and local muscular endurance) are more likely to develop the functional capacities that will enable them to pursue a variety of health-enhancing PA as an ongoing lifestyle choice.[3,12,13] The specific effects of resistance training on performance enhancement and injury risk reduction in athletes highlight the importance of exposing modern day youth to well-designed interventions that include resistance training exercises.[14–18]

Researchers and practitioners have expanded our understanding of the effects of resistance exercise on children and adolescents and a growing number of school-age youth are participating in resistance-training programmes in schools, fitness facilities, and sport centres. The qualified acceptance of youth resistance training by medical, fitness, and sports organizations has become widespread, and public health objectives now aim to increase the number of children and adolescents who regularly perform PA that enhances muscular fitness.[2,19–21] In response to the growing need to develop healthy, capable, and resilient young athletes, the International Olympic Committee (IOC) recognizes the importance of resistance training early in life to develop fitness, enhance athleticism, and foster positive skill development.[19] This chapter uses the term resistance training to mean a specialized method of conditioning that involves the progressive use of a wide range of resistive loads, different movement velocities, and a variety of training modalities, including weight machines, free weights (barbells and dumbbells), medicine balls, elastic bands, and body weight.

Resistance training and physical development

A contemporary corollary of the sedentariness among modern day youth is a lower level of muscular fitness and motor skill development.[22–25] Research examining secular trends in muscular fitness in English children showed declines in bent arm hang, sit-up performance, and handgrip strength over a 10-year period.[22] Similar trends were observed in selected measures of motor fitness (e.g. shuttle run and plate tapping) in Dutch primary school children[23] and muscular power (e.g. long jump and vertical jump) in Spanish adolescents.[24] Australian researchers reported low levels of motor skill competence in school-age youth and noted a clear and consistent association between low competency in motor skills and inadequate levels of cardiorespiratory fitness.[25] Although cross-sectional data from a random sample of school-age youth were used to analyse secular trends in physical fitness in these reports, these data illustrate the troubling impact of modern-day lifestyles on selected measures of muscular fitness and motor skill performance in school-age youth.

Without interventions that target deficits in muscular fitness early in life, these trends will likely continue and the gap between youth with low and high levels of motor skill competence will widen across developmental time.[11,26,27] This divergence in physical performance during the growing years may prevent relatively weaker youth from catching up with peers who possess average or high levels of relative strength and motor skill prowess.[28,29] In support of this contention, a 2-year investigation of 501 children between 6 and 10 years of age found that low motor-competent children participated less in sports and had fewer opportunities for developing motor abilities and physical fitness.[9] Others reported that children with a low or average rate of change in their developmental pathways of fitness and motor competence were several times more prone to become overweight or obese at the end of primary school, independent of sex and body mass index at baseline.[27]

Many chronic diseases that become clinically evident during adulthood originate in childhood when lifestyle habits such as PA (and physical inactivity) are established and engrained.[30,31] These findings highlight the need to re-focus efforts on the prevention of adverse health outcomes early in life before youth become resistant to targeted interventions later in life. Youth with inadequate levels of muscular strength and movement skill competency may be less likely to participate in school- and community-based exercise and sport programmes with energy, interest, and enthusiasm.[9,32–34]

Moreover, children at the highest risk of injury during physical education, leisure-time activities, or sport tend to have the lowest levels of habitual PA.[35] Without regular opportunities to engage in structured (e.g. exercise class) and unstructured (e.g. outdoor play) strength-building activities with ongoing support from teachers, coaches, parents, and peers, children and young people will be more likely to experience negative health outcomes, and less likely to enhance their long-term physical development.

Effectiveness of youth resistance training

An understanding of the effectiveness of resistance exercise will assist in the design of training programmes that optimize long-term adaptations. Provided that resistance training programmes are of sufficient intensity, volume, and duration, children and adolescents can significantly improve their muscular fitness above and beyond growth and development.[2,36,37] Research shows that boys and girls have benefited from participation in a resistance-training programme and different combinations of programme variables have proven to be effective.[38–44] Well-designed youth exercise programmes grounded in resistance training may help fill the critical need for children and adolescents to maximize long-term physical development while minimizing the risk of activity-related injury.

It can be expected that active children and adolescents will show noticeable gains in height, weight, and measures of physical fitness during the developmental years, even without participation in a structured resistance-training programme. For example, muscular strength normally increases from childhood through the early adolescent years, at which time there is a marked acceleration in strength in boys and a general plateau in strength in girls.[45] However, a child or adolescent who participates in a resistance-training programme will have better strength performance at any age when compared to an age-matched peer who does not participate in this type of training.[41,44,46–49] Moreover, youth fitness programmes that include exercises that are purposely designed to enhance muscle fitness will likely set the stage for even greater gains in strength and power later in life.

Physiological mechanisms for strength development

Data from several research studies indicate that neuromuscular adaptations (i.e. a trend towards increased motor unit activation and changes in motor unit coordination, recruitment, and firing) and possibly intrinsic muscle adaptations (as evidenced by increases in twitch torque) appear to be primarily responsible for training-induced strength gains during preadolescence.[50–52] Others found a decrease in electromechanical delay (time between the onset of muscle activity and force) following 8 weeks of progressive resistance training in children,[49] and improvements in leg stiffness in response to a 4-week plyometric training intervention.[43] Gains in motor-skill performance and the coordination of the involved muscle groups may also play a significant role because both neural and mechanical factors influence force production in children.[53]

Improvements in movement coordination are likely a more important contributor to training-induced gains if the exercises include complex movements (e.g. weightlifting exercises) rather than isolated muscle actions. Although there is a possibility that training-induced anabolism may contribute to observed strength gains during preadolescence, it appears that children appear to experience more difficulty increasing their muscle mass in response to resistance training.[51,52] Muscle hypertrophy is more common following resistance training in adolescent males because testosterone and other hormonal influences on muscle hypertrophy would be operant.[54]

Most studies examining changes in muscle size in youth have used anthropometric techniques and have provided no evidence of training-induced hypertrophy in children.[50–52] Although some earlier findings are at variance with this observation,[55,56] children appear to experience more difficulty increasing their muscle mass in response to a training programme due to inadequate levels of circulating androgens. It is possible, however, that higher training loads, longer study durations, and more sensitive measuring techniques that are ethically appropriate for the paediatric population may be needed to partition the effects of resistance training on fat-free mass from expected gains due to growth and development.

Detraining and persistence of training-induced gains

The temporary or permanent reduction of the training stimulus is referred to as detraining.[57] Most children and adolescents will undergo periods of reduced training because of programme design factors, travel plans, examination schedules, school vacations, or decreased motivation. The concept of detraining in youth is relatively complex, because any loss in strength and power due to a reduction in training may be masked by the growth-related increase in muscle performance that will occur during the detraining period. Training-induced gains in muscular strength and power are impermanent and tend to regress towards untrained control group values during the detraining period.[42,57–60] In one report, the effects of an 8-week training programme followed by an 8-week detraining period were evaluated in boys and girls ages 7–12 years.[58] While significant gains in upper and lower body strength were observed following the training period, strength gains regressed towards untrained control group values during the detraining period at a rate of 3% per week. It was speculated that changes in neuromuscular functioning and possibly a loss of motor coordination could be at least partly responsible for the detraining response observed in youth.

It is possible that maturity status as well as the design of the resistance training programme could influence the adaptations as well as the regressions that take place during the detraining period. Following 8 weeks of detraining, researchers reported the greatest loss of strength and power in the pre-peak height velocity (PHV) group as compared to the mid- and post-PHV groups.[42] The degree of muscular fitness or neuromuscular skill required to perform selected exercises may also influence the detraining response in children. Regressions towards baseline values were found in some, but not all, fitness tests following an 8-week training programme in 7-year-old children that focused on enhancing muscular fitness and fundamental movement skills.[57] Some of the neuromuscular mechanisms that underpin changes in performance during the detraining period may be influenced by the intensity of the exercise, the type of exercise, and the complexity of the skill. Only a limited number of resistance training studies have evaluated the effects of training frequency on strength maintenance in youth. A 1 day·week^{-1} maintenance programme was just as effective as a 2 day·week^{-1} maintenance programme in retaining the strength gains made after 12 weeks of resistance training in a group of pubescent male athletes.[61] Others reported that school children[62] and young athletes[63,64] who completed a resistance training programme were able to maintain training-induced gains in muscular fitness following several weeks of reduced training. The importance of youth regularly engaging in resistance training throughout the year, or some type of maintenance training at an appropriate intensity, to enhance or preserve training-induced gains in muscular fitness is an important consideration for youth fitness and sport programmes.

Risks and concerns

Despite a compelling body of supportive evidence, resistance training was not always recommended for children and adolescents due to the presumed high risk of injury associated with this type of training as well as the alleged lack of training-induced benefit. A common misperception was that this type of training would be injurious to the physis or growth plate in a young lifter's body, which could result in time lost from training, significant discomfort, and growth disturbances. However, in the vast majority of prospective research studies, no overt clinical injuries were reported in training programmes where qualified supervision, safe equipment, and adherence to developmentally appropriate training guidelines were followed.[65–67]

While injury to the developing skeleton of young weightlifters was a traditional concern in the 1970s and 1980s, injury to the growth cartilage has not been reported in any prospective youth resistance training study and there is no evidence to suggest that resistance training will negatively impact growth during childhood and adolescence.[65,67,68] Of note, most of the forces that youth are exposed to in various sports (e.g. gymnastics) and recreational activities (e.g. tag games) are likely to be far greater, both in exposure time and magnitude, than resistance exercise.[69] For example, jumping and landing activities during competitive sports and play have been found to induce ground reaction forces greater than twice body mass depending upon age and jumping technique.[70,71] Others reported peak landing forces of up to five times body mass in children who performed 12 different jumps with one foot or two feet.[72]

Maximum strength testing

Of potential relevance, one repetition maximum (1 RM) strength and power testing has been found to be a safe and reliable testing procedure for children and adolescents.[73–75] Researchers assessed 1 RM performance on the chest press and leg press weight machine exercises in 96 children (6 to 12 years of age) and no adverse consequences or complaints of muscle soreness were reported.[73] In other paediatric research studies, children and adolescents safely performed 1 RM strength tests using free weights.[76–79] Although data on 1 RM test-retest reliability in youth is limited, intra-class correlation coefficients between 0.93[80] and 0.98[74] have been reported for maximal strength and power testing, respectively, which compare favourably to other tests of physical performance in youth. Therefore, technique-driven 1 RM testing has a high degree of reproducibility in youth and can be safely evaluated provided standard testing procedures are followed.

As with most physical activities, resistance training does carry with it some degree of inherent risk of musculoskeletal injury, yet this risk is no greater than many other sports or recreational activities in which children and adolescents regularly participate. Although data directly comparing the relative safety of resistance training with other sports and activities are limited, in one retrospective evaluation of injury rates in adolescents it was revealed that resistance training was markedly safer than many other sports and activities.[81] These researchers also reported that participation in the sport of weightlifting (which involves the performance of the snatch, and clean and jerk exercises) resulted in fewer injuries than other sports, including soccer and rugby.[81] In support of these observations, others reported significant gains in strength and power without any report of injury when weightlifting movements (e.g. modified cleans, pulls, and presses) were incorporated into youth training programmes.[40,76,82,83] Although weightlifting movements have become popular among youth coaches,[84] professionals who teach these lifts to children and adolescents should be knowledgeable of the stepwise progression from basic exercises (e.g. front squat/overhead squat), to skill transfer exercises (e.g. hang clean/drop snatch) and finally to the competitive lifts (e.g. full squat clean/full snatch).

If youth resistance training guidelines are not followed, there is the potential for injury. Researchers reported that two-thirds of resistance training injuries sustained by 8- to 13-year-old patients who reported to emergency rooms in the United States were to the hand and foot and were most often related to 'dropping' and 'pinching' in the injury descriptions.[85] It is noteworthy that 77% of the reported injuries in this age group were categorized as accidental.[85] These observations are supported by epidemiological findings from Kerr and colleagues[86] who found that children aged 12 years and younger suffered a larger proportion of hand and foot injuries than older participants while engaged in strength and conditioning activities. Collectively, these findings suggest that a majority of injuries are the result of accidents that appear to be preventable with qualified supervision, careful selection of exercise equipment, and adherence to safety guidelines. Although there have not been any preventive trials that have focused specifically on measures to prevent resistance-training injuries in children and adolescents, modifiable risk factors associated with youth resistance training injuries are outlined in Table 36.1.[87]

In order to reduce the risk of accidents and injury, participants should receive safety instructions on appropriate starting weights, correct exercise technique, and the proper handling of barbells, dumbbells, and plates. Without qualified supervision and instruction, youth are more likely to attempt to lift weights that exceed their abilities or perform an excessive number of repetitions with improper exercise technique. In addition, professionals who work with children and adolescents should monitor individual responses to training sessions, allow for adequate recovery between vigorous workouts, and ensure resistance training skill competency is maintained throughout the training programme.[16,88] In addition to evaluating the 'quantity' of the resistance exercise performance (i.e. how much weight was lifted), it is equally important to provide constructive feedback on the 'quality' of the movement. Technique-driven instruction not only enhances participant safety and enjoyment of the training experience; but also direct supervision of resistance-training programmes has been shown to improve programme adherence and training-induced gains in performance.[89,90]

It is vital that professionals are aware of the individual responses to resistance exercise and that they may need to identify participants who may warrant more attention and/or a modification of their training programme. Although higher levels of muscular fitness and physical qualities are associated with a reduced risk of injury, undesirable outcomes may occur if the demands of the training programme (and possibly sport practice and competition) exceed the physical abilities of the participant.[91–93] While chronic

Table 36.1 Modifiable risk factors associated with resistance-training injuries in children and adolescents which can be reduced (or eliminated) with qualified supervision and instruction.

Risk factor	Example	Modification by qualified professional
Unsafe exercise environment	Insufficient clear space between equipment and lifting platforms	Adequate training space and proper equipment layout
Improper equipment storage	Dumbbells and barbells not placed back on storage rack	Secure storage of exercise equipment
Unsafe use of equipment	Safety clips not used on barbells	Instruction on safety rules in the training area
Excessive load & volume	Child attempting to perform a high volume set of back squats without consideration for technical competency	Prescription and progression of training programme driven by technical performance of prescribed exercise movement
Poor exercise technique	Poor spinal alignment during a deadlift exercise	Clear instruction and feedback on exercise movements
Poor trunk control	Lack of pelvic control during an overhead push press	Targeted neuromuscular training
Muscle imbalances	Upper body muscular development biased towards anterior muscle groups	Training programme prioritizes/targets opposing muscle groups
Previous injury	Recovery from anterior cruciate ligament injury	Communicate with treating clinician and modify programme
Sex-specific growth	Lack of neuromuscular spurt in young females	Targeted training to address deficits
Inadequate recuperation	Multiple consecutive training days or repeated exposure to resistance training immediately following a competition	Incorporate active rest and consider lifestyle factors such as proper nutrition and adequate sleep

low-training loads may result in suboptimal gains in physical development, the potential for overtraining and overuse injuries in youth should be recognized. Therefore, qualified professionals should systematically prescribe training programmes and regularly monitor training stress.[21]

Potential benefits of youth resistance training

New insights into the design of youth physical development programmes have highlighted the importance of enhancing muscular fitness early in life to alter PA trajectories, reduce associated injury risks, and enhance long-term health.[3,4,6,7,94] In addition to increasing muscular strength and power, regular participation in a well-designed resistance training programme can increase bone mineral density, improve cardiovascular risk factors, fuel metabolic health, facilitate weight control, enhance psychosocial well-being, and prepare youth for the demands of daily PA and competitive sport.[2,3,16,18] Moreover, participation in a school- or community-based resistance training programme provides all boys and girls with an opportunity to gain the knowledge, motivation, and confidence needed to engage in physical activities for life.

In a prospective study of over one million male adolescents age 16–19 years who were followed over a period of 24 years, low muscular strength was recognized as an emerging risk factor for major causes of death, including cardiovascular disease.[95] Others reported that young athletes are at greater risk of a sports-related injury if they are not prepared for the demands of sports practice and competition.[14,15,94,96] Collectively, these findings emphasize the importance of early recognition of low muscle strength in youth and highlight the value of regular resistance training throughout childhood and adolescence. The potential health- and fitness-related benefits of youth resistance training are described in Figure 36.1.

Bone health

Childhood and adolescence may be the opportune time for the bone remodelling process to respond to the tensile and compressive forces associated with resistance exercise.[97,98] Since youth with low muscle strength are at an increased risk of fracture,[99] weight-bearing activities, particularly resistance training and jumping exercises, may be most beneficial during the growing years because the mechanical stress from this type of training may act synergistically with growth-related increases in bone mass.[100–102] Of interest, adolescent weightlifters who regularly train with heavy loads have been found to have levels of bone mineral density and bone mineral content well above values of age-matched controls.[103,104] While peak bone mass is strongly influenced by genetics, it appears that muscular forces which must act on bone to perform a desired movement with a moderate to heavy load are a potent osteogenic stimulus for new bone formation in certain individuals.[102,105,106]

No evidence indicates that regular participation in a structured training programme that includes weight-bearing activities will have an adverse effect on bone growth and development.[69,107,108] While the responses to resistance training will vary among individuals, it appears that activity-induced gains in bone health early in life will likely influence bone health later in life.[109] These observations are supported by data from a 20-year follow-up study which found that the main physical fitness component at adolescence related to adult bone mineral content was muscular fitness.[110] Others found that training-induced benefits on bone mass early in life were still present 30 years after retirement from sport.[111] Health care providers, physical education teachers, and youth coaches should value the importance of weight-bearing PAs, including resistance exercise, during childhood and adolescence in order to maximize the development of bone mass and reduce the risk of skeletal fracture. (Readers interested in a more detailed discussion of PA and bone health are referred to Chapter 18).

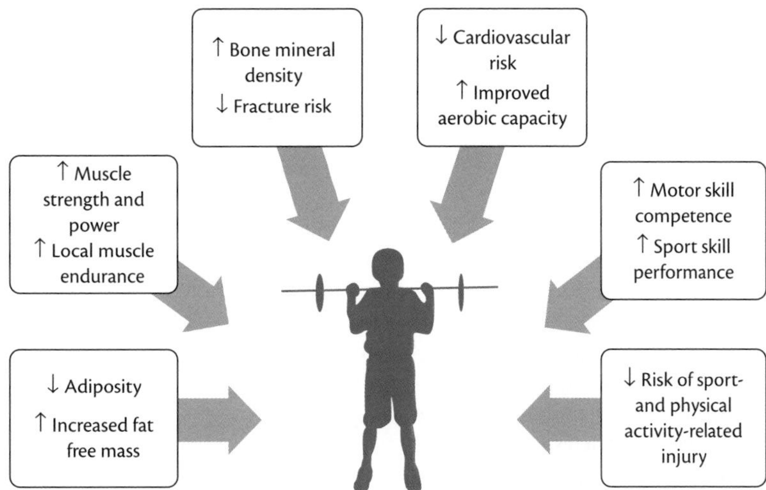

Figure 36.1 The multiple benefits of resistance training for youth.
Based on data from references 2, 13, 15, 16, 18, 46, 98, 99, 120, 122, and 125.

Adiposity and metabolic health

The prevalence of paediatric overweight and obesity continues to increase worldwide and weight-related cardiovascular and metabolic problems are being seen in youth at an increased rate.[112,113] In addition to traditional cardiovascular disease risk factors (e.g. hypertension and dyslipidaemia), low levels of muscular strength early in life appear to be an emerging risk factor for cardiometabolic risk in youth.[114–117] Based on data from a sample of 1642 youth between 9 and 15 years, researchers found that muscular strength, endurance, and power were inversely associated with clustered cardiovascular disease risk.[118] While there is not one programme of proven efficacy that professionals can use to manage weight-related cardiovascular and metabolic problems, participation in exercise programmes that enhance muscular fitness may improve the metabolic efficiency of muscle (i.e. lipid oxidation and glucose transport capacity) and increase spontaneous PA.[3,48]

Favourable changes in body composition, metabolic measures, and endothelial function have been observed in overweight and obese youth following resistance training.[119–125] Sigal and colleagues[122] randomized 304 obese adolescents to an aerobic training, resistance training, or a combined training group. Following 22 weeks of training, the combined training group had greater changes in percent body fat as compared to the aerobic group but not the resistance training group. These findings are supported by other researchers who reported significant improvements in body composition, endothelial function, metabolic profiles, and physical fitness in nondiabetic obese adolescents following 12 weeks of resistance training.[121] Along with favourable changes in psychological health following resistance training in overweight and obese youth,[123,126] the beneficial effects of resistance training or combined aerobic and resistance training on adiposity and metabolic health may offer an alternative to aerobic training alone.

Motor skills and sports performance

Although the ability of youth to adapt to training is influenced by a nexus of anatomical and physiological processes at each stage of development, meta-analytical findings indicate that children show greater training-induced gains in jumping, running, and throwing following structured resistance training than adolescents.[13] The first few years of life are characterized by rapid changes in myelination of the central nervous system and brain development.[127,128] Consequently, training that is designed to enhance motor skill performance may be most effective and enduring when participants are most sensitive to skill-based training.[6] Since training adaptations are specific to the movement pattern and the velocity, type, and magnitude of muscle contractions, training programmes that include complex movements may be more likely to result in favourable changes in motor skill performance. Of note, researchers reported that the combination of resistance training and plyometric training may actually be synergistic in youth with their combined effect being greater than each programme performed in isolation.[41,129–132]

A high level of muscular fitness contributes to effective performance ability in young athletes, and a multidimensional strength and conditioning programme can improve performance on a wide range of physiological and motor skill assessments.[4,16,133] Existing research indicates that various forms of resistance training can elicit performance improvements in muscular fitness,[17,37] running velocity,[134] tennis serve velocity,[135] ball shooting speed,[132] change of direction speed,[136] aerobic endurance,[132] dynamic balance,[137] and flexibility[77] in children and adolescents. In addition to increasing muscular strength, regular participation in a structured resistance training programme for 2 years improved sprint performance up to 6% in elite youth soccer players compared to a group of age-matched peers who only played soccer.[39,138] Collectively, these findings suggest that stronger young athletes will be better prepared to learn complex movements, master sport tactics, and withstand the demands of long-term sports training and competition.

Since motor performance skills are essential components of sport movements, there is a unique opportunity during childhood and adolescence to build a strong foundation that can be augmented with more advanced training strategies as competence and confidence to perform resistance exercise develops over time.[16] An accumulation of learned skills and reinforced abilities early in life will provide aspiring young athletes with the physical prowess and perceived confidence to engage regularly in a variety of sport-related activities. Data from cross-sectional and longitudinal studies indicate that motor competence is positively associated with multiple aspects of health[29] and therefore targeted interventions that include some type of resistance exercise should begin early in life.

Injury reduction in youth sport

Regardless of sporting success, young athletes who do not address strength deficits early in life are less likely to sustain high-level performance and more likely to suffer a 'preventable' sports injury.[14,15] A certain level of force production and force attenuation is required to perform all athletic movements, and therefore the importance of enhancing muscular fitness should be considered the foundation to athletic development.[4,16] This type of intervention may be particularly valuable for modern-day young athletes who unfortunately may specialize in one sport at an early age at the expense of enhancing general physical fitness and learning diversified sport skills. Early sports specialization limits the opportunity to 'sample' different sports during childhood and acquire the foundational physical, psychological, and cognitive skills that are critical for long-term physical development and sport success.[139,140]

Regular resistance training will enhance sports performance, aid in the prevention of injury, and help support participation in daily MVPA as an ongoing lifestyle choice.[21,96] This is of particular importance for the alarmingly high number of youth who fail to meet global PA recommendations and consequently present with muscular weaknesses and neuromuscular deficits.[16,141] Participation in sport alone does not ensure that youth will attain a level of muscular fitness that is consistent with long-term physical development. Reports indicate that youth sport practice may not provide an adequate amount of MVPA because a large amount of time is spent in sedentary or light activities.[142,143] An integrative approach to conditioning grounded in resistance exercise is needed to maximize athletic performance and reduce the risk of sports-related injuries.

Although the total elimination of sports-related injuries is an unrealistic goal, a meta-analysis on exercise interventions to prevent sports injuries found that resistance training reduced sports injuries by almost 70%.[14] Others found that training interventions with strengthening and proximal control exercises significantly reduced anterior cruciate ligament injury incidences in young female athletes compared to interventions without those exercise components.[15] While intrinsic risk factors such as previous injury, muscle imbalances, and growth are noteworthy considerations, professionals should not overlook the value of targeting deficits in muscular fitness as a preventative health measure.[144] Multi-faceted interventions have proven to be an effective strategy for reducing sports-related injuries in adolescent athletes,[145–147] and it seems that similar effects could be observed in children if the training programme was integrative, progressive, and technique driven. Owing to neuromuscular plasticity during the developmental years,[6,148] it seems prudent to start education and instruction on proper training techniques early in life in order to optimize outcomes and stimulate an ongoing interest in this type of conditioning.[149]

Enhancing muscular fitness should be a priority in any athletic development programme, since the right 'dose' of resistance exercise can improve performance on a wide range of physiological and skill assessments. A majority of the available data indicates that regular participation in a well-designed and supervised conditioning programme that includes resistance training may enhance muscular fitness, improve neuromuscular control, and lessen the likelihood of sports-related injuries in young athletes.[18,94,150] These findings underline a potential synergistic adaptation whereby the prescribed training stimulus complements naturally occurring adaptations. Without structured interventions, coaches at all levels will eventually need to address neuromuscular limitations which become harder to 'fix' when ingrained motor control patterns develop over time. Evidence for the effectiveness of resistance training in the reduction of youth sport injuries supports the implementation and ongoing maintenance of these programmes in schools and sport centres.

Youth resistance-training guidelines

If the benefits of resistance exercise during childhood and adolescence are to be realized, specific details of the intervention need to be properly prescribed by qualified professionals and the 'dose' of exercise must be developmentally appropriate, meaningful, and enjoyable. An 'overdose' of training can result in non-functional overreaching, overtraining, or injury.[91,92,151] Consequently, the systematic progression of different training variables, along with individual monitoring of stress tolerance, will determine the long-term training-induced adaptations that take place. In addition, cautionary measures (e.g. pre-screening and qualified supervision) need to be considered before children and adolescents participate in a resistance-training programme. A medical examination prior to participation in a resistance-training programme is not mandatory for healthy youth, although caution should be used for children and adolescents with a pre-existing medical condition.[152]

All participants should be given an opportunity to understand fundamental training principles and establish a sound strength base before progressing to more intense training regimens with heavier loads. A basic level of resistance training skill competency along with an understanding of youth resistance training guidelines and safety procedures (e.g. sensible starting weights and the proper storage of equipment) are intrinsic during an introductory class. For youth with low resistance training skill competency, qualified professionals should prescribe a range of basic exercises that enhance muscular strength while developing competence and confidence to perform a variety of resistance exercises. This type of programme involves the ongoing evaluation of movement patterns that are considered essential for mastery of a particular exercise. For participants with high resistance training skill competency, dynamic qualities can be enhanced with more advanced resistance training exercises that are designed to optimize specific physiological and performance outcomes.[16]

The concept of resistance training skill competency does not imply that all youth will achieve a high level of technical competence on all exercises, but rather suggests that all participants should have the opportunity to learn and practice the desired skills in a controlled environment.[88] This type of coaching and instruction provides a needed opportunity for all participants, especially those with deficient muscle strength, to learn task-related activities and perform resistance exercise. While most children can learn basic movements that require squatting, pushing, and pulling, their ability to progress to more complex movements will be influenced by the amount of time they have practised basic skills with a qualified professional. Children as young as 5 and 6 years of age have benefitted from participation in a resistance training programme,[153,154] although an age of 7–8 years is when most children are ready for some type of structured resistance training.[2,155]

The programme variables that should be considered when designing a youth resistance training programme include the following: i) choice and order of exercise, ii) training intensity, iii) training volume, iv) repetition velocity, v) rest intervals between sets and exercises, and vi) training frequency. Resistance training guidelines from the International Consensus Statement on youth resistance training are outlined in Figure 36.2.[2]

Choice and order of exercises

It is important to select exercises that are appropriate for a participant's body size, fitness level, and resistance training skill competency. Children and adolescents in schools and sport programmes have used body weight exercises, free weights (barbells and dumbbells), weight machines, elastic bands, and medicine balls.[38,40,41,44,46,156,157] It is reasonable to start with relatively simple movements and gradually progress to more advanced exercises as confidence and competence improve. Multi-joint exercises, including weightlifting movements, can be incorporated into youth conditioning programmes provided that qualified instruction is available.[76,82,83,132]

For most youth, multiple exposures to total body workouts over the course of a week will provide an adequate stimulus. However, more advanced programming may be more appropriate for young athletes with greater training history. In general, multi-joint exercises should be performed before single-joint exercises. Adopting this exercise order should allow heavier loads to be used on the multi-joint exercises because fatigue will be less of a factor. It is also important to perform more challenging exercises earlier in the workout when the neuromuscular system is less fatigued, e.g. when learning a back squat exercise, the child will be able to perform the movement with less fatigue if the exercise is done near the beginning of the programme.[158] Extreme conditioning protocols have been found to alter barbell squat mechanics in trained adults,[159] and therefore this type of exhaustive metabolic training would not be expected to optimize resistance training skill competency in youth with less training experience.

Training intensity and volume

Training *intensity* typically refers to the amount of weight used for an exercise, whereas training *volume* generally refers to the total amount of work performed in a training session. While both are important training variables, training intensity is one of the more important factors in the design of a resistance-training programme. Of note, a significant positive correlation was found between gains in motor performance skills and the mean intensity (% 1 RM) of the youth resistance-training programme.[13] Therefore, once youth develop proper exercise technique using light and moderate loads, the training programme should be advanced to the use of greater loads on the proviso that the individual can maintain the ability to properly perform the desired movements. By periodically varying the training stimulus with periods of low-, moderate-, and high-intensity training, it is likely that long-term performance gains will be optimized, boredom will be reduced, and the risk of overuse injuries will decrease.[77]

Different combinations of sets and repetitions may be effective, although meta-analytical data suggest that the average resistance training programme consists of two to three sets of 8–15 repetitions with loads between 60% and 80% of the 1 RM on six to eight exercises.[37] One approach for a beginner may be to start resistance training with one or two sets of 8–12 repetitions with a moderate load (50–70% 1 RM) on six to ten exercises, and then gradually progress the training programme depending on training goals and objectives. When prescribing an appropriate training intensity for youth it seems reasonable to first establish a repetition range and then change the training load to maintain the desired training stimulus. By closely monitoring exercise technique as well as the level of perceived muscular exertion, youth should be able to make noticeable gains in muscular fitness.

The number of repetitions performed per set, the number of sets performed per exercise, and the weight lifted all influence the training volume, which is often expressed as the 'volume-load'.[160] It is

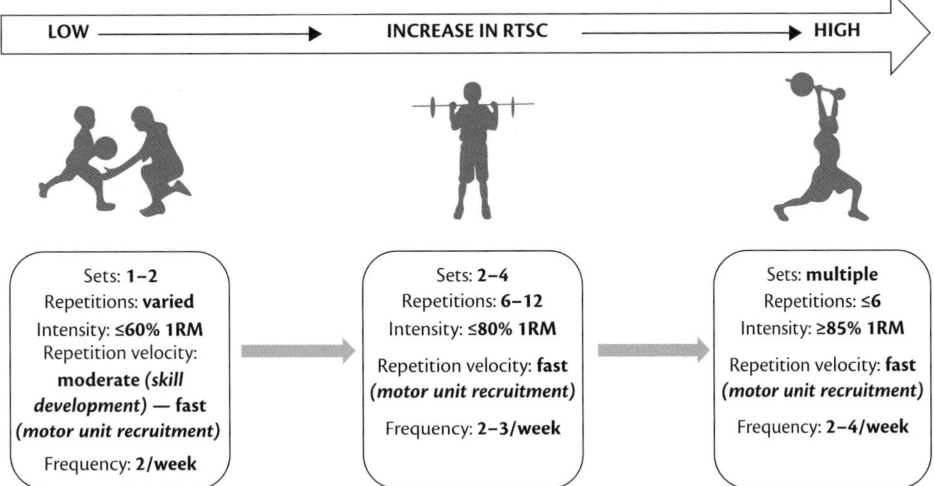

Figure 36.2 Youth resistance training guidelines with progression based on each participant's resistance training skill competency.

Reprinted from Faigenbaum A, Lloyd R, MacDonald J, Myer G. Citius, Altius, Fortius: beneficial effects of resistance training for young athletes: Narrative review. Br J Sports Med. 2015; 50: 3–7.

important to remember that every training session does not need to be characterized by the same number of sets, repetitions, and exercises. In general, it is reasonable to begin resistance training with one or two sets on a variety of exercises, and then gradually progress to two- or three-set protocols following the first few weeks of training. The systematic manipulation of programme variables (primarily intensity and volume) will allow participants to make even larger gains because the body will be challenged to adapt to increased demands.[40,42,77]

Rest interval between sets and exercises

The length of the rest interval between sets and exercises is an important training variable since acute force and power production may be compromised if the rest interval is too short. While a rest interval of 2–3 min for primary, multi-joint exercises is typically recommended for adults, this recommendation may not be consistent with the needs and abilities of younger populations due to growth and maturation-related differences in the response to physical exertion.[161] It appears that children and adolescents can resist fatigue to a greater extent than adults during several repeated bouts of resistance exercise.[78,162,163] (Fatigue resistance is reviewed in Chapter 9).

In one study examining the lifting performance of children, adolescents, and adults following different rest intervals, the researchers found that adults may need rest intervals of at least 3 min between sets, adolescents may require rest intervals of 2 min, while children may only require rest intervals of 1 min to minimize loading reductions and attain the highest lifting performance.[78] These observations are consistent with others who found that children had less neuromuscular fatigue and recovered faster than adults from low- and high-intensity resistance training.[163] Although additional study is warranted, possible factors contributing to a faster recovery in children include less muscle mass, a lower reliance on glycolysis, faster phosphocreatine re-synthesis, better acid-base regulation, increased fatigue resistance due to a lower power output, and differential motor unit activation.[164,165] Consequently, a shorter rest interval (e.g. 1–2 min) between sets and exercises may suffice in children and adolescents when performing moderate-intensity resistance training. Youth with resistance training experience who perform more advanced programmes that require higher levels of strength and power may require longer rest intervals to maintain muscle performance.[2]

Repetition velocity

The velocity or cadence at which an exercise is performed can affect the adaptations to a training programme. It is generally recommended that untrained youth initially perform resistance exercises with a light to moderate load in a controlled manner maintaining a relatively low to moderate velocity (i.e. low cadence). However, different training cadences may be used depending on the choice of exercise and programme goals. For example, the warm-up phase (including low load movement preparation exercises) may consist of slower, controlled movements, while the main strength and power exercises (inclusive of weightlifting and plyometric exercises) will need to be performed at a high velocity. The development of high velocity movement may be especially important during the growing years when neural plasticity and motor coordination are most sensitive to change.[166] Although additional research is needed, it is likely that the performance of different training velocities within a resistance training programme may provide the most effective training stimulus.[41,129,131]

Training frequency

A training frequency of two to three times$\cdot$week^{-1} on non-consecutive days is recommended for most children and adolescents.[37] Limited evidence indicates that 1 day$\cdot$week^{-1} of resistance training may be suboptimal for enhancing muscular strength in youth.[167] A training frequency of twice or thrice weekly, on non-consecutive days, will allow for adequate recovery between sessions (48–72 h between sessions) and will be effective for enhancing musculoskeletal strength and performance. Although some young athletes may train more than 3 days$\cdot$week^{-1} (e.g. split routine training), factors such as the weekly training volume, nutritional intake, and sleep habits should also be considered, as these factors may influence one's ability to recover from and adapt to the training programme.[21]

Long-term physical development

While additional data are needed to validate the design of long-term physical development programmes, the available evidence indicates that interventions targeting children should begin early in life, as PA behaviours tend to track into the adult years.[12,29,30] Troubling trends in PA and obesity among youth worldwide highlight the importance of developmentally appropriate interventions for modern day youth.[141,168] Of note, the decline in levels of muscular fitness in school-age youth over the past few years will likely have a direct impact on the design of any long-term physical development model since coordinated muscular strength is an essential component of motor skill performance.[22,24]

In addition to enhancing the physical development of inactive youth, proper year-round training can be especially beneficial to young athletes who may not have had adequate exposure to developmental fitness activities. While deliberate practice and sports training are necessary for athletic success, they appear to be inadequate for optimizing performance and minimizing the risk of injury.[142,143] Consequently, the primary emphasis of long-term physical development should be on the development of muscular strength and movement competency to develop robust and resilient young athletes who can tolerate the loadings associated with competitive sports.[4,5] While practitioners will likely adopt their preferred philosophy of periodization (e.g. progressive cycling of various aspects of training), planning sequential blocks of training are important for optimizing training-induced adaptations.[77,169]

Both the IOC and the National Strength and Conditioning Association recognize that youth conditioning is a long-term process that should involve the sensible integration of different training methods and the periodic manipulation of programme variables over time.[19,21] It seems reasonable for young children entering a long-term physical development model to devote a majority of their time to general preparatory training and the development of gross movement skills.[170] However, as a young athlete moves through the developmental pathway a greater emphasis may be placed on competition, so that by the time they reach adulthood they will potentially spend 25–35% of their time in training and 65–75% of their time in competition. While these ratios are estimates and do not account for individual differences, the notion of prioritizing general conditioning, inclusive of resistance training, during childhood is essential.

An example of a long-term approach to physical development is illustrated within the Youth Physical Development (YPD) model for males and females (Figures 36.3a and 36.3b).[7] Within the 'physical qualities' section of the YPD model, training emphasis is highlighted by font size, i.e. the larger the font size, the greater the emphasis of a particular fitness component. Although literature shows that all fitness components can be trained during all stages of development, the enduring importance of muscular strength throughout childhood and adolescence is underscored within the model.[7] In addition, the YPD model showed that while both children and adolescents can make worthwhile gains in a range of fitness components, the mechanisms, magnitude, and tempo of adaptation for youth of varying maturity will differ. For example, while muscle strength and motor skill competence should be targeted during the early years, other fitness components that possess a high neuromuscular demand (i.e. power, speed, and agility) should also be trained owing to the neural plasticity associated with childhood.

The level of technical competency and training history should ultimately dictate the design and rate of progression and/or regression within a programme. For example, from an athletic development perspective, a 15-year-old adolescent boy with a low-training age and poor technical competency should not commence a high-intensity, highly skilled resistance-training programme without first developing a broad range of fundamental movement skills and primal levels of muscular strength. Similarly, a 10-year-old prepubertal girl who possesses innate athleticism and high levels of technical competency should not be restricted to training modes typically associated with very inexperienced children. Irrespective of stage of maturation, muscular strength, and motor skill competency should remain key components for any long-term physical development programme for the child to gain well-established performance enhancement and injury prevention benefits. While the YPD model provides a framework that attempts to integrate training and maturation, all models should be recognized as flexible guidelines as opposed to stringent blueprints. More research is needed to better understand the interactions between growth, maturation, and training throughout childhood and adolescence.

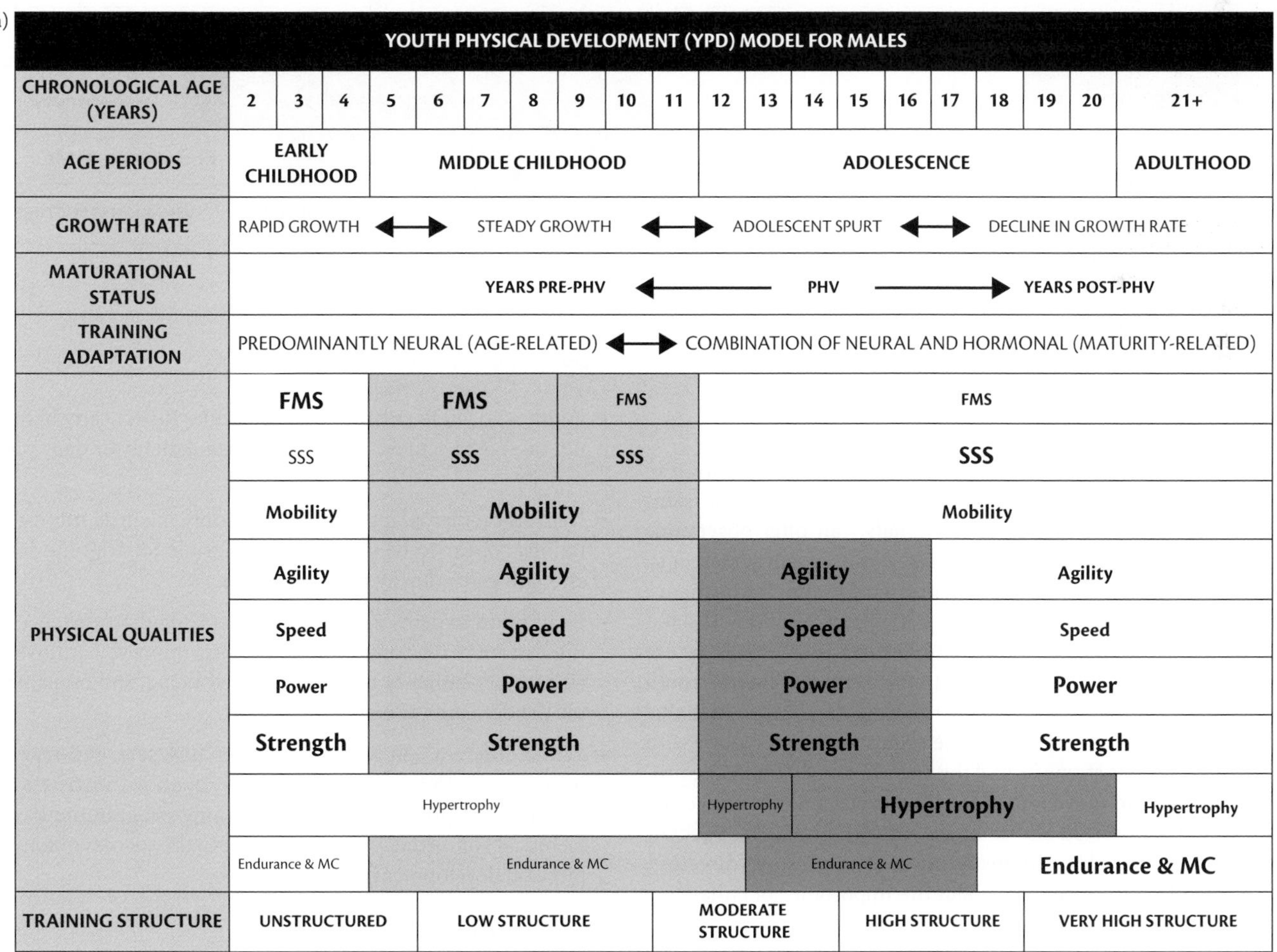

Figure 36.3a The youth physical development model for males.

The font size refers to importance; light purple boxes refer to preadolescent periods of adaptation, dark purple boxes refer to adolescent periods of adaptation.

PHV = peak height velocity; FMS = fundamental movement skills; SSS = sport-specific skills; MC = metabolic conditioning.

Lloyd R, Oliver J. The youth physical development model: A new approach to long-term athletic development. Strength Cond J. 2012; 34: 61–72.

(b)

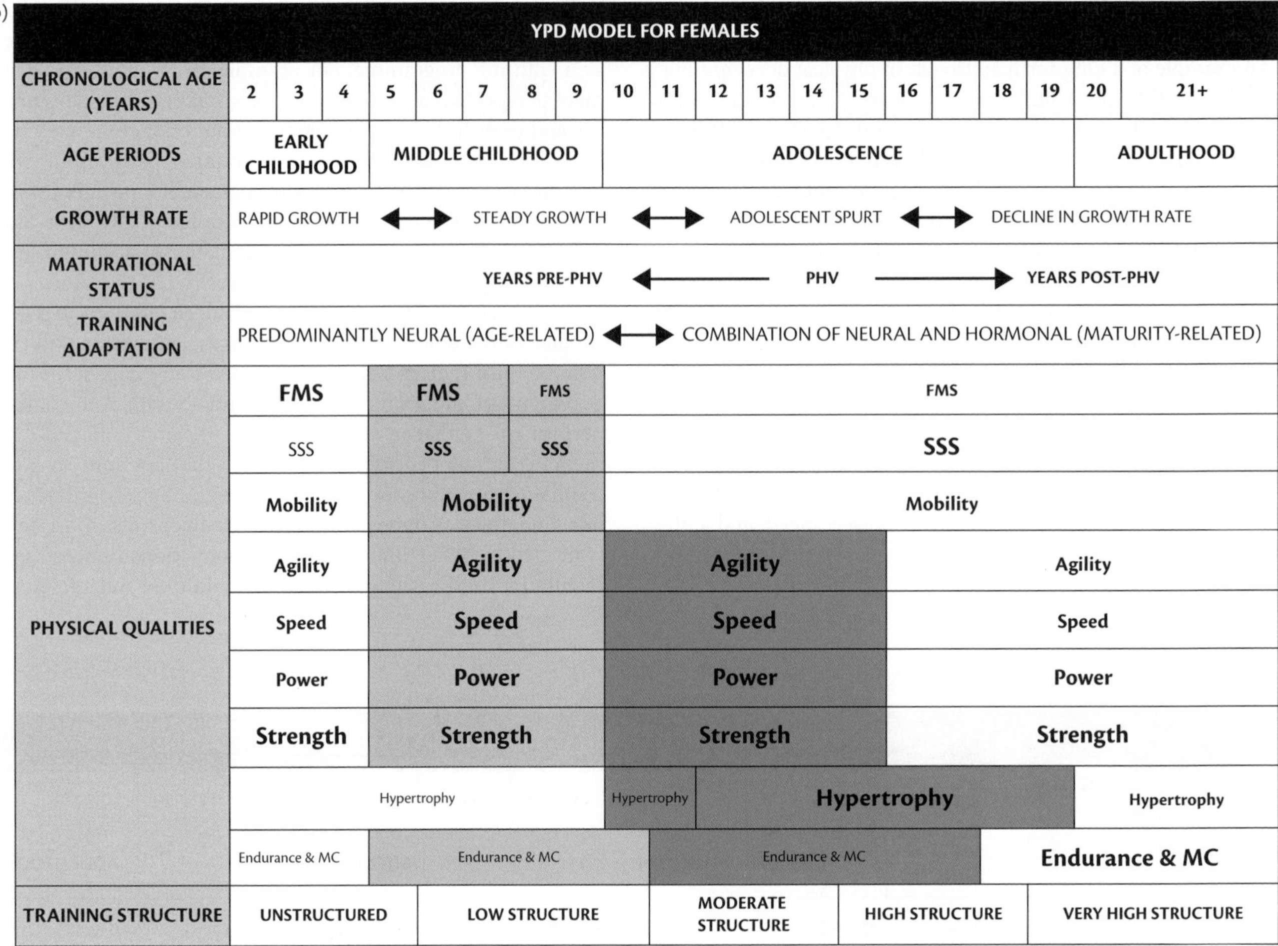

Figure 36.3b The youth physical development model for females.

The font size refers to importance; light purple boxes refer to preadolescent periods of adaptation, dark purple boxes refer to adolescent periods of adaptation.

PHV = peak height velocity; FMS = fundamental movement skills; SSS = sport-specific skills; MC = metabolic conditioning.

Lloyd R, Oliver J. The youth physical development model: A new approach to long-term athletic development. Strength Cond J. 2012; 34: 61–72.

Conclusions

A compelling body of data indicates that regular participation in well-designed and developmentally appropriate resistance training, supervised by qualified professionals, can offer observable health, fitness, and performance value to children and adolescents. Gains in muscular fitness can enhance motor skill performance and stronger young athletes will be better prepared to withstand the demands of sports training and competition. While future research investigating the potential long-term benefits of youth resistance training is warranted, existing data show that due consideration must be given to the identification of youth with inadequate muscle strength, and the promotion of sustainable programmes that can prevent the cascade of adverse health outcomes later in life. Concerted efforts by health care providers, paediatric researchers, school administrators, and youth sport directors, are needed to raise awareness about the importance of enhancing muscular fitness early in life.

Summary

- A compelling body of evidence indicates that regular participation in a youth resistance-training programme offers observable health and fitness benefits to children and adolescents.
- Youth who fail to enhance their muscular fitness early in life may not be able to achieve global recommendations for daily physical activity.
- Neuromuscular adaptations and possibly intrinsic muscle adaptations appear to be primarily responsible for training-induced strength gains during preadolescence.
- In addition to gains in muscular fitness, regular resistance training can increase bone mineral density, improve cardiovascular risk factors, enhance psychosocial well-being, and prepare youth for the demands of competitive sport.
- While different combinations of exercises, sets, and repetitions have proven to be safe and effective, qualified instruction and a systematic progression of the training programme based on technical competency are paramount to the success of long-term physical development.

References

1. Faigenbaum A, Lloyd R, Myer G. Youth resistance training: Past practices, new perspectives and future directions. *Pediatr Exerc Sci.* 2013; 25: 591–604.
2. Lloyd R, Faigenbaum A, Stone M, *et al.* Position statement on youth resistance training: the 2014 International Consensus. *Brit J Sports Med.* 2014; 48: 498–505.

3. Smith J, Eather N, Morgan P, Plotnikoff R, Faigenbaum A, Lubans D. The health benefits of muscular fitness for children and adolescents: A systematic review and meta-analysis. *Sports Med.* 2014; 44: 1209–1223.
4. Lloyd R, Oliver J, Faigenbaum A, *et al.* Long-term athletic development-Part 1: A pathway for all youth. *J Strength Cond Res.* 2015; 29: 1439–1450.
5. Lloyd R, Oliver J, Faigenbaum A, *et al.* Long-term physical development: Barriers to success and potential solutions-Part 2. *J Strength Cond Res.* 2015; 29: 1451–1464.
6. Myer G, Faigenbaum A, Edwards E, Clark. J., Best T, Sallis R. 60 minutes of what? A developing brain perspective for activation children. *Br J Sports Med.* 2015; 49: 1510–1516.
7. Lloyd R, Oliver J. The youth physical development model: A new approach to long-term athletic development. *Strength Cond.* 2012; 34: 61–72.
8. Faigenbaum A, Myer G. Exercise deficit disorder in youth: Play now or play later. *Curr Sports Med Rep.* 2012; 11: 196–200.
9. Fransen J, Deprez D, Pion J, *et al.* Changes in physical fitness and sports participation among children with different levels of motor competence: a 2-year longitudinal study. *Pediatr Exerc Sci.* 2014; 26: 1–21.
10. Lopes V, Rodriques L, Maia A, Malina R. Motor coordination as a predictor of physical activity in childhood. *Scand J Med Sci Sport.* 2011; 21: 663–669.
11. Hands B. Changes in motor skill and fitness measures among children with high an low motor competence: A five year longitudinal study. *J Sci Med Sport.* 2008; 11: 155–162.
12. Cattuzzo M, Dos Santos HR, Ré A, *et al.* Motor competence and health related physical fitness in youth: A systematic review. *J Sci Med Sport.* 2015; 19: 123–129.
13. Behringer M, Vom Heede A, Matthews M, Mester J. Effects of strength training on motor performance skills in children and adolescents: a meta-analysis. *Pediatr Exerc Sci.* 2011; 23: 186–206.
14. Lauersen J, Bertelsen D, Andersen L. The effectiveness of exercise interventions to prevent sports injuries: a systematic review and meta-analysis of randomised controlled trials. *Br J Sports Med.* 2014; 48: 871–877.
15. Sugimoto D, Myer G, Barber Foss K, Hewett T. Specific exercise effects of preventive neuromuscular training intervention on anterior cruciate ligament injury risk reduction in young females: meta-analysis and subgroup analysis. *Br J Sports Med.* 2015; 49: 282–289.
16. Faigenbaum A, Lloyd R, MacDonald J, Myer G. Citius, Altius, Fortius: beneficial effects of resistance training for young athletes: Narrative review. *Br J Sports Med.* 2015; 50: 3–7.
17. Harries S, Lubans D, Callister R. Resistance training to improve power and sports performance in adolescent athletes: a systematic review and meta-analysis. *J Sci Med Sport.* 2012; 15: 532–540.
18. Soomro N, Sanders R, Hackett D, *et al.* The efficacy of injury prevention programs in adolescent team sports: A meta-analysis. *Am J Sports Med.* 2015; 44: 2415–2424.
19. Bergeron M, Mountjoy M, Armstrong N, *et al.* International Olympic Committee consensus statement on youth athletic development. *Br J Sports Med.* 2015; 49: 843–851.
20. World Health Organization. *Global recommendations on physical activity for health.* Geneva: WHO Press; 2010.
21. Lloyd R, Cronin J, Faigenbaum A, *et al.* The National Strength and Conditioning Association position statement on long-term athletic development. *J Strength Cond Res.* 2016; 30: 1491–1509.
22. Cohen D, Voss C, Taylor M, Delextrat A, Ogunleye A, Sandercock G. Ten-year secular changes in muscular fitness in English children. *Acta Paediatr.* 2011; 100: e175–e177.
23. Runhaar J, Collard DC, Singh A, Kemper HC, van Mechelen W, Chinapaw M. Motor fitness in Dutch youth: Differences over a 26-year period (1980-2006). *J Sci Med Sport.* 2010; 13: 323–328.
24. Moliner-Urdiales D, Ruiz J, Ortega FB, *et al.* Secular trends in health-related physical fitness in Spanish adolescents: the AVENA and HELENA studies. *J Sci Med Sport.* 2010; 13: 584–588.
25. Hardy L, Barnett L, Espinel P, Okely A. Thirteen-year trends in child and adolescent fundamental movement skills: 1997-2010. *Med Sci Sports Exerc.* 2013; 45: 1965–1970.
26. D'Hondt E, Deforche B, Gentier I, *et al.* A longitudinal analysis of gross motor coordination in overweight and obese children versus normal-weight peers. *Int J Obesity.* 2013; 37: 61–67.
27. Rodrigues L, Stodden D, Lopes V. Developmental pathways of change in fitness and motor competence are related to overweight and obesity status at the end of primary school. *J Sci Med Sport.* 2016; 19: 87–92.
28. Myer G, Faigenbaum A, Ford K, Best T, Bergeron M, Hewett T. When to initiate integrative neuromuscular training to reduce sports-related injuries and enhance health in youth? *Curr Sports Med Rep.* 2011; 10: 155–166.
29. Robinson L, Stodden D, Barnett L, *et al.* Motor competence and its effect on positive developmental trajectories of health. *Sports Med.* 2015; 45: 1273–1284.
30. Telama R, Yang X, Leskinen E, *et al.* Tracking of physical activity from early childhood through youth into adulthood. *Med Sci Sports Exerc.* 2014; 46: 955–962.
31. Rowland T. Promoting physical activity for children's health. *Sports Med.* 2007; 37: 929–936.
32. Hardy L, Reinten-Reynolds T, Espinel P, Zask A, Okely A. Prevalence and correlates of low fundamental movement skill competency in children. *Pediatrics.* 2012; 130: e390–e398.
33. Ruas C, Punt C, Pinto R, Oliveira M. Strength and power in children with low motor performance scores: A descriptive analysis. *Braz J Motor Behav.* 2014; 8: 1–8.
34. O'Neill J, Williams H, Pfeiffer K, *et al.* Young children's motor skill performance: Relationships with activity types and parent perception of athletic competence. *J Sci Med Sport.* 2014; 17: 607–610.
35. Bloemers F, Collard D, Paw M, Van Mechelen W, Twisk J, Verhagen E. Physical inactivity is a risk factor for physical activity-related injuries in children. *Br J Sports Med.* 2012; 46: 669–674.
36. Faigenbaum A, Myer G. Pediatric resistance training: Benefits, concerns and program design considerations. *Curr Sports Med Rep.* 2010; 9: 161–168.
37. Behringer M, vom Heede A, Yue Z, Mester J. Effects of resistance training in children and adolescents: A meta-analysis. *Pediatrics.* 2010; 126: e1199–e1210.
38. Faigenbaum A, Bush J, McLoone R, *et al.* Benefits of strength and skill based training during primary school physical education. *J Strength Cond Res.* 2015; 29: 1255–1262.
39. Sander A, Keiner M, Wirth K, Schmidtbleicher D. Influence of a 2-year strength training programme on power performance in elite youth soccer players. *Eur J Sport Sci.* 2013; 13: 445–451.
40. Chaouachi A, Hammami R, Kaabi S, Chamari K, Drinkwater E, Behm D. Olympic weightlifting and plyometric training with children provides similar or greater performance improvements than traditional resistance training. *J Strength Cond Res.* 2014; 28: 1483–1496.
41. Lloyd R, Radnor J, De Ste Croix M, Cronin J, Oliver J. Changes in sprint and jump performance following traditional, plyometric and combined resistance training in male youth pre- and post-peak height velocity. *J Strength Cond Res.* 2016; 30: 1239–1247.
42. Meylan C, Cronin J, Oliver J, Hopkins W, Contreras B. The effect of maturation on adaptations to strength training and detraining in 11–15-year-olds. *Scand J Med Sci Sport.* 2014; 24: e156–164.
43. Lloyd R, Oliver J, Hughes M, Williams C. Effects of 4-weeks plyometric training on reactive strength index and leg stiffness in male youths. *J Strength Cond Res.* 2012; 26: 2812–2819.
44. Faigenbaum AD, Loud RL, O'Connell J, Glover S, Westcott WL. Effects of different resistance training protocols on upper-body strength and endurance development in children. *J Strength Cond Res.* 2001; 15: 459–465.
45. Malina R, Bouchard C, Bar-Or O. *Growth, maturation and physical activity,* 2nd ed. Champaign, IL: Human Kinetics: 2004.
46. Alves A, Marta C, Neiva H, Izquierdo M, Marques M. Concurrent training in prepubescent children: the effects of eight weeks of strength

and aerobic training on explosive strength and $\dot{V}O_2$max. *J Strength Cond Res.* 2016; 30: 2019–2032.
47. Faigenbaum A, Zaichkowsky L, Westcott W, Micheli L, Fehlandt A. The effects of a twice per week strength training program on children. *Pediatr Exerc Sci.* 1993; 5: 339–346.
48. Meinhardt U, Witassek F, Petrò R, Fritz C, Eiholzer U. Strength training and physical activity in boys: a randomized trial. *Pediatrics.* 2013; 132: 1105–1111.
49. Waugh C, Korff T, Fath F., Blazevich A. Effects of resistance training on tendon mechanical properties and rapid force production in prepubertal children. *J Appl Physiol.* 2014; 117: 257–266.
50. Ozmun JC, Mikesky AE, Surburg PR. Neuromuscular adaptations following prepubescent strength training. *Med Sci Sports Exerc.* 1994; 26: 510–514.
51. Ramsay JA, Blimkie CJ, Smith K, Garner S, MacDougall JD, Sale DG. Strength training effects in prepubescent boys. *Med Sci Sports Exerc.* 1990; 22: 605–614.
52. Granacher U, Goesele A, Roggo K, *et al.* Effects and mechanisms of strength training in children. *Int J Sports Med.* 2011; 32: 357–364.
53. Waugh C, Korff T, Fath F, Blazevich A. Rapid force production in children and adults: mechanical and neural contributions. *Med Sci Sports Exerc.* 2013; 45: 762–771.
54. Falk B, Eliakim A. Endocrine response to resistance training in children. *Pediatr Exerc Sci.* 2014; 26: 404–422.
55. Mersch F, Stoboy H. Strength training and muscle hypertrophy in children. In: Oseid S, Carlsen K (eds.) *Children and exercise XIII.* Champaign, IL: Human Kinetics; 1989. p. 165–182.
56. Fukunaga T, Funato K, Ikegawa S. The effects of resistance training on muscle area and strength in prepubescent age. *Am Physiol Anthrop.* 1992; 11: 357–364.
57. Faigenbaum A, Farrell A, Fabiano M, *et al.* Effects of detraining on fitness performance in 7-year-old children. *J Strength Cond Res.* 2013; 27: 323–330.
58. Faigenbaum A, Westcott W, Micheli L, *et al.* The effects of strength training and detraining on children. *J Strength Cond Res.* 1996; 10: 109–114.
59. Ingle L, Sleap M, Tolfrey K. The effect of a complex training and detraining programme on selected strength and power variables in early prepubertal boys. *J Sport Sci.* 2006; 24: 987–997.
60. Tsolakis CK, Vagenas GK, Dessypris AG. Strength adaptations and hormonal responses to resistance training and detraining in preadolescent males. *J Strength Cond Res.* 2004; 18: 625–629.
61. DeRenne C, Hetzler RK, Buxton B, Ho KK. Effects of training frequency on strength maintenance in pubescent baseball players. *J Strength Cond Res.* 1996; 10: 8–14.
62. Mayorga-Vega D, Viciana J, Cocca A. Effects of a circuit training program on muscular and cardiovascular endurance and their maintenance in school children. *J Hum Kin.* 2013; 37: 153–160.
63. Diallo O, Dore E, Duche P, Van Praagh E. Effects of plyometric training followed by a reduced training program on physical performance in prepubescent soccer players. *J Sports Med Phys Fit.* 2001; 41: 342–348.
64. Santos E, Janeira M. Effects of reduced training and detraining on upper and lower body explosive strength in adolescent male basketball players. *J Strength Cond Res.* 2009; 23: 1737–1744.
65. Faigenbaum A, Myer G. Resistance training among young athletes: Safety, efficacy and injury prevention effects. *Br J Sports Med.* 2010; 44: 56–63.
66. Johnson B, Salzberg C, Stevenson D. A systematic review: plyometric training programs for young children. *J Strength Cond Res.* 2011; 25: 2623–2633.
67. Malina R. Weight training in youth-growth, maturation, and safety: an evidence-based review. *Clin J Sport Med.* 2006; 16: 478–487.
68. Falk B, Eliakim A. Resistance training, skeletal muscle and growth. *Pediatr Endocrinol Rev.* 2003; 1: 120–127.
69. Malina R, Baxter-Jones A, Armstrong N, *et al.* Role of intensive training in the growth and maturation of artistic gymnasts. *Sports Med.* 2013; 43: 783–802.
70. McNitt-Gray J, Hester D, Mathiyakom W, Munkasy B. Mechanical demand on multijoint control during landing depend on orientation of the body segments relative to the reaction force. *J Biomech.* 2001; 34: 1471–1482.
71. Streckis V, Skurvydas A, Ratkevicius A. Children are more susceptible to central fatigue than adults. *Muscle Nerve.* 2007; 36: 357–363.
72. McKay H, Tsang G, Heinonen A, MacKelvie K, Sanderson D, Khan KM. Ground reaction forces associated with an effective elementary school based jumping intervention. *Br J Sports Med.* 2005; 39: 10–14.
73. Faigenbaum A, Milliken L, Westcott W. Maximal strength testing in healthy children. *J Strength Cond Res.* 2003; 17: 162–166.
74. Faigenbaum A, McFarland J, Herman R, *et al.* Reliability of the one-repetition-maximum power clean test in adolescent athletes. *J Strength Cond Res.* 2012; 26: 432–437.
75. Fry A, Irwin C, Nicoll J, Ferebee D. Muscular strength and power in 3- to 7-year-old children. *Pediatr Exerc Sci.* 2015; 27: 345–354.
76. Channell BT, Barfield JP. Effect of Olympic and traditional resistance training on vertical jump improvement in high school boys. *J Strength Cond Res.* 2008; 22: 1522–1527.
77. Moraes E, Fleck S, Ricardo Dias M, Simão R. Effects on strength, power, and flexibility in adolescents of nonperiodized vs. daily nonlinear periodized weight training. *J Strength Cond Res.* 2013; 27: 3310–3321.
78. Faigenbaum A, Ratamess N, McFarland J, *et al.* Effect of rest interval length on bench press performance in boys, teens, and men. *Pediatr Exerc Sci.* 2008; 20: 457–469.
79. Ignjatovic A, Markovic Z, Radovanovic D. Effects of 12-week medicine ball training on muscle strength and power in young female handball players. *J Strength Cond Res.* 2012; 26: 2166–2173.
80. Faigenbaum A, Westcott W, Long C, Loud R, Delmonico M, Micheli L. Relationship between repetitions and selected percentages of the one repetition maximum in healthy children. *Pediatr Phys Ther.* 1998; 10: 110–113.
81. Hamill B. Relative safety of weight lifting and weight training. *J Strength Cond Res.* 1994; 8: 53–57.
82. Faigenbaum A, McFarland J, Johnson L, *et al.* Preliminary evaluation of an after-school resistance training program for improving physical fitness in middle school-age boys. *Percept Motor Skills.* 2007; 104: 407–415.
83. Gonzales-Badillo J, Gorostiaga E, Arellano R, Izquierdo M. Moderate resistance training produces more favorable strength gains than high or low volume during a short-term training cycle. *J Strength Cond Res.* 2005; 19: 689–697.
84. Duehring M, Feldmann CR, Ebben WP. Strength and conditioning practices of United States high school strength and conditioning coaches. *J Strength Cond Res.* 2009; 23: 2188–2193.
85. Myer G, Quatman C, Khoury J, Wall E, Hewett T. Youth vs. adult 'weightlifting' injuries presented to United States Emergengy Rooms: Accidental vs. non-accidental injury mechanisms. *J Strength Cond Res.* 2009; 23: 2054–2060.
86. Kerr Z, Collins C, Comstock R. Epidemiology of weight training-related injuries presenting to United States emergency departments, 1990 to 2007. *Am J Sports Med.* 2010; 38: 765–771.
87. Faigenbaum A, Myer G, Naclerion F, Casas A. Injury trends and prevention in youth resistance training. *Strength Cond.* 2011; 33: 36–41.
88. Barnett L, Reynolds J, Faigenbaum A, Smith J, Harries S, Lubans D. Rater agreement of a test battery designed to assess adolescents' resistance training skill competency. *J Sci Med Sport.* 2015; 18: 72–76.
89. Coutts A, Murphy A, Dascombe B. Effect of direct supervision of a strength coach on measures of muscular strength and power in young rugby league players. *J Strength Cond Res.* 2004; 18: 316–323.
90. Gentil P, Bottaro M. Influence of supervision ratio on muscle adaptations to resistance training in nontrained subjects. *J Strength Cond Res.* 2010; 24: 639–643.
91. Difiori J, Benjamin H, Brenner J, *et al.* Overuse injuries and burnout in youth sports: a position statement from the american medical society for sports medicine. *Clin J Sports Med.* 2014; 24: 3–20.

92. Matos N, Winsley R, Williams C. Prevalence of nonfunctional overreaching /overtraining in young English athletes. *Med Sci Sports Exerc.* 2011; 43: 1287–1294.
93. Gabbett T. The training-injury prevention paradox: should athletes be training smarter and harder? *Br J Sports Med.* 2016; 50: 273–280.
94. Emery C, Roy T, Whittaker J, Nettel-Aguirre A, van Mechelen W. Neuromuscular training injury prevention strategies in youth sport: a systematic review and meta-analysis. *Br J Sports Med.* 2015; 49: 865–870.
95. Ortega F, Silventoinen K, Tynelius P, Rasmussen F. Muscular strength in male adolescents and premature death: cohort study of one million participants. *BMJ.* 2012; 345: e7279.
96. Valovich McLeod T, Decoster L, Loud K, *et al.* National Athletic Trainers' Association position statement: prevention of pediatric overuse injuries. *J Athl Train.* 2011; 46: 206–220.
97. Ishikawa S, Kim Y, Kang M, Morgan D. Effects of weight-bearing exercise on bone health in girls: a meta-analysis. *Sports Med.* 2013; 43: 875–892.
98. Behringer M, Gruetzner S, McCourt M, Mester J. Effects of weight-bearing activities on bone mineral content and density in children and adolescents: a meta-analysis. *J Bone Min Res.* 2014; 29: 467–478.
99. Clark E, Tobias J, Murray L, Boreham C. Children with low muscle strength are at an increased risk of fracture with exposure to exercise. *J Musculoskel Neuron Inter.* 2011; 11: 196–202.
100. Heinonen A, Sievänen H, Kannus P, Oja P, Pasanen M, Vuori I. High-impact exercise and bones of growing girls: a 9-month controlled trial. *Osteoporos Int.* 2000; 11: 1010–1017.
101. Nogueira R, Weeks B, Beck B. Targeting bone and fat with novel exercise for peripubertal boys: the CAPO kids trial. *Pediatr Exerc Sci.* 2015; 27: 128–139.
102. Bernardoni B, Thein-Nissenbaum J, Fast J, *et al.* A school-based resistance intervention improves skeletal growth in adolescent females. *Osteoporos Int.* 2014; 25: 1025–1032.
103. Conroy BP, Kraemer WJ, Maresh CM, *et al.* Bone mineral density in elite junior Olympic weightlifters. *Med Sci Sports Exerc.* 1993; 25: 1103–1109.
104. Virvidakis K, Georgiu E, Korkotsidis A, Ntalles A, Proukakis C. Bone mineral content of junior competitive weightlifters. *Int J Sports Med.* 1990; 11: 244–246.
105. Morris F, Naughton G, Gibbs J, Carlson J, Wark J. Prospective ten-month exercise intervention in premenarcheal girls. *J Bone Min Res.* 1997; 12: 1453–1462.
106. Ward K, Roberts S, Adams J, Mughal M. Bone geometry and density in the skeleton of prepubertal gymnasts and school children. *Bone.* 2005; 26: 1012–1018.
107. Erlandson M, Sherar L, Mirwald R, Maffulli N, Baxter-Jones A. Growth and maturation of adolescent female gymnasts, swimmers, and tennis players. *Med Sci Sports Exerc.* 2008; 40: 34–42.
108. Jackowski S, Baxter-Jones A, Gruodyte-Raciene R, Kontulainen S, Erlandson M. A longitudinal study of bone area, content, density, and strength development at the radius and tibia in children 4–12 years of age exposed to recreational gymnastics. *Osteoporos Int.* 2015; 26: 1677–1690.
109. Meyer U, Ernst D, Zahner L, *et al.* 3-Year follow-up results of bone mineral content and density after a school-based physical activity randomized intervention trial. *Bone.* 2013; 55: 16–22.
110. Barnekow-Bergkvist M, Hedberg G, Pettersson U, Lorentzon R. Relationships between physical activity and physical capacity in adolescent females and bone mass in adulthood. *Scand J Med Sci Sports.* 2006; 16: 447–455.
111. Tveit M, Rosengren B, Nilsson J, Karlsson M. Exercise in youth: High bone mass, large bone size, and low fracture risk in old age. *Scand J Med Sci Sport.* 2015; 25: 453–461.
112. McCrindle B. Cardiovascular consequences of childhood obesity. *Can J Cardiol.* 2015; 31: 124–130.
113. Hannon T, Arslanian S. The changing face of diabetes in youth: lessons learned from studies of type 2 diabetes. *Ann New York Acad Sci.* 2015; 1353: 113–137.
114. Peterson M, Zhang P, Saltarelli W, Visich P, Gordon P. Low muscle strength thresholds for the detection of cardiometabolic risk in adolescents. *Am J Prev Med.* 2016; 50: 593–599.
115. Grøntved A, Ried-Larsen M, Christian Møller N, *et al.* Muscle strength in youth and cardiovascular risk in young adulthood (the European Youth Heart Study). *Br J Sports Med.* 2015; 49: 90–94.
116. Artero E, Ruiz J, Ortega F, *et al.* Muscular and cardiorespiratory fitness are independently associated with metabolic risk in adolescents: the HELENA study. *Pediatr Diabetes.* 2011; 12: 704–712.
117. Steene-Johannessen J, Anderssen S, Kolle E. Low muscle fitness is associated with metabolic risk in youth. *Med Sci Sports Exerc.* 2009; 41: 1361–1367.
118. Magnussen C, Schmidt M, Dwyer T, Venn A. Muscular fitness and clustered cardiovascular disease risk in Australian youth. *Eur J Appl Physiol.* 2012; 112: 3167–3171.
119. Shaibi GQ, Cruz ML, Ball GD, *et al.* Effects of resistance training on insulin sensitivity in overweight Latino adolescent males. *Med Sci Sports Exerc.* 2006; 38: 1208–1215.
120. Van der Heijden G, Wang Z, Chu Z, *et al.* Strength exercise improves muscle mass and hepatic insulin sensitivity in obese youth. *Med Sci Sports Exerc.* 2010; 42: 1973–1980.
121. Dias I, Farinatti P, de Souza M, *et al.* Effects of resistance training on obese adolescents. *Med Sci Sports Exerc.* 2015; 47: 2636–2644.
122. Sigal R, Alberga A, Goldfield G, *et al.* Effects of aerobic training, resistance training, or both on percentage body fat and cardiometabolic risk markers in obese adolescents: the healthy eating aerobic and resistance training in youth randomized clinical trial. *JAMA Pediatr.* 2014; 168: 1006–1014.
123. Goldfield G, Kenny G, Alberga A, *et al.* Effects of aerobic training, resistance training, or both on psychological health in adolescents with obesity: The HEARTY randomized controlled trial. *J Consult Clin Psych.* 2015; 83: 1123–1135.
124. Alberga A, Prud'homme D, Kenny G, *et al.* Effects of aerobic and resistance training on abdominal fat, apolipoproteins and high-sensitivity C-reactive protein in adolescents with obesity: the HEARTY randomized clinical trial. *Int J Obesity.* 2015; 39: 1494–1500.
125. Dietz P, Hoffmann S, Lachtermann E, Simon P. Influence of exclusive resistance training on body composition and cardiovascular risk factors in overweight or obese children: a systematic review. *Obesity Facts.* 2012; 5: 546–560.
126. Schranz N, Tomkinson G, Parletta N, Petkov J, Olds T. Can resistance training change the strength, body composition and self-concept of overweight and obese adolescent males? A randomised controlled trial. *Br J Sports Med.* 2013; 48: 1482–1488.
127. Gogtay N, Giedd J, Lusk L, *et al.* Dynamic mapping of human cortical development during childhood through early adulthood. *Proc Nat Acad Sci USA.* 2004; 101: 8174–8179.
128. Gogtay N, Thompson P. Mapping gray matter development: implications for typical development and vulnerability to psychopathology. *Brain Cog.* 2010; 72: 6–15.
129. Faigenbaum A, McFarland J, Keiper F, *et al.* Effects of a short term plyometric and resistance training program on fitness performance in boys age 12 to 15 years. *J Sports Sci Med.* 2007; 6: 519–525.
130. Santos E, Janeira M. Effects of complex training on explosive strength in adolescent male basketball players. *J Strength Cond Res.* 2008; 22: 903–909.
131. Faigenbaum A, Farrell A, Fabiano M, *et al.* Effects of integrated neuromuscular training on fitness performance in children. *Pediatr Exerc Sci.* 2011; 23: 573–584.
132. Wong P, Chamari K, Wisloff U. Effects of 12-week on-field combined strength and power training on physical performance among U-14 young soccer players. *J Strength Cond Res.* 2010; 24: 644–652.

133. Gabbett T, Whyte D, Hartwig T, Wescombe H, Naughton G. The relationship between workloads, physical performance, injury and illness in adolescent male football players. *Sports Med.* 2014; 44: 989–1003.
134. Mikkola J, Rusko H, Nummela A, Pollari T, Häkkinen K. Concurrent endurance and explosive type strength training improves neuromuscular and anaerobic characteristics in young distance runners. *Int J Sports Med.* 2007; 28: 602–611.
135. Behringer M, Neuerburg S, Matthews M, Mester J. Effects of two different resistance-training programs on mean tennis-serve velocity in adolescents. *Pediatr Exerc Sci.* 2013; 25: 370–384.
136. Thomas K, French D, Hayes P. The effect of two plyometric training techniques on muscular power and agility in youth soccer players. *J Strength Cond Res.* 2009; 23: 332–335.
137. DiStefano L, Padua DA, Blackburn J, Garrett W, Guskiewicz KM, Marshall S. Integrated injury prevention program improves balance and vertical jump height in children. *J Strength Cond Res.* 2010; 24: 332–342.
138. Keiner M, Sander A, Wirth K, Schmidtbleicher D. Long-term strength training effects on change-of-direction sprint performance. *J Strength Cond Res.* 2014; 28: 223–231.
139. Myer G, Jayanthi N, DiFiori J, *et al.* Sport specialization, Part I: Does early sports specialization increase negative outcomes and reduce the opportunity for success in young athletes? *Sports Health.* 2015; 7: 437–442.
140. Myer G, Jayanthi N, DiFiori J, *et al.* Sports specialization, Part II: Alternative solutions to early sport specialization in youth athletes. *Sports Health.* 2015; 8: 65–73.
141. Tremblay M, Gray C, Akinroye K, *et al.* Physical activity of children: A global matrix of grades comparing 15 countries. *J Phys Act Health.* 2014; 11(Supp 1): S113–S125.
142. Leek D, Carlson J, Cain K, *et al.* Physical activity during youth sports practices. *Arch Pediatr Adolesc Med.* 2010; 165: 294–299.
143. Guagliano J, Rosenkranz R, Kolt G. Girls' physical activity levels during organized sports in Australia. *Med Sci Sports Exerc.* 2013; 45: 116–122.
144. Carter C, Micheli L. Training the child athlete: physical fitness, health and injury. *Br J Sports Med.* 2011; 45: 880–885.
145. Emery CA, Meeuwisse W. The effectiveness of a neuromuscular prevention strategy to reduce injuries in youth soccer: a cluster-randomised controlled trial. *Br J Sports Med.* 2010; 44: 555–562.
146. Wingfield K. Neuromuscular training to prevent knee injuries in adolescent female soccer players. *Clin J Sports Med.* 2013; 23: 407–408.
147. LaBella C, Huxford M, Grissom J, Kim K, Peng J, Christoffel K. Effect of neuromuscular warm-up on injuries in female soccer and basketball athletes in urban public high schools: cluster randomized controlled trial. *Arch Pediatr Adolesc Med.* 2011; 165: 1033–1040.
148. Ungerleider L, Doyon J, Karni A. Imaging brain plasticity during motor skill learning. *Neurobiol Learn Mem.* 2002; 78: 553–564.
149. Myer G, Sugimoto D, Thomas S, Hewett T. The influence of age on the effectiveness of neuromuscular training to reduce anterior cruciate ligament injuries in female athletes: A meta analysis. *Am J Sports Med.* 2013; 41: 203–215.
150. Sugimoto D, Myer G, Bush H, Klugman M, Medina McKeon J, Hewett T. Compliance with neuromuscular training and anterior cruciate ligament injury risk reduction in female athletes: a meta-analysis. *J Athl Train.* 2012; 47: 714–723.
151. Meeusen R, Duclos M, Foster C, *et al.* Prevention, diagnosis, and treatment of the overtraining syndrome: joint consensus statement of the European College of Sport Science and the American College of Sports Medicine. *Med Sci Sports Exerc.* 2013; 45: 186–205.
152. American Academy of Pediatrics. Strength training by children and adolescent. *Pediatrics.* 2008; 121: 835–840.
153. Annesi JJ, Westcott WL, Faigenbaum AD, Unruh JL. Effects of a 12-week physical activity protocol delivered by YMCA after-school counselors (Youth Fit for Life) on fitness and self-efficacy changes in 5–12-year-old boys and girls. *Res Q Exerc Sport.* 2005; 76: 468–476.
154. Faigenbaum AD, Westcott WL, Loud RL, Long C. The effects of different resistance training protocols on muscular strength and endurance development in children. *Pediatrics.* 1999; 104: e5.
155. Myer G, Lloyd R, Brent J, Faigenbaum A. How young is too young to start training? *ACSM's Health Fit J.* 2013; 17: 14–23.
156. Lubans D, Sheaman C, Callister R. Exercise adherence and intervention effects of two school-based resistance training programs for adolescents. *Prev Med.* 2010; 50: 56–62.
157. Faigenbaum A, Mediate P. The effects of medicine ball training on physical fitness in high school physical education students. *Phys Educ.* 2006; 63: 160–167.
158. Balsamo S, Tibana R, Nascimento DC, *et al.* Exercise order influences number of repetitions and lactate levels but not perceived exertion during resistance exercise in adolescents. *J Strength Cond Res.* 2013; 21: 293–304.
159. Hooper D, Szivak T, Comstock B, *et al.* Effects of fatigue from resistance training on barbell back squat biomechanics. *J Strength Cond Res.* 2014; 28: 1127–1134.
160. Stone M, Stone M, Sands W. *Principles and practice of resistance training.* Champaign, IL: Human Kinetics; 2007.
161. Falk B, Dotan R. Child-adult differences in the recovery from high-intensity exercise. *Exerc Sport Sci Rev.* 2006; 34: 107–112.
162. Zafeiridis A, Dalamitros A, Dipla K, Manou N, Galanis N, Kellis S. Recovery during high intensity intermittent anaerobic exercise in boys, teens and men. *Med Sci Sports Exerc.* 2005; 37: 505–512.
163. Murphy J, Button D, Chaouachi A, Behm D. Prepubescent males are less susceptible to neuromuscular fatigue following resistance exercise. *Eur J Appl Physiol.* 2014; 114: 825–835.
164. Ratel S, Duché P, Williams C. Muscle fatigue during high-intensity exercise in children. *Sports Med.* 2006; 36: 1031–1065.
165. Dotan R, Mitchell C, Chohen R, Klentrou P, Gabriel D, Falk B. Child-adult differences in muscle activation—a review. *Pediatr Exerc Sci.* 2012; 24: 2–21.
166. Casey B, Tottenham N, Liston C, Durston S. Imaging the developing brain: what have we learned about cognitive development? *Trend Cog Sci.* 2005; 9: 104–110.
167. Faigenbaum A, Milliken L, Loud R, Burak B, Doherty C, Westcott W. Comparison of 1 and 2 days per week of strength training in children. *Res Q Exerc Sport.* 2002; 73: 416–424.
168. Katzmarzyk P, Barreira T, Broyles S, *et al.* Physical activity, sedentary time, and obesity in an international sample of children. *Med Sci Sports Exerc.* 2015; 47: 2062–2069.
169. Harries S, Lubans D, Callister R. Comparison of resistance training progression models on maximal strength in sub-elite adolescent rugby union players. *J Sci Med Sport.* 2016; 19: 163–169.
170. Haff G. Periodization strategies for youth development. In: Lloyd R, Oliver J (eds.) *Strength and conditioning for young athletes: Science and application.* Oxford: Routledge; 2014. p. 149–168.

CHAPTER 37

Speed and agility training

Jon L Oliver and Rhodri S Lloyd

Introduction

Natural play activities in children are characterized by fundamental movement skills that include agility and speed, which are also determinants of success in youth sport.[1–3] It has also been suggested that speed and agility may be important components of health-related fitness, with some limited evidence suggesting they may be an important marker of bone health.[4–6] As a result, sprint and agility tests have become both popular assessments in youth sport[3,7–10] as well as components of health-related fitness test batteries for children and adolescents.[4,6] While linear sprinting and agility both require the ability to move at speed it has been shown that they each represent independent locomotor qualities in youth athletes.[11] Therefore, it is pertinent to consider speed and agility as separate entities.

Sprinting is a linear skill, with an individual propelling themselves forward as rapidly as possible. A sprint can be divided into four phases; first step quickness, acceleration, maximal speed, and deceleration.[12] Typically, measurements in youth have considered acceleration and speed. Although acceleration and maximal speed (hereafter referred to as speed) are related to one another, they are not the same.[10,13] Time taken to cover the first 10 m of a sprint is often used as a measure of acceleration, which incorporates first step quickness (0–5 m).[12] Speed is normally measured over longer distances of 30–40 m, often with the split times recorded from 10 m onwards to remove the acceleration phase, although the actual point of transition from acceleration to maximal speed will vary between individuals and across populations.[12] In a large sample of 11- to 16-year-old boys it has been shown that maximal speed in a single stride occurs between 15 and 30 m.[14] This chapter discusses the natural development and trainability of speed and agility in children and adolescents.

Until the last decade agility had largely been considered as the ability to rapidly change direction.[15] More recently the definition of agility has been extended to incorporate that rapid changes of direction occur in response to a stimulus.[16] Consequently, agility has both a physical perspective reflecting change-of-direction-speed and a cognitive perspective reflecting perceptual and decision-making skills. Given the difficulty of measuring perceptual skills in context-specific scenarios, most (if not all) of the literature about research in this area with regard to children and adolescents has assessed change-of-direction-speed rather than agility, per se.[3,7–10] Our current understanding of the development and trainability of agility to the physical determinants of change-of-direction-speed are therefore limited, although evidence of perceptual development from the broader literature is available.

Speed

Sprinting is considered a fundamental movement skill (FMS) that is important for both free-play activities and sport participation. Speed can be a distinguishing and desirable physical characteristic, and is also known to be a determinant of success in youth sports, distinguishing between playing levels and age groups in sports such as football,[8] rugby league,[17] and basketball.[9] Consequently, talent identification in youth sports will often include measures of speed as key performance indicators.[3,17,18] This may be problematic; although speed is associated with sports performance it is influenced by age, maturation, and growth. For instance, it has been suggested that peak rates of improvements in speed occur around the time of peak height velocity (PHV),[19] and that these gains will be influenced by changes in body mass and lower limb length,[20] as well as qualitative changes in muscle-tendon structure and function that accompany maturation.[21] It has also been suggested that these developmental processes may influence the responsiveness to speed training throughout childhood and adolescence.[22]

Natural development of speed

Given that sprinting is a key FMS[1] and can be a determinant of success in adult[7,23] and youth sports,[2,3] it is surprising that relatively few studies describe the natural development of sprint speed during childhood and adolescence. Previous large-cohort studies have used plate tapping and shuttle run tests as a form of speed assessment,[24,25] with only a few studies directly examining sprint speed.[14,26] It has been suggested that both boys and girls exhibit similar sprint speed in the first decade of life,[27,28] with both sexes experiencing more rapid natural gains in speed between the ages of 5–9 years; this phenomenon has been termed the 'preadolescent spurt'.[29] A second 'adolescent spurt' occurs with maturation, with peak gains coinciding with puberty[27] and the timing of peak PHV.[14,19] However, it has also been suggested that this spurt in speed development occurs in the early phase of the growth spurt.[30] With maturation, sex differences in speed become more apparent. From the age of 12 years the rate of progression of speed development is dramatically reduced in females when compared to males.[31] It has been suggested that the arrival of the fourth puberty stage (interested readers are referred to Chapter 1 for an analysis of the assessment of biological maturity) marks the end of maximal speed development in girls not involved in sport. [32] Natural speed development, on the other hand, continues into full maturity in males.[29] This disparity between the sexes is attributed to maturational changes in circulating androgens, body dimensions, and body composition.[21,24,29,33]

Development of sprint speed in boys and girls between the ages of 9 and 15 years is shown in Figure 37.2. It is clear that improvements in speed are observed across the age range for all percentiles in boys, and most percentiles in girls. For a given percentile boys are always faster than girls, but the relative difference between the sexes changes with age. Girls demonstrate a more rapid rate of speed development up until the age of 12 years, whereas boys demonstrate a more rapid rate of speed development from the age of 12 years onwards. The differential timing of periods of rapid development when comparing the sexes supports a maturational effect on speed development. The timing of rapid speed development shown in Figure 37.1, which is based on data from Catley and Tomkinson,[34] occurs prior to the expected age of PHV in the population. This observation supports the longitudinal monitoring of speed in a small cohort of boys and girls, where peak gains in speed occurred prior to PHV.[30] In another longitudinal study of a small sample of boys, peak gains in speed were suggested to occur around the timing of PHV; according to Philippaerts *et al.*,[19] participants actually became slower in the 18 months prior to PHV, and the subsequent increase in speed may simply have reflected a long-term correction to speed.[35] The observation that some youths become slower around the onset of the growth spurt has been attributed to adolescent awkwardness and temporarily disrupted co-ordination during periods of rapid limb growth.[19,24] When comparing boys of different maturity status, Rumpf and colleagues[36] found that maximal speed could be largely explained by power and horizontal force in both pre- and post-PHV boys. However, this was not the case for boys circa PHV, which again may have been related to this group experiencing some level of awkwardness. Increases in maximal running speed in boys of advancing age have been shown to disappear when data are adjusted for somatic maturity,[2,36] confirming that speed gains are maturation dependent. From cross-sectional examination of a large cohort of 11- to 16-year-old boys, data show that speed remains relatively stable from approximately 3 years to 1 year prior to PHV, with significant gains in speed observed from the timing of PHV onwards.[14] While there is clearly an influence of maturation on speed development, it is not entirely clear whether peak gains in speed coincide with the timing of PHV, or the start of the growth spurt.

It is difficult to understand the mechanisms that underpin the natural development of speed during different stages of growth and maturation, given the contribution and integration of a number of different factors. These include quantitative changes in body size, muscle cross-sectional area and length, biological and metabolic changes, morphological alterations to the muscle and tendon, and neural/motor development as well as biomechanical and co-ordination factors[21] (interested readers are referred to Chapter 3 and Chapter 4 for a discussion of motor development and biomechanical coordination). There is a suggested link between the observed preadolescent spurt in sprint speed and the development of the central nervous system and improved co-ordination.[27,29] This theory is supported by the rapid growth of the central nervous system during the first 7 years of life,[28] the peak maturation of brain regions which control movement (at 7.5 years and 10 years of age in girls and boys, respectively),[37] and the observation that mature stride dynamics are achieved somewhere between the ages of 7 and 11–14 years of age.[31,38]

Changes in height, leg length, and muscle size during adolescence support a maturational influence on speed development, although Butterfield *et al.*[33] found no association between longitudinal growth rates of height and weight and improved running speed in children aged 11–13 years. Metabolic factors can influence maximal sprint speed, and it may be that immature children have lower muscle phosphocreatine (PCr) stores,[39] although children and adults have been shown to break down adenosine triphosphate (ATP) and PCr at similar rates.[40] Maturation of the glycolytic system is likely to be more pronounced, but this would likely have more of an effect on prolonged high-intensity running, rather than maximal speed. Maturation of muscle-tendon architecture and inherent characteristics are likely to have a substantial influence on the development of sprint speed. Ovalle[41] reported marked increases in the surface area of the muscle-tendon junction from childhood into adulthood; this change was accompanied by a reduced number of Golgi organs in the mature state. Partly as a consequence of these changes in the biomechanical properties of muscle and connective tissue, a tenfold increase in muscle-tendon stiffness has been observed in the first two decades of life.[42] Changes in muscle stiffness will also be influenced by neural factors, with firing rates,[31] twitch times,[42]

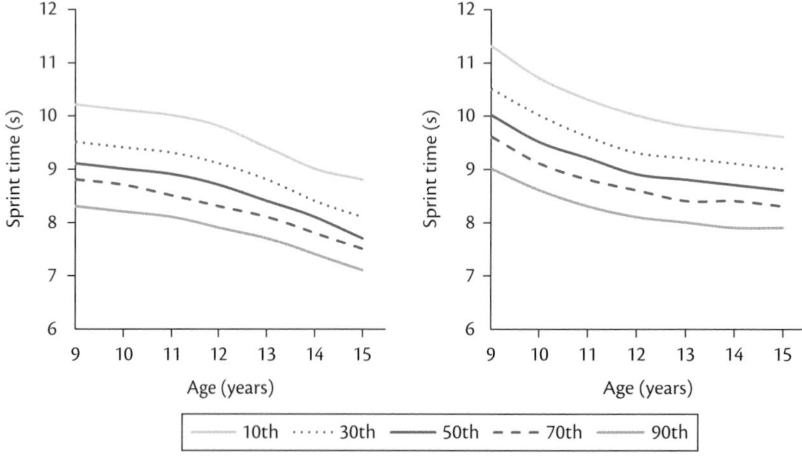

Figure 37.1 Fifty-metre sprint time percentiles in 9- to 15-year-old Australian boys and girls. Boys on the left and girls on the right.
Data from Catley MJ, Tomkinson GR. Normative health-related fitness values for children: analysis of 85347 test results on 9–17-year-old Australians since 1985. Br J Sports Med. 2013; 47: 98–108.

preactivation,[43,44] reflex muscle activity,[45,41] and coactivation[42,46] all shown to develop through childhood in a manner that would favour increased speed production. Greater muscle-tendon and leg stiffness will theoretically enhance sprint performance by enabling the lower limbs to resist large vertical displacement of the centre of mass as well as increasing rate of force development during ground contact.[47] Leg stiffness has been shown to be a predictor of maximal sprint speed in adolescent boys.[48] When examining sprint speed on a non-motorized treadmill, Rumpf *et al.*[49] noted that maximal speed, relative vertical stiffness, and relative leg stiffness all increased from pre-, to circa-, to post-PHV in boys; however, these differences disappeared when maturation was statistically controlled. These findings support a role of maturation and stiffness in the development of sprint speed.

Growth, maturation, and spatio-temporal determinants of speed

Running speed is a product of stride frequency and length.[50] Stride frequency is a function of ground contact time and flight time and stride length is determined by a combination of the distance covered while in contact with the ground and the distance covered while in flight. Understanding these spatio-temporal determinants of speed can help provide insight into the process of speed development in children and adolescents. In an early study Schepens *et al.*[26] examined the sprint mechanics of 2- to 16-year-old youths, concluding that step frequency changes little with age and that age-related changes in maximal speed are almost entirely due to proportional increases in stride length. However, a trend for decreasing step frequency was apparent in the data and the lack of a statistically significant change was likely due to the small sample sizes in each group (n = 6–8). Recently Meyers *et al.*[14] examined spatio-temporal determinants of speed in a large cohort of circa-adolescent boys (n = 336). The authors reported significant decreases in stride frequency across boys classified from approximately 3- to 1-year prior to PHV; during this time, stride length significantly increased and there was no net change in speed. Stride frequency then stabilized in boys around PHV and 1 year post-PHV, while continued gains in stride length in these boys resulted in increased maximal speed. Similar to Schepens *et al*,[26] Meyers *et al.*[14] concluded that increased stride length is the primary determinant of maximal speed, as this variable explained 57% of the reported variance. This contrasts with adult data, with data showing faster runners achieving longer strides through greater application of ground reaction forces during a reduced ground-contact period.[51,52] In comparison, paediatric data suggest that through adolescence children increase ground-contact times, which reduces stride frequency; however, this is more than compensated for by relatively larger increases in stride length. It is also worth noting that flight times remain unchanged with maturation,[14] which is consistent with comparisons of adult sprinters of different abilities.[51,52]

A recent study by Meyers *et al.*[20] demonstrated that spatio-temporal determinants of speed are maturity dependent. In boys pre-PHV, stride frequency accounted for the greatest amount of variability (58%) in maximal speed, whereas in boys circa- and post-PHV, stride length explained the greatest amount of variance (54%) in speed. In elite adult sprinters it has been suggested that those with lower levels of strength are more stride-*frequency* reliant and those with greater strength levels are more stride-*length* reliant.[53] This theory can be applied to the development of speed; immature children with lower muscle mass and lower strength, but who have a well-developed somatic nervous system, appear to be more reliant on a quick turnover of their legs to generate speed. Conversely, maturation-related improvements in strength and power output observed around the time of PHV[54,55] result in an ability to generate large relative forces and a shift to where adolescents become more stride length reliant when generating speed. Indeed, when comparing maximal sprinting in boys pre-, circa- and post-PHV, data show that relative force production increases alongside stride length and speed.[36] This suggests that with the onset of maturation, increases in mass, muscle size, and relative strength allow adolescents to become more stride-length reliant when generating speed.

Physical growth also influences speed development. Data suggest that increasing body mass as a result of maturation is related to increased contact times that reduce stride frequency.[14,20] However, both greater relative levels of strength[36] and increases in stature and leg length may compensate for this, and increased leg length with advancing maturation has been shown to influence sprint performance,[2,19,20,26] with recent research reporting a correlation of r = 0.60 ($p < 0.01$) between leg length and stride length at maximal speed in 11- to 15-year-old boys.[14] A longer leg may allow for a greater distance to be covered while in contact with the ground; this has been suggested in adult sprinters.[51] The role of increasing limb length would support a developmental spurt in speed during the early phase of the growth spurt, when long bones of the body are experiencing rapid growth. It should be noted that our understanding of the development of spatio-temporal determinants of speed is limited to research with boys.

Speed training

There has been debate over recent years regarding how age and maturation interact with training responsiveness in children and adults. The 'trigger hypothesis'[56] suggests children do not respond to training until after the onset of puberty. Similarly, a popular coaching model suggests that 'windows of opportunity' exist when training gains in speed are maximized at specific ages in boys and girls, and that a failure to fully utilize those windows will limit future potential.[57] However, this belief has been strongly refuted due to a lack of supporting empirical evidence.[21,58] More recently, it has been suggested that training-induced gains in sprint speed can be made throughout childhood and adolescence, although the mechanisms that underpin those gains, as well as the types of training that are most effective, might differ with maturation.[1,22]

Short-term speed training interventions

Sprint speed can be improved through a variety of training modes, including sprint training, technical training, strength training, and plyometric training. Sprint training involves participants completing maximal sprint efforts, which can be modified to include various forms of both resisted (e.g. sled towing) and assisted (e.g. downhill) training. Given that specificity is a key principle of training it is surprising that few studies have focused on the efficacy of free, resisted, or assisted sprint training to improve speed in youths.[22] Likewise, a recent systematic review highlighted that only a handful of free, resisted, and assisted sprint training studies have been done in adults.[59] While training interventions to improve speed may employ some sprint work, they typically involve either plyometric or strength training, or a combination of these. Table 37.1 provides an overview of sprint training studies in boys and highlights the

Table 37.1 An overview of training studies that have assessed maximal sprint speed in boys aged 10–17-years-old.

Reference	Age	Mode	Total sessions	Test distance(s)	% Change
Rumpf *et al.*[62]	10.4 ± 0.8	Res Sprint	16	0–30	1.0
Venturelli *et al.*[63]	11.0 ± 0.5	Sprint	24	0–20	2.4
Venturelli *et al.*[63]	11.0 ± 0.5	Combined	24	0–20	2.2
Kotzamanidis[64]	11.1 ± 0.5	Sprint	20	10–20	5.5
Kotzamanidis[65]	11.1 ± 0.5	Plyometric	10	10–20	3.5
Pettersen and Mathisen[66]	11.5 ± 0.3	Sprint	6	0–20	1.8
Chelly *et al.*[67]	11.7 ± 1.0	Plyometric	30	Vmax	3.7
Ingle *et al.*[68]	11.8 ± 0.4	Combined	36	0–40	3.2
Diallo *et al.*[69]	12.3 ± 0.4	Plyometric	30	0–20	2.8
Wong *et al.*[70]	13.5 ± 0.7	Strength	24	0–30	2.3
Chaouachi *et al.*[71]	13.3 ± 0.7	Combined	24	0–30	2.8
Chaouachi *et al.*[71]	13.7 ± 0.8	Plyometric	24	0–30	3.4
Christou *et al.*[60]	13.8 ± 0.4	Strength	32	0–30	2.6
Rumpf *et al.*[62]	15.2 ± 1.6	Res Sprint	16	0–30	5.8
Coutts *et al.*[72]	16.6 ± 1.2	Strength	18–36	0–20	≤0.9
Chelly *et al.*[73]	17.0 ± 0.3	Strength	16	35–40	10.9
Kotzamanidis[74]	17.0 ± 1.1	Combined	39	0–30	3.5
Kotzamanidis[74]	17.1 ± 1.1	Strength	39	0–30	0.5
Thomas *et al.*[75]	17.3 ± 0.4	Plyometric	12	0–20	≤0.3
Maio Alves *et al.*[76]	17.4 ± 0.6	Combined	6–12	0–15	≤7.0

The dashed lines separate the table in to age groups that approximate to pre- (top), circa- (middle), and post- (bottom) peak height velocity.
A positive % change represents an improvement in sprint performance.
Res Sprint = Resisted Sprint (sled towing), Vmax = maximum velocity.

different forms of training employed across studies; they examined training programmes lasting from 6 to 16 weeks with between one and three training sessions per week. Changes in speed in Table 37.1 are reported for sprint distances ≥15 m, to reflect changes in speed rather than acceleration. All studies report on positive improvements in speed following training. Most studies show the level of improvement as > the level of expected noise (coefficient of variation = 0.83%) reported for 12- to 15-year-olds completing a 30 m sprint.[60] Additionally, training-related gains in performance are generally greater than those that would be expected from growth and maturation. Williams *et al.*[35] have reported that 30-m sprint times improve at a rate of 2.7% per year in 11- to 16-year-old football players, which would equate to gains of approximately 0.3–0.8% over the period of the training studies included in Table 37.1. While there are much fewer data available for girls, the existing research does suggest that girls can also improve their speed with sprint training.[61]

In a systematic review of training studies, Rump *et al.*[22] concluded that plyometric training and combined training are the most effective methods to improve speed for pre- and post-PHV boys, respectively; there were limited data available for boys who were circa-PHV. However, it should be noted those conclusions were based on measures of both acceleration and speed. Additionally, these data are from studies where maturity was not directly classified. The findings of Rumpf *et al.*[22] and the results presented in Table 37.1 support the notion that children and adolescents can be responsive to training. The fact that pre- and post-PHV participants may be more responsive to different types of training has been linked to natural development.[1,22] From studies identified in Table 37.1, boys who would be expected to be in a pre-PHV age range (<13 years old) respond to training that includes a plyometric stimulus, either in isolation or combined with other training. Boys in a post-PHV age range respond most to interventions that include a strength stimulus (either in isolation or combined). These responses may be facilitated by high neural plasticity in immature children and the greater propensity of mature youth to experience hormone-mediated changes in muscle size and architecture, although direct evidence is needed to confirm this. While there are limited data available on boys who are circa-PHV, the evidence from Table 37.1 suggests that boys around the age of PHV (~13.5–14 years old) can make speed gains via a variety of training methods. The similar success across a range of studies and interventions in this age group may be related to the fact that all studies included a reasonable and consistent dosage of two sessions per week, for either 12 or 16 weeks.

Direct investigations of maturation and training interactions

Studies that have directly examined the interaction of age and maturation with training provide further insight into responsiveness.

Rumpf *et al.*[62] compared gains in sprint speed in 10- and 15-year-old boys after 6 weeks of sled tow (resistance) training. While younger boys showed no changes in performance, older boys significantly improved sprint performance, stride frequency, stride length, leg and vertical stiffness, force, and power production. Both groups followed the same training programme pulling loads of between 2.5–10% of body mass. However, data show that when pulling relative loads, pre-PHV children are 50% slower than post-PHV children during resisted sprints.[77] Therefore, it may be that lower levels of strength, excessive resistance, and an immature biological state combined to prevent the younger boys from experiencing any speed gains. In a recent study, Meylan *et al.*[78] reported that pre-PHV boys experienced small gains (2.1%) in sprint speed following 8 weeks of strength training, compared to moderate gains for both circa-PHV (3.6%) and post-PHV (3.1%) boys. Following the intervention, the post-PHV group achieved large gains in strength compared to only small gains in other groups; this suggests that more mature youth may be able to achieve greater gains in force production following strength training.[79]

Lloyd *et al.*[80] examined the influence of maturation and mode of training on speed development, comparing the responses of pre- and post-PHV boys between control, plyometric, strength, and combined (strength and plyometric) training groups. Twenty-metre sprint speed demonstrated small gains in performance for both the pre- and post-PHV groups following either plyometric or combined training, but with no gains in the control or strength training groups. As strength training did transfer benefits to other performance markers, including concentric strength and acceleration (post-PHV only), gains are therefore most likely to be observed when testing is specific to training. Both Lloyd *et al.*[80] and Thomas *et al.*[75] exposed post-PHV boys to plyometric interventions that included two sessions per week for 6 weeks, with both studies exposing participants to a similar volume of ground contacts. While Lloyd *et al.*[80] reported significant gains in speed, Thomas *et al.*[75] noted no change in speed. The disparity in findings between these similar studies can most likely be accounted for by considering the sample characteristics. Lloyd *et al.*[80] recruited a population of previously untrained boys, while Thomas *et al.*[75] examined youth with at least 4 years of football training history. For the latter, the training load of 80–120 ground contacts per session may have been too low given their training history. This may be significant, especially when considering that another plyometric training study with adolescent football players used a training load of 200 contacts per session.[81] However, it should also be noted that a systematic review of plyometric training in youth recommends that volume should not exceed 120 contacts per session to help prevent overuse injuries.[82] Alternatively, Table 37.1 and the work of Lloyd *et al.*[80] suggest that combining strength and plyometric training is an effective way to promote speed development for youth of all ages and maturation. Furthermore, it can provide the variety of training that should be central to any long-term athletic development programme.[1]

Longitudinal monitoring of speed in sporting populations

There is limited research available relating to the effectiveness of long-term, systematic training on speed development in childhood and adolescence. What information does exist comes largely from longitudinal investigations of the development of male youth soccer players. Gravina *et al.*[8] reported that 11- to 14-year-old soccer players who are regularly selected to play improve their sprint time by approximately 5% over the course of a season, compared to improvements of only 1% in reserve players. These findings may reflect the fact that selected players are exposed to a greater training stimulus through more game time, or there may be a likely selection bias towards those experiencing early maturation and rapid gains in speed.[8] Williams *et al.*[35] observed 12–16-year-old boys in a soccer centre of excellence over a 3-year period and found boys improved 30-m sprint times at a rate of 2.7% per year. Vanttinen *et al.*[83] used longitudinal and cross-sectional data to compare the development of 11- to 17-year-old soccer players and controls. While soccer players were faster than controls in each age group, the rate of improvement in 30-m sprint performance was similar in both cohorts, with improvements of approximately 19% over the 6-year period. In another study of young soccer players, academy players were found to improve 30-m sprint times significantly more than controls over a 3-year period (~9% versus ~4%).[84] Sander *et al.*[85] examined the influence of strength training in youth soccer players, comparing 13-, 15-, and 17-year-old players. Players were split into a control group, and a strength-training programme group for a 2-year period. Strength-training groups routinely made gains in speed significantly greater than controls, and the magnitude of gains decreased with advancing age; 30 m sprint times in the strength-training groups improved by 5.8% in the youngest group, 4.6% in the 15-year-olds, and 1.5% in the oldest group. Therefore, it appears that systematic long-term training in a soccer academy setting can promote enhanced speed development. However, although sometimes significant, the magnitude of the difference between gains in experimental and control groups in longitudinal studies is relatively modest;[83–85] similar gains have been observed in intervention studies of much shorter terms.[64,73] To the authors' knowledge, no long-term training studies have been specifically designed to improve maximal speed in children and adolescents.

Agility

Previously accepted definitions of agility suggested the ability to 'change direction rapidly';[15] however, it is now accepted that this paints an overly simplistic view of what is an intricate, multifactorial physical quality.[16] Regardless of the setting, movement occurs in response to external stimuli, e.g. an obstacle or an opposition player. Therefore, the more recent definition describes agility as rapid, whole-body movements that require the changing of direction, velocity, or both, in response to a stimulus.[16] Figure 37.2 (adapted from Sheppard and Young[16]) provides a schematic representation of the change-of-direction-speed and perceptual and decision-making skill sub-components of agility. This definition better represents true agility performance, and recognizes both *change-of-direction-speed* and *perceptual and decision-making processes*, and the multi-factorial nature of each component. For example, a child performing an agility-based movement will i) initially observe their external environment, ii) process relevant cues, and then iii) recruit and employ the relevant motor control strategy in response to the task. Therefore, while change-of-direction-speed variables (e.g. technique, sprinting ability, leg muscle qualities, and anthropometry) will ultimately affect the witnessed movement output, these cannot be used without first receiving and interpreting external stimuli. This process is further confounded by the manner in which children learn and perform motor skills. How a combined interaction of individual constraints, environmental constraints, and task constraints influences motor skill development has been thoroughly examined.[86] Therefore, it should be noted that the perfect agility technique does not exist, as the child will invariable modify their technique based on the interaction between individual (e.g. height), task (e.g. degree of challenge), and environmental (e.g. floor surface) constraints.

Agility is a key FMS,[87] which children need in order to maintain adequate physical fitness later in life.[88] Agility is also recognized as an integral component of successful sports performance, and research highlights its importance for success in multidirectional, intermittent invasion sports such as lacrosse,[89] basketball,[90] and soccer.[91] Furthermore, it has been shown that agility performance can differentiate between elite and novice player status across a range of sports.[17,92,93] Yet, despite the obvious importance of agility to general health and sports performance, it remains one of the most under-researched physical fitness components within the paediatric literature.[94]

Testing agility

As both change-of-direction-speed and perceptual and decision-making skills comprise true agility performance, it becomes evident that a number of existing protocols used to test agility instead test change-of-direction-speed. Examples previously used within paediatric research include the quadrant jump test,[95] 5 × 10 m test,[19] the zigzag test,[9] Balsom agility test,[96] 10 × 5 m test,[18] line drill, T-test,[97] and the 5-0-5 agility test.[75] All of these test protocols involve pre-planned movements and do not necessitate responding to an external stimulus, which is the true discerning quality of agility. This has connotations for our understanding of both the way in which agility performance develops naturally as a result of growth and maturation, as well as how, as a physical quality, it can be augmented with relevant training interventions.

Natural development of agility

Minimal literature exists that explores the way in which growth and maturation interact with the development of agility. Consequently, how and why agility performance changes as a result of the unique developmental processes associated with both childhood and adolescence remain unclear. Due to both the existing limitations within the

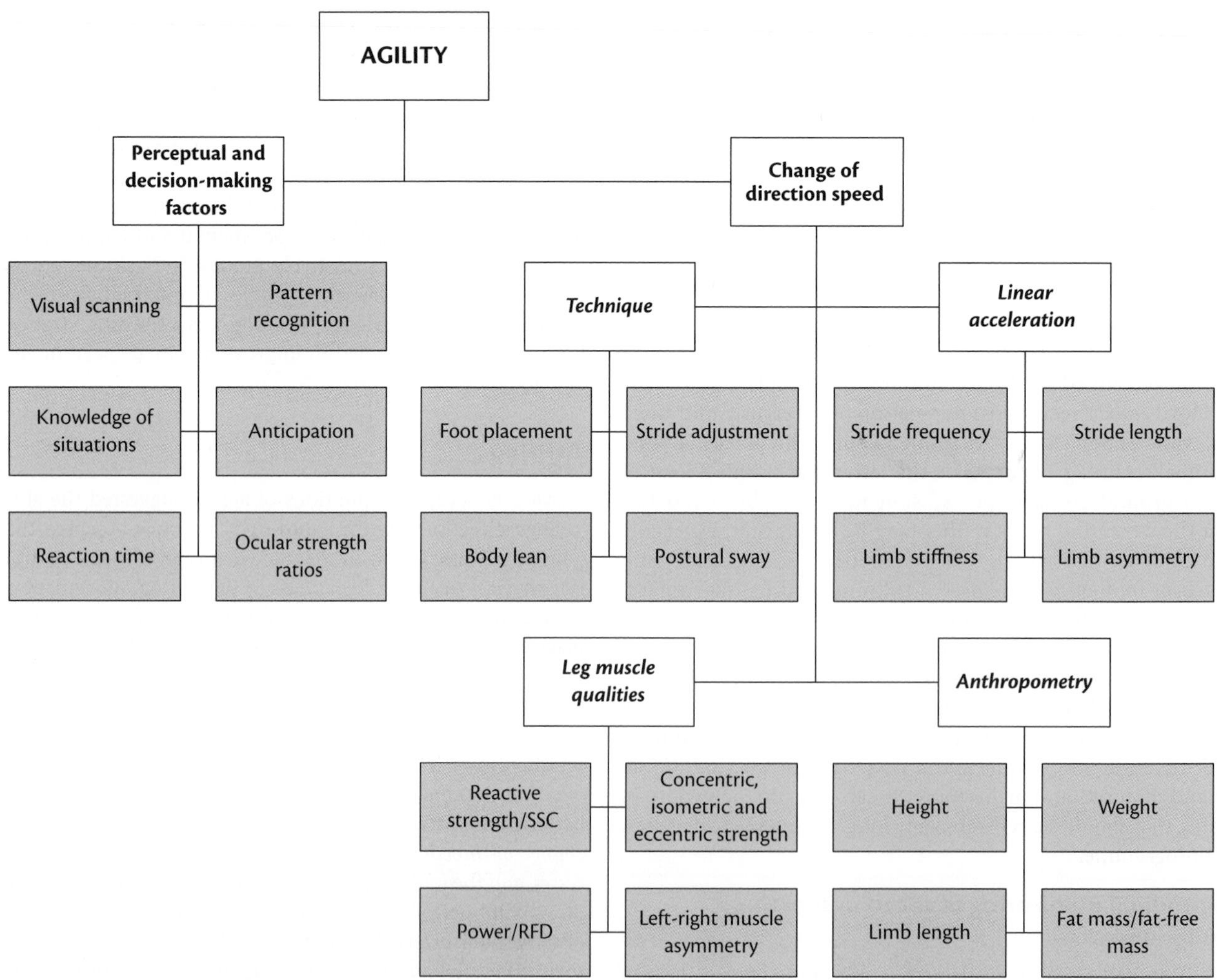

Figure 37.2 Components of agility performance.
Adapted from Sheppard JM, Young WB. Agility literature review: classifications, training and testing. J Sports Sci. 2006; 24: 919–932.

agility development literature and the multifactorial nature of agility performance, we must examine how both change-of-direction-speed and perceptual and decision-making skills develop independently.[94]

Change-of-direction-speed

Small amounts of existing longitudinal data, as well as some cross-sectional studies, show that change-of-direction-speed develops naturally in a non-linear fashion throughout childhood and adolescence.[83,95,98] Research also shows that sex differences only become apparent at the onset of puberty. Specifically, Eisenmann and Malina[95] studied change-of-direction-speed performance in the quadrant jump test in a sample of boys and girls over a 5-year period (Figure 37.3). Their data showed that prepubertal boys and girls performed similarly in the quadrant jump test, although sex-associated differences were apparent during the adolescent growth spurt. Notably, during puberty and into late adolescence boys, continued to improve change-of-direction-speed performance, while girls' rate of improvement plateaued. The influence of puberty on change-of-direction-speed has also been highlighted in more recent research. Jakovljevic *et al.*[9] showed that change-of-direction-speed, as measured by performance in the zigzag test, was significantly better in 14-year-old boys than in 12-year-old boys, while Philippaerts *et al.*[19] revealed that the greatest rate of change in the 5 × 10 m test occurred approximately around the time of PHV. Similarly, a group of regional male youth soccer players were routinely tested on the eight figure test over a 2-year period. Data showed that the greatest relative improvement in change-of-direction-speed was evident in those boys who transitioned from 13 to 14 years of age.[83] Cumulatively, these data suggest that natural development of change-of-direction-speed: i) is better in adolescents than children, ii) occurs in a non-linear fashion, and iii) is similar in both girls and boys prior to puberty, but sex differences emerge as a result of the adolescent growth spurt.

While the determinants of natural development of change-of-direction-speed remain unclear, an understanding of the determinants of change-of-direction-speed performance (Figure 37.2) and key physiological principles of paediatric exercise science may help explain potential age- and maturity-related changes in performance. Sheppard and Young[16] highlight that *anthropometrics* are potentially an influencing factor in change-of-direction-speed performance. While very little is known about the influence of limb lengths, centre-of-mass orientation, and the ratio of fat mass versus fat-free mass on change-of-direction-speed in youth, intuitively, when comparing two individuals of the same maturity status, the individual with shorter relative limb length, lower centre of gravity, lower levels of fat mass, and higher amounts of fat-free mass would be expected to outperform a taller, fatter, and less muscled peer. While an increase in limb length will likely increase speed into, and out of, a change-of-direction task, greater limb lengths will also increase the height of centre of mass, which makes changing direction more challenging. Conceivably, the positive effect of increased limb length in combination with greater force production from natural increases in muscle mass will likely offset any detrimental effects of an increase in height of centre-of-mass on change-of-direction-speed performance.

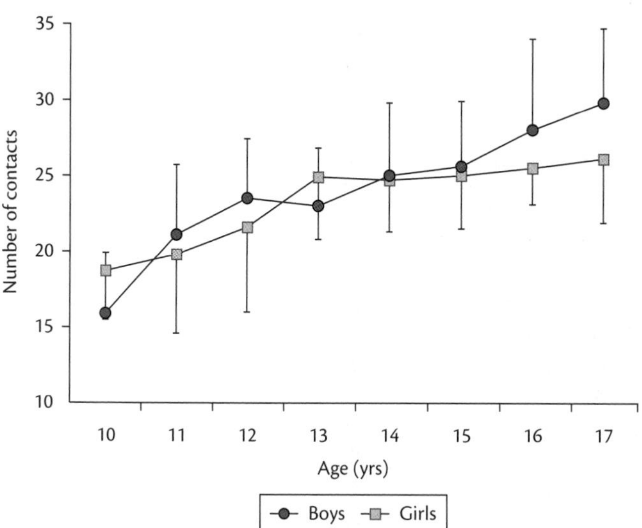

Figure 37.3 Development of change-of-direction-speed as measured from the quadrant jump test in boys and girls, the test measures the number of valid contacts made in 10 s.

Data from Eisenmann JC, Malina RM. Age- and sex-associated variation in neuromuscular capacities of adolescent distance runners. J Sports Sci. 2003; 21: 551–557.

More significantly, leg muscle qualities have also been associated with successful change-of-direction-speed performance.[16] Children and adolescents require appropriate levels of concentric, isometric, and eccentric strength to effectively decelerate, transition, and reaccelerate respectively. Increased relative muscular strength and power, as well as a more effective utilization of the stretch-shortening cycle action ultimately enables the child or adolescent to attenuate and produce greater forces and rates-of-force-development during the act of changing direction. Recent research emphasizes the importance of muscular strength for effective change-of-direction performance, especially when strength is normalized to body mass.[99–101] The importance of relative strength and power for effective change-of-direction-speed performance, combined with underpinning paediatric muscle physiology, to some degree, helps explain the natural development of change-of-direction speed in youth. Prepubertal boys and girls perform similarly in change-of-direction-speed tasks,[95] which mirrors the comparatively similar linear development of muscle strength in both boys and girls during childhood.[102] Noticeable improvements in change-of-direction-speed are evident as children reach the onset of puberty and experience the adolescent growth spurt, which is commensurate with the concomitant non-linear gains in muscle strength.[103] During adolescence, males experience accelerated gains in muscle strength, while females are less likely to experience on-going improvements.[104] This likely explains the associated sex differences witnessed in change-of-direction-speed following the adolescent growth spurt.[95]

Perceptual and decision-making processes

Within the agility literature, there is a lack of empirical research examining the natural development of perceptual and decision-making processes during childhood and adolescence. Thus it remains unclear how growth and maturation interact upon the development of these vital sub-components of agility performance. However, developmental motor control literature has shown that childhood is an opportune time to develop cognitive processes because of the heightened neural plasticity associated with childhood.[105,106] Specifically, strengthening of synaptic pathways,[107] further neural myelination,[108] and the process of synaptic pruning[109] all mediate faster stimulus-response times and overall increased cognitive capacity in children. Therefore, theoretically, while greater maturity-related natural developments in force-producing capacity would be expected in adolescents compared to children, the age-related plasticity of neural pathways may lead to more adaptable perceptual and decision-making processes in children when compared to adolescents. However, it should be noted that further research is required to validate this speculative theory.

Agility training

Effect of targeted training on change-of-direction-speed

While there is now a compelling body of evidence supporting the trainability of physical qualities including strength, power, speed, and endurance in youth, research examining the trainability of agility performance remains scarce. Owing to the limitations surrounding the various definitions and testing modalities for agility, previous studies that have attempted to monitor training-induced changes in agility have rather typically only examined the effects of training on change-of-direction-speed. Within the literature, a range of short-term training interventions have proven successful in augmenting positive changes in change-of-direction-speed performance in youth, including strength training,[110,111] plyometric training,[75,112,113] combined training,[96,114] change-of-direction sprints,[115] and small-sided games.[115,116] Typically, the duration of these interventions has ranged from as little as 3 weeks up to 16 weeks. Therefore, little is known about the long-term effects of training on change-of-direction speed ability. Of the available evidence, Keiner *et al.*[117] recently examined the effects of a 2-year strength training intervention on change-of-direction-speed performance in young soccer players. The study showed that under 15, under 17, and under 19 players all made significant improvements in change-of-direction-speed following exposure to the training programme. Interestingly, changes in change-of-direction-speed performance showed moderate to strong correlations with changes in relative strength levels (as determined by one repetition maximum front and back squats). This latter finding highlights the relative importance of force-producing capacities for successful performance in change-of-direction tasks. Table 37.2 provides a summary of the training interventions targeted towards enhancing change-of-direction-speed performance, and shows that improvements in change-of-direction can be achieved through a variety of training means. However, the majority of studies examined adaptations in adolescents, and thus there is a lack of research examining training effects in immature, prepubertal youth. Similarly, there is a lack of data relating to the responsiveness of change-of-direction-speed to training in girls.

Effect of targeted training on perceptual and decision-making processes

Very little research exists into the trainability of perceptual and decision-making determinants of agility performance, especially in paediatric populations. Therefore, the manner in which

Table 37.2 Summary of training studies targeting change-of-direction-speed in boys aged 12–17 years old.

Reference	Age	Duration	Test	Mode	% Change
Söhnlein *et al.*[113]	12.3 ± 0.8	16 weeks	Hurdle agility test	Control	0.5
	13.0 ± 0.9			Plyometric	6.0
Meylan and Malatesta[112]	13.1 ± 0.6	8 weeks	10 m zigzag agility test	Control Plyometric	−2.8
	13.3 ± 0.6				9.6
Faigenbaum *et al.*[114]	13.4 ± 0.9	6 weeks	Pro-agility test	Combined Resistance	3.8
	13.6 ± 0.7				0.3
Gabbett *et al.*[111]	14.1	10 weeks	5-0-5 agility test	Strength/RSA	2.1
Chaouachi *et al.*[115]	14.2 ± 0.9	6 weeks	Zigzag test	SSG	2.5
				COD	5.0
				Control	2.6
Garcia-Pinillos *et al.*[96]	15.5 ± 1.3	12 weeks	Balsom agility test	Contrast	5.1
	16.4 ± 1.5			Control	0.3
Gabbett *et al.*[111]	16.9 ± 0.3	10 weeks	5-0-5 agility test	Strength/RSA	1.0
Thomas *et al.*[75]	17.3 ± 0.4	6 weeks	5-0-5 agility test	CMJ	11.4
				DJ	7.0
Young and Rogers[116]	17.3 ± 0.5	7 weeks	Planned AFL test	CODS	0.1
	17.5 ± 0.8		Video-based RAT	SSG	0
			Planned AFL test		0.8
			Video-based RAT		3.8

The dashed lines separate the table into age groups that approximate to pre- (top), circa- (middle) and post- (bottom) peak height velocity; a positive % change represents an improvement in change-of-direction-speed performance.

RSA = repeated sprint ability; SSG = small-sided games; CODS = change-of-direction-speed; CMJ = countermovement jump; DJ = drop jump; AFL = Australian Football League; RAT = reactive agility test.

growth, maturation, and training interact to develop these qualities remains unclear. Of the minimal evidence available, one study has attempted to determine the effects of a short-term (3-week) reactive agility training programme on the perceptual and decision-making components of agility in youth rugby players; however, this programme comprised players aged between 18–20 years old.[118] Participants were allocated to either a control group that continued with regular training, or an experimental group that participated in reactive agility training exercises. These exercises required players to perform movements in reaction to video footage projected onto a large screen. Measures of performance on a reactive agility test and a change-of-direction-speed test were collected before and after the intervention period. While the control group showed no performance changes, the experimental group significantly improved reactive agility performance. Interestingly, while significant changes were reported in reactive agility performance, change-of-direction-speed performance remained unaffected by the intervention. This would suggest that improvements in reactive agility were a result of perceptual and decision-making skills rather than change-of-direction-speed variables. While these novel findings provide some evidence for the trainability of perceptual and decision-making skills, the research was recognized as a preliminary study; therefore, these results should be interpreted with caution. Additionally, while the study used participants from a national youth rugby league competition, the ages of the participants involved means that any understanding of how children and adolescents would respond to similar training interventions during different stages of maturation remains unclear.

Interestingly, while research suggests that repeated exposure to a given stimulus will enhance faster response times, for the health and well-being of youth, and especially young athletes, it should be noted that development of the key perceptual and decision-making determinants identified by Sheppard and Young[16] can be developed with varied practice. Specifically, generic pattern recognition, hand-eye coordination, and decision-making skills can be enhanced when youth are exposed to a variety of activities,[119] additional research shows that a cumulative exposure to a breadth of sporting experiences may promote selective transfer of pattern recall, and ultimately facilitate expert performance.[120] Such an approach would reduce the need for a specialized and narrow approach to the development of sporting talent, which is indicative of the experiences of those children who concentrate on a single sport from a young age. The notion of sport specialization has recently been highlighted as a major concern for young athletes, given the associated risks of overuse injury, overtraining, and eventual dropout from the sport.[121]

Conclusions

Speed and agility are recognized as unique and fundamental movement skills that form the basis of many physical activities, contribute to sports performance, and may be important markers of health in children and adolescents. Unfortunately, our understanding of agility in youth is primarily limited to the physical development of change-of-direction-speed, with limited information available on the perceptual factors that contribute to agile movements in real-world situations. It is clear that speed and change-of-direction-speed develop naturally with growth and maturation in both boys and girls. Similarly, both speed and change-of-direction-speed appear to be sensitive to training in children and adolescents, with a variety of different training methods all shown to promote positive gains in performance. However, there are still considerable gaps in our knowledge; much less information is available regarding the interaction of maturity and training in girls when compared to boys and there is a general lack of well-controlled long-term intervention studies.

Summary

- Speed and agility are fundamental movement skills that contribute to natural play activities, determine success in youth sports, and may be related to health-related fitness. However, speed and agility are independent qualities and should be considered separately.
- A maturational influence on the development of speed is evidenced by the differential timing of periods of rapid development when comparing boys and girls, as well as from longitudinal data which align speed with growth rates. However, it is not entirely clear whether peak gains in speed coincide with peak height velocity or the start of the growth spurt.
- With maturation, sprint mechanics alter, ground contact times increase, and stride frequency is reduced. These changes are more than compensated for by increases in stride length, which drive gains in sprint speed.
- There is minimal literature available on the development and trainability of agility in paediatric populations. The available research has focused on the physical component of change-of-direction-speed, with limited attention given to the perceptual component of agility.
- While speed and change-of-direction-speed are independent qualities they demonstrate similar, non-linear developmental progress; boys and girls perform similarly at a young age, but sex differences become more apparent with the onset of puberty.
- Natural improvements in both speed and change-of-direction-speed are related to growth-related changes in size, as well as qualitative changes in neural-muscle-tendon structure and function.
- Available evidence suggests that gains in both speed and change-of-direction-speed can be achieved using a variety of different short-term training interventions in both children and adolescents, although more research is needed with girls.
- Limited evidence suggests youth involved in sports programmes involving long-term systematic training will improve their speed and change-of-direction-speed more than those not involved in such programmes.
- The type of training and the underpinning adaptations that promote the greatest gains in speed may differ between children and adolescents. Combining strength and plyometric training appears to be an effective method for improving speed in both children and adolescents.
- From the limited evidence available, natural development and training-induced gains in change-of-direction-speed appear to be associated with gains in relative strength.

References

1. Lloyd RS, Oliver JL. The Youth Physical Development Model: A new approach to long-term athletic development. *Strength Cond J*. 2012; 34: 61–72.

2. Mendez-Villanueva A, Buchheit M, Kuitunen S, *et al.* Age-related differences in acceleration, maximum running speed, and repeated-sprint performance in young soccer players. *J Sports Sci.* 2011; 29: 477–484.
3. Reilly T, Williams AM, Nevill A, Franks A. A multidisciplinary approach to talent identification in soccer. *J Sports Sci.* 2000; 18: 695–702.
4. Ortega FB, Cadenas-Sanchez C, Sanchez-Delgado G, *et al.* Systematic review and proposal of a field-based physical fitness-test battery in preschool children: the PREFIT battery. *Sports Med.* 2015; 45: 533–555.
5. Ortega FB, Ruiz JR, Castillo MJ, Sjostrom M. Physical fitness in childhood and adolescence: a powerful marker of health. *Int J Obes (Lond).* 2008; 32: 1–11.
6. Ruiz JR, Castro-Pinero J, Espana-Romero V, *et al.* Field-based fitness assessment in young people: the ALPHA health-related fitness test battery for children and adolescents. *Br J Sports Med.* 2011; 45: 518–524.
7. Gabbett TJ, Kelly JN, Sheppard JM. Speed, change of direction speed, and reactive agility of rugby league players. *J Strength Cond Res.* 2008; 22: 174–181.
8. Gravina L, Gil SM, Ruiz F, *et al.* Anthropometric and physiological differences between first team and reserve soccer players aged 10–14 years at the beginning and end of the season. *J Strength Cond Res.* 2008; 22: 1308–1314.
9. Jakovljevic ST, Karalejic MS, Pajic ZB, Macura MM, Erculj FF. Speed and agility of 12- and 14-year-old elite male basketball players. *J Strength Cond Res.* 2012; 26: 2453–2459.
10. Vescovi JD, Rupf R, Brown TD, Marques MC. Physical performance characteristics of high-level female soccer players 12–21 years of age. *Scand J Med Sci Sports.* 2011; 21: 670–678.
11. Vescovi JD, McGuigan MR. Relationships between sprinting, agility, and jump ability in female athletes. *J Sports Sci.* 2008; 26: 97–107.
12. Rumpf MC, Cronin JB, Oliver JL, Hughes M. Assessing youth sprint ability-methodological issues, reliability and performance data. *Pediatr Exerc Sci.* 2011; 23: 442–467.
13. Little T, Williams AG. Specificity of acceleration, maximum speed, and agility in professional soccer players. *J Strength Cond Res.* 2005; 19: 76–78.
14. Meyers RW, Oliver JL, Hughes MG, Cronin JB, Lloyd RS. Maximal sprint speed in boys of increasing maturity. *Pediatr Exerc Sci.* 2015; 27: 85–94.
15. Bloomfield J, Ackland TR, Elliot BC. *Applied anatomy and biomechanics in sport.* Melbourne: Blackwell Scientific; 1994.
16. Sheppard JM, Young WB. Agility literature review: classifications, training and testing. *J Sports Sci.* 2006; 24: 919–932.
17. Gabbett TJ. Physiological characteristics of junior and senior rugby league players. *Br J Sports Med.* 2002; 36: 334–339.
18. Hirose N, Seki T. Two-year changes in anthropometric and motor ability values as talent identification indexes in youth soccer players. *J Sci Med Sport.* 2016; 19: 158–162.
19. Philippaerts RM, Vaeyens R, Janssens M, *et al.* The relationship between peak height velocity and physical performance in youth soccer players. *J Sports Sci.* 2006; 24: 221–230.
20. Meyers RW, Oliver JL, Hughes MG, Lloyd RS, Cronin JB. The influence of age, maturity and body size on the spatiotemporal determinants of maximal sprint speed in boys. *J Strength Cond Res.* 2015; doi: 10.1519/JSC.0000000000001310
21. Ford PA, De Ste Croix MBA, Lloyd. RS, *et al.* The long-term athlete development model: problems with its physiological application. *J Sports Sci.* 2011; 29: 389–402.
22. Rumpf MC, Cronin JB, Pinder SD, Oliver J, Hughes M. Effect of different training methods on running sprint times in male youth. *Pediatr Exerc Sci.* 2012; 24: 170–186.
23. Salaj S, Markovic G. Specificity of jumping, sprinting, and quick change-of-direction motor abilities. *J Strength Cond Res.* 2011; 25: 1249–1255.
24. Beunen G, Malina RM. Growth and physical performance relative to the timing of the adolescent spurt. *Exerc Sport Sci Rev.* 1988; 16: 503–540.
25. Lefevre J, Beunen G, Steens G, Claessens A, Renson R. Motor performance during adolescence and age thirty as related to age at peak height velocity. *Ann Hum Biol.* 1990; 17: 423–435.
26. Schepens B, Willems PA, Cavagna GA. The mechanics of running in children. *J Physiol.* 1998; 509 (Pt 3): 927–940.
27. Borms J. The child and exercise: an overview. *J Sports Sci.* 1986; 4: 3–20.
28. Malina RM, Bouchard C, Bar-Or O. *Growth, matuation and physical activity.* Champaign, IL: Human Kinetics: 2004.
29. Viru A, Loko J, Harrow M, *et al.* Critical periods in the development of performance capacity during childhood and adolescence. *Eur J Phys Educ.* 1999; 4: 75–119.
30. Yague PH, De La Fuente JM. Changes in height and motor performance relative to peak height velocity: A mixed-longitudinal study of Spanish boys and girls. *Am J Hum Biol.* 1998; 10: 647–660.
31. Whithall J. Development of locomotor co-ordination and control in children. In: Savelsberg GJP, Davids K, Van Der Kamp J (eds.) *Development of movement co-ordination in children.* London: Routledge; 2003. p. 251–270.
32. Szczesny S, Coudert J. Changes in running speed and endurance among girls during puberty. In: Day JAP, Duguet JW (eds.) *Kinanthropometry IV.* London: Routledge; 1993. p. 268–284.
33. Butterfield SA, Lehnhard R, Lee J, Coladarci T. Growth rates in running speed and vertical jumping by boys and girls ages 11–13. *Percept Mot Skills.* 2004; 99: 225–234.
34. Catley MJ, Tomkinson GR. Normative health-related fitness values for children: analysis of 85347 test results on 9–17-year-old Australians since 1985. *Br J Sports Med.* 2013; 47: 98–108.
35. Williams CA, Oliver JL, Faulkner J. Seasonal monitoring of sprint and jump performance in a soccer youth academy. *Int J Sports Physiol Perform.* 2011; 6: 264–275.
36. Rumpf MC, Cronin JB, Oliver J, Hughes M. Kinematics and kinetics of maximum running speed in youth across maturity. *Pediatr Exerc Sci.* 2015; 27: 277–284.
37. Lenroot RK, Giedd JN. Brain development in children and adolescents: insights from anatomical magnetic resonance imaging. *Neurosci Biobehav Rev.* 2006; 30: 718–729.
38. Hausdorff JM, Zemany L, Peng C, Goldberger AL. Maturation of gait dynamics: stride-to-stride variability and its temporal organization in children. *J Appl Physiol.* 1999; 86: 1040–1047.
39. Eriksson O, Saltin B. Muscle metabolism during exercise in boys aged 11 to 16 years compared to adults. *Acta Paediatr Belg.* 1974; 28(Suppl): 257–265.
40. Berg A, Kim SS, Keul J. Skeletal muscle enzyme activities in healthy young subjects. *Int J Sports Med.* 1986; 7: 236–239.
41. Ovalle WK. The human muscle-tendon junction. A morphological study during normal growth and at maturity. *Anat Embryol (Berl).* 1987; 176: 281–294.
42. Lin JP, Brown JK, Walsh EG. Soleus muscle length, stretch reflex excitability, and the contractile properties of muscle in children and adults: a study of the functional joint angle. *Dev Med Child Neurol.* 1997; 39: 469–480.
43. Lloyd RS, Oliver JL, Hughes MG, Williams CA. Age-related differences in the neural regulation of stretch-shortening cycle activities in male youths during maximal and sub-maximal hopping. *J Electromyogr Kinesiol.* 2012; 22: 37–43.
44. Oliver JL, Smith PM. Neural control of leg stiffness during hopping in boys and men. *J Electromyogr Kinesiol.* 2010; 20: 973–979.
45. Grosset JF, Mora I, Lambertz D, Perot C. Changes in stretch reflexes and muscle stiffness with age in prepubescent children. *J Appl Physiol.* 2007; 102: 2352–2360.
46. Lambertz D, Mora I, Grosset JF, Perot C. Evaluation of musculotendinous stiffness in prepubertal children and adults, taking into account muscle activity. *J Appl Physiol.* 2003; 95: 64–72.
47. Brughelli M, Cronin J. Influence of running velocity on vertical, leg and joint stiffness: modelling and recommendations for future research. *Sports Med.* 2008; 38: 647–657.
48. Chelly SM, Denis C. Leg power and hopping stiffness: relationship with sprint running performance. *Med Sci Sports Exerc.* 2001; 33: 326–333.

49. Rumpf MC, Cronin JB, Oliver JL, Hughes MG. Vertical and leg stiffness and stretch-shortening cycle changes across maturation during maximal sprint running. *Hum Mov Sci.* 2013; 32: 668–676.
50. Hunter JP, Marshall RN, McNair PJ. Interaction of step length and step rate during sprint running. *Med Sci Sports Exerc.* 2004; 36: 261–271.
51. Weyand PG, Sandell RF, Prime DN, Bundle MW. The biological limits to running speed are imposed from the ground up. *J Appl Physiol.* 2010; 108: 950–961.
52. Weyand PG, Sternlight DB, Bellizzi MJ, Wright S. Faster top running speeds are achieved with greater ground forces not more rapid leg movements. *J Appl Physiol.* 2000; 89: 1991–1999.
53. Salo AI, Bezodis IN, Batterham AM, Kerwin DG. Elite sprinting: are athletes individually step-frequency or step-length reliant? *Med Sci Sports Exerc.* 2011; 43: 1055–1062.
54. Forbes H, Bullers A, Lovell A, *et al.* Relative torque profiles of elite male youth footballers: effects of age and pubertal development. *Int J Sports Med.* 2009; 30: 592–597.
55. Ramos E, Frontera WR, Llopart A, Feliciano D. Muscle strength and hormonal levels in adolescents: gender related differences. *Int J Sports Med.* 1998; 19: 526–531.
56. Katch VL. Physical conditioning of children. *J Adolesc Health Care.* 1983; 3: 241–246.
57. Balyi I, Hamilton A. *Long-term athlete development: trainability in childhood and adolescence, windows of opportunity, optimal trainability.* Victoria: National Coaching Institute British Columbia and Advanced Training and Performance Ltd; 2004.
58. Bailey R, Collins D, Ford P, *et al.* Participant development in sport: An academic review. *Sports Coach UK.* 2010: 1–134.
59. Rumpf MC, Lockie RG, Cronin JB, Jalilvand F. The effect of different sprint training methods on sprint performance over various distances: a brief review. *J Strength Cond Res.* 2015; 30: 1767–1785.
60. Christou M, Smilios I, Sotiropoulos K, *et al.* Effects of resistance training on the physical capacities of adolescent soccer players. *J Strength Cond Res.* 2006; 20: 783–791.
61. Mathisen GE, Pettersen SA. The effect of speed training on sprint and agility performance in female youth. *J Phys Educ Sport.* 2015; 15: 395–399.
62. Rumpf MC, Cronin JB, Mohamad IN, *et al.* The effect of resisted sprint training on maximum sprint kinetics and kinematics in youth. *Eur J Sport Sci.* 2015; 15: 374–381.
63. Venturelli M, Bishop D, Pettene L. Sprint training in preadolescent soccer players. *Int J Sports Physiol Perform.* 2008; 3: 558–562.
64. Kotzamanidis C. The effect of sprint training on running performance and vertical jump in pre-adolescent boys. *J Hum Mov Studies.* 2003; 44: 225–240.
65. Kotzamanidis C. Effect of plyometric training on running performance and vertical jumping in prepubertal boys. *J Strength Cond Res.* 2006; 20: 441–445.
66. Pettersen SA, Mathisen GE. Effect of short burst activities on sprint and agility performance in 11- to 12-year-old boys. *J Strength Cond Res.* 2012; 26: 1033–1038.
67. Chelly MS, Hermassi S, Shephard RJ. Effects of in-season short-term plyometric training program on sprint and jump performance of young male track athletes. *J Strength Cond Res.* 2015; 29: 2128–2136.
68. Ingle L, Sleap M, Tolfrey K. The effect of a complex training and detraining programme on selected strength and power variables in early pubertal boys. *J Sports Sci.* 2006; 24: 987–997.
69. Diallo O, Dore E, Duche P, Van Praagh E. Effects of plyometric training followed by a reduced training programme on physical performance in prepubescent soccer players. *J Sports Med Phys Fitness.* 2001; 41: 342–348.
70. Wong PL, Chamari K, Wisloff U. Effects of 12-week on-field combined strength and power training on physical performance among U-14 young soccer players. *J Strength Cond Res.* 2010; 24: 644–652.
71. Chaouachi A, Othman AB, Hammami R, Drinkwater EJ, Behm DG. The combination of plyometric and balance training improves sprint and shuttle run performances more often than plyometric-only training with children. *J Strength Cond Res.* 2014; 28: 401–412.
72. Coutts AJ, Murphy AJ, Dascombe BJ. Effect of direct supervision of a strength coach on measures of muscular strength and power in young rugby league players. *J Strength Cond Res.* 2004; 18: 316–323.
73. Chelly MS, Fathloun M, Cherif N, *et al.* Effects of a back squat training program on leg power, jump, and sprint performances in junior soccer players. *J Strength Cond Res.* 2009; 23: 2241–2249.
74. Kotzamanidis C, Chatzopoulos D, Michailidis C, Papaiakovou G, Patikas D. The effect of a combined high-intensity strength and speed training program on the running and jumping ability of soccer players. *J Strength Cond Res.* 2005; 19: 369–375.
75. Thomas K, French D, Hayes PR. The effect of two plyometric training techniques on muscular power and agility in youth soccer players. *J Strength Cond Res.* 2009; 23: 332–335.
76. Maio Alves JM, Rebelo AN, Abrantes C, Sampaio J. Short-term effects of complex and contrast training in soccer players' vertical jump, sprint, and agility abilities. *J Strength Cond Res.* 2010; 24: 936–941.
77. Rumpf MC, Cronin JB, Mohamad IN, *et al.* Acute effects of sled towing on sprint time in male youth of different maturity status. *Pediatr Exerc Sci.* 2014; 26: 71–75.
78. Meylan CM, Cronin JB, Oliver JL, Hopkins WG, Contreras B. The effect of maturation on adaptations to strength training and detraining in 11–15-year-olds. *Scand J Med Sci Sports.* 2014; 24: e156–e164.
79. Behringer M, Vom Heede A, Yue Z, Mester J. Effects of resistance training in children and adolescents: a meta-analysis. *Pediatrics.* 2010; 126: e1199–1210.
80. Lloyd RS, Radnor JM, De Ste Croix MB, Cronin JB, Oliver JL. Changes in sprint and jump performance following traditional, plyometric and combined resistance training in male youth pre- and post-peak height velocity. *J Strength Cond Res.* 2015; 30: 1239–1247.
81. Saez de Villarreal E, Suarez-Arrones L, Requena B, Haff GG, Ferrete C. Effects of plyometric and sprint training on physical and technical skill performance in adolescent soccer players. *J Strength Cond Res.* 2015; 29: 1894–1903.
82. Bedoya AA, Miltenberger MR, Lopez RM. Plyometric training effects on athletic performance in youth soccer athletes: A systematic review. *J Strength Cond Res.* 2015; 29: 2351–2360.
83. Vanttinen T, Blomqvist M, Nyman K, Hakkinen K. Changes in body composition, hormonal status, and physical fitness in 11-, 13-, and 15-year-old Finnish regional youth soccer players during a two-year follow-up. *J Strength Cond Res.* 2011; 25: 3342–3351.
84. Wrigley RD, Drust B, Stratton G, Atkinson G, Gregson W. Long-term soccer-specific training enhances the rate of physical development of academy soccer players independent of maturation status. *Int J Sports Med.* 2014; 35: 1090–1094.
85. Sander A, Keiner M, Wirth K, Schmidtbleicher D. Influence of a 2-year strength training programme on power performance in elite youth soccer players. *Eur J Sport Sci.* 2013; 13: 445–451.
86. Gallahue DL, Ozmun JC, Goodway JD. *Understanding motor development.* New York: McGraw-Hill; 2012.
87. Lubans DR, Morgan PJ, Cliff DP, Barnett LM, Okely AD. Fundamental movement skills in children and adolescents: review of associated health benefits. *Sports Med.* 2010; 40: 1019–1035.
88. Stodden D, Langendorfer S, Roberton MA. The association between motor skill competence and physical fitness in young adults. *Res Q Exerc Sport.* 2009; 80: 223–229.
89. Enemark-Miller EA, Seegmiller JG, Rana SR. Physiological profile of women's lacrosse players. *J Strength Cond Res.* 2009; 23: 39–43.
90. Delextrat A, Cohen D. Physiological testing of basketball players: toward a standard evaluation of anaerobic fitness. *J Strength Cond Res.* 2008; 22: 1066–1072.
91. Stolen T, Chamari K, Castagna C, Wisloff U. Physiology of soccer: an update. *Sports Med.* 2005; 35: 501–536.
92. Sheppard JM, Young WB, Doyle TL, Sheppard TA, Newton RU. An evaluation of a new test of reactive agility and its relationship to sprint speed and change of direction speed. *J Sci Med Sport.* 2006; 9: 342–349.
93. Farrow D, Young W, Bruce L. The development of a test of reactive agility for netball: a new methodology. *J Sci Med Sport.* 2005; 8: 52–60.

94. Lloyd RS, Read P, Oliver JL, *et al.* Considerations for the development of agility during childhood and adolescence. *Strength Cond J.* 2013; 35: 2–11.
95. Eisenmann JC, Malina RM. Age- and sex-associated variation in neuromuscular capacities of adolescent distance runners. *J Sports Sci.* 2003; 21: 551–557.
96. Garcia-Pinillos F, Martinez-Amat A, Hita-Contreras F, Martinez-Lopez EJ, Latorre-Roman PA. Effects of a contrast training program without external load on vertical jump, kicking speed, sprint, and agility of young soccer players. *J Strength Cond Res.* 2014; 28: 2452–2460.
97. Vanderford ML, Meyers MC, Skelly WA, Stewart CC, Hamilton KL. Physiological and sport-specific skill response of olympic youth soccer athletes. *J Strength Cond Res.* 2004; 18: 334–342.
98. Chiodera P, Volta E, Gobbi G, *et al.* Specifically designed physical exercise programs improve children's motor abilities. *Scand J Med Sci Sports.* 2008; 18: 179–187.
99. Delaney JA, Scott TJ, Ballard DA, *et al.* Contributing factors to change-of-direction ability in professional rugby league players. *J Strength Cond Res.* 2015; 29: 2688–2696.
100. Spiteri T, Newton RU, Binetti M, *et al.* Mechanical determinants of faster change of direction and agility performance in female basketball athletes. *J Strength Cond Res.* 2015; 29: 2205–2214.
101. Spiteri T, Nimphius S, Hart NH, *et al.* Contribution of strength characteristics to change of direction and agility performance in female basketball athletes. *J Strength Cond Res.* 2014; 28: 2415–2423.
102. Branta C, Haubenstricker J, Seefeldt V. Age changes in motor skills during childhood and adolescence. *Exerc Sport Sci Rev.* 1984; 12: 467–520.
103. Parker DF, Round JM, Sacco P, Jones DA. A cross-sectional survey of upper and lower limb strength in boys and girls during childhood and adolescence. *Ann Hum Biol.* 1990; 17: 199–211.
104. Beunen GP, Malina RM. Growth and biological maturation: relevance to athletic performance. In: Hebestreit H, Bar-Or O (eds.) *The young athlete.* Oxford: Blackwell Publishing; 2008. p. 3–17.
105. Gogtay N, Giedd JN, Lusk L, *et al.* Dynamic mapping of human cortical development during childhood through early adulthood. *Proc Natl Acad Sci.* 2004; 101: 8174–8179.
106. Myer GD, Faigenbaum AD, Edwards NM, *et al.* Sixty minutes of what? A developing brain perspective for activating children with an integrative exercise approach. *Br J Sports Med.* 2015; 49: 1570–1576.
107. Casey BJ, Giedd JN, Thomas KM. Structural and functional brain development and its relation to cognitive development. *Biol Psychol.* 2000; 54: 241–257.
108. Paus T, Zijdenbos A, Worsley K, *et al.* Structural maturation of neural pathways in children and adolescents: in vivo study. *Science.* 1999; 283: 1908–1911.
109. Casey BJ, Tottenham N, Liston C, Durston S. Imaging the developing brain: what have we learned about cognitive development? *Trends Cogn Sci.* 2005; 9: 104–110.
110. Jullien H, Bisch C, Largouet N, *et al.* Does a short period of lower limb strength training improve performance in field-based tests of running and agility in young professional soccer players? *J Strength Cond Res.* 2008; 22: 404–411.
111. Gabbett TJ, Johns J, Riemann M. Performance changes following training in junior rugby league players. *J Strength Cond Res.* 2008; 22: 910–917.
112. Meylan C, Malatesta D. Effects of in-season plyometric training within soccer practice on explosive actions of young players. *J Strength Cond Res.* 2009; 23: 2605–2613.
113. Sohnlein Q, Muller E, Stoggl TL. The effect of 16-week plyometric training on explosive actions in early to mid-puberty elite soccer players. *J Strength Cond Res.* 2014; 28: 2105–2114.
114. Faigenbaum AD, McFarland JE, Keiper FB, *et al.* Effects of a short-term plyometric and resistance training program on fitness performance in boys age 12 to 15 years. *J Sports Sci Med.* 2007; 6: 519–525.
115. Chaouachi A, Chtara M, Hammami R, *et al.* Multidirectional sprints and small-sided games training effect on agility and change of direction abilities in youth soccer. *J Strength Cond Res.* 2014; 28: 3121–3127.
116. Young W, Rogers N. Effects of small-sided game and change-of-direction training on reactive agility and change-of-direction speed. *J Sports Sci.* 2014; 32: 307–314.
117. Keiner M, Sander A, Wirth K, Schmidtbleicher D. Long-term strength training effects on change-of-direction sprint performance. *J Strength Cond Res.* 2014; 28: 223–231.
118. Serpell BG, Young WB, Ford M. Are the perceptual and decision-making components of agility trainable? A preliminary investigation. *J Strength Cond Res.* 2011; 25: 1240–1248.
119. Baker J, Cote J, Abernethy B. Sport-specific practice and the development of expert decision-making in team ball sports. *J Appl Psychol.* 2003; 15: 12–25.
120. Abernethy B, Baker J, Cote J. Transfer of pattern recall skills may contribute to the development of sport expertise. *Appl Cognit Psychol.* 2005; 19: 705–718.
121. DiFiori JP, Benjamin HJ, Brenner J, *et al.* Overuse injuries and burnout in youth sports: a position statement from the American Medical Society for Sports Medicine. *Clin J Sport Med.* 2014; 24: 3–20.

CHAPTER 38

Overtraining syndrome

Richard J Winsley

Introduction

Children's participation in organized sport remains as popular as ever. In the United States it is estimated that between 30 and 45 million children aged between 16–18 years take part in some form of organized sport.[1,2] Similarly, data from the United Kingdom indicate that between 70 and 80% of children aged 5–10 years old take part in sport organized outside of the school on at least a weekly basis.[3] These figures are to be celebrated, as sport can play a positive formative role in the physiological, psychological, and social development of the child. But what happens when sport involvement has a negative influence, where it not only stops being enjoyable, but also negatively affects the health of the child?

The issue of overtraining has been relatively well researched in adults and our understanding of this phenomenon in the young athlete is also developing. Our understanding largely derives from adolescent athletes playing their sport at a national or international level, but recent data are now available for younger athletes and at lower representative levels, such as club standard; no data are available for children younger than 11 years of age. What we currently understand reveals some worrying parallels between children and adults, as well as some unique factors that need to be considered.

Clarity among complexity

Overtraining is complex. Uncertainty and disagreement exists around the definition, its duration, its causes, and its prevention and treatment. Although team physicians, coaches, and athletes would welcome a simple list of agreed symptoms and causes that would allow for diagnosis, treatment, and prevention, the reality is that this has proved impossible. Overtraining effects each individual differently, and we must treat each individual, and their circumstances, separately. Therefore, it is important to take a holistic view of the condition to ensure both the recovery and future prevention for that particular athlete, regardless of his/her age.

Why we should care about overtraining in the young athlete

A significant minority of young athletes experience overtraining at some point during their sporting careers. Thousands, if not tens of thousands, of young people worldwide are not receiving the appropriate duty of care from sporting organizations, nor from their coaches, teachers, and parents. Any child who experiences an episode of overtraining has arguably been failed by the adults involved. The young athlete who is overtrained will not be performing to the best of his/her abilities; therefore, avoiding overtraining will mean the coach has a fully fit squad to work with. Finally, long-term prevention of overtraining should result in a greater number of children who are healthy and motivated. This motivation will help them develop their sport, benefit from coaching expertise, and increase their potential career success. Furthermore, they increase their chances of entering the pool of talent from which elite adult squads subsequently select.

Definition of overtraining

There is currently no universally accepted definition of overtraining; however, the recent 2013 consensus statement from the European College of Sport Science (ECSS) and the American College of Sports Medicine (ACSM)[4] provides some welcome clarity and guidance. Importantly, there are no unique definitions used for children and therefore adult terminology must be employed.

Overtraining describes both a process and an end point—both an action and a state of being. To differentiate between the two, the term overtraining syndrome (OTS) better represents the end-state of the condition and also acknowledges the multi-factorial nature of the problem.[4] However, as our understanding of the condition has grown, it is clear that the condition is comprised of related conditions,[5] including:

- Functional overreaching (FOR)
- Non-functional overreaching (NFOR)
- Overtraining syndrome (OTS)
- Active burnout
- Burnout

After a typical training session, it is not uncommon for the athlete to feel acute fatigue due to the overload experience, which may reduce performance in subsequent sessions. However, this is short lived—from a few hours to a few days—and with adequate recovery, performance is ultimately improved, in keeping with the principle of supercompensation.[6]

Functional overreaching arises when the detriment in performance lasts slightly longer. For example, an athlete may attend a training camp where he/she is intentionally exposed to an intensified training period. This intense training leaves the athlete tired, and he/she exhibits reduced performance in the days following the camp. The reduction in performance may last between a few days to 2 weeks. However, the athlete ultimately recovers and experiences enhanced performance when compared to that prior to the camp.[7] If the detriment or stagnation in performance lasts more than 2 weeks, or extends to months, the athlete is then defined as being

NFOR.[4,8] Importantly, the upper limit of NFOR is vaguely termed 'months', and no agreed upper threshold has been set. Finally, if the decrease in performance lasts, in combination with other markers of chronic fatigue, from months to years, then the athlete would be defined as having OTS.

A reduction in performance is central in defining and diagnosing overtraining.[5,9] A measurable decrease in performance may be relatively straightforward to quantify in sports like swimming, track cycling, or athletics. but what would constitute a decreased performance in soccer, field hockey, or water-polo, for example? Other issues arising from the ECSS/ACSM consensus statement[4] include using stagnation of performance as a criterion to define the athlete as being NFOR. If an athlete's performance is decreased and remains depressed over the defined time period, this criterion is helpful in diagnosis of NFOR. However, it is less useful if the athlete's performance simply does not increase in parallel with other athletes. Finally, although the 2-week limit for FOR gives welcome delineation, the precise number of months that need to pass before NFOR becomes OTS remains uncertain.

Although there is an increase in severity of the condition between these categories, and the recovery time is longer for each, an athlete does not necessarily always face a downhill slide from one to the other—an athlete may experience one episode of NFOR and this may never be repeated, whereas another may experience repeated episodes of NFOR, which finally conclude into a sustained bout of OTS. Ultimately, however, it is vital that athletes understand OTS can be successfully overcome; therefore, it should not be considered a career-ending condition.

Burnout is a psychological syndrome resulting in an athlete experiencing exhaustion, reduced accomplishment, and depersonalization.[10] This phenomenon has been reported in professionals from a range of careers, including the airline industry, business, armed forces, and caring professions.[10] However, it is also seen in both adult and young athletes. Athletic burnout is a negative response to chronic stress experienced by the young athlete, changing a previously enjoyable activity into a highly demanding and damaging stressor.[11] A critical difference between the athlete who has OTS and that with burnout is motivation. An athlete with OTS continues to train and compete, where the athlete suffering from burnout has lost their motivation and is likely to quit the sport.[12] Although the symptoms of athletic burnout are strikingly similar to those seen in other professions, the context of the stressors in athletic burnout is unique to athletes. Athletic burnout features physical/emotional exhaustion, reduced athletic accomplishment, and sports devaluation.[13] Overtraining syndrome has been defined as both a stepping stone towards burnout and as a parallel endpoint.[14,15] However, OTS arises from maladaptation to excessive training, where burnout has a greater psychosocial emphasis, and arises from perceptions of high external pressure, lack of control, and feelings of entrapment.[16]

Overtraining, in its broadest sense, involves both training and non-training stressors, and we must acknowledge that for the athlete, there is a unique blend of physical, mental, and social dimensions to the problem. The distinction between OTS and burnout may lie in the duration of the condition, the length of recovery, the motivation to continue, and whether or not the athlete is still participating.

Finally, active burnout can occur when the athlete, displaying the symptoms of chronic fatigue and performance decline, has lost the motivation to keep participating in their sport, but continues to do so based on their situation[12] (financial commitments, parental pressure etc.) (see section on Active burnout and entrapment).

Other definitions that have been historically used to describe this condition include staleness (i.e. OTS), drop-out (i.e. burnout),[15] and Unexplained Underperformance Syndrome.[17] The latter term has been coined in recognition of the difficulty in identifying the causes of overtraining for the individual athlete.

Prevalence rates

In adults, overtraining prevalence rates have been reported between 10 and 60%[4,14,18] with a clustering at ~25–30%. Prevalence rates are higher over a longer time frame surveyed, for OTS than Burnout, if NFOR and OTS are combined, and in individual compared to team sport athletes. In young athletes prevalence rates are similar to those seen in adults, with prevalence of OTS at ~30–35% and burnout at about 5–10% (see Table 38.1).

Many of these data come from older children, typically teenagers to young adults, and therefore work assessing overtraining prevalence in younger children would be valuable. Matos *et al.*[19] sampled children aged 11–18 years old, and reported that NFOR/OTS athletes were slightly older (15.3 ± 1.9 years) than those who had never experienced NFOR/OTS. Interestingly, there was no significant difference between the groups in years of training and competing, which supports the findings of Raglin *et al.*[20] a decade earlier

Children competing in individual sports appear to show a greater incidence of staleness: general: individual (48%) vs team (30%);[21] NFOR/OTS: individual (37%) vs team (17%);[19] and burnout: individual (11%) vs team (5%).[12] It has been proposed that team sports provide a social support buffer, leading to fewer instances of NFOR/OTS,[22] but it may be the breadth of friendship groups, rather than the total number of friends, that are more critical for the young athlete.

Whether there is a gender difference in OTS prevalence is not clear. Some studies have shown the prevalence of staleness and NFOR to be greater in girls,[19,20] while other studies report no such difference.[11,21]

Signs and symptoms of overtraining syndrome in children

Caveats accepted, a persistent and marked reduction in performance is the most widely accepted criterion used to identify OTS in the young athlete. However, performance reduction should not be used in exclusion, and additional markers should also be considered. Again, complexity exists, with over 90 different symptoms being reported in athletes with OTS. Symptoms range from physiological and psychological to performance-based symptoms.[14,23] It appears that each athlete presents with a unique set of signs and symptoms,[9] making individual diagnosis very difficult, or to compile a comprehensive set of diagnostic criteria for coaches and team physicians to use.

However, certain symptoms are more frequently reported—in both adults and children—including:[22,23]

- Increased perception of effort during exercise
- Feelings of muscle heaviness
- Frequent upper respiratory tract (URTI) infections

Table 38.1 Prevalence of overtraining syndrome in young athletes.

Study	Age group (n)	Sport	Definition	Prevalence
Raedeke[13]	13–18 years (n = 236)		Active burnout + high burnout rating on ABQ	11%
Raglin *et al.*[20]	13–18 years (n = 231)	Swimmers	Staleness	35%
Kentta *et al.*[21]	16–20 years (n = 272)	Junior national athletes from 16 different sports	Staleness	37%
Gustafsson *et al.*[12]	16–21 years (n = 980)	Swedish sport school athletes from 29 sports	High burnout scores on ABQ	1–9%
Black and Smith[37]	13–22 years (n = 182)	Swimmers	High burnout rating on ABQ	5%
Smith *et al.*[11]	16–19 years (n = 205)	Sport school athletes	High burnout rating on ABQ	6%
Schmikli *et al.*[31]	16 years (n = 77 soccer/n = 52 runners)	Elite soccer players and middle-long distance runners	Performance decrement lasting > 1 month over a season	6%
Matos *et al.*[19]	11–18 years (n = 376)	19 different sports	NFOR + OTS	29%
Hill[48]	13–16 years (n = 167)	English academy soccer players	Symptoms of burnout at least once in their careers	25%

ABQ = Athlete Burnout Questionnaire; NFOR = Non-functional overreaching; OTS = Overtraining syndrome.

- Persistent muscle soreness
- Mood changes
- Sleep disturbance
- Loss of appetite

Crucially, if there exists any doubt about the young athlete, he/she should be referred to a family doctor to screen and rule out any medical condition that may explain the presence of these symptoms.[4]

Other symptoms indicating OTS that have been reported in young athletes include increased conflicts with family/ coaches, decreased interest in training, less motivation to compete, personal frustration with training, lower self-confidence, shortness in temper, increased feelings of sadness, and depression.[24,25]

A wealth of studies looking at the signs, symptoms, and proposed mechanisms of OTS in adults have been completed,[4,8,14] with conflicting findings and recommendations as to their usefulness as a diagnostic tool. Fewer studies have been performed in children, largely stemming from the fact that it is unethical to deliberately overreach/overtrain a child for research purposes. Thus, the data available come from either retrospective recall or longitudinal profiling over a competitive season.

Markers of overtraining syndrome in young athletes

The incidence of URTIs and 'flu-like illness' have been reported to be higher in adolescents (soccer players aged 15–18 years) who had the highest Recovery Stress Questionnaire (REST-Q) scores (indicating a poorer recovery[26]) and training loads in the week before the illness[27]. Matos and Winsley[19] also noted that 44% of NFOR/OTS young athletes reported frequently getting UTRIs, compared to just 15% of their healthy peers.

Testosterone:Cortisol (T:C) ratio has not been assessed in younger athletes due to the low levels of circulating testosterone in prepubertal children.[28] However, a decrease in T:C ratio was seen in adolescent male rugby players, arising from a lower level of circulating testosterone in the players reporting the highest fatigue scores.[29] No correlation was noted between resting cortisol levels and fatigue indices. Higher resting levels of cortisol are seen in NFOR adult athletes[30], whereas the OTS athlete may demonstrate a reduction in cortisol production secondary to hypothalamic-pituitary-adrenal axis dysfunction. A blunted adrenocorticotropic hormone (ACTH) response to exercise is thought to be in evidence in the OTS athlete,[30] resulting in the lower cortisol production. In the few studies to have investigated this in young athletes, Nederhof *et al.*[18] observed an 'excessive' ACTH response in the single NFOR athlete in their case study (with resultant high cortisol levels). Conversely, Schmikli *et al.*[31] saw no difference in resting ACTH levels in NFOR youth soccer players compared to their healthy peers, and thus no differences in resting cortisol as a consequence.

Markers of autonomic nervous system over-activation have been observed in adult athletes with OTS, but again there is limited evidence for children. A higher resting blood pressure, heart rate, and levels of circulating catecholamines have been recorded in young athletes with NFOR /high Athlete Burnout Questionnaire (ABQ) scores,[32] along with a higher submaximal exercise heart rate.[31]

Characteristic patterns have also been reported in psychological profiles. Non-functional overreaching young athletes and those recovering from a recent episode of NFOR had REST-Q profiles indicative of a poorer recovery and profile of mood states that were suggestive of a worse mood state.[33] These findings were supported by Schmikli *et al.*,[31] who reported young soccer players with NFOR demonstrating greater levels of anger and depression. Finally, higher self-ratings of emotional and physical exhaustion, sports devaluement, and reduced accomplishment were seen in those young athletes with long-term performance reductions.[12]

One criticism of the overtraining research literature is the disproportional focus on injury, implying that overtraining is purely about physical injury. This paradigm is also evident in research and opinion papers about young athletes, where commentaries about overuse injuries, epiphyseal plate damage, and altered growth and maturation issues abound.

This is not to dismiss the link between injury and exposure risk. It is suggested that up to 50% of all paediatric sports injuries are due to overuse,[1,2] and higher injury rates are noted in those children who spend the greatest time participating in sport activities, as this increases their exposure time risk[34] (interested readers are referred to Chapter 40 for further discussion). A strong association exists between high training volumes and overuse injury across a range of youth sports from basketball to gymnastics,[1] with the injury risk highest when training volume exceeds 16 $h \cdot week^{-1}$.[34] It is logical to link overuse injury rates and training loads, but is important to define if injury in children is a symptom or a cause of OTS. Brink *et al*.'s [27] study of young soccer players showed that the players who sustained a traumatic injury during the season reported more feelings of training monotony and higher session ratings of perceived exertion in the week preceding the injury (see Chapter 15 for a discussion of ratings of perceived exertion). This suggests that injury may be a result of an OTS profile in young athletes. Similarly, those children who accumulated the least amount of sleep each week had the highest rates of injury.[35] In this case it is unclear whether tiredness contributed to sustaining the injury or the pain of the injury resulted in a poorer night's sleep. Therefore, injury should be seen as an important, but not exclusive, factor in profiling OTS in the young athlete.

Causes

Are training loads responsible?

There is evidence both to support and refute the theory that high training volumes are associated with OTS.

Kentta *et al*.[21] revealed that young athletes classed as being stale spent the greatest amount of time training, typically 3–5 $h \cdot day^{-1}$, compared to their non-stale peers. Additionally, recent evidence from 1245 young Swiss athletes (aged 16–20 years) indicated that those doing more than 17.5 $h \cdot week^{-1}$ practice had the lowest well-being scores.[36] However, no association was seen between training load and burnout in young Swedish athletes,[12] between training yardage and high ABQ scores (reduced accomplishment, sports devaluation),[37] between weekly training hours and burnout[11] ($r = 0.1$–0.2), or differences in training load (both hours and days per week) between NFOR/OTS and healthy young athletes.[19] Interestingly, Hartwig *et al*.[38] not only showed that stress scores (REST-Q) in youth rugby players were no higher than average in the players performing the greatest training loads, but also that of the 55 players sampled, only one showed the anticipated high training volume/high perceived stress/low recovery combination. This indicates that the direct link between these factors might be weaker than believed.

Overtraining syndrome is also seen in young athletes participating in low-physical demand sports. Kentta *et al*.[21] observed an 18% incidence of staleness in athletes participating in such sports, and this position was recently supported by a study of young English athletes whereby the incidence of NFOR/OTS was significantly higher (34 vs 25%) in low physical demand sports (<6 METS—e.g. netball, 3-day eventing, golf, and gymnastics)[19] compared to high-demand sports, once again underlining how other pressures clearly play their part in OTS.

It may be that training too much is the cause of the problem for some young athletes, but it would be wrong to think that this is the only cause of every case of OTS, as it can also be caused by a combination of factors. Indeed, even if it was the most important factor, we should ask the question why the young athlete was training so much in the first place. What pressures have made the child train so much that it ends up hurting them?

Quite often, the amount of weekly/yearly training and competing done by young athletes is overlooked. A promising young athlete may be training with or representing a number of teams from school to national level. Coaches can be guilty of just thinking about the training load they impose on their players without considering other training commitments the enthusiastic young player may be trying to balance. More often than not, training and competing across various sports causes seasonal activities to blend with each other creating a non-stop state of activity.[1] In addition, sports like soccer have long competitive seasons, and there is little downtime during the season for the young athlete.[39] The American Academy of Pediatrics[2] recommends at least 2–3 months off from sport each year to let injuries heal and to refresh the mind and body; this recommendation is often ignored.

It has been suggested that young athletes playing at the highest level may be somewhat more protected from excessive training loads. They no longer play and train with lower level squads, and their elite coaches take more control over scheduling. Data from 14- to 18-year-old rugby union players showed that the highest training loads were being undertaken by those in the 'representative' group (607 $min \cdot week^{-1}$) compared to the more elite 'talent' squad (424 $min \cdot week^{-1}$),[38] suggesting that it is the promising middle-standard group who, in an effort to attain elite levels of competition, may be in danger of training excessively and thus may be most at risk.

Both training and non-training stressors are considered as important factors in the development of OTS.[4] However, an understanding of the latter in the context of the young athlete is equally important as the former.

Coach and parent pressure

Good coaching and supportive parents can produce an environment for the young athlete that is nurturing, productive, and enjoyable. In contrast, parents and coaches may also unknowingly increase stress and pressure in the young athlete, thereby creating a need in the athlete to train too much, potentially resulting in OTS.

A number of factors can create this negative situation. If the young athlete receives or perceives to receive more praise or love from their coach and/or parent if they train harder, longer, or win, this can increase the pressure on them to do more training. This 'conditional love' is a powerful influence on young people, who frequently mention it in questionnaires designed to diagnose OTS/burnout in young athletes.[14,19]

Parents who over-emphasize winning, have unrealistic expectations, or openly criticize their child[40] help to create or perpetuate an ego-orientated participation environment. This environment teaches the child that only superior ability is recognized and praised, and that mistakes only draw negative attention. This parental over-emphasis on success is linked with greater levels of performance anxiety in young athletes.[41] A study of young swimmers who had burned out and dropped out from their sport described how high levels of parental expectations and criticism reduced their enjoyment of swimming and increased their anxiety, both of which contributed to the decision to leave the sport.[42] The same study also noted that coaches who provided poor social support (i.e. pressure, unrealistic expectations, lack of empathy, and lack of confidence in the athlete) and led with an autocratic style resulted in decreased motivation and greater incidences of burnout in the athletes they were training.

Parental and/or coach pressure may be out of proportion for various reasons. Both parties may be guilty of vicarious living, making the young athlete's talent and potential a proxy of their own unfulfilled ambitions.[2] Some excellent narrative case studies are available to illustrate the issue.[14] Additionally, the lure of lucrative sponsorship deals, professional accolades, fame, and reflected glory can be strong motivators for the adults involved, resulting in an increase in pressure on the young athlete to succeed. Parents and families can also inadvertently create a suffocating environment for their sporting child. In an effort to support their child's talent and ambitions, parents often invest large amounts of time and money in the pursuit of success. Investments may include money spent on equipment, coaching, travel, and registration, and time spent transporting the young athlete to training at all times of the day and night; often, family holidays are sacrificed in order to support the child.[41] Conversely, once these types of investments are made, parents may hesitate to reduce them, for fear the child will interpret this as though they have failed. A young athlete is very aware of the family's emotional and financial investment, and many feel a pressure to repay these investments through sporting success.

Lack of perceived control

Over-zealousness in a coach, teacher, or parent can disenfranchise the young athlete from having control over their sporting lives. In a study of 182 young swimmers (aged 13–22 years), the lack of perceived control explained 13% of the variance in resultant burnout,[37] which supports the conclusions of Coakley[43] and Raedeke[13] from a decade earlier.

Often this lack of autonomy results from well-intended adult efforts to help the athlete succeed, resulting in the athlete having little or no control over training, competition scheduling, sponsors negotiations, diet, and travel plans. What may be perceived by the adult as helpful may leave the child feeling frustrated and impotent.[44] This disempowerment may result in stress, anxiety, and resentment of both the adult and the situation. Data have shown that chronic exposure to stress may make children more susceptible to burnout.[37]

Active burnout and entrapment

One of the key differentiators between OTS and burnout is whether motivation to continue training and competing remains in the athlete. If the athlete loses motivation, drop-out from the sport usually quickly follows. However, even after the loss of motivation, a young athlete may find him/herself trapped in a state of active burnout.[13] Awareness is key criterion in diagnosing a state of active burnout. Children and adolescents who experience active burnout are acutely aware of the investment in time and money that their parents and/or coaches have made to support them. Additionally, they feel unable to communicate the desire to quit, and often remain involved in the sport so as not to disappoint the adults. This predicament in which they find themselves may only heighten their anxiety and stress, but their entrapment in the sporting world they used to embrace remains real.

Single identity

Another important factor of active burnout in young athletes relates to single identity. Training volume data show that many talented young athletes spend 15–20 $h \cdot week^{-1}$ training for and competing in their sport. This amount of time, coupled with school commitments leaves little time for involvement with non-sport activities or with non-sport friendship groups. Kentta *et al.*[21] reported that 20% of stale athletes spend fewer than 5 $h \cdot week^{-1}$ involved in activities outside their sport, and that 40% of these athletes only participated in their sport and attended school. These findings were echoed more recently by Matos *et al.*,[19] whose study data also indicated that 24% of NFOR/OTS young athletes—compared to 10% of normal peers—spent fewer than 5 $h \cdot week^{-1}$ on hobbies outside of their sport. This exclusivity results in limited chances for the young athlete to form different groups of friends; typically their friendship groups comprise other young athletes from training and competition events. It has been suggested that having different friendship groups may provide a cushion for the stresses of training and performance, which may offer the young athlete more life balance and better coping mechanisms for stress.[43] This is particularly so for younger athletes who may have less-developed coping strategies,[45] and therefore rely more heavily on social support.

Secondly, many child athletes rarely do or are given the chance to do something unrelated to their sport, which prevents them from developing new skills, meeting new people, or having a break from their sporting existence. This lack of opportunity to do things outside of sport may act as a component to identity foreclosure, and thus the development of a single identity.[43] Identities are claimed and constructed through the social relationships experienced through life,[46] and therefore if sport and/or training provides the sole opportunity for social interaction, it is unsurprising that a single identity may result.

Self-worth and self-esteem can become entwined with sporting success and achievement in the young athlete. Recognition, adulation, and social status as a result of their sporting talent and abilities may result in a young athlete feeling defined by the sport itself. The young athlete may thrive during times of success, but reduction in performance or change in team hierarchy may have the opposite effect. Here a perceived solution is for the young athlete to channel self-pressure into training even more;[14] however, it can also result in an increase in anxiety coupled with a reduction in self-esteem (which may be performance based).[12] Both of these psychological stressors can be potential factors in the development of OTS.

Gustaffsson[12] reported that young athletes suffering from burnout frequently cited unidimensional identity and feelings of entrapment, but their link to active burnout is also clear. Feelings of entrapment can result from not having a sense of self outside of sport, a fear of filling hours previously spent in training, a fear of having no friends outside of sport, as well as a serious concern of others' potential judgments regarding a decision to leave training and competing. For a child or adolescent, maintaining the status quo regarding sports participation and training may be a far easier solution, despite the stress.[11]

Perfectionist traits

Perfectionism is broadly defined as the compulsive pursuit of high standards and to be overly harsh and critical of one's accomplishments.[47] There are two forms of perfectionism; self-oriented and socially prescribed perfectionism. In self-oriented perfectionism, the individual sets the standards of achievement, but they are overly self-critical. Socially prescribed perfectionism involves the athlete attempting to attain standards perceived as set by others, and that any criticism comes from an external source.

The limited evidence available suggests that external pressures, rather than self-imposed pressure, may exert a greater influence on the young athlete. Recent work involving 206 15-year-old athletes reported that those with the highest ABQ scores also exhibited the highest socially prescribed perfectionist traits.[47,48] This evidence sustains the idea that children strive to meet the standards and performance expectations of their coaches and parents.[19] Failure to meet these standards can result in the child receiving (real or imagined) criticism (i.e. conditional love) and may greatly reduce their self-esteem. The desire to succeed may result in more training, but may also result in anxiety or avoidance coping (e.g. running away from the sport).[48] Although the external perfectionist pressures may be a negative influence, the studies by Appleton *et al.*[47] and Hill *et al.*[48] indicated that children with the highest self-oriented perfectionist ratings employed more problem-focused coping strategies, and had lower ABQ scores.

Early specialization

Early specialization is associated with incidence of higher rates of injury, increased psychological stress, and dropout.[1] This arises as a result of an increased pressure to train and also contributes to the development of a single identity.

There is a positive relationship between the number of hours spent practicing and the level of achievement in youth sports.[34] The myth of expertise as a result of '10 000 of deliberate practice' has been ingested by society as fact, regardless that data show some elite young athletes reach their goals with as few as 4000 h.[49] A recent study of elite adult athletes revealed that the majority trained less in childhood and only slowly increased training volumes in later adolescence.[50] There is external and/or internal pressure on the young athlete to achieve this prescribed (and mythical) number of training hours target in the belief that it is the route to success. Additionally, early success may trigger an inner pressure to train more.[12] Both external and self-imposed pressures can inevitably contribute to chronic fatigue, and reduce the opportunity for children and adolescents to participate in things outside of the sporting environment.

In fact, there is increasing evidence that suggests later specialization may be advisable. Swimmers who specialized later retired later in their elite careers.[42] Other studies revealed that the majority of elite adult athletes did not specialize in a sport until after age 15 years, and that they had sampled a range of different sports before settling on their chosen sport.[50] The Developmental Model of Sport Participation follows the journey in subjects between the ages of 6 and 18 years from play through sampling to final specialization in sport. The model advocates experiencing and sampling a wide range of different activities during childhood to develop the basic physical literacy, with specialization occurring only after age 13 years. This late specialization results in an athlete who has a wider repertoire of motor skills and superior decision-making qualities when he/she eventually enters their adult sport specialty.[42] The other consequence of following this structure is that the breadth provides variety of experience, reduces the intensity of focus on one sport, and allows the young athlete to meet new people in different environments, thus guarding against the development of the single identity.

Moreover, the American Academy of Pediatrics[2] advocates that, as a preventative strategy against burnout, children should be encouraged to participate in a wide range of sports rather than just one.

It is clear that a number of interrelated factors may exist in young athletes' lives to produce an environment in which they become overreached, overtrained, or burned out. This is reflected in published case study narratives of overtrained young athletes or the retrospective recollections of those who dropped out from their sports.[42,51] Fraser-Thomas *et al.*[42] interviewed young swimmers who had dropped out; the following factors were the most commonly cited as influencing the decision to drop-out:

- Few chances to be involved in extra-curricular activities at school or college, except for sports.
- Less time in unstructured play as a young child.
- Started training earlier in their lives.
- Had earlier success in their clubs.
- Had fewer 'breaks' from swimming over their careers.
- Perceived that they used to get more one-on-one coaching from their coaches, and had a close bond with their coach.
- Were more likely to have had parents who were decent standard athletes.
- Were often the youngest in their training group.

Recovery and prevention

The recent ECSS/ACSM[4] consensus statement provides sound advice in its recommendation of 'Treat OTS with rest'. However, the process of recovery begins only when the cause(s) of the OTS are identified. Because OTS is multifactorial in nature, rest alone may not be adequate for recovery.

As both training and non-training related stressors may be causative factors in OTS, a holistic approach to recovery will result in a greater chance of getting to the root of the problem. The following list of potential factors leading to OTS is not exhaustive or exclusive but can act as a framework to identify possible causes:

- Training load—how much training is the young athlete doing on a daily to yearly basis?
- Rest—how much rest and time away from sport do they experience each week, month, and year?
- Healthy living—are they eating, sleeping, and drinking adequately and healthily?
- Competition load—are the number and importance of the competitions reasonable?
- Single identity—what do they do outside of sport? How important is sport in their lives? What other interests do they have?
- Friendship groups—do they have a wide range of friends both within and outside of sport?
- Covert extra training—do they do extra training outside of the scheduled sessions? Are they a self-critical perfectionist?
- Study/sport/home life balance—what competing time and task demands are they juggling? Are they coping?
- Power relationships and voice—are they involved in making decisions about their sporting lives?

- Conditional love—are the coaches and parents guilty of this?
- Injury—are illnesses and injury hidden in order to keep participating? How many recent URTIs have they had?
- Entrapment—Does the athlete's environment increase the potential for entrapment?

By continuously considering these as possible factors for OTS, parents and coaches can screen young athletes for OTS, and engage in early preventative measures to help young athletes reach their full potential, whether in elite sports, or simply at a recreational level.

Conclusions

The seeds of overtraining can be planted in childhood with episodes of NFOR and shorter-duration OTS being overlooked or misinterpreted by both young athletes and adults involved. Through ignorance of the symptoms and their causes, poor training habits and weak support structures can become embedded and create an environment where the young athlete can become overtrained. Increasing awareness of this problem through targeted education initiatives by the sport governing bodies and coach education programmes should result in a wider support and prevention network, thereby reducing the current incidence rates. As a result, young athletes will experience sustained sporting success and achievement from childhood through to adulthood.

Summary

- Overtraining is not a single condition but rather a continuum of related entities namely—overreaching, overtraining syndrome (OTS), active burnout, and burnout.
- Prevalence rates of overreaching/OTS in young athletes are ~30–35% and burnout about 5–10%, indicating that a significant minority of young athletes are affected at some time in their sporting careers.
- No agreed list of symptoms exists, with presenting symptoms varying considerably between each young athlete. The most commonly reported being a sustained reduction or stagnation in performance, increased perception of effort during exercise, feelings of muscle heaviness, frequent upper respiratory tract infections, persistent muscle soreness, mood changes, sleep disturbance, and loss of appetite.
- Excessive training is not always the cause of overtraining.
- Each case is unique, as are the causes of overtraining; therefore, both training and non-training stressors need to be considered.
- Power imbalances, single identity, early specialization, coach and/or parent pressure, conditional love, perfectionism, and entrapment appear particularly influential factors in explaining overtraining in childhood and adolescence.
- Screening and prevention strategies should take a holistic approach and consider the physical, organizational, sociological, and psychological aspects of the young athlete's sporting environment to ensure that these support the continued enjoyment and development in their chosen sport(s).

References

1. DiFiori JP, Benjamin HJ, Brenner JS, *et al.* Overuse injuries and burnout in youth sports: a position statement from the American Medical Society for Sports Medicine. *Br J Sports Med.* 2014; 48: 287–288.
2. Brenner JS; American Academy of Pediatrics Council on Sports Medicine and Fitness. Overuse injuries, overtraining, and burnout in child and adolescent athletes. *Pediatrics.* 2007; 119: 1242–1245.
3. Department for Culture Media and Sport. *Taking Part 2013/14: Sport.* UK Government; 2013.
4. Meeusen R, Duclos M, Foster C, *et al.* Prevention, diagnosis and treatment of the overtraining syndrome: Joint consensus statement of the European College of Sport Science and the American College of Sports Medicine. *Eur J Sport Sci.* 2013; 13: 1–24.
5. Halson SL, Jeukendrup AE. Does overtraining exist? An analysis of overreaching and overtraining research. *Sports Med.* 2004; 34: 967–981.
6. Viru A. The mechanism of training effects: a hypothesis. *Int J Sports Med.* 1984; 5: 219–227.
7. Meeusen R, Duclos M, Gleeson M, Rietjens G, Steinacker JM, Urhausen A. Prevention, diagnosis and treatment of the Overtraining Syndrome. *Eur J Sport Sci.* 2006; 6: 1–14.
8. Kreher JB, Schwartz JB. Overtraining syndrome: a practical guide. *Sports Health.* 2012; 4: 128–138.
9. Urhausen A, Kindermann W. Diagnosis of overtraining: what tools do we have? *Sports Med.* 2002; 32: 95–102.
10. Maslach C. *Burnout: the cost of caring.* New York: Prentice Hall; 1982.
11. Smith A, Gustafsson H, Hassmen P. Peer motivational climate and burnout perceptions of adolescent athletes. *Psych Sport and Exerc.* 2010; 11: 453–460.
12. Gustafsson H, Kentta G, Hassmen P, Lundqvist C. Prevalence of burnout in competitive adolescent athletes. *Sport Psych.* 2007; 20: 21–37.
13. Raedeke TD. Is athlete burnout more than just stress? A sport commitment perspective. *J Sport Exerc Psych.* 1997; 19: 396–417.
14. Richardson SO, Andersen MB, Morris T. *Overtraining athletes: Personal journeys in sport.* Champaign, IL: Human Kinetics; 2008.
15. Silva JM. An analysis of training stress syndrome in competitive athletes. *J App Sports Psych.* 1990; 2: 5–20.
16. Raedeke TD, Smith AL. Coping resources and athlete burnout: A examination of stress mediated and moderation hypotheses. *J Sport Exerc Psych.* 2004; 26: 525–541.
17. Budgett R, Newsholme E, Lehmann M, *et al.* Redefining the overtraining syndrome as the unexplained underperformance syndrome. *Br J Sports Med.* 2000; 34: 67–68.
18. Nederhof E, Lemmink KA, Visscher C, Meeusen R, Mulder T. Psychomotor speed: possibly a new marker for overtraining syndrome. *Sports Med.* 2006; 36: 817–828.
19. Matos NF, Winsley RJ, Williams CA. Prevalence of nonfunctional overreaching/overtraining in young English athletes. *Med Sci Sports Exerc.* 2011; 43: 1287–1294.
20. Raglin J, Sawamura S, Alexiou S, Hassmen P, Kentta G. Training practices and staleness in 13–18-year-old swimmers: A cross-cultural study. *Pediatr Exerc Sci.* 2000; 12: 61–70.
21. Kentta G, Hassmen P, Raglin JS. Training practices and overtraining syndrome in Swedish age-group athletes. *Int J Sports Med.* 2001; 22: 460–465.
22. Matos N, Winsley RJ. Trainability of young athletes and overtraining. *J Sports Sci Med.* 2007; 6: 353–367.
23. Fry RW, Morton AR, Keast D. Overtraining in athletes. An update. *Sports Med.* 1991; 12: 32–65.
24. Hollander D, Meyers M, LeUnes A. Psychological factors associated with overtraining:Implications for youth sport coaches. *J Sport Behav.* 1995; 18: 3–15.
25. Winsley R, Matos N. Overtraining and elite young athletes. *Med Sport Sci.* 2011; 56: 97–105.
26. Kellmann M. Preventing overtraining in athletes in high-intensity sports and stress/recovery monitoring. *Scand J Med Sci Sports.* 2010; 20: 95–102.
27. Brink MS, Visscher C, Arends S, Zwerver J, Post WJ, Lemmink KA. Monitoring stress and recovery: new insights for the prevention of injuries and illnesses in elite youth soccer players. *Br J Sports Med.* 2010; 44: 809–815.

28. Kushnir MM, Rockwood AL, Roberts WL, *et al.* Performance characteristics of a novel tandem mass spectrometry assay for serum testosterone. *Clin Chem.* 2006; 52: 120–128.
29. Maso F, Lac G, Filaire E, Michaux O, Robert A. Salivary testosterone and cortisol in rugby players: correlation with psychological overtraining items. *Br J Sports Med.* 2004; 38: 260–263.
30. Meeusen R, Nederhof E, Buyse L, Roelands B, de Schutter G, Piacentini MF. Diagnosing overtraining in athletes using the two-bout exercise protocol. *Br J Sports Med.* 2010; 44: 642–648.
31. Schmikli SL, Brink MS, de Vries WR, Backx FJ. Can we detect non-functional overreaching in young elite soccer players and middle-long distance runners using field performance tests? *Br J Sports Med.* 2011; 45: 631–636.
32. Wyller VB, Saul JP, Walloe L, Thaulow E. Sympathetic cardiovascular control during orthostatic stress and isometric exercise in adolescent chronic fatigue syndrome. *Eur J Appl Physiol.* 2008; 102: 623–632.
33. Nederhof E, Zwerver J, Brink M, Meeusen R, Lemmink K. Different diagnostic tools in nonfunctional overreaching. *Int J Sports Med.* 2008; 29: 590–597.
34. Jayanthi N, Pinkham C, Dugas L, Patrick B, Labella C. Sports specialization in young athletes: evidence-based recommendations. *Sports Health.* 2013; 5: 251–257.
35. Luke A, Lazaro RM, Bergeron MF, Keyser L, *et al.* Sports-related injuries in youth athletes: is overscheduling a risk factor? *Clin J Sport Med.* 2011; 21: 307–314.
36. Merglen A, Flatz A, Belanger RE, Michaud PA, Suris JC. Weekly sport practice and adolescent wellbeing. *Arch Dis Child.* 2014; 99: 208–210.
37. Black JM, Smith A. An examination of Coakley's perspective on identity, control and burnout among adolescent athletes. *Int J of Sport Psych.* 2007; 38: 417–436.
38. Hartwig TB, Naughton G, Searl J. Load, stress, and recovery in adolescent rugby union players during a competitive season. *J Sports Sci.* 2009; 27: 1087–1094.
39. Saether SA, Aspvik NP. Seasonal variation in objectively assessed physical activity among young Norwegian talented soccer players: A description of daily physical activity level. *J Sports Sci Med.* 2014; 13: 964–968.
40. Gould D, Collins K, Lauer L, Chung Y. Coaching life skills: A working model. *Sport Exerc Psych Rev.* 2006; 2: 4–11.
41. Bean CN, Fortier M, Post C, Chima K. Understanding how organized youth sport maybe harming individual players within the family unit: a literature review. *Int J Environ Res Public Health.* 2014; 11: 10226–10268.
42. Fraser-Thomas J, Cote J, Deakin J. Examining adolescent sport dropout and prolonged engagement from a developmental perspective. *J App Sport Psych.* 2008; 20: 318–333.
43. Coakley J. Burnout among adolescent athletes—a personal failure or social problem? *Sociol of Sport J.* 1992; 9: 271–285.
44. Udry E, Gould D, Bridges D, Tuffey S. People helping people? Examining the social ties of athletes coping with burnout and injury stress. *J Sport Exerc Psych.* 1997; 19: 368–395.
45. Tamminen KA, Holt NL. A meta-study of qualitative research examining stressor appraisals and coping among adolescents in sport. *J Sport Sci.* 2010; 28: 1563–1580.
46. Thoits PA. Multiple identities and psychological well being—a reformation and test of the social isolation hypothesis. *Amer Sociol Rev.* 1983; 48: 174–187.
47. Appleton PR, Hall HK, Hill AP. Relations between multidimensional perfectionism and burnout in junior-elite male athletes. *Psych Sport Exerc.* 2009; 10: 457–465.
48. Hill AP, Hall HK, Appleton PR. Perfectionism and athlete burnout in junior elite athletes: the mediating role of coping tendencies. *Anxiety Stress Coping.* 2010; 23: 415–430.
49. Capranica L, Millard-Stafford ML. Youth sport specialization: how to manage competition and training? *Int J Sports Physiol Perform.* 2011; 6: 572–579.
50. Moesch K, Elbe AM, Hauge ML, Wikman JM. Late specialization: the key to success in centimeters, grams, or seconds (cgs) sports. *Scand J Med Sci Sports.* 2011; 21: e282–e290.
51. Lidstone JE, Amundson ML, Amundson LH. Depression and chronic fatigue in the high school student and athlete. *Prim Care.* 1991; 18: 283–296.

CHAPTER 39

Physiological monitoring of elite young athletes

Neil Armstrong and Alan R Barker

Introduction

Youth competitive sport is performed at several distinct levels which are best described using a performance pyramid. Figure 39.1 shows the pyramid model, with mass participation at school/community level at the base, and increasingly rigorous selection procedures and greater drop-out as the pyramid narrows. At the peak of the performance pyramid sit a highly selected group of elite young athletes, those who have superior athletic talent, undergo specialized training, receive expert coaching, and are regularly exposed to high level competition at national and international events.[1]

The physiological monitoring of elite adult athletes as a means of promoting the enhancement of performance is well established,[2] but literature solely reviewing the physiological monitoring of elite young athletes is sparse. Clear rationales and laboratory protocols for the physiological assessment of both healthy[3] and clinical[4] populations of children and adolescents have been documented for decades, but elite young athletes have received much less attention[5]. Even texts wholly devoted to the young athlete seldom address adequately the physiological monitoring of elite young athletes, and instead focus on the assessment of healthy young people with little or no reference to the special needs of elite young athletes.[6]

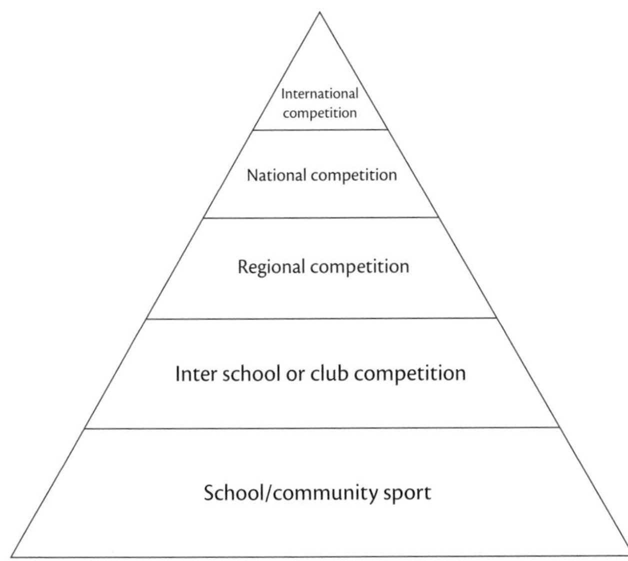

Figure 39.1 Performance pyramid. Levels of participation and competition in youth sport.

Elite athletes are young athletes who have experienced a range of sports and have specialized in a sport in which they have been identified as leading performers. With the exception of participants in early specialization sports such as gymnastics, elite young athletes are likely to be in late adolescence or biologically mature.[7] They might, however, still experience significant growth and performance development. Elite young athletes under 18 years of age are, in most countries, legally minors. While they are well aware of the demands of their sport, they are less likely than adults to cope with sport-life balance and the stresses related to intensive training, family and peer pressure, educational demands, extensive travel, and regular competition.[8]

This chapter presents a rationale for physiological monitoring, examines the ethics of physiological testing of minors, analyses the challenges of developing a physiological monitoring programme, comments on the assessment of the principal physiological determinants of sport performance, and explores the relationship between scientists, coaches, and elite young athletes.

Rationale for physiological monitoring

Physiological monitoring should be an integral component of regular and continuing scientific support for elite young athletes. The overarching rationale for physiological monitoring rests in its ability to develop knowledge and understanding of the exercise capabilities of the participant in order to maximize their present and future sporting performance. A comprehensive physiological monitoring programme should:

- Assess strengths and weaknesses in performance of the athlete's sport;
- Inform design and implementation of training programmes;
- Analyse effectiveness of training programmes;
- Determine current state of preparedness to perform;
- Contribute towards prevention of overuse injuries and unexplained underperformance syndrome (overtraining);
- Assess health status and readiness to resume training following injury, illness, or overtraining;
- Provide motivation by helping to set achievable short-term goals;
- Monitor progress towards short- and long-term goals;
- Improve athletes' and coaches' knowledge and understanding of the physiological demands of their sport; and
- Enhance present and future sport performance.

Ethics of physiological monitoring

The ethics and legalities of research including the physiological assessment of children and adolescents (legally minors) have been debated at length.[9–11] The prevailing view is that experimental procedures must place a young person at no more than negligible risk of harm. Negligible risk has been defined by the UK Medical Research Council (MRC)[11] to mean that, 'the risks of harm anticipated in the proposed research are not greater, considering the probability and magnitude of physiological or psychological harm or discomfort, than those normally encountered in daily life or during the performance of routine physical or psychological examinations or tests'.[11(pp14–15)] In defining procedures involving negligible risk, the MRC includes observation of behaviour, non-invasive physiological monitoring, developmental assessments and physical examinations, changes in diet, and obtaining blood and urine specimens.

Sport physiologists working with young people must adhere to professional codes of conduct, institutional (or regional) ethical regulations, and national laws. Moreover, some countries require background checks on adults prior to them working with young people. For example, in England sport physiologists (and coaches) must have a Disclosure and Disbarring Service Certificate to work with minors.

In many nations, athletes under the age of 18 years cannot provide legal consent to participate in exercise physiology tests. To protect all parties, it is advisable to obtain both written informed parental/guardian consent and assent from the young athlete. Before testing can begin, the purpose, procedures, potential benefits, and risks of the tests must be explained in a form appropriate to the athlete's and guardian's culture and level of comprehension. Additionally, it is advisable that a contract clearly outlining the role the sport physiologist will play is agreed and signed by all parties. For elite athletes and national teams, signatories should include a representative of the national governing body as well as the coach.

For a detailed analysis of ethics in paediatric sport science, interested readers are directed to a comprehensive discussion paper by Jago and Bailey.[12] However, there are some specific issues worthy of note in the current context. For example, for consent to be provided freely there must be an absence of implied pressure. Sport physiologists must therefore be aware of factors such as power differentials and coercion in the recruitment process. It is unlikely that elite young athletes will refuse to participate in a monitoring programme if their coach insists on providing proxy permission on their behalf. Parents may feel obliged to consent to tests in order to sustain a good relationship with the coach or, perhaps to ensure (or at least not threaten) selection.[10] As physiological monitoring involves regular testing, the young athlete must also retain the option to withdraw from the testing programme at their discretion without fear of penalty (e.g. being cut from the team). Similarly, data are confidential and the physiologist should ensure that parental consent and athlete assent are obtained before disclosing any test results to a third party, e.g. a coach.

Development of a physiological monitoring programme

Laboratory assessment of young people's responses to exercise is well documented[13–15] and there is a growing consensus on the appropriate interpretation of data in relation to body size and biological maturation.[16] There is a surfeit of field tests of young people's fitness.[17] However, much less attention has been accorded to the development of sport-specific monitoring of elite young athletes.[5]

Most young athletes identified as 'elite' are likely to be in late adolescence or biologically mature, but their performance capabilities (e.g. muscle strength) may still be developing. In contrast, in some sports (e.g. artistic gymnastics) success is associated with later maturation.[18] The timing and tempo of the process of biological maturation can have dramatic effects on sport performance[19] and assessing biological maturity is complex[20] (interested readers are referred to Chapter 1 for an an analysis of the assessment of biological maturity). To effectively interpret data sports physiologists must therefore have a comprehensive understanding of the developmental exercise physiology of both male[21] and female[22] athletes.

All tests employed in a physiological monitoring programme must be valid and reliable, regardless of the subjects undergoing the testing. However, physiological tests which satisfy these criteria with non-athletic, young people often lack the sport specificity and measurement sensitivity necessary to monitor adequately the exercise responses of elite young athletes. Even if a test provides a valid measure of a variable, it must be determined as to whether a change in the physiological variable makes a worthwhile difference to sport performance.

Validity

Validity is the extent to which a test actually measures the physiological variable it is intended to assess. For example, a physiologist may deduce that aerobic fitness is an important component of performance in a particular sport. With both healthy[23] and clinical[15] populations of young people, peak oxygen uptake (peak $\dot{V}O_2$) determined by running to exhaustion on a treadmill is recognized as a valid test of aerobic fitness. However, if the sport physiologist is specifically interested in the aerobic fitness of elite young swimmers, peak $\dot{V}O_2$ determined running on a treadmill lacks specificity, does not exercise the major muscle groups involved in propulsion specific to the sport, and is therefore not an ecologically valid test of aerobic fitness. To provide an ecologically valid test several simulated swimming ergometers have been developed[24] and used, with mixed success,[25] to assess aerobic fitness in the laboratory and the swimming pool.

Reliability

Reliability refers to the consistency of test scores and can be defined as the amount of measurement error that has been deemed acceptable for the effective practical use of a measurement tool.[26] There is a lively debate among statisticians about which statistical tests best describe reliability or measurement error.[26–28] (Interested readers are referred to Chapter 21 for further discussion of the assessment and interpretation of validity and reliability). There is a clear consensus, however, that the minimization of measurement error is particularly important in elite sport, where winning margins can be extremely small and relatively small changes in performance can result in a worthwhile improvement in finishing position.

Hopkins *et al.*[29] examined the within-athlete variability of performances in elite 100-metre races and calculated that the minimum change in performance required for a change in finishing position could be as little as 0.3%. This is known as the 'smallest worthwhile change' or 'minimal worthwhile effect', and is often in conflict with traditional statistical techniques. It is conventional in paediatric exercise science to accept a physiological test with a coefficient of variation below 5% as reliable, but this might not be meaningful with young athletes. When monitoring elite young athletes physiologists should focus on reducing measurement error as much as possible and evaluating whether an intervention (e.g. training) is having the desired effect by using the smallest worthwhile change in performance.[30,31] For a detailed discussion of measurement theory, interested readers are referred to an excellent review by Atkinson and Nevill.[32]

Physiological variables and sport performance

In some sports (e.g. the US National Football League [NFL]), batteries of tests are given a great deal of credence by those involved in selection for the sport. This has been reported to result in coaches training young players specifically to be successful in the NFL Combine battery of tests, rather than preparing them to compete in the sport.[33] This is not the role of physiological monitoring, which is normally designed to inform the coach and athlete about changes in sport performance, rather than be an end product in itself.

Even if the determination of a physiological variable is deemed to be valid, the degree to which changes in the variable influence sport performance must be considered carefully before inclusion in a monitoring programme. A study by Murphy and Wilson[34] clearly demonstrates the dilemma. In their study, they reasoned that resistance training would enhance muscle strength and power, which would result in improvements in sport performance. In conflict with their hypothesis, their results showed no relationship between changes in measures of muscle function and training-induced changes in performance. Moreover, if there is a relationship between a laboratory measure and performance, it may not be linear. This has been demonstrated in cycling, where the relationship between power and speed is non-linear with, at high power outputs, smaller changes in cycling speed resulting from a given change in power output.[35] In adults, a 5% change in power output has been predicted to result in a ~2% improvement in time in a 50 km time trial.[32] The precise influence (if any) of a change in a single physiological variable on subsequent sport performance during youth is unknown.

Again, a single change in a physiological variable may have little (or no) effect on sport performance, and it has been demonstrated in adult athletes that it is often instead an *accumulation* of related changes that enhance performance. It may be necessary for one physiological variable to be maintained (e.g. peak $\dot{V}O_2$) in parallel with an improvement in a related variable (e.g. running economy) for performance in a specific event (e.g. running a marathon) to improve. These changes may take several years of training.

World marathon record-holder Paula Radcliffe provides a fascinating case study of the complexity of responses to a sustained, high-quality training programme and the challenges to her scientific support team. Paula was regularly monitored from being an 18-year-old elite young athlete. Her maximal oxygen uptake ($\dot{V}O_2$ max), which is used herein as synonymous with peak $\dot{V}O_2$, remained remarkably stable, albeit at an exceptionally high, level of ~70 $mL \cdot kg^{-1} \cdot min^{-1}$, for 11 years. In contrast, her running economy improved by 15% enabling her running speed at $\dot{V}O_2$ max (or any given fraction thereof) to significantly increase in the later years of her career. It was speculated that changes in flexibility (a decrease) and muscle strength (an increase) contributed to her marked improvement in running economy, and her subsequent enhanced marathon performance.[36]

Identification and selection of physiological tests

To be effective and retain the confidence of all parties, physiological monitoring should be as sport-specific as possible. A sound understanding of the physiological requirements of the athlete's sport and, where appropriate, the demands of different positions in a team is required in order to design individualized monitoring programmes. The physiologist should discuss with the coach and athlete the merits and limitations of the tests, including their relevance to sport performance, before selecting and incorporating them into the testing programme.

Sport performance is multifactorial and identification of the physiological determinants of performance is the first step in selecting appropriate tests. A good starting point in devising a monitoring programme is to identify the energy system(s), the muscle group(s), and the movement patterns employed in specific sports, but this can be challenging.

Energy systems

Superficially, the identification of the predominant energy system used in a sport appears reasonably straight forward. In the case of single events, e.g. endurance running,[37] it is, but it becomes more perplexing in multi-event activities (we will use artistic gymnastics[38] as an appropriate example throughout the chapter) and in team games with different positional demands (we will use soccer[39] as an appropriate example).

In middle- and long-distance running, the aerobic system predominates. Jones[37] has speculated that with elite adult athletes the 800 m event requires the energetic equivalent of ~120% $\dot{V}O_2$ max; the 1500 m ~110% $\dot{V}O_2$ max; the 5000 m ~96% $\dot{V}O_2$ max; the 10 000 m ~92% $\dot{V}O_2$ max; and the marathon ~85% $\dot{V}O_2$ max. It is therefore apparent that anaerobically generated energy becomes progressively less important as the race distance increases. These estimates are probably reasonable for elite young athletes who have well-developed aerobic energy systems.[21,22] However, although $\dot{V}O_2$ max (or peak $\dot{V}O_2$) is an important determinant of middle- and long-distance running, as distances increase other aerobic performance variables such as running economy[36] (but see the section on Exercise economy) and lactate threshold (T_{LAC})[40] become progressively more important.

In gymnastics, floor routines and rhythmic gymnastics are predominantly dependent on aerobic metabolism, but vaults, pommel horse, and bars routines are principally reliant on anaerobic metabolism. During the vaults, the main source of energy comes directly from the breakdown of phosphocreatine (PCr) in the muscle, with a small contribution from glycolysis and a minute contribution from aerobic metabolism. The pommel horse and bar routines are primarily supported through glycolysis following an initial contribution from high energy phosphates, with the aerobic contribution increasing with the length of the routine.[38] The differently sized muscle groups used (legs vs arms) increase the complexity of designing an appropriate physiology monitoring programme. Gymnasts tend to mature later than athletes in other sports[7] and the asynchronous development of the physiological variables underpinning aerobic and anaerobic performance during youth further confound the problem.[41]

Aerobic metabolism is the predominant energy system in competitive soccer, but anaerobic metabolism primarily supports activities such as sprinting, jumping, tackling, and dribbling. The physiological demands of soccer vary with position, and analysis of soccer matches has shown positional differences in distances run both with and without the ball. Midfield players tend to cover the greatest distance, followed by strikers, full backs, and centre backs. Total distance run has been shown to be consistent with the distribution of aerobic fitness, but total distance run is only one factor, as strikers have been reported to sprint more often than midfield players.[42] Differentiation in energy use indicates clearly the need for position-specific physiological monitoring with players in team games.

Muscle groups

Identification of the principal muscle groups involved in a sport is a prerequisite of any physiological monitoring programme. It has, for example, been demonstrated that arm exercise, but not leg exercise, can discriminate aerobic fitness between trained and untrained prepubertal girl swimmers.[43] Sport performance is, however, seldom reliant on a single muscle group, and although primary muscle groups are generally emphasized, a comprehensive monitoring programme should identify and include an evaluation of the relative contribution of a range of additional muscle groups that may support performance.

Success in many sports is, at least partially, dependent on the production by the muscles of high levels of force (strength) and the rate at which force is applied (power). In interpreting changes in muscle function, however, the physiologist and coach need to be cognizant of the biological development of muscle strength and power which, particularly in males, may continue into the third decade of life.[44,45]

The significance of the strength and power of the muscle groups involved in sport performance is well recognized, but a direct relationship between improvements in muscle function and sport performance is contentious, partially through a lack of specificity in assessing muscle function.[34] It is important that any test of muscle function adheres to the movement patterns and velocities of contraction that closely replicate the young athlete's event.

Movement patterns

The greatest challenge to the paediatric sport physiologist is perhaps the design of tests which both reproduce the sport-specific movement patterns of young athletes and enable reliable monitoring of key physiological functions. Reasonable laboratory simulation of the movement patterns of middle- and long-distance runners can be provided through running on a treadmill. Simple modifications, such as setting the treadmill gradient to 1% to compensate for the lack of air resistance in the laboratory, have been shown to adjust the energy cost of running to equivalent to that when running outdoors.[46]

In contrast, gymnastic movement patterns are extremely difficult to replicate in a laboratory during the monitoring of physiological variables. The drive to replicate sport-specific movement patterns in a laboratory has led to the development of a plethora of purpose-built ergometers,[42] but current test batteries used to monitor gymnasts lack the specificity required for confident extrapolation to gymnastics performances.[47]

Valid laboratory assessment of the physiological determinants of performance in team games is also problematic. Treadmill protocols to simulate soccer match play have been developed but are unable to accommodate sideways and backwards movements, jumping, and tackling, which are frequently experienced in a game.[48] In youth team sports, more specific field tests are growing in popularity.[49–51]

Primary components of physiological monitoring programmes

It is the responsibility of the sport physiologist, in consultation with the coach and athlete, to identify the specific physiological determinants of the athlete's sport, event(s), or team position, select the appropriate variables to examine, and design a battery of ecologically valid and reliable tests. Numerous sport-specific ergometers have been developed for laboratory assessment of adult athletes,[2] and with minor modifications they are often appropriate for monitoring elite young athletes.[52–54] Few studies of elite young athletes, however, report reliability data[55] and measurement error needs to be determined for each test prior to inclusion in a physiology monitoring programme.

Sport-specificity of testing is the overriding priority but with elite young athletes there are, in addition, essential components of performance which, for health and well-being reasons, warrant general monitoring regardless of the sport. These variables include body composition, muscle strength, anaerobic fitness, and aerobic fitness. For example, aerobic fitness might not appear to be an important component of performance in a specific sport, but the scientific support team might decide that it is worth monitoring because of the health-related benefits that can be attributed to a high level of general aerobic fitness. The nature of the sport will dictate the relative importance of a physiological variable and whether a sport-specific analysis should be supplemented with a general fitness appraisal.

Body composition

In sports categorized by weight and in sports in which the power/body mass ratio influences performance, body composition is particularly important and requires frequent monitoring. Moreover, in some sports where negative energy balance and eating disorders are common (e.g. gymnastics), body composition should be scrutinized carefully and on a regular basis.[56]

Numerous laboratory and field methods are available to measure and monitor body composition, but procedures are largely dependent on predictive equations that were not developed on elite young athletes.[57] The sport physiologist is normally concerned with monitoring changes in body size, body mass, lean mass, and fat mass. Therefore, measures of stature, body mass, and surface anthropometry will in most cases be the assessments of choice.[58] The collection of raw anthropometric data by a suitably trained physiologist will suffice for monitoring, as the subsequent use of prediction equations to estimate % body fat is surplus to requirements and likely to introduce errors.

Muscle strength

Muscle strength is the ability of muscles to exert force, either for the purpose of resisting or moving external loads, or to propel objects (including one's own body) against gravity. Muscle strength can act in a direct manner by providing the increased force necessary in many sports to differentiate the elite young athlete from the less-successful performer. It can also act permissively by providing increased joint stability, minimizing the risk of musculoskeletal injuries, and facilitating re-entry into sport following injury. The development and assessment of aspects of muscle strength during youth have been widely reported[59–61] (interested readers are referred to Chapter 7 for further discussion), but less emphasis has been placed on the specific effects of changes in muscle strength on the sport performance of elite young athletes.

Isometric strength

Isometric strength testing requires the production of maximum force or torque against an immovable resistance with no change in joint angle. Force or torque can be measured by strain gauge, cable tensiometer, load cell, force platform, or isokinetic dynamometry at zero velocity. Few sports involve the expression of maximum isometric force and the relationship between isometric muscle strength and sport performance is weak. Similarly, isometric tests are generally insensitive to training-induced changes in isokinetic or isoinertial strength.[61]

Isokinetic strength

The assessment of isokinetic strength needs a dynamometer to control the velocity of movement while maximal force is exerted against a moving lever arm. The controlled conditions under which isokinetic strength is assessed facilitate minimal measurement error, but the limitations of isokinetic dynamometry restrict the applicability of the assessment to sport. Isokinetic dynamometry cannot replicate the strength-shortening cycle that typifies most sport activities, and isokinetic measures are therefore not generally sensitive to changes in sport performance.[60]

Isoinertial strength

Isoinertial strength tests use free weights or fixed resistance machines to quantify the greatest resistance moved over a specified range of motion. Fixed resistance machines share similar issues of specificity as isokinetic dynamometers, and assessment with free weights is generally considered the strength testing mode most applicable to monitoring changes in sport performance. Rigorously determined isoinertial strength assessments are sensitive to training-induced changes in isoinertial strength, power, and sprint training.[62]

Anaerobic fitness

High-intensity exercise is primarily reliant on anaerobic metabolism, although the relative contribution from aerobic metabolism will increase with the duration of the task. High-intensity exercise is fundamental to most sports, but the rigorous assessment of anaerobic fitness has challenged sport physiologists for decades. With young athletes, the problem is further confounded by the ethical issues surrounding invasive investigations with minors. Attempts have been made to estimate anaerobic energy contribution during exhaustive exercise using techniques such as measurement of post-exercise blood lactate[63] or maximal accumulated oxygen debt,[64] but most laboratory estimates of anaerobic fitness employ performance tests.[65]

The Wingate anaerobic test (WAnT) allows the determination of peak and mean power output through maximal pedalling cadence against a fixed braking force, and has emerged as the 'all-purpose' laboratory test of anaerobic performance.[66] (The advantages and limitations of the WAnT are reviewed in Chapter 8). The WAnT is robust, but it has numerous flaws and data cannot be readily extrapolated to sports other than cycling.[5] Nevertheless, several variants of the WAnT have provided a foundation for useful testing protocols. For example, British Cycling has developed a procedure in which maximal power output is determined using a six-second maximal pedalling test from a standing start on a SRM ergometer.[67]

Maximal sprint tests on a non-motorized treadmill are more appropriate for sports where body mass is transported.[68] A single 'all out' sprint on a treadmill is, however, unlikely to replicate the physiological requirements of team sports, and a test monitoring performance over multiple sprints with short recovery periods is a more useful protocol.[69] This has been demonstrated by Oliver *et al.*,[70] who devised a protocol of multiple sprints on a non-motorized treadmill. These authors then further developed this concept into a prolonged test of sprinting, running, jogging, and walking interspersed with rest periods designed to reflect the physiological demands over one half of a soccer match. The physiological stress of the test, estimated from heart rate and blood lactate, was comparable to previously reported data in young people during soccer matches.[71]

There is no gold standard laboratory technique for the assessment of anaerobic fitness, but sport-specific tests of elite young athletes using laboratory apparatus are only limited by the ingenuity of the scientific support.

Aerobic fitness

Aerobic fitness is the ability to deliver oxygen to the muscles and to utilize it to generate energy to support muscle activity during exercise. Peak $\dot{V}O_2$ limits the rate at which oxygen can be provided during exercise, and a high peak $\dot{V}O_2$ is a prerequisite of elite performance in several sports. Numerous studies have reported that trained young athletes of both sexes have significantly higher peak $\dot{V}O_2$ than their untrained peers, although whether this is due to initial selection, training, or both is equivocal.[72] Peak $\dot{V}O_2$ does not, however, describe all aspects of aerobic fitness.[73] Other aerobic fitness measures of interest to the sport physiologist include exercise economy,[36] blood lactate accumulation and associated thresholds,[40] and pulmonary $\dot{V}O_2$ (p$\dot{V}O_2$) kinetics.[74]

Components of aerobic fitness are comprehensively discussed in Chapter 12 and Chapter 13, and aerobic trainability is reviewed in Chapter 34; therefore, only specific issues related to monitoring will be addressed here.

Peak oxygen uptake

The laboratory assessment of young people's peak $\dot{V}O_2$ has been extensively documented,[15,75,76] and for a general analysis of aerobic fitness a continuous, incremental treadmill test to voluntary exhaustion within 8–12 min is the conventional protocol.[15] The duration of each incremental stage may vary according to whether or not steady-state measures of p$\dot{V}O_2$ and blood lactate are required. A steady-state in p$\dot{V}O_2$ during moderate intensity exercise can be achieved in 2 min, but 3 min stages are required for blood lactate accumulation to reflect the exercise intensity.[77]

Laboratory cycling ergometer protocols are also well established,[77] but as treadmill running engages a larger muscle mass than cycling, the peak $\dot{V}O_2$ obtained is more likely to be limited by central (cardiopulmonary) factors than peripheral (local muscle) factors. Peak $\dot{V}O_2$ is therefore about 8–10% higher on a treadmill than on a cycle ergometer.[23] Cyclists often achieve higher peak $\dot{V}O_2$ on a cycle ergometer, and personal bicycles, which can be easily adapted for laboratory use in peak $\dot{V}O_2$, endurance, and power tests, are the ergometers of choice with elite young cyclists.[55]

It is imperative that young athletes whose sport relies predominantly on arm exercise should be tested appropriately. For example, a study of elite young swimmers reported mean cycle ergometer determined peak $\dot{V}O_2$ to be 91% of treadmill values and peak $\dot{V}O_2$ determined on a biokinetic swim bench to be 67% of treadmill and 74% of cycle ergometer values. Pearson product moment correlations between peak $\dot{V}O_2$ scores on the different ergometers were high ($r = 0.86$–0.89), indicating that any of the ergometers would be appropriate for a general description of the group's aerobic fitness. However, the most elite young swimmer (a national champion) recorded a biokinetic swim bench peak $\dot{V}O_2$ which was higher than his cycle ergometer score, clearly illustrating the need for sport-specific testing with elite young athletes.[52]

Having determined peak $\dot{V}O_2$, physiologists need to explain and subsequently monitor the result. In non-body-mass-supporting sports such as rowing, expressing peak $\dot{V}O_2$ in absolute terms ($L \cdot min^{-1}$) appears most appropriate.[79] Peak $\dot{V}O_2$ is, however, strongly correlated with body mass ($r = \sim 0.80$), and physiologists have conventionally attempted to control for body mass differences by dividing peak $\dot{V}O_2$ by body mass, and expressing it as the simple ratio $mL \cdot kg^{-1} \cdot min^{-1}$. The use of ratio values has clouded the physiological understanding of peak $\dot{V}O_2$ during growth and maturation, as rather than removing the influence of body mass, ratio scaling 'over scales' and results in favouring light individuals and penalizing heavy individuals. Compelling arguments have demonstrated that a more appropriate method of controlling for body mass is through the use of allometric scaling techniques.[16] Nevertheless, with athletes who carry their body mass, such as track runners, expressing peak $\dot{V}O_2$ in $L \cdot min^{-1}$ and $mL \cdot kg^{-1} \cdot min^{-1}$ is appropriate.[80] It is prudent for sport physiologists to analyse and interpret all variables related to body mass in absolute, ratio, and allometric terms for a full picture of changes over time. (Interested readers are referred to Chapter 12 where the assessment and interpretation of peak $\dot{V}O_2$ are comprehensively discussed).

Exercise economy

Exercise economy (or efficiency) is the oxygen cost of exercise at a given speed or power output. A lower oxygen cost signifies better economy. Running economy has been shown to be an important determinant of middle-distance running independent of peak $\dot{V}O_2$ in both trained young runners[81] and elite young athletes.[36] Similarly, the oxygen cost of swimming has been reported to be an important predictor of performance and national ranking in elite adolescent swimmers.[82]

In the moderate intensity exercise domain (i.e. exercise intensity below the T_{LAC}) a steady state in $p\dot{V}O_2$ can be achieved after ~2 min. Running economy can therefore be determined by measuring the oxygen cost of the third minute of running on a treadmill at a fixed speed. Running economy is usually expressed in relation to body mass and treadmill velocity ($mL \cdot kg^{-1} \cdot km^{-1}$). As discussed in Chapter 12 and Chapter 13, the initiation of a slow component of $p\dot{V}O_2$ at exercise intensities above the T_{LAC} confounds the rigorous determination of exercise economy during heavy-intensity exercise.[83]

A useful extension of the concept of exercise economy is to calculate the running speed corresponding to peak $\dot{V}O_2$ (v-peak $\dot{V}O_2$) by extrapolating, via linear regression, the submaximal relationship between running speed and $p\dot{V}O_2$ to peak $\dot{V}O_2$ as shown in Figure 39.2. Despite the limitations of this type of extrapolation of submaximal to maximal values, the v-peak $\dot{V}O_2$ has been reported to be a strong predictor of middle-distance running in trained adolescents, exceeding the independent contributions of running economy and peak $\dot{V}O_2$.[81]

Blood lactate accumulation

Blood lactate accumulation has been used to monitor young endurance athletes as it reflects the ability to sustain submaximal exercise, but sport physiologists should be cognizant of the methodological challenges of assessing and interpreting blood lactate accumulation during youth.[84] (Interested readers are referred to Chapter 12 for further detail).

Elite young athletes present lower blood lactate accumulation than their untrained peers at the same submaximal exercise intensity.[85] Endurance training moves the blood lactate accumulation curve to the right and T_{LAC} occurs at a higher percentage of peak $\dot{V}O_2$ following training,[86] as shown in Figure 39.3. The T_{LAC} therefore provides a sensitive means of evaluating improvements in muscle oxidative capacity with endurance training, often in the absence

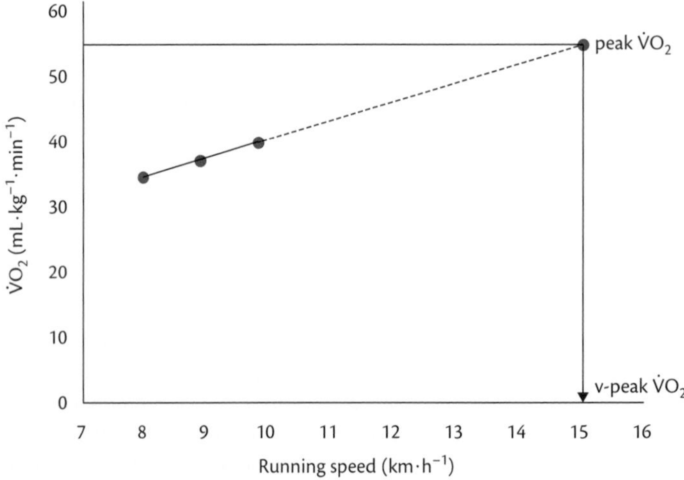

Figure 39.2 Determination of v-peak oxygen uptake. Relationship between submaximal oxygen uptake and running speed determined over three treadmill speeds with the linear relationship (solid line) extrapolated (dotted line) to peak oxygen uptake to reveal the v-peak oxygen uptake.
In this case peak oxygen uptake is 55 $mL \cdot kg^{-1} \cdot min^{-1}$ and v-peak oxygen uptake is 15 $km \cdot h^{-1}$.

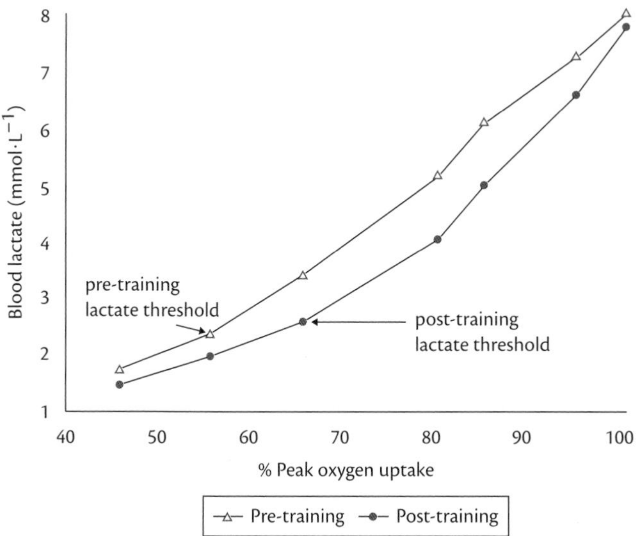

Figure 39.3 Blood lactate and % peak oxygen uptake pre- and post-training.
Endurance training moves the blood lactate accumulation curve to the right. In this case the lactate threshold occurs at a higher % peak $\dot{V}O_2$ post-training (~65%) than pre-training (~57%).
Figure drawn from data stored in the Children's Health and Exercise Research Centre, University of Exeter, database.

of changes in peak $\dot{V}O_2$. The T_{LAC} is normally determined using a discontinuous, incremental protocol with 3 min stages for young athletes. The incremental exercise protocol is designed so that five or six blood samples can be obtained and blood lactate accumulation is plotted against treadmill speed, power output, or % peak $\dot{V}O_2$. The T_{LAC} is the first inflection or 'breakpoint' on the lactate accumulation curve[87] (~65% of peak $\dot{V}O_2$ post-training in Figure 39.3).

The highest exercise intensity that can be sustained without incurring a progressive blood lactate accumulation is defined as the maximal lactate steady state (MLSS). Exercise can be sustained for prolonged periods at or below the MLSS, and it therefore has the potential to be a useful monitor of performance and training intensity.[77] However, the determination of the MLSS is time consuming and demanding, consisting of at least four 20 min constant speed treadmill runs at or near the lower threshold of very heavy-intensity exercise.[88] Secure data from young people are not available and no study appears to have examined rigorously the relationship between MLSS and performance in elite young athletes.

To avoid taking multiple blood samples from young people, non-invasive alternatives to the T_{LAC} and MLSS have become popular. Robust laboratory methods have been developed to determine the ventilatory threshold[89] (or V-slope[90]) to replace the T_{LAC}. The V-slope can be rigorously determined during a ramp test to determine peak $\dot{V}O_2$.[78] Critical power (CPo, the highest metabolic rate at which $p\dot{V}O_2$ can be stabilized below peak $\dot{V}O_2$)[91] has emerged as a substitute for the MLSS but, although promising, more data from elite young athletes are required before it can be confidently included in a sport-specific monitoring programme.

Pulmonary oxygen uptake kinetics

Peak $\dot{V}O_2$ is recognized as the best single measure of aerobic fitness and a high peak $\dot{V}O_2$ is an asset in many sports. However, some athletes and coaches might consider it to be merely a laboratory variable of investigative convenience, as in several sports the ability to engage in rapid changes in exercise intensity is at least as important as peak $\dot{V}O_2$. Under these circumstances, it is the transient kinetics of $p\dot{V}O_2$ which best reflect the effective integrated response of the pulmonary, circulatory, and muscle metabolic systems. Furthermore, in young people peak $\dot{V}O_2$ is not related to the $p\dot{V}O_2$ kinetics response at the onset of exercise.[83]

In the laboratory, $p\dot{V}O_2$ kinetics are analysed from a step transition where a period of very low-intensity exercise, such as unloaded pedalling on a cycle ergometer, is followed by a sudden increase in exercise intensity to a predetermined level. The $p\dot{V}O_2$ kinetics response to the step change in exercise intensity is interpreted in relation to four exercise intensity domains. The upper threshold of the moderate-intensity domain is the T_{LAC} which also serves as the lower threshold of the heavy-exercise intensity domain. The upper marker of the heavy-exercise intensity domain is the MLSS or, more often in young people, CPo. Exercise above MLSS or CPo, but below peak $\dot{V}O_2$, is in the very heavy-exercise domain, and exercise above peak $\dot{V}O_2$ is in the severe-exercise domain.[74]

The $p\dot{V}O_2$ response to a step transition has three phases. At the onset there is an immediate increase in cardiac output which occurs prior to the arrival at the lungs of venous blood from the exercising muscles. This cardiodynamic phase (phase I) which, in children, lasts ~20 s is independent of $\dot{V}O_2$ at the muscle and reflects an increase in pulmonary blood flow with exercise. Phase II, the primary component, is a rapid exponential increase in $p\dot{V}O_2$ that arises with hypoxic and hypercapnic blood from the exercising muscles arriving at the lungs. Phase II kinetics are described by the time constant (τ), which is the time taken to achieve 63% of the change in $p\dot{V}O_2$. In phases I and II, ATP re-synthesis cannot be fully supported by oxidative phosphorylation and the additional energy requirements of the exercise are met from body oxygen stores, PCr, and anaerobic glycolysis. During moderate-intensity exercise with children, $p\dot{V}O_2$ reaches a steady state (phase III) within ~2 min. In the heavy-intensity exercise domain, the primary phase II oxygen cost is similar to that observed during moderate-intensity exercise, but the overall oxygen cost of exercise increases over time. This is due to a slow component of $p\dot{V}O_2$ being superimposed upon the primary component, and the achievement of a steady state might be delayed by ~10 min (see Figure 12.3). Rigorously determined and analysed data in youth are predominantly from the moderate- (i.e. below the T_{LAC}) and heavy- (i.e. above the T_{LAC} but below the MLSS or CPo) exercise domains, and have been discussed in detail[92] and reviewed in Chapter 13.

Data on young athletes are sparse. Trained prepubertal[43] and pubertal[93] girl swimmers have been reported to exhibit faster $p\dot{V}O_2$ kinetics at the onset of a transition to heavy-intensity exercise than untrained girls. Similarly, trained male[94] and female[95] soccer players have presented faster $p\dot{V}O_2$ kinetics at the onset of a transition to moderate-intensity exercise than their untrained peers. However, all testing has taken place on cycle or arm ergometers. The development of suitable sport-specific protocols to monitor $p\dot{V}O_2$ kinetics remains a primary challenge for the sport physiologist.

Training interventions that either speed the primary τ (reducing the oxygen deficit) or attenuate the slow component (reducing the oxygen cost) will improve exercise tolerance. In adults the primary τ and the slow component have been shown to respond positively and rapidly to training, but the optimal training programme in youth remains to be determined. Despite the potential of $p\dot{V}O_2$ kinetics to provide insights into changes in performance, there are, to date, no published data on either prospective training studies or sustained monitoring of elite young athletes.

Field tests

The principal distinction between laboratory and field tests lies in the concept of specificity. Laboratory testing provides a gold standard for the measurement of physiological variables and allows close control over extraneous factors that might influence results. Laboratory testing enables the reliable monitoring of physiological variables, but it is difficult to match the exact movement patterns and limb velocities compared with actual sports performance, even when using sport-specific ergometers. In contrast, field testing allows better replication of appropriate movement patterns and therefore offers greater ecological validity, but field tests tend to be less reliable than laboratory tests.

Field tests have been developed for most sports, but they are regularly recommended without an understanding of their limitations.[96] It is not always possible to meaningfully assess physiological variables (e.g. peak $\dot{V}O_2$) in the field. The 20 m shuttle run[97] (20MST) has been used extensively to predict peak $\dot{V}O_2$ and monitor the aerobic fitness of young people, but a recent meta-analysis[98] resolved that 'it is simply an estimation and not a direct measure of aerobic fitness'.[98(p545)] Furthermore, it was concluded that the criterion-related validity of the 20MST was considerately less with children and adolescents than with adults.[98]

Data from field tests are often misleading. For example, 20MST scores suggest that there has been a large decline in young people's aerobic fitness over the last 40 years. But, there is no compelling evidence to suggest that over the same period young people's peak $\dot{V}O_2$ has declined, perhaps because increases in body fatness explain ~50–70% of the decline in 20MST performance.[72] Similarly, although the 20MST is widely used to monitor the fitness of young soccer players, a recent study noted no significant difference in the 20MST performance of English soccer academy scholars and recreational soccer players.[99] This is not surprising as the continuous, progressively faster running speeds of the 20MST do not replicate the intermittent sprint activity of soccer. More soccer-specific tests have evolved from standard shuttle runs,[100] but their ability to predict the peak $\dot{V}O_2$ of young soccer players is low to moderate.[50] In contrast, a modified Hoff test with 15-year-old soccer players was shown to be sensitive to changes induced by 8 weeks of interval training.[51] However, a recent review of the development of aerobic fitness in young team players concluded that performance during intermittent shuttle run tests can be improved by various training methods without a concomitant increase in peak $\dot{V}O_2$.[101] Field tests must therefore be selected with clear objectives in mind and used cautiously.[102]

Field tests are less expensive and less time consuming than laboratory assessments. They are, therefore, generally more conducive to team sports where testing may involve large squads of young players. The tests are often perceived by team players to be more relevant to performance and more convenient and less stressful than visiting a sophisticated laboratory. It has been argued that this engenders greater compliance and motivation among team players, which therefore improves the chance of consistent and maximal efforts when testing is repeated over a prolonged period.[33]

The development of a comprehensive physiological monitoring programme is likely to involve both laboratory and field assessments. Decisions on the balance of testing and interpretation of data are best made on a sport-by-sport basis.

Scientist, coach, and athlete relationship

A successful physiological monitoring programme is based on rigorous ethical, scientific, and sport-specific procedures with all parties agreeing to a realistic contract. The aims and objectives need to be established at the beginning of the monitoring programme, with the young athlete's safety, health, and well-being the prime considerations. In some cases, physiologists may be part of a large scientific support team working cooperatively with professionals from other disciplines such as psychology, biomechanics, medicine, nutrition, and physiotherapy. If so, they need to be absolutely clear about their role in the team, the confidentiality and storage of data, and the lines of communication to the athlete and coach.

The relationship between the scientist, coach, and young athlete is an essential component of a successful monitoring programme. The coach and young athlete must have confidence in the physiologist and the contribution that physiological monitoring can make to optimizing performance. Retention of the confidence of the coach and athlete in the data and its interpretation in relation to current and subsequent sport performance are vital ingredients of a successful relationship. Renshaw and Gorman[103] outline an occasion where confidence between scientific support and coaching teams broke down through a perceived use of inappropriate testing. Sport scientists working with the UK national table tennis team devised a reaction-time speed test to distinguish between players. When the best player achieved the lowest scores on the test, the players lost confidence in the scientists and the contract was terminated.

It has been recommended that physiological assessments of adult Olympic athletes should be scheduled every 3 months.[79] There are no established protocols for physiological assessment schedules for young people, but testing should be constructed around key periods in the young athlete's training and competition schedule, which will vary with both athlete and sport. The frequency of testing should be decided in advance and in partnership with the coach and athlete. When establishing the testing programme, recognition should be given to the sport-life balance of elite young athletes, as they will have commitments in addition to training and competing, often including school or college attendance. Special allowance needs to be made for additional monitoring if a young athlete is recovering from injury[104] or gradually returning to a full training programme following a period of illness or overtraining.[105]

Regularity and confidentiality of feedback and the format of its presentation should be agreed from the onset of the programme. Following the physiological assessment, verbal feedback to the coach and athlete should be prompt and free of scientific jargon. The initial verbal feedback should be followed within 48 h with a written report that contains an explanation of the tests performed, their purpose, an analysis of the data obtained, and, where possible, a comparison with previous data recorded by the same young athlete.[79] A comprehensive written report can then serve as a basis for discussion with the coach and athlete about performance progression, implications for future training, and the scheduling of competitions.

Conclusions

To optimize the development of elite young athletes and to improve their preparation to compete, and to achieve and sustain success at the highest level, a comprehensive scientific support team is required. Regular physiological assessment and data interpretation are essential components of scientific support. The development and implementation of a physiological monitoring programme requires paediatric sport physiologists to:

- Behave ethically in relation to demands made on young athletes who are often legally minors
- Prioritize the health and well-being of young athletes
- Be cognizant of and up-to-date with developmental exercise physiology
- Identify the physiological determinants of the sport, event, or position in the team
- Select, with the coach and young athlete, the physiological variables to assess
- Be aware of the limitations of current testing equipment and protocols
- Adopt or design ecologically valid and reliable tests for use in the laboratory and/or the field
- Understand measurement error and the concept of minimal worthwhile effect
- Determine the appropriate frequency of physiological monitoring, often on an individual basis
- Evaluate test data and, if necessary, devise new tests, procedures and protocols
- Work closely and cooperatively with other members of the scientific support team
- Interpret and communicate results to coach and young athlete in a user-friendly manner, in relation to sport performance; and
- Maintain appropriate confidential data records and reports.

The overall merit of a physiological monitoring programme is ultimately judged by the extent that it contributes to knowledge and understanding of the exercise capabilities of elite young athletes in order to maximize their present and future sporting performance.

Summary

- Elite young athletes have superior athletic talent, undergo specialized training, receive expert coaching, and are regularly exposed to high-level competition at national and international events.
- Physiological monitoring of elite young athletes is a key component of their scientific support and should contribute to the enhancement of current and future sport performance.
- Many elite young athletes are legally minors, and sports physiologists need to be cognizant of and adhere to ethical guidelines in accord with national laws and professional codes of conduct.
- The sports physiologist must have a sound understanding of the physiological determinants of the elite young athlete's sport in order to identify and select or design ecologically valid tests.
- A range of sport-specific ergometers are commercially available, but the resourcefulness of sport physiologists has enabled many laboratories to design and produce custom made ergometers for the monitoring of elite athletes.
- Both laboratory and field tests have strengths and weaknesses and decisions on their individual and/or combined use should be made on a sport-by-sport basis.
- Physiological tests must be reliable. Success in elite competitive sport is dependent on small differences in performance and measurement error should be minimized in accord with the concept of minimal worthwhile effect.
- Retention of the confidence of the coach and young athlete are essential constituents of a successful relationship. The physiologist should therefore discuss with the coach and young athlete the merits and limitations of tests before including them in a monitoring programme.
- Monitoring results should be rapidly communicated to coach and young athlete free of scientific jargon. They should serve as a basis for discussion about performance progression, implications for future training, and scheduling of competitions.

References

1. Mountjoy M, Armstrong N, Bizzini L, *et al.* International Olympic Committee consensus statement: Training the elite child athlete. *Br J Sports Med.* 2008; 42: 163–164.
2. Tanner RK, Gore CJ (eds.) *Physiological tests for elite athletes*, 2nd ed. Champaign, IL: Human Kinetics; 2013.
3. Docherty D (ed.) *Measurement in pediatric exercise science.* Champaign, IL: Human Kinetics; 1996.
4. Rowland TW (ed.) *Pediatric laboratory exercise testing: Clinical guidelines.* Champaign, IL: Human Kinetics; 1993.
5. Barker AR, Armstrong, N. Exercise testing elite young athletes. *Med Sport Sci.* 2011; 56: 106–125.
6. Hebestreit H, Bar-Or O (eds.) *The young athlete.* Oxford: Blackwell; 2008.
7. Malina RM. Baxter-Jones ADG, Armstrong N, *et al.* The role of intensive training in the growth and maturation of artistic gymnasts. *Sports Med.* 2013; 43: 783–802.
8. Armstrong N, McManus AM (eds.) *The elite young athlete.* Basel: Karger; 2011.
9. Nicholson RH. *Medical research with children.* Oxford: Oxford University Press; 1986.
10. Oliver S. Ethics and physiological testing. In: Winter EM, Jones AM, Davison RC, Bromley PD, Mercer TH (eds.) *Sport and exercise physiology testing guidelines. Volume 1 Sport testing.* London: Routledge; 2007. p. 30–37.
11. Working Party on Research in Children. *The ethical conduct of research on children.* London: Medical Research Council; 1991.
12. Jago R, Bailey R. Ethics and paediatric exercise science: Issues and making a submission to a local ethics and research committee. *J Sports Sci.* 2001; 19: 527–533.
13. Gaul CA. Muscular strength and endurance. In: Docherty D (ed.) *Measurement in paediatric exercise science.* Champaign, IL: Human Kinetics; 1996. p. 225–258.
14. Van Praagh E. Anaerobic fitness tests: What are we measuring? *Med Sports Sci.* 2007; 50: 26–45.
15. McManus AM, Armstrong N. Maximal oxygen uptake. In: Rowland TW (ed.) *Cardiopulmonary exercise testing in children and adolescents.* Champaign, IL: Human Kinetics; 2017. In press.
16. Welsman J, Armstrong N. Scaling for size: Relevance to understanding effects of growth on performance. In: Hebestreit, H, Bar-Or O (eds.) *The young athlete.* Oxford: Blackwell; 2008. p. 50–62.
17. Castro-Pinero J, Artero EG, Espana-Romero V, *et al.* Criterion-related validity of field-based fitness tests in youth: A systematic review. *Br J Sports Med.* 2010; 44: 934–943.
18. Baxter-Jones ADG, Mundt C. The young athlete. In: Armstrong N (ed.) *Paediatric exercise physiology.* Edinburgh: Churchill Livingstone; 2007. p. 299–324.
19. Armstrong N. Sport and children. In: White GP, Loosemore M, Williams C (eds.) *ABC of sport and exercise medicine*, 4th ed. Chichester: Wiley; 2015. p. 97–102.

20. Malina RM, Beunen G. Growth and maturation: Methods of monitoring. In: Hebestreit H, Bar-Or O (eds.) *The young athlete*. Oxford: Blackwell; 2008. p. 430–442.
21. Armstrong N, McManus AM. Physiology of elite young male athletes. *Med Sport Sci*. 2011; 56: 1–22.
22. McManus AM, Armstrong N. Physiology of elite young female athletes. *Med Sport Sci*. 2011; 56: 23–46.
23. Armstrong N, Welsman JR. Assessment and interpretation of aerobic fitness in children and adolescents. *Exerc Sport Sci Rev*. 1994; 22: 435–476.
24. Thompson KG, Taylor SR. Swimming. In: Winter EM, Jones AM, Davison RC, Bromley PD, Mercer TH (eds.) *Sport and exercise physiology testing guidelines. Volume 1 Sport testing*. London: Routledge; 2007. p. 184–190.
25. Dalamitros AA, Manou V, Pelarigo JG. Laboratory based tests for swimmers: Methodology, reliability, considerations and relationships with front crawl swimming. *J Hum Sport Exerc*. 2014; 9: 172–184.
26. Atkinson G, Nevill AM, Statistical methods in assessing measurement error (reliability) in variables relevant to sports medicine. *Sports Med*. 1998; 26: 217–238.
27. Hopkins W. Measures of reliability in sports medicine and science. *Sports Med*. 2000; 30; 1–15.
28. Atkinson G, Nevill AM. Typical error versus limits of agreement. *Sports Med*. 2000; 30: 375–377.
29. Hopkins WG, Hawley JA, Burke LM. Design and analysis of research on sport performance enhancement. *Med Sci Sports Exerc*. 1999; 31: 472–485.
30. Atkinson G. What is this thing called measurement error? In: Reilly T, Marfell-Jones M (eds.) *Kinanthropometry VIII*. London: Routledge; 2003. p. 3–14.
31. Atkinson G, Nevill AM. Method agreement and measurement error in the physiology of exercise. In: Winter EM, Jones AM, Davison RC, Bromley PD, Mercer TH (eds.) *Sport and exercise physiology testing guidelines. Volume 1 Sport testing*. London: Routledge; 2007. p. 41–48.
32. Atkinson G, Nevill AM. Selected issues in the design and analysis of sport performance research. *J Sport Sci*. 2001; 19: 811–827.
33. Gamble P. *Strength and conditioning for team sports*, 2nd ed. Oxford: Routledge; 2013.
34. Murphy AJ, Wilson GJ. The ability of tests of muscular function to reflect training induced changes in performance. *J Sports Sci*. 1997; 15: 191–200.
35. Martin JC, Milliken DL, Cobb JE, McFadden KL, Coggan AR. Validation of a mathematical model for road cycling power. *J Appl Biomech*. 1998; 14: 276–291.
36. Jones AM. The physiology of the world record holder for the women's marathon. *Int J Sports Sci Coach*. 2006; 1: 101–116.
37. Jones AM. Middle and long distance running. In: Winter EM, Jones AM, Davison RC, Bromley PD, Mercer TH (eds.) *Sport and exercise physiology testing guidelines. Volume 1 Sport testing*. London: Routledge; 2007. p. 147–154.
38. Armstrong N, Sharp NCC. Gymnastics physiology. In: Caine DJ, Russell K, Lim L (eds.) *Gymnastics*. Chichester: Wiley-Blackwell; 2013. p. 85–96.
39. Deprez D, Fransen J, Boone J, Lenior M, Philippaerts R, Vaeyens R. Characteristics of high-level youth soccer players: variation by playing position. *J Sports Sci*. 2015; 33: 243–254.
40. Pfitzinger P, Freedson P. Blood lactate responses to exercise in children: Part 2. Lactate threshold. *Pediatr Exerc Sci*. 1997; 9: 299–307.
41. Armstrong N, Barker AR, McManus AM. Muscle metabolism changes with age and maturation: How do they relate to youth sport performance? *Br J Sports Med*. 2015; 49: 860–864.
42. Reilly T, Morris T, Whyte G. The specificity of training prescription and physiological assessment: A review. *J Sports Sci*. 2009; 27: 575–589.
43. Winlove MA, Jones AM, Welsman JR. Influence of training status and exercise modality on pulmonary O_2 uptake kinetics in pre-pubertal girls. *Eur J Appl Physiol*. 2010; 108: 1169–1179.
44. Jones DA, Round JM. Muscle development during childhood and adolescence. In: Hebestreit H, Bar-Or O (eds.) *The young athlete*. Oxford: Blackwell; 2008. p. 18–26.
45. Inbar O, Chia M. Development of maximal anaerobic performance: An old issue revisited. In: Hebestreit H, Bar-Or O (eds.) *The young athlete*. Oxford: Blackwell; 2008. p. 27–38.
46. Jones AM, Doust JH. A 1% treadmill gradient most accurately reflects the energetic effects of outdoor running. *J Sports Sci*. 1996; 14: 321–327.
47. Brevik SL. Artistic gymnastics. In: Winter EM, Jones AM, Davison RC, Bromley PD, Mercer TH (eds.) *Sport and exercise physiology testing guidelines. Volume 1 Sport testing*. London: Routledge; 2007. p. 220–224.
48. Drust B, Reilly T, Cable T. Physiological responses to laboratory-based soccer-specific intermittent and continuous exercise. *J Sports Sci*. 2000; 18: 885–892.
49. Williams CA, Oliver JL, Faulkner J. Seasonal monitoring of sprint and jump performance in a soccer youth academy. *Int J Sports Physiol Perf*. 2001; 6: 264–275.
50. Chamari K, Hachana Y, Ahmed YB, *et al*. Field and laboratory testing in young elite soccer players. *Br J Sports Med*. 2004; 38: 191–196.
51. Chamari K, Hachana Y, Kaouech F, Jeddi R, Moussa-Chamari I, Wisloff U. Endurance training and testing with the ball in young elite soccer players. *Br J Sports Med*. 2005; 39: 24–28.
52. Armstrong N, Davies B. An ergometric analysis of age-group swimmers. *Br J Sports Med*. 1981; 15: 20–26.
53. Sharp NCC. The exercise physiology of children. In: Maffulli N (ed.) *Color atlas and text of sports medicine in childhood and adolescence*. London: Mosby-Wolfe; 1995. p. 51–64.
54. Gibson PB, Szimonisz SM, Rowland TW. Rowing ergometry for assessment of aerobic fitness in children. *Int J Sports Med*. 2000; 21: 579–582.
55. Steiger VM, Williams CA, Armstrong N. The reliability of an endurance performance test in adolescent cyclists. *Eur J Appl Physiol*. 2005; 94: 618–625.
56. Sundgot-Borgen J, Garthe I, Meyer N. Energy needs and weight management for gymnasts. In: Caine DJ, Russell K, Lim L (eds.) *Gymnastics*. Chichester: Wiley-Blackwell; 2013. p. 51–59.
57. Lohman TG, Going SB, Herrin BR. Body composition assessment in the young athlete. In: Hebestreit H, Bar-Or O (eds.) *The young athlete*. Oxford: Blackwell; 2008. p. 415–429.
58. Stewart AD, Eston RG. Surface anthropometry. In: Winter EM, Jones AM, Davison RC, Bromley PD, Mercer TH (eds.) *Sport and exercise physiology testing guidelines. Volume 1 Sport testing*. London: Routledge; 2007. p. 76–83.
59. Farpour-Lambert NJ, Blimkie CJR. Muscle strength. In: Armstrong N, van Mechelen W (eds.) *Paediatric exercise science and medicine*, 2nd ed. Oxford: Oxford University Press; 2008. p. 37–53.
60. De Ste Croix MBA, Deighan MA, Armstrong N. Assessment and interpretation of isokinetic strength during growth and maturation. *Sports Med*. 2003; 33: 727–743.
61. Lloyd RS, Oliver JL (eds.) *Strength and conditioning for young athletes: Science and application*. London: Routledge; 2014.
62. Blazevich AJ, Cannavan D. Strength testing. In: Winter EM, Jones AM, Davison RC, Bromley PD, Mercer TH (eds.) *Sport and exercise physiology testing guidelines. Volume 1 Sport testing*. London: Routledge; 2007. p. 130–137.
63. Welsman JR, Armstrong N. Assessing postexercise lactates in children and adolescents. In: Van Praagh E (ed.) *Pediatric anaerobic performance*. Champaign, IL: Human Kinetics; 1998. p. 137–153.
64. Carlson JS, Naughton GA. Assessing accumulated oxygen deficit in children. In: Van Praagh E (ed.) *Pediatric anaerobic performance*. Champaign, IL: Human Kinetics; 1998. p. 119–136.
65. Van Praagh E. Testing anaerobic performance. In: Hebestreit H, Bar-Or O (eds.) *The young athlete*. Oxford: Blackwell; 2008. p. 453–468.
66. Bar-Or O. Anaerobic performance. In: Docherty D (ed.) *Measurement in paediatric exercise science*. Champaign, IL: Human Kinetics; 1996. p. 161–182.
67. Davison RC, Wooles AL. Cycling. In: Winter EM, Jones AM, Davison RC, Bromley PD, Mercer TH (eds.) *Sport and exercise physiology testing guidelines. Volume 1 Sport testing*. London: Routledge; 2007. p. 160–164.
68. Sutton NC, Childs DJ, Bar-Or O, Armstrong N. A non-motorized treadmill test to assess children's short-term power output. *Pediatr Exerc Sci*. 2000; 12: 91–100.

69. Meckel Y, Machnai O, Eliakim A. Relationship among repeated sprint tests, aerobic fitness, and anaerobic fitness in elite adolescent soccer players. *J Strength Cond Res*. 2009; 23: 163–169.
70. Oliver JL, Williams CA, Armstrong N. Reliability of a field and laboratory test of repeated sprint ability. *Pediatr Exerc Sci*. 2006; 18: 339–350.
71. Oliver JL, Armstrong N, Williams CA. Reliability and validity of a soccer-specific test of prolonged repeated sprint ability. *Int J Sports Physiol Perf*. 2007; 2: 137–149.
72. Armstrong N, Tomkinson GR, Ekelund U. Aerobic fitness and its relationship to sport, exercise training and habitual physical activity during youth. *Br J Sports Med*. 2011; 45: 849–858.
73. Armstrong N, Welsman JR. Aerobic fitness: What are we measuring? *Med Sports Sci*. 2007; 50: 5–25.
74. Fawkner SG, Armstrong N. Oxygen uptake kinetic response to exercise in children. *Sports Med*. 2003; 33: 651–669.
75. Leger L. Aerobic performance. In: Docherty D (ed.) *Measurement in pediatric exercise science*. Champaign, IL: Human Kinetics; 1996. p. 183–224.
76. Hebestreit H, Beneke R. Testing for aerobic capacity. In: Hebestreit H, Bar-Or O (eds.) *The young athlete*. Oxford: Blackwell; 2008. p. 443–452.
77. Williams JR, Armstrong N. Relationship of maximal lactate steady state to performance at fixed blood lactate reference values in children. *Pediatr Exerc Sci*. 1991; 3: 333–341.
78. Barker AR, Williams CA, Jones AM, Armstrong N. Establishing maximal oxygen uptake in young people during a ramp test to exhaustion. *Br J Sports Med*. 2011; 45: 498–503.
79. Davison RC, Somerson KA, Jones AM. Physiological monitoring of the Olympic athlete. *J Sport Sci*. 2009; 27: 1433–1442.
80. Nevill A, Rowland TW, Goff D, Martell L, Ferrone L. Scaling or normalizing maximum oxygen uptake to predict 1-mile run time in boys. *Eur J Appl Physiol*. 2004; 92: 285–288.
81. Almarwaey OA, Jones AM, Tolfrey K. Physiological correlates with endurance running performance in trained adolescents. *Med Sci Sports Exerc*. 2003; 35: 480–487.
82. Unnithan VB, Holohan J, Fernhall B, Wylegala J, Rowland TW, Pendergast DR. Aerobic cost in elite female adolescent swimmers. *Int J Sports Med*. 2009; 30: 194–199.
83. Armstrong N, Barker AR. Oxygen uptake kinetics in children and adolescents. A review. *Pediatr Exerc Sci*. 2009; 21: 130–147.
84. Williams JR, Armstrong N, Kirby BJ. The influence of the site of sampling and assay medium upon the measurement and interpretation of blood lactate responses to exercise. *J Sports Sci*. 1992; 10: 95–107.
85. Armstrong N, Barker AR. Endurance training and elite young athletes. *Med Sport Sci*. 2011; 56: 59–83.
86. Armstrong N, Welsman JR. *Young people and physical activity*. Oxford: Oxford University Press; 1997.
87. Spurway N, Jones AM. Lactate testing. In: Winter EM, Jones AM, Davison RC, Bromley PD, Mercer TH (eds.) *Sport and exercise physiology testing guidelines. Volume 1 Sport testing*. London: Routledge; 2007. p. 112–119.
88. Almarwaey OA, Jones AM, Tolfrey K. Maximal lactate steady state in trained adolescent runners. *J Sport Sci*. 2004; 22: 215–225.
89. Mahon AD, Cheatham CR. Ventilatory threshold in children. A review. *Pediatr Exerc Sci*. 2002; 14: 16–29.
90. Fawkner SG, Armstrong N, Childs DJ, Welsman JR. Reliability of the visually identified ventilatory threshold and V-slope in children. *Pediatr Exerc Sci*. 2002; 14: 189–193.
91. Fawkner SG, Armstrong N. Assessment of critical power with children. *Pediatr Exerc Sci*. 2002; 14: 259–268.
92. Fawkner SG, Armstrong N. Can we confidently study $\dot{V}O_2$ kinetics in young people? *J Sports Sci Med*. 2007; 6: 277–285.
93. McNarry MA, Jones AM, Welsman JR. Influence of training status and exercise modality on pulmonary O_2 kinetics in prepubertal girls. *Eur J Appl Physiol*. 2011; 111: 621–631.
94. Marwood S, Roche D, Rowland TW, Garrard M, Unnithan VB. Faster pulmonary oxygen uptake kinetics in trained versus untrained male adolescents. *Med Sci Sports Exerc*. 2010; 42: 127–134.
95. Unnithan VB, Roche DM, Garrard M. Oxygen uptake kinetics in trained and untrained adolescent females. *Eur J Appl Physiol*. 2015; 115: 213–220.
96. Winter EM, Jones AM, Davison RC, Bromley PD, Mercer TH (eds.) *Sport and exercise physiology testing guidelines. Volume 1 Sport testing*. London: Routledge; 2007.
97. Leger LA, Lambert J. A maximal multistage 20m shuttle run test to predict $\dot{V}O_2$ max. *Eur J Appl Physiol*. 1982; 49: 1–12.
98. Mayorga-Vega D, Aguiler-Soto P, Viciana J. Criterion-related validity of the 20-m shuttle run test for estimating cardiorespiratory fitness: A meta-analysis. *J Sports Sci Med*. 2015; 14: 536–547.
99. Durst B, Gregson W. Fitness testing. In: Williams AM (ed.) *Science and soccer*, 3rd ed. London: Routledge; 2013. p. 43–64.
100. Bangsbo J, Lindquist F. Comparison of various exercise tests with endurance performance during soccer in professional players. *Int J Sports Med*. 1992; 13: 125–132.
101. Harrison CB, Gill ND, Kinugasa T, Kilding AE. Development of aerobic fitness in young team sport athletes. *Sports Med*. 2015; 45: 969–983.
102. Paul D, Nassis GP. Physical fitness testing in youth soccer: Issues and considerations regarding reliability, validity, and sensitivity. *Pediatr Exerc Sci*. 2015; 27: 301–313.
103. Renshaw I, Gorman AD, Challenges to capturing expertise in field settings. In: Baker J, Farrow D (eds.) *Routledge handbook of sport expertise*. London: Routledge, 2015. p. 282–294.
104. Emory CA, Thierry-Olivier R, Whittaker JL, Nettel-Aguirre A, van Mechelen W. Neuromuscular training injury prevention strategies in youth sport: a systematic review and meta-analysis. *Br J Sports Med*. 2015; 49: 865–870.
105. Winsley RJ, Matos N. Overtraining and elite young athletes. *Med Sports Sci*. 2011; 56: 97–105.

PART 4

Sport medicine

CHAPTER 40

Epidemiology and prevention of sports injuries

Joske Nauta, Willem van Mechelen, and Evert ALM Verhagen

Introduction

The many beneficial effects of a physically active lifestyle in children are extensively addressed in Chapter 16, Chapter 17, Chapter 18, and Chapter 19. Being physically active does, however, have one negative consequence, which is that active children are at risk of sustaining an injury. Children are not only at increased injury risk during organized sport participation, but also spend a substantial part of their time in unorganized physical activities.[1,2] The risk of a child sustaining an injury while being active has been estimated to be between 0.40 and 0.59 injuries per 1000 h of physical activity participation[3]. These are rather abstract figures, but consider this: if 100 children are active for 1 year, then between 15 and 23 of them will sustain some sort of injury.

Luckily, injuries sustained by children are usually not life threatening, but they do result in pain, short-term disability, school absence, and in the long term, possibly osteoarthritis.[4,5] Although sports injuries in children are a given, effective prevention programmes, based on results from epidemiological studies conducted on incidence, severity, and aetiology of sports injuries, should be implemented. Furthermore, the effectiveness of preventive measures needs to be assessed, and the implementation of a programme closely evaluated. In Chapter 41, Chapter 42, and Chapter 43, various authors describe these aspects of sports and physical activity related injuries for specific sports. This chapter briefly summarizes the current concepts used to develop and evaluate sport injury prevention programmes as a means of introduction into sports injury research in children. In this chapter, children are defined as aged 5–18 years old. This is because children usually start participating in sports and or physical education after they enter primary school.

Conceptual models for sports injury prevention

Sequence of prevention

In the field of injury research, a widely used conceptual model to guide the development of preventive measures is the sequence of prevention (Figure 40.1).[6] The first step in the development of a preventive programme is a thorough description of the injury in terms of incidence and severity. Next, the factors and mechanisms that play a part in the occurrence of sports injuries need to be identified.

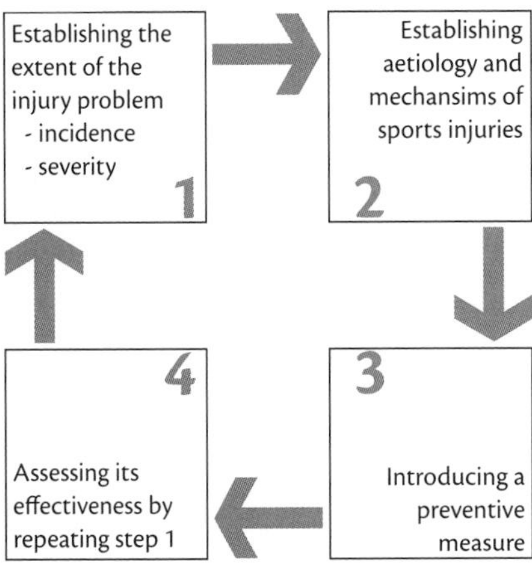

Figure 40.1 The sequence of prevention of sports injuries.
van Mechelen W, Hlobil H, Kemper HCG. Incidence, severity, aetiology and prevention of sports injuries. Sports Med. 1992; 14: 82–99.

The third step is to introduce measures that are likely to reduce the future risk and/or severity of sports injuries. Such measures should be based on the aetiology and the mechanisms as identified in the second step. Finally, the effect of the measure must be evaluated by repeating the first step, which leads to so-called time-trend analysis of injury patterns. Ideally, the preventive programme is evaluated performing a randomized controlled trial (RCT) in which half of the participants receive the programme and the other half do not. This type of research was, until recently, quite scarce in the sports injury prevention field, especially in children. However, the number of high quality studies is increasing.

Models for sports injury aetiology

According to the sequence of prevention, establishing the aetiology and mechanisms of sports injuries is the second step in the development of a preventive measure. The word aetiology is derived from the Greek word aitiologia, which means 'giving reason for', and aetiology is, therefore, the study of causation. In injury prevention, the most important causes are usually divided into two main categories: characteristics of the individual that influence injury risk (intrinsic risk factors), and characteristics that are not related to the individual (extrinsic, or environmental risk factors).[6] Examples of intrinsic risk factors are age, gender, and physical fitness. Extrinsic

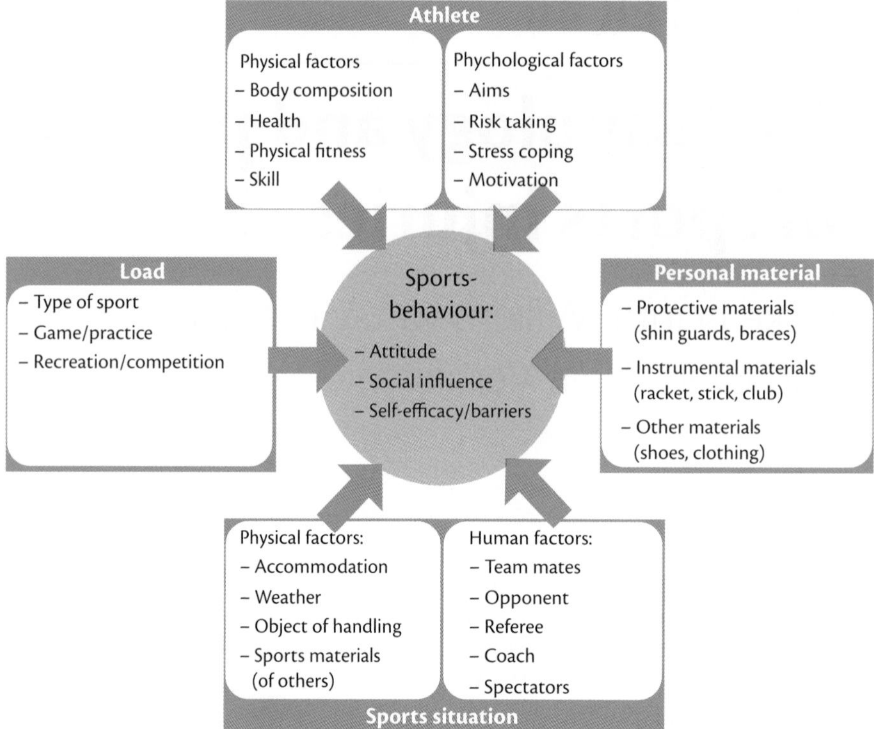

Figure 40.2 Risk indicators for sports injuries and determinants of sports and preventive behaviour.
van Mechelen W, Hlobil H, Kemper HCG. Incidence, severity, aetiology and prevention of sports injuries. Sports Med. 1992; 14: 82–99.

risk factors include, for example, the type of sports and the use of protective equipment. The combination of intrinsic and extrinsic risk factors makes up the susceptibility of a child to sustain an injury. It is essential in sports injury prevention that not only a risk factor is established, but also that the underlying injury mechanism is understood.

The probability of a child experiencing an injury is dependent on the interaction between the child, his/her personal characteristics, and the sports environment. Many conceptual models are available to describe the interaction between risk factors and the occurrence of injuries. One of those is depicted in Figure 40.2 (model of risk indicators); the determinants of sports behaviour model. According to this model, many risk factors will influence the child's sports behaviour and subsequent injury risk by influencing the determinants of behaviour (i.e. attitude, social influences, and self-efficacy).[7] Despite the multi-causal nature of sports injuries, many studies in the field of sports injury prevention have concentrated on identifying single internal and external risk indicators from a medical, mono-causal point of view, rather than from a multi-causal point of view. Another problem arises when a model includes an inciting event as a component of the causal pathway, for example, the model of Bahr and Krosshaug.[8] Most children will repeatedly have an 'inciting' event that, however, does not result in an injury.

According to Meeuwisse *et al.*,[9] the linear approach that contains a start point and an end point does not reflect the true nature of injury in sport. Therefore, they developed a dynamic model that describes the interplay between different factors along the path to injury (Figure 40.3). Their model clearly postulates that an injury is the result of a recursive complex interaction between internal and external risk factors, and is not exclusively caused by the inciting event that is generally associated with the onset of injury. The model classifies the (intrinsic) child-related factors as predisposing factors that are *necessary* to produce injury, but seldom *sufficient*.[9] Extrinsic risk factors, on the other hand, act on the predisposed child from without, as enabling factors that facilitate the manifestation of an injury. It is the sum of these risk factors and the interaction between them that 'prepare' the athlete for an injury to happen, at a given place, in a given sports situation. Due to the cyclic nature of the model, the child can enter in the injury chain at any point, and the occurrence of an injury is not necessarily the finite end-point.

Translation research into injury prevention practice framework

Although the four stages of the sequence of prevention are useful to guide research in injury prevention, the sequence also has its limitations. The major flaw is that no attention is paid to the actual implementation of a preventive measure. Because effectiveness is often established in a controlled setting, preventive exercises are usually guided by trained personnel, participants usually receive incentives when they comply with the study protocol, or preventive measures are distributed for free. Direct implementation, however, of such an intervention is likely to fail, because certain fundamental support is missing. To overcome this gap Finch[10] proposed the Translation Research into Injury Prevention Practice (TRIPP) framework. The TRIPP framework builds on the four stages of the sequence of prevention. The underlying thought is that the introduction of preventive measures implies a change or modification of behaviours of the athlete and/or others involved in the athlete's care. It may be that the desired preventive behaviour conflicts with the actual sports behaviour, for instance, because it is believed by the athlete that the preventive behaviour will negatively affect sports performance.

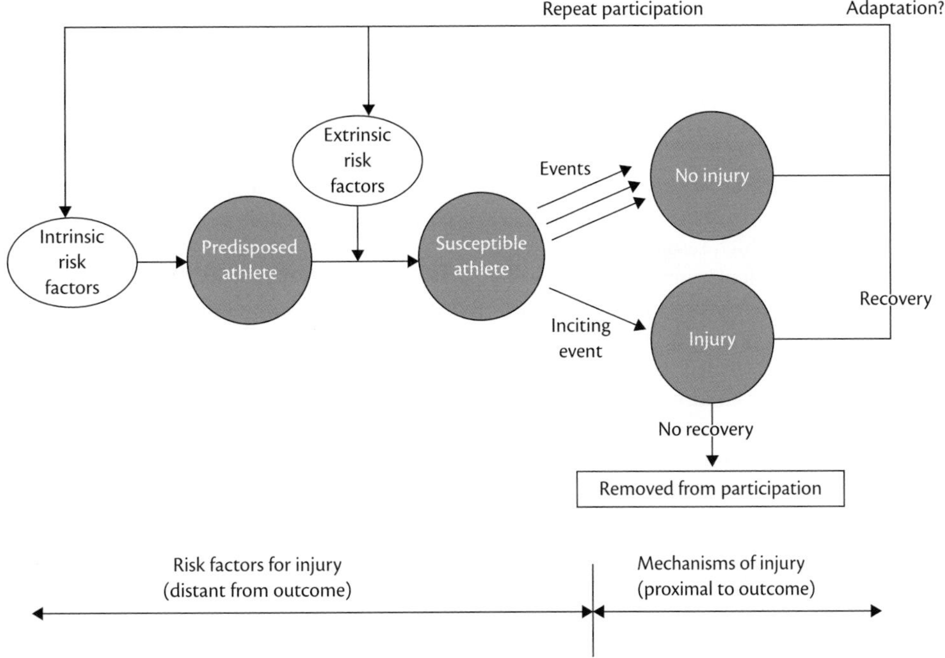

Figure 40.3 A dynamic, recursive model of aetiology in sport injury.
Meeuwisse WH, Tyreman H, Hagel B, Emery C. A dynamic model of etiology in sport injury: the recursive nature of risk and causation. Clin J Sport Med. 2007; 17: 215–219.

When introducing preventive measures and when evaluating the effect of such measures, it is therefore necessary to have knowledge of the determinants of the acting behaviours. Stage 5 of the TRIPP framework, therefore, focuses on understanding how an effective intervention can be translated into actions that can be actually implemented in the real-world context of on-field sports behaviours.[10] This includes the identification of facilitators and barriers. The last step of the TRIPP framework involves the implementation of the intervention in a real-world context, and the evaluation of the effectiveness of the implementation.

Knowledge transfer scheme

More recently, Verhagen *et al.*[11] recognized that most implementation frameworks are research driven: knowledge gathered through science is subsequently top-down translated into practice. However, a preventive measure is more likely to be adopted if sports participants themselves recognize the problem. To guide such a bottom-up approach, the Knowledge Transfer Scheme (KTS) has been developed. The KTS, displayed in Figure 40.4, can start with a problem postulated by practice or research, but will not proceed to the next phase if consensus is not reached between practice and science on the scope of the problem. Key in the KTS is that the end users are involved from the outset in the development of any preventive measure. Knowledge transfer groups are established, consisting of key stakeholders, practitioners and researchers, with expertise on the injury problem and/or practical experience in the sport. Such KTS groups have a shared responsibility for the development of the preventive approach and the assessment of the effectiveness of implementation.

Research in sports injuries

There are a number of methodological issues that must be addressed while researching injury epidemiology and prevention. This is especially important while interpreting the outcomes of different studies.

Defining sports injury

The first issue of importance is the definition of sports injury. In general, sports injury is a collective name for all types of damage that can occur in relation to sporting activities. Various studies of incidence define the term sports injury in different ways. In some studies, a sports injury is defined as any injury sustained during sporting activities for which an insurance claim is submitted; in others, the definition is confined to injuries treated at a hospital casualty/emergency department, or other medical department[6]. In

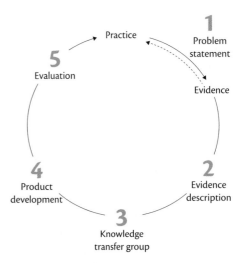

Figure 40.4 The five-step Knowledge Transfer Scheme.
Verhagen E, Voogt N, Bruinsma A, Finch CF. A knowledge transfer scheme to bridge the gap between science and practice: an integration of existing research frameworks into a tool for practice. Br J Sports Med. 2014; 48: 698–701.

children, the term 'medically treated' is also rather broad; it can include injuries treated by a parent, but also injuries seen by a medical specialist. Since differences in definitions used reflect injuries of varying severity, this might partially explain incidence figures reported in the literature.[3] Thus, caution is warranted when comparing sports injury incidence surveys.

Another problem arises when injuries are recorded through medical channels. A common method to collect injury data is at emergency departments of hospitals, which results in a fairly large percentage of serious, predominantly acute, injuries. This results in a partial description of the total injury problem, since less serious and/or overuse injuries are not recorded. This 'tip-of-the-iceberg' phenomenon is commonly described in epidemiological research.[12] This holds especially true for children, since overuse as well as 'minor' acute injuries are relatively common in youth.[1]

To make sports injury surveys comparable and to avoid the 'tip-of-the-iceberg' phenomenon as much as possible, an unambiguous, universally applicable definition of sports injury is the first prerequisite. This definition must be based on a concept of health other than that customary in standard medicine, and should, for instance, take incapacitation for sports or school into account. However, even if a single uniform definition of sports injury is applied, the need remains for uniform agreement on other issues as well.

Sports injury incidence

One way of getting an impression of the extent of the sports injury problem is by counting the absolute number of injuries. For example, when these numbers are compared with the number of road accidents or the number of injuries sustained during leisure time activities, the relative extent of the sports injury problem can be revealed. However, such a comparison is unable to reveal the true risk of a certain activity. One can only sustain a road accident when participating in traffic. Even so, one can only sustain a sports injury when participating in sports. Therefore, a comparison of absolute injury numbers is an inferior strategy from an epidemiological perspective.

When the scope of the research is to describe the spread of disease in (a section of) the population, incidences are calculated. If disease is substituted by 'sports injury' or 'sports accident', incidence can be defined as the number of new sports injuries or accidents sustained during a particular period, divided by the total number of sports persons at the start of the period (i.e. the population at risk). Incidence thus defined also gives an estimate of risk. If the obtained figure is multiplied by 100, the resulting figure is the incidence percentage rate.[13] Expressed in this way, sports injury incidence figures give insight into the extent of the sports injury problem in a particular population-at-risk. It is clear from this definition of incidence that it can only be assessed properly if both a clear definition of sports injury, as well as of the population-at-risk, are used. Another way to assess sports injury risk is by calculating the number of new sports injuries during a particular period (e.g. 1 year), divided by the total number of sports persons at the start of that period (population-at-risk). To interpret and compare incidence rates of different studies, one should not only compare the used injury definition, but also evaluate the comparability of the population-at-risk.

In these examples, the injury incidence is expressed as the number of injuries in a specific type of sports participant, per season or year. Sometimes the number of injuries per player per match is calculated. The difficulty with these examples is that differences in actual exposure are not taken into account. Currently, studies in injury prevention usually express the incidence per number of hours during which the sports participant was actually at risk. Incidence figures that do not take exposure into account are no longer considered a good indicator of the 'true' risk. For example, in some soccer injury research, it is even deemed necessary to calculate separate injury incidences for training and competition, because of differences in injury risk.[14]

The severity of sports injuries

Information consisting of injury incidence alone is not enough to guide injury prevention. The total burden of sports injuries is based on both the injury incidence and injury severity. This injury severity can be described by six main criteria.[15]

Nature of sports injuries

Sports injuries usually affect the musculoskeletal system and can be the result of an inciting event (acute injuries), or have a more gradual onset (overuse injuries). Describing the nature of these injuries, either in terms of medical diagnosis or injury location, is essential to guide injury prevention. For adults, sports injury classification systems are in use to improve sports injury surveillance.[16] The injuries sustained by youth sports participants are different from those reported in adults. A specific youth sports injury classification systems is, however, not available. Therefore, the International Classification of Disease[17] has been used to classify injuries in children.[1]

The most common youth sport injuries are described in detail in Chapter 42 and Chapter 43. For acute injuries, the medical diagnoses that are common are sprains of joint capsule and ligaments, strains of muscle or tendon, contusions (also known as bruising), dislocations or subluxations, and bone fractures. Overuse injuries in children often affect the soft tissue, but primarily include Sever's lesions (inflammation of the growth plate of the heel) and Sinding-Larsens disease (traction injury patellar tendon). Osgood-Schlatter (inflammation of patellar tendon attachment) is another overuse injury that is often reported[1]. Most injuries sustained in active youth are located in the lower extremities,[1,2] although most upper extremity injuries occur during (unorganized) physical activity.[2]

Duration and nature of treatment

Data on the duration and nature of treatment can be used to determine exactly the severity of an injury, especially if it is a question of what medical bodies are involved in the treatment and what therapies are used.

Sports time loss

It is important for a child to be able to take up his or her sport again as soon as possible after an injury. Sport and exercise are an essential part in a child's free time and thus influence their mental wellbeing. The loss of sporting time gives the most precise indication of the consequences of an injury to a sports person.[6] Injury severity can be defined based on the number of days a child could not participate in sports. For soccer, consensus has been reached that absence from sports for 1–7 days is a mild injury, absence for 8–28 days is a moderate injury, and sports time loss for more than 29 days is a severe injury.[14]

Working or school time loss

Calculating the duration of absence from work is, notwithstanding the direct medical costs, a measure for the costs of a sports injury at a societal level. For children, these costs will usually involve the absence from work of their parents or caregivers. The data of working days lost can be used to compare the cost to society of sports injuries with that of other situations involving risks, such as traffic accidents.

Permanent damage

The vast majority of sports injuries in children heal without permanent disability. Serious injuries, such as fractures, ligament, tendon and intra-articular injuries, spinal injuries, and eye injuries, can leave permanent damage and result in residual symptoms. Excessive delay between the occurrence of an injury and medical assistance can aggravate the injury and should therefore be avoided. If the residual symptoms are minor, they may cause the individual to modify his/her level of sporting activity. In some cases, however, the young athlete may have to choose another sport, or worse, give up sport altogether.[18] When taking precautions, priority should be given to sports in which serious injuries are common, even if the particular sport itself is characterized by low sports injury incidence and/or a low absolute number of participants.

Costs of sports injuries

The calculation of the costs of sports injuries essentially involves the expression of the five categories of seriousness of sports injuries in economic terms. The economic costs can be divided into:

i) direct costs, i.e. the cost of medical treatment (e.g. diagnostic expenses such as X-rays, doctor's fee, cost of medicines, admission costs, etc.); and

ii) indirect costs, i.e. the costs incurred by parents who were absent from paid work, the presence of a caregiver, and transportation to and from daily activities in a different way than usual as a result of the injury. In extreme cases, this also involves the costs of death or a handicap.

Research design

There are many factors that influence the internal validity of research. In this section, the most important issues that influence the quality of a study are summarized. It is important to note that these factors are not only important while designing a study, but can also be used to assess the quality of a study.

Collecting data

The methods used to collect data highly influence the quality of the results of a study. In the past, the method of choice to register both injuries and time-at-risk was self-reporting. In self-reporting, participants are generally asked to recall what they did last week, last month, or even last year. It is difficult to adequately answer such questions, even for adults, and children and adolescents may find it even harder. The so-called recall bias usually results in an overestimation of physical activity participation.[19,20] The use of modern techniques has increased the possibilities to prospectively collect injury and sports exposure data. Examples are the use of accelerometers to estimate time-at-risk and mobile phones for online injury registration systems.[1,21]

Clinical cases are a type of research often presented in sports medicine journals. Conclusions are drawn from these case studies regarding the incidence and the risk of sustaining sports injuries. However, this type of study usually does not provide information about the population-at-risk and may not include a control group. A consequence of such flaws in research design is that no valid or applicable conclusions can be drawn from case studies.[22]

Representativeness of the sample

For valid estimations of injury incidence, the sample used in a study must be representative for the population-at-risk. It is, therefore, important to clearly identify the population-at-risk. The performance level varies between children of different ages, as do physical and psychological characteristics. In children, who are still growing, the injury incidences reported are higher during and shortly after a growth spurt. Other variables that influence injury incidence is the type of sport,[23] with high-contact sports usually resulting in more acute injuries compared to non-contact sports.

Conclusions

Over the years, several conceptual models have been designed to guide injury prevention. In these models, the actual effectiveness in a real-life setting has become increasingly important. To establish the aetiology and mechanisms of injuries in children, research of appropriate quality is necessary. This should include a clear injury definition, a representative sample of the population-at-risk, and a well-designed data collection protocol.

Summary

- The aetiology of sports injuries is highly multi-causal and recursive. This fact, as well as the sequence of events leading to a sports injury, should be accounted for when studying the aetiology of sports injuries and when trying to prevent them.
- It is important to take the determinants of different behaviours (e.g. sports and preventive behaviour) into account when attempting to solve the sports injury problem.
- The outcome of research on the extent of the sports injury problem is highly dependent on the definitions of 'sports injury', 'sports injury incidence', and 'sports participation'.
- The severity of sports injuries can be expressed by taking six indices into consideration, i.e. nature of sports injuries, duration and nature of treatment, sports time loss, working or school time loss, permanent damage, and costs of sports injuries.
- The outcome of sports epidemiological research depends on the research design and methodology, the representativeness of the sample, and whether or not exposure time was considered when calculating incidence.

References

1. Jespersen E, Rexen CT, Franz C, Møller NC, Froberg K, Wedderkopp N. Musculoskeletal extremity injuries in a cohort of schoolchildren aged 6-12: A 2.5-year prospective study. *Scand J Med Sci Sports.* 2015; 25: 251–258.
2. Verhagen EALM, Collard DC, Chin A Paw, MJM, van Mechelen W. A prospective cohort study on physical activity and sports-related injuries in 10–12-year-old children. *Br J Sports Med.* 2009; 43: 1031–1035.
3. Nauta J, Martin-Diener E, Martin BW, van Mechelen W, Verhagen EALM. Injury risk during different physical activity behaviours in children: a systematic review with bias assessment. *Sports Med.* 2015; 45: 327–336.
4. Caine D, Maffulli N, Caine C. Epidemiology of injury in child and adolescent sports: injury rates, risk factors, and prevention. *Clin Sports Med.* 2008; 27: 19–50, vii.

5. Maffulli N, Longo UG, Gougoulias N, Caine D, Denaro V. Sport injuries: a review of outcomes. *Br Med Bull.* 2011; 97: 47–80.
6. van Mechelen W, Hlobil H, Kemper HCG. Incidence, severity, aetiology and prevention of sports injuries. *Sports Med.* 1992; 14: 82–99.
7. Kok G, Bouter LM. On the importance of planned health education. Prevention of ski injury as an example. *Am J Sports Med.* 1990; 18: 600–605.
8. Bahr R, Krosshaug T. Understanding injury mechanisms: a key component of preventing injuries in sport. *Br J Sports Med.* 2005; 39: 324–329.
9. Meeuwisse WH, Tyreman H, Hagel B, Emery C. A dynamic model of etiology in sport injury: the recursive nature of risk and causation. *Clin J Sport Med.* 2007; 17: 215–219.
10. Finch C. A new framework for research leading to sports injury prevention. *J Sci Med Sport.* 2006; 9: 3–9.
11. Verhagen E, Voogt N, Bruinsma A, Finch CF. A knowledge transfer scheme to bridge the gap between science and practice: an integration of existing research frameworks into a tool for practice. *Br J Sports Med.* 2014; 48: 698–701.
12. Walter SD, Sutton JR, McIntosh JM, Connolly C. The aetiology of sport injuries. A review of methodologies. *Sports Med.* 1985; 2: 47–58.
13. Chambers RB. Orthopaedic injuries in athletes (ages 6 to 17). Comparison of injuries occurring in six sports. *Am J Sports Med.* 1979; 7: 195–197.
14. Fuller CW, Ekstrand J, Junge A, *et al.* Consensus statement on injury definitions and data collection procedures in studies of football (soccer) injuries. *Clin J Sport Med.* 2006; 16: 97–106.
15. van Mechelen W. Etiology and prevention of sports injuries in youth. In: Froberg K, Pedersen P, Steen Hansen H, Blimkie CJR (eds.) *Exercise and fitness—children and exercise.* Denmark: Odense. University Press; 1997. p. 209–228.
16. Orchard J, Rae K, Brooks J, *et al.* Revision, uptake and coding issues related to the open access Orchard Sports Injury Classification System (OSICS) versions 8, 9 and 10.1. *Open Access J Sports Med.* 2010; 1: 207–214.
17. World Health Organization. *International Classification of diseases and health related problems (ICD-10),*10th edition. Geneva: World Health Organization; 2016. p. S00–T98.
18. Hubbard-Turner T, Turner MJ. Physical activity levels in college students with chronic ankle instability. *J Athl Train.* 2015; 50: 742–747.
19. Klesges RC, Eck LH, Mellon MW, Fulliton W, Somes GW, Hanson CL. The accuracy of self-reports of physical activity. *Med Sci Sports Exerc.* 1990; 22: 690–697.
20. Pate RR, Freedson PS, Sallis JF, *et al.* Compliance with phsycial acitvity guidelines: prevalence in a population of children and youth. *Ann Epidemiol.* 2002; 12: 303–308.
21. Martin-Diener E, Wanner M, Kriemler S, Martin BW. Associations of objectively assessed levels of physical activity, aerobic fitness and motor coordination with injury risk in 7–9 year old school children: A cross-sectional study. *BMJ Open.* 2013; 3(8): pii: e003086.
22. Borchers JR, Best T. Study designs. In: Verhagen EALM, van Mechelen W (eds.) *Sports injury research.* New York: Oxford University Press; 2010. p. 9–18.
23. Beachy G, Rauh M. Middle school injuries: a 20-year (1988–2008) multisport evaluation. *J Athl Train.* 2014; 49: 493–506.

CHAPTER 41

Epidemiology and prevention of injuries in physical education

Dorine CM Collard, Joske Nauta, and Frank JG Backx

Introduction

All school-aged children participate in physical education (PE) at school, and it is aimed at all-round physical conditioning by employing a diversity of human movements. Physical education has the potential to make distinctive contributions to the development of children's fundamental movement skills and physical competencies. These are necessary precursors of physical activity (PA) and sports participation in later life.[1] However, the frequency and duration of PE classes is relatively small, and diminishes as children grow older. In the Netherlands, 75% of primary school children (6–12 years old) receive 2 h PE per week.[2] In secondary school children (13–18 years old), only 53% receive 2 h PE per week.[3] This short time spent in PE classes is not desirable, especially as research has shown a decrease in physical and neuromotor fitness performance in children over the last few decades.[4,5] Physical education classes can not only increase children's physical and neuromotor fitness, but also can contribute to improvements in the social, cognitive, and affective domains, given the right social contextual and pedagogical circumstances.[6] Another benefit of participating in PE classes is that children are more likely to reach recommended daily PA levels. According to international guidelines, children and young people aged 5–17 years should accumulate at least 60 min of moderate- to vigorous-intensity PA daily.[7] In the Netherlands, a study found that PE lessons were responsible for 30% of the total PA energy expenditure in adolescents on a school day.[8] This indicates that PE does contribute significantly to total daily PA. Moreover, this provides a certain amount of PA to all children, which is especially important for children with very low levels of PA. Traditionally, one of the primary goals of PE is to motivate children to participate in sports over a lifetime. Negative experiences like injuries sustained during PE will adversely affect the achievement of this objective. Data concerning injuries in PE classes are mostly obtained indirectly from large epidemiological studies that do not specifically address the issue. Consequently, there are only limited specific data on the topic. Furthermore, data concerning the role of the PE teacher in injury prevention are scarce. This chapter summarizes the available information on the epidemiology and prevention of injuries sustained during PE classes.

Injury incidence

The physical and physiological differences between children and adults mean children may be more vulnerable to specific (growth-related) injuries. Thus, results from studies of adults cannot be used to describe the extent of and risk factors for injuries in children. With respect to children, little has been published about sports-, leisure time-, or PE-related injuries. Few studies on sports injuries in children and adolescents have outlined the incidence and type of injuries in PE classes.[9–12] Pitfalls and problems in the registration of injuries during PE are comparable with those reported for sports-related injuries in Chapter 40. Comparison between studies is hindered by the lack of a uniform injury definition, limited reliability of collected data, and insufficient information on exposure.[13] Definitions of injuries include criteria such as the occurrence of a new symptom or complaint, or the need to visit an emergency department. If injuries are only recorded through the medical channels, less-serious injuries will not be recorded. This is often described as the 'tip-of-the-iceberg' phenomenon (interested readers are referred to Chapter 40 for further discussion). Overuse injuries are a specific problem that applies to the registration of injuries within a PE setting. These injuries are characterized by a gradual onset and are the result of repeated microtrauma.[14] Although PE classes are unlikely to cause overuse injuries, this type of injury could mistakenly be reported during PE. Most primary or secondary schools do not maintain good injury records. Therefore, to assess injury incidence, children themselves are required to fill in an injury registration form. The self-reporting of injuries, sometimes with assistance of a PE teacher, can lead to inadequate data. Furthermore, data on injuries are often collected retrospectively, thereby introducing recall-bias, resulting in under- or over-recording. Finally, it is difficult to collect adequate information on exposure time. Injury incidence refers to the number of new injuries during a particular period of time (i.e. during 1000 h of PE). Insight into the exposure time is therefore important. Total time of PE classes is generally known. However, the exact number of minutes that children are physically active during a PE class is usually unknown. As a result of several differences in definitions of injury, the locus of measurement, and the content of PE classes, it is not surprising that injury rates are difficult to obtain and vary widely between studies. Another factor that might have an impact on the injury risk, especially during PE, is the PE teacher. The quality of the teacher, and the ability of the teacher to properly support a child during an exercise, will influence the risk of sustaining an injury. The selection of exercises is also the responsibility of the teacher. Some teachers may include more dangerous activities in their classes, which could result in a higher injury risk. Although

Table 41.1 Number of injuries occurring during physical education and needing medical treatment.

	Primary school (4–12 y)	%	Secondary school (13–18 y)	%	Total[a]	%
Injuries	41 000	100	140 000	100	220 000	100
Medical treatment[b]	30 000	73	46 000	33	90 000	41
Emergency department treatment	8500	21	8100	6	17 000	8
Hospital admittance	470	1	240	<1	710	<1

[a] For many injuries, the specific activity during which the injury occurred is unclear; therefore, the numbers do not add up; [b] including paramedical treatment.

Based on Consumer Safety Institute. Physical education: Injury rates. Consumer Safety. 2012 (in Dutch).

PE teachers have a major role in controlling the injury risk during their classes, relevant evidence is non-existent.

Risk of injury in physical education classes

In the Netherlands, injury data are collected on a national level in two separate injury registries. The first injury registry is a continuous registry of injuries treated at selected emergency departments all around the Netherlands. The other registration is based on a yearly questionnaire on unintentional injuries, which is sent out to 10 000 Dutch citizens. The data from both injury registration systems are utilized in Table 41.1. According to these data, PE ranks fourth on the prevalence of injury list. Only soccer, running, and fitness caused more injuries on an annual basis.[15] The high ranking of PE is at least partially caused by the fact that PE is obligatory in the Netherlands. When expressed as injuries per 1000 h of participation, the odds of sustaining an injury during PE is comparable with badminton, tennis, and martial arts.[15] The number of PE-related injuries in the Netherlands is summarized in Table 41.1. These numbers clearly show that the majority of injuries are sustained by children aged 13 years and older. The proportion of injuries that need medical treatment is, however, relatively higher in younger children. The injury risk of sustaining an injury during PE has been reported in three studies. The incidence of an injury requiring medical treatment varied from 0.21[10] to 2.2[9] per 1000 h of PE. In a Danish study, 0.14 injuries per 1000 h of PE were clinically diagnosed.[11] When evaluating emergency department treatments of injuries caused by incidents during PE classes, an increase of 150% was registered over an 11-year period in the United States.[16] The same trend, although less striking, was registered in Dutch emergency departments, where both primary school children (<12 years of age) and secondary school children (13–18 years of age) showed an increase of 20% over a period of 4 years in PE-related injury treatments.[15] Although the reason for the increase in injuries remains unclear, the same pattern was registered in sports injuries and private accidents. The importance of a physically active lifestyle has been documented in Chapter 16, Chapter 17, Chapter 18, and Chapter 19. Increasing the number of PE classes has the potential to increase PA levels in children. In a Danish study[11] injury rates were compared between normal schools (1.5 h of PE per week) and schools with increased PE participation (4.5 h of PE per week). The study showed that increasing the number of hours of PE resulted in an increased acute lower extremity injury risk (Odds 1.6). No differences were reported for overuse injuries or injuries to the upper extremity.[11] The teachers in this study received education on training children in a biologically relevant manner, depending on the physical and physiological maturity of the children.[17] It remains unclear if the training of the teachers actually affected the content of the PE classes.

Physical education versus (un-)organized sport

Physical activity in children can be categorized into three main activities: PE, organized (sport), and leisure time. All children are obliged to participate in PE classes in school. Besides that, 20% of Dutch children (aged 6–12 years) participate in leisure time PA each day.[18] In the Netherlands, children aged 6–11 years are more often members of sport clubs than children aged 12–17 years old (respectively 83% and 70% in 2013). Since the character of each type of activity varies enormously, different injury risks can be expected. Unorganized PA is usually expected to have an increased risk because of the lack of supervision. For soccer, at least, more injuries were treated in an emergency department for injuries occurring during unorganized soccer, compared to soccer in an organized setting.[19]

Also, during unorganized PA, children are more likely to wear inadequate footwear and play on irregular surfaces. Both PE and sports are performed in supervised settings. There are two major differences between PE and sports, which also have their effect on injury risk: PE is both obligatory and less competitive than sport. Less-intense competition arguably results in reduced risky behaviour and thus fewer injuries. The fact that PE is obligatory for all children, even children with low fitness levels, is expected to increase the number of injuries.[20,21] The most valuable information on differences in injury incidence between PA modalities is derived from studies that report on all three physical activities (i.e. PE, sports, and unorganized PA). There are currently only two relevant studies (see Figure 41.1). Both studies[10,11] prospectively collected injury data from young children (<12 years). Unexpectedly, reported injury rates were lower for unorganized PA than for sports (0.37–0.57 injuries per 1000 h of unorganized PA versus 0.6–1.57 injuries per 1000 h of sport).[10,11] Regarding the risk of PE, results were conflicting. In the Danish cohort, only 0.14 injuries were reported per 1000 h of PE[11] while in the Dutch cohort the injury risk was not statistically different from the sports-related injury risk (0.50 injuries per 1000 h of PE).[10]

A Swedish study focused solely on the injury risk during PE and reported an injury risk as high as 2.2 injuries per 1000 h of PE.[9] When all research on the risk of PA is compiled, it remains unclear how risky PE is, compared to other PA behaviours.[22] Sports were reported to be most risky (range 0.20–0.67 medically treated

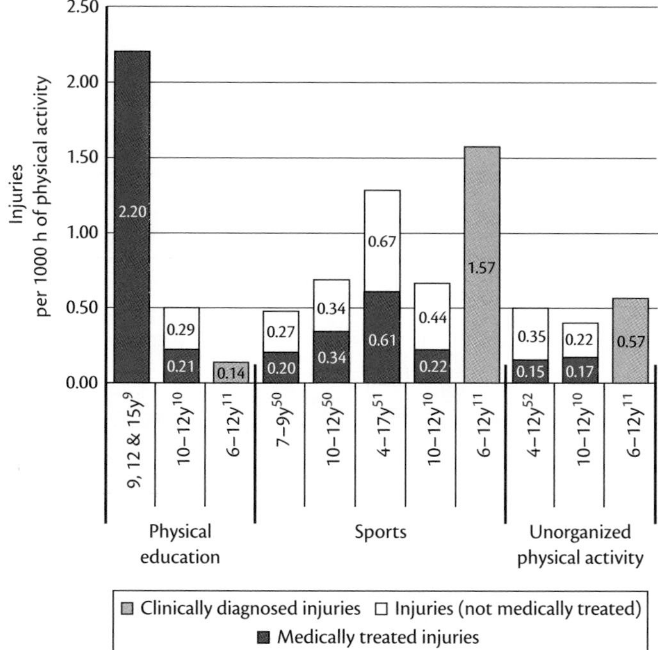

Figure 41.1 Reported injury incidence rates expressed per 1000 h of physical education, sports, and unorganized physical activity.
y = age of participants in calendar years. Bold superscript = reference number of original source.
Nauta J, Martin-Diener E, Martin BW, van Mechelen W, Verhagen EALM. Injury risk during different physical activity behaviours in children: a systematic review with bias assessment. Sports Med. 2015; 45: 327–336.

injuries) compared to unorganized PA (range 0.15–0.17 medically treated injuries).[22] When absolute numbers of injuries are counted, 46–56% of all injuries were registered during unorganized PA, compared to 8–21% during PE.[10,11]

Gender

Gender differences in injury risk are frequently reported. In children, many studies report a higher injury risk for girls than for boys.[9,10,20,21] Verhagen *et al.*[10] reported that the higher injury risk in girls was mainly due to a more than twofold higher injury incidence resulting from leisure time physical activities. Sundblad *et al.*[9] reported that almost twice as many girls as boys were injured during PE classes. Their results can possibly be explained by the reporting behaviour of girls and boys, and the fact that boys are less likely to report a minor injury. From the literature it is also clear that girls have an increased risk of hypermobility[23] and anterior cruciate ligament (ACL) injuries. Anterior cruciate ligament injury rates are low in young children and increase sharply during puberty, especially in girls, who have higher rates of non-contact ACL injuries than boys do in similar sports.[24] There are different explanations for this higher risk, including anatomical, hormonal, and neuromuscular factors.[25] However, boys are reported to have a higher risk of sports injuries as they are more aggressive, have larger body mass, participate more often in vigorous exercise, have higher exposure time, and experience greater contact compared to girls in the same sports activities.[26] During PE classes, boys and girls in primary school have the same risk for (medically treated) injuries[20]. In the Netherlands, both sexes are treated equally in the hospital due to injuries in PE classes in primary school.[10,15] Boys and girls both participate in PE classes in comparison with organized sports, where boys and girls participate separately. It is important for PE teachers to know how to organize their classes and their choices for activities, to make sure that both boys and girls are able to participate without injury.

Age

Naturally, the distribution of injuries relative to age depends substantially on the type of activities planned and instructed by PE teachers. Nevertheless, there are differences between children in primary and secondary school in injuries sustained.[27,28] In primary school (4–12 years), the children aged 10–12 years have the highest risk of injury.[29] In secondary school, the youngest group (13–14 years) has the highest risk of getting injured. In all sports, adolescents (>13 years) are at a greater risk of injury than younger children.[26] Besides acute injuries occurring during PE classes, injuries primarily attributable to biological growth are also included. Focusing on severity of injuries, there is no consensus on the influence of age (or gender) on hospital admission. Results on the relationship between age and injuries are not well described, mainly because many studies have focused on a narrow age range. This makes it difficult to observe a possible association between age and injury incidence.[26]

Aerobic fitness, weekly physical activity, and body composition

Children (aged 7–9 years) with low levels of aerobic fitness as assessed with the 20 m shuttle run test (20MST) are at increased injury risk compared to children with medium and high levels of aerobic fitness.[21] During PE classes all children participate, including those with a low level of aerobic fitness. Less fit children are at greater risk of injury. Bloemers *et al.*[20] found that injury risk in overall physical activities significantly declined with an increase in weekly exposure. The most active children (ages 10–12 years) had the lowest injury risk. This was also found for leisure time injuries. Martin-Diener *et al.*[21] concluded that levels of objectively assessed PA were not associated with injury risk in school children (aged 7–9 years). Studies of the association between body composition and injuries are conflicting. Different studies used different methods to characterize body composition, such as stature and body mass, lean muscle mass, body-fat content, and BMI.[25] Taller and heavier children may be more susceptible to injury due to greater forces being absorbed through soft tissues and joints[26]. However, Warsh *et al.*[30] and Kemler *et al.*[31] found that BMI status is not an effect modifier of the relationship between PA and PA-related injuries in youth. Jespersen[32] reported that when comparing two different measures of overweight, overweight by total body fat percentage was a greater risk factor than overweight by BMI. This suggests that a high proportion of adiposity is more predictive of lower extremity injuries, possibly due to a lower proportion of lean muscle mass.

Location of injury

The part of the body that will most likely be injured is heavily dependent on the PA that is employed during PE classes. Injuries to hands and fingers are more likely during ball games, while activities that require fast twisting motions increase the risk of ankle and knee injuries. As mentioned before, the teacher will usually decide

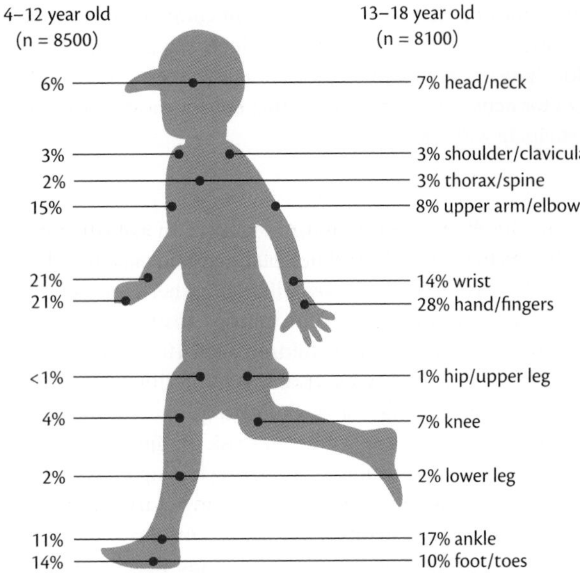

Figure 41.2 Percentage distribution of 16 600 physical education related injuries over body areas in 4- to 12-year-olds and 13- to 18-year-olds.
Based on Consumer Safety Institute. Physical education: Injury rates. Consumer Safety. 2012 (in Dutch).

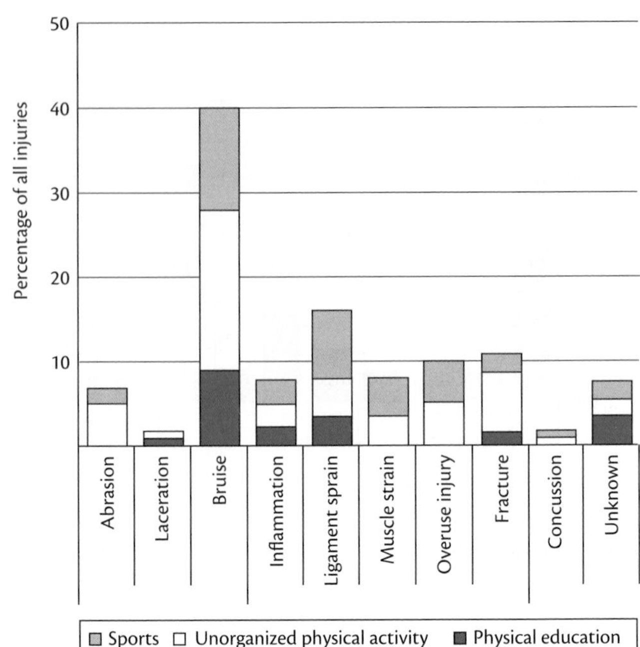

Figure 41.3 Injury type within different modalities of physical activity, presented as a percentage of all injuries.
n =104 injuries.
Data from Verhagen EALM, Collard DC, Chin A Paw MJM, van Mechelen W. A prospective cohort study on physical activity and sports-related injuries in 10- to 12-year-old children. Br J Sports Med. 2009; 43: 1031–1035.

on the environmental context and the programme, and can thereby influence the injury risk. During PA in general, the lower extremities are most often injured,[10–12] although head injuries have also been reported to be an important injury location in very young children (7–9 years old).[9] Figure 41.2 summarizes injuries treated at Dutch emergency departments after an incident during PE. These data suggest that the majority of the injuries involve the upper extremities. Note that the data include only relatively severe injuries that need hospital treatment. When less-severe injuries are also included, lower extremities injuries account for over half of the injuries.[10,12] Compared to young children, older children more frequently injure their hand and/or fingers and ankle. In addition, younger children have a higher incidence of wrist and elbow injuries.[15]

Type of injury and injury mechanism

Acute injuries

Figure 41.3 shows the distribution of injury type over the three main PA behaviours in children. Most injuries are soft tissue injuries like bruises, strains, sprains, and contusions. The occurrence of a fracture during PE is relatively uncommon.[9,10,33] Emergency department studies include the more severe injuries, and therefore more fractures are expected. In Dutch emergency departments, 39% of PE-related injuries treated in children under 18 years are fractures.[15] This proportion is in sharp contrast with the consideration that fractures are uncommon during PE. This could be partially explained by the Dutch medical system requiring a patient to first be screened by a general practitioner before seeking treatment at an emergency department. Thus, relatively minor injuries are treated elsewhere. To put these data into perspective, the number of fractures caused by a sports accident in children under the age of 14 years was reported to be as high as 49%. The proportion of fractures is higher in children under 12 years of age, mostly caused by a higher number of arm and wrist fractures.[15]

Physical education classes containing activities such as gymnastics and ball games (basketball, soccer, volleyball) provoke the most damage.[9,15] In primary school-age children, gymnastics account for the majority of injuries.[15] When children get older, the proportion of injuries as a result of ball games increases, and reported proportions range from 26–62%.[9,15] Again, these figures are heavily dependent on the activities PE teachers choose for their PE classes. Most of the injuries during PE classes are caused by the pupils themselves through falls or twisting movements.[9,15,33] Other common causes of injuries are collisions with another pupil, or being hit by a loose object.[9,15]

Overuse injuries

Overuse injuries are characterized by a gradual onset caused by repeated microtrauma.[14] Up to 50% of all paediatric injuries are overuse injuries.[34] The majority of these overuse injuries are growth-related injuries, such as Osgood-Schlatter's disease, Sever's disease, Sinding-Larsen-Johansson's disease, and jumper's knee (these conditions are described in more detail in Chapter 45). The lack of an identifiable event responsible for the injury and being caused by accumulating different types of PA makes it difficult to study overuse injuries within a specific sports context. In a Danish primary school cohort, the effect of additional PE classes (4.5 $h \cdot week^{-1}$ instead of 1.5 $h \cdot week^{-1}$) on injuries was studied.[34] Over 2.5 years, all injuries were diagnosed by a health care professional on a weekly basis. Of 1416 injuries reported, 1062 were overuse injuries, including 454 growth-related injuries. Not school type, but volume of organized PA (PE and organized sport) was reported to increase overuse injury risk by a factor of 1.29, and growth-related injury risk by a factor of 1.38.[34] Physical education lessons are usually more diverse than training sessions for a specific sport. Since repetition is one of the mechanisms that can cause an overuse injury, it is more likely that an overuse injury originates from sports participation than from PE.

Severity of injuries

Injuries can cause unnecessary suffering, and pain can be associated with prolonged periods of disability. Long-term effects are particularly frequent after acute injuries to the knee or ankle. It is suggested that the long-term effect of an injury sustained at a young age has a negative influence on participation in health-enhancing PA and sports.[33] There are different factors of importance to describe the severity of injuries in an efficient and practical manner. The severity of injuries can be described based on the nature of the injury, nature of the treatment, costs of the treatment, and time lost from sport or school.

Nature of the injury

Very serious PE accidents in youth, leading to permanent handicap or death, are exceptional.[9] Because of the frequency and potential for adverse long-term health outcomes three types of potentially serious injuries in youth need to be addressed: ACL injury, concussion, and physeal injury. Researchers have noted an increase in the numbers of ACL injuries over the past two decades.[35] Reasons for the increase in ACL injury rate include the growing number of children and adolescents participating in organized sports, and an increased participation in high-demand sports at an earlier age. An ACL injury may increase the risk of osteoarthritis in the future.[35] Concussion is not reported often during PE classes, but it can have a huge impact on children's cognitive development during their formative years, and potentially impair scholastic achievements. It is therefore important to prevent these injuries. Growth plate injury is an injury unique to the paediatric population, which can have negative effect on growth and the ability to participate in sports.

Nature of the treatment

Data from a Dutch study of primary school children indicate that 40% of all injuries in children required medical treatment.[10] This resulted in an incidence of 0.19 (para-)medically treated injuries per 1000 h of exposure (95% CI:0,13–0.25). If an injury was medically treated, the children mostly visited the general practitioner, physical therapist, or the emergency department. In the Netherlands, of the injured school-aged children (4–18 years) visiting emergency departments, 3–6% of children (4–12 years) and 3% of adolescents (13–18 years) needed hospitalization.[29] One study showed that the incidence of (para-)medically treated injuries was divided equally between different modalities of physical activities. The injury incidence for (para-medically treated injuries occurred during PE classes was 0.21 (95% CI: 0.07–0.34).[10]

Costs of the treatment

Medically treated injuries are associated with high health care costs. However, health care costs are not often assessed for sport-related injuries in children. In the Netherlands in 2013, the economic burden of sport injuries was estimated at 530 million euros. From this, 140 million euro was as a result of PA related injuries in children (<18 years old).[36] Also costs of injuries can be used to determine the severity of injuries. The use of health care and the associated annual costs as a result of PE-related injuries in children has seldom been examined. Collard *et al.*[37] reported on the economic burden of injuries occurring during organized sports, unorganized PA, and PE classes. All direct (i.e. health care costs) and indirect (i.e. costs associated with absenteeism, care-taker costs etc.) costs were registered from the moment of injury onwards, until recovery. The mean direct and indirect costs for injuries that occurred during PE classes were 182 euros (±269). The total costs for upper extremities injuries occurred during organized sports, unorganized PA, and PE classes were significantly higher than the total costs for lower extremities injuries (316 ± 401 euros and 75 ± 232 euros). Additionally, Meerding *et al.*[38] found that upper extremities injuries in terms of health care costs are relatively high during childhood.

Time lost from (un-)organized sport or school

The number of days elapsed until the child returns to PA is often reported as a measure of injury severity. Injuries occurring in children are mostly classified as minor, according to the abbreviated injury scale (AIS). This scale has three different grades: one (return within a week), two (absence for more than a week but less than a month) and three (absence for more than a month). Sundblad *et al.*[9] showed that 70% of children could return to PA at school within a week after they were injured during PA in school. The severity of an injury can also be defined as the amount of time lost in school. School absenteeism as an outcome parameter was studied in earlier studies. Children who were injured during PE classes had more time loss of total school days in comparison with those whose injuries were sustained during club sports.[12] Focusing on PA-related injuries in children, but not specifically PE-related injuries, Verhagen *et al.*[10] reported a sport absence of 1 week in 45% of all cases of injury, 29% resulted in an absence of 2 weeks, and 26% resulted in an absence of 3 weeks or more. They also concluded that 14% of the children who sustained a PA-related injury reported absence from regular school activities, with a mean loss of 1.8 school days per injury (±1.3). It must be noted that the duration of sports or school absenteeism can be influenced by bias. Bias can easily be caused by factors such as the individual's tolerance to pain, type of treatment, parents, and PE teacher or coach. Therefore, these estimates of injury severity are more practical than valid parameters.

Aetiology

Aetiology is the study of causation. In injury prevention, the most important causes are usually divided into two main categories: characteristics of the individual that influence injury risk (intrinsic risk factors), and characteristics that are not related to the individual (extrinsic or environmental risk factors). Intrinsic risk factors for PA-related injuries in children include among others: (aerobic) fitness, flexibility, strength, joint stability, balance/proprioception, previous injury, age, and gender. The latter three are non-modifiable risk factors.[26] Extrinsic risk factors for PA-related injuries in children include among others: sport played (contact/non-contact), rules, playing time, playing surface (type/condition), and equipment (protective/footwear).[26] The combination of intrinsic and extrinsic risk factors makes up the susceptibility of a child to sustain an injury. The susceptibility will determine if a child will be injured after an inciting event or not.[39] Knowledge of the causes of injuries is, therefore, necessary for the development of preventive measures.[40,41] Some extrinsic and intrinsic risk factors are difficult to change, and it is important that a PE teacher acknowledges this, while also identifying risk factors that are potentially modifiable. For example, the PE teacher needs to make sure that the equipment (including protective) available is well maintained and properly used. Additionally, he/she must insure that the playing surface is in good condition. He/she can also modify the rules, or replace a contact activity with a non-contact activity in order to decrease the risk of injury. Of special concern is the risk of a recurrent injury incident. If a pupil has been injured, decisions concerning return-to-play remain difficult not only for a medical doctor but also for a PE teacher. Expert consensus guidelines recommend that injured children should not be returned to competition or PE class until they have recovered completely. There is currently no gold standard for injuries related to recovery processes.[42] It is, however, certain that for both PE classes and sport, premature return-to-play after an injury leads to high risk of recurrence. Establishing criteria for return-to-PE classes after an injury is essential for injury management, particularly regarding the prevention of recurrent injuries.

Prevention

Despite the potential benefits of sport- and PE-related exercise on health, it is paramount that injury prevention plays a major role in any exercise programme. One of the strategies in the battle against injuries is aimed at behaviour modification of the participants during sporting activities. Health education as a tool in realizing behavioural change can be implemented in school curricula and, consequently, should be taught by well-educated PE teachers. The need for PE teachers to become involved in the field of sports injury prevention may vary from one country to another, depending on the number of other groups of professionals working in the same area. Involving PE teachers can ensure aspects such as:

- Creating an environment for safe and fair play;
- Checking appropriate equipment and good condition of the playing site;
- Screening of physical limitations to participate;
- Including experience and qualification in sports medicine and injury prevention; and
- Raising public awareness.

In our view, the primary tasks of the physical educator must not be limited to a stimulating role in the development of skills, or to applying preventive measures for safety in PE classes. The PE teacher should be, at a minimum, a message mediator to educate school-aged children in practical and theoretical aspects of injury prevention, which will also be valuable for out-of-school sports activities. Although the effects of health education still have to be proven in this specific area, there are strong indications that in the short term it can be beneficial in improving knowledge, raising awareness on injury prevention, and reducing the number of PA-related injuries

Table 41.2 Description and effectiveness of injury prevention programmes implemented in physical education classes.

Authors	Backx *et al.*[12]	Collard *et al.*[43,44]	Nauta *et al.*[45]
Year of publication	1991	2010	2013
Main aim	To determine the interrelationship between knowledge and attitude towards injury prevention on the one hand, and the injured and non-injured school children on the other hand.	Improve injury preventing behaviour and motor fitness and prevent PA-related injuries.	Improve fall skills and prevent (severe) fall-related injuries.
Target group	Secondary school children (12–18 years).	Primary school children (10–12 years) and their parents.	Primary school children (7–12 years).
Intervention programme	PE lessons aimed at warming up, stretching exercises, cooling down, exercises for ankle stabilization and general coordination, and techniques to fall correctly. In addition, biology lessons concerning adequate sporting shoes, protective materials, and first aid in sports.	Monthly newsletters for children and parents, posters in the school and exercises (to improve strength, speed, flexibility, and coordination) during PE classes.	Exercises during PE classes to teach children to distribute the impact energy associated with a fall over a larger contact area and to convert the fall into a rolling motion.
Duration of the programme	24 PE lessons and six biology lessons in 4 months.	8 months	8 weeks
Outcome	Success was achieved by improving knowledge and attitude about injury prevention. The programme had a favourable influence on injury incidence, even though the explained variance was minimal. No reduction in the severity of sports injuries was seen.	The programme did significantly improve knowledge and attitude. A small non-significant improvement in motor fitness was found. There was a substantial and relevant reduction (not significant) in physical activity-related injuries, only in the least active children (OR = 0.47: 95%CI 0.21–1.06).	Significant improvements were found for self-reported fall skills. A trend (not significant) was shown suggesting that the educational programme was effective in decreasing fall-related injury risk, but only in the least active children (IDR = 0.44: 95%CI 0.25–0.77). No significant difference were reported for injury severity.

(in specific subgroups). Long-range effects are only speculative. To do so, it is, however, necessary to compose a post-academic course for PE teachers, in order to optimize their role in the prevention of sports injuries. Before implementing a newly developed preventive intervention in PE classes, it is necessary to assess the effectiveness in a controlled setting. By creating an ideal environment for the intervention, information on the evidence base of an intervention can be collected.

To our knowledge, there are three studies that have investigated the effect of an injury-prevention programme implemented by a PE teacher during PE classes. Table 41.2 describes the interventions and their results. It can be speculated that if the interventions had been executed more frequently and for a longer period of time, the effectiveness of the educational programmes would have been larger. Because of the encouraging results of these health educational programmes, especially for children who were less active, the advice is to implement this kind of health education intervention into the school curriculum on a more regular basis. In addition, ingredients from effective injury-prevention programmes in sports clubs can be implemented in PE classes. For example, the 11+ warm up programme for football players. This warm-up programme reduced injuries among male and female football players aged 14 years and older. Children who performed the 11+ exercises at least twice a week had 30–50% less risk for an injury.[46] Such a programme can also be implemented in PE classes. Additionally, literature showed that not wearing protective equipment is also a risk factor for injuries.[26] It is recommended to encourage children to wear protective equipment (during PE class, but also during organized and unorganized sport activities) that is effective in decreasing injuries such as ankle brace or tape,[47] elbow protectors,[48] and a helmet.[49]

Conclusions

The risk of a child sustaining an injury during PE classes is relatively small. But since so many children participate in (obligatory) PE, the absolute number of injuries is high. Not much is currently known about risk factors for PE-related injuries in children, and how to influence injury risk. However, it is evident that PE teachers can play a large role in the prevention of injuries by creating a safe environment for play.

Summary

- The number of injuries occurring in physical education (PE) classes might be much higher than observed, as many schools do not maintain good injury records.
- 3–6% of school children (4–18 years) seek help from emergency departments or need hospitalization.
- Sprains are considered the most common type of injury, and wrist and hand the most frequently injured body areas.
- Physical education classes give rise to relatively more upper extremity injuries.
- Physical education lessons containing activities such as gymnastics and team ball games (soccer, basketball, volleyball, baseball) provoke most damage.
- The complexity of games (those that include sprinting, twisting, and jumping) can cause a higher risk for injuries and accidents.
- Falls or twisting movements of the students themselves cause most of the injuries during PE classes. It is advisable to start with fall clinics in primary schools.
- The PE teacher should be a message mediator by educating school-aged children in practical and theoretical aspects of injury prevention.

References

1. Bailey R. Physical education and sport in schools: a review of benefits and outcomes. *J Sch Health*. 2006; 76: 397–401.
2. Reijgersberg N, van der Werff H, Lucassen J. [Baseline measurement of physical education in primary schools]. Utrecht: Mulier Institute (in Dutch); 2014.
3. Reijgersberg N, Lucassen J, Beth J, van der Werff H. [Baseline measurement of physical education in secondary schools]. Utrecht: Mulier Institute (in Dutch); 2014.
4. Tomkinson GR, Olds TS. Secular changes in pediatric aerobic fitness test performance: the global picture. *Med Sport Sci*. 2007; 50: 46–66.
5. Runhaar J, Collard DC, Singh AS, Kemper HC, van Mechelen W, Chin A Paw MJM. Motor fitness in Dutch youth: differences over 26-year period (1980–2006). *J Sci Med Sport*. 2010; 13: 323–328.
6. Bailey R, Armour K, Kirk D, Jess M, Pickup I, Sandford R. The educational benefits claimed for physical education and school sport: an academic review. *Res Papers Educ*. 2009; 24: 1–27.
7. World Health Organization. *Global recommendations on physical activity for health*. Geneva: WHO Press; 2010.
8. Slingerland M, Borghouts LB, Hesselink MKC. Physical activity energy expenditure in Dutch adolescents: Contribution of active transport to school, physical education, and leisure time activities. *J Sch Health*. 2012; 82: 225–232.
9. Sundblad G, Saartok T, Engstrom LM, Renstrom P. Injuries during physical activity in school children. *Scand J Med Sci Sports*. 2005; 15: 313–323.
10. Verhagen EALM, Collard DC, Chin A Paw MJM, van Mechelen W. A prospective cohort study on physical activity and sports-related injuries in 10–12-year-old children. *Br J Sports Med*. 2009; 43: 1031–1035.
11. Jespersen E, Rexen CT, Franz C, Møller NC, Froberg K, Wedderkopp N. Musculoskeletal extremity injuries in a cohort of schoolchildren aged 6–12: A 2.5-year prospective study. *Scand J Med Sci Sports*. 2015; 25: 251–258.
12. Backx FJG, Beijer HJM, Bol E, Erich WBM. Injuries in high-risk persons and high-risk sports, a longitudinal study of 1818 school children. *Am J Sports Med*. 1991; 19: 124–130.
13. Collard DC, Verhagen EA, Chin A Paw MJM, van Mechelen W. Acute physical activity and sports injuries in children. *Appl Physiol Nutr Metab*. 2008; 33: 393–401.
14. Fuller CS, Ekstrand J, Junge A, *et al*. Consensus statement on injury defenitions and data collection procedures in studies of football (soccer) injuries. *Br J Sports Med*. 2006; 40: 193–201.
15. Consumer Safety Institute. *Physical education: Injury rates*. Amsterdam: Consumer Safety Institute (in Dutch); 2012.
16. Nelson NG, Alhaij M, Yard E, Comstrock D, McKenzie LB. Physical education class injuries treated in emegency departments in the US in 1997–2007. *Pediatrics*. 2009; 124: 918–925.
17. Klakk H. Body composition and cardiovascular health in school-aged children. The childhood health, activity and motor performance school study Denmark. An evaluation on the health effect of sport schools in the Svendborg project. PhD [Thesis]. Odense, Denmark: University of Southern Denmark; 2013.
18. Snel N. [Quality of playing environment in own neighborhood]. Available from: http://www.jantjebeton.nl/.../Onderzoek-Buitenspelen-4702013-TNS-NIPO.pdf Utrecht: TNS Nipo/Jantje Beton (in Dutch); 2013.
19. Gianotti M, Al-Sahab B, McFaull S, Tamim H. Epidemiology of acute soccer injuries in canadian children and youth. *Pediatr Emerg Care*. 2011; 27: 81–85.

20. Bloemers F, Collard DC, Chin A Paw MJM, van Mechelen W, Twisk JWR, Verhagen EALM. Physical inactivity is a risk factor for physical activity-related injuries in children. *Br J Sports Med.* 2011; 46: 669–674.
21. Martin-Diener E, Wanner M, Kriemler S, Martin BW. Associations of objectively assessed levels of physical activity, aerobic fitness and motor coordination with injury risk in 7–9 year old school children: A cross-sectional study. *BMJ Open.* 2013; 3: doi:10.1136/bmjopen-2013-003086.
22. Nauta J, Martin-Diener E, Martin BW, van Mechelen W, Verhagen EALM. Injury risk during different physical activity behaviours in children: a systematic review with bias assessment. *Sports Med.* 2015; 45: 327–336.
23. Qvindesland A1, Jónsson H. Articular hypermobility in Icelandic 12-year-olds. *Rheumatology.* 1999; 38: 1014–1016.
24. LaBella CR, Hennrikus W, Hewett TE. Anterior cruciate ligament injuries: diagnosis, treatment, and prevention. *Pediatrics.* 2014; 133: 1437–1450.
25. Murphy DF, Connolly DA, Beynnon BD. Risk factors for lower extremity injury: a review of the literature. *Br J Sports Med.* 2003; 37: 13–29.
26. Emery C.A. Risk factors for injury in child and adolescent sport: a systematic review of the literature. *Clin J Sport Med.* 2003; 13: 256–268.
27. Linakis JG, Amanullah S, Mello MJ. Emergency department visits for injury in school-aged children in the United States: a comparison of nonfatal injuries occurring within and outside of the school environment. *Acad Emerg Med.* 2006; 13: 567–570.
28. Videmsek M, Karpljuk D, Mlinar S, Mesko M, Stihec J. Injuries in primary school pupils and secondary school students during physical education classes and in their leisure time. *Coll Antropol.* 2010; 34: 973–980.
29. Onderwijsconsument. Available from: http://www.onderwijsconsument.nl/jaarlijks-13-500-ongevallen-in-gymles/ (in Dutch). 2009. [Accessed 11 February 2016].
30. Warsh J, Pickett W, Janssen I. Are overweight and obese youth at increased risk for physical activity injuries? *Obese Facts.* 2010; 3: 225–230.
31. Kemler E, Vriend I, Paulis WD, Schoots W, van Middelkoop M, Koes B. Is overweight a risk factor for sports injuries in children, adolescents, and young adults? *Scand J Med Sci Sports.* 2015; 25: 259–264.
32. Jespersen E, Verhagen E, Holst R *et al.* Total body fat percentage and body mass index and the association with lower extremity injuries in children: a 2.5-year longitudinal study. *Br J Sports Med.* 2013; 47: 1–6.
33. Kelm J, Ahlhelm F, Pape D, Pitsch W, Engel C. School sports accidents: analysis of causes, modes, and frequencies. *J Pediatr Orthop.* 2001; 21: 165–168.
34. Rexen CT, Andersen LB, Ersbøll AK, Jespersen E, Franz C, Wedderkopp N. Injuries in children with extra physical education in primary schools. *Med Sci Sports Exerc.* 2015; 46: 745–752.
35. Caine DJ, Golightly YM. Osteoarthritis as an outcome of paediatric sport: an epidemiological perspective. *Br J Sports Med.* 2011; 45: 52–56.
36. Bernaards C, Valkenberg H, Proper K, Chorus A. *Trendrapport Bewegen en Gezondheid (in Dutch), 2000–2014.* Leiden: TNO; 2015.
37. Collard DC, Verhagen EA, van Mechelen W, Heymans MW, Chinapaw MJ. Economic burden of physical activity-related injuries in Dutch children aged 10–12. *Br J Sports Med.* 2011: 45: 1058–1063.
38. Meerding WJ, Mulder S, van Beeck EF. Incidence and costs of injuries in the Netherlands. *Eur J Public Health.* 2006; 16: 272–278.
39. Meeuwisse WH, Tyreman H, Hagel B, Emery CA. Dynamic model of etiology in sport injury: The recursive nature of risk and causation. *Clin J Sports Med.* 2007; 17: 215–219.
40. van Mechelen W, Hlobil H, Kemper HC. Incidence, severity. aetiology and prevention of sports injuries. A review of concepts. *Sports Med.* 1992; 14: 82–99.
41. Finch, C. A new framework for research leading to sports injury prevention. *J Sci Med Sport.* 2006; 9: 3–9.
42. Shrier I, Safai P, Charland L. Return to play following injury: whose decision should it be? *Br J Sports Med.* 2014; 48: 394–401.
43. Collard DC, Chinapaw MJ, Verhagen EA, Bakker I, van Mechelen W. Effectiveness of a school-based physical activity-related injury prevention program on risk behavior and neuromotor fitness a cluster randomized controlled trial. *Int J Behav Nutr Phys Act.* 2010; 28: 7–9.
44. Collard DC, Verhagen EA, Chinapaw MJ, Knol DL, van Mechelen W. Effectiveness of a school-based physical activity injury prevention program: a cluster randomized controlled trial. *Arch Pediatr Adolesc Med.* 2010; 164: 145–150.
45. Nauta J, Knol DL, Adriaensens L, Klein Wolt K, van Mechelen W, Verhagen EA. Prevention of fall-related injuries in 7-year-old to 12-year-old children: a cluster randomised controlled trial. *Br J Sports Med.* 2013; 47: 909–913.
46. Soligard T, Myklebust G, Steffen K, *et al.* Comprehensive warm-up program to prevent injuries in young female footballers: cluster randomised controlled trial. *BMJ.* 2008; 337: a2469.
47. Kemler E, van de Port I, Backx F, van Dijk CN. A systematic review on the treatment of acute ankle sprain: Brace versus other functional treatment types. *Sports Med.* 2011; 41: 185–197.
48. Vriend M. Hoofwijk P, den Hartog C. [Effectiveness of injury prevention in sport]. Amsterdam: Consumer Safety (in Dutch); 2001.
49. Russell K, Christie J, Hagel BE. The effect of helmets on the risk of head and neck injuries among skiers and snowboarders: a meta-analysis. *Clin Med Am J.* 2010; 182: 333–340.
50. Spinks AB, MacPherson AK, Bain C, McClure RJ. Injury risk from popular childhood physical activities: results from an Autralian primary school cohort. *Inj Prev.* 2006; 12: 390–394.
51. Schmikli SL, Backx FJG, Kemler HJ, van Mechelen W. National survey on sports injuries in the Netherlands: target populations for sports injury prevention programs. *Clin J Sports Med.* 2009; 19: 101–106.
52. Spinks AB, McClure RJ, Bain C, MacPherson AK. Quantifying the association between physical activity and injury in primary school-aged children. *Pediatrics.* 2006; 118: e43.

CHAPTER 42

Epidemiology and prevention of injuries in competitive contact sports

Joske Nauta and Evert ALM Verhagen

Introduction

The theoretical framework regarding the aetiology and prevention of sports injures, as well as the aetiology and prevention of physical education-related injuries, has been discussed in Chapter 40 and Chapter 41. This chapter focuses on sport-specific injuries in contact sports. A number of sports that include common or intentional contact with the opponent have been selected.

Each sport is covered in a systematic manner by describing some practical information concerning the particular sport, as well as the epidemiology and aetiology of sport-specific injuries, and by summarizing preventive strategies. Where possible, trends that can be drawn from the literature are provided to give a reasonable basis on which to develop and promote prevention strategies.

In general, sports injuries in contact sports are more frequent than in non-contact sports.[1,2] One should, however, keep in mind that a large proportion of sports pathology is common to both contact and non-contact sports where similar movements are involved that potentially can lead to injury, e.g. running and cutting.

Soccer

An estimated 265 million people worldwide play soccer.[3] This staggering number of players suggests that it is the world's most popular sport. Soccer is, by nature, a very physical sport, with regular and intense contact with the ball and other players. The physical component, combined with the hard cuts and sharp turns off a planted foot,[4] make soccer players vulnerable to injury. Since over 30% of all soccer players are under the age of 18 years,[5] specific knowledge of injury mechanisms in children is warranted. Although more and more is known about soccer-related injury patterns in youth, research in injuries in the very young (<13 years of age) is still scarce.

Epidemiology of soccer injuries

Although soccer injuries are common, the sport is usually considered fairly safe.[6] According to North American data, fewer than 2% of soccer-related emergency department treatments in children needed hospitalization.[7,8] The same two studies calculated that 2 out of 1000 paediatric injuries treated at an emergency department in the US were caused by a soccer-related incident. It is important to note that such population-based estimations are heavily influenced by the number of children that play soccer. It is preferable to express the number of injuries per 1000 h of exposure. More specifically, in soccer-related injury research it is common practice to report separately on competition and training-related injuries.[9]

For paediatric soccer injuries, injury incidence data were compiled in an extensive review of 21 studies.[10] Most of the included studies were based in Europe (except for two). All but a few of the studies focused on injuries in 13- to 18-year-old children and the majority of studies focused on boys. The summarized results were reported separately for training and competition. In 13- to 19-year-olds, 1 to 5 injuries per 1000 h of training can be expected.[10,11] During competition, the risk generally increases three to sixfold.[10] Soccer-related injury rates increased with age, and this was especially evident for injuries during competition, where injury rates increased from 9 to 11 injuries per 1000 h competition in the under 13 group, up to 15–20 injuries per 1000 h of competition in 15- to 19-year-olds.[10]

Besides acute injuries, i.e. injuries that have a sudden onset, young soccer players are also prone to overuse injury. An overuse injury, i.e. tissue damage as a result of repetitive demands over the course of time,[9] has been estimated to account for 10–40% of all soccer-related injuries.[10]

Injury location

The nature of the game of soccer includes not only running, twisting, turning, and jumping,[12] but also intensive contact with the ball and other players. This makes the player vulnerable for an injury to the lower extremities. Not surprisingly, the lower extremities are, with 80% of all injuries, most frequently affected by an acute soccer-related injury.[10] The thigh and hip area is the most common injury site (~24% of all injuries), closely followed by the ankle (~23% of all injuries), and the knee (17% of all injuries).[10]

Three decades ago, Keller *et al.*[13] recognized that youth soccer players were at increased upper extremity injury risk. More recent findings suggest that the turning point could be near the age of 14 years. Below this age, an increased upper body injury risk has been reported (20–29% vs. 11–21%).[10] It is believed that younger children are more prone to sustain an upper extremity injury because they fall more frequently on outstretched hands, and have increased fragility of the upper extremity epiphyses.

About 5% of injuries affect the head or face[10]. Since heading the ball is part of the game of soccer, one might expect that this is also the mechanism that causes most concussions. The evidence regarding soccer-related concussions was compiled by Maher *et al.*[14] Their results showed that concussions were most often caused by player-to-player contact (53–85% of concussions), followed by player-to-ball contact (8–26%). The remaining concussions were caused by player-to-surface contact (6–23%).[14]

Risk factors

In children from the general population, it is known that girls are at increased injury risk compared to boys.[15] In soccer, the same risk patterns are only seen in concussion risk.[14] No relevant gender differences in overall soccer-related injury risk could be reported after compiling evidence from 21 studies.[10]

For age, it was pointed out that younger children are at increased upper extremity injury risk. The overall risk of sustaining an injury during soccer is, however, lower in younger soccer players. There could be a link to maturity status here. Although the study of maturity status in soccer players so far has some methodological pitfalls, it has been reported that early-maturing soccer players have higher injury rates compared to later-maturing players.[10] This could be caused by the reported spike in injury risk during the year of peak height velocity.[16]

Another suggested risk factor for injuries is the level of play. The four studies that were included by Faude *et al.*[10] reported that injury incidences of elite youth soccer players (aged 13–18 years) were in the upper range of reported values for sub-elite players. When the comprehensive medical service of elite teams is taken into account, a similar injury risk was expected for elite soccer players.

Playing on artificial turf has been shown in the past to increase injury risk in youth soccer players.[17,18] However, the mechanisms alleged to increase injury risk, such as hardness of the field and excessive heat retention,[19] have been addressed by the industry. Newer (generation three and four) artificial surfaces have now comparable rates of injury to natural turf.[10,20]

When an adult soccer player is injured, the risk of sustaining a recurrent injury is increased.[21] The same risk factor is recognized in youth soccer players, where a history of (lower extremity) injury resulted in a twofold greater risk to sustaining an injury compared to players without an injury history.[22] For players with multiple previous injuries, the risk was increased threefold.[22]

Preventative strategies

To target soccer-related injuries in youth, a neuromuscular warm-up programme was developed by the International Federation of Football Associations (FIFA) in cooperation with international experts called 'FIFA 11+'. The programme is comprised of a combination of exercises to increase core stability, eccentric exercises of the thigh muscles, proprioceptive exercises, exercises to increase dynamic stabilization, and plyometric drills performed with good postural alignment. This programme has proven to be successful in reducing injuries in young soccer players.[23] The effectiveness in children under the age of 12 years has yet to be determined.

An important role in the prevention of injuries in youth lies with the coaches and the referees. Coaches not only have a large influence over how young players embrace injury-prevention programmes,[24] but they are also responsible for the reduction of on-field aggressiveness such as shirt pulling, deliberate 'take downs', and tackling from behind. Such behaviours should not be tolerated, since they increase the number of injuries. Additionally, the role of a good referee is to keep the game under tight control, and prevent dangerous behaviour on the field.[25]

There are two issues that need more attention from those involved in the development of soccer-related injury prevention. These are the increased risk of upper extremity injuries in young players, and the fact that sustaining an injury increases the risk of a recurrent injury. Tackling those two issues has great potential to relieve the burden of injuries in soccer.

American football

American football, also called tackle football, is a collision sport which is extremely popular in the US. Although approximately 2.8 million children aged 6–14 years still participate in organized American football,[26] popularity is declining. The reason for this decline might be related to the relatively high injury risk.

Given that football is a collision sport, it would be expected that most football injuries are acute, as opposed to overuse or gradual onset injuries. Most research on football injury risk in youth describes the risk during high school football.

Epidemiology of American football injuries

Many parents withdraw their child from organized football participation because of the relatively high risk of sustaining an injury. Compared to other competitive sports like basketball and wrestling, football has the highest percentage of medically treated injuries.[2] Furthermore, six separate studies[27] reported the risk of sustaining a concussion was highest in American football.

Emergency department registries have been used to calculate injury risk in retrospect. The overall risk was 6.2–9.5 injuries per 1000 players, with the risk of sustaining an injury increasing as children got older (>12 years).[28,29] Although injury rates are frequently reported per 1000 players, this does not include the varying practice and competition sessions for each player. Moreover, as indicated, injuries treated in emergency departments are relatively severe injuries.

More information is provided by three studies that used a broader injury definition, and expressed the number of injuries as a ratio of the time at risk. Overall, the reported injury risk was 4.4–17.8 injuries per 1000 athletic exposures.[30,31,32] The wide range is probably the result of the differences used in injury definitions. The proportion of minor injuries reported ranged from 49–64%.[30,31,32] Ten per cent of the injuries were so severe that the career or season ended for the player.[32]

Injury location

Tackling and blocking, and thus collision, is an essential part of football. During these manoeuvres, the chance of sustaining a concussion is relatively high. It is no surprise that, compared to other sports, the risk of sustaining a concussion during American football is highest.[33] The distribution of percentage of injuries per body area as reported by six studies is provided in Table 42.1. One in every six injuries that are treated in an emergency department are in the head/neck region.[28,29] Also, of all injuries treated in emergency departments, arm injuries account for the majority of cases.[28,29] The number of leg injuries increases when a broader injury definition is used.[30,32,34,35]

Table 42.1 Location of injury in youth football players.

	Stuart[34]	Dompier[30]	Mello[28*]		Nation[29*]	Turbeville[35]	Shankar[32]
	9–13 years	9–14 years	7–11 years	12–17 years	6–17 years	10–15 years	< 14 years
Head/neck	7	7	17	19	16	5	12
Ribs/back	14	10	14	17	8	3	12
Upper extremity	25	37	43	37	49	44	29
Lower extremity	51	38	24	27	26	39	47

*Results based on emergency department visits and expressed in percentages.

Contusions, strains, and sprains account for 54–76% of all football-related injuries,[28,29,30,35] and 27–30% of the treated injuries are fractures.[28,29,35] The mechanism of injury being 'contact with another player' is listed in 48–77% of the cases,[28,32,36] the majority of these being the result of a tackle or being tackled. In 13–15% of the cases, the injury was caused by a fall.[28,32,36]

Risk factors

Players will be more aggressive during games than during practice. As a consequence, the risk of sustaining an injury during a game is between two and five times as high as the risk during practice.[30–32,35,36] During competition, most injuries are caused while a player is tackling or being tackled. In contrast, during practice more injuries occur while running.[32] During games, different injury patterns have been identified. The proportion of severe injuries is, for example, highest at the beginning and the middle of the play compared to the end.[36]

Since American football is usually not played by girls, gender has not been identified as a risk factor. Compared to boys, girls more often injure their arm and are twice as likely to get injured while playing football at home.[29]

Age is another risk factor for football injuries, with children over 12 years of age being at highest risk.[30,34,37] The odds that a child treated for a football injury in an emergency department is over 12 years of age is 40% higher than in younger children.[28,29] Also, football players under 12 years of age are more likely to injure their arm, while older players more often sustain a leg injury.[28,29]

In contrast to what might be expected, height, weight, and physical strength have not been identified as risk factors for football-related injuries in children.[31,34,35] This is probably caused by the weight restrictions that are operative in youth football, which reduces the risk of a heavy player from running into a lighter defensive player.[31]

Because younger football players commonly play many different positions, it is difficult to accurately calculate injury rates by player position. Nevertheless, the majority of the injuries occur while players are on the offence, with running backs and linemen most frequently injured.[32,35] There are, however, more linemen on the field and thus correction is necessary to assess the actual injury risk.

Preventative strategies

The effectiveness of three football injury prevention programmes for children has been established in children with a mean age of 11 years. The first programme, called P.R.E.P.A.R.E., included gradual activity recommendations, water breaks every 10–20 min, gradual warm-up, instructions on stretching routine and a check of the first aid kit.[38] A decline in overall football injury incidence was reported both during competition and playing games (8.94 vs 12.56 per 1000 h of athletic exposure). When only the more severe injuries were taken into account, no differences were reported between children receiving the P.R.E.P.A.R.E. training and children receiving regular training.[38] It should be noted that this study was performed in a controlled setting. The effectiveness of the programme in the real world, the last two stages of the TRIPP model[24,39] (interested readers are referred to Chapter 40 for further discussion), remains unclear.

Two less-invasive extensive initiatives are the 'Heads Up Football' programme and the Pop Warner guidelines. In the Heads Up Football programme, coaches receive training on proper equipment fitting, proper tackling techniques, strategies for reducing player-to-player contact, and education on concussion, heat illness, and cardiac events. In the Pop Warner guidelines, contact between players is restricted: no full-speed head-on blockings are allowed, as in tackling when players are lined up more than 3 yards (~2.8 m) apart. Furthermore, a maximum of one-third of the practice time is spent in contact drills.[37] A combination of both the Heads Up Football programme and the Pop Warner guidelines proved most effective in decreasing injuries during both practice and games. Compared to usual training, the Heads Up Football programme was only effective in reducing injury risk during practice.

Another preventive strategy shown to be effective in decreasing the incidence of acute ankle injuries in adolescents is the use of an ankle brace.[40] Wearing a lace-up ankle brace did, however, not decrease the number of severe ankle injuries, knee injuries, or other lower extremity injuries.

Ice hockey

In ice hockey, high skating speeds, individual flare for stick handling, and accurate puck shooting are combined with team play. Ice hockey enjoys an enthusiastic worldwide following and is played by athletes of all ages. Since intentional high-energy collision, i.e. body checking, is part of the game, the risk of injury is always present.

Epidemiology of ice hockey injuries

Although ice hockey is a popular sport in Canada, Czech Republic, Finland, Russia, Sweden, and the US, comparisons of injury risk between ice hockey and other sports are uncommon.[1,2] Such comparisons have only been made for concussions. The number of concussions during ice hockey is 0.41–0.54 concussions per 1000 playing hours.[33] These numbers are on the high end of the reported concussions risks, and comparable to the number of concussions reported during American football.

Overall injury rates for ice hockey vary between 12 and 34 injuries per 1000 h of play,[41] suggesting that ice hockey is more dangerous than American football (4–18 injuries per 1000 h of play)[2,31,32] and soccer (15–20 injuries per 1000 h of play).[10] Comparison should, however, be done with caution as injury definitions and data collection methods heavily bias such outcomes.

Injury location

Before full facial protection was mandatory, head injuries accounted for over 59% of all youth ice hockey injuries.[42] Wearing head protection has resulted in a decline in the number of head injuries, but 22–31% of injuries are generally still reported in the head/neck area.[42,43,44] Two-thirds of these injuries are traumatic brain injuries.[44] Especially in very young ice hockey players (<8 years of age), face and mouth injuries are fairly common,[43] usually because of falling on the ice or being hit by a stick.

No matter how injuries are defined, the upper extremities are most often injured in youth ice hockey play.[42,43] Upper extremity injuries also tend to be more serious in nature, since the reported injury frequency is even higher in emergency department studies.[43] Two distinct mechanisms of upper extremities injuries can be recognized: elbow/lower extremities injuries are usually caused by a fall, and shoulder/upper arm injuries are most often the result of contact with the boarding.[43]

Lower extremities injuries account for 20–34% of all ice hockey injuries.[42,43] Over one-third of the injuries to the lower extremities are non-contact injuries,[43] most likely caused by the explosive muscle contractions that are needed during the skating stride.

Risk factors

Although the number of female ice hockey players has increased over the last decade, the majority of ice hockey players is still male (86–93%).[45] A difference in injury risk, at least for adolescent players, is probably caused by differences in rules. In female hockey, intentional body contact like body checking is not permitted at any level. In young adult players, no gender differences were reported regarding injury risk. Male players did, however, sustain more severe injuries than female players.[42,46] A large study of emergency department childhood ice hockey injuries (8–18 years) reported that soft tissue injuries are more common in girls compared to boys. Boys over 11 years of age are, on the other hand, more likely to sustain a fracture. The proportion of head injuries (concussion and minor brain injuries) is highest in young boys (<11 years) but changes over time eventually result in a higher percentage of head injuries for girls (>12 years).[45]

Body checking, and other forms of intentional contact like bumping, shoving, or pushing[45] have been identified as a risk factor for injuries. Youth players in leagues in which intentional physical contact is permitted have a higher risk of sustaining an injury.[41,47] Differences in experience with body checking have been reported to not change overall ice hockey-related injury risk, but to decrease the risk of a more severe injury in boys.[48]

While some studies do not report age as a risk factor, increasing age is usually reported to increase ice hockey-related injury risk.[41,43] The increased injury risk can, at least partially, be explained by the fact that body checking is allowed for older players.

Having sustained a concussion has repeatedly been identified as a risk factor for sustaining a recurrent concussion.[41,47,49] Other risk factors for concussion are reported headaches and neck pain at the beginning of the season.[49]

The influence of height and body weight on injury risk remains unclear since results are conflicting. It may very well be that the size of the player does influence the probability of a specific location. Smaller players have, for example, a higher risk of sustaining a concussion,[49] while heavier players are reported to have an increased shoulder injury risk.[41]

Preventative strategies

Body checking is a crucial injury risk, and therefore body checking should have a strong justification.[47,50] The age at which body checking is allowed has been increased in some leagues to 14 years. But increasing the age boundary may not be enough, given that a low level of experience with body checking increases the risk of a severe injury.[48] Proper introduction of body checking techniques and adequate training could be an effective measure to prevent severe injuries.

An overview of preventive measures in ice hockey players has been provided by Cusimano *et al.*[51] Changes to mandatory rules were noted to be most effective in reducing the number of penalties for aggressive acts and injuries related to aggression among ice hockey players. The effectiveness of education and cognitive behavioural interventions on injury rates were less clear.[51]

Basketball

Basketball has long been considered as a non-contact sport, but has evolved to a game where contact is inevitably part of the game. Modern basketball is an intense, fast-paced game that involves jumping, hard cuts, sharp turns of a planted foot, and intense contact with the ball and other players. Basketball continues to grow in popularity with players at all levels of play. As the number of players increases, so does the number of injuries. Much of the data related to basketball are found in studies comparing various sports.

Epidemiology of basketball injuries

In the US, several multisport injury registration systems have been used to assess the risk of different sports.[1,2] The reported basketball related injury risk ranged from 7.3–9.2 injuries per 1000 h of play.[1,2] When listing injury risks for several sports, basketball was ranked between soccer and indoor track,[2] with playing golf ranked as least risky and field hockey and lacrosse ranked as most risky. Another multisport cohort showed that basketball was more risky than the calculated average risk for all sports combined.[1]

The number of emergency department treatments due to an incident during basketball decreased in US youth by over 20% between 1997 and 2007.[52] Despite this decline in overall basketball-related injury risk, the proportion of all injuries that accounted for concussions in boys doubled in the same period. Moreover, for girls, the reported proportion of concussions tripled.[52]

Injury location

The information regarding basketball-related injuries has been based on the compilation of results in ten separate studies as reviewed by Harmer.[27] The majority of the basketball-related injuries affect the lower extremities. The ankle/foot region is the most often injured (17–44% of reported injuries[27]) area of the leg, followed by the knee (5–20%). Within the upper extremities, the hand

and fingers are the most often damaged during basketball.[27] The most often-reported injuries are strains and sprains,[27,52] followed by fractures and dislocations.[52] A large proportion of the fractures and dislocations is located in the hand/fingers, probably due to contact with the ball.

Risk factors

According to two reviews conducted a few years ago, girls playing basketball are at increased injury risk, particularly for knee and ankle injury,[27,52] which has been confirmed in more recent studies.[52,54,55] These injuries tend to be more serious, in particular because knee injuries more often need surgery or involve the anterior cruciate ligament.[27,53] The injury risk seems to increase with increasing age,[27,52,55] but it remains unclear if this increase is caused by advancing age, increased physical development, or pubertal age[27]. Specifically, for ankle injuries, balance deficits have been identified as a risk factor in high-school basketball players.[53,56]

Preventative strategies

The majority of the preventive measures suggested in basketball are 'common sense' and include advice for officials to stimulate fair play or improve the physical capacities of the players.[27]

Since balance has been identified as a predictor of acute injuries,[4] improving balance has been the focus of basketball-specific injury prevention strategies. Such programmes with home-based exercises or a warm-up routine, have been shown to decrease the risk of acute injuries in high-school basketball players.[56,57]

Another preventive strategy that has proven effective in preventing both first time and recurrent ankle sprains in high-school basketball players is the use of external support of the ankle.[58] The use of an ankle brace did, however, not influence the total number of lower extremities injuries in high-school basketball players.

Martial arts

Participation in martial arts has become increasingly popular in Western countries. Martial arts is an umbrella term for oriental combat sports. There are several varieties of martial arts, but the main stream martial arts are karate, Taekwondo, and judo. All three have different characteristics. Karate is characterized by stances, punches, kicks, and knee/elbow strikes.[59] In Taekwondo, youth perform strikes and blocks while emphasizing high kicks. Judo involves no punching or kicking. Judo techniques have their goal in working the opponent to the ground. This involves physical contact, but differently to karate and Taekwondo. Competitors in all three forms of martial arts compete in divisions according to age, sex, experience, and bodyweight.

Epidemiology of martial arts injuries

Very few studies have focused on the risk of sustaining an injury during martial arts, especially in children. The most recent estimates from Canada have shown that the risk of sustaining an injury during martial arts is 4.4–4.8 injuries per 10 000 persons.[60] No other descriptive studies are available that report on the risk of youth participation in martial arts. Furthermore, no youth studies are available comparing the risk of each of the mainstream martial arts.

The studies that have been conducted have reported on injury risk for a specific type of martial arts. Of the three mainstream martial arts, the risk of judo is the only one that has been compared to other types of sport in children. In the US, the reported judo-related injury risk was lower than the average risk of all sports combined (4.5–6.8 vs. 6.7–7.7).[1] A Swiss study, however, reported an injury incidence as low as 0.23 injuries per 1000 h of judo participation.

Studies that report injury risk of karate have focused on match-related injuries. Since karate involves physical contact, it is reasonable to expect that the number of injuries during combat exceed those that occur during training sessions. In Finnish competition, 0.28 injuries per competition bout occurred during the national karate championship.[61] In the Dutch national youth competition, 100–115 injuries per 1000 athletic exposures were reported in children under 15 years of age.[62]

Taekwondo is considered the most violent of the three martial arts described here. During competition, players wear head gear, a chest and abdomen protector, a groin guard, and shin and forearm guards. This does, of course, not prevent all injuries. An estimated 7.4–11.4 time-loss injuries per 1000 h of Taekwondo still occur during competition.[63] Other research has reported that per 100 players in a youth tournament, 3.4 will sustain an injury.[64]

Injury location

In an emergency department study in the US, Yard *et al.*[59] registered the mechanism of injury and injury location for all three mainstream martial arts. We do stress, yet again, that these figures only describe the relatively severe injuries that need emergency treatment.

The nature of judo is very different from both karate and Taekwondo, where other injury locations and mechanisms of injury are recorded. Being kicked is the number one injury mechanism in both karate and Taekwondo,[59] followed by falling, and giving a kick (i.e. kicking). Kicking or being kicked is typically not part of judo, and therefore no such injuries are registered. In judo, being thrown or flipped over is the number one cause of injury,[59] followed by falling. During karate and Taekwondo, children sustain injuries in the same body parts: most injuries occur in the lower leg (31–32%), followed by hand/wrist injuries (28–23%) and injuries to the face (10–11%).[59] In judoka, who are more likely to fall or be flipped over, shoulder injuries are frequently reported (19%), followed by lower leg, foot, and ankle injuries (16%). The lower arm is the third ranking injury location in judo (15%).[59]

Risk factors

Participation in competition, especially in karate, has been identified as an injury risk factor. In children 7–15 years of age, injury rates during competition have been reported to be as high as 100–115 injuries per 1000 athletic exposures.[62] This is in stark contrast with injury rates reported in 6- to 16-year-olds who were trained at a karate school that did not partake in competition and at which training did not involve free sparring. At this karate school, no time-loss injuries were reported during 1 year.[65] In competition, injury rates during Taekwondo have been reported to be lower than in karate,[62] arguably due to the use of protective equipment.

Another risk factor for injury, again established in karate, is experience. Injury risk tends to rise with increasing experience in terms of years.[65] Additionally, pupils with a brown belt (high experience level) are more than six times as likely to sustain an injury compared to children with a lower-level belt.[65]

Preventative strategies

Suggestions for preventive strategies specifically for children in martial arts have yet to be established. The following recommendations are drawn from research with adult participants. Referees should have an appropriate amount of competition experience to better assess the nature of blows being exchanged in the ring and other aspects of the bout.[66] According to Pieter *et al.*,[67] the current course for Taekwondo referees mainly consists of learning standard hand signals and game regulations. To minimize the damage after sustaining an injury, coaches should have basic injury prevention and management skills to reduce the burden after injury.

It has been recommended that athletes beginning karate or Taekwondo should not be allowed to engage in free exchange of blows.[64] In Taekwondo, the increase of blocking skills has been suggested as a possible strategy to preventing injury, as deficient blocking skills are still among the most frequent mechanisms of both general and severe injuries.[67] Modification of the rules in karate and Taekwondo such that blows to the head are prohibited, at least in children, might help to reduce serious injuries such as concussions.

Wrestling

Wrestling is a popular sport in the US at both the youth and high school levels.[68] Most of its popularity is ascribed to the fact that athletes of all sizes and ages can compete in the sport. There are three different styles of wrestling, but each style requires similar training techniques despite the differences in competition. The competitive season is long and practices are frequent, long, and intense. Furthermore, in wrestling there is contact 100% of the time, which increases the effective exposure period. Therefore, although wrestlers are at the same risk for injury as other contact sport athletes, the exposure for an individual wrestler is high.

Epidemiology of wrestling injuries

Wrestling-related injuries usually focus on high school pupils.[2,69–71] An emergency department study of over 170 000 wrestling-related injuries in youth showed that wrestlers aged 12–17 years had a tenfold higher number of injuries compared to younger wrestlers.[68] This difference was only partially caused by the difference in youth participating in wrestling. If the injuries were expressed per 1000 h of exposure, youth over 12 years of age had an injury incidence of nearly 30 injuries per 1000 h of wrestling. Younger wrestlers, on the other hand, had an injury incidence of 6.5 injuries per 1000 h of wrestling.[68]

Different (i.e. lower) injury incidence numbers have been reported, e.g. when an injury is recorded where medical treatment was provided by an athletic trainer or physician. This broader injury definition resulted in injury incidences ranging from 2.5–11.6 injuries per 1000 h of athletic exposure.[2,69,70,71]. The one study that focused on middle school sports with participants aged between 12–15 years reported an injury incidence of ten injuries per 1000 h of wrestling.[1]

Three studies compare the injury incidence of wrestling with other high school sports. According to these studies, the risk of sustaining an injury during wrestling is comparable[70] or slightly increased[1,2] compared to other popular high school sports. The percentage of injuries that cause time lost from sports is, however, relatively high in youth wrestlers. Time-loss injuries are reported to account for 21.5–43.2% of all wrestling injuries.[1,2]

Injury location

The majority of the injuries sustained during wrestling affect the upper extremity and head/neck region. These body areas account for 56–82% of the injuries.[68,69,71] The distribution of injuries does not vary between relatively minor and severe injuries. Muscle strains and joint sprains account for the majority of the wrestling-related injuries.[68,69,71] Brain injuries or concussions account for 5–13% of the injuries. This seems a large proportion, but five studies reported the risk expressed per athletic exposure to be below the average of contact sports.[33]

A classic wrestling injury is acute or recurrent auricular haematoma resulting in 'cauliflower ear' or 'wrestler's ear'.[72] The wrestler's headgear is designed to minimize the risk of these injuries,[73] but studies reporting on headgear wear, performed over 30 years ago, have shown low compliance.[72,73] When treated on time, a chronic cauliflower ear can be prevented. The treatment is, however, painful and might therefore be avoided by athletes. Another possible reason for athletes avoiding treatment is a cauliflower ear is considered as mark of distinction that identifies them immediately as wrestler.[73]

Risk factors

Injuries to the head, mainly concussions, are predominantly caused by head-knee or head-head collisions during takedowns, i.e. working the opponent to the ground. Concussions can also be caused by contact with the mat. Sprains and strains in the neck region are frequently encountered in wrestling.[73] These injuries can occur when a wrestler drives the opponent with his neck and hyperextends it. Lower back injuries commonly occur during takedowns.[71] During a match wrestlers pull and push with the lumbar spine in mild hyperextension. This extension together with twisting results in injuries.[69] Chest injuries can be caused in different manners, from direct trauma during takedowns or when direct pressure is applied (i.e. 'bear hug').[73] Shoulder injuries can be caused when being thrown on the mat from a standing position. A wrestler may attempt to break a fall with an extended arm, imparting force to the shoulder girdle; if unable to extend the arm, the fall is taken directly on the shoulder.[73]

Lower extremity injuries are usually caused by the moves used in different wrestling manoeuvres. When a move is not executed correctly or when the opponent makes a countermove unnatural twisting and stretching of ligaments might occur, resulting in injuries.[73] For instance, meniscus injuries occur frequently via a twisting injury to a weight-bearing extremity, and a varus or valgus force to the weight-bearing extremity is commonly the cause of collateral ligament sprains. The same goes for ankle injuries. For example, when a wrestler attempts to throw his opponent, he rises onto his toes and twists. Loss of balance will cause the wrestler to invert his ankle.

The absolute number of injuries is usually reported highest during practice, which is logical considering the large amount of time spent in practice. When the incidence rate is expressed per 1000 h of wrestling, the number of injuries is higher during competition.[1,69] Furthermore, the injury rates increase with an increase in level of wrestling.[69]

The wrestling mat is, by far, the largest piece of equipment used in wrestling. Since driving the opponent onto the mat is common, it is essential that the mat is of good condition. Beside the condition, i.e. good shock absorbing qualities, the mat must also be clean. Without daily disinfection, counts of microorganisms on the mat will theoretically increase, and increase the chance of transmission of dermatological infections from mat to wrestler.[72]

Wrestlers with higher body weights are injured more often, possibly due to the greater forces exerted by heavier wrestlers.[73] The 'weight class system' decreases the risk of injury by reducing discrepancies in weight, size, and strength between athletes. This system is also the reason that wrestlers generally lose large amounts of weight in a short period of time prior to certification or competition.[72] Rapid weight loss can be a risk factor for injury in itself, but also the weaker of the two wrestlers has a greater risk of injury.

Preventative strategies

Weight reduction for competition should be limited in wrestling. If there is a discrepancy in strength between two wrestlers, this difference can the risk of injury for the weaker athlete. Furthermore, in reducing weight a wrestler loses a lot of water and can become dehydrated. An athlete should, therefore, drink in moderation before, during, and after exercise.[72]

For safe competition with inexperienced wrestlers, close attention to proper technique is essential. It has been recommended that coaches teach wrestlers to keep their heads up when performing shooting or takedowns to avoid axial compression or flexion of the spine, which can lead to serious injury.[74]

Dermatological illnesses and bacterial infections are commonly seen in wrestling. Dermatological illnesses are transmitted by contact with the opponent, and bacteria are commonly found on the mats. Proper hygiene by the wrestler, e.g. daily washing of clothes after training and daily showering after training, should reduce dermatological illnesses. Proper cleaning of the mat should reduce bacterial illnesses.

The use of headgear decreases the injury risk. The role of other protective equipment, e.g. kneepads, shoes, or mouth guards, has not been evaluated.[73] In other sports, however, these measures have been effective in preventing injuries.[72]

Conclusions

Although research in injury prevention has evolved over the last decades, the knowledge of injury mechanisms and aetiology in youth is still lagging behind that in adults. Very little is known of injury risk when the very young (<12 years of age) are participating in contact sports. One injury that is of special concern in those contact sports that involve intentional physical contact is concussion. Prevention of concussions in the young, underdeveloped, brain should be a prime area of research focus.

Summary

- Although a large proportion of sports pathology is common to both contact and non-contact sports, in general, sports injuries in contact sports are more frequent than in non-contact sports.
- Injuries in contact sports are generally sport specific. Nevertheless, especially in young children, injuries to the upper extremities and head are a point of concern in injury prevention.
- In youth, the risk of sustaining an injury during contact sports generally increases with increasing age.
- For certain contact sports, few data are available on children and adolescents to serve as a basis for aetiology and prevention. As children are not miniature adolescents, more research is needed specifically on young children in sports.
- Since injury risk is increased during games, the role of coaches and referees are considered key in the reduction of aggression and foul play on the field, which can thereby decrease the number of injuries during sports matches.

References

1. Beachy G, Rauh M. Middle school injuries: a 20-year (1988–2008) multisport evaluation. *J Athl Train.* 2014; 49: 493–506.
2. Dompier TP, Marshall SW, Kerr ZY, Hayden R. The national athletic treatment, injury and outcomes network (NATION): Methods of the surveillance program, 2011–2012 through 2013–2014. *J Athl Train.* 2015; 50: 862–869.
3. FIFA Communications Division, Information Services. *FIFA Big Count 200.* Available from: http://www.fifa.com/mm/document/fifafacts/bcoffsurv/bigcount.statspackage_7024.pdf. 2007. [Accessed 27 October 2015].
4. Larson M, Pearl AJ, Jaffet R, Rudawsky A. Soccer. In: Caine DJ (ed.) *Epidemiology of sports injuries.* Campaign, IL: Human Kinetics; 1996. p. 387–397.
5. Esquivel AO, Bruder A, Ratkowiak K, Lemos SE. Soccer-related injuries in children and adults aged 5 to 49 years in US emergency departments from 2000 to 2012. *Sports Health.* 2015; 7: 366–370.
6. Schiff MA, Mack CD, Polissar NL, Levy MR, Dow SP, O'Kane JW. Soccer injuries in female youth players: comparison of injury surveillance by certified athletic trainers and internet. *J Athl Train.* 2010; 45: 238–242.
7. Adams AL, Schiff MA. Childhood soccer injuries treated in US emergency departments. *Acad Emerg Med.* 2006; 13: 571–574.
8. Leininger RE, Knox CL, Comstock RD. Epidemiology of 1.6 million pediatric soccer-related injuries presenting to US emergency departments from 1990 to 2003. *Am J Sports Med.* 2007; 35: 288–293.
9. Fuller CW, Ekstrand J, Junge A, *et al.* Consensus statement on injury definitions and data collection procedures in studies of football (soccer) injuries. *Clin J Sport Med.* 2006; 16: 97–106.
10. Faude O, Rossler R, Junge A. Football injuries in children and adolescent players: are there clues for prevention? *Sports Med.* 2013; 43: 819–837.
11. Tourny C, Sangnier S, Cotte T, Langlois R, Coquart J. Epidemiologic study of young soccer player's injuries in U12 to U20. *J Sports Med Phys Fitness.* 2014; 54: 526–535.
12. Wong P, Hong Y. Soccer injury in the lower extremities. *Br J Sports Med.* 2005; 39: 473–482.
13. Keller CS, Noyes FR, Buncher CR. The medical aspects of soccer injury epidemiology. *Am J Sports Med.* 1987; 15: 230–237.
14. Maher ME, Hutchison M, Cusimano M, Comper P, Schweizer TA. Concussions and heading in soccer: a review of the evidence of incidence, mechanisms, biomarkers and neurocognitive outcomes. *Brain Inj.* 2014; 28: 271–285.
15. Nauta J, Martin-Diener E, Martin BW, van Mechelen W, Verhagen E. Injury risk during different physical activity behaviours in children: a systematic review with bias assessment. *Sports Med.* 2015; 45: 327–336.
16. van der Sluis A, Elferink-Gemser MT, Coelho-e-Silva MJ, Nijboer JA, Brink MS, Visscher C. Sport injuries aligned to peak height velocity in talented pubertal soccer players. *Int J Sports Med.* 2014; 35: 351–355.
17. Agel J, Evans TA, Dick R, Putukian M, Marshall SW. Descriptive epidemiology of collegiate men's soccer injuries: National Collegiate Athletic Association Injury Surveilance System, 1988–1989 through 2002–2003. *J Athl Train.* 2007; 42: 270–277.

18. Ekstrand J, Nigg B. Surface-related injuries in soccer. *Sports Med.* 1989; 8: 56–62.
19. Aoki H, Kohno T, Fujiya H, *et al.* Incidence of injury among adolescent soccer players: a comparative study of artificial and natural grass turfs. *Clin J Sport Med.* 2010; 20: 1–7.
20. Williams S, Hume PA, Kara S. A review of football injuries on third and fourth generation artificial turfs compared with natural turf. *Sports Med.* 2011; 41: 903–923.
21. Hägglund M, Walden M, Ekstrand J. Previous injury as a risk factor for injury in elite football: a prospective study over two consecutive seasons. *Br J Sports Med.* 2006; 40: 767–772.
22. Kucera KL, Marshall SW, Kirkendall DT, Marchak PM, Garrett WE Jr. Injury history as a risk factor for incident injury in youth soccer. *Br J Sports Med.* 2005; 39: 462–466.
23. Bizzini M, Dvorak J. FIFA 11+: an effective programme to prevent football injuries in various player groups worldwide-a narrative review. *Br J Sports Med.* 2015; 49: 577–579.
24. Finch CF, White P, Twomey D, Ullah S. Implementing an exercise-training programme to prevent lower-limb injuries: considerations for the development of a randomised controlled trial intervention delivery plan. *Br J Sports Med.* 2011; 45: 791–796.
25. Kibler BW. Injuries in adolescent and preadolescent soccer players. *Med Sci Sports Exerc.* 1993; 25: 1330–1332.
26. Alic S. USA Football releases preliminary data in study examining youth football player health and safety. Available from: http://usafootball.com/health-safety/usa-football-releases-preliminary-date-study-examining-youth-football-player-health-an. [Accessed 28 October 2015].
27. Harmer PA. Basketball injuries. *Med Sport Sci.* 2005; 49: 31–61.
28. Mello MJ, Myers R, Christian JB, Palmisciano L, Linakis JG. Injuries in youth football: national emergency department visits during 2001–2005 for young and adolescent players. *Acad Emerg Med.* 2009; 16: 243–248.
29. Nation AD, Nelson NG, Yard EE, Comstock RD, McKenzie LB. Football-related injuries among 6- to 17-year-olds treated in US emergency departments, 1990–2007. *Clin Pediatr (Phila).* 2011; 50: 200–207.
30. Dompier TP, Powell JW, Barron MJ, Moore MT. Time-loss and non-time-loss injuries in youth football players. *J Athl Train.* 2007; 42: 395–402.
31. Malina RM, Morano PJ, Barron M, Miller SJ, Cumming SP, Kontos AP. Incidence and player risk factors for injury in youth football. *Clin J Sport Med.* 2006; 16: 214–222.
32. Shankar PR, Fields SK, Collins CL, Dick RW, Comstock RD. Epidemiology of high school and collegiate football injuries in the United States, 2005–2006. *Am J Sports Med.* 2007; 35: 1295–1303.
33. Harmon KG, Drezner J, Gammons M, *et al.* American Medical Society for Sports Medicine position statement: concussion in sport. *Clin J Sport Med.* 2013; 23: 1–18.
34. Stuart MJ, Smith AM, Nieva JJ, Rock MG. Injuries in youth ice hockey: a pilot surveillance strategy. *Mayo Clin Proc.* 1995; 70: 350–356.
35. Turbeville SD, Cowan LD, Asal NR, Owen WL, Anderson MA. Risk factors for injury in middle school football players. *Am J Sports Med.* 2003; 31: 276–281.
36. Yard EE, Comstock RD. Effects of field location, time in competition, and phase of play on injury severity in high school football. *Res Sports Med.* 2009; 17: 35–49.
37. Kerr ZY, Yeargin S, Valovich McLeod TC, *et al.* Comprehensive coach education and practice contact restriction guidelines result in lower injury rates in youth American football. *Orthop J of Sports Med.* 2015; 3: doi: 10.1177/2325967115594578
38. Barron MJ, Branta CF, Powell JW, Ewing ME, Gould DR, Maier K. Effects of an injury prevention program on injury rates in American youth football. *Int J of Sports Sci Coach.* 2014; 9: 1227–1240.
39. Finch C. A new framework for research leading to sports injury prevention. *J Sci Med Sport.* 2006; 9: 3–9.
40. McGuine TA, Hetzel S, Wilson J, Brooks A. The effect of lace-up ankle braces on injury rates in high school football players. *Am J Sports Med.* 2012; 40: 49–57.
41. Emery CA, Hagel B, Decloe M, Carly M. Risk factors for injury and severe injury in youth ice hockey: a systematic review of the literature. *Inj Prev.* 2010; 16: 113–118.
42. MacCormick L, Best TM, Flanigan DC. Are there differences in ice hockey injuries between sexes? *Orthop J Sports Med.* 2014; 2: doi: 10.1177/2325967113518181.
43. Deits J, Yard EE, Collins CL, Fields SK, Comstock RD. Patients with ice hockey injuries presenting to US emergency departments, 1990–2006. *J Athl Train.* 2010; 45: 467–474.
44. Polites SF, Sebastian AS, Habermann EB, Iqbal CW, Stuart MJ, Ishitani MB. Youth ice hockey injuries over 16 years at a pediatric trauma center. *Pediatrics.* 2014; 133: e1601–e1607.
45. Forward KE, Seabrook JA, Lynch T, Lim R, Poonai N, Sangha GS. A comparison of the epidemiology of ice hockey injuries between male and female youth in Canada. *Paediatr Child Health.* 2014; 19: 418–422.
46. Schick DM, Meeuwisse WH. Injury rates and profiles in female ice hockey players. *Am J Sports Med.* 2003; 31: 47–52.
47. Emery CA, Kang J, Shrier I, *et al.* Risk of injury associated with body checking among youth ice hockey players. *JAMA.* 2010; 303: 2265–2272.
48. Emery C, Kang J, Shrier I, *et al.* Risk of injury associated with bodychecking experience among youth hockey players. *Can Med Assoc J.* 2011; 183: 1249–1256.
49. Schneider KJ, Meeuwisse WH, Kang J, Schneider GM, Emery CA. Preseason reports of neck pain, dizziness, and headache as risk factors for concussion in male youth ice hockey players. *Clin J Sport Med.* 2013; 23: 267–272.
50. Emery CA, Meeuwisse WH. Injury rates, risk factors, and mechanisms of injury in minor hockey. *Am J Sports Med.* 2006; 34: 1960–1969.
51. Cusimano MD, Nastis S, Zuccaro L. Effectiveness of interventions to reduce aggression and injuries among ice hockey players: a systematic review. *Can Med Assoc J.* 2013; 185: E57–E69.
52. Randazzo C, Nelson NG, McKenzie LB. Basketball-related injuries in school-aged children and adolescents in 1997–2007. *Pediatrics.* 2010; 126: 727–733.
53. Caine D, Maffulli N, Caine C. Epidemiology of injury in child and adolescent sports: injury rates, risk factors, and prevention. *Clin. Sports Med.* 2008; 27: 19–50, vii.
54. Borowski LA, Yard EE, Fields SK, Comstock RD. The epidemiology of US high-school basketball injuries, 2005–2007. *Am J Sports Med.* 2008; 36: 2328–2335.
55. Pappas E, Zazulak BT, Yard EE, Hewett TE. The epidemiology of pediatric basketball injuries presenting to US emergency departments: 2000–2006. *Sports Health.* 2011; 3: 331–335.
56. McGuine TA, Keene JS. The effect of a balance training program on the risk of ankle sprains in high-school athletes. *Am J Sports Med.* 2006; 34: 1103–1111.
57. Emery CA, Rose MS, McAllister JR., Meeuwisse WH. A prevention strategy to reduce the incidence of injury in high-school basketball: a cluster randomized controlled trial. *Clin J Sport Med.* 2007; 17: 17–24.
58. McGuine TA, Brooks A, Hetzel S. The effect of lace-up ankle braces on injury rates in high-school basketball players. *Am J Sports Med.* 2011; 39: 1840–1848.
59. Yard EE, Knox CL, Smith GA, Comstock RD. Pediatric martial arts injuries presenting to Emergency Departments, United States 1990–2003. *J Sci Med Sport.* 2007; 10: 219–226.
60. McPherson M, Pickett W. Characteristics of martial art injuries in a defined Canadian population: a descriptive epidemiological study. *BMC Public Health.* 2010; 10: 795.
61. Tuominen R. Injuries in national karate competitions in Finland. *Scand J Med Sci Sports.* 1995; 5: 44–48.
62. Pieter W. Competition injury rates in young karate athletes. *Sci Sports.* 2010; 25: 32–38.

63. Beis K, Pieter W, Abatzides G. Taekwondo techniques and competition characteristics involved in time-loss injuries. *J Sports Sci Med.* 2007; 6: 45–51.
64. Oler M, Tomson W, Pepe H, Yoon D, Brandoff R, Branch J. Morbidity and mortality in the martial arts: a warning. *Trauma.* 1991; 31: 251–253.
65. Zetaruk MN, Violan MA, Zurakowski D, Micheli LJ. Karate injuries in children and adolescents. *Accid Analys Prev.* 2000; 32: 421–425.
66. McLatchie GR. Injuries in combat sports. In: Reilly T (ed.) *Sports fitness and sports injuries.* London: Faber and Faber; 1981. p. 168–174.
67. Pieter W, Fife GP, O'Sullivan DM. Competition injuries in taekwondo: a literature review and suggestions for prevention and surveillance. *Br J Sports Med.* 2012; 46: 458–491.
68. Myers RJ, Linakis SW, Mello MJ, Linakis JG. Competitive wrestling-related injuries in school-aged athletes in US emergency departments. *Western J Emerg Med.* 2010; 11: 442–449.
69. Pasque CB, Hewett TE. A prospective study of high school wrestling injuries. *Am J Sports Med.* 2000; 28: 509–515.
70. Rechel JA, Yard EE, Comstock RD. An epidmeiologic comparison of high school sports injureis sustained in practice and competition. *J Athl Train.* 2008; 43: 197–204.
71. Yard EE, Comstock RD. A comparison of pediatric freestyle and Greco-Roman wrestling injuries sustained during a 2006 US national tournament. *Scand J Med Sci Sports.* 2007; 18: 491–497.
72. Hewett TE, Pasque C, Heyl R, Wroble R. Wrestling injuries. *Med Sport Sci.* 2005: 49: 152–178.
73. Wroble RR. Wrestling. In: Kordi R (ed.) *Combat sports medicine.* Springer Science + Business Media; 2009. p. 215–245.
74. Boden BP, Lin W, Young M, Mueller FO. Catastrophic injuries in wrestlers. *Am J Sports Med.* 2002; 30: 791–795.

CHAPTER 43

Epidemiology and prevention of injuries in competitive non-contact sports

Luiz Carlos Hespanhol Junior, Saulo Delfino Barboza, and Per Bo Mahler

Introduction

The global approach to aetiology and prevention of sports injuries has been discussed in Chapter 40. Therefore, this chapter concentrates on sport-specific problems and, in particular, those of non-contact sports. A number of sports where no intentional contact with an opponent occurs has been selected based on their worldwide popularity.[1] Each sport is covered in a systematic manner, including information about the practice of the sport, epidemiology and aetiology of sport-specific injuries, risk factors (intrinsic and extrinsic), and preventative strategies. Because of similarities, skiing and snowboarding are grouped and discussed together, as are tennis and badminton. Certain sports that are less universally practised, or that are country specific, are beyond the scope of this chapter.

In general, injuries in non-contact sports are less frequent than in contact sports, and often fall in the overuse group.[2–5] However, it is important to emphasize that a large proportion of sports pathology is common to both contact and non-contact sports where similar biomechanical factors are involved (running, cutting, etc.). It is noteworthy that little information is available on children and adolescents in certain sports.[6–8] Therefore, data from adults have been used to extrapolate findings when appropriate. Taking this into consideration, this chapter underlines certain trends that can be drawn from the literature and that give a reasonable basis to develop and promote prevention programmes appropriate to children and adolescents.

Bicycling

Apart from being a popular sport, cycling is an equally popular means of transport and leisure activity. It is therefore difficult to differentiate between sports-related and sports-independent injuries, as multiple risk factors are present in both activities. Special emphasis will be placed on competitive cycling injuries when possible.

Epidemiology of cycling injuries

In the emergency department of the British Columbia Children's Hospital, 13.5% of all paediatric sports injuries (14.7% in boys and 11.3% in girls) recorded from 1992–2005 were bicycle related.[9] The annual injury rate of paediatric bicycle injuries varies from 2.36–5.01 injuries per 1000 children.[10,11] Emergency departments in Brisbane registered an annual injury rate of fatal injuries (accidents involving vehicles) by 0.018 per 1000 children for boys, and 0.007 per 100 000 children for girls.[11] Dutch hospitals have registered an annual increase of paediatric bicycle injuries by 3.8% (95% confidence interval [CI] 2.8–4.8%) from 2001–2009 (from around 38/100 000 injuries in 2001 to around 58/100 000 injuries in 2009).[12]

Injuries can be divided into acute (including accidents) and overuse (gradual onset) injuries. Bicycle injuries resulting from accidents occur frequently in the face (15%), head (13%), and forearm (12%).[9] The types of injury include abrasions/lacerations (63%), fractures (16%), closed head injuries, and concussions (2%).[13] In the overuse group, bicycle injuries in professional competitive adult athletes frequently occur in the lower back/pelvis/sacrum, knee, shoulder/clavicle, lower leg / Achilles tendon, thigh, and neck/cervical spine.[14] The types of bicycle injuries include anterior and lateral knee pain,[15] neck and low back pain,[16] ischial pain and pudendal nerve palsy,[17] microtrauma to the scrotal contents,[18] ulnar nerve pain,[19] and stenotic thickening of the external iliac artery.[20]

Aetiology of cycling injuries

Factors associated with a higher risk of cycling injuries can be found in Table 43.1. Falls are the most frequent source of accidental injuries, followed by hitting a stationary object, hitting or being hit by a motor vehicle, hitting another cyclist, pedestrian, or animal, and bicycle malfunction.[21] Motor vehicles are involved in a minority of accidents (10–35%), but are responsible for about 90% of fatalities.[11,21] Accidents also correlate with the type of road (more fatal accidents on high speed limit roads), damaged or slippery roads, the availability of cycle tracks, excessive speed, sharp curves, downhill riding, uneven surfaces, and unexpected obstacles such as waste or rough fragments of stone, brick, concrete, etc.[21,22]

The non-use of helmets has been shown to be a major risk factor for head and brain injuries in cyclists.[23–25] The age group from 10 to 14 years is at higher risk of bicycle injuries compared to other children and adolescents age groups.[9,12,13] Musculoskeletal

Table 43.1 Risk factors for cycling injuries.

Intrinsic risk factors	Extrinsic risk factors
Age (10–14 years at higher risk)[9,12,13]	Protective equipment (helmets)[23–25]
Gender (boys at higher risk)[9,10,12,28]	Exposure[16,22,27]
Low level of general conditioning[22,26]	Training quality (progression, programme)[16,22,27]
Behaviour (unrealistic perceived skills and unsafe riding)[11,22]	Type of roads, intersections, cycle tracks[10,22]
Inexperience[22]	Bicycle fit[16,22,27]
Cycling technique[22]	Mechanical malfunction of the bicycle[21,22]

immaturity may partly explain this finding, because approximately 15% of all sports injuries in children can be attributed to inadequate bone growth, skeletal development, and musculoskeletal imbalance.[22] Other risk factors for bicycle injuries may include inexperience, low level of general conditioning (such as strength, flexibility, and neuromuscular control), and risk behaviour.[22,26] With regard to behaviour, younger cyclists are less likely to wear helmets because of peer pressure that results in the belief that the use of helmets is 'uncool'.[22] In addition, unrealistic perceived skills and lack of knowledge about safe riding also contribute to bicycle accidents.[11,22]

Overuse injuries seem to be linked to biomechanical and training factors. As in other sports, training volume and progression are very important. Bicycle fit (e.g. saddle position, foot clips, frame size, and handlebars) should be carefully evaluated and re-evaluated in the case of injury.[16,22,27] Cycling technique (foot, hip, and arm position) should also be analysed.[22]

Preventative strategies

Accidents are responsible for the most serious injuries and their prevention should therefore receive special attention. The Haddon Matrix,[13] which identifies modifiable risk factors and divides them into three phases (pre-impact, during impact, and post-impact), is a valuable model for cycling injury prevention. Important factors like helmet use, cyclist education, bicycle design, road/path design, emergency services, and rehabilitation should be stressed.

The use of helmets decreases head injuries by up to 80%.[23] However, some debate still exists about the evidence to enforce helmet use, because one could argue that the compulsory use of helmets without education training could lead cyclists to believe that they are safer than they actually are, leading to an increase in risk behaviours.[29] Therefore, the use of helmets should be recommended, followed by education and training, including how to use helmets and ride safely.[11]

Overuse injuries mostly occur due to bicycle-rider misfit or training errors; hence bicycle choice (accessories) and adjustment should be carried out by a professional and adapted to growth. Exercise-based prevention programmes are effective in preventing sports injuries in children and adolescents.[26] These exercises are usually aimed at enhancing general conditioning (e.g. strength, flexibility, and neuromuscular control) and they can be done as a training routine, preseason conditioning programme, or during warm-up exercises.[26]

Dance

Dance in its various forms (ballet, jazz, breakdance, flamenco, etc.) can be compared with other sports when considering athletic qualities required, methodical training programmes, and risk of injuries.[30] Dancing is a popular activity among youth and often requires intensive involvement in training at young age.[30,31]

Epidemiology of dance injuries

Systematic reviews have shown that the point-prevalence of dance injuries varies from 51–85%,[31] and the average incidence rate is 1.33 injuries per 1000 h of dancing (range of 0.18–4.70) or 1.93 injuries per dancer per year (range of 0.05–6.83).[32] Prospective studies have shown that the incidence rate of ballet injuries varies from 0.9[33] to 1.38 (95% CI 1.24–1.52)[34] injuries per 1000 h of dancing. In professional dancers, 16% of injuries occur in class, 28% in rehearsals, and 33% during performances.[35]

Dance injuries mostly fall into the overuse group.[34,36] Studies with ballet dancers have shown that about 75% of all ballet injuries are caused by overuse.[34,36] Body regions most affected are foot/ankle (35–53%, especially in ballet), knee (13–29%), shin/calf (22%), spine (9–17%), hip/groin (10%), shoulder (15%, especially in breakdance), and wrist/hand (10%, especially in breakdance).[34,36–41] The types of dance injuries most frequently reported are muscle/tendon injuries (13–32%), joint/ligament injuries (25%), bone stress/fractures (5–12%), and contusions (2%).[38,39]

Aetiology of dance injuries

Factors associated with a higher risk of dance injuries can be found in Table 43.2. The main mechanisms of dance injuries described by Campoy *et al.*[41] were repetitive movements with an insufficient time to recover (44% in classical ballet; 37% in jazz/contemporary dance; 41% in street dance; and 65% in tap/folk dance); dynamic overload (43% in classical ballet; 46% in jazz/contemporary dance; 36% in street dance; and 20% in tap/folk dance); and direct traumatic impact (13% in classical ballet; 18% in jazz/contemporary dance; 23% in street dance; and 16% in tap/folk dance). These results corroborate with Ojofeitimi *et al.*,[39] who reported 50% of hip hop injuries were caused by overuse mechanisms, followed by landing (42%), twisting (36%), and slipping (31%). Dancing on inadequate floor (slippery, hard, or sticky) has been described as a contributor to dance injuries.[39,42]

Sports exposure influences the incidence of sports injuries. Kadel *et al.*[43] found that the risk of sustaining a stress fracture increased

Table 43.2 Risk factors for dance injuries.

Intrinsic risk factors	Extrinsic risk factors
Previous injury[45]	Exposure[37,38,43]
Irregular menstrual cycles[43,50–52]	Inadequate dance surface[39,42]
Amenorrhea[43]	Overstretching[53]
Low BMI (nutrition)[51]	Training factors[44]
Foot pronation[36,48]	Organizational factors[44]
Hyperflexed forefoot[54]	Environmental factors[44]
Insufficient plantar flexion[36]	

significantly in professional dancers who practised over 5 h·day^{-1}. Steinberg *et al.*[38] found that an additional hour of dancing per week increased the risk of dance injuries by 28%. Norwegian ballet dancers have reported in a prospective study that they believe that training, organizational, and environmental characteristics are risk factors for dance injuries.[44]

Previous injuries have been associated with the occurrence of new dance injuries in prospective[45] and retrospective[36] studies. Reduced functional turnout has been shown to be related to a higher risk of dance injuries.[46,47] Dancing 'en pointe' or 'demi-pointe', and foot pronation have been suggested to be related to ankle injuries, resulting in tendinitis of the flexor hallucis longus and Achilles tendon, osteochondral fractures of the talus, sprains, and anterior impingement syndromes of the ankle.[48,49]

Some dancers can be at higher risk of bone injuries because of their extreme nutritional habits (to minimize body fat) and intensive training loads, which when combined can lead to hormonal perturbations, delayed bone growth, and irregular menstrual cycles including amenorrhea.[43,50–52] Kadel *et al.*[43] found that dancers with stress fractures had a significantly longer duration of amenorrhea than those with no stress fractures.

Preventative strategies

A preventative approach to reduce dance injuries may include proper treatment of injuries, careful monitoring of individual stretching routines (avoiding overstretching), good nutritional counselling with follow-up, close monitoring of any menstrual irregularities, and the constant re-evaluation of training load and floor conditions.[55,56]

Exercise-based intervention programmes are promising in reducing dance injuries.[26,55,57] A 3-year prospective study has shown that an individualized conditioning programme consisting of neuromuscular control, specific muscle training, and functional activities (e.g. jumping) significantly reduced the annual incidence rate of dance injuries.[57]

The management and monitoring of dance injuries should also be considered in prevention programmes. A healthcare programme implemented in a modern dance company in New York (Alvin Ailey) was effective in reducing the incidence of dance injuries by 34%, the number of workers' compensation claims by 66%, the number of days lost from dance by 56%, and saved $860.76 (benefit-cost ratio of 3.98) in workers compensation premiums (direct plus indirect costs) after 6 years from its implementation.[58,59]

Gymnastics

Gymnastics is an increasingly popular sport in certain countries and requires early involvement (6–9 years of age) in intensive training.[60] Training volume can reach 40 h or more per week for elite gymnasts, and generates significant loads to both upper and lower extremities, which potentially may result in injury.

Epidemiology of gymnastics injuries

Injury rates vary considerably between studies depending on competitive level, club or school structure, gender, and data processing. Injury rates for girls vary between 1.4 to 3.7 injuries per 1000 h of exposure at club level.[60] In female collegiate gymnasts, the incidence rate can reach 22.7 injuries per 1000 h of gymnastics.[61] A study that investigated gender-specific injury rates in collegiate gymnasts reported 8.78 (95% CI 7.67–9.89) injuries per 1000 athlete-exposures in men, and 9.37 (8.07–10.66) in women.[62]

Most gymnastics injuries are of sudden onset (acute injuries), representing 52–83% of all gymnastics injuries.[60] However, the difficulty in distinguishing between an acute injury and an acute injury superimposed on a predisposing overuse injury may bias this conclusion.[63] Also, injury type tends to be limb specific, with more overuse injuries being observed at the upper extremity and low back in comparison to the lower extremity.[60,64]

The lower limb is the most frequently involved body part (54–70%), followed by the spine/trunk (14–44%) and the upper extremity (14–25%).[60] The ankle (15–31%) is the anatomical region most frequently injured in the lower limb, followed by knee (9–20%) and upper leg (3–4%).[60,65,66] The wrist (5–10%), elbow (4–9%), and hands/fingers (1–5%) are the most frequently involved body regions in the upper extremity.[60,65,66] The lower back (5–20%) is the most often involved body region in injuries to the spine/trunk.[60] Male gymnasts tend to have more injuries in the upper extremities (shoulder and wrist) compared to other body regions, indicating that the injury location is gender-specific.[60] Sprains (16–44%) and strains (6–32%) are consistently the most frequently observed injury mechanisms in women and men.[60]

Aetiology of gymnastics injuries

The high-impact loads and extreme biomechanics seen in gymnastics certainly contribute to both overuse and accidental injuries. Vault take-offs have been shown to produce ground reaction forces of up to 5.1 times body weight to the lower limb,[67] whereas forces of 8.8–14.4 times body weight were found on landing.[68] Extreme biomechanics involving hyperflexion, rotation, and hyperextension of the trunk can also be considered causative factors.[69] The upper limb is also exposed to large loads, ranging from 1.6 times body weight in vaulting[67] to 9.2 times body weight in still rings.[70] Few catastrophic injuries have been reported in gymnastics and are mainly related to trampoline (trampette) exercises.[71–74]

Numerous factors shown to be associated with gymnastics injuries are summarized in Table 43.3. Anthropometric factors such as body size, body weight, and puberty are closely related to injury in girls.[75–77] Early maturation, rapid growth, large body size, and weight have been described as risk factors for gymnastics

Table 43.3 Risk factors for gymnastics injuries.

Intrinsic risk factors	Extrinsic risk factors
Large body size and weight[75–77]	Event (floor condition, uneven parallel bars, vault, balance beam)[61,62,66,80–82]
Previous injury[65,66]	Inappropriate use of safety and personal protective equipment[83–85]
High competitive level (severe injuries)[75,79]	Exposure (especially training ≥8 h·day^{-1})[65]
Early maturation (higher body fat)[75–77]	Training errors[86]
Rapid growth[75–77]	Period of the sports season[75]
	Stressful life events[87]

injuries.[75–77] Previous injury, which is consistent through most sports,[78] is also an intrinsic risk factor for gymnastics injuries.[65,66]

Exposure,[65] competitive level,[75,79] and the type of event[61,62,66,80–82] have been associated with gymnastics injuries. Floor condition has been observed to be the source of most acute traumatic injuries (31–42%), followed by uneven parallel bars (8–32%), vault (10–27%), and balance beam (12–17%).[66,80] The first half hour of practice and certain periods of the season (e.g. following interruptions, intensive preparation, pre-competition, and during competition) have also been described as risk factors.[75]

Preventative strategies

Prevention programmes should start with education of gymnasts and coaches concerning sport-specific preparation, injuries, preventative measures, treatment, nutrition, and coach/child/family interaction.[84,86,88] Continuing education of coaches should be mandatory,[89] and alternate loading, quality of training, motivation, individualization, general conditioning (e.g. strength, flexibility, and neuromuscular training), growth, and interpersonal skills should all be covered.[26,84] Correct technique, landing strategies, and adequate body posture have been suggested as essential in gymnastics injury prevention.[60,84] Appropriate use of safety and personal protective equipment have also been advised in order to reduce the risk of gymnastics injuries.[83–85]

A large proportion of gymnasts (51%) seem to compete despite pain.[90] Learning to differentiate between exertional soreness and pain owing to injury might help prevent subsequent injuries.[91] Medical support becomes important when children reach competitive level. Preseason screening and post-injury medical evaluation are important to re-evaluate risk factors and guide the gymnast and his/her support 'team'. Therefore, it has been suggested that continuous musculoskeletal screening for injury prevention should be done periodically, and corrective actions should be implemented to address identified problems.[84]

Running

Running is a widespread activity and is common to a multitude of both contact and non-contact sports. Running is also a popular way to motivate and engage children and adolescents in physical activity,[92] and it is commonly used to maintain and/or train general conditioning components in other sports.

Epidemiology of running injuries

The incidence of running injuries in high-school runners varies from 16% in 1 month[93] to 39% during a season.[94] Incidence rates vary from 9.4–17.0 injuries per 1000 athlete-exposures, and girls present a higher incidence (11.4–19.6 injuries per 1000 athlete-exposures) than boys (7.8–15.0 injuries per 1000 athlete-exposures).[93,94] Once injured, the incidence rate of a subsequent injury (new or recurrent injury) was found in a prospective study to be 50 injuries per 1000 athlete-exposures.[94]

Most running injuries are of an overuse nature,[93,95,96] representing 84% of all running injuries in high-school cross-country runners.[93] The body regions most affected are the shin (28%), knee (28%), ankle (16%), and hip (13%).[93,94] The most common injuries reported in children and adolescents are medial tibial stress syndrome, i.e. shin splints (39%), ankle sprain (30%), patellofemoral pain syndrome (19%), stress fracture (5–14%), Achilles tendinopathy (7%), iliotibial band syndrome (6%), and plantar fasciitis (4%).[93,97]

Aetiology of running injuries

Table 43.4 provides a summary of intrinsic and extrinsic risk factors for running injuries in children and adolescents. The main intrinsic risk factor for running injuries reported in the literature is previous injury.[94,97,98] Rauh *et al.*[94] showed that high-school cross-country runners with a previous history of running injuries may be 80% more likely to have a new running injury.

Prospective studies have found that girls are at 30–40% higher risk for running injuries than boys.[93,94] Younger chronological age, younger age at menarche, and reduced whole-body bone mineral content were found to be risk factors for stress fractures among young female cross-country runners.[97] Quadriceps angle (Q-angle) ≥20° and right-left Q-angle difference ≥4° have also been associated with running injuries in prospective studies.[94,99]

Malisoux *et al.*[100] suggested that exposure (running practice) is a necessary cause of running injuries. A retrospective study found that higher weekly running distances were associated with running injuries in high-school runners.[96] A prospective study found that high-school cross-country runners who did not frequently alternate short and long running distances on different days, and who ran more than 33% of the time on predominantly hilly or irregular terrains, were at higher risk for running injuries.[93]

Preventative strategies

Adequate information should be given to the runner with respect to injury risk, risk factors, and acknowledgement of early symptoms of injury. Intrinsic and extrinsic risk factors for running injuries (Table 43.4) should be identified and corrected when possible. Young runners should be encouraged to increase running volume progressively and slowly. Additionally, young runners should run on alternate days, alternate short and long running distances on different days, alternate the running terrain, perform a proper warm-up, include a regular general conditioning programme (e.g. strength, flexibility, and neuromuscular training), be aware of injury symptoms, seek appropriate treatment when injured, and return to running progressively after an interruption.

Pre-participation evaluation by healthcare professionals and/or trainers should be encouraged if intensive participation is

Table 43.4 Risk factors for running injuries.

Intrinsic risk factors	Extrinsic risk factors
Previous injury[94,97,98]	Exposure[93,96,101]
Gender (girls at higher risk)[93,94]	Do not alternate short and long running distance on different days[93]
Younger age (chronological and at menarche) for stress fractures[97]	Running more than 33% of the time on predominantly hilly terrains[93]
Reduced whole-body bone mineral content for stress fractures[97]	Running more than 33% of the time on irregular terrains[93]
Quadriceps angle (Q-angle) ≥20° [94,99]	Higher weekly running distance[96]
Right-left Q-angle difference ≥4° [99]	

considered. Jakobsen *et al.*[102] found that a clinical examination followed by education on injury prevention (such as avoiding rapid increase in running distance, the importance of warm-up, and getting treatment for overuse symptoms), and an individualized training programme based on a repeated running test over time was significantly effective in reducing running injuries in adult long-distance runners.

Skiing and snowboarding

Skiing and snowboarding have become increasingly popular over the last decades because of the facilitated access and increased capacity of ski areas. It is estimated that there are about 200 million leisure skiers worldwide.[103] Snowboarding has also contributed to the popularity of alpine sports, adding a 'fun' dimension, which has attracted numerous youngsters.

Epidemiology of skiing and snowboarding injuries

During the first Winter Youth Olympic Games 2012, which included athletes aged 14–18 years, alpine skiing and snowboarding were responsible for 25% of all registered injuries.[104] A total of 47% of injuries occurred during training and 49% during competition. Lower extremity was most affected (36%), followed by trunk (33%), upper extremity (18%), and head (13%). The most frequent injury types reported were contusions (40%), sprains (22%), strains (15%), and concussion (9%).

Kim *et al.*[105] prospectively registered skiing and snowboarding injuries over 18 seasons (1988–2006). In children and adolescents (≤16 years old), lower extremity contusion was the most common skiing injury registered (18% of all injuries), followed by medial collateral ligament injury of the knee (7%), metacarpophalangeal-ulnar (MCP-ulnar) collateral ligament tear of the thumb (7%), concussions (5%), tibia fractures (5%), wrist injuries (5%), upper body lacerations (4%), shoulder soft tissue injuries (4%), anterior cruciate ligament tears (3%), and ankle sprains (3%). The injury trend from 1988–2006 showed a significant decrease in thumb MCP-ulnar collateral ligament and knee medial collateral ligament sprains, while the remaining injury types did not change over time.[105]

In child and adolescent snowboarders, wrist injuries (including contusions, sprains, distal radius/ulna fractures, and carpal fractures) represented 38% of all injuries registered by Kim *et al.*,[105] followed by lower extremity contusions (6%), concussions (5%), clavicle fractures (5%), shoulder soft tissue injuries (3%), knee medial collateral ligament sprains (3%), ankle sprains (3%), upper body lacerations (3%), tibial fractures (1%), and ankle fractures (1%). Clavicle fractures significantly increased over time (from 1988–2006) while a decrease in knee medial collateral ligament and ankle injuries was observed.[105]

Aetiology of skiing and snowboarding injuries

The main causes of skiing and snowboarding injuries in the first Winter Youth Olympic Games 2012 were attributed to non-contact trauma (47%), contact with a fixed object (24%), overuse (16%), weather conditions (4%), contact with another athlete (2%), and contact with moving objects (2%).[104]

The contact with objects and other athletes may explain lower leg contusions in skiers. The thumb MCP-ulnar collateral ligament injury happens when the skier's hand is driven into the snow still grasping the pole.[105] Injuries to the head and spine are often due to loss of control, collisions with other skiers or trees, incorrect landings after jumps,[106] and negligible helmet use.[107] Five mechanisms, involving rotational and translation forces in the knee, have been described by Feagin *et al.*[108] for anterior cruciate injuries.

As snowboarders have their feet fixed on the board, they are more likely to fall when they lose balance, particularly those with less experience.[105] When falling, the most common reaction is to break the fall with an outstretched hand, which may lead to a wrist injury.[105] Clavicle fractures are associated with jumping activities, and consequently these injuries occur more often in experienced athletes.[105] Snowboard manoeuvres (e.g. aerials) have become popular, which may explain the increasing trend in clavicle fractures over time.[105] Snowboarding injuries vary as a function of the activity (e.g. more head, face, and spinal injuries in aerial manoeuvres), type of boots (more severe injuries with stiff boots), and snow conditions (66% of injuries on icy and hard slopes).[107,109,110] A summary of the risk factors for skiing and snowboarding injuries can be found in Table 43.5.

Preventative strategies

Educating athletes through video presentations has been effective in reducing skiing injuries.[121,122] Using knee braces is recommended for skiers, wrist guards for snowboarders,[111] and both skiers and snowboarders should be strongly encouraged to use helmets.[111,123] These strategies can be useful in injury prevention programmes, especially for novice athletes, who are at higher risk of injury than their more experienced counterparts (Table 43.5).[111]

Information on types of exercises (e.g. strength, flexibility, and neuromuscular training), warming up and cooling down can be helpful and should be integrated in educational strategies. Exercise-based injury prevention programmes in children and adolescents have been shown to be effective.[26] Recommendations should be made in order to encourage novice athletes to attend ski schools where body skills (e.g. physical conditioning, balance, and coordination) can be trained and improved.[124]

Swimming

Swimming is a very popular leisure and competitive sport worldwide. Participants often begin at a young age, and swimmers who reach competitive level quickly progress to intensive training, which leads to increased loads, especially to the upper extremities.[125]

Table 43.5 Risk factors for skiing and snowboarding injuries.

Intrinsic risk factors	Extrinsic risk factors
Novice athletes[107,110–112]	Poor visibility[111]
Gender (girls at higher risk)[111]	Inappropriate equipment[111]
Age (children > adolescents > adults)[113,114]	Binding adjustment[103]
	Helmets[115,116]
	Snow conditions and weather (avalanches)[109,117,118]
	Wrist guards (snowboarding)[119,120]

Epidemiology of swimming injuries

Chase *et al.*[125] reported an injury incidence rate of 3.04 per 1000 h of swimming in collegiate competitive athletes prospectively followed-up during a season. Most injuries concerned the shoulder (39%), followed by the trunk (16%), knee (13%), ankle (13%), upper leg (10%), groin (7%), and neck (3%). Most injuries were classified as tendinopathies (58%), while 36% were strains and 7% were sprains. Overuse injuries represented 58% of the total.

Pollard *et al.*[126] reported swimming injuries treated in US emergency departments over 19 years (1990–2008). Most injuries (61%) were reported by individuals younger than 17, and the annual injury rate was higher for individuals aged 7–17 years (18.78 injuries per 10 000 participants) than for individuals over 17 (9.15 injuries per 10 000 participants). Head and neck were the most affected body regions (37%), followed by the lower extremities (33%).

Aetiology of swimming injuries

Most authors agree that repetitive loads and high training volume, leading to about two million strokes per year in elite swimmers, are the main sources of injury.[127] Injury incidence has been shown to correlate with exposure and performance,[128,129] and medal winners seem to present a higher incidence of injury.[130]

Injury types vary between strokes. Shoulder injuries are most common in free-style, back-stroke, and butterfly swimming,[127] while knee and groin injuries are more common in breast stroke.[131,132] This can be explained by differences in biomechanics between the strokes, which stress different structures. Shoulder problems mainly result from sub-acromial impingement and labral pathology, which are linked to repetitive overhead motion.[133] This scenario may be worsened by muscle imbalance between internal and external rotators, shoulder instability,[134,135] and acromial shape.[136] Shoulder injuries have also been related to improper technique, strength training at a premature age, and the use of devices such as the pull buoy and paddles.[127]

Knee problems are mainly linked to patellofemoral dysfunction during kicking or medial collateral ligament stress, which is more specific to breast stroke. Malalignment of the lower extremity and patellar instability have been suggested as risk factors.[137]

Back pain can be linked to repeated flexion and twisting during flip turns, torsional strain if the body is not rolled as a whole unit during the stroke, or to swimming techniques that lead to lumbosacral hyperextension (e.g. breast stroke and butterfly).[138] Risk factors for swimming injuries are summarized in Table 43.6.

Preventative strategies

Emphasis should be placed on proper stroke biomechanics, and training sessions should start very progressively and terminate at the first signs of fatigue (perturbed biomechanics). Strength training should begin in skeletally mature swimmers, when proper swimming biomechanics have been acquired, and it should start with high-repetition and low-resistance exercises.[127]

Behaviour is considered a key factor to be addressed in order to prevent sport injuries in real-life situations.[139] Adolescent swimmers engaged in high-school competitive clubs tend to believe that shoulder pain is a normal part of training and should be tolerated.[140] Therefore, educational strategies involving athletes, trainers, and medical staff might contribute to change these beliefs and behaviours, reducing the number of athletes training with shoulder pain.[140]

Table 43.6 Risk factors for swimming injuries.

Intrinsic risk factors	Extrinsic risk factors
Previous injury[125]	Exposure[128,129]
Poor technique[127,138]	Using a pull buoy or paddles[127]
Shoulder muscle imbalance[134]	Premature or not-adjusted strength training[127]
Shoulder instability[135]	Type of stroke[127,131,132]
Acromial shape[136]	
Malalignment of the lower extremity[137]	
Patellar instability[137]	

Tennis and badminton

Because of similarities in injury profile and biomechanics, tennis and badminton are discussed together. These sports have become increasingly popular among youths, leading to early specialization and intensified training programmes. This has resulted in an increasing number of tennis and badminton injuries in the younger population.[141]

Epidemiology of tennis and badminton injuries

Pluim *et al.*[142] reported an average weekly prevalence of 3.0% (95% CI 2.3–3.7%) for acute injuries and 12.1% (95% CI 10.9–13.3%) for overuse injuries in elite junior tennis players prospectively followed-up during a season. Overuse injuries were generally of longer duration than acute injuries, and had a higher impact on hampering training volume and performance. Ankle/foot were mostly affected by acute injuries (36%), followed by hip/groin (25%), knee (12%), wrist/hand (8%), and fingers (8%). For overuse injuries, the knee (18%), followed by back/spine (17%), shoulder (16%), ankle/foot (13%), wrist/hand (9%), elbow (8%), leg (8%), and hip/groin (5%) were the most affected regions.[142] Similarly, most injuries in badminton are classified as overuse (74%) and involve mainly the lower extremity (83%).[143]

Garrick and Requa[144] reported an incidence proportion of 3% of tennis injuries in high-school girls, and 7% in high-school boys during a 2-year follow-up period. The same study found that the incidence of badminton injuries was 6% in high-school girls.[144] Maquirriain and Ghisi[145] reported a particularly high incidence (13%) of stress fractures in young elite tennis players. Shoulder subluxation, labral tears, Osgood-Schlatter's disease of the shoulder, slipped capital humeral epiphysis, and stress fractures of the humeral epiphysis have been described in junior tennis and badminton athletes.[146,147] Eye injuries[148] and neurological injuries involving the suprascapular nerve[149] have also been described.

Aetiology of tennis and badminton injuries

Most tennis and badminton injuries are due to repetitive microtrauma.[142,150] The overuse mechanism is often attributed to poor technique, repetitive unnatural and dynamic movements,[151] fatigue,

Table 43.7 Risk factors for tennis and badminton injuries.

Intrinsic risk factors	Extrinsic risk factors
Previous injury[159]	Exposure[159]
Low flexibility[141,157]	Inappropriate equipment use (racquet, grip, cord tension, balls)[152,153]
Low fitness level[141]	Inappropriate training programmes[152,153]
Insufficient shoulder strength[160]	
Muscle imbalance[158]	

lack of coordination, inappropriate equipment, and improper training programmes.[152,153] Lower extremity injuries are related to the constant pounding, accelerations, and decelerations during games,[154] as well as to the high eccentric loads which can lead to muscle tears and tendon injuries.[155,156] In badminton, however, injuries are often sustained while players stumble when trying to play a stroke.[143] Range of motion may also influence the predisposition to injury. For example, internal rotation has been shown to be limited in the dominant arm of tennis athletes.[157] Muscle imbalances and shortness observed in the shoulder, forearm, and trunk are also considered to predispose the athlete to injury.[158] A higher exposure to matches, as shown by Kibler *et al.*,[141] may contribute to a higher risk of injuries in tennis. Risk factors for tennis and badminton injuries are summarized in Table 43.7.

Preventative strategies

Prevention programmes for tennis and badminton injuries should start by educating players, coaches, and healthcare professionals regarding the risks of injury linked to the sport, injury treatment, and preventative measures. A good basic fitness level, specific strengthening,[26] regular stretching exercises (e.g. internal rotation of the dominant arm),[161] and adequate equipment[162] should be encouraged. Proper warm-up and cool-down exercises should also be incorporated in training and competition activities.[163]

Volleyball

Volleyball has progressively become one of the most popular sports for both boys and girls, and it is widely practised around the world.[164] Volleyball has also become more attractive to children, with the introduction of mini-volleyball and beach volleyball.

Epidemiology of volleyball injuries

Backx *et al.*[3] found an injury incidence rate of 6.7 per 1000 h of volleyball. A different result came from Zaricznyj *et al.*,[165] who found an injury incidence of 0.13 per 1000 h of volleyball. Backx *et al.*[3] found that most volleyball injuries were sustained during training and were recorded at the beginning of a season. Data from the 2nd and 3rd Dutch national volleyball divisions showed an incidence rate of 2.6 volleyball injuries per 1000 h of volleyball during a season.[166] Injuries during training seem to be more frequent than during competitions.[3,167,168] Volleyball has become a highly competitive sport with high training volumes. This may have contributed to the increasing number of injuries observed over the last decades.[169]

In school volleyball, 50% of injuries concern hands and fingers, 20% the ankles, and 6% the knees.[165,170] However, in adult elite volleyball, around 83% of acute injuries concern the lower limb, and ankle sprains are the most frequent injuries (41% of all volleyball injuries).[166] Knobloch *et al.*[170] found that 41% of volleyball injuries were sprains or strains, 17% were fractures, and 16% were bruises.

Nationwide records of the emergency departments in US have registered volleyball injuries from 1990 through 2009, resulting in an annual injury rate of 6.23 injuries per 1000 participants.[171] The annual volleyball injury rate was 7.49 injuries per 1000 participants aged 12–17 years, and 2.68 per 1000 participants aged 7–11 years.[171] Upper extremities were more affected (48%) than lower extremities (39%). In the upper extremities, fingers were most affected (48%), while ankles were the most affected body region in the lower extremities (65%). Head and trunk injuries represented 9% and 4% of volleyball injuries, respectively. Strains and sprains were the most common injury mechanism in lower and upper extremities (43% and 57%, respectively), with ankles representing 79% of lower extremity sprains/strains, and fingers and wrists representing 46% and 35% of upper extremity sprains/strains, respectively. Fractures and dislocations were mostly found in the upper extremities, with lacerations mostly in the head, face, and neck.[171]

Aetiology of volleyball injuries

Landing (after offensive and defensive plays) and numerous contacts between the knee and the playing surface (during defensive plays) are considered to be responsible for most of the injuries around the knee.[3,172] Jumping and landing with the knees in a valgus position,[173] landing with a twisting motion of the knee,[174] taking-off with one leg, and landing with one leg[175] seem to increase the risk of volleyball injuries. Ankle injuries are mostly sustained during jumping,[171] collisions between players, and often with the opponent under the net.[176] Verhagen *et al.*[166] found that previous ankle sprain is a major risk factor for re-injuries, especially during the first year post injury. Shoulder injuries, including supraspinatus tendinopathy, impingement, and nerve entrapment, are due to the extreme biomechanical loads involved with spiking and jump serve.[177] Fingers are mainly at risk during blocking, and the head during contact with net/pole.[171]

Extrapolating data from adult literature, blocking seems to be responsible for the largest number of volleyball injuries, followed by spiking and defence manoeuvres.[178] However, in school volleyball, collisions between opponents (60%), the landing phase (9%), and striking the ball (7%) seem to be the main sources of injury.[170] Risk factors for volleyball injuries are summarized in Table 43.8.

Table 43.8 Risk factors for volleyball injuries.

Intrinsic risk factors	Extrinsic risk factors
Previous injury[166]	Exposure[166,172,174,179]
Gender (boys at higher risk)[179]	Position (offensive > defensive)[176]
Younger age group[180]	Inappropriate training[181]
Growth spurt[182]	Collision with opponent[176]
Poor jumping technique[173–175]	

Preventative strategies

Specific attention should be given to children's growth phases and adapting training loads to the individual. Malalignment and muscle imbalance should be identified and corrected when possible. As in other sports, educational strategies involving athletes, coaches/trainers, and healthcare professionals are encouraged to properly implement preventative and management strategies. Jumping and landing techniques have been shown to be important and, when well trained, can have a protective effect, especially on ankle injuries. Special attention should be given to jumping and landing training techniques during preparation periods.[183] Neuromuscular training and the use of protective braces are strongly recommended to prevent ankle sprains.[164,184,185] Premature return to sport should be avoided for injured athletes until treatment and recovery are complete.

Conclusions

Paediatric sports injuries in non-contact sports have been shown to be a substantial burden for young athletes, teams, healthcare systems, and society. This chapter has presented the epidemiology, aetiology, and preventative strategies for such injuries. Although paucity of evidence on injury prevention in some sports may challenge practical approaches, implementing preventative measures discussed here may help to prevent injuries in children and adolescents. This knowledge should be implemented in real-life situations in order to encourage children and adolescents to participate in sports, and to allow them to experience the well-known health benefits of sports participation with the lowest risk possible.

Summary

- Although scientific evidence on paediatric sports injuries in non-contact sports is plagued by numerous methodological issues and paucity of data, similarities do exist in epidemiological trends, injury risk factors, and preventative strategies.
- In general, informing coaches, athletes, and healthcare professionals about sports injury prevention, risk factors, adapting the training load to growth, doing appropriate warm-up and cool-down exercises, maintaining an appropriate and continuous general conditioning training programme (e.g. strength, flexibility, and neuromuscular control), taking a proper recovery and/or healing time, treating injuries properly, using protective equipment, and ensuring adequate nutrition and hydration must be encouraged in all sports.
- Assigning least responsibility to the child and the most to sports organizations and government is noteworthy and stresses the need for structured preventative measures.[89]
- It is the right of all children and adolescents to benefit from a safe environment, a healthy sports practice, and a proper application of the Children's Bill of Rights in Sport.[186]

References

1. DeKnop P, Engström L, Skirstad B, Weiss M. *World-wide trends in youth sport*. Champaign, IL: Human Kinetics; 1996.
2. De Loës M, Goldie I. Incidence rate of injuries during sport activity and physical exercise in a rural Swedish municipality: incidence rates in 17 sports. *Int J Sports Med*. 1988; 9: 461–467.
3. Backx FJ, Beijer HJ, Bol E, Erich WB. Injuries in high-risk persons and high-risk sports. A longitudinal study of 1818 school children. *Am J Sports Med*. 1991; 19: 124–130.
4. Kujala UM, Taimela S, Antti-Poika I, *et al*. Acute injuries in soccer, ice hockey, volleyball, basketball, judo, and karate: analysis of national registry data. *BMJ*. 1995; 311: 1465–1468.
5. Van Mechelen W, Twisk J, Molendijk A, *et al*. Subject-related risk factors for sports injuries: a 1-yr prospective study in young adults. *Med Sci Sports Exerc*. 1996; 28: 1171–1179.
6. MacKay M, Scanlan A, Olsen L, *et al*. Looking for the evidence: a systematic review of prevention strategies addressing sport and recreational injury among children and youth. *J Sci Med Sport*. 2004; 7: 58–73.
7. Emery CA. Injury prevention and future research. *Med Sport Sci*. 2005; 49: 170–191.
8. Steffen K, Engebretsen L. More data needed on injury risk among young elite athletes. *Br J Sports Med*. 2010; 44: 485–489.
9. Pakzad-Vaezi K, Singhal A. Trends in paediatric sport- and recreation-related injuries: An injury surveillance study at the British Columbia Children's Hospital (Vancouver, British Columbia) from 1992 to 2005. *Paediatr Child Health*. 2011; 16: 217–221.
10. Lykissas MG, Eismann EA, Parikh SN. Trends in pediatric sports-related and recreation-related injuries in the United States in the last decade. *J Pediatr Orthop*. 2013; 33: 803–810.
11. Acton CH, Thomas S, Nixon JW, *et al*. Children and bicycles: what is really happening? Studies of fatal and non-fatal bicycle injury. *Inj Prev*. 1995; 1: 86–91.
12. Janssens L, Holtslag HR, Leenen LPH, *et al*. Trends in moderate to severe paediatric trauma in Central Netherlands. *Injury*. 2014; 45: 1190–1195.
13. Baker S, Fowler C, Dannenberg A. *Injuries to bicyclists: A national perspective*. Baltimore, MD: The Johns Hopkins University Injury Prevention Centre; 1993.
14. Clarsen B, Krosshaug T, Bahr R. Overuse injuries in professional road cyclists. *Am J Sports Med*. 2010; 38: 2494–2501.
15. Holmes JC, Pruitt AL, Whalen NJ. Lower extremity overuse in bicycling. *Clin Sports Med*. 1994; 13: 187–205.
16. Mellion MB. Neck and back pain in bicycling. *Clin Sports Med*. 1994; 13: 137–164.
17. Weiss BD. Clinical syndromes associated with bicycle seats. *Clin Sports Med*. 1994; 13: 175–186.
18. Frauscher F, Klauser A, Hobisch A, Pallwein L, Stenzl A. Subclinical microtraumatisation of the scrotal contents in extreme mountain biking. *Lancet*. 2000; 356: 1414.
19. Richmond DR. Handlebar problems in bicycling. *Clin Sports Med*. 1994; 13: 165–173.
20. Rousselet MC, Saint-Andre JP, L'Hoste P, *et al*. Stenotic intimal thickening of the external iliac artery in competition cyclists. *Hum Pathol*. 1990; 21: 524–529.
21. Friede AM, Azzara C V, Gallagher SS, Guyer B. The epidemiology of injuries to bicycle riders. *Pediatr Clin North Am*. 1985; 32: 141–151.
22. Aleman KB, Meyers MC. Mountain biking injuries in children and adolescents. *Sports Med*. 2010; 40: 77–90.
23. Thompson DC, Patterson MQ. Cycle helmets and the prevention of injuries. Recommendations for competitive sport. *Sports Med*. 1998; 25: 213–219.
24. Macpherson AK, To TM, Macarthur C, *et al*. Impact of mandatory helmet legislation on bicycle-related head injuries in children: a population-based study. *Pediatrics*. 2002; 110: e60.
25. Mock CN, Maier R V, Boyle E, Pilcher S, Rivara FP. Injury prevention strategies to promote helmet use decrease severe head injuries at a level I trauma center. *J Trauma*. 1995; 39: 29–33; discussion 34–35.
26. Rössler R, Donath L, Verhagen E, *et al*. Exercise-based injury prevention in child and adolescent sport: a systematic review and meta-analysis. *Sports Med*. 2014; 44: 1733–1748.
27. Burke ER. Proper fit of the bicycle. *Clin Sports Med*. 1994; 13: 1–14.
28. Kronisch RL, Pfeiffer RP, Chow TK, Hummel CB. Gender differences in acute mountain bike racing injuries. *Clin J Sport Med*. 2002; 12: 158–164.

29. Robinson DL. No clear evidence from countries that have enforced the wearing of helmets. *BMJ*. 2006; 332: 722–725.
30. Colvin AC, Lynn A. Sports-related injuries in the young female athlete. *Mt Sinai J Med*. 2010; 77: 307–314.
31. Hincapié CA, Morton EJ, Cassidy JD. Musculoskeletal injuries and pain in dancers: A systematic review. *Arch Phys Med Rehabil*. 2008; 89: 1819–1829.
32. Allen N, Ribbans W, Nevill A, Wyon M. Musculoskeletal injuries in dance: A systematic review. *Int J Phys Med Rehabil*. 2014; 03: 1–8.
33. Reid DC, Burnham RS, Saboe LA, Kushner SF. Lower extremity flexibility patterns in classical ballet dancers and their correlation to lateral hip and knee injuries. *Am J Sports Med*. 1987; 15: 347–352.
34. Ekegren CL, Quested R, Brodrick A. Injuries in pre-professional ballet dancers: Incidence, characteristics and consequences. *J Sci Med Sport*. 2014; 17: 271–275.
35. Bowling A. Injuries to dancers: prevalence, treatment, and perceptions of causes. *BMJ*. 1989; 298: 731–734.
36. Gamboa JM, Roberts LA, Maring J, Fergus A. Injury patterns in elite preprofessional ballet dancers and the utility of screening programs to identify risk characteristics. *J Orthop Sports Phys Ther*. 2008; 38: 126–136.
37. Steinberg N, Siev-Ner I, Peleg S, *et al*. Injury patterns in young, non-professional dancers. *J Sports Sci*. 2011; 29: 47–54.
38. Steinberg N, Aujla I, Zeev A, Redding E. Injuries among talented young dancers: findings from the UK Centres for Advanced Training. *Int J Sports Med*. 2014; 35: 238–244.
39. Ojofeitimi S, Bronner S, Woo H. Injury incidence in hip hop dance. *Scand J Med Sci Sports*. 2012; 22: 347–355.
40. Kauther MD, Wedemeyer C, Wegner A, Kauther KM, von Knoch M. Breakdance injuries and overuse syndromes in amateurs and professionals. *Am J Sports Med*. 2009; 37: 797–802.
41. Campoy FAS, Coelho LR de O, Bastos FN, *et al*. Investigation of risk factors and characteristics of dance injuries. *Clin J Sport Med*. 2011; 21: 493–498.
42. Wanke EM, Mill H, Wanke A, *et al*. Dance floors as injury risk: analysis and evaluation of acute injuries caused by dance floors in professional dance with regard to preventative aspects. *Med Probl Perform Art*. 2012; 27: 137–142.
43. Kadel NJ, Teitz CC, Kronmal RA. Stress fractures in ballet dancers. *Am J Sports Med*. 1992; 20: 445–449.
44. Byhring S, Bø K. Musculoskeletal injuries in the Norwegian National Ballet: A prospective cohort study. *Scand J Med Sci Sports*. 2002; 12: 365–370.
45. Wiesler ER, Hunter DM, Martin DF, Curl WW, Hoen H. Ankle flexibility and injury patterns in dancers. *Am J Sports Med*. 1996; 24: 754–757.
46. Negus V, Hopper D, Briffa NK. Associations between turnout and lower extremity injuries in classical ballet dancers. *J Orthop Sports Phys Ther*. 2005; 35: 307–318.
47. Coplan JA. Ballet dancer's turnout and its relationship to self-reported injury. *J Orthop Sports Phys Ther*. 2002; 32: 579–584.
48. Stoller SM, Hekmat F, Kleiger B. A comparative study of the frequency of anterior impingement exostoses of the ankle in dancers and nondancers. *Foot Ankle*. 1984; 4: 201–203.
49. Scheller AD, Kasser JR, Quigley TB. Tendon injuries about the ankle. *Clin Sports Med*. 1983; 2: 631–641.
50. Benson JE, Geiger CJ, Eiserman PA, Wardlaw GM. Relationship between nutrient intake, body mass index, menstrual function, and ballet injury. *J Am Diet Assoc*. 1989; 89: 58–63.
51. Warren MP, Brooks-Gunn J, Hamilton LH, Warren LF, Hamilton WG. Scoliosis and fractures in young ballet dancers. Relation to delayed menarche and secondary amenorrhea. *N Engl J Med*. 1986; 314: 1348–1353.
52. Castelo-Branco C, Reina F, Montivero AD, Colodrón M, Vanrell JA. Influence of high-intensity training and of dietetic and anthropometric factors on menstrual cycle disorders in ballet dancers. *Gynecol Endocrinol*. 2006; 22: 31–35.
53. Askling C, Lund H, Saartok T, Thorstensson A. Self-reported hamstring injuries in student-dancers. *Scand J Med Sci Sports*. 2002; 12: 230–235.
54. Micheli LJ, Sohn RS, Solomon R. Stress fractures of the second metatarsal involving Lisfranc's joint in ballet dancers. A new overuse injury of the foot. *J Bone Joint Surg Am*. 1985; 67: 1372–1375.
55. Russell JA. Preventing dance injuries: current perspectives. *Open Access J Sports Med*. 2013; 4: 199–210.
56. Reid DC. Prevention of hip and knee injuries in ballet dancers. *Sports Med*. 1988; 6: 295–307.
57. Allen N, Nevill AM, Brooks JHM, Koutedakis Y, Wyon MA. The effect of a comprehensive injury audit program on injury incidence in ballet: a 3-year prospective study. *Clin J Sport Med*. 2013; 23: 373–378.
58. Bronner S, Ojofeitimi S, Rose D. Injuries in a modern dance company: effect of comprehensive management on injury incidence and time loss. *Am J Sports Med*. 2003; 31: 365–373.
59. Ojofeitimi S, Bronner S. Injuries in a modern dance company effect of comprehensive management on injury incidence and cost. *J Dance Med Sci*. 2011; 15: 116–122.
60. Caine DJ, Nassar L. Gymnastics injuries. *Med Sport Sci*. 2005; 48: 18–58.
61. Sands WA, Shultz BB, Newman AP. Women's gymnastics injuries. A 5-year study. *Am J Sports Med*. 1993; 21: 271–276.
62. Westermann RW, Giblin M, Vaske A, Grosso K, Wolf BR. Evaluation of men's and women's gymnastics injuries: A 10-year observational study. *Sports Health*. 2015; 7: 161–165.
63. Bahr R. No injuries, but plenty of pain? On the methodology for recording overuse symptoms in sports. *Br J Sports Med*. 2009; 43: 966–972.
64. Dixon M, Fricker P. Injuries to elite gymnasts over 10 yr. *Med Sci Sports Exerc*. 1993; 25: 1322–1329.
65. Purnell M, Shirley D, Nicholson L, Adams R. Acrobatic gymnastics injury: Occurrence, site and training risk factors. *Phys Ther Sport*. 2010; 11: 40–46.
66. Marshall SW, Covassin T, Dick R, Nassar LG, Agel J. Descriptive epidemiology of collegiate women's gymnastics injuries: National Collegiate Athletic Association Injury Surveillance System, 1988–1989 through 2003–2004. *J Athl Train*. 2007; 42: 234–240.
67. Takei Y. A comparaison of techniques used in performing the men's compulsory gymnastic vault at the 1988 Olympics. *Int J Sport Biomech*. 1991; 7: 54–75.
68. Panzer V, Wood G, Bates B, Mason B. Lower extremity loads in landings of elite gymnasts. In: de Groot G, Hollander A, Huijing P, van Ingen Schenau G (eds.) *Biomechanics XI-B*. Amsterdam: Free University Press; 1988. p. 727–735.
69. Hall SJ. Mechanical contribution to lumbar stress injuries in female gymnasts. *Med Sci Sports Exerc*. 1986; 18: 599–602.
70. Sands W, Cheltham P. Velocity of the vault run: junior elite female gymnasts. *Technique*. 1986; 6: 10–14.
71. Leonard H, Joffe AR. Children presenting to a Canadian hospital with trampoline-related cervical spine injuries. *Paediatr Child Health*. 2009; 14: 84–88.
72. Brown PG, Lee M. Trampoline injuries of the cervical spine. *Pediatr Neurosurg*. 2000; 32: 170–175.
73. Loder RT, Schultz W, Sabatino M. Fractures from trampolines: results from a national database, 2002 to 2011. *J Pediatr Orthop*. 2014; 34: 683–690.
74. Torg JS. Trampoline-induced quadriplegia. *Clin Sports Med*. 1987; 6: 73–85.
75. Caine D, Cochrane B, Caine C, Zemper E. An epidemiologic investigation of injuries affecting young competitive female gymnasts. *Am J Sports Med*. 1989; 17: 811–820.
76. De Smet L, Claessens A, Lefevre J, Beunen G. Gymnast wrist: an epidemiologic survey of ulnar variance and stress changes of the radial physis in elite female gymnasts. *Am J Sports Med*. 1994; 22: 846–850.
77. Meeusen R, Borms J. Gymnastic injuries. *Sports Med*. 1992; 13: 337–356.
78. Fuller CW, Bahr R, Dick RW, Meeuwisse WH. A framework for recording recurrences, reinjuries, and exacerbations in injury surveillance. *Clin J Sport Med*. 2007; 17: 197–200.

79. Kolt GS, Kirkby RJ. Epidemiology of injury in elite and subelite female gymnasts: a comparison of retrospective and prospective findings. *Br J Sports Med.* 1999; 33: 312–318.
80. Caine D, Knutzen K, Howe W, *et al.* A three-year epidemiological study of injuries affecting young female gymnasts. *Phys Ther Sport.* 2003; 4: 10–23.
81. Léglise M. Limits on young gymnast's involvement in high-level sport. *Technique.* 1998; 18: 8–14.
82. Lueken J, Stone J, Wallach B. Olympic training center report men's gymnastics injuries. *Gymnast Saf Update.* 1993; 8: 4–5.
83. Caine D, Roy S, Singer KM, Broekhoff J. Stress changes of the distal radial growth plate. A radiographic survey and review of the literature. *Am J Sports Med.* 1992; 20: 290–298.
84. Daly RM, Bass SL, Finch CF. Balancing the risk of injury to gymnasts: how effective are the counter measures? *Br J Sports Med.* 2001; 35: 8–18; quiz 19.
85. Gremion G, Bielinski R, Vallotton J, *et al.* [Gymnastic world championship in Lausanne: medical staffing]. *Rev Med Suisse Romande.* 1998; 118: 709–711.
86. Sands W, Crain R, Lee K. Gymnastics coaching survey. *Technique.* 1990; 10: 22–27.
87. Minden H. Psychological factors related to the occurrence of athletic injuries. *J Sport Exerc Psychol.* 1988; 10: 167–173.
88. Smith A, Andrish J, Micheli L. Current comment from the American College of Sports Medicine. August 1993–'The prevention of sport injuries of children and adolescents'. *Med Sci Sports Exerc.* 1993; 25: 1–7.
89. Emery CA, Hagel B, Morrongiello BA. Injury prevention in child and adolescent sport: whose responsibility is it? *Clin J Sport Med.* 2006; 16: 514–521.
90. Harringe ML, Lindblad S, Werner S. Do team gymnasts compete in spite of symptoms from an injury? *Br J Sports Med.* 2004; 38: 398–401.
91. Nemeth RL, von Baeyer CL, Rocha EM. Young gymnasts' understanding of sport-related pain: a contribution to prevention of injury. *Child Care Health Dev.* 2005; 31: 615–625.
92. Mehl AJ, Nelson NG, McKenzie LB. Running-related injuries in school-age children and adolescents treated in emergency departments from 1994 through 2007. *Clin Pediatr (Phila).* 2011; 50: 126–132.
93. Rauh MJ. Summer training factors and risk of musculoskeletal injury among high-school cross-country runners. *J Orthop Sport Phys Ther.* 2014; 44: 793–804.
94. Rauh MJ, Koepsell TD, Rivara FP, Margherita AJ, Rice SG. Epidemiology of musculoskeletal injuries among high school cross-country runners. *Am J Epidemiol.* 2006; 163: 151–159.
95. Lopes AD, Hespanhol Junior LC, Yeung SS, *et al.* What are the main running-related musculoskeletal injuries? A systematic review. *Sports Med.* 2012; 42: 891–905.
96. Tenforde AS, Sayres LC, McCurdy ML, *et al.* Overuse injuries in high school runners: lifetime prevalence and prevention strategies. *PMR.* 2011; 3: 125–131.
97. Kelsey JL, Bachrach LK, Procter-Gray E, *et al.* Risk factors for stress fracture among young female cross-country runners. *Med Sci Sports Exerc.* 2007; 39: 1457–1463.
98. Saragiotto BT, Yamato TP, Hespanhol Junior LC, *et al.* What are the main risk factors for running-related injuries? *Sport Med.* 2014; 44: 1153–1163.
99. Rauh MJ, Koepsell TD, Rivara FP, Rice SG, Margherita AJ. Quadriceps angle and risk of injury among high school cross-country runners. *J Orthop Sports Phys Ther.* 2007; 37: 725–733.
100. Malisoux L, Nielsen RO, Urhausen A, Theisen D. A step towards understanding the mechanisms of running-related injuries. *J Sci Med Sport.* 2014; 18: 523–528.
101. Nielsen RØ, Parner ET, Nohr EA, *et al.* Excessive progression in weekly running distance and risk of running-related injuries: an association which varies according to type of injury. *J Orthop Sports Phys Ther.* 2014; 44: 739–47.
102. Jakobsen BW, Krøner K, Schmidt SA, Kjeldsen A. Prevention of injuries in long-distance runners. *Knee Surg Sports Traumatol Arthrosc.* 1994; 2: 245–249.
103. Burns TP, Steadman JR, Rodkey WG. Alpine skiing and the mature athlete. *Clin Sports Med.* 1991; 10: 327–342.
104. Ruedl G, Schobersberger W, Pocecco E, *et al.* Sport injuries and illnesses during the first Winter Youth Olympic Games 2012 in Innsbruck, Austria. *Br J Sport Med.* 2012; 46: 1030–1037.
105. Kim S, Endres NK, Johnson RJ, Ettlinger CF, Shealy JE. Snowboarding injuries: trends over time and comparisons with alpine skiing injuries. *Am J Sports Med.* 2012; 40: 770–776.
106. Reid DC, Saboe L. Spine fractures in winter sports. *Sports Med.* 1989; 7: 393–399.
107. Shorter NA, Jensen PE, Harmon BJ, Mooney DP. Skiing injuries in children and adolescents. *J Trauma.* 1996; 40: 997–1001.
108. Feagin JA, Lambert KL, Cunningham RR, *et al.* Consideration of the anterior cruciate ligament injury in skiing. *Clin Orthop Relat Res.* 1987; Mar: 13–18.
109. Bladin C, McCrory P. Snowboarding injuries. An overview. *Sports Med.* 1995; 19: 358–364.
110. Chow TK, Corbett SW, Farstad DJ. Spectrum of injuries from snowboarding. *J Trauma.* 1996; 41: 321–325.
111. Hume PA, Lorimer A V, Griffiths PC, Carlson I, Lamont M. Recreational snow-sports injury risk factors and countermeasures: A meta-analysis review and Haddon Matrix evaluation. *Sports Med.* 2015; 45: 1175–1190.
112. Berghold F, Seidl AM. [Snowboarding accidents in the Alps. Assessment of risk, analysis of the accidents and injury profile]. *Schweiz Z Sportmed.* 1991; 39: 13–20.
113. Blitzer CM, Johnson RJ, Ettlinger CF, Aggeborn K. Downhill skiing injuries in children. *Am J Sports Med.* 1984; 12: 142–147.
114. Xiang H, Kelleher K, Shields BJ, Brown KJ, Smith GA. Skiing- and snowboarding-related injuries treated in US emergency departments, 2002. *J Trauma.* 2005; 58: 112–118.
115. Hagel BE, Pless IB, Goulet C, Platt RW, Robitaille Y. Effectiveness of helmets in skiers and snowboarders: case-control and case crossover study. *BMJ.* 2005; 330: 281.
116. Sulheim S, Holme I, Ekeland A, Bahr R. Helmet use and risk of head injuries in alpine skiers and snowboarders. *JAMA.* 2006; 295: 919–924.
117. Pigozzi F, Santori N, Di Salvo V, Parisi A, Di-Luigi L. Snowboard traumatology: an epidemiological study. *Orthopedics.* 1997; 20: 505–509.
118. Rønning R, Rønning I, Gerner T, Engebretsen L. The efficacy of wrist protectors in preventing snowboarding injuries. *Am J Sports Med.* 2001; 29: 581–585.
119. O'Neill DF. Wrist injuries in guarded versus unguarded first time snowboarders. *Clin Orthop Relat Res.* 2003; 409: 91–95.
120. Machold W, Kwasny O, Gässler P, *et al.* Risk of injury through snowboarding. *J Trauma.* 2000; 48: 1109–1114.
121. Jłrgensen U, Fredensborg T, Haraszuk JP, Crone KL. Reduction of injuries in downhill skiing by use of an instructional ski-video: A prospective randomised intervention study. *Knee Surg Sports Traumatol Arthrosc.* 1998; 6: 194–200.
122. Ettlinger CF, Johnson RJ, Shealy JE. A method to help reduce the risk of serious knee sprains incurred in alpine skiing. *Am J Sports Med.* 1995; 23: 531–537.
123. Russell K, Christie J, Hagel BE. The effect of helmets on the risk of head and neck injuries among skiers and snowboarders: A meta-analysis. *CMAJ.* 2010; 182: 333–340.
124. Meyers MC, Laurent CM, Higgins RW, Skelly W. Downhill ski injuries in children and adolescents. *Sport Med.* 2007; 37: 485–499.
125. Chase KI, Caine DJ, Goodwin BJ, Whitehead JR, Romanick MA. A prospective study of injury affecting competitive collegiate swimmers. *Res Sports Med.* 2013; 21: 111–123.
126. Pollard KA, Gottesman BL, Rochette LM, Smith GA. Swimming injuries treated in US EDs: 1990 to 2008. *Am J Emerg Med.* 2013; 31: 803–809.
127. Ciullo J V, Stevens GG. The prevention and treatment of injuries to the shoulder in swimming. *Sports Med.* 1989; 7: 182–204.

128. Ciullo J V. Swimmer's shoulder. *Clin Sports Med.* 1986; 5: 115–137.
129. Stocker D, Pink M, Jobe FW. Comparison of shoulder injury in collegiate- and master's-level swimmers. *Clin J Sport Med.* 1995; 5: 4–8.
130. Bak K, Bue P, Olsson G. [Injury patterns in Danish competitive swimming]. *Ugeskr Laeger.* 1989; 151: 2982–2984.
131. Costill D, Maglischo E, Richardson A. *Swimming.* Oxford: Backwell Science; 1992.
132. Grote K, Lincoln TL, Gamble JG. Hip adductor injury in competitive swimmers. *Am J Sports Med.* 2004; 32: 104–108.
133. Brushøj C, Bak K, Johannsen H V, Faunø P. Swimmers' painful shoulder arthroscopic findings and return rate to sports. *Scand J Med Sci Sports.* 2007; 17: 373–377.
134. McMaster WC. Swimming injuries. An overview. *Sports Med.* 1996; 22: 332–336.
135. Bak K, Magnusson SP. Shoulder strength and range of motion in symptomatic and pain-free elite swimmers. *Am J Sports Med.* 1997; 25: 454–459.
136. Fowler P, Webster-Bogaert M. Swimming. In: Reider B (ed.) *Sports medicine, the school-age athlete.* Philadelphia: Saunders Company; 1991. p. 429–446.
137. Fowler PJ, Regan WD. Swimming injuries of the knee, foot and ankle, elbow, and back. *Clin Sports Med.* 1986; 5: 139–148.
138. Kenal KA, Knapp LD. Rehabilitation of injuries in competitive swimmers. *Sports Med.* 1996; 22: 337–347.
139. Verhagen EALM, van Stralen MM, van Mechelen W. Behaviour, the key factor for sports injury prevention. *Sports Med.* 2010; 40: 899–906.
140. Hibberd EE, Myers JB. Practice habits and attitudes and behaviors concerning shoulder pain in high school competitive club swimmers. *Clin J Sport Med.* 2013; 23: 450–455.
141. Kibler WB, McQueen C, Uhl T. Fitness evaluations and fitness findings in competitive junior tennis players. *Clin Sports Med.* 1988; 7: 403–416.
142. Pluim BM, Loeffen FGJ, Clarsen B, Bahr R, Verhagen EALM. A one-season prospective study of injuries and illness in elite junior tennis. *Scand J Med Sci Sports.* 2015; 26: 564–571.
143. Krøner K, Schmidt SA, Nielsen AB, *et al.* Badminton injuries. *Br J Sports Med.* 1990; 24: 169–172.
144. Garrick JG, Requa RK. Injuries in high school sports. *Pediatrics.* 1978; 61: 465–469.
145. Maquirriain J, Ghisi JP. The incidence and distribution of stress fractures in elite tennis players. *Br J Sports Med.* 2006; 40: 454–459; discussion 459.
146. Gregg JR, Torg E. Upper extremity injuries in adolescent tennis players. *Clin Sports Med.* 1988; 7: 371–385.
147. Boyd KT, Batt ME. Stress fracture of the proximal humeral epiphysis in an elite junior badminton player. *Br J Sports Med.* 1997; 31: 252–253.
148. Larrison WI, Hersh PS, Kunzweiler T, Shingleton BJ. Sports-related ocular trauma. *Ophthalmology.* 1990; 97: 1265–1269.
149. Black KP, Lombardo JA. Suprascapular nerve injuries with isolated paralysis of the infraspinatus. *Am J Sports Med.* 1990; 18: 225–228.
150. Kibler W Ben, Safran M. Tennis injuries. *Med Sport Sci.* 2005; 48: 120–137.
151. Van der Hoeven H, Kibler WB. Shoulder injuries in tennis players. *Br J Sports Med.* 2006; 40: 435–440; discussion 440.
152. Nirschl R, Sobel J. Tennis. In: Reider B (ed.) *Sports medicine, the school-age athlete.* Philadelphia: Saunders Company; 1991. p. 664–672.
153. Beillot J, Parier J. Tennis: Technological factors and epicondylitis. *J Traumatol du Sport.* 1998; 15: 1S62–1S69.
154. Gecha SR, Torg E. Knee injuries in tennis. *Clin Sports Med.* 1988; 7: 435–452.
155. Miller WA. Rupture of the musculotendinous juncture of the medial head of the gastrocnemius muscle. *Am J Sports Med.* 1977; 5: 191–193.
156. Silva RT, Takahashi R, Berra B, Cohen M, Matsumoto MH. Medical assistance at the Brazilian juniors tennis circuit–A one-year prospective study. *J Sci Med Sport.* 2003; 6: 14–18.
157. Ellenbecker TS, Roetert EP, Piorkowski PA, Schulz DA. Glenohumeral joint internal and external rotation range of motion in elite junior tennis players. *J Orthop Sports Phys Ther.* 1996; 24: 336–341.
158. Bylak J, Hutchinson MR. Common sports injuries in young tennis players. *Sports Med.* 1998; 26: 119–132.
159. Hjelm N, Werner S, Renstrom P. Injury risk factors in junior tennis players: a prospective 2-year study. *Scand J Med Sci Sports.* 2012; 22: 40–48.
160. Ellenbecker TS, Davies GJ, Rowinski MJ. Concentric versus eccentric isokinetic strengthening of the rotator cuff. Objective data versus functional test. *Am J Sports Med.* 1988; 16: 64–69.
161. Kibler WB, Chandler TJ. Range of motion in junior tennis players participating in an injury risk modification program. *J Sci Med Sport.* 2003; 6: 51–62.
162. Knudson D V. Factors affecting force loading on the hand in the tennis forehand. *J Sports Med Phys Fitness.* 1991; 31: 527–531.
163. Herman K, Barton C, Malliaras P, Morrissey D. The effectiveness of neuromuscular warm-up strategies, that require no additional equipment, for preventing lower limb injuries during sports participation: A systematic review. *BMC Med.* 2012; 10: 1–12.
164. Reeser JC, Verhagen E, Briner WW, Askeland TI, Bahr R. Strategies for the prevention of volleyball related injuries. *Br J Sports Med.* 2006; 40: 594–600; discussion 599–600.
165. Zaricznyj B, Shattuck LJ, Mast TA, Robertson R V, D'Elia G. Sports-related injuries in school-aged children. *Am J Sports Med.* 1980; 8: 318–324.
166. Verhagen EALM, Van der Beek AJ, Bouter LM, Bahr RM, van Mechelen W. A one season prospective cohort study of volleyball injuries. *Br J Sports Med.* 2004; 38: 477–481.
167. Kujala UM, Taimela S, Antti-Poika I, *et al.* Acute injuries in soccer, ice hockey, volleyball, basketball, judo, and karate: analysis of national registry data. *BMJ.* 1995; 311: 1465–1468.
168. Ferrari G, Turra S, Fama G, Gigante C. Traumatic injury to the hand and wrist in volleyball, and its evolution. *J Sport Traumatol Relat Res.* 1990; 12: 95–99.
169. Aagaard H, Jørgensen U. Injuries in elite volleyball. *Scand J Med Sci Sports.* 1996; 6: 228–232.
170. Knobloch K, Rossner D, Gössling T, Richter M, Krettek C. [Volleyball sport school injuries]. *Sportverletz Sportschaden.* 2004; 18: 185–189.
171. Pollard KA, Shields BJ, Smith GA. Pediatric volleyball-related injuries treated in US emergency departments, 1990–2009. *Clin Pediatr (Phila).* 2011; 50: 844–852.
172. Ferretti A, Puddu G, Mariani P, Neri M. Jumpers knee: An epidemiological study of volleyball players. *Phys Sportsmed.* 1984; 12: 97–106.
173. Sommer HM. Patellar chondropathy and apicitis, and muscle imbalances of the lower extremities in competitive sports. *Sports Med.* 1988; 5: 386–394.
174. Ferretti A, Papandrea P, Conteduca F, Mariani PP. Knee ligament injuries in volleyball players. *Am J Sports Med.* 1992; 20: 203–207.
175. Van Soest AJ, Roebroeck ME, Bobbert MF, Huijing PA, van Ingen Schenau GJ. A comparison of one-legged and two-legged countermovement jumps. *Med Sci Sports Exerc.* 1985; 17: 635–639.
176. Schafle MD, Requa RK, Patton WL, Garrick JG. Injuries in the 1987 national amateur volleyball tournament. *Am J Sports Med.* 1990; 18: 624–631.
177. Sturbois XS. Biomechanics and instability of the shoulder in volleyball. *Hermes (Belgium).* 1990; 21: 423–430.
178. Lindner K, Ferretti A. Volleyball. In: Caine D, Caine C, Lindner K (eds.) *Epidemiology of sports injuries.* Champaign, IL: Human Kinetics; 1996. p. 399–416.
179. Visnes H, Bahr R. Training volume and body composition as risk factors for developing jumper's knee among young elite volleyball players. *Scand J Med Sci Sports.* 2013; 23: 607–613.
180. DeHaven KE, Lintner DM. Athletic injuries: comparison by age, sport, and gender. *Am J Sports Med.* 1986; 14: 218–224.

181. Bobbert MF. Drop jumping as a training method for jumping ability. *Sports Med.* 1990; 9: 7–22.
182. Backx FJ, Erich WB, Kemper AB, Verbeek AL. Sports injuries in school-aged children. An epidemiologic study. *Am J Sports Med.* 1989; 17: 234–240.
183. Bahr R, Lian O, Bahr IA. A twofold reduction in the incidence of acute ankle sprains in volleyball after the introduction of an injury prevention program: a prospective cohort study. *Scand J Med Sci Sports.* 1997; 7: 172–177.
184. Janssen KW, Hendriks MRC, van Mechelen W, Verhagen E. The cost-effectiveness of measures to prevent recurrent ankle sprains: Results of a 3-arm randomized controlled trial. *Am J Sports Med.* 2014; 42: 1534–1541.
185. Janssen KW, van Mechelen W, Verhagen EALM. Bracing superior to neuromuscular training for the prevention of self-reported recurrent ankle sprains: A three-arm randomised controlled trial. *Br J Sports Med.* 2014; 48: 1235–1239.
186. Mahler P, Bizzini L, Marti M, Bouvier P. [The bill of rights for children in sport: a tool to promote the health and protect the child in sport]. *Rev Med Suisse.* 2006; 2: 1774–1777.

CHAPTER 44

Upper extremity and trunk injuries

Christopher M Shaw, Akin Cil, and Lyle J Micheli

Introduction

Injuries to the trunk and upper extremity in young athletes are increasingly common as a result of expanded participation and higher competitive levels in youth sports. Injury patterns are unique to the growing musculoskeletal system and specific to the demands of the involved sport. Recognition of injury patterns with early activity modification and the initiation of efficacious treatment can potentially prevent future deformity or disability and return the youth athlete to sport.

This chapter reviews the diagnosis and management of common upper extremity and trunk injuries in the paediatric athlete.

Upper extremity injuries

Shoulder injuries

General

The shoulder complex involves four articulations and multiple ossification centres. The secondary centre of ossification of the proximal humeral epiphysis is usually radiographically evident near 6 months of age. Additional ossification centres appear at the greater tuberosity between 7 months and 3 years of age and at the lesser tuberosity 2 years later. Between 5 and 7 years of age, these centres coalesce to form the proximal humeral epiphysis. The proximal humeral physis contributes approximately 80% of the longitudinal growth of the humerus and usually fuses between 19 and 22 years of age. The proximal humeral physis is extra-articular, except medially where the capsule extends beyond the anatomic neck, inserting on the medial metaphysis. The clavicle forms by intramembranous ossification in its central portion by the sixth gestational week. The medial secondary ossification centre appears between 12 and 19 years of age and fuses to the shaft between 22 and 25 years of age. The lateral epiphysis is inconsistent: appearing, ossifying, and fusing over a period of a few months around age 19 years. The scapula appears as a cartilaginous anlage in the first gestational week at the C4–C5 level, and gradually descends to its adult position overlying the first to fifth ribs. Failure of the scapula to descend results in persistent elevation and limited glenohumeral motion, a condition termed Sprengel's deformity. The scapula ossifies via intramembranous ossification with multiple remaining secondary ossification centres. The ossification centre of the coracoid process appears around age 1 year, coalescing with the ossification centre of the upper glenoid by 10 years of age. The acromion ossifies by multiple (from one to four) ossification centres, which usually appear at the time of puberty and fuse by 22 years of age. Failure of fusion of one of these ossification centres may result in an os acromionale. Various other scapular malformations may occur, including bipartite coracoid, acromion duplication, glenoid dysplasia, and scapular clefts.

Injury patterns to the paediatric athlete's shoulder tend to be sport specific. In American football, the shoulder ranks second only to the knee in number of overall injuries.[1–3] Injury patterns in rugby are similar. These injuries tend to result from macrotrauma and include glenohumeral dislocation, acromioclavicular separation, and clavicle fractures.

Bicycling is another popular recreational and sporting activity among children and adolescents. About 60% of all bicycle injuries occur in children between the ages of 5 and 14 years, and 85% of injuries involve the upper extremity.[4,5] A common injury pattern during bicycling involves lateral clavicle fracture or acromioclavicular separation from landing on the point of the shoulder when thrown from the bicycle.

Shoulder injuries during alpine skiing and snowboarding are being seen with increased frequency and account for approximately 40% of upper extremity injuries and 10% of all injuries.[6] In wrestling, 30% of injuries occur in the upper extremity, with the shoulder being the most commonly involved location.[7] Injury to the acromioclavicular joint is frequent, resulting from a direct blow of the shoulder against the mat.[7,8]

Overuse injuries to the shoulder, resulting from repetitive overhead use, are becoming more common in the paediatric age group. In baseball, injury to the paediatric shoulder from throwing is a result of microtrauma from repetitive motions of large rotational forces.[9–11] The proximal humeral physis is particularly vulnerable to these large, repetitive forces, resulting in a chronic physeal stress fracture termed Little League shoulder.[10–17] The shoulder in tennis is similarly subjected to repetitive overhead motions involving large torques; impingement and depression of the shoulder, called tennis shoulder, may occur.[18] Repetitive microtrauma also frequently leads to shoulder dysfunction in swimmers.[19] The risk of injury is related to the level of competition and the type of event. Injuries include impingement syndrome and glenohumeral instability. Multidirectional instability is often seen and is related to the underlying ligamentous laxity common in swimmers. Similarly, multidirectional instability can be seen in gymnasts who also frequently demonstrate generalized ligamentous laxity. Additional shoulder injuries unique to gymnasts include cortical hypertrophy at the pectoralis major insertion, ringman's shoulder, and supraspinatus tendonitis.[20–22]

Sternoclavicular joint injury

True sternoclavicular joint dislocations are rare in the skeletally immature. The characteristic injury involves a physeal fracture of the medial clavicle, most commonly a Salter–Harris I or II injury as the medial clavicular physis does not fuse until the early twenties.[23,24] The epiphysis stays attached to the sternum via the robust sternoclavicular ligaments and the medial clavicular shaft displaces posteriorly or anteriorly (Figure 44.1). Medial clavicular injury often results from an indirect force transmitted along the clavicle from a direct blow during contact sports to the lateral shoulder. If the shoulder is driven forward, posterior displacement of the medial clavicle occurs. Conversely, if the shoulder is driven posteriorly, anterior displacement of the medial clavicle occurs. The patient often describes a pop in the region of the sternoclavicular joint and there is tenderness to palpation of the medial clavicle. The direction of displacement may be obscured by marked swelling. Posterior displacement can be a medical emergency as the medial clavicle can impinge on vital mediastinal structures including the innominate great vessels, trachea, or oesophagus.[25,26] Venous congestion, diminished pulses, dysphagia, or dyspnoea should alert the clinician to the possibility of such injury. Standard anteroposterior radiographs of the chest or sternoclavicular joint are often hard to interpret given the overlapping spinal, thoracic, and mediastinal structures. A tangential X-ray taken in a 40° cephalad directed manner, the serendipity view, may aid in visualization of the medial clavicle displacement. Bilateral images should be obtained regularly for comparison purposes. Definitive delineation of the fracture pattern and direction of displacement is provided by computed tomography (CT scan).[27]

Minimally displaced fractures heal readily. Attempted reduction of anteriorly displaced fractures can be accomplished under local anaesthesia or sedation by placing the patient supine with a bolster between the scapulae. The arm is abducted 90° and then extended with gentle posterior pressure directly over the medial clavicle followed by protraction of the shoulder. After reduction, the shoulder is immobilized in a figure-of-eight dressing or shoulder immobilizer and a gentle range of motion exercise regimen is started as pain allows. Most fractures heal in 4–6 weeks, with return to sport after return of full painless range of motion and strength. Unstable fractures usually heal and remodel rapidly. Posteriorly displaced medial clavicular fractures with impingement of mediastinal structures require emergent reduction with thoracic surgery standby for the rare but potential injury of the major thoracic vessels.[28] Addressing these injuries is performed under general anaesthesia with the patient supine, traction is applied to the arm with the shoulder extended, and a towel clip can be used to reduce the medial clavicle. Patients with acute posterior physeal injuries, which are seen within the first 10 days, should have an attempted closed reduction.[29] However, if a patient persists beyond that time and does not show any signs of compromise of the mediastinal structures, they can be treated non-operatively with close observation.[29] There is occasionally need for open reduction and internal fixation of irreducible medial clavicular physeal fractures. Care should be taken with internal fixation and pins should never be used, as catastrophic complications of pin migration from hardware about the sternoclavicular joint have been reported.[30] Open reduction and stabilization of the torn periosteum and ligamentous structures with heavy non-absorbable suture should be attempted initially.

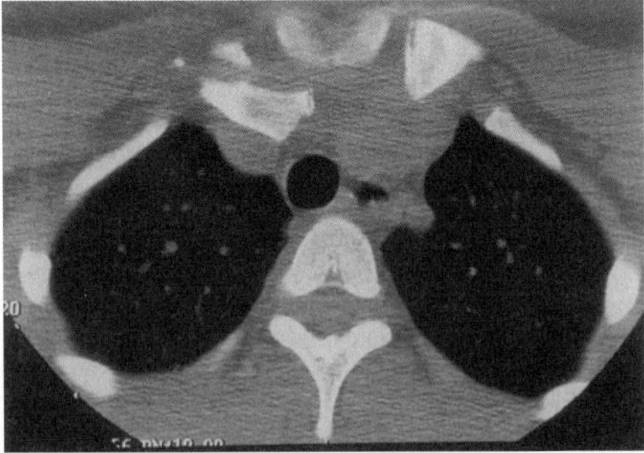

Figure 44.1 Sternoclavicular joint injury. Axial CT scan demonstrating physeal fracture/separation of the medial clavicle with compression of the innominate vein in a 16-year-old female.

Clavicle fracture

In children, the clavicle is the most commonly fractured bone in the shoulder region, accounting for 10–15% of all children's fractures, with 90% occurring in the midshaft.[31,32] The clavicular shaft is vulnerable to injury from direct blows during contact sports. In addition, indirect forces on the outstretched arm may lead to clavicular fracture. The clavicular shaft is mechanically vulnerable as a strut given its S-shaped configuration and the strong ligamentous bindings at each end. With fracture, there is limited shoulder motion, tenderness over the fracture site, and in some cases tenting of the overlying skin, which can lead to skin and soft tissue compromise. The proximal fragment may be elevated superiorly due to spasm of the sternocleidomastoid or trapezius muscles. Consequential neurovascular injury is rare, but should be assessed clinically, given the proximity of the subclavian vessels and the brachial plexus. Plain radiographs are usually sufficient for diagnosis and management. Younger children may exhibit a greenstick fracture or plastic deformation.[33]

The prognosis of clavicular shaft fractures in children is excellent. Immobilization is accomplished by a figure-of-eight bandage or shoulder immobilizer. Slings that exert significant pressure to affect a reduction should be avoided. Even displaced fractures typically heal readily with a bump of healing callous, which remodels over a period of 6–12 months. One study reported only 15 patients who had surgery for a clavicle fracture in a 21-year period.[34] Return to sport is allowed when the clavicle is non-tender; there is radiographic evidence of union and motion and strength are full. This usually occurs by 4–6 weeks in younger children and 6–10 weeks in the adolescent. Significant malunion which does not remodel and non-union of clavicular shaft fractures in the skeletally immature are rare, but can occur.[31] Open reduction and internal fixation is indicated for open fractures, fractures with neurovascular compromise, threatened skin from fracture displacement, and floating shoulder injuries.[35,36]

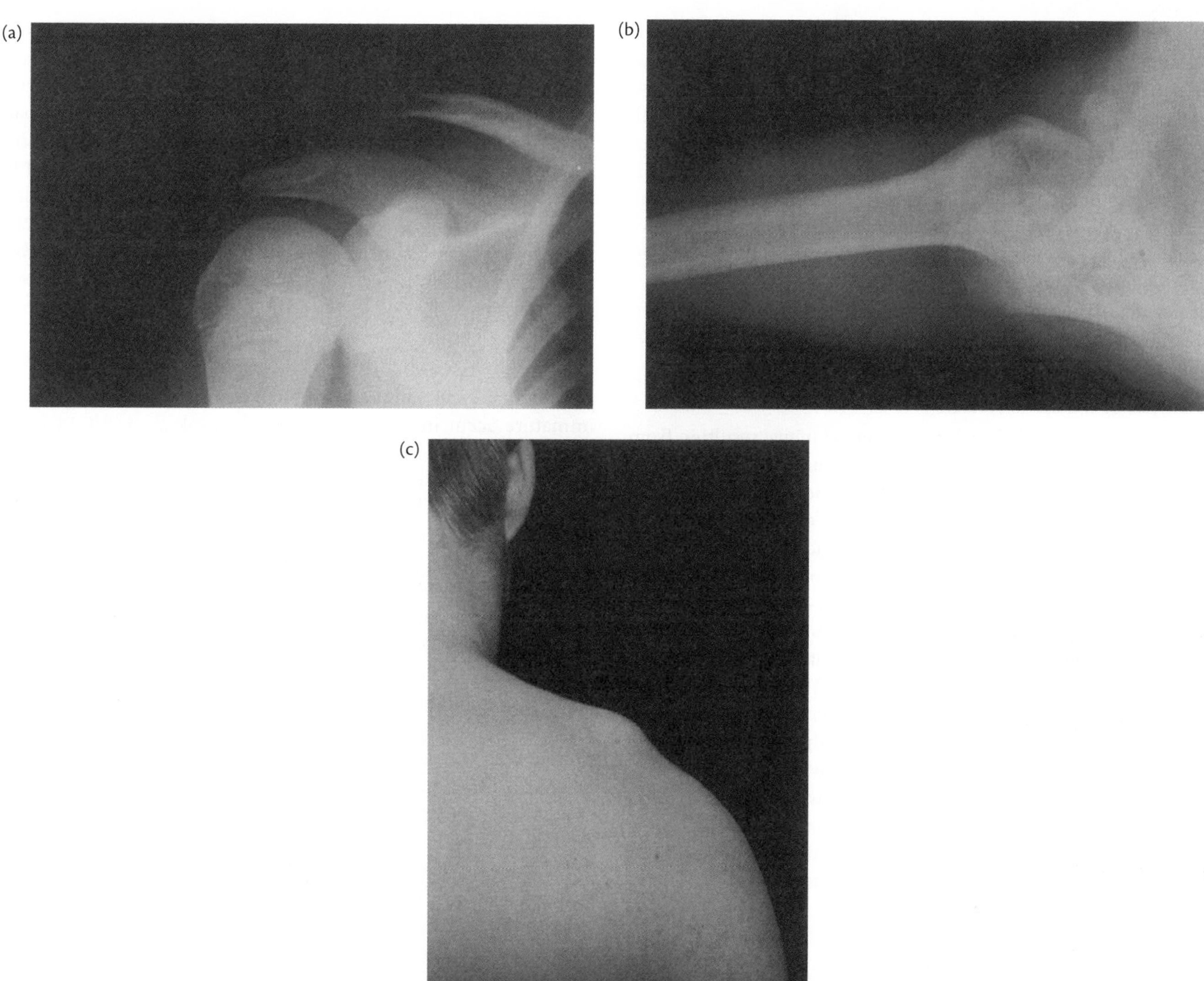

Figure 44.2 Type IV acromioclavicular injury. (a) AP X-ray, (b) axillary lateral view demonstrating posterior displacement, and (c) photograph showing posterior prominence of lateral clavicle in a 16-year-old male.

Acromioclavicular joint injury

A fall on the point of the shoulder usually results in acromioclavicular separation in the adult and older adolescent, but often results in physeal fracture of the lateral clavicle in prepubescents.[37–42] With lateral clavicle fracture and true acromioclavicular separation in the paediatric patient, displacement of the proximal clavicle occurs superiorly through a tear in the thick periosteal tube surrounding the distal clavicle. The lateral clavicular epiphysis, along with the acromioclavicular and coracoclavicular ligaments, usually remains continuous with the periosteal tube. In the case of the paediatric athlete with lateral clavicle physeal fracture or acromio-clavicular injury, the injury usually occurs after a fall or contact to the point of the shoulder. Pain and deformity are localized to the acromioclavicular joint. Plain radiographs are usually sufficient to evaluate the injury, or stress radiographs with 2.3–4.6 kg of traction may also aid in delineating the degree of instability. An axillary lateral radiograph can delineate anteroposterior displacement. Similar to adult acromioclavicular injuries, Rockwood[42] has classified paediatric acromioclavicular injuries based on the position of the lateral clavicle and the accompanying injury to the periosteal tube.

Type I injuries involve mild sprain of the acromioclavicular ligaments, without disruption of the periosteal tube. Type II injuries involve partial disruption of the dorsal periosteal tube, with slight widening of the acromioclavicular joint. Type III injuries involve a large dorsal disruption of the periosteal tube, with gross instability of the distal clavicle. Type IV injuries (Figure 44.2) involve disruption of the periosteal tube with posterior displacement of the lateral clavicle. Type V injuries involve periosteal tube disruption with >100% superior subcutaneous displacement of the lateral clavicle. Type VI injuries involve an inferior sub-coracoid dislocation of the lateral clavicle.

Non-operative management of acromioclavicular injuries in boys under 13 years of age is the mainstay of treatment as these injuries almost always represent a physeal fracture rather than a true acromioclavicular joint dislocation.[37–42] Thus, these injuries exhibit a great potential for healing and remodelling as the periosteal tube usually remains in continuity with the epiphyseal fragment and acromioclavicular and coracoclavicular ligaments. For type IV, V, and VI injuries with large displacement, operative stabilization may be indicated. Repair of the periosteal tube with or without internal fixation is usually performed. As with sterno-clavicular injury, hardware should be removed 6 weeks after repair to avoid complications of pin migration. For late adolescent and adult-type true acromioclavicular joint separations, non-operative management results in good outcomes for type I and II injuries, while operative management is indicated for type IV, V, and VI injuries. The management of type III injuries in the athlete remains controversial, with many recommending initial non-operative management.[43–45]

Osteolysis of the distal clavicle

Osteolysis of the distal clavicle is an overuse injury resulting from repetitive microtrauma, most commonly identified in young adult weightlifters. It has also been described as a potential sequelae following traumatic injury to the distal clavicle or acromioclavicular joint. In addition, this entity is being identified in other sports as cross-training has become more popular among younger athletes, who are weight training year-round for higher-level sports. Patients complain of an aching discomfort about the acromioclavicular joint after workouts, which progresses to interfere with training and eventually with activities of daily living. There is tenderness to palpation of the distal clavicle and pain with cross-chest adduction. Treatment consists of rest, particularly from weight training, and anti-inflammatory medications. For those who fail conservative treatment or who are unable to refrain from weight training, distal clavicle resection usually results in resolution of pain and return to sport.[46,47] Operative treatment should be delayed until skeletal maturity, if possible, to lessen the risk of re-ossification.

Little League shoulder

As a result of repetitive microtrauma from the large rotational moments involved in throwing, chronic stress fracture of the proximal humeral physis can occur. This entity has been termed Little League shoulder and is most commonly seen in high-performance male baseball pitchers between 11 and 13 years of age.[10–17,48] In addition to age and the large rotational forces of pitching, poor throwing mechanics may predispose to injury. In an extensive study of Little League pitchers, Albright[12] found that those who had poor pitching mechanics were more likely to be symptomatic. Patients complain of shoulder pain and there is typical widening of the proximal humeral physis on radiographs in addition to demineralization, sclerosis of the metaphysis, and fragmentation of the lateral aspect of the proximal humeral metaphysis. Often, comparative radiographs of the unaffected side are required to detect subtle physeal changes. Good results can usually be obtained by enforcing rest from pitching for the remainder of the season with a vigorous pre-season conditioning programme in the subsequent year. Excessive volume of throwing is the most likely risk factor. Proper throwing mechanics should be stressed with an emphasis on control instead of speed and intensity. Despite the absence of definitive evidence-based guidelines concerning throwing volume and pitch types, following guidelines from a recent study can serve as a baseline.[49] In order to minimize complaints of shoulder and elbow pain, pitchers between 9 and 14 years of age should not throw the curve ball or slider. These pitchers should use the fastball and change-up exclusively. Baseball organizations may consider limiting pitchers in this age group to 75 pitches in a game and 600 pitches in a season. Alternatively, the number of batters faced during a game and season could be limited to 15 and 120, respectively. Furthermore, pitchers should not be allowed to circumvent pitch limits by participating in more than one league at a time. Full-effort pitching should be limited, and all organized throwing sessions should be monitored closely by a responsible coach or parent. The recommended limits refer to full-effort, competitive game pitches and do not include warm-up pitches, practice pitches, throwing from other positions, and throwing drills, all of which are vital to a pitcher's development.[49]

Proximal humerus fracture

Approximately 20% of proximal humeral fractures in the skeletally immature occur in sporting events. The peak age is 10–14 years. Two-thirds involve the proximal humeral metaphysis and one-third involves the proximal humeral physis. Approximately one-fourth of fractures in this region occur through unicameral bone cysts.[50] Salter–Harris type I proximal humeral epiphyseal fractures occur primarily in neonates and children younger than 5 years of age. Metaphyseal fractures are seen mostly between 5 and 11 years of age. In older children, Salter–Harris type II fractures are predominant. With physeal fracture, the distal fragment usually displaces anteriorly and laterally through a relatively weaker area of periosteum, and the proximal fragment rotates into abduction and forward flexion due to its intact rotator cuff attachments; patients present with shoulder pain, limited motion, and tenderness to palpation. Routine roentgenograms are usually sufficient to demonstrate the fracture pattern, amount of displacement, or presence of a unicameral bone cyst.[50–56]

Non-displaced or minimally angulated metaphyseal or physeal fractures can usually be treated adequately with a shoulder immobilizer. Since most of these fractures are intrinsically stable, shoulder motion can be initiated early. There is great potential for remodelling of proximal humerus fractures due to the physis being very active. Thus, many moderately displaced, angulated, or bayoneted fractures can be accepted in less-than anatomic alignment with satisfactory functional outcomes, particularly in younger children. However, in young athletes involved in overhead sports, anatomic reduction must be attained and maintained to prevent loss of abduction and external rotation. Reduction is usually achieved by bringing the distal shaft fragment into flexion, abduction, and external rotation to align it with the proximal fragment. If stable after reduction, the fracture can be immobilized next to the chest. If unstable, the reduction must be held immobilized by a shoulder spica cast or shoulder spica brace. These require experience in application and may be poorly tolerated by patients and parents. Percutaneous pinning of the anatomically reduced fracture may allow the arm to be put in a sling after reduction, but maintenance of reduction must be monitored closely with radiographs (Figure 44.3). Rarely, open reduction is indicated as a result of interposed periosteum, deltoid, capsule, or more frequently, the long head of the biceps and can result in poor outcomes.[50–56] Despite this, there is literature support demonstrating that achieving and maintaining reduction in severely displaced proximal humeral epiphyseal fractures can be safely performed and results in excellent long-term shoulder function, especially in the older adolescent who has minimal potential for remodelling.[57]

(a)

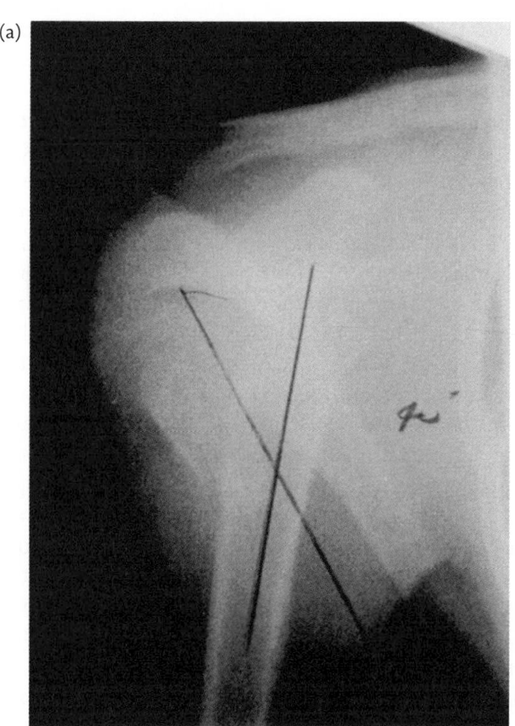

(b)

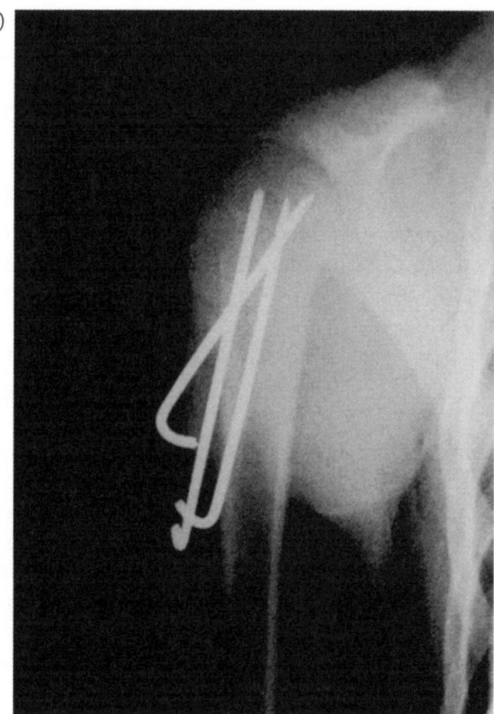

Figure 44.3 Proximal humerus fracture.
(a) Oblique view and (b) oblique view after reduction and percutaneous pinning in a 16-year-old male.

Glenohumeral instability

The glenohumeral joint is the most commonly dislocated large joint in adolescents and adults, but is less commonly involved in children before skeletal maturity. In large series of patients with glenohumeral instability, the proportion of skeletally immature patients ranges from 1 to 5%.[58–63] Traumatic anterior dislocation is by far the most common type of instability seen in adolescent athletes; however, multidirectional instability, posterior subluxation, and recurrent subluxation are being recognized with increasing frequency, particularly in gymnasts, swimmers, and throwing athletes. The patient with a traumatic anterior dislocation presents with pain, limited motion, and deformity. The humeral head may be palpated anteriorly, or in the axilla, and the arm is typically held in a slightly abducted, externally rotated position. Careful examination, particularly of the axillary nerve, is essential to rule out neurovascular injury. In the setting of posterior dislocation, the coracoid process may be prominent anteriorly, and the arm is often held in internal rotation and adduction. Anteroposterior and lateral views of the glenohumeral joint demonstrate the dislocation and identify associated fractures or Hill-Sachs lesions. Posterior dislocations are frequently missed emergently because of inadequate lateral images. Gentle reduction of an anterior dislocation is performed by one of several techniques including traction–counter traction, Stimson manoeuvre, or abduction manoeuvres. After a brief period of immobilization, a rehabilitation programme focused on rotator cuff strengthening and avoiding the evocative position is initiated.

Reported rates of recurrent instability after traumatic dislocation in adolescents and young adults vary between 25% and 90% in various series.[59,64–66] Rowe[61,62] reported 100% recurrence in children less than 10 years old and 94% recurrence in patients in the age group of 11 to 20 years. Rockwood[42] reported a recurrence rate of 50% in adolescent patients between 14 and 16 years of age and Marans *et al.*[60] reported a 100% recurrence rate in children between 4 and 15 years of age with open physes at the time of dislocation. Most recently Deitch *et al.*[67] evaluated adolescent patients and found recurrent instability in 75% of patients, which led to 50% of them requiring surgical stabilization. Management of the adolescent patient with significant recurrent instability is usually surgical involving capsulorraphy or a Bankart-type repair for capsulo-ligamentous disruption. Both arthroscopic and open techniques have been utilized with success rates of arthroscopic repair reaching the open repair in recent studies.[68] In addition to younger age, return to contact sports has also recently been noted to be associated with increased risk of recurrence.

Atraumatic instability can be seen in the paediatric athlete without a clear history of trauma, and may occur with throwing, hitting, swimming, or overhead serving. There is usually a lack of pain with these episodes of subluxation with spontaneous reduction. Clinical examination often reveals signs of generalized ligamentous laxity including hyper-extensibility of the elbows, knees, and metacarpophalangeal joints.[69] Examination may also show signs of multidirectional instability, including the sulcus sign, as well as excessive translation with anterior and posterior drawer tests or the load and shift test. A vigorous rehabilitation programme stressing rotator cuff strengthening is successful in most patients.[65] In those patients who fail non-operative management, a capsular shift reconstruction is recommended.[70]

Rotator cuff injury

Much less common than in adults, rotator cuff tendonitis and subacromial impingement can occur in the paediatric overhead athlete. Repetitive microtrauma in high-intensity overhead sports such as

Table 44.1 Timing of secondary centres of ossification about the elbow.

Site	Appearance	Epiphyseal Coalescence
Capitellum	18 months	14 years
Radial head	4 years	16 years
Medial epicondyle	5 years	15 years
Trochlea	8 years	14 years
Olecranon	10 years	14 years
Lateral epicondyle	12 years	16 years

swimming, baseball, and tennis can lead to tendonitis, secondary muscle weakness, mechanical imbalance, and secondary instability. In the paediatric athlete with joint laxity, true extrinsic impingement with compromise of the sub-acromial space is uncommon. Rather, impingement secondary to muscle imbalance and anterior instability is seen.[17,71–74] The usual symptom is pain with overhead activities progressing to constant pain or night pain.

Throwing athletes describe having pain on warm-up that does not improve. The pain tends to be the worst at the top of the throwing motion when the arm is in full external rotation or in deceleration after the ball is released. As the process continues, range of motion and strength may be diminished with loss of internal rotation. Hypermobility of the scapula with diminished periscapular strength is common. Impingement may be elicited with forward elevation or secondary to provocative instability tests. Magnetic resonance imaging (MRI) may be useful to assess the integrity of the rotator cuff; however, full-thickness tears in the paediatric or adolescent shoulder are uncommon.

In competitive swimmers, a variant of impingement syndrome can be seen, which is called the swimmer's shoulder. This involves anterior impingement associated with multidirectional instability and posterior subluxation.

Treatment of rotator cuff impingement consists of rest, non-steroidal anti-inflammatory medications, and a rehabilitation programme emphasizing restoration of range of motion, rotator cuff strengthening, and scapular stabilization with the goal of restoring dynamic joint stability. For cases refractory to non-operative management, shoulder arthroscopy may be of benefit to rule out associated intra-articular pathology. Sub-acromial decompression is rarely indicated in the paediatric athlete.[17,71–74]

Elbow injuries

General

The elbow joint has three major articulations: humero-radial, humero-ulnar, and proximal radio-ulnar joints. Delineating injury patterns in children can be challenging given the cartilaginous composition of the distal humerus and the multiple ossification centres. A site-specific clinical examination and radiographs of the contralateral uninjured elbow can prove useful in identifying injury. There are six major secondary centres of ossification, which appear and unite with the epiphysis at characteristic ages (see Table 44.1). Except for the medial and lateral epicondyles, the remaining ossification centres are intra-articular. The clinical carrying angle of the elbow averages 7° valgus alignment. There are several radiographic lines that are useful in assessing post-injury alignment. Bauman's angle, the angle between the capitellar physeal line and a line perpendicular to the humeral shaft, is a guide to the varus attitude of the distal humerus and should be within 5–8° of the contralateral elbow. On the lateral X-ray, the capitellum forms an angle flexed forward 30–40° from the humeral shaft, with the anterior humeral line bisecting the capitellum. Elbow stability is provided by congruous articular surfaces and soft-tissue constraint via capsular and ligamentous structures.

Elbow injury patterns in the paediatric athlete are dependent on the age-related stage of elbow development and the sport-specific mechanism of injury. Acute macro-traumatic injuries often result in fractures about the elbow. In younger children, supracondylar and lateral condyle fractures predominate. In adolescence and near- skeletal maturity, epicondylar and olecranon fractures are more common. In addition, elbow dislocations, ligamentous injuries, and muscular avulsions about the elbow can occur.

Repetitive microtraumatic injuries are often sport-specific involving upper extremity overuse. Repetitive throwing places high demands on the vulnerable developing elbow. Tension overload of the medial elbow restraints occurs during late cocking and can lead to medial epicondyle fragmentation, ulnar collateral ligament strain, flexor muscle strains, and traction ulnar neuritis. Compression overload of the lateral articulation also occurs during late cocking and can lead to chondral injuries and growth disturbances of the capitellum or radial head. Posteromedial shear overload of the posterior articular surface occurs during follow through and can lead to posterior spurs, olecranon apophysitis or avulsion, and spurs of the coronoid process.[75] In gymnastics, the elbow becomes a weight-bearing joint often subjected to repetitive large loads. Medial epicondyle traction injuries, partial tears of the flexor-pronator mass origin, ulnar collateral ligament strains, subluxation/dislocation often with medial epicondyle avulsion, osteochondral fractures of the capitellum, and posterior elbow spurring have been described.[2,22,76] Osteochondritis dissecans of the capitellum occurs with presentation similar to throwing injuries.

Supracondylar fracture

Supracondylar humerus fractures are the most common elbow fracture in children, accounting for approximately 75% of injuries. The mechanism of injury is usually an acute hyperextension load on the elbow from falling on an outstretched arm. The injury typically occurs in children aged 5–10 years because of thin bony architecture in the supracondylar region and ligamentous laxity. The distal fragment displaces posteriorly in over 95% of cases and the fracture is classified according to displacement: minimally displaced (type I), posterior angulation hinged on an intact posterior cortex (type II), and completely displaced (type III) (Figure 44.4). With complete displacement, rotational malalignment often occurs and can lead to cubitus-varus deformity if unreduced. Injury to the anterior interosseous nerve, radial nerve, median nerve, and brachial artery has been reported in 10–18% of displaced fractures.[77,78]

Treatment of supracondylar fractures is dictated by fracture type. Type I fractures are treated in a long-arm cast for 3 weeks with the elbow flexed 90° to 100°. Type II fractures can be treated with closed reduction and casting alone; however, the elbow should be flexed beyond 90° to maintain reduction, and this position may not be tolerated secondary to vascular insufficiency and swelling.

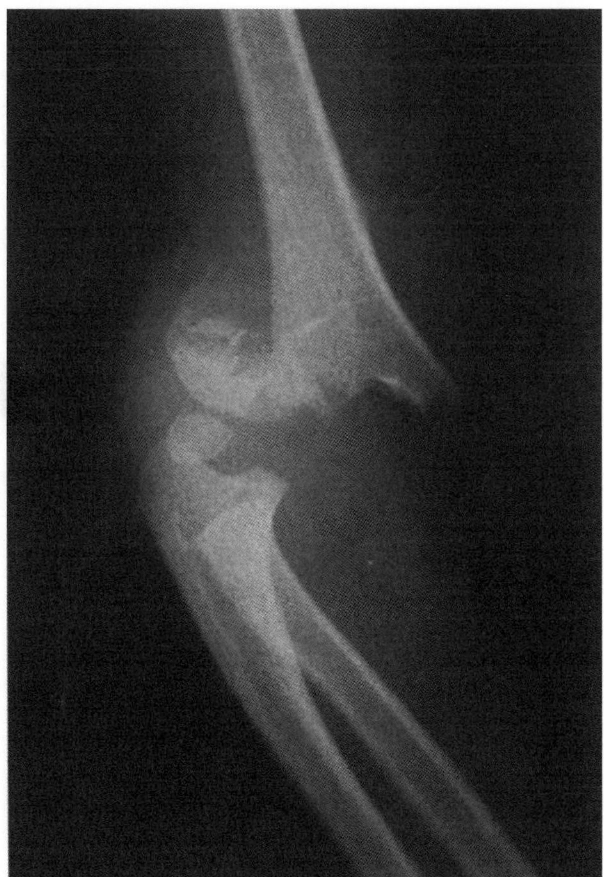

Figure 44.4 Supracondylar humerus fracture.
Oblique view of type III displaced fracture in a 6-year-old child.

Thus, closed reduction and percutaneous pinning with two lateral pins is now most often the treatment of choice. Closed reduction and percutaneous pinning is the preferred method of treatment for type III fractures, obviating the problems of ischaemic contracture (compartment syndrome) and cubitus varus deformity seen with closed treatment. Reduction is accomplished by extension of the elbow, followed by correction of medial–lateral translation, followed by traction and flexion of the elbow with anterior force on the olecranon. For fractures with medial displacement, the forearm is pronated which tightens the reduction against the intact medial periosteum while closing the lateral column. Systematic review of the literature suggests that the most biomechanically stable pin configuration involves medial and lateral pins crossing above the fracture line.[79] However, more recent randomized clinical trials have demonstrated that both lateral-entry pin fixation and medial- and lateral-entry pin fixation are effective in the treatment of completely displaced (type III) extension supracondylar fractures of the humerus in children, while minimizing the risk of neurological complications associated with surgical stabilization.[80] Motion is begun after the pins are removed at 3–4 weeks.[77,78] In cases with excessive comminution or other associated extremity injuries, skeletal traction with an olecranon pin may be beneficial.

Lateral condyle fracture

Lateral condyle fractures are the second most common elbow fractures in children and occur typically between 6 and 10 years of age. The mechanism of injury is often a valgus compressive force from the radial head or a varus tensile force on a supinated forearm from the extensor longus and brevis muscles, and collateral ligament.

There is a slightly increased risk of this fracture in children with a pre-existing cubitus varus.[81] A significant portion of the fragment is unossified, leaving often only a thin lateral metaphyseal rim of bone to herald the injury. This fracture involves both the physis and the articular surface, making anatomic reduction essential. Lateral condyle fractures are classified by the Milch system as either type I or type II, depending on where the fracture line exits at the articular surface. Milch I fractures occur at the capitellotrochlear groove and correspond to classic Salter–Harris type IV fractures. These fractures also tend to leave the elbow joint more stable. Milch II fractures extend into the apex of trochlea and although they resemble Salter–Harris type II fractures, it is still an articular fracture, and hence, a Salter–Harris type IV. Displacement and rotation are common due to the lateral extensor muscle mass. Treatment depends on the degree of displacement and fragment stability. Minimally displaced fractures, i.e. <3 mm, which are demonstrated to be stable by clinical examination, are treated with cast immobilization for approximately 3–4 weeks. Follow-up radiographs (particularly the oblique view) are essential 1 week after injury to rule out further displacement. Any fracture with associated elbow instability should be anatomically reduced and fixated. Fractures with initial displacement of 3–4 mm are at risk of late displacement and non-union; thus, many recommend percutaneous pinning to stabilize these fractures. Fractures with over 4 mm of displacement are often also rotated, necessitating open reduction and internal fixation to restore articular continuity. Complications of lateral condyle fractures include nonunion, progressive valgus deformity, and tardy ulnar neuritis.[78]

Radial head/neck fracture

Proximal radius injuries in the skeletally immature athlete are either physeal fractures of the radial head or fractures of the radial neck. These fractures occur most commonly in children over the age of 9 years as the result of valgus stress with longitudinal force on an outstretched arm. Treatment depends on the degree of angulation, amount of displacement, age of child, and associated fractures (Figure 44.5). Children younger than 10 years old can tolerate up to 40–45° of angulation of the radial neck due to expected remodelling, if articular step-off is not more than 1 mm. In older children, less angulation (15–20°) is acceptable due to the decreased potential for remodelling. In fractures with acceptable angulation, cast immobilization with early motion at 10–14 days is recommended. Closed reduction can be performed by direct pressure over the radial head with a varus stress and rotation. Alternatively, a percutaneous pin can be used to manipulate the proximal fragment, the so-called joystick technique. Indications for open reduction include complete displacement of the radial head, irreducible angulation over 45°, or a displaced Salter–Harris type IV fracture. Radial head fractures with significant displacement should be anatomically reduced and fixated. Radial head excision is contraindicated as proximal radial migration, radial deviation of the hand, and valgus deviation of the elbow can occur.[78,82,83] Complications of this fracture include limitations of motion and radio-ulnar synostosis.

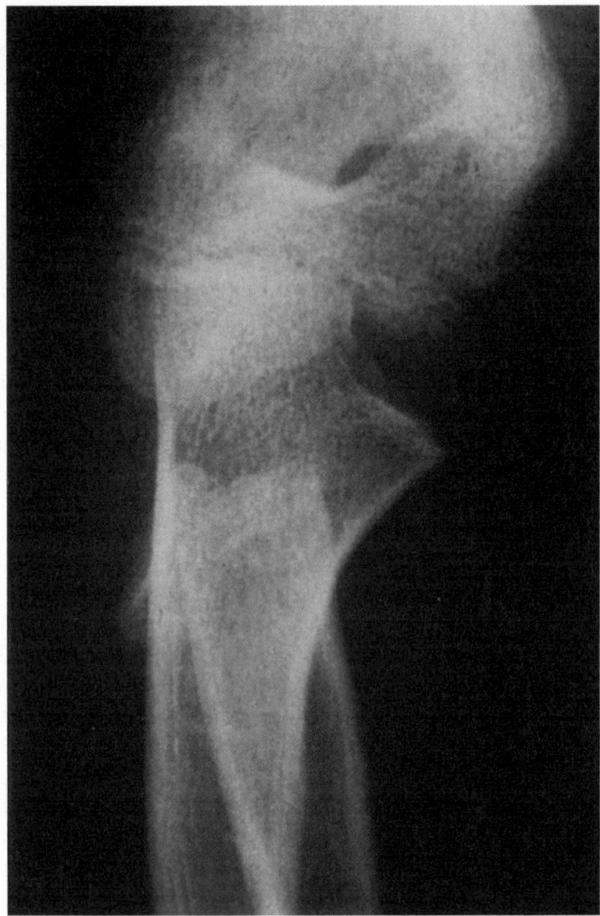

Figure 44.5 Radial head fracture.
AP view demonstrating angulation and displacement of proximal radial physeal fracture in a 12-year-old boy.

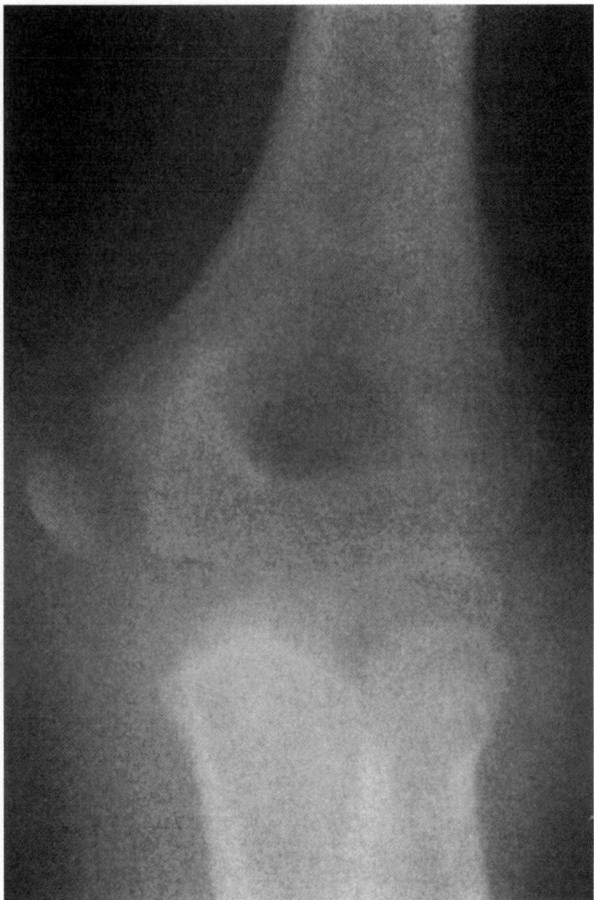

Figure 44.6 Medial epicondyle avulsion.
AP view of a displaced medial epicondyle avulsion fracture in a 14-year-old male pitcher.

Medial epicondyle fracture

The medial epicondyle can be avulsed from a valgus load applied to the extended elbow (Figure 44.6). The flexor origin and the ulnar collateral ligament play a role in fracture displacement. These fractures occur typically in children 10–14 years old. Almost 50% of these injuries are thought to occur concomitantly with elbow dislocation (Figure 44.7). For the general paediatric population, many advocate closed treatment of this injury, particularly when there is less than 5 mm of displacement. Some literature suggests they all do well without immediate or delayed sequelae, regardless of the amount of displacement.[84] Although non-union may occur, it is often asymptomatic or can be treated with fragment excision when symptomatic.

Relative indications for open reduction and fixation include competitive athletes with >2 mm displacement or valgus instability to restore the integrity of the medial collateral ligament and retention of the forearm flexors. An absolute indication for open reduction and internal fixation is medial epicondylar entrapment within the joint associated with elbow dislocation (Figure 44.7). A common complication of medial epicondyle fracture is joint stiffness. Internal fixation allows for early post-operative range of motion at 2–3 weeks.[78,85–87]

Elbow dislocation

Elbow dislocation is relatively uncommon in the child athlete as the peak incidence is in the second decade. However, elbow dislocation may be encountered in the adolescent athlete in contact sports such as football or wrestling, or in non-contact sports such as gymnastics. The most common pattern of injury is posterolateral displacement without disruption of the proximal radio-ulnar joint. The injury may also involve disruption of the anterior capsule, tearing of the brachialis muscle, avulsion of the medial epicondyle, injury to the ulnar collateral ligament, brachial artery compromise, or nerve injury to the median or ulnar nerves. Clinical presentation is that of a grossly swollen and deformed elbow with pain on attempt at movement. Median or ulnar nerve injuries occur in up to 10% of dislocations, and a thorough neurovascular examination is crucial prior to an attempt at reduction. Prompt and gentle reduction is performed under sedation. Non-concentric reduction should alert the clinician to the possibility of interposed soft tissue or medial epicondyle avulsion (Figure 44.7). For simple elbow dislocations, a posterior splint is used for the acute phase of pain and swelling for 10–14 days, followed by assisted range of motion and physical therapy.[78,88] Immobilization beyond 3 weeks is contraindicated due to stiffness.

Little League elbow

The term Little League elbow describes a group of pathologic entities about the elbow joint in young throwers. Originally, these findings were noted in baseball pitchers; however, the throwing motion is common to the non-pitcher's throw, the tennis serve, the javelin throw, the cricket bowl, and the football pass. The entity includes

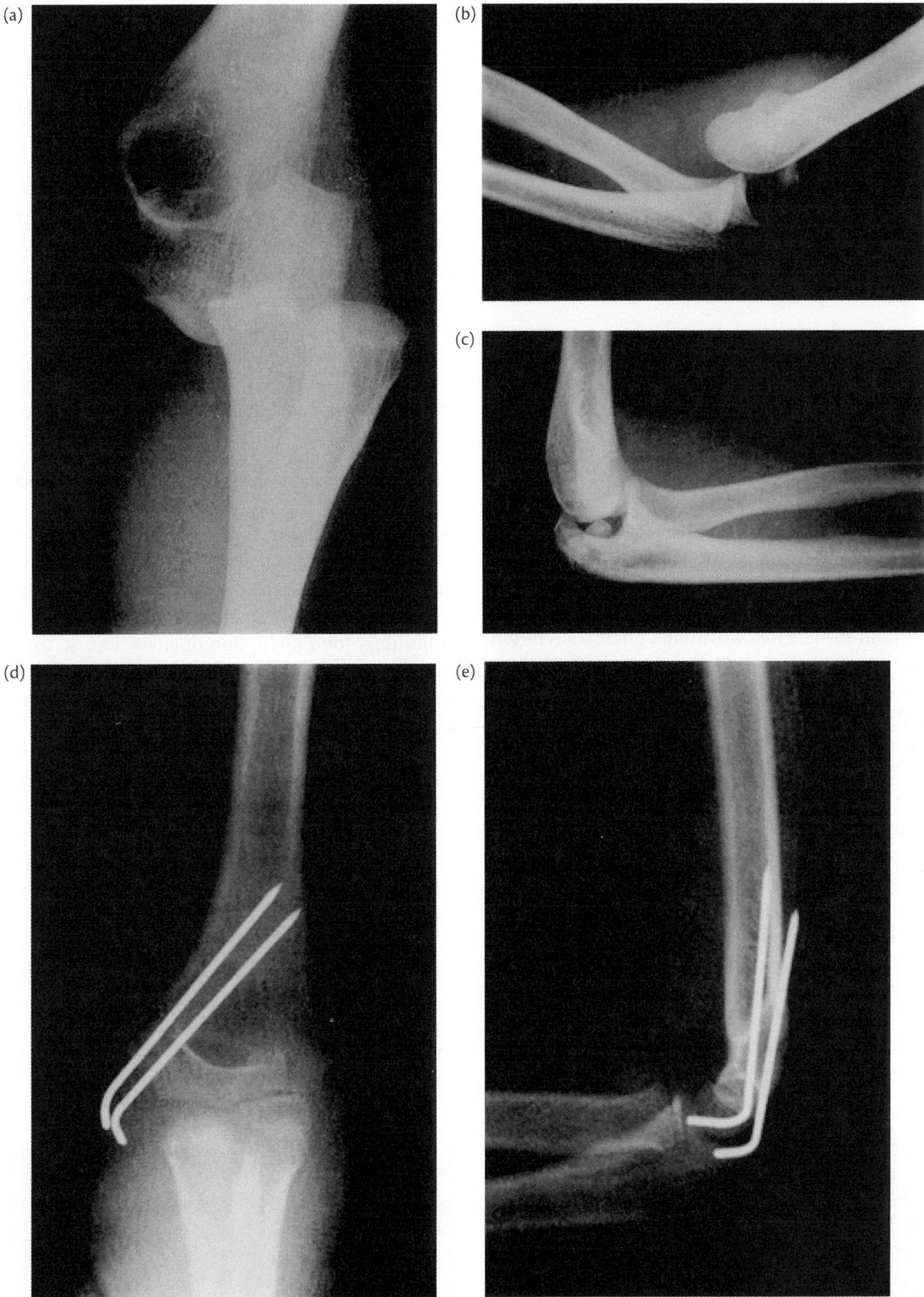

Figure 44.7 Elbow dislocation with medial epicondyle avulsion.

(a) AP and lateral (b) views demonstrating elbow dislocation with medial epicondyle avulsion in a 13-year-old female gymnast, and (c) entrapped medial epicondyle fragment, (d) AP and lateral, and (e) views after open reduction and internal fixation.

medial epicondyle fragmentation and avulsion (Figure 44.6), growth alteration of the medial epicondyle, Panner disease (osteochondritis of the capitellum), deformation or osteochondritis of the radial head, hypertrophy of the ulna, and olecranon apophysitis. Osteochondritis of the capitellum may also be seen in high-performance female gymnasts.[89] Most cases of Little League elbow present with medial elbow complaints, including medial pain and decreased throwing effectiveness/distance. Medial tension overload results from repetitive valgus stress and flexor forearm pull.

The changes seen with Little League elbow are age dependent. During childhood, irregular appearance of the secondary centres of ossification of the medial epicondyle may be seen. In adolescence with increasing muscle strength, avulsion fracture of the medial epicondyle may occur. After fusion of the medial epicondyle in young adulthood, injuries of the ulnar collateral ligament and flexor muscle origin become more apparent. Laterally, repetitive valgus compression may lead to damage of the radiocapitellar articulation. Panner disease is a benign form of osteochondritis dissecans of the capitellum in younger children. It is thought to be in the spectrum between normal ossification and a true osteochondritis dissecans. Osteochondritis dissecans can affect both the capitellum and the radial head. Changes include chondromalacia with softening and fissuring of the articular surface, subchondral collapse, and bony eburnation.

Osteochondritis dissecans of the capitellum can present with wide variations in radiographic appearance depending on the extent of osteonecrosis and the presence of loose bodies. Availability of MRI has given opportunity for early diagnosis, prior to radiographic changes. Pain, tenderness, and contracture dominate the clinical presentation. Additional lateral injuries seen during throwing in the skeletally immature athlete include lateral apophysis avulsion from traction during follow-through and radial physeal injury from repetitive valgus overload. Posterior elbow pain in throwers is frequently due to the powerful contraction of the triceps in the early acceleration phase, coupled with the impaction of the olecranon into its humeral fossa in the late follow-through phase. Olecranon apophysitis, avulsion fracture (Figure 44.8), posteromedial osteophytes, and loose bodies may form.[10,12,16,17,75,90–95]

Treatment of Little League elbow is directed at removing the recurrent microtrauma. Cessation of all throwing until the elbow is asymptomatic, followed by reassessing throwing mechanics and number of pitches thrown, is essential. More than 300 full effort throws per week may predispose to injury. Range-of-motion exercises and dynamic splinting may be useful for contractures. Triceps strengthening with stretching of the anterior capsule is helpful for avoidance of contracture. Arthroscopy or open surgery is useful for assessing chondral injury, removal of loose bodies, and management of osteochondritis dissecans through drilling or fragment fixation in unstable lesions.[96] Open reduction of displaced medial epicondyle fractures is indicated in the throwing athlete. Results of treatment of Little League elbow are generally favourable when instituted early.[10,12,16,17,75,90–95]

Wrist and hand injuries

General

In most sports, the hand and wrist are exposed, and thus are vulnerable to injury. Injury patterns are sport specific, with macrotraumatic injury or repetitive microtraumatic injury depending upon the demands placed on the upper extremity.

Injuries are also age specific, i.e. related to the stage of skeletal development. In several large series of paediatric and adolescent athletic injuries studies, hand and wrist injury rates vary from 15 to 65% of all injuries in paediatric and adolescent athletes depending on the sport involved.[97–99] Injuries to the hand are particularly common during basketball, American football, boxing, 16-inch (41 cm) softball, skateboarding, and alpine skiing. Repetitive stress injuries, particularly of the wrist, are common in gymnasts. Injuries are relatively infrequent during swimming and soccer.[100–102]

Distal radius fractures

Distal radial metaphyseal fracture is the most common fracture of childhood.[103] If treated properly, these fractures usually heal without residual disability. Initial management consists of splinting and careful neurovascular evaluation of the hand. X-rays are usually sufficient to define the fracture and its angulation/displacement (Figure 44.9). This fracture may occur in association with distal radio-ulnar joint disruption or elbow injury. Torus and greenstick fractures are often relatively stable and may be treated in a short-arm cast in older children and a long-arm cast in children younger than 5 years of age.

The completely displaced distal radial metaphyseal fracture often requires intravenous sedation or general anaesthesia for reduction followed by long-arm casting with an appropriate mould. In the child younger than 8 years of age, bayonet apposition may be accepted. In the rare irreducible fracture, an open reduction may be necessary through a volar approach, which allows for release of the carpal canal. The position of immobilization of this fracture is controversial, with advocates of pronation, neutral, and supination positioning. Approximately 10–30% of distal third radius fractures re-displace and angulate to an unacceptable position (>20°) requiring repeat closed manipulation. For the healing fracture, acceptable limits of angulation are wider. In a child aged under 8 years, up to 30° may be acceptable due to remodelling potential with an

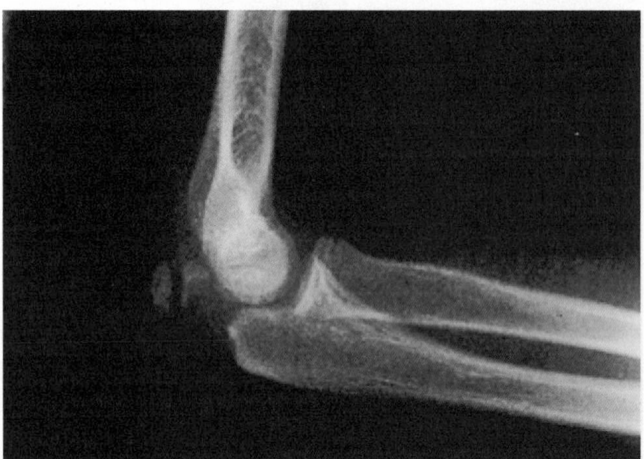

Figure 44.8 Olecranon avulsion.
Lateral view demonstrating olecranon apophysis avulsion in a 12-year-old male pitcher.

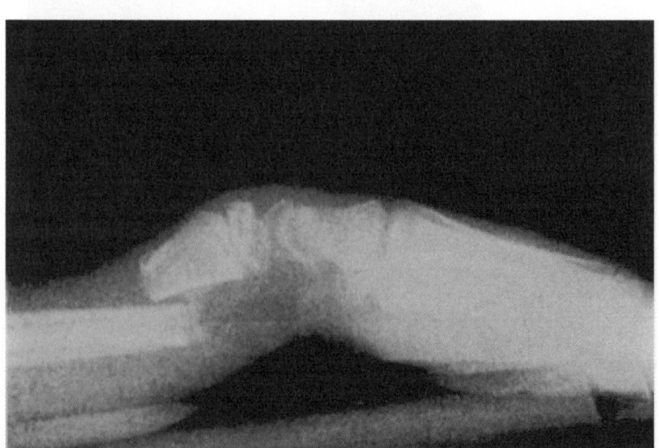

Figure 44.9 Distal radius fracture.
Lateral view in a 6-year-old boy.

estimated correction of $1° \cdot month^{-1}$.[104] In the child aged above 12 years, these fractures become increasingly unstable with less remodelling potential leading to treatment similar to that of an adult.

Galeazzi fractures are fractures of the distal radius with disruption of the radio-ulnar joint. Children may have separation of the ulnar physis instead of true disruption of the radio-ulnar joint.[105] They can be managed with closed reduction in younger children. Older children, like adults, require an open reduction.[106]

Physeal fractures of the distal radius occur most commonly in the adolescent. Salter–Harris type I and type II fracture patterns predominate. The distal fragment is usually dorsally displaced with an intact dorsal periosteum. This fracture may be associated with acute carpal tunnel syndrome or compartment syndrome. Reduction should be as atraumatic as possible to avoid further injury to the physis. The fracture should be immobilized in the position of stability as determined during reduction. Intraepiphyseal fracture extension, such as in Salter–Harris type III or IV injuries, is uncommon but should be treated with anatomical reduction of the articular surface and intraepiphyseal or transphyseal fixation.

Wrist injuries

Wrist pain has become extremely common in young, highly competitive gymnasts, and is usually related to chronic, repetitive upper-extremity weight-bearing during growth and development. Chronic repetitive stress injury to the distal radial and ulnar physes was described by Roy and colleagues in young, highly competitive gymnasts who practised ~36 $h \cdot week^{-1}$.[107] The presenting symptoms were stiffness and dorsiflexion pain. Radiographs showed widened physes, cystic changes, and distal metaphyseal beaking. Nearly all patients returned to competitive gymnastics without growth arrest after treatment with rest, and with or without casting. Subsequently, others have reported acquired Madelung's deformity and increased ulnar variance in young, competitive gymnasts.[108,109] A spectrum of pathologic entities may be found on clinical examination, radiographs, MRI, and arthroscopy, including stress changes of the distal radial-ulnar physes, articular cartilage changes of the wrist/carpal joints, distal radio-ulnar joint injury, triangular fibrocartilage complex (TFCC) tears, and ganglion cysts. Management is primarily non-operative with rest, immobilization, if necessary, and activity modification.

Distal radio-ulnar joint injuries in the child and adolescent athlete are rare. Acute dislocations present with pain and deformity of the joint. Acute dislocations are treated with long-arm cast immobilization with the wrist in supination for dorsal dislocations and pronation for volar dislocations. Fibrocartilage injuries are increasingly being recognized in patients with repetitive wrist loading, particularly gymnasts. Patients typically present with ulnar-sided wrist pain and injury may be demonstrated on MRI arthrogram or arthroscopy. For patients who fail non-operative management, patients with neutral or negative ulnar variance can be treated by arthroscopic debridement and patients with positive ulnar variance can be treated by ulnar shortening and/or debridement. In a child or adolescent with significant growth remaining, bony procedures should be delayed until growth ceases.[110]

The scaphoid fracture is the most common carpal fracture in children with a peak incidence between 12 and 15 years of age. In the skeletally immature, the majority of fractures are minimally displaced. The blood supply to scaphoid enters at the distal pole, and the ossification follows the pattern of blood supply. Because of the early ossification and stout soft tissue attachments that protect its proximal pole, fractures of the scaphoid in children are often distal pole.[111] However, with increased athletic participation at increasingly intense competitive levels by children and adolescents, more adult-type displaced wrist fractures are being seen. Patients present with wrist pain, limited motion, and tenderness in the anatomic snuff box. Management of minimally displaced fractures involves a short-arm thumb spica cast for 6 weeks for distal pole fractures, and a long-arm thumb spica cast for 4 weeks for waist fractures, followed by short-arm casting until union occurs. Occult fractures can be diagnosed with bone scanning. Acute displaced fractures should be treated with open reduction and internal fixation. Scaphoid non-union usually requires bone grafting with or without excision (Figure 44.10).[112–114] Scaphoid malunion or non-union can lead to degenerative changes of the wrist in the long term. Stress fracture of the scaphoid waist can be seen particularly in competitive gymnasts.[115,116] Initial X-rays are often negative, with follow-up X-rays revealing a stress fracture. MRI is diagnostic.

Ligamentous injuries of the wrist are unusual in children, but are being seen with increased frequency in the adolescent athlete engaged in high-level sports. The volar intercarpal ligaments, particularly the radioscapholunate and radioscaphocapitate ligament, are important stabilizers of the wrist. Patients present with wrist pain and limited motion. Radiographs may reveal widening of the scapholunate interval or alteration of the scapholunate angle (normal 30–60°). Dorsal intercalated segment instability (DISI) can result from scaphoid fracture or scapholunate dissociation, resulting in an increased scapholunate angle. Volar intercalated segment

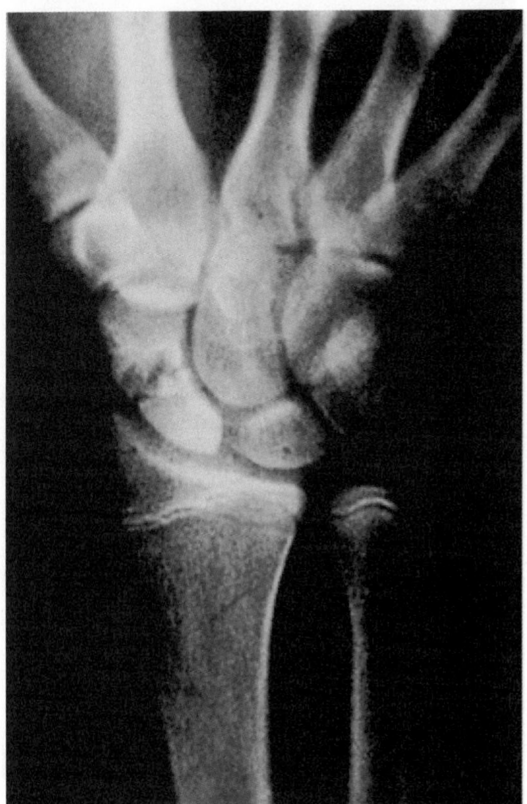

Figure 44.10 Scaphoid nonunion.

instability (VISI) can result from disruption of the radiocarpal ligaments on the ulnar side of the wrist, resulting in a decreased scapholunate angle. Wrist arthrography, MRI, and arthroscopy can be used to further delineate the extent of ligamentous injury. Partial injuries are treated with immobilization. Acute complete ligamentous injuries are treated with ligament repair and K-wire fixation. Chronic carpal instability is usually treated with limited carpal fusions or proximal row carpectomy, often with unpredictable results.

Hand injuries

The thumb metacarpal-phalangeal joint is commonly injured, particularly during skiing. These injuries result from excessive radial deviation during a fall on the outstretched hand with the thumb in abduction. In adults and older adolescents, injury to the ulnar collateral ligament of the thumb metacarpal-phalangeal joint occurs ('gamekeeper's or skier's thumb'). In children and adolescents, physeal fracture at the base of the proximal phalanx is more common. The ulnar collateral ligament inserts onto the proximal phalangeal epiphysis, thus predisposing to a Salter–Harris type III fracture, which may involve a large portion of the articular surface (Figure 44.11). Non-displaced fractures and partial ulnar collateral ligament injuries are treated with 4–6 weeks of immobilization in a short-arm thumb spica cast. Displaced fractures are treated with open reduction and internal fixation. Complete ligamentous injuries (>35–40° opening in flexion without a firm end point) and Stener's lesions (interposition of the adductor aponeurosis) are treated with ligament repair.[117–121]

The 'jammed finger' is the most common joint injury in the child and adolescent athlete's hand. Axial compressive forces applied to the end of the finger can result in proximal interphalangeal joint (PIP) hyperextension with subluxation or dislocation of the joint. This injury is common in ball-catching sports such as basketball or American football. Reduction of the dislocated joint is accomplished by linear traction. Volar plate injury/avulsion or volar Salter–Harris type III fracture may be associated, but rarely requires fixation. Treatment involves a very brief period of immobilization (dorsal alumifoam splint) followed by oedema control (elastoplast wrapping) and motion (buddy-taping to adjacent digit) to avoid stiffness and a fixed flexion deformity. Most athletes can return to sports (with buddy-taping) in 1–2 weeks, although some pain and swelling may persist for months. Axial loading of the finger may also result in boutonniere deformity (PIP flexion, distal interphalangeal joint (DIP) extension) secondary to rupture of the central slip or a dorsally displaced Salter–Harris type III fracture at the base of the middle phalanx. Acute injuries should be splinted in full extension for 4–5 weeks. Chronic reconstruction results in less reliable outcomes.[117–121]

Mallet finger is the most common injury occurring at the DIP joint, resulting from hyperflexion injury producing either extensor tendon (terminal tendon) rupture or Salter–Harris type III avulsion of the distal phalangeal epiphysis (Figure 44.12). The patient is unable to actively extend the DIP joint; however, there is full passive motion. Unless there is significant displacement of a substantial epiphyseal fragment, the DIP joint should be splinted with a dorsal splint in full extension for approximately 6 weeks. Terminal tendon

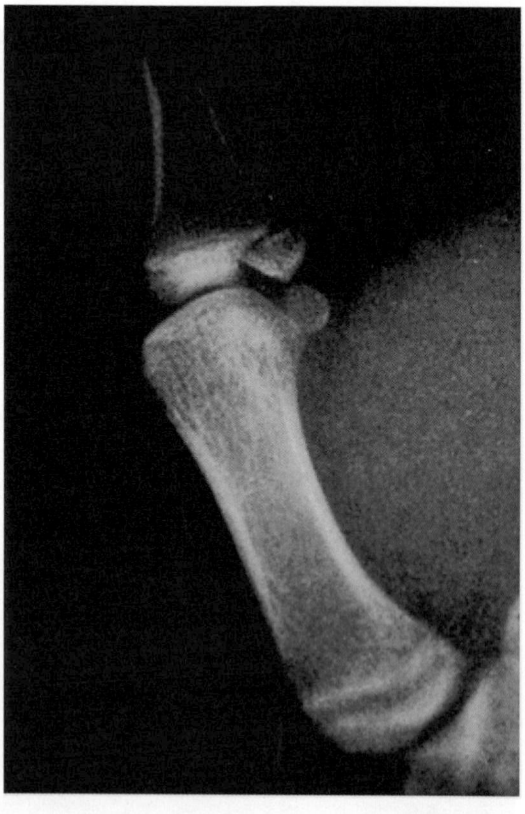

Figure 44.11 Gamekeeper's thumb.
Salter–Harris type III injury in a 10-year-old male.

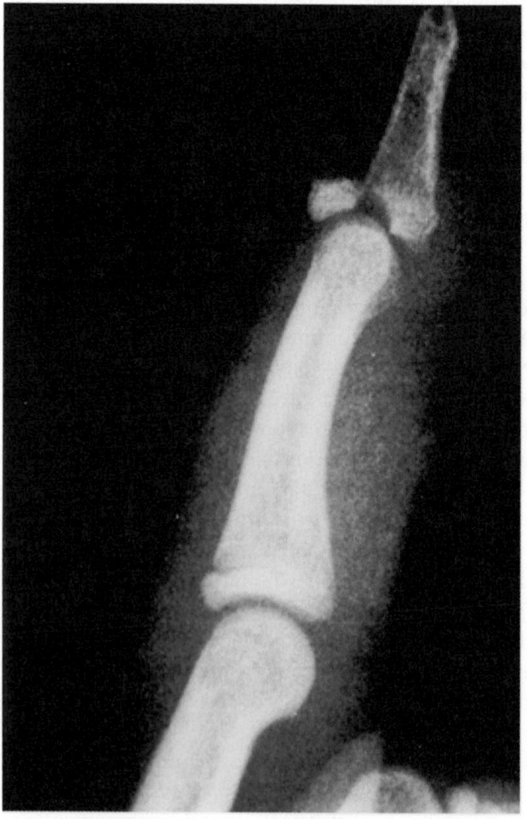

Figure 44.12 Mallet fracture.

repair may be necessary if an extensor lag persists after 10 weeks, although this is unusual.[117–121]

Hyperextension of the DIP joint may result in a dorsal DIP dislocation or avulsion of the flexor digitorum profundus (FDP). Flexor digitorum profundus avulsion most commonly involves the ring finger and occurs during American football or rugby as the finger catches on the opposing player's shirt ('jersey finger'). If identified early, the injury can be successfully treated. Missed diagnosis occurs when the patient does not recognize a significant injury or the care provider believes that the inability to flex the DIP joint is secondary to pain and swelling. Direct repair to the distal phalanx is accomplished if possible. With late diagnosis, direct repair is usually not possible as the tendon retracts and fibrosis occurs. In these cases, tendon grafts may be necessary.[122]

Hand fractures are common athletic injuries in children. Fractures involving the physis are frequent, accounting for approximately 40% of hand fractures in the skeletally immature.[101] Ossific nuclei appear in the metacarpals and phalanges by 3 years of age and fuse between 14 and 17 years of age. Remodelling potential exists for fractures near the epiphysis in the plane of motion; however, there is minimal remodelling of rotational deformity. The vast majority of hand fractures in children can be managed non-operatively with splinting of non-displaced fractures and closed reduction of angulated or displaced fractures. Fingertip crush injuries occur in tackling and collision sports. These injuries often involve a nailbed laceration and tuft fracture requiring splinting and nailbed repair. Phalangeal neck fractures typically occur between 5 and 10 years of age and involve the proximal phalanx. These fractures may re-displace after reduction and may have substantial rotation not appreciated on plain radiographs, and therefore require careful clinical examination. Metacarpal fractures in children are less common than adults. Little finger metacarpal neck fractures (boxer's fracture) can usually be managed by closed reduction and cast immobilization for 3 weeks. Thumb metacarpal fractures often involve a Salter–Harris type II fracture through the base of the metacarpal.[117–121]

Trunk injuries

General

Back pain and injuries to the thoracolumbar spine are not infrequent in the school-aged athlete. Spine-related complaints constitute almost 10% of athletes' medical problems and approximately 75% of high-performance athletes have some sort of back pain, at some point.[27]

In particular, sports that require repetitive or high-velocity twisting or bending, such as gymnastics, dancing, football, and rowing, have a predilection for back injuries.[101,123–132] With the increasing number of young athletes pursuing rigorous training and intense competition in some of these sports at an early age, the prevalence of back pain in the young athlete may be expected to increase. Effective clinical management of back pain in the child and adolescent athlete requires an accurate diagnosis and a specific treatment plan. Accurate diagnosis necessitates an understanding of the differing aetiologies of back pain in the young athlete in contradistinction to back pain in the adult.[133] In the adult, mechanical back pain, degenerative disorders, and disc disease predominate, with symptomatology sometimes related to secondary gains, including disability and psychologic issues. In the young athlete with back pain, a specific diagnosis should be sought, such as spondylolysis, spondylolisthesis, apophysitis, tumour, or infection. Macrotrauma and microtrauma must be distinguished. The former involves a single-tissue overload while the latter represents cumulative trauma. Macrotrauma is typically seen in high-energy contact sports, such as rugby or football. Microtrauma is more commonly seen in athletes participating in sports requiring high-energy repetitive bending, twisting, or rotation, such as gymnasts, dancers, or football lineman. The growing athlete has several unique risk factors relevant to the adolescent spine. The growth cartilage of the vertebral end plates and apophyses are more susceptible to injury. Musculotendinous imbalances are quite common because of periods of rapid longitudinal growth. Eating disorders with irregular menstruation and osteoporosis are not uncommon in adolescent gymnasts and dancers, a condition termed the female athletic triad. In addition, extrinsic factors such as poor technique, grouping of children by similar age despite differing abilities, and insufficient conditioning may predispose to injury.

Major anatomic differences of the spine in the skeletally immature include an increased cartilage to bone ratio and the presence of secondary centres of ossification at the vertebral end plates, which normally fuse to the vertebral bodies by maturity. Unlike adults who often have asymptomatic pre-existing degenerative changes in the fibrocartilaginous disc, intervertebral discs in the child are generally well hydrated and tightly adhered to the cartilaginous plate. The apophyseal ring is thinner in the middle than the periphery; thus, axial compression with forward flexion may force the disc through the end plates into the cancellous bone of the vertebral body as opposed to through the annulus towards the spinal canal as seen in adults. In addition, compressive and bending forces tend to fracture the weaker vertebral end plate rather than producing annulus failure and disc herniation.

A thorough history and discerning physical examination are essential in the assessment of spine injuries in child and adolescent athletes. The athlete's age, sex, pattern of complaints, location and radiation of pain, and chronology of symptoms are essential facts to obtain. Attention should be directed toward the mechanics of the sport producing the pain, such as walkovers in gymnasts, butterfly stroke in swimmers, and hyperextension and loading in American football linemen. A family history is implicated in scoliosis and spondylolisthesis. Night pain suggests tumour, morning stiffness associated with sacroiliac pain may be the presenting symptoms of juvenile ankylosing spondylitis, and systemic symptoms such as fever and chill suggest infection. Neurologic symptoms such as paraesthesia, weakness, and bowel/bladder dysfunction require immediate attention. The physical examination should include an assessment of gait and leg lengths. The frontal and sagittal contour of the spine should be examined both standing and bending to evaluate any asymmetry or deformity. Range of motion should be measured and localized areas of tenderness elicited. Provocative tests such as hyperextension or straight leg raise testing should be performed. Hip range of motion, muscle tightness, and generalized laxity should be assessed. Finally, a thorough neurologic examination of muscle strength, sensation, and reflexes should be performed. Radiographs and further diagnostic studies such as MRI, computed tomography (CT), and radionuclide scanning should be individualized, depending on the differential diagnosis and symptomatology.

Spondylolysis and spondylolisthesis

Mechanical injury to the pars interarticularis is a common source of discomfort in young athletes involved in competitive sports and is probably the most frequently diagnosed anatomic lesion in young people with back pain. Spondylolysis refers to a bony defect in the pars interarticularis, and spondylolisthesis refers to translation of a vertebral body relative to an adjacent body in the sagittal plane. Fracture of the pars interarticularis occurs as a consequence of activity and is usually an overuse injury. Spondylolytic defects are rare in young children, have not been reported in newborns, are absent in other primates, and are not seen in patients who have not assumed an upright posture.[134] Nearly 50% of patients with spondylolysis relate the onset of symptoms to competitive sports training.[135] In a series of 177 male high-school and college athletes, approximately 21% showed radiographic evidence of spondylolysis, far exceeding the incidence of spondylolysis in the general population which is estimated at approximately 4% in the adolescents, increasing to 6% in adulthood.[136,137,138] Many inactive individuals are asymptomatic. The average age of diagnosis in the symptomatic school-age athletic population is between 15 and 16 years. LaFond[139] noted that 23% of spondylolysis patients in his series experienced the onset of symptoms before 20 years of age; however, only 9% of them had severe enough symptoms to seek medical attention. Approximately 85% of spondylolysis occurs at the L5 level.

It is postulated that spondylolysis and isthmic spondylolisthesis represent acquired fatigue fractures as a result of repeated microtrauma. Shear stresses of 400–600 N due to hyperextension, flexion, and torsion are concentrated across the pars interarticularis, an area calculated to be only 0.75 cm^2 at L5.[140,141] Repetitive hyperextension loading sports such as gymnastics, blocking in American football, hurdling, ballet dancing, volleyball spiking, competitive diving, tennis serving, weight lifting, and swimming turns have all been associated with spondylolysis. Pars defects occur four times more frequently in young female gymnasts than the general female population.[128] However, given the same demands within the same sport, it is difficult to determine why one athlete is predisposed to spondylolysis while another avoids injury. Genetic predisposition of spondylolytic defects has been documented.[142,143] Anatomic variations such as transitional vertebrae, spina bifida occulta, and an elongated pars may be seen. In addition, poor technique, inadequate supervision, poor conditioning, poor flexibility, and hyperlordotic posture may predispose to injury.

Diagnosis and initiation of protective treatment as early as possible is essential. The onset of symptoms typically coincides with the adolescent growth spurt and with the onset of strenuous, repetitive training. In athletes, symptoms are usually insidious aching low back pain without radiation. Initially, the pain is elicited by strenuous activity; however, the pain often becomes progressively more severe and becomes associated with activities of daily living. L5 radicular symptoms may arise from foraminal encroachment, fibrocartilaginous callus at the healing pars, or forward displacement of L5 on S1. Physical examination may demonstrate paraspinal tenderness, limited motion, hyperlordosis, and hamstring tightness.[144] In many cases, pain can be reproduced with hyperextension and occasionally can be localized with ipsilateral hyperextension. Initial diagnostic work-up includes radiographs of the lumbosacral spine. Slippage through a pars defect may be seen on the standing lateral view, allowing for measurement of the percent slippage and slip angle (Figures 44.13 and 44.14). A 25–45° oblique view may demonstrate the spondylolytic defect (Figure 44.13). Acutely, the defect appears as a narrow gap with irregular edges. Over time, the edges become rounded and smooth. Reactive sclerosis and hypertrophy of the opposite pars or lamina can be seen in unilateral spondylolysis and occasionally confused with osteoid osteoma. If spondylolysis is suspected but not demonstrated on plain Alms, single photon emission computed tomography (SPECT) scanning is particularly sensitive in detecting pars defects (Figure 44.13).[145]

More important, several studies have found that a positive bone scan or SPECT correlates with a painful pars lesion.[146] Early diagnosis with SPECT is of great practical significance as fresh pars defects may heal with early effective immobilization.[147] Computed tomography has significant limitations as a primary diagnostic tool, as an early stress reaction in pars without overt fracture results in a normal CT. However, oblique linear tomography or CT scanning may demonstrate the established pars lesion. With radicular symptoms, MRI is useful in demonstrating the aetiology of root compression. The limitations of MRI in terms of correctly grading the pars lesions are particularly apparent in patients with stress reaction in the pars without a clear fracture line.[148]

Management must consider the athlete's age, type of sport activity, severity of symptoms, and risk of progression. Risk factors for slip progression include slip percentage >50%, high slip angle, spina bifida, convex sacral contour, ligamentous laxity, and the adolescent age group.[149–153] The asymptomatic individual should be periodically followed clinically and radiographically if there are risk factors for progression. The symptomatic adolescent athlete can initially be treated with restriction of athletic activity and a core (abdominal, back and hip) strengthening programme. We treat this as a stress fracture with activity modification and immobilization, using a rigid polypropylene lumbosacral brace constructed with 0° of lumbar flexion (anti-lordosis). The main effect of bracing appears to be restriction in gross body motion, and a brace may act as a means of restricting activity rather than stabilizing the fractures in these patients, as compliance with activity restriction is difficult to achieve in the active athletic youth, but it is critical to successful management.[154] We advocate full-time brace use for approximately 3 months. Braced patients are allowed to resume limited activities several weeks after initiation of brace wear, when most patients have become asymptomatic. Results are promising with this treatment. In our series, 32% of 75 patients achieved bony union and 88% were able to return to previously painful sports, even if the pars defect had not healed.[155,156] A recent update from our institution revealed that a favourable clinical outcome can be achieved in 80% with bracing. However, the success of bracing depends on the type of sports participated in, in addition to acute onset of pain and hamstring tightness, which were found to be associated with a worse outcome. For this reason, hip range of motion and hamstring stretching are a vital portion of the overall core strengthening regimen. With this regimen and with the brace treatment, the young athlete can return to sports in as little as 4–6 weeks.[157]

Bone scans or CT scans may be helpful in following the status of a lesion.[138,158,159] A positive bone scan usually indicates that the defect is healing or has the potential to heal; however, a cold scan should not be taken as a contraindication to bracing.[147] Hamstring tightness is also an indicator of the success of treatment. Patients who fail to improve after an appropriate

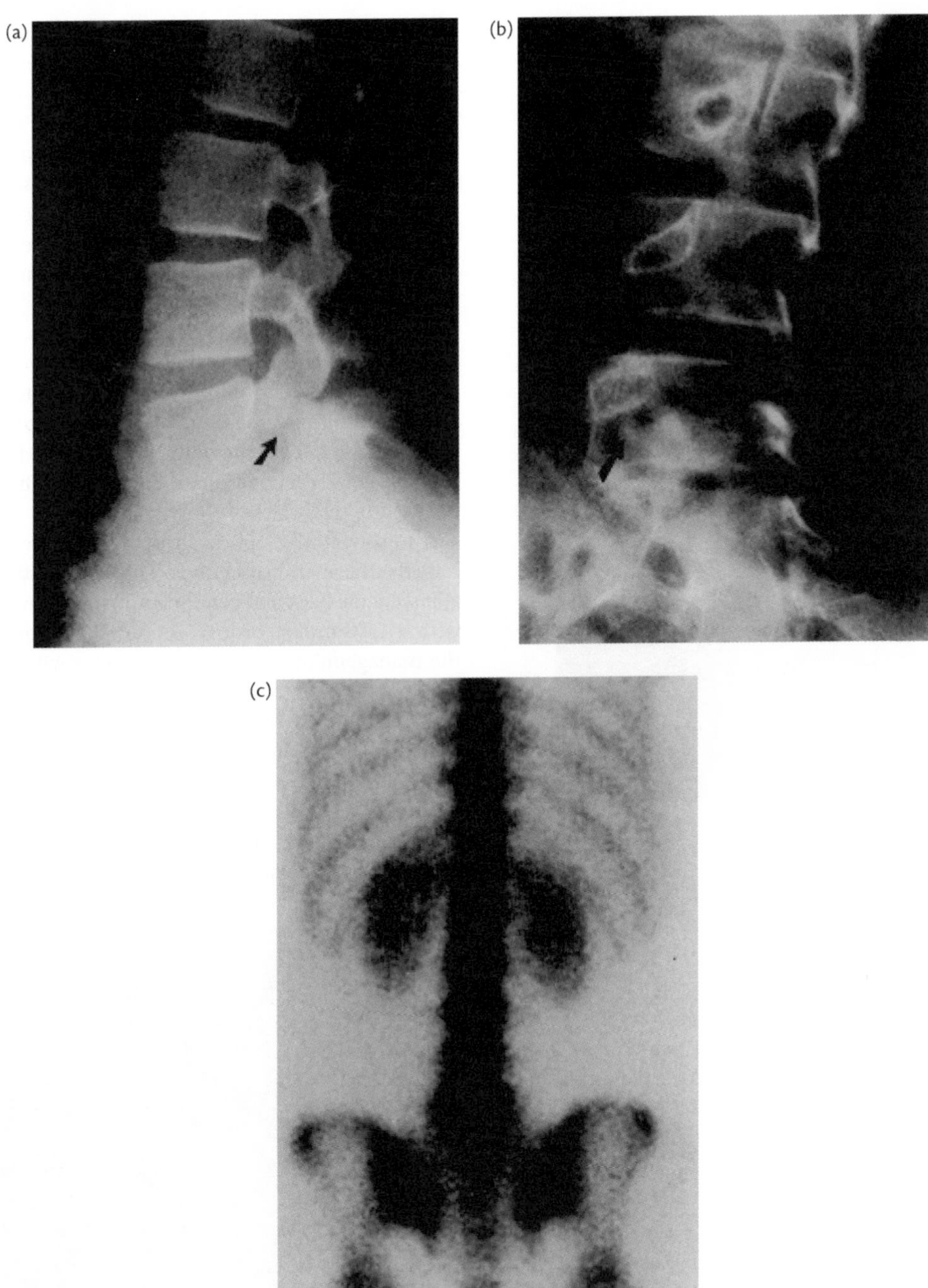

Figure 44.13 Spondylolysis.
(a) Lateral, (b) Oblique, and (c) SPECT scan in a 14-year-old female gymnast.

bracing regimen or who are unable to be weaned from the brace may require surgery. Posterolateral in situ fusion of L5–S1 is usually performed for L5 spondylolysis with post-operative bracing until fusion for up to 6 months. For spondylolysis of L4 or above, direct repair of the pars defect with wiring or osteosynthesis can be attempted, maintaining a motion segment and allowing earlier return to activity.[160–162] Management of the spondylolisthesis in the adolescent athlete depends on the degree of slippage and the severity of symptoms. Fortunately, it is rare to see progressive listhesis in the adolescent onset stress fracture pars defect seen in young athletes. For patients who remain symptomatic despite bracing, posterolateral in situ fusion of L5–S1 with post-operative bracing is performed.[150,152,163,164] Fusion should be extended to L4 for slips >50%. A slip of over 50% in the immature spine should be stabilized, even in an asymptomatic individual, because of the high risk of progression.[152,163,164] The asymptomatic athlete with <25% spondylolisthesis should be allowed to participate in all sports, including contact sports, while being followed periodically for progression (Figure 44.14).[165] Asymptomatic athletes with 25–50% slippage fall into a controversial category. Some advocate observation for progression, some advocate avoidance of contact sports, and some advocate surgical management if the patient wishes to return to competitive sports. It is rare that an individual with high-grade slippage and severe lumbosacral

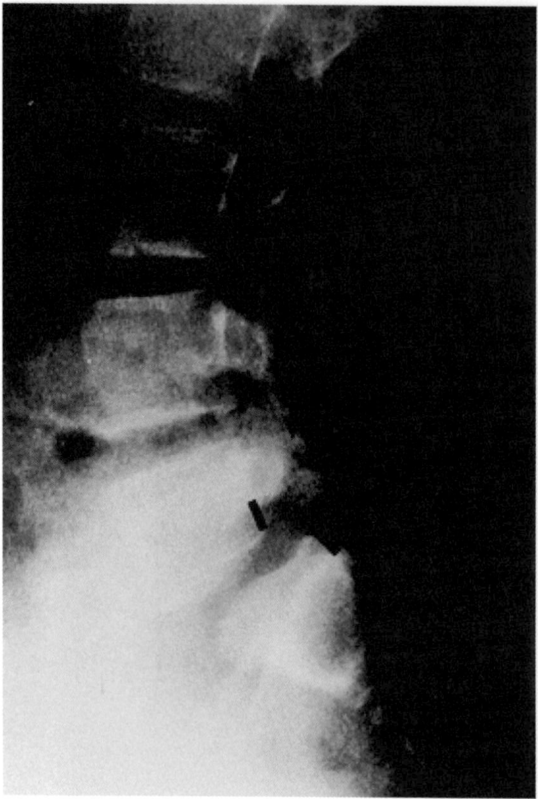

Figure 44.14 Spondylolisthesis.
Lateral view in a 17-year-old male football lineman.

kyphosis may benefit from reduction and fusion as opposed to in situ fusion; however, reduction is associated with a higher risk of neurologic complications.[166] Decompression in conjunction with fusion is reserved for a clear neurologic deficit and a readily discernible lesion such as the hypertrophied fibrocartilaginous mass at the level of the pars defect, irritating the L5 root. With high-grade slips, the sacral dome may stretch the thecal sac and sacral nerve roots.

Discogenic disorders

Although much less common in adolescents than adults, disc herniation and degenerative disc disease can occur in the young adolescent athlete. The true incidence is unknown, although it is estimated that between 1 and 4% of all disc herniations occur in the paediatric population, and less than 10% of young athletes' back pain is discogenic.[142,167,168–171] The natural history of disc disease in this population is not well understood, although some studies have suggested that these patients continue to have back problems as adults.[172] Acute macrotrauma may result in acute disc herniation, e.g. in collision-sport athletes and weightlifters, while repetitive microtrauma may result in degenerative disc disease or insidious herniation, e.g. in gymnasts. In contrast to adults with pre-existing degenerative disc changes, disc tissue in adolescents is usually noted to be firm, well hydrated, and solidly attached to the cartilaginous end plate.[171–175] These anatomic differences may predispose to disc herniation into the vertebral body or through an end-plate fracture rather than the classic extruded or sequestered disc through the annulus seen in adults. Disc herniations have been associated with sports with repetitive flexion and axial loading of the lumber spine, such as gymnastics, running, American football, weight lifting, basketball, soccer, and tennis.

The diagnosis can be difficult to determine clinically, because the presentation can be quite different from the classic radicular symptomatology of the adult. In the adolescent with a ruptured disc, the most frequent complaint is low back pain with radiation confined to the buttock. There may be a decrease in hamstring flexibility, limited motion, abnormal gait or running pattern, asymmetric paravertebral spasm, or subtle 'sciatic' scoliosis. Neurologic findings of altered reflexes, muscle weakness, and atrophy are rare. In cases of severe pain and systemic symptoms, white blood cell count, sedimentation rate, and bone scan should be performed to rule out occult disc-space infection. Work-up includes lumbosacral spine films that may show end-plate fracture. Disc-space narrowing is unusual. Magnetic resonance imaging confirms the presence of a neurocompressive lesion (Figure 44.15).

A non-operative approach is the mainstay of management for both disc herniation and discogenic pain. Initial treatment is aimed at resting the back and avoiding sporting activities. Brace treatment with a 15° lumbar lordosis module has been a useful adjunct to the management of adolescent athletes with discogenic pain that does not respond to rest.[155] In our experience, rigid bracing is more effective than use of a soft corset and allows the athlete to return to daily activities and a light training programme. If the athlete is still symptomatic at 8–12 weeks, epidural corticosteroids are considered.[176] For those who fail non-operative management or have evidence of cauda equina syndrome or severe motor loss, discectomy may be necessary. In general, surgical intervention in this age

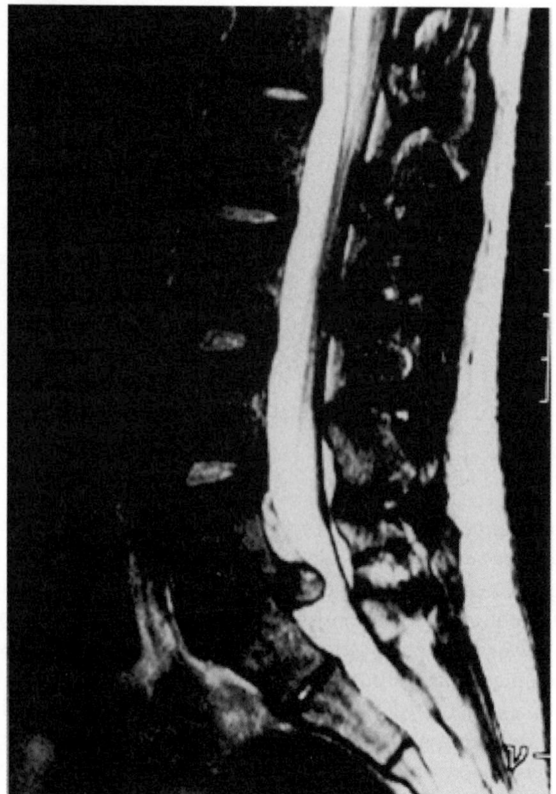

Figure 44.15 Herniated disc.
Sagittal MRI in a 17-year-old gymnast.

group has good short-term results; however, return to high-level competitive sports may not be possible.[156,167,172,177]

In addition, the risk of long-term sequelae such as degenerative changes at the involved level or herniation at a different level is not well understood. A condition that is almost indistinguishable from a herniated lumbar disc is a slipped vertebral apophysis or end-plate fracture.[174,178] This condition is often associated with heavy lifting and typically involves displacement of the posterior inferior apophysis of L4 with its disc attachment into the vertebral canal. Patients present with signs of a herniated disc with neurologic findings. Radiographs reveal the avulsion fragment and MRI reveals an extradural mass. Treatment consists of excision of both the cartilaginous disc and the bony fragment with relief of symptoms.

Scoliosis

Idiopathic scoliosis generally does not cause pain and does not interfere with sports. Scoliotic curves are often detected by asymmetry noted by parents, coaches, or screening. Forward bending accentuates the deformity by revealing the rotational deformity associated with coronal plane curvature. After a thorough history and examination to rule out associated abnormalities, full-length standing spine radiographs are obtained and the curve measured. Full-time bracing is initiated for progressive curves or, in general, curves over 25° in a child with substantial growth remaining. The braced patient is allowed to participate in sports out of the brace, and there is no evidence that sports participation increases the risk of curve progression. On the contrary, physical activity and strengthening are an essential aspect of brace management of scoliosis. After growth is complete, bracing is discontinued and no restrictions are placed on the adolescent with idiopathic scoliosis. Patients with progressive curves despite bracing or curves over 50° have a high incidence of progression after maturity and are treated with spinal instrumentation and fusion. Post-operatively, sports are restricted until the fusion mass heals and matures. Following fusion for scoliosis, contact sports and vigorous gymnastics are restricted due to risks of pseudarthrosis, hardware failure, and degenerative changes about the fused levels.[179]

Scheuermann's disease

Scheuermann's disease consists of kyphosis of the thoracic spine with anterior vertebral wedging, Schmorl's nodes, and vertebral end-plate deformity. Radiographic criteria include wedging of 5° or more of three consecutive vertebrae.[180] The aetiology is unknown, although repetitive flexion microtrauma and fatigue failure are implicated. Patients typically present due to deformity without pain. On physical examination, patients have a kyphotic deformity with increased lumbar lordosis in the standing position. Most are unable to correct this deformity with forced hyperextension. The hamstrings are invariably tight. Treatment of Scheuermann's kyphosis consists of postural training, pelvic control, abdominal strengthening, and flexibility exercises to address the tight hamstrings and lumbodorsal fascia. Progressive kyphosis over 50° in an immature child is an indication for bracing and progression to curves beyond 70° is an indication for spinal fusion. Idiopathic kyphosis without radiographic changes of Scheuermann's disease is seen about the adolescent growth spurt in children with tight lumbodorsal fascia and hamstrings which subsequently compensate for this pelvic tilt with thoracic kyphosis. In general, this is a flexible kyphosis that can be managed with posture, strength, and flexibility training. Atypical Scheuermann's disease consists of degenerative changes of the disc and vertebral end plates at the thoracolumbar junction. This is seen in adolescent athletes involved in vigorous flexion–extension activity of the spine such as gymnastics, diving, and rowing. Irregularities of the ring apophysis, end-plate wedging, and Schmorl's nodes may be seen on radiographs. These changes are often accompanied by pain and are thought to result from microtrauma with resultant end-plate fractures or disc herniation through the anterior ring apophysis with secondary bony deformation of the vertebrae.[170] Typically, the adolescent with atypical Scheuermann's has a flat back with thoracic hypokyphosis and lumbar hypolordosis. Pain is accentuated by forward flexion and relieved with rest. Our treatment utilizes full-time bracing with a moulded thoracolumbar orthosis of 15° extension advanced to 30° if tolerated. Abdominal strengthening, hamstring stretching, and pelvic control are also initiated. The gymnast is often able to slowly return to activity in 3–6 months.

Fractures

Fractures of the thoracolumbar spine in child and adolescent athletes are quite rare. Most reports of spinal injuries with neurologic deficit in children involve the cervical spine.[181,182] It takes considerable force to result in thoracolumbar fracture in the adolescent athlete and the absence of a major force should prompt a search for a pathologic lesion. The classification and stability of compression fractures can be conceptualized in Denis's three column model where the anterior column consists of the anterior longitudinal ligament and the anterior half of the vertebral body, the middle column consists of the posterior half of the vertebral body and the posterior longitudinal ligament, and the posterior column consists of the posterior elements and ligamentous structures. Instability is inferred when two columns are disrupted. Evaluation of these injuries includes a thorough history and physical examination, including neurologic, cardiopulmonary, and abdominal assessment. Anteroposterior and lateral radiographs of the spine are obtained and further studies are performed as needed, such as CT to define the extent of bony injury, and MRI to evaluate neurologic involvement or disc injury. Stable compression fractures of less than 50% can be treated in a molded thoracolumbar orthosis or hyperextension brace for 6–12 weeks, depending on healing and symptoms (Figure 44.16). Return to sports is allowed when the athlete is pain free and has full strength and flexibility. Unstable fracture dislocations, fractures with neurologic compromise, and fractures with significant deformity may require spinal fusion with possible neurologic decompression.

Apophyseal avulsion injuries resulting from rapid flexion, extension, and torsion are specific to the adolescent. Transverse process fractures may occur with contact sports. Associated intrathoracic, abdominal, and retroperitoneal injuries are the initial concerns. Management of these injuries consists of rest, followed by gradually increased range of motion and strength. Temporary bracing may be helpful. Return to gymnastics and contact sports is allowed when normal flexibility and strength are obtained.

Mechanical back pain

Mechanical back pain secondary to acute or chronic musculoligamentous strains and sprains is rare in the young athlete and should be a diagnosis of exclusion in children with low back pain. Such

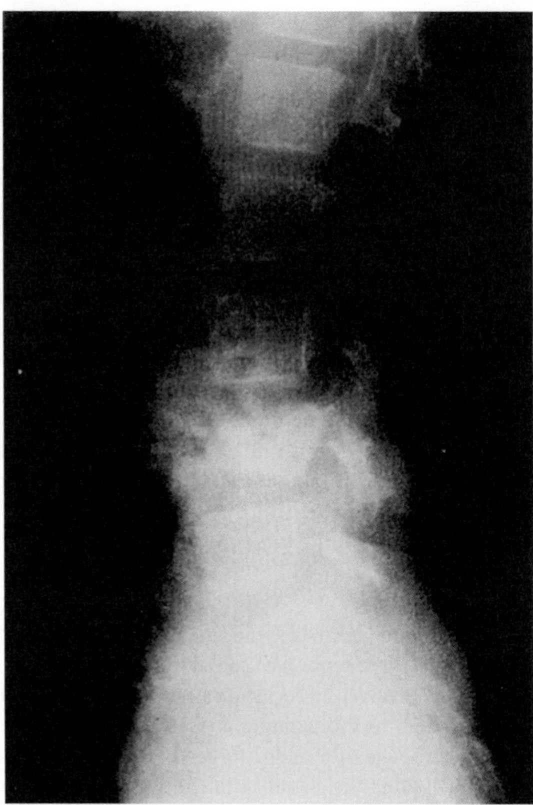

Figure 44.16 Compression fracture.
Lateral view in a 10-year-old female child.

back pain is thought to represent overuse or stretch injuries of the soft tissues including the muscle-tendon unit, ligaments, joint capsules, and facets. This is more commonly seen in the older age group and may be related to the adolescent growth spurt. Young athletes with mechanical back pain may be predisposed to injury due to weak abdominal musculature, tight lumbodorsal fascia, tight hamstrings, limited lumbar motion, and poor training technique.[183] The pain is often nondescript, exacerbated by activity, and relieved by rest. Physical examination reveals paraspinal muscle tenderness, decreased flexibility, and limited spinal motion. Radiographs are normal. Acutely, treatment consists of rest. Massage, NSAIDs, and phonophoresis may be helpful. Once the acute phase has resolved, a rehabilitation programme consisting of postural control, abdominal strengthening, and flexibility is initiated. Return to sport is gradually allowed with resolution of pain and return of strength and flexibility. Proper technique, conditioning, and stretching are emphasized.

Conclusions

In conclusion, injuries to the trunk and upper extremity are being seen more frequently in children and adolescent athletes in recent years due to expanded participation in organized sports, increased training time, and competition in this age group. Additionally, increased awareness of athletic injuries by physicians and trainers will result in more reporting of these injuries. Hopefully, with early identification of these injuries chronic deformity and disability can be prevented and full return to sport can be accomplished.

Summary

- Children and adolescents are not smaller adults. Injury patterns in children and adolescents are unique to the growing musculoskeletal system.
- Injuries to the trunk and upper extremity are being seen more frequently in recent years due to expanded participation in organized sports, increased training time, and competition in this age group. In addition, increased awareness of athletic injuries by physicians and trainers will result in more reporting of these injuries.
- Early recognition of injuries prevents deformity formation and facilitates full return to sports.

References

1. Goldberg B, Rosenthal PP, Nicholas JA. Injuries in youth football. *Phys Sports Med.* 1984; 12: 122–132.
2. Olson OC. The Spokane study: high-school football injuries. *Phys Sports Med.* 1979; 7: 75–82.
3. Consumer Product Safety Commission: Bicycle related injuries: Data from the National Electronic Injury Surveillance System. *JAMA.* 1987; 257: 34–37.
4. Kirburz D, Jacobs R, Reckling F, *et al.* Bicycle accidents and injuries among adult cyclists. *Am J Sports Med.* 1986; 14: 416–419.
5. Culpepper MI, Niemann KMW. High school football injuries in Birmingham, Alabama. *S Med J.* 1983; 76: 873–878.
6. Kocher MS, Feagin JA, Jr. Shoulder injuries during alpine skiing. *Am J Sports Med.* 1996; 24: 665–669.
7. Requa R, Garrick JG. Injuries in interscholastic wrestling. *Phys Sports Med.* 1981; 9: 44–51.
8. Snook GA. Injuries in intercollegiate wrestling: A 5-year study. *Am J Sports Med.* 1982; 10: 142–144.
9. Gainor BM, Piotrowski G, Puhl J, Allen WC, Hagen R. The throw: Biomechanics and acute injury. *Am J Sports Med.* 1980; 8: 114–118.
10. Tullos HS, Fain RH. Little league shoulder: Rotational stress fracture of proximal humeral epiphysis. *J Sports Med.* 1974; 2: 152–153.
11. Tullos HS, King JW. Lesions of the pitching arm in adolescents. *JAMA.* 1972; 220: 264–271.
12. Albright JA, Jokl P, Shaw R, *et al.* Clinical study of baseball pitchers: Correlation of injury to the throwing arm with method of delivery. *Am J Sports Med.* 1978; 6: 15–21.
13. Barnett LS. Little league shoulder syndrome: Proximal humeral epiphysis in adolescent baseball pitchers. *J Bone Joint Surg.* 1985; 67A: 495–496.
14. Cahill BR, Tullos HS. Little league shoulder. *Sports Med.* 1974; 2: 150–153.
15. Dotter WE. Little leaguer's shoulder: A fracture of the proximal epiphyseal cartilage of the humerus due to baseball pitching. *Guthrie Clinic Bull.* 1953; 23: 68–72.
16. Lipscomb AB. Baseball injuries in growing athletes. *J Sports Med.* 1975; 3: 25–34.
17. Torg JS, Pollack H, Sweterlitsch P. The effect of competitive pitching on the shoulders and elbows of preadolescent baseball players. *Pediatrics.* 1972; 49: 267–272.
18. Priest JD, Nagel DA. Tennis shoulder. *Am J Sports Med.* 1976; 4: 28–42.
19. Richardson AB, Jobe FW, Collins HR. The shoulder in competitive swimming. *Am J Sports Med.* 1980; 8: 159–163.
20. Fulton NN, Albright JP, El-Khoury GY. Cortical desmoid-like lesion of the proximal humerus and its occurence in gymnasts. *Am J Sports Med.* 1979; 7: 57–61.
21. Goldberg MJ. Gymnastic injuries. *Orthop Clin North Am.* 1980; 11: 717–732.
22. Snook GA. Injuries in women's gymnastics: A 5-year study. *Am J Sports Med.* 1979; 7: 242–244.

23. Brooks AL, Henning GD. Injury to the proximal clavicular epiphysis. *J Bone Joint Surg*. 1972; 54A: 1347–1351.
24. Denham RH, Dingley AF. Epiphyseal separation of the medial clavicle. *J Bone Joint Surg*. 1967; 49A: 1179–1183.
25. Lewonowski K, Bassett GS. Complete posterior retrosternal epiphyseal separation: A case report and review of the literature. *Clin Orthop*. 1992; 281: 84–88.
26. Winter J, Sterner S, Maurer D, *et al*. Retrosternal epiphyseal disruption of medial clavicle: Case and review in children. *J Emerg Med*. 1989; 7: 9–13.
27. Destouet JM, Gilula LA, Murphy WA, *et al*. Computed tomography of the sternoclavicular joint and sternum. *Radiology*. 1981; 138: 123–128.
28. Selesnick FH, Jablon M, Frank C, *et al*. Retrosternal dislocation of the clavicle. *J Bone Joint Surg*. 1984; 66A: 287–291.
29. Wirth MA, Rockwood CA. Acute and traumatic injuries of the sternoclavicular joint. *J Am Acad Orthop Surg*. 1996; 4: 268–278.
30. Clark RL, Milgram JW, Yawn DH. Fatal aortic perforation and cardiac tamponade due to Kirschner wire migrating from the right sternoclavicular joint. *South Med J*. 1974; 67: 316–318.
31. Nogi J, Heckman JD, Hakala M, *et al*. Non-union of the clavicle in a child: A case report. *Clin Orthop*. 1975; 110: 19–21.
32. Nordquist A, Petersson C. The incidence of fractures of the claviculae. *Clin Orthop*. 1994; 300: 127–132.
33. Bowen A. Plastic bowing of the clavicle in children: A report of two cases. *J Bone Joint Surg*. 1983; 65A: 403–405.
34. Kubiak R, Slongo T. Operative treatment of clavicle fractures in children: A review of 21 years. *J Pediatr Orthop*. 2002; 22: 736–739.
35. Howard FM, Shafer SJ. Injury to the clavicle with neurovascular complications: A study of fourteen cases. *J Bone Joint Surg*. 1965; 47A: 1335–1346.
36. Zenni EJ, Krieg JK, Rosen MJ. Open reduction and internal fixation of clavicular fractures. *J Bone Joint Surg*. 1981; 63A: 147–151.
37. Black GB, McPherson JA, Reed MH. Traumatic pseudodislocation of the acromioclavicular joint in children. *Am J Sports Med*. 1991; 19: 644–666.
38. Eidman DK, SiB SJ, Tullos HS. Acromioclavicular lesions in children. *Am J Sports Med*. 1981; 9: 150–154.
39. Falstie-Jensen S, Mikkelsen P. Pseudodislocation of the acromioclavicular joint. *J Bone Joint Surg*. 1982; 64B: 368–369.
40. Havranek P. Injuries of the distal clavicular physis in children. *J Pediatr Orthop*. 1989; 9: 213–215.
41. Ogden JA. Distal clavicular physeal injury. *Clin Orthop*. 1984; 188: 68–73.
42. Rockwood CA. Fractures of outer clavicle in children and adults. *J Bone Joint Surg*. 1982; 64B: 642–649.
43. Bjerneld H, Hovelius L, Torling J. Acromioclavicular separations treated conservatively. *Acta Orthop Scand*. 1983; 54: 743–745.
44. Galpin RD, Hawkins RJ, Grainger RW. A comparative analysis of operative versus nonoperative management of grade III acromioclavicular separations. *Clin Orthop*. 1985; 193: 150–155.
45. Larsen E, Bjerg-Nielsen A, Christensen P. Conservative or surgical treatment of acromioclavicular dislocation. *J Bone Joint Surg*. 1986; 68A: 552–555.
46. Cahill BR. Atraumatic osteolysis of the distal clavicle: A review. *Sports Med*. 1992; 13: 214–222.
47. Scavenius M, Iversen BF. Nontraumatic clavicular osteolysis in weight lifters. *Am J Sports Med*. 1992; 20: 463–467.
48. Larson RL, Singer KM, Bergstrom R, *et al*. Little League survey: The Eugene study. *Am J Sports Med*. 1976; 4: 201–209.
49. Lyman S, Fleisig G, Andrews JR, *et al*. Effect of pitch type, pitch count, and pitching mechanics on risk of elbow and shoulder pain in youth baseball pitchers. *Am J Sports Med*. 2002; 30: 463–468.
50. Kohler R, Trillaud JM. Fracture and fracture separation of the proximal humerus in children: Report of 136 cases. *J Pediatr Orthop*. 1983; 3: 326–332.
51. Baxter MP, Wiley J. Fractures of the proximal humeral epiphysis: Their influence on humeral growth. *J Bone Joint Surg*. 1986; 68B: 570–573.
52. Dameron TB, Reibel DB. Fractures involving the proximal humeral epiphyseal plate. *J Bone Joint Surg*. 1969; 51A: 289–297.
53. Neer CS, Horowitz BS. Fractures of the proximal humeral epiphyseal plate. *Clin Orthop*. 1965; 41: 24–31.
54. Nilsson S, Svartholm F. Fracture of the upper end of the humerus in children. *Acta Chir Scand*. 1965; 130: 433–439.
55. Sherk H, Probst C. Fractures of the proximal humeral epiphysis. *Orthop Clin North Am*. 1975; 6: 401–413.
56. Williams DJ. The mechanisms producing fracture separation of the proximal humeral epiphysis. *J Bone Joint Surg*. 1981; 63B: 102–107.
57. Dobbs MB, Luhmann SL, Gordon JE, *et al*. Severely displaced proximal humeral epiphyseal fractures. *J Pediatr Orthop*. 2003; 23: 208–215.
58. Asher MA. Dislocations of the upper extremity in children. *Orthop Clin North Am*. 1976; 7: 583–591.
59. Hovelius L. Anterior dislocation of the shoulder in teenagers and young adults. *J Bone Joint Surg*. 1987; 69A: 393–399.
60. Marans HJ, Angel KR, Schemitsch EH, *et al*. The fate of traumatic anterior dislocation of the shoulder in children. *J Bone Joint Surg*. 1992; 74A: 1242–1244.
61. Rowe CR. Anterior dislocation of the shoulder: Prognosis and treatment. *Surg Clin North Am*. 1963; 43: 1609–1614.
62. Rowe CR. Prognosis in dislocation of the shoulder. *J Bone Joint Surg*. 1956; 38A: 957–977.
63. Wagner KT, Lyne ED. Adolescent traumatic dislocations of the shoulder with open epiphysis. *J Pediatr Orthop*. 1983; 3: 61–62.
64. Aronen JG, Regan K. Decreasing the incidence of recurrence of First time anterior shoulder dislocation with rehabilitation. *Am J Sports Med*. 1984; 12: 283–291.
65. Burkhead WZ, Rockwood CA. Treatment of instability of the shoulder with an exercise program. *J Bone Joint Surg*. 1992; 74A: 890–896.
66. Simonet WT, Cofeld RH. Prognosis in anterior shoulder dislocation. *Am J Sports Med*. 1984; 12: 19–24.
67. Deitch J, Mehlman CT, Foad SL, *et al*. Traumatic anterior shoulder dislocation in adolescents. *Am J Sports Med*. 2003; 31: 758–763.
68. Jones KJ, Wiesel B, Ganley TJ, *et al*. Functional outcomes of early arthroscopic bankart repair in adolescents aged 11 to 18 years. *J Pediatr Orthop*. 2007; 27: 209–213.
69. Carter C, Sweetnam R. Recurrent dislocation of the patella and the shoulder: Their association with familial joint laxity. *J Bone Joint Surg*. 1960; 42B: 721–727.
70. Neer CS, Foster DR. Inferior capsular shift for involuntary inferior and multidirectional instability of the shoulder. *J Bone Joint Surg*. 1980; 62A: 897–908.
71. Bigliani LU, D'Alessandro DF, Duralde XA, *et al*. Anterior acromioplasty for subacromial impingement in patients younger than 40 years of age. *Clin Orthop*. 1989; 246: 111–116.
72. Hawkins RJ, Kennedy JC. Impingement syndrome in athletes. *Am J Sports Med*. 1980; 8: 151–157.
73. Tibone JE. Shoulder problems of adolescence. *Clin Sports Med*. 1983; 2: 423–426.
74. Tibone JE, Elrod B, Jobe FW, *et al*. Surgical treatment of tears of the rotator cuff in athletes. *J Bone Joint Surg*. 1986; 68A: 887–891.
75. Pappas AM. Elbow problems associated with baseball during childhood and adolescence. *Clin Orthop*. 1982; 164: 30–41.
76. Aronem JG. Problems of the upper extremity in gymnastics. *Clin Sports Med*. 1985; 4: 61–71.
77. Otsuka NY, Kasser JR. Supracondylar fractures of the humerus in children. *J Am Acad Orthop Surg*. 1997; 5: 19–26.
78. Skaggs DL. Elbow fractures in children: diagnosis and management. *J Am Acad Orthop Surg*. 1997; 5: 303–312.
79. Brauer CA, Lee BM, Bae DS, *et al*. A systematic review of medial and lateral entry pinning versus lateral entry pinning for supracondylar fractures of the humerus. *J Pediatr Orthop*. 2007; 27: 181–186.
80. Kocher MS, Kasser JR, Waters PM, *et al*. Lateral entry compared with medial and lateral entry pin fixation for completely displaced supracondylar humeral fractures in children. A randomized clinical trial. *J Bone Joint Surg Am*. 2003; 89: 706–712.

81. Davids J, Maguire M, Mubarak S, *et al.* Lateral condylar fracture of the humerus following posttraumatic cubitus varus. *J Pediatr Orthop.* 1994; 14: 466–470.
82. Bernstein SM, McKeever P, Bernstein L. Percutaneous reduction of displaced radial neck fractures in children. *J Pediatr Orthop.* 1993; 13: 85–88.
83. Gill TJ, Micheli LJ. The immature athlete: Common injuries and overuse syndromes of the elbow and wrist. *Clin Sports Med.* 1996; 15: 401–423.
84. Farsetti P, Potenza V, Caterini R, *et al.* Long term results of treatment of fractures of the medial humeral epicondyle in children. *J Bone Joint Surg Am.* 2007; 83: 1299–1305.
85. Dias J, Johnson G, Hoskinson J, *et al.* Management of severely displaced medial epicondyle fractures. *J Orthop Trauma.* 1987; 1: 59–62.
86. Josefsson PO, Danielsson LG. Epicondylar elbow fracture in children: 35-year follow-up of 56 unreduced cases. *Acta Orthop Scand.* 1986; 57: 313–315.
87. Woods GW, Tullos HS. Elbow instability and medial epicondyle fractures. *Am J Sports Med.* 1977; 5: 23–30.
88. Carlioz H, Abols Y. Posterior dislocation of the elbow in children. *J Pediatr Orthop.* 1984; 4: 8–12.
89. Jackson DW, Silvino N, Reiman P. Osteochondritis in the female gymnasts's elbow. *Arthroscopy.* 1989; 5: 129–136.
90. Brogdon BG, Crow NE. Little Leaguer's elbow. *Am J Roentgenel.* 1960; 83: 671–675.
91. Gugenheim JJ, Stanley RF, Wood GW, *et al.* Little League survey: The Houston study. *Am J Sports Med.* 1976; 4: 189–200.
92. Hang YS. Little League elbow: A clinical and biomechanical study. *Int Orthop.* 1982; 3: 70–78.
93. Slager RF. From Little League to the big league, the weak spot is the arm. *Am J Sports Med.* 1977; 5: 37–48.
94. Smith MGH. Osteochondritis of the humeral capitellum. *J Bone Joint Surg.* 1964; 46B: 50–54.
95. Tiynon MC, Anzel SH, Waugh TR. Surgical management of osteochondritis dissecans of the capitellum. *Am J Sports Med.* 1976; 4: 121–128.
96. Takahara M, Mura N, Sasaki J, *et al.* Classification, treatment, and outcome of osteochondritis dissecans of the humeral capitellum. *J Bone Joint Surg Am.* 2007; 89: 1205–1214.
97. Chambers RB. Orthopedic injuries in athletes (ages 6 to 17). *Am J Sports Med.* 1979; 7: 195–197.
98. Watson AW. Sports injuries during one academic year in 6,799 Irish school children. *Am J Sports Med.* 1984; 12: 65–71.
99. Zaricznyj B, Shattuck LJ, Mast TA, *et al.* Sports-related injuries in school-aged children. *Am J Sports Med.* 1980; 8: 318–324.
100. Blitzer CM, Johnson RJ, Ettlinger CF, *et al.* Downhill skiing injuries in children. *Am J Sports Med.* 1984; 12: 142–147.
101. Garrick JF, Regua RK. Epidemiology of women's gymnastic injuries. *Am J Sports Med.* 1980; 8: 261–264.
102. Sullivan JA, Gross RH, Grana WA, *et al.* Evaluation of injuries in youth soccer. *Am J Sports Med.* 1980; 8: 325–327.
103. Mann DC, Rajmaira S. Distribution of physeal and non-physeal fractures in 2650 long bone fractures in children aged 0–16 years. *J Pediatr Orthop.* 1990; 10: 713–716.
104. Friberg K. Remodeling after distal forearm fractures. *Acta Orthop Scand.* 1970; 50: 731–750.
105. Landfried MJ, Stenclik M, Sui JG. Variant of Galeazzi fracture-dislocation in children. *J Pediatr Orthop.* 1991; 11: 332–335.
106. Rodriguez-Merchan EC. Pediatric fractures of the forearm. *Clin Orthop.* 2005; 432: 65–72.
107. Roy S, Caine D, Singer KM. Stress changes of the distal radius epiphysis in young gymnasts. *Am J Sports Med.* 1985; 13: 301–308.
108. Mandelbaum BR, Bartolozzi AR, Davis CA, *et al.* Wrist pain syndrome in the gymnast. Pathogenetic, diagnostic, and therapeutic considerations. *Am J Sports Med.* 1989; 17: 305–317.
109. Vender MI, Watson HK. Acquired Madelung-like deformity in a gymnast. *J Hand Surg.* 1988; 13A: 19–21.
110. Terry CL, Waters PM. Triangular Fibrocartilage injuries in pediatric and adolescent patients. *J Hand Surg.* 1998; 23A: 626–634.
111. Fabre O, De Boeck H, Haentjens P. Fractures and nonunions of the carpal scaphoid in children. *Acta Orthop Belg.* 2001; 67: 121–125.
112. Mintzer CM, Waters PM, Simmons BP. Nonunion of the scaphoid in children treated with Herbert screw fixation and bone grafting. A report of five cases. *J Bone Joint Surg.* 1995; 77B: 98–100.
113. Riester JN, Baker BE, Mosher JF, *et al.* A review of scaphoid fracture healing in competitive athletes. *Am J Sports Med.* 1985; 13: 154–161.
114. Southcott R, Rosman MA. Non-union of carpal scaphoid fractures in children. *J Bone Joint Surg.* 1977; 59B: 20–23.
115. Hanks GA, Kalenak A, Bowman LS, *et al.* Stress fractures of the carpal scaphoid. A report of four cases. *J Bone Joint Surg.* 1989; 71A: 938–941.
116. Manzione M, Pizzutillo PD. Stress fracture of the scaphoid waist. *Am J Sports Med.* 1981; 9: 268–269.
117. Burton RI, Eaton RG. Common hand injuries in the athlete. *Orthop Clin North Am.* 1973; 4: 809–838.
118. Hastings H, Simmons BP. Hand fractures in children. *Clin Orthop.* 1984; 188: 120–130.
119. McCue FC, Baugher WH, Kulund DN, *et al.* Hand and wrist injuries in the athlete. *Am J Sports Med.* 1979; 7: 275–286.
120. Posner MA. Injuries to the hand and wrist in athletes. *Orthop Clin North Am.* 1977; 8: 593–617.
121. Simmons BP, Lovallo JL. Hand and wrist injuries in children. *Clin Sports Med.* 1988; 7: 495–512.
122. Leddy JP, Packer JW. Avulsion of the profundus tendon insertion in athletes. *J Hand Surg.* 1977; 2: 66–69.
123. Ciullo JV, Jackson DW. Pars interarticularis stress reaction, spondylolysis, and spondylolisthesis in gymnasts. *Clin Sports Med.* 1985; 4: 95–110.
124. Ferguson RH, McMaster JF, Stanitski CL. Low back pain in college football linemen. *Am J Sports Med.* 1974; 2: 63–69.
125. Hall SJ. Mechanical contribution to lumbar stress injuries in female gymnasts. *Med Sci Sports Exerc.* 1986; 18: 599–602.
126. Howell DW. Musculoskeletal profile and incidence of musculoskeletal injuries in lightweight women rowers. Am *J Sports Med.* 1984; 12: 278–281.
127. Ireland ML, Micheli LJ. Bilateral stress fracture in the lumbar pedicle in a ballet dancer. *J Bone Joint Surg.* 1987; 69A: 140–142.
128. Jackson DW, Wiltse LL, Cirincione RJ. Spondylolysis in the female gymnast. *Clin Orthop.* 1976; 117: 68–73.
129. McCarroll JR, Miller JM, Ritter MA. Lumbar spondylolysis and spondylolisthesis in college football players. *Am J Sports Med.* 1986; 14: 404–406.
130. Micheli LJ. Back injuries in dancers. *Clin Sports Med.* 1983; 2: 473–484.
131. Micheli LJ. Back injuries in gymnastics. *Clin Sports Med.* 1985; 4: 85–93.
132. Semen RL, Spengler D. Significance of lumbar spondylolysis in college football players. *Spine.* 1981; 6: 172–174.
133. Micheli LJ. Low back pain in the adolescent: Differential diagnosis. *Am J Sports Med.* 1979; 7: 362–364.
134. Rosenberg NJU, Bargar WL, Friedman B. The incidence of spondylolysis and spondylolisthesis in nonambulatory patients. *Spine.* 1981; 6: 35–38.
135. O'Neill DB, Micheli LJ. Post-operative radiographic evidence for fatigue fracture as the etiology of spondylolysis. *Spine.* 1989; 14: 1342–1355.
136. Hoshina H. Spondylolysis in athletes. *Phys Sports Med.* 1980; 8: 75–78.
137. Baker DR, McHolick W. Spondylolysis and spondylolisthesis in children. *J Bone Joint Surg.* 1956; 38A: 933–934.
138. Collier BD, Johnson RP, Carrera GF. Painful spondylolysis or spondylolisthesis studied by radiography or single photon emission computed tomography. *Radiology.* 1985; 154: 207–211.
139. LaFond G. Surgical treatment of spondylolisthesis. *Clin Orthop.* 1962; 22: 175–9.

140. Hutton WC, Stott JRR, Cyron BM. Is spondylolysis a fatigue fracture? *Spine*. 1977; 2: 202–229.
141. Letts M, Smallman T, Afanasiev R, *et al*. Fracture of the pars interarticularis in adolescent athletes: A clinical-biomechanical analysis. *J Pediat Orthop*. 1986; 6: 40–46.
142. Fredrickson BE, Baker D, McHolick WJ, *et al*. The natural history of spondylolysis and spondylolisthesis. *J Bone Joint Surg*. 1984; 66A: 699–707.
143. Winney-Davies R, Scott JHS. Inheritance and spondylolisthesis–a radiographic family survey. *J Bone Joint Surg*. 1979; 61B: 301–305.
144. Phalen GS, Dickson JA. Spondylolisthesis and tight hamstrings. *J Bone Joint Surg*. 1961; 43A: 505–512.
145. Bellah RD, Summerville DA, Treves ST, *et al*. Low-back pain in adolescent athletes: Detection of stress injury to the pars interarticularis with SPECT. *Radiology*. 1991; 180: 509–512.
146. Staendert CJ, Herring SA. Spondylolysis: a critical review. *Br J Sports Med* 2000; 34: 415–442.
147. Morita T, Ikata T, Katoh S, *et al*. Lumbar spondylolysis in children and adolescents. *J Bone Joint Surg*. 1995; 77B: 620–625.
148. Campbell RS, Grainger AJ, Hide IG, *et al*. Juvenile spondylolysis: A comparative analysis of CT, SPECT, and MRI. *Skeletal Radiol*. 2005; 34: 63–73.
149. Saraste H. Prognostic radiologic aspects of spondylolisthesis. *Acta Radiol*. 1984; 25: 427–434.
150. Saraste H. Long-term clinical and radiographic follow-up of spondylolysis and spondylolisthesis. *J Pediatr Orthop*. 1987; 7: 631–638.
151. Turner R, Bianco A. Spondylolysis and spondylolisthesis in children and teenagers. *J Bone Joint Surg*. 1971; 53A: 1298–1306.
152. Wiltse LL, Jackson DW. Treatment of spondylolisthesis and spondylolysis in children. *Clin Orthop*. 1976; 117: 92–100.
153. Wiltse LL, Widell EH, Jackson DW. Fatigue fracture: The basic lesion in isthmic spondylolisthesis. *J Bone Joint Surg*. 1974; 57A: 17–22.
154. Calmels P, Fayolle-Minon I. An update on orthotic devices for the lumbar spine based on a review of the literature. *Rev Rheum (Engl Ed)*. 1996; 63: 285–291.
155. Micheli LJ, Hall JE, Miller ME. Use of modified Boston back brace for back injuries in athletes. *Am J Sports Med*. 1980; 8: 351–356.
156. Micheli LJ, Steiner ME. Treatment of symptomatic spondylolysis and spondylolisthesis with the modified Boston brace. *Spine*. 1985; 10: 937–943.
157. d'Hemecourt PA, Zurakowski D, Kriemler S. Spondylolysis: Returning the athlete to sports participation with brace treatment. *Orthopedics*. 2002; 25: 653–657.
158. Congeni J, McCulloch J, Swanson K. Lumbar spondylolysis. A study of natural progression in athletes. *Am J Sports Med*. 1997; 25: 248–253.
159. Papanicolaou N, Wilkinson RH, Emans JB, *et al*. Bone scintigraphy and radiography in young athletes with low back pain. *Am J Roentgenol*. 1985; 145: 1039–1044.
160. Bradford DS, Iza J. Repair of the defect in spondylolysis or minimal degrees of spondylolisthesis by segmental fixation and bone grafting. *Spine*. 1985; 10: 673–679.
161. Buck J. Direct repair of the defect in spondylolisthesis. *J Bone Joint Surg*. 1970; 52B: 432–437.
162. Buring K, Fredensborg N. Osteosynthesis of spondylolysis. *Acta Orthop Scand*. 1973; 44: 91–97.
163. Boxall D, Bradford D, Winter R, *et al*. Management of severe spondylolisthesis in children and adolescents. *J Bone Joint Surg*. 1979; 61A: 479–495.
164. Hensinger R, Lang J, MacEwen G. Surgical management of spondylolisthesis in children and adolescents. *Spine*. 1976; 1: 207–214.
165. Muschik M, Hahnel H, Robinson PN, *et al*. Competitive sports and the progression of spondylolisthesis. *J Pediatr Orthop*. 1996; 16: 364–369.
166. Bradford DS. Treatment of severe spondylolisthesis: A combined approach for reduction and stabilization. *Spine*. 1979; 4: 423–429.
167. Borgesen SE, Vang PS. Herniation of the lumbar intervertebral disk in children and adolescents. *Acta Orthop Scand*. 1974; 45: 540–549.
168. Epstein JA, Epstein NE, Marc J, *et al*. Lumbar intervertebral disk herniation in teenage children: Recognition and management of associated anomalies. *Spine*. 1984; 9: 427–432.
169. Garrido E, Humphreys RP, Hendrick EB, *et al*. Lumbar disc disease in children. *Neurosurgery*. 1978; 2: 222–226.
170. Swärd L, Hellström M, Jacobsson B, *et al*. Acute injury of the vertebral ring apophysis and intervertebral disc in adolescent gymnasts. *Spine*. 1990; 15: 144–148.
171. Swärd L, Hellström M, Jacobsson B, *et al*. Disc degeneration and associated abnormalities of the spine in elite gymnasts. *Spine*. 1991; 16: 437–443.
172. DeOrio JK, Bianco AJ. Lumbar disc excision in children and adolescents. *J Bone Joint Surg*. 1982; 64A: 991–995.
173. Kurihara A, Kataoka O. Lumbar disc herniation in children and adolescents. A review of 70 operated cases and their minimum 5-year follow-up studies. *Spine*. 1980; 5: 443–451.
174. Lippitt AB. Fracture of a vertebral body end plate and disk protrusion causing subarachnoid block in an adolescent. *Clin Orthop*. 1976; 116: 112–115.
175. Resnick D, Niwayama G. Intravertebral disk herniation: cartilaginous (Schmorl's) nodes. *Radiology*. 1978; 126: 57–65.
176. Jackson DW, Rettig A, Wiltse LL. Epidural cortisone injections in the young athletic adult. *Am J Sports Med*. 1980; 8: 239–243.
177. Day AL, Friedman WA, Indelicato PA. Observations on the treatment of lumbar disk disease in college football players. *Am J Sports Med*. 1987; 15: 72–75.
178. Techakapuch S. Rupture of the lumbar cartilage plate into the spinal canal in an adolescent. A case report. *J Bone Joint Surg*. 1981; 63A: 481–482.
179. Micheli LJ. Sports following spinal surgery in the young athlete. *Clin Orthop*. 1985; 198: 152–157.
180. Sorenson HK. *Scheuermann's juvenile kyphosis*. Copenhagen: Munksgaard; 1964.
181. Hubbard DD. Injuries of the spine in children and adolescents. *Clin Orthop*. 1974; 100: 56–65.
182. Kewalramani MD, Tori JA. Spinal cord trauma in children: neurological patterns, radiologic features, and pathomechanics of injury. *Spine*. 1980; 5: 11–18.
183. Kujala UM, Taimela S, Oksanen A, *et al*. Lumbar mobility and low back pain during adolescence. A longitudinal three-year follow-up study in athletes and controls. *Am J Sports Med*. 1997; 25: 363–368.

CHAPTER 45

Lower limb injuries

Umile Giuseppe Longo and Nicola Maffulli

Introduction

Physical activity plays a significant role in the well-being of a child.[1] Long-term health benefits depend on continuation of the physical activity, thus enhancing well-being and favouring balanced development during childhood and adolescence.[2–4] Injuries can counter the beneficial effects of sports participation if a child is unable to continue to participate because of the residual effects of injury.

Prevention of sports injuries in young people has been largely implemented in the last few years.[5,6] For example, the injury prevention programme 'The 11', developed with the support of the Federation Internationale de Football Associations (FIFA), aims to reduce the impact of intrinsic injury risk factors in soccer, and it has been validated in that sport.[7,8] A subsequent modified version of 'The 11' ('The 11+') has been shown to be effective in preventing injuries in young female soccer players.[9] The FIFA 11+ provided more than a 40% reduction in the risk of injury.[9] We conducted a cluster randomized controlled trial to examine the effect of the FIFA 11+ on rates of injuries in elite male basketballers.[5] A subgroup analysis of the children included in the study showed that the programme is effective in reducing the rates of injuries in young male basketballers.[5]

Several factors can be related to the risk of injury during sport. Therefore, different exercises or factors might have been responsible for efficacy of the FIFA 11+ to prevent injuries. The programme was found to be ineffective in preventing the following injuries: ankle, anterior thigh, posterior thigh (hamstring), hip/groin, sprains, strains, fractures, and anterior lower leg pain (periostitis). On the other hand, the programme was effective in preventing knee injuries, lower extremity injuries, overall injuries, severe injuries, and overuse injuries such as lower extremity tendon pain and low back pain. Mechanism of injury data in soccer,[10,11] basketball,[12] handball,[13] rugby,[14] and alpine skiing,[15] indicate that the success of the programme could be related to running exercises to obtain proper knee control and core stability during cutting and landing, exercises to improve dynamic and static balance, neuromuscular control and proprioception (particularly of the knee and the hip), and exercises increasing hamstring muscle strength to prevent injuries to the anterior cruciate ligament.

The lower extremity is under specific biomechanical demands important in the context of the increasing numbers of athletes in soccer, skiing, and running.[16]

The musculoskeletal system in childhood

The growing musculoskeletal system has some peculiarities. Tendons and ligaments are relatively stronger than the epiphyseal plate, and considerably more elastic. Therefore, in severe trauma, the epiphyseal plate, being weaker than the ligaments, gives way.[3] Hence, growth plate damage is more common than ligamentous injuries.

In children, bones and muscles show increased elasticity[17] and heal faster.[18] Weight bearing is beneficial for the skeleton, but excessive strains may produce serious injuries to joints.[17] Low-intensity training can stimulate bone growth, but high-intensity training can inhibit it.[19] There are adaptive changes to sport activity, and up to puberty muscular strength is similar in girls and boys.

Different metabolic and psychological aspects of childhood in sport

Children produce more heat relative to body mass, have a low sweating capacity, and also tend not to drink enough compared to adults. Therefore, heat prostration and exhaustion, especially in hot climates, is more likely than in adults. (Interested readers are referred to Chapter 14 for a detailed discussion of temperature regulation.)

Young competitors may have the same chronological age, but not necessarily the same biological age, and children need to be more closely matched with the other competitors by both chronological and biological age.[20,21] It is also possible that parents and coaches push children too hard,[18,22] not appreciating that time is needed to develop high-performance abilities. Children may also develop psychological complications following injuries.[23]

Endogenous risk factors

There are a number of well-established risk factors for paediatric musculoskeletal injury in sport.[24–29] Imbalances in the musculoskeletal system may influence the rate of occurrence of injuries.[18] Common conditions such as pes cavus, pes planus, and calcaneus valgus may play a role in the aetiology of some injuries.[18] Anatomical factors have been hypothesized in the aetiology of injuries where overuse is common, such as in patellofemoral stress syndrome, ileotibial band syndrome, medial tibial stress syndrome, and plantar fasciitis. Compared to adults, children have decreased strength and endurance, which has to be taken into account when planning training and competition.

With growth spurts, there is a decrease in flexibility due to relative bone lengthening. This predisposes to injury in the absence of appropriate stretching exercises, prior to commencing sport. Studies in adults have shown that stretching prior to exercise does not reduce the incidence of injury,[30,31] although this has not yet been shown in children. Training in improper environments or with incorrect footwear can also result in injury. Cross training and gradual change in training schedules is good practice. Players should ideally be matched with appropriate body protection and supervision. Balanced nutrition is vital: the amenorrhoeic, anorexic female with reduced bone mineral density is at higher risk of injury. High-resistance training may also predispose children to an increased risk of injury if not properly supervised.[32]

Epidemiology of lower limb injuries

The actual incidence of injury in children's sports is very difficult, if not impossible, to determine.[1,33–35] Published studies vary significantly in terms of populations studied, methodology used, and types and severity of injuries reported. In addition, because of the different criteria used to define an injury, comparisons between reports are difficult, and any such comparisons should be interpreted with caution.

Approximately 3–11% of school children are injured per year while participating in sport. Twice as many boys as girls sustain sports-related injuries, although some authors report a similar incidence between the genders.[36, 37] Boys, however, still sustain more severe injuries, possibly because they are more aggressive. For certain sports, such as horse riding, injuries are four times more common in females. Sports involving contact and jumping have the highest injury levels, with football in particular accounting for the majority of injuries. Elite athletes, however, have lower injury rates than the general sporting population.[38] Using a mixed longitudinal study design, an incidence rate of less than 1 injury per 1000 h of training in 453 elite young British athletes was reported.[39] In general, the incidence of sports injuries seems to increase with age, with injuries in older children approaching the incidence rate of more senior players.

Schmidt and Höllwarth[40] compared the frequency of sport injuries according to their location. They found that 43.8% of all injuries occur in the upper extremity, 16% in the head, and 34.5% in the lower extremity, with a peak at age 12 years. Sprains, contusions, and lacerations account for the majority (60%) of injuries.[41,42]

In the lower extremity, the knee joint is most often involved.[43] In adults, knee injuries are responsible for 20%[44] of all football (soccer) injuries, and 13%[45] of all American football injuries. Ankle injuries are frequent as well, and in a study of gymnastics[46] and tennis,[47] they were reported to be even more common than knee injuries.

Traumatic injuries are often typical of a specific sport. The pattern of injury has changed over the years, and is related to sporting equipment. Currently, an increased number of overuse injuries are being reported. Overuse or chronic injuries as a result of repetitive microtrauma manifest as bursitis, tendinopathy, stress fracture, chondromalacia patellae, osteochondritis dissecans, and traction apophysitis, and are more common in the lower extremity. Risk factors may include training errors, muscle-tendon imbalance, anatomical alignments, footwear, and nutritional factors.

Injury characteristics and severity

Injuries can either occur acutely, and are associated with a macrotraumatic event, such as fractures and sprains, or arise gradually due to a repetitive microtraumatic event, such as stress fracture, osteochondritis dissecans, apophysitis, or tendinopathies.[48] Presentation for macrotrauma is invariably not delayed. There is typically a good clear history and mechanism of injury. On examination, there will be pain and, depending on the area of the body, swelling and deformity. This allows the examiner to determine a likely diagnosis and whether any further investigations are warranted. Luckily, the majority of injuries are minor and require a short period of rest, analgesia, and compression prior to graduated formal rehabilitation. Microtrauma or overuse injuries invariably give a more insidious onset of symptoms that are typically related to activity. These symptoms will obviously depend very much on the anatomical location. In the younger individual, they may present purely with reduced performance or a limp. Exact identification of the anatomical area injured can be difficult. History and examination are vital. The type of sport played may give extra clues to the likely diagnosis, although further investigations may be required to confirm the diagnosis. Management generally requires a period of relative rest, with the child partaking in a different sport to allow healing while maintaining general condition. If this fails, then rest must be absolute, and referral for specialist assessment is advisable. Coaches are appropriately advised to observe attitude, behaviour, and development, which may suggest neglect or abuse. This may be evident acutely or present as a chronic injury.

The severity of injuries spans broadly from sprains and contusions to death, and certain types of injury occur more commonly in specific sports. For example, spiral fractures of the tibia are the most common fracture in children with skiing injuries, and in ankle injuries are the most common injury seen in basketball. Fortunately, the vast majority of sports injuries are minor and do not require medical attention. Very serious sports accidents in youth, such as brain or spinal cord damage, lesions of the heart, or submersions leading to invalidity or death, are exceptional.[49]

Ligament, muscle, and tendon injuries

Ligaments in youth are considerably more elastic than in adults.[18] Sprains are common, especially in lax individuals, and are normally well tolerated. Ankle sprains are more common in patients with weak and deconditioned peroneal muscles and pes cavus varus deformity.[50,51] In general, they should be managed conservatively with the use of orthotics if the hindfoot is in varus. The first line management in chronic ankle instability should be strengthening and proprioceptive training.[18,52] The prophylactic effect of external stabilization with strapping remains doubtful, and one study reported no effect of high-top shoes in preventing ankle sprains in 622 college basketball players.[53]

Chronic compartment syndrome occurs even in young athletes, and is typical in running. In these patients, compartment pressure monitoring, modification of activity, and fasciotomy should be considered.

Muscle injuries

Quadriceps contusions may produce local muscle bleeds associated with injury.[17,54] As in other muscle injuries, the injury may occur from a direct blow, sudden explosive action, or occasionally from a more trivial action. Management includes rest, ice, compression, elevation, and analgesia.[55,56] Restriction of sport is essential, followed by a graduated return to sport. Healing with fibrous tissue, the area may be prone to further injury. Occasionally a lump is palpable, and, if there are any concerns, magnetic resonance imaging (MRI) is useful to exclude neoplasia.

Ligament injuries

Injuries of the knee most often result in physeal injuries because ligaments are stronger than growth plates. In one study, 90% of young athletes over the age of 12 years with anterior cruciate ligaments (ACL) disruptions were found to have intrasubstance tears.[57] A MRI scan may be performed to ascertain whether an ACL tear has indeed occurred. Although MRI has a good ability to predict ACL disruption with a specificity of 95% and a sensitivity of 88%, clinical examination is still paramount.[58–61] Conservative management of ACL rupture leads to severe instability and poor knee function, and carries the risk of sustaining secondary injuries such as meniscal tears. However, operative reconstruction of the ACL in skeletally immature patients has the potential to cause growth arrest or result in leg length discrepancy due to physeal damage. Complications such as femoral valgus deformity with arrest of the lateral femoral physis, tibial recurvatum with arrest of the tibial tubercle apophysis, genu valgum without arrest, and leg length discrepancy have been reported.[62] As a result, several authors have advised delayed surgery, allowing time for skeletal maturity prior to reconstructing the ACL.

Several studies have reported on ACL reconstruction in skeletally immature patients.[43,58] Soft tissue grafts seem to have no influence on epiphyseal growth. Smith and Tao[16] recommend hamstring tendon grafts using central tibial tunnel placement. Lo[63] found no leg-length discrepancy in five patients, aged between 8 and 14 years, who underwent ACL reconstruction. More recently, in a series of 47 knees that underwent ACL reconstruction with a four-strand hamstrings graft, no leg length discrepancy or growth arrest occurred.[64] Leg length discrepancies after ACL reconstruction may represent anatomically normal variants. Despite this, it is essential that the risks and benefits of ACL reconstruction be analysed prior to surgery in skeletally immature patients.[62,65]

Medial cruciate ligament (MCL) and lateral collateral ligament (LCL) injuries are managed non-operatively as in adults. Rarely, children may sustain tears in the posterolateral corner of the knee, and in such situations surgery is indicated. Injuries of the posterior cruciate ligament, however, can be managed conservatively or operatively after the growth plates have closed.[16]

Tendinopathy

Tendinopathy is a common overuse injury of the lower extremity.[29,66,67] Most affected is the site of tendon insertion, the apophysis. In most patients, partial rest and strapping are sufficient. Absolute immobilization leads to musculoskeletal atrophy.[18] Over the past few years, various new therapeutic options have been proposed for the management of tendinopathy.[68] Despite the morbidity associated with tendinopathy, management is far from scientifically based, and many of the therapeutic options described and in common use lack hard scientific background.[69] Physical therapy, rest, training modification, splintage, taping, cryotherapy, electrotherapy, shock wave therapy, hyperthermia, pharmaceutical agents such as non-steroidal anti-inflammatory drugs, and various peritendinous injections have been proposed. Most essentially follow the same principles. Management methods that have been investigated with randomized controlled trials include nonsteroidal anti-inflammatory medication, eccentric exercise, glyceryl trinitrate patches, electrotherapy (microcurrent and microwave), sclerosing injections, and shock wave treatment. Despite this abundance of therapeutic options, very few randomized prospective, placebo-controlled trials exist to assist in choosing the best evidence-based management in children with tendinopathy[70]. A brief overview of the most common tendinopathies of the lower limb is provided in Table 45.1.

Table 45.1 Common forms of soft tissue injury of the lower limb.

Type	Reason	Remarks	Conservative management
Snapping hip	Stenosing tenosynovitis of the iliopsoas tendon	May be subluxation of the hip joint	Exercises to strengthen the hip extensors and abductors
Shin splint syndrome = medial tibial stress syndrome	Overuse of the soleus muscle on its attachment to the tibia	Often in runners	Rest, orthotics to prevent hyperpronation, running on soft surfaces
Posterior tibial tendinopathy	Repetitive excessive traction (with hyperpronation)	Often associated with excessive midfoot pronation	Orthotics to control excessive pronation, cortisone injection, physiotherapy
Achilles tendinopathy	Excessive eccentric weight loading	Often bilateral and associated with calcaneal apophysitis	Conservative, eccentric exercises, Shock wave therapy
Peroneal tendinopathy	Impingement in the excessively pronated foot		Orthotics, cortisone injections
Tibialis anterior tendinopathy	Direct pressure in skates or ski boots		Alter footwear, Vaseline, pad to reduce friction
Extensor hallucis longus tendinopathy	Tight heel cords with lack of ankle dorsiflexion results in increased activity of the extensor hallucis tendon		Heel lifts and orthotics to support the forefoot
Plantar fasciitis	Predisposition: pes cavus or pes planus		Physiotherapy, orthotics, cortisone injections, alteration of activity Shock wave therapy

Table supported by references[18,52,71,72].

Joint injuries

Hip

Direct forces such as dashboard injuries may dislocate the hip and fracture the acetabulum, and such fracture-dislocations are usually posterior. After emergency reduction, patients should be kept in traction for 3–6 weeks. A haematoma can be evacuated. Magnetic resonance imaging is recommended to exclude soft tissue interposition, and later to identify vascular necrosis of the femoral head.

The long-term consequences of hip dislocations can be serious: 50% of patients develop avascular necrosis of the femoral head, and, if the acetabular limbus is torn, the stability of the hip joint can be seriously impaired.

Knee

Patellar subluxation or dislocation occurs in one in 1000 children aged between 9 and 15 years of age (Figure 45.1). A common cause is a twisting injury, when the femur is twisted medially with the foot planted on the ground, or direct trauma. Patella alta, in which the patella rides high in the femoral groove, predisposes to patellar instability,[17,73–76] and may be accompanied by chronic low-grade knee pain due to patellofemoral stress syndrome.[71] Spontaneous reduction is possible, and the patient may present with an effusion at times due to injury of the ACL. Management consists of immediate reduction of the dislocated patella. However, one in six patients will develop recurrent dislocations, and will require realignment surgery. Skyline radiographs are recommended to exclude marginal osteochondral fractures, which can result in loose bodies.[17]

Giving way of the knee on twisting should be considered of patellar origin until proved otherwise. Although meniscal problems in this age group are unusual, and are generally associated with a discoid meniscus with a painless clonking noise before the tear, meniscal lesions in adolescents need to be considered, and warrant arthroscopy.[77] In the case of meniscal injuries, repair of torn menisci is recommended because of the extremely poor long-time results following meniscectomy in children.

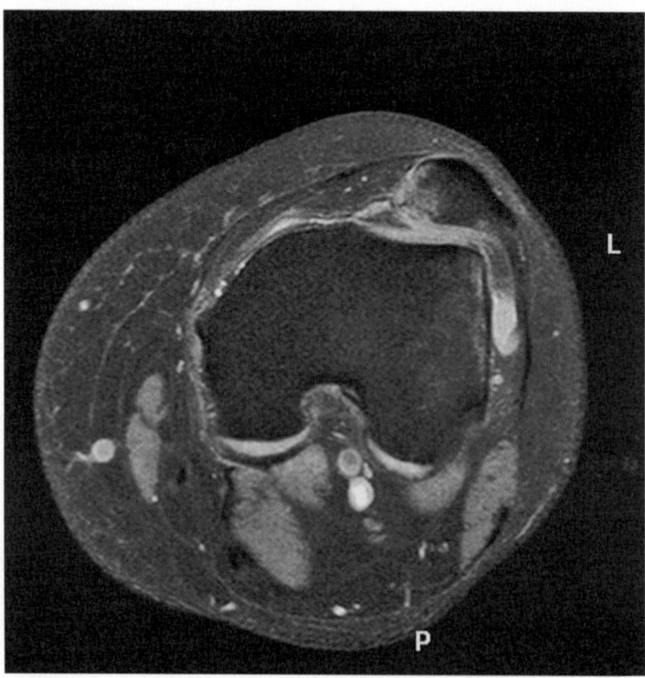

Figure 45.1 Patellar subluxation.

Haemarthrosis of the knee is often accompanied by severe ligamentous or meniscal injury. In 70 young patients with haemarthrosis after acute trauma, Stanitski[78] found that 47% had ACL tears and 47% a meniscal tear. In adolescents (13–18 years), the rate was 65% and 45%, respectively.

Foot

Pain in the first metatarsal-cuneiform joint is rare, and most often relates to hypermobility of the joint due to hindfoot or subtalar joint pronation. Orthotics limiting such hypermobility may be successful.

Problems of the first metatarso-phalangeal joint in children differ from those in adults due to the lack of arthritic changes. These can occur in children with pes planus and hallux valgus, when a bunion rubs against the shoe. This appears to be a congenital abnormality rather than the results of poorly fitting shoes. Management consists of orthotics and wider fitting shoes, and, if symptoms persist, surgery after the growth plate has closed.

Bone injuries

Epiphyseal injuries

The growing parts of the bone include the physis and the epiphysis. Two types of epiphyses are found in the extremities: traction and pressure.[79] Traction epiphyses (or apophyses) are located at the site of attachment of major muscle tendons to bone and are subjected primarily to tensile forces. The apophyses contribute to bone shape, but not to longitudinal growth. As a result, acute or chronic injuries affecting traction growth plates are not generally associated with disruption of longitudinal bone growth.[79]

Pressure epiphyses are situated at the end of long bones and are subjected to compressive forces. The epiphyses of the distal femur and proximal tibia are examples of pressure epiphyses. The growth plate or physis is located between the epiphysis and metaphysis and is the essential mechanism of endochondral ossification.[79,80] In contrast with traction growth plates, injury to pressure epiphyses and their associated growth plates may result in growth disturbance. These are weaker areas, and therefore predisposed to injury. Injuries of the epiphyseal plates have been classified into five types.[81]

Type I injuries show a complete separation of the epiphysis from the metaphysis without any bone fracture. The germinal cells of the growth plate remain with the epiphysis, and the calcified layer remains with the metaphysis. In type II, the most common physeal injuries, the line of separation extends along the growth plate, then out through a portion of the metaphysis, producing a triangular shaped metaphyseal fragment sometimes referred to as the Thurston Holland sign. Type III, which is intra-articular, extends from the joint surface to the weak zone of the growth plate and then extends along the plate to its periphery (Figures 45.2a and b). In type IV, often involving the distal humerus, a fracture extends from the joint surface through the epiphysis, across the full thickness of the growth plate and through a portion of the metaphysis, thereby producing a complete split. In type V, a relatively uncommon injury, there is compression of the growth plate, thereby extinguishing further growth.

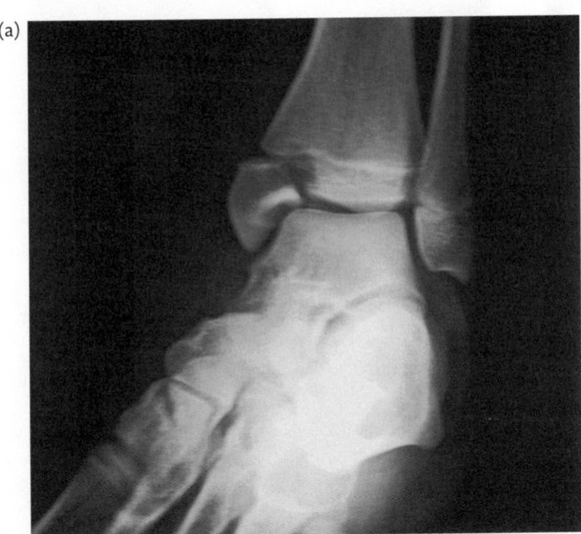

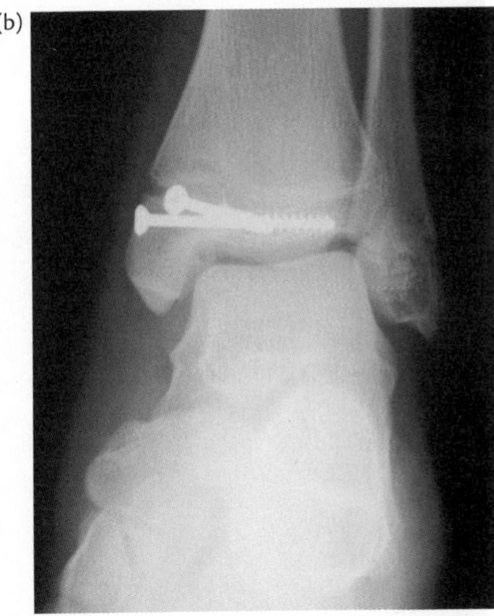

Figure 45.2 (a) A type III injury of the distal tibia. (b) Open reduction and internal fixation of type III injury of the distal tibia, without damage to the cartilage plate.

Prognosis for types I and II fractures is good if the germinal cells remain with the epiphysis, and circulation is unchanged. However, these injury types are not as innocuous as originally believed, and can be associated with risk of growth impairment. Type III injuries have a good prognosis if the blood supply in the separated portion of the epiphysis is still intact and the fracture is not displaced. Surgery can be necessary to restore the joint surface to normal. In type IV injuries, surgery is needed to restore the joint surface to normal and to perfectly align the growth plate. Type IV injuries have a poor prognosis unless the growth plate is completely and accurately realigned. A diagnosis of Salter V injury can be difficult at the time of injury. Growth can be disturbed, and, given the nature of the injury, may only become obvious at a later stage. Physeal injuries can be difficult to diagnose by radiographs. Therefore, if clinically suspected, protection of the limb with a cast and repeat radiographs and examination after 2 weeks are useful.

Fractures

Pelvis, femur, patella, and tibia

Pelvic fractures are mostly found in polytrauma patients, and require careful investigation of internal organs and, in most patients, external fixation. In children, they occur rarely in sports. Similarly, physeal fractures of the proximal femur and acetabulum are seldom associated with sports, and are often a result of high-energy trauma. Open reduction and internal fixation with pins across the epiphysis is recommended. Patients and their families should be counselled regarding the high risk of avascular necrosis of the femoral head and of premature closure of the epiphysis in such injuries.

Slipping of the upper femoral epiphysis occurs mainly in overweight boys with underdeveloped gonads, and in tall thin children during the growth spurt, between 10 and 16 years. The child frequently presents after an injury in which the thigh has apparently become suddenly painful. Close questioning often reveals some premonitory discomfort. Knee pain is often the presenting complaint because of the nerve supply of the hip, and many children are referred to an orthopaedic clinic with a painful knee for unknown causes. The physical signs consist of loss of internal rotation or even fixed external rotation and shortening of the leg, with external rotation of the foot while standing. With the child supine on the couch, internal rotation is restricted or impossible. Such physical signs demand a radiograph of the hip. The deformity is much easier to see in the lateral view. Surgical management to prevent further displacement consists of internal fixation of the upper femoral epiphysis in situ without attempting to reduce it. Despite appropriate and prompt management, avascular necrosis and chondrolysis may ensue, putting an end to an athletic career, and the hip at risk of secondary osteoarthritis. Hypothyroidism and renal osteodystrophy may be associated with epiphysiolysis, and should be excluded. Operative management is generally performed on an emergency basis and pinning in situ is recommended.

Femoral fractures can often be managed conservatively, especially in younger children. Shaft fractures are often managed with the application of a spica cast after an initial period of traction, because deviation of the femoral axis will correct spontaneously. In older children and adolescents, however, operative management with external fixation, plating, or intramedullary nailing is indicated.[82] Femoral nailing carries a risk of femoral head necrosis; therefore, some authors prefer external fixation or flexible unreamed nails. In anatomically reduced femoral shaft fractures, leg length discrepancy is also possible because of the increased blood supply to the fracture area, which results in increased growth of the fractured limb.

Tibial shaft fractures are the most common fractures in skiing. Management should be conservative for closed fractures, while for open or complicated fractures, anatomical reposition and stable fixation is necessary (Figures 45.3a and b). Osteochondral fractures around the knee are accompanied mostly by severe haemarthrosis.

Table 45.2 provides an overview of the different pattern and management possibilities of femoral, tibial, and patellar fractures.

Ankle

Symptomatic medial malleolar ossifications should be considered in the differential diagnosis of ankle pain in young athletes. On radiographs, spherical ossicles are visible, and conservative management is appropriate.

Ankle fractures are caused by major violence and, if undisplaced, they do not need internal fixation. Tillaux-Chaput fractures are Salter-Harris type III fracture of the distal tibia, with an epiphyseal fragment

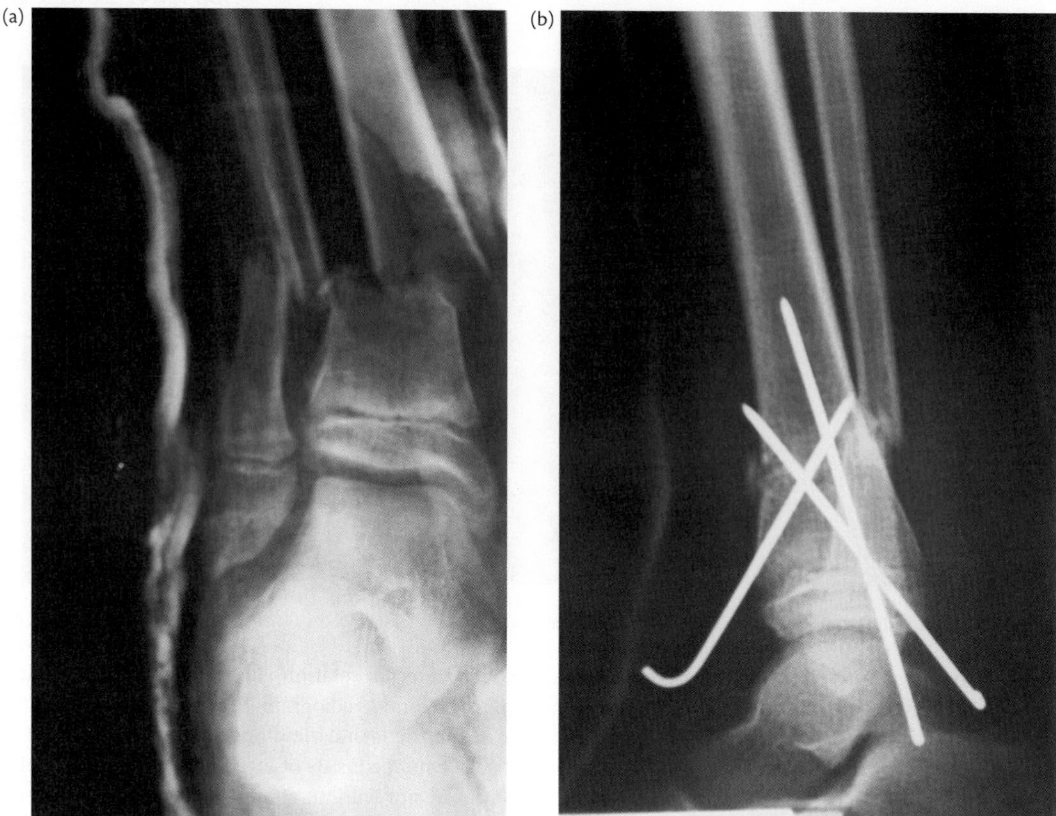

Figure 45.3 (a) Fracture of the distal diaphysis of tibia and fibula. (b) The surgical management of the fracture of the distal diaphysis of the tibia and fibula.

Table 45.2 Common fractures and epiphyseal injuries of femur, patella, and tibia.

Type	Cause	Remarks	Management
Proximal femur fractures	Direct trauma	High risk of femoral head necrosis, pseudarthrosis and coxa vara	ORIF and non-weight bearing for 3–6 months
Femoral stress fractures	Repetitive overload	Rare crescendo pain initial radiographs may be normal	Reduction of activity to a pain-free level
Distal femoral physeal fracture	High velocity trauma	Uncommon in sports often Salter V fractures with disturbance of leg length growth	ORIF for Salter III and IV
Patellar fractures	Direct trauma or avulsion		ORIF in the case of patellar surface disruption
Sleeve fractures of the patella	Periosteum is stripped downwards in continuity with the tendon results in double patella appearance	Diagnosis usually missed	Early surgery
Proximal tibia fracture	Direct trauma	Often with an avulsion fracture of the patellar tendon, injury to peroneal nerve possible	ORIF if displaced
Tibial shaft fracture	Direct or twisting trauma		Conservative, if displaced or open: ORIF
Tibial stress fractures	Repetitive overload	Crescendo pain initial radiographs may be normal	Reduction of activity to a pain-free level for 8–12 weeks
Tibial eminence fracture (avulsion of tibial spine)	Direct trauma or forceful hyperextension with rotation	Complication: ACL laxity	ORIF for displaced fractures
Tibial tuberosity fracture	Intensive jumping	Predisposition from Osgood-Schlatter`s lesion	ORIF in displaced fractures

ORIF: open reduction and internal fixation.

Supported by references[17,83,84].

connected to the syndesmosis. This fracture occurs in young athletes close to the end of puberty, and requires internal fixation.

The most common fractures of the ankle after twisting are type I or II Salter injuries with an open distal fibular epiphysis.[17,85] These fractures often close up, leaving only tenderness over the epiphysis with normal radiographs. Stress radiographs, however, usually reveal the underlying pathology, and, according to the age of the patient, internal fixation should be considered.[17,18,82,86,87] An overview of ankle fractures is provided in Table 45.3.

Foot

The most common complaint is heel pain due to Sever's lesion. Forefoot problems are common, especially after chronic overload. Osteochondroses typically occur around the tarsal and metatarsal bones of the foot. Freiberg's lesion consists of collapse of the articular surface and subchondral bone of the metatarsal head. Most commonly the second metatarsal is affected (68%), but it is also found in the third (27%) or fourth (5%) metatarsal. The collapse is related to reduced blood supply caused by mechanical overload. The main principle of management is to redistribute load, with help from orthotics if necessary. Late surgery in adulthood can also be considered for resistant cases. Köhler's lesion, i.e. vascular necrosis of the tarsal navicular bone, results in localized pain. It is diagnosed by radiographic increased density of the navicular. Management is usually conservative with orthotics or a period in plaster.[88,89] Generally, it takes 2–3 years to return to normal. An overview of the most common bony injuries of the foot is provided in Table 45.4.

Table 45.3 Ankle fractures and epiphyseal injuries.

Type	Predisposing factors	Conservative management	Operative management
Epiphyseal fracture	Weak and deconditioned tendons Pes cavus Tarsal coalition	Early motion/taping, casting, Aircast splint	ORIF for Salter III and IV
Osteochondral fractures		Early motion, non-weight bearing	Occasionally but possible, normally undisplaced detached fragment: ORIF
Chronic osteochondral fracture (without displacement)		Casting	Failure of non-surgical management: surgical debridement, forage, grafting
Isolated fibula fracture	Varus deformity of the hindfoot	Casting or splint	Displaced: ORIF
Fibular fracture with medial malleolus fracture		Casting in anatomical position	Unstable fracture needs ORIF
Ankle mortis fracture without displacement			Unstable fracture needs ORIF
Triplane fracture of the distal tibia			ORIF required

ORIF: open reduction and internal fixation.

Supported by references[17,18].

Table 45.4 Bony foot injuries.

Type	Predisposition	Conservative management	Operative management
Sesamoiditis of the first metatarsal	Pes cavus	Orthotics, metatarsal pad	
Metatarsalgia of the metatarsophalangeal joints	Morton's foot with a short first ray	Modified activity, metatarsal pad	
Freiberg's lesion	Long second metatarsal	Modified activity, insert to unload the metatarsal head, rigid soled shoes	Late surgery
Fracture of the metatarsal		Plaster casting	
Stress fracture of 2nd to 4th metatarsals	Pes cavus	Decrease activity, modify footwear	
Navicular stress fracture	Kohler's lesion cricket bowling	Activity reduction, casting for 4–6 weeks	Occasionally screw-fixation
Jones fracture of the fifth metatarsal		Plaster casting	Surgery for non-union
Painful tarsal coalition	Bony or cartilaginous bar in the hindfoot	Physiotherapy, alteration of activity or footwear	Late surgery

Supported by references[17,18,72,83].

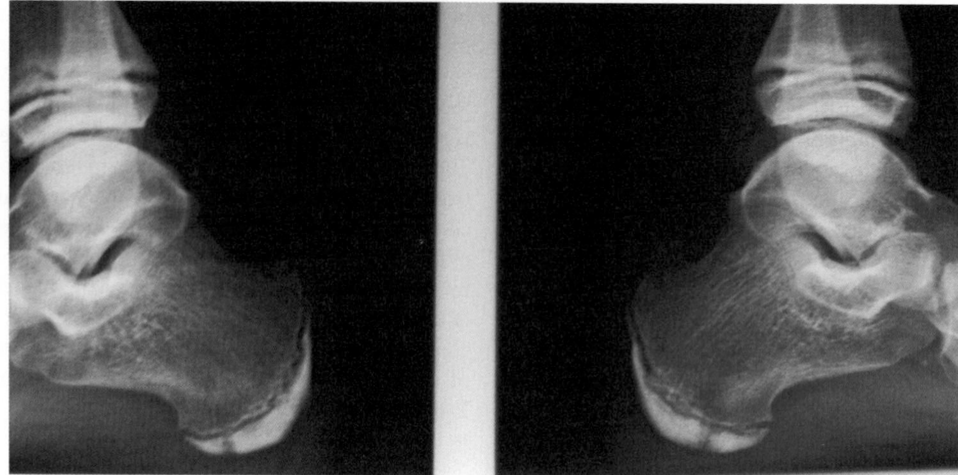

Figure 45.4 Bilateral Sever's disease.

Avulsion fractures and apophysitis

Avulsion fractures are common. They arise because of sudden intense muscular traction exerted on the immature skeleton. Tendons are relatively stronger than bones and avulsion fractures of growth plates are the result of chronic or acute traction.

Tibial avulsion fractures and apophysitis

Osgood-Schlatter lesion, a traction apophysitis of the tibial tubercle, and Sever's lesion, a traction apophysitis of the calcaneal apophysis, are the most common traction apophysitis[48]. They are common in boys around the time of growth spurts[71]. The onset of pain is commonly induced by a higher than normal amount of physical activity. Conservative management is normally sufficient.

A mature tibial tubercle forms from ossification centres in the epiphysis. The pulling action of the patellar tendon may cause inflammation and pain, resulting in Osgood-Schlatter's lesion, which occurs between 8 and 13 years in girls, and 10 and 15 years in boys. Boys are nearly twice as commonly affected as girls, possibly because of their higher activity levels. The onset of pain is commonly induced by a higher than normal amount of physical activity. Conservative management is normally sufficient.

Sever's lesion (Figure 45.4) presents with well-localized, activity-related pain at the tip of the heel and radiographic fragmentation of the calcaneal apophysis. Sever's lesion may result from intensive training and improper footwear.[71] Some authors consider Sever's lesion to be a form of stress fracture, but there is often a similar radiographic appearance of the other asymptomatic side. Severs's lesion is often bilateral.[71] The pain responds to rest and a shock absorber under the heel (Table 45.5).

Table 45.5 Avulsion injuries of the lower extremity.

Location		Remarks	Management
Pelvis and hip	Anterior inferior iliac spine Lesser trochanter Iliac crest Whole ischium	Caused by m. psoas Caused by m. psoas Caused by m. sartorius, Abductors and hamstrings	Conservative: non-weight bearing for 3 weeks Operative: considered when long fragments are displaced
Knee	Osgood-Schlatter: traction apophysitis of the tibial tubercle		Conservative Operative: when pain persists with excision of intratendinous ossicles
	Sinding-Larsen-Johannson: lower patella pole		Conservative
Ankle and foot	Avulsion of a bony fragment of the anterior tibio-fibular ligament from the distal tibial epiphysis	= Tillaux fracture	Internal fixation
	Iselin's lesion: apophysitis of the fifth metatarsal	Rare	Conservative
	Sever's lesion	Excessive tensile loads in tension. Predisposition: tight heel cord, often associated with Achilles tendinopathy, age usually 8 to 13 years	Conservative (shock absorber), avoid barefoot walking: physiotherapy, stretching and strengthening, casting if persistent

Supported by references[17,63,90].

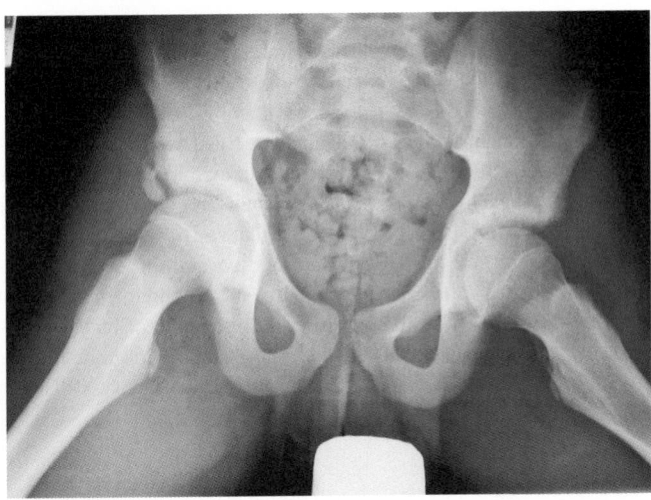

Figure 45.5 Avulsion of the anterior inferior iliac spine.

Iliac spine avulsion fractures

The anterior inferior iliac spine (AIIS) tends to fail during football when the kicking foot is suddenly blocked, as happens in a tackle (Figure 45.5). More often, when the foot hits the ground, the AIIS is pulled off by the reflected head of rectus femoris. In similar circumstances, the psoas muscle can avulse the lesser trochanter. The whole apophyseal plate of the ischium can separate through the powerful pull of the hamstrings. This can happen in cross-country running when the ditch being jumped is wider than expected, and the leading leg is overstretched. More rarely, the anterior superior iliac spine (ASIS) can be avulsed by the action of musculus sartorius in a bad gymnastics vault landing. The whole iliac crest apophysis can also be pulled off by the abdominal muscles, although displacement is uncommon.

Typically, the young athlete presents a history of severe, immediate, and well-localized pain, and the appropriate radiographic views confirm the diagnosis. As the avulsions are deep, cryotherapy is unhelpful, and oral analgesia is the preferred option for pain relief, with rest and gradual return to activity as pain permits. Immediate surgery is not indicated, and late surgery is rarely required despite occasional dramatic radiographic changes.

Patellar avulsion fractures

Sinding-Larsen-Johansson lesion is a syndrome of tenderness and radiographic fragmentation localized at the inferior pole of the patella. The lesion can be considered a calcific tendinopathy in an avulsed portion of the patellar tendon, and is self limiting.

Osteochondritis dissecans

Osteochondritis dissecans (OCD) can be due to intense physical activity causing repetitive microtrauma. This can be shown by the rate of OCD being three times more prevalent in active boys than girls around puberty, and also in competitive sports involving jumping. Osteochondritis dissecans usually occurs in the lateral aspect of the medial femoral condyle, femoral head and middle third of the lateral border of the talus. The radiographic diagnosis can be confirmed by MRI, and, if necessary, definitive management can be performed by arthroscopy. In general, management is conservative in stable lesions, and, with larger fragments, arthroscopic removal of intraarticular loose bodies or fixation is recommended. The long-term prognosis associated with excision of the fragment is poor because of an increased risk of osteoarthritis.

Stress fractures

Stress fractures are difficult to diagnose,[91] and are often associated with training errors. Endogenous factors such as body size, sex, diet, hormonal status, and anatomical factors are important as well, but difficult to prove. Stress fractures occur more often in women, in particular amenorrhoeic athletes with decreased bone density.[92,93] Stress fractures occur more often in organized sports.

Typical locations are the metatarsals, the middle and proximal tibia, the proximal femur, and the calcaneus. A study of 320 stress fractures reported that 49% of them occur in the tibia, 25% in the tarsal bones, and 9% in the metatarsals. Varus alignment seems to play an important role in lower extremity stress fractures. Stress fractures of the navicular are associated with a short first metatarsal, metatarsal adductus, and limited ankle dorsiflexion and subtalar motion.

Diagnosis may be difficult on plain radiographs taken at the time of onset of pain, and therefore should be repeated 2–3 weeks later. At this stage, however, the rapid periosteal response can be confused with infections or tumours. Magnetic resonance imaging or computed tomography (CT) may be helpful. If the clinical picture is not typical, a technetium-scan is indicated. Primary management consists of immobilization with exercise within the limitations of pain.

Legg-Calve-Perthes disease

Legg-Calve-Perthes disease is a form of avascular necrosis of the femoral head that occurs mainly between 5 and 10 years of age. The condition is probably due to two or more episodes of raised intra-articular pressure,[94] although the influence of sports is doubtful.[17] It presents as an irritable hip with sclerosis of the femoral head. In general, the more complete the lesion, the worse the outcome. On the other hand, the earlier its onset, the better the outcome. If Legg-Calve-Perthes disease does occur in a young athlete, a temporary interruption or limitation of sports activities is necessary. In the early phases of Legg-Calve-Perthes disease, plain radiographs may be normal, but bone scanning may show decreased uptake in the femoral head. Magnetic resonance imaging does provide better evaluation of involvement in the early stages of Legg-Calve-Perthes disease than plain radiography, but its cost effectiveness needs to be assessed.[95] Management is either conservative or surgical, depending on various indications and the stage of the disease.[96] Despite its benignity, investigations are mandatory to exclude the rare cases of tuberculosis or bone tumour that may present as an irritable hip. A larger joint effusion is generally a sign of sepsis, usually caused by *Staphylococcus aureus*. In this instance, the young athlete will generally present with pyrexia, malaise, and severe fatigue. Bone scanning shows increased uptake at both sides of the joint. If pus is aspirated, the hip should be explored surgically, and antibiotics started.

Tarsal coalitions and sinus tarsi problems

Tarsal coalitions can cause pain associated with physical activity, and should be suspected after a history of multiple ankle sprains and subtalar stiffness on examination.[90] Most commonly, the subtalar joint is affected, followed by coalition between the calcaneus and navicular.[97] The coalition can be fibrous, cartilaginous, or osseous, and is accompanied by loss of supination. Management consists of casting in the painful stage, and surgery for the calcaneal navicular coalition for young children at a later stage.[72]

Sinus tarsi syndrome often occurs after starting a new activity.[72] Patients show tenderness in the sulcus of the sinus tarsi, with, at times, swelling. Management should consist of limiting pronation by orthotics, and, if the pain persists, surgery is indicated[98].

Navicular problems

Navicular pain in young athletes is common, and is often accompanied by irritation of the tibialis posterior tendon insertion. It can also be caused by an accessory navicular bone. Excessive pronation can be limited by the use of orthotics.[72]

Prevention

The epidemiological approach in sports traumatology aims to quantify the occurrence of sports injuries in relation to who is affected by injuries, where and when these injuries have occurred, and what is their outcome (descriptive approach). Efforts are also made to explain why and how such injuries occur, to develop strategies to limit their occurrence, and to prevent them (analytical approach).[99] Preventing sports injuries in young individuals is important to reduce the short- and long-term social and economic consequences.[100] The epidemiological approach implies that injuries do not happen purely by chance.[101]

Most of the preventive measures suggested in the literature have arisen from descriptive research, and have not been derived from risk factors that have been substantiated as defensible injury predictors through correlational or experimental research.[99] Not only will children have their own risk factors, but so will their particular sports. There has already been widespread involvement in assessing general risks and trends that result in children's injuries.[102,103] Once the analytical evidence points to an association between certain risk factors and injury, thereby establishing a degree of predictability for those participants who are likely to sustain an injury, a method of intervention can be devised for prevention.[104] Intervention can be either therapeutic, using tapes or braces to an injured area resulting in reduction in re-injuries, or preventive, in which an agent or procedure is tried on athletes free from injury and is evaluated by recording the reduction of risk of injury.

Sports-specific studies, for example skiing, baseball, skating, tennis, or gymnastics, all have similar conclusions regarding safety barriers or run-offs, adequate supervision, appropriate warm ups, and protective equipment.[36,105–108] Up to approximately one-third of injuries may be preventable. Many of these parallel adult sporting common sense issues. Perceived insight into injury risk has not been reported. Issues specific to children include more fair matching of size, weight, and height, appropriate supervision, properly fitting equipment for young individuals, and limiting external pressure imposed by parents and coaches. This is a difficult balance to achieve.

Pre-participation screening limits the participation of the most susceptible individuals, and its value continues to be evaluated.[109,110] Balance, for example, can be used as a predictor of future ankle injury.[109] Prevention is based on defining the fitness and flexibility required, as well as the general medical status. These variables need to be measured appropriately and advice given to maintain or improve physical status. Pre-season conditioning works well to reduce early season injuries[111]. Well-reported successful cases of injury prevention have followed a number of important working parties. Perhaps the most well-known examples include reduction in the rates of quadriplegia following the banning of spearing in American football, the use of appropriate head and face guards in ice hockey, breakaway bases in baseball[112], appropriate ball selection, limiting repetitive actions, e.g. in throwing and bowling sports, and appropriate fluid management in hot weather. However, not all such interventions are entirely successful. For example, while the use of chest protectors in baseball does give extra protection, cases of commotio cordis have still been reported[113].

Conclusions

Overall, injuries in children are uncommon, and, although their incidence increases with age, most are self-limiting and have no long-term effects. Any sport can cause musculoskeletal injuries, and the specific pattern and location of injuries of each sport should be known by health professionals. Training programmes and performance standards should take into account the biological age of the participants, and their physical and psychological immaturity, more than their chronological age. A deep knowledge of the different aspects of training, including duration, intensity, frequency, and recovery, are needed to avoid serious damage to the musculoskeletal system of athletic children.

Physical injury is an inherent risk in sports participation and, to a certain extent, must be considered an inevitable cost of athletic training and competition. However, coaches and parents can minimize the risk of injury by ensuring the proper selection of sporting events, using appropriate equipment, enforcing rules, using safe playing conditions, and providing adequate supervision. Although injuries in young athletes are sustained, it is important to balance the negative effects of sports injuries with the many social, psychological, and physical health benefits that result from a serious commitment to sport.

Summary

- The actual incidence of injury in children's sports is very difficult, if not impossible, to determine.
- Imbalances in the musculoskeletal system of children may influence the rate of occurrence of injuries. Common conditions such as pes cavus, pes planus, and calcaneus valgus may play a role in the aetiology of some injuries.
- With growth spurts, there is a decrease in flexibility due to relative bone lengthening. This predisposes to injury in the absence of appropriate stretching exercises, prior to commencing sport.
- Sports-related injuries of the lower limb in children mainly concern the following diagnosis: ligament injuries, fractures, epiphyseal injuries, and apophysitis. The most frequent approaches for the management of these injuries include: conservative management for undisplaced fractures or partial ligamentous ruptures. Surgery is recommended for displaced fractures or complete ligamentous injuries.

- Most injuries in children are self-limiting and have no long-term effects.
- Any sport can cause lower limb musculoskeletal injuries, and the specific pattern and location of injuries of each sport should be known by health professionals.
- Training programmes and performance standards should take into account the biological age of the participants, and their physical and psychological immaturity, more than their chronological age. A deep knowledge of the different aspects of training, including duration, intensity, frequency, and recovery, are needed to avoid serious damage to the musculoskeletal system of athletic children.

References

1. Maffulli N, Longo UG, Gougoulias N, Loppini M, Denaro V. Long-term health outcomes of youth sports injuries. *Br J Sports Med.* 2010; 44: 21–25.
2. Shephard RJ. Physical activity and the child. *Sports Med.* 1984; 1: 205–233.
3. Maffulli N, Longo UG, Spiezia F, Denaro V. Aetiology and prevention of injuries in elite young athletes. *Med Sport Sci.* 2011; 56: 187–200.
4. De Mozzi P, Longo UG, Galanti G, Maffulli N. Bicuspid aortic valve: a literature review and its impact on sport activity. *Br Med Bull.* 2008; 85: 63–85.
5. Longo UG, Loppini M, Berton A, Marinozzi A, Maffulli N, Denaro V. The FIFA 11+ program is effective in preventing injuries in elite male basketball players: a cluster randomized controlled trial. *Am J Sports Med.* 2012; 40: 996–1005.
6. Longo UG, Loppini M, Cavagnino R, Maffulli N, Denaro V. Musculoskeletal problems in soccer players: current concepts. *Clin Cases Miner Bone Metab.* 2012; 9: 107–111.
7. Tegnander A, Olsen OE, Moholdt TT, Engebretsen L, Bahr R. Injuries in Norwegian female elite soccer: a prospective one-season cohort study. *Knee Surg Sports Traumatol Arthrosc.* 2008; 16: 194–198.
8. Steffen K, Myklebust G, Olsen OE, Holme I, Bahr R. Preventing injuries in female youth football—a cluster-randomized controlled trial. *Scand J Med Sci Sports.* 2008; 18: 605–614.
9. Soligard T, Myklebust G, Steffen K, *et al.* Comprehensive warm-up programme to prevent injuries in young female footballers: cluster randomised controlled trial. *BMJ.* 2008; 9; 337: a2469.
10. Mjolsnes R, Arnason A, Osthagen T, Raastad T, Bahr R. A 10-week randomized trial comparing eccentric vs. concentric hamstring strength training in well-trained soccer players. *Scand J Med Sci Sports.* 2004; 14: 311–317.
11. Arnason A, Andersen TE, Holme I, Engebretsen L, Bahr R. Prevention of hamstring strains in elite soccer: an intervention study. *Scand J Med Sci Sports.* 2008; 18: 40–48.
12. Krosshaug T, Nakamae A, Boden BP, *et al.* Mechanisms of anterior cruciate ligament injury in basketball: video analysis of 39 cases. *Am J Sports Med.* 2007; 35: 359–367.
13. Olsen OE, Myklebust G, Engebretsen L, Bahr R. Injury mechanisms for anterior cruciate ligament injuries in team handball: a systematic video analysis. *Am J Sports Med.* 2004; 32: 1002–1012.
14. Longo UG, Huijsmans PE, Maffulli N, Denaro V, De Beer JF. Video analysis of the mechanisms of shoulder dislocation in four elite rugby players. *J Orthop Sci.* 2011; 16: 389–397.
15. Bere T, Florenes TW, Krosshaug T, *et al.* Mechanisms of anterior cruciate ligament injury in World Cup alpine skiing: a systematic video analysis of 20 cases. *Am J Sports Med.* 2011: 39: 1421–1429.
16. Smith AD, Tao SS. Knee injuries in young athletes. *Clin Sports Med.* 1995; 14: 629–650.
17. Maffulli N, Baxter-Jones AD. Common skeletal injuries in young athletes. *Sports Med.* 1995; 19: 137–149.
18. Stanish WD. Lower leg, foot, and ankle injuries in young athletes. *Clin Sports Med.* 1995; 14: 6516–6568.
19. Tipton CM, Matthes RD, Maynard JA, Carey RA. The influence of physical activity on ligaments and tendons. *Med Sci Sports.* 1975; 7: 165–175.
20. Baxter-Jones AD. Growth and development of young athletes. Should competition levels be age related? *Sports Med.* 1995; 20: 59–64.
21. Baxter-Jones AD, Helms P, Maffulli N, Baines-Preece JC, Preece M. Growth and development of male gymnasts, swimmers, soccer and tennis players: a longitudinal study. *Ann Hum Biol.* 1995; 22: 381–394.
22. Baxter-Jones AD, Maffulli N. Parental influence on sport participation in elite young athletes. *J Sports Med Phys Fitness.* 2003; 43: 250–255.
23. Pillemer FG, Micheli LJ. Psychological considerations in youth sports. *Clin Sports Med.* 1988; 7: 679–689.
24. Wilkins K. The uniqueness of the young athlete: musculoskeletal injuries. *Am J Sports Med.* 1980; 8: 377–382.
25. Micheli LJ, Glassman R, Klein M. The prevention of sports injuries in children. *Clin Sports Med.* 2000; 19: 821–834.
26. Purvis JM, Burke RG. Recreational injuries in children: Incidence and prevention. *J Am Acad Orthop Surg.* 2001; 9: 365–374.
27. Baxter-Jones AD, Maffulli N. Intensive training in elite young female athletes. Effects of intensive training on growth and maturation are not established. *Br J Sports Med.* 2002; 36: 13–15.
28. Ahmad CS, Redler LH, Ciccotti MG, Maffulli N, Longo UG, Bradley J. Evaluation and management of hamstring injuries. *Am J Sports Med.* 2013: 41: 2933–2947.
29. Maffulli N, Longo UG, Maffulli GD, Khanna A, Denaro V. Achilles tendon ruptures in elite athletes. *Foot Ankle Int.* 2011; 32: 9–15.
30. Pope RP, Herbert RD, Kirwan JD, *et al.* A randomized trial of preexercise stretching for prevention of lower-limb injury. *Med Sci Sports Exerc.* 2000; 32: 271–277.
31. Shrier I. Stretching before exercise: an evidence based approach. *Br J Sports Med.* 2000; 34: 324–325.
32. Faigenbaum AD. Strength training for children and adolescents. *Clin Sports Med.* 2000; 19: 593–619.
33. Caine DJ, Maffulli N. Epidemiology of children's individual sports injuries. An important area of medicine and sport science research. *Med Sport Sci.* 2005; 48: 1–7.
34. Maffulli N, Caine D. The epidemiology of children's team sports injuries. *Med Sport Sci.* 2005; 49: 1–8.
35. Maffulli N, Longo UG, Gougoulias N, Caine D, Denaro V. Sport injuries: a review of outcomes. *Br Med Bull.* 2011; 97: 47–80.
36. Castiglia PT. Sports injuries in children. *J Pediatr Health Care.* 1995; 9: 32–33.
37. Sahlin Y. Sport accidents in childhood. *Br J Sports Med.* 1990; 24: 40–44.
38. Baxter-Jones A, Maffulli N, Helms P. Low injury rates in elite athletes. *Arch Dis Child.* 1993; 68: 130–132.
39. Maffulli N, King JB, Helms P. Training in elite young athletes (the Training of Young Athletes (TOYA) Study): injuries, flexibility and isometric strength. *Br J Sports Med.* 1994; 28: 123–136.
40. Schmidt B, Höllwarth ME. Sportunfälle im kindes- und jugendalter. *Zeitschrift für Kinderchirurgie.* 1989; 44: 357–362.
41. Cotta H, Steinbrück K. *Sportverletzungen und sportschäden im breitensport.* Köln: Kongreßband Deutscher-Sportärzte-Kongreß; 1982.
42. Bridgman SA, Clement D, Downing A, Walley G, Phair I, Maffulli N. Population based epidemiology of ankle sprains attending accident and emergency units in the west midlands of England, and a survey of UK practice for severe ankle sprains. *Emerg Med J.* 2003; 20: 508–510.
43. Longo UG, King JB, Denaro V, Maffulli N. Double-bundle arthroscopic reconstruction of the anterior cruciate ligament: does the evidence add up? *J Bone Joint Surg Br.* 2008; 90: 995–999.
44. Ekstrand J, Gillquist J. Soccer injuries and their mechanisms: a prospective study. *Med Sci Sports Exerc.* 1983; 15: 267–270.
45. Pritchett JW. A statistical study of knee injuries due to football in high-school athletes. *J Bone Joint Surg Am.* 1982; 64: 240–242.

46. Lindner KJ, Caine DJ. Injury patterns of female competitive club gymnasts. *Can J Sport Sci.* 1990; 15: 254–261.
47. Hutchinson MR, Laprade RF, Burnett QM, 2nd, Moss R, Terpstra J. Injury surveillance at the USTA Boys' Tennis Championships: a 6-yr study. *Med Sci Sports Exerc.* 1995; 27: 826–830.
48. Maffulli N. Intensive training in young athlete. The orthopaedic surgeons viewpoint. *Sports Med.* 1990; 9: 229–243.
49. Longo UG, Denaro L, Campi S, Maffulli N, Denaro V. Upper cervical spine injuries: indications and limits of the conservative management in Halo vest. A systematic review of efficacy and safety. *Injury.* 2010; 41: 1127–1135.
50. Longo UG, Loppini M, Romeo G, van Dijk CN, Maffulli N, Denaro V. Bone bruises associated with acute ankle ligament injury: do they need treatment? *Knee Surg Sports Traumatol Arthrosc.* 2013; 21: 1261–1268.
51. McCollum GA, Calder JD, Longo UG, *et al.* Talus osteochondral bruises and defects: diagnosis and differentiation. *Foot Ankle Clin.* 2013; 18: 35–47.
52. Bernhardt DT, Landry GL. *Sport injuries in young athletes.* St Louis: Mosby-Year Book; 1995.
53. Barrett JR, Tanji JL, Drake C, Fuller D, Kawasaki RI, Fenton RM. High- versus low-top shoes for the prevention of ankle sprains in basketball players. A prospective randomized study. *Am J Sports Med.* 1993; 21: 582–585.
54. Maffulli N. The growing child in sport. *Br Med Bull.* 1992; 48: 561–568.
55. Lippi G, Longo UG, Maffulli N. Genetics and sports. *Br Med Bull.* 2010; 93: 27–47.
56. Longo UG, Loppini M, Berton A, Spiezia F, Maffulli N, Denaro V. Tissue engineered strategies for skeletal muscle injury. *Stem Cells Int.* 2012; 2012: 175038.
57. Kellenberger R, von Laer L. Nonosseous lesions of the anterior cruciate ligaments in childhood and adolescence. *Prog Pediatr Surg.* 1990; 25: 123–131.
58. Maffulli N, Longo UG, Denaro V. Anterior cruciate ligament tear. *N Engl J Med.* 2009; 360: 1463; author reply: 63.
59. Longo UG, Rizzello G, Frnaceschi F, Campi S, Maffulli N, Denaro V. The architecture of the ipsilateral quadriceps two years after successful anterior cruciate ligament reconstruction with bone-patellar tendon-bone autograft. *Knee.* 2014; 21: 721–725.
60. Rizzello G, Longo UG, Petrillo S, *et al.* Growth factors and stem cells for the management of anterior cruciate ligament tears. *Open Orthop J.* 2012; 6: 525–530.
61. Capuano L, Hardy P, Longo UG, Denaro V, Maffulli N. No difference in clinical results between femoral transfixation and bio-interference screw fixation in hamstring tendon ACL reconstruction. A preliminary study. *Knee.* 2008; 15: 174–179.
62. Kocher MS, Saxon HS, Hovis WD, *et al.* Management and complications of anterior cruciate ligament injuries in skeletally immature patients: a survey of the Herodicus Society and The ACL Study Group. *J Pediatr Orthop.* 2002; 22: 452–457.
63. Lo IK, Kirkley A, Fowler PJ, Miniaci A. The outcome of operatively treated anterior cruciate ligament disruptions in the skeletally immature child. *Arthroscopy.* 1997; 13: 627–634.
64. Aichroth PM, Patel DV, Zorrilla P. The natural history and treatment of rupture of the anterior cruciate ligament in children and adolescents. A prospective review. *J Bone Joint Surg (Am).* 2002; 84B: 38–41.
65. Paletta GA. Special considerations. Anterior cruciate ligament reconstruction in the skeletally immature. *Orthop Clin North Am.* 2003; 34: 65–77.
66. Maffulli N, Wong J, Almekinders LC. Types and epidemiology of tendinopathy. *Clin Sports Med.* 2003; 22: 675–692.
67. Maffulli N, Longo UG, Loppini M, Spiezia F, Denaro V. New options in the management of tendinopathy. *Open Access J Sports Med.* 2010; 1: 29–37.
68. Maffulli N, Longo UG, Ronga M, Khanna A, Denaro V. Favorable outcome of percutaneous repair of achilles tendon ruptures in the elderly. *Clin Orthop Relat Res.* 2010; 468: 1039–1046.
69. Franceschi F, Longo UG, Ruzzini L, Rizzello G, Maffulli N, Denaro V. The Roman Bridge: a 'double pulley—suture bridges' technique for rotator cuff repair. *BMC Musculoskelet Disord.* 2007; 8: 123.
70. Longo UG, Lamberti A, Petrillo S, Maffulli N, Denaro V. Scaffolds in tendon tissue engineering. *Stem Cells Int.* 2012; 2012: 517165.
71. O'Neill DB, Micheli LJ. Overuse injuries in the young athlete. *Clin Sports Med.* 1988; 7: 591–610.
72. Santopietro FJ. Foot and foot-related injuries in the young athlete. *Clin Sports Med.* 1988; 7: 563–589.
73. Oliva F, Ronga M, Longo UG, Testa V, Capasso G, Maffulli N. The 3-in-1 procedure for recurrent dislocation of the patella in skeletally immature children and adolescents. *Am J Sports Med.* 2009; 37: 1814–1820.
74. Garau G, Rittweger J, Mallarias P, Longo UG, Maffulli N. Traumatic patellar tendinopathy. *Disabil Rehabil.* 2008; 30: 1616–1620.
75. Longo UG, Rizzello G, Ciuffreda M, *et al.* Elmslie-Trillat, Maquet, Fulkerson, Roux Goldthwait, and other distal realignment procedures for the management of patellar dislocation: systematic review and quantitative synthesis of the literature. *Arthroscopy.* 2016; 32: 929–43.
76. Ronga M, Oliva F, Longo UG, Testa V, Capasso G, Maffulli N. Isolated medial patellofemoral ligament reconstruction for recurrent patellar dislocation. *Am J Sports Med.* 2009; 37: 1735–1742.
77. Binfield PM, Maffulli N, Good CJ, King JB. Arthroscopy in sporting and sedentary children and adolescents. *Bull Hosp Jt Dis.* 2000; 59: 125–130.
78. Stanitski CL, Harvell JC, Fu F. Observations on acute knee hemarthrosis in children and adolescents. *J Pediatr Orthop.* 1993; 13: 506–510.
79. Caine D, DiFiori J, Maffulli N. Physeal injuries in children's and youth sports: reasons for concern? *Br J Sports Med.* 2006; 40: 749–760.
80. Maffulli N. Epiphyseal injuries of the proximal phalanx of the hallux. *Clin J Sport Med.* 2001; 11: 121–123.
81. Salter RB, Harris WR. Injuries involving the epiphyseal plate. *J Bone Joint Surg (Am).* 1963; 45: 587–622.
82. England SP, Sundberg S. Management of common pediatric fractures. *Ped Clin N Am.* 1996; 43: 991–1012.
83. Buckley SL. Sports injuries in children. *Curr Opin Pediatr.* 1994; 6: 80–84.
84. Albiñana J. Pediatric orthopaedic problems in lower limbs. *Curr Opin Orthop.* 1997; 8: 10–15.
85. Ogden JA. Skeletal injury in the child. Philadelphia: Lea & Febinger; 1982.
86. Ertl JP, Barrack RL, Alexander AH, VanBuecken K. Triplane fracture of the distal tibial epiphysis. Long-term follow-up. *J Bone Joint Surg Am.* 1988; 70: 967–976.
87. Maffulli N. Radial overgrowth and deformity after metaphyseal fracture fixation in a child. *Clin Orthop Relat Res.* 2006; 443: 350; author reply: 50.
88. Ippolito E, Ricciardi Pollini PT, Falez F. Kohler's disease of the tarsal navicular: long-term follow-up of 12 cases. *J Pediatr Orthop.* 1984; 4: 416–417.
89. Williams GA, Cowell HR. Kohler's disease of the tarsal navicular. *Clin Orthop Relat Res.* 1981; 158: 53–58.
90. Griffin LY. Common sports injuries of the foot and ankle seen in children and adolescents. *Orthop Clin North Am.* 1994; 25: 83–93.
91. Martinez de Albornoz P, Khanna A, Longo UG, Forriol F, Maffulli N. The evidence of low-intensity pulsed ultrasound for in vitro, animal and human fracture healing. *Br Med Bull.* 2011; 100: 39–57.
92. Jones BH, Bovee MW, Harris JM3rd, Cowan DN. Intrinsic risk factors for exercise-related injuries among male and female army trainees. *Am J Sports Med.* 1993; 21: 705–710.
93. Barrow GW, Saha S. Menstrual irregularity and stress fractures in collegiate female distance runners. *Am J Sports Med.* 1988; 16: 209–216.
94. Quain S, Catterall A. Hinge abduction of the hip. Diagnosis and treatment. *J Bone Joint Surg Br.* 1986; 68: 61–64.
95. Henderson RC, Renner JB, Sturdivant MC, Greene WB. Evaluation of magnetic resonance imaging in Legg-Perthes disease: a prospective, blinded study. *J Pediatr Orthop.* 1990; 10: 289–297.

96. Evans IK, Deluca PA, Gage JR. A comparative study of ambulation-abduction bracing and varus derotation osteotomy in the treatment of severe Legg-Calve-Perthes disease in children over 6 years of age. *J Pediatr Orthop*. 1988; 8: 676–682.
97. Harris RI, Beath T. Etiology of peroneal spastic flat foot. *J Bone Joint Surg (Br)*. 1948; 30B: 624–634.
98. O'Neill DB, Micheli LJ. Tarsal coalition. A followup of adolescent athletes. *Am J Sports Med*. 1989; 17: 544–549.
99. Caine CG, Caine DJ, Lindner KJ. *Epidemiology of sports injuries*. Champaign, IL: Human Kinetics; 1996.
100. Tursz A, Crost M. Sports-related injuries in children. A study of their characteristics, frequency, and severity, with comparison to other types of accidental injuries. *Am J Sports Med*. 1986; 14: 294–299.
101. Duncan DF. *Epidemiology. Basis for disease prevention and health; promotion*. New York: Macmillan; 1988.
102. Hackam DJ, Kreller M, Pearl RH. Snow-related recreational injuries in children: assement of morbidity and management strategies. *J Pediatr Surg*. 1999; 34: 65–69.
103. Helms PJ. Sports injuries in children: should we be concerned? *Archiv Dis Childhood*. 1997; 77: 161–163.
104. Meeuwisse WH. Predictability of sports injuries. What is the epidemiological evidence? *Sports Med*. 1991; 12: 8–15.
105. Kocher MS, Waters PM, Micheli LJ. Upper extremity injuries in the paediatric athlete. *Sports Med*. 2000; 30: 117–135.
106. Zetaruk MN. The young gymnast. *Clin Sports Med*. 2000; 19: 757–780.
107. Stevenson MR, Hamer P, Finch CF, *et al*. Sport-, age- and sex-specific incidence of sports injuries in Western Australia. *Br J Sports Med*. 2000; 3: 188–194.
108. Coulon L, Lackey G, Mok M, Nile D. A profile of Little League athletes injuries and the prevention methods used. *J Sci Med Sport*. 2001; 4: 48–58.
109. Metzel JD. The adolescent preparticipation physical examination. Is it helpful. *Clin Sports Med*. 2000; 19: 577–592.
110. Reed FE. Improving the preparticipation exam process. *J S C Med Assoc*. 2001; 97: 342–346.
111. Heidt RS, Sweeterman LM, Carlonas RL, *et al*. Avoidance of soccer injuries with preseason conditioning. *Am J Sports Med*. 2000; 28: 659–662.
112. Janda DH, Bir C, Kedrosle B. A comparison of standard vs. breakaway: an analysis of a preventative intervention for softball and baseball for and ankle injuries. *Foot Ankle Int*. 2001; 22: 810–816.
113. Viano DC, Bir CA, Cheney AK, *et al*. Prevention of commotio cordis in baseball: an evaluation of chest protectors. *J Trauma*. 2000; 49: 1023–1028.

CHAPTER 46

Injuries to the head and cervical spine

Robert V Cantu and Robert C Cantu

Introduction

Although traumatic brain or cervical injury can occur in many sports, Box 46.1 lists those with the highest risk. Some sports seem obvious as far as risk for head or neck injury, such as boxing or auto racing. Other sports may have an overall low risk of serious head injury, but have a certain position or event that is considered higher risk. One example is soccer, where although concussion is not uncommon, more severe head injury is quite low in most positions except for the goal keeper. Similarly, most track and field athletes have a low risk for head injury, except for pole vaulters. Most cases of serious head injury in pole vaulters have occurred when the head did not land on the safety pad but instead hit the surrounding hard surface. This was the case in a review conducted between 1982–1998 of pole vaulters, where 16 out of 34 of pole vaulters reviewed were seriously injured or died.[1] The authors recommended an increase in the size of the landing pad and to ensure the surrounding surface is a soft material.

Box 46.1 Sports with the highest risk for injury to head and cervical spine

1. Auto racing
2. Boxing
3. Cheerleading
4. Cycling
5. Diving
6. Equestrian
7. Football
8. Gymnastics
9. Hang gliding
10. Ice hockey

According to statistics from the National Center for Catastrophic Sports Injury Research, the three common school sports with the highest risk of head and cervical spine injury per 100 000 participants are American football, gymnastics, and ice hockey. Although the rate is slightly higher in cheerleading, due to the fact over 1.5 million youths play football annually, the absolute numbers are highest in football.

In many sports, the risk of moderate to severe head or neck injury increases as athletes mature from the youth to adolescent level. American football is an example where the risk of severe injury is low in the youngest age groups, but increases through junior high and high school. The main reason is the participants at the younger age groups are smaller and slower and cannot typically generate the forces seen by high-school or collegiate players. These older, more physically mature athletes can generate greater force which results in greater impact. In youth baseball, however, the use of aluminium bats has been associated with head injuries in pitchers, as the ball speed coming off the bat is substantially higher than with wooden bats. In a study from 1982–2002, 11 out of 14 cases of head injury in pitchers occurred when they were struck by a ball hit by an aluminium bat;[2] in the other three cases the type of bat was not known. It has been recommended that aluminium bats not be used in youth baseball and that pitchers wear head protection.

Health professionals providing game coverage where athletes could sustain head or neck injury should make certain organizational decisions before the season begins. First, a 'captain' of the medical team responsible for supervising on the field management of the injured athlete should be designated. Although this captain will usually be the team physician, in certain localities it may be the athletic trainer or an emergency medical technician. Second, all necessary emergency equipment for the head- or spine-injured athlete should be on the sidelines. At a minimum, this would include equipment for immobilization of the injured athlete and the initiation and maintenance of cardiopulmonary resuscitation (CPR).

Types of head injury

The differential diagnosis for an athlete with a head injury includes, concussion, intracranial haemorrhage, axonal shear, second-impact syndrome or malignant brain oedema, and post-concussion syndrome. Prompt recognition and treatment is important as severe head injury has a mortality rate as high as 50% and survivors often have persistent cognitive, motor, and memory deficits.

Concussion

The word concussion is derived from the Latin *concussus*, which means to 'to shake violently'.[3] The Committee on Head Injury Nomenclature of the Congress of Neurological Surgeons defines concussion as a 'clinical syndrome characterized by immediate and transient post-traumatic impairment of neural function, such as alteration of consciousness, disturbance of vision, equilibrium, etc.

due to brainstem involvement'.[4] It has also been stated that a concussion is a 'trauma-induced alteration in mental status that may or may not involve loss of consciousness'.[4] The American Orthopaedic Society for Sports Medicine defines concussion as 'any alteration in cerebral function caused by a direct or indirect (rotation) force transmitted to the head resulting in one or more of the following acute signs and symptoms: a brief loss of consciousness, light-headedness, vertigo, cognitive and memory dysfunction, tinnitus, blurred vision, difficulty concentrating, amnesia, headache, nausea, vomiting, photophobia, or balance disturbance'.[4] Delayed signs and symptoms may also include sleep irregularities, fatigue, personality changes, inability to perform usual daily activities, depression, or lethargy.

Concussion is the most common athletic head injury, with one in five high-school American football players suffering one annually. A player who has already sustained one concussion in football is four to six times more likely to sustain a second compared, to an athlete who had never been concussed.[5] The true incidence of concussion is difficult to ascertain, as many go unrecognized or unreported, but estimates at all levels in American football have been as high as 250 000 per year.[6] The annual incidence of all sport and recreation traumatic brain injuries in the US has been estimated to be 3.8 million.[7]

Previously, a concussion has been described as a physiologic disturbance without structural damage, but more recent animal and human studies have shown that neurochemical and structural changes with loss of brain cells can occur.[8] Additionally, a neurochemical cascade begins within minutes following a concussion and can continue for days. Disruption of the neuronal cell membrane, stretching of axons, and opening of potassium channels lead to an efflux of potassium out of affected neurons.[9] Depolarization of neurons leads to release of glutamate, which further induces an efflux of potassium. The extra-cellular potassium leads to a release of excitatory amino acids and further depolarization, both serving to further increase extra-cellular potassium. Increased adenosine triphosphate (ATP) is required to restore the imbalance in potassium and the membrane potential. Glucose utilization increases, leading to a state of hyperglycolysis that in rat studies lasts several hours, but in humans may last substantially longer. It is during this period that neurons remain in a vulnerable state, susceptible to minor changes in cerebral blood flow, increases in intracranial pressure, and anoxia. Animal studies have shown that during this susceptible period, a decrease in cerebral blood flow that normally would have little consequence can produce extensive neuronal cell death.[8]

Several attempts have been made to classify concussions based on their severity, with guidelines for return to play. The most commonly used classifications have three grades, with a type 1 described as mild, type 2 as moderate, and type 3 as severe. The classification schemes have some variation, but are all based on the clinical presentation of the athlete, and especially with the Cantu Grading System, the duration of symptoms.[3] (Table 46.1).

The late effects of repeated head injury, even at the concussive or sub-concussive levels, can lead to anatomic patterns of chronic brain injury with correlating signs and symptoms. Martland first described the term 'punch drunk' in 1928, which also has been called dementia pugilistica.[10] Although this term was first used to describe the effects of repetitive head injury in boxers, any athlete who has sustained repeated blows to the head can develop what is now referred to as chronic traumatic encephalopathy (CTE). The characteristic signs and symptoms of CTE include the gradual appearance of a euphoric dementia with emotional lability, with the victim displaying little insight into his deterioration. Speech and thought become progressively slower and memory deteriorates considerably. Simple fatuous cheerfulness is the most common prevailing mood, though sometimes depression with paranoia can occur. Wide mood swings may occur with intense irritability, sometimes leading to uninhibited violent behaviour. From the clinical standpoint, the neurologist may encounter almost any combination of pyramidal, extrapyramidal, and cerebellar signs.

Table 46.1 Cantu Grading System for concussion.

Grade 1	Grade 2	Grade 3
No LOC*	LOC < 1min,	LOC > 1 min
PTA**/PCCS*** < 30 min	PTA > 30min but < 24 h,	PTA > 24h
	PCCS > 30min but < 7 days	PCCS > 7days

* Loss of consciousness (LOC), ** Post-traumatic amnesia (PTA), *** Post-concussion signs/symptoms (PCCS).

Characteristic patterns of cerebral change have been described on autopsy results of men who had been boxers.[11] Corsellis *et al.* reported changes seen in the middle of the brain, which in some cases was essentially sheared into two layers.[11] Destruction of the limbic system, a portion of the brain that governs emotion and plays a role in memory and learning, was also described. A characteristic loss of cells in the cerebellum, part of the brain regulating balance and coordination, was also seen. Microscopic changes were seen throughout the brain, resembling changes seen with Alzheimer's disease. Neurofibrillary tangles, but not senile plaques, were observed, suggesting they were a distinct finding unique to subjects who had suffered multiple blows to the head.

Post-concussion syndrome

While both the American Psychiatric Association and the World Health Organization have defined post-concussion syndrome (Box 46.2), most clinicians recognize this as the persistence of concussion symptoms lasting more than 1 month.[12,13] Symptoms typically include headache (especially with exertion), dizziness, fatigue, irritability, and impaired memory and concentration. The persistence of these symptoms reflects altered

Box 46.2 International classification of diseases, 10th revision: clinical criteria for post-concussion syndrome

A. Head injury usually severe enough to cause loss of consciousness within 4 weeks of symptom onset.

B. Pre-occupation with symptoms and fear of brain damage with hypochondrial concern and adaptation of sick role.

C. Three from below:
Headache, dizziness, malaise, noise intolerance, irritability, depression, anxiety, emotional lability, concentration, memory, or intellectual deficit without neuropsychological evidence of deficit, insomnia.

neurotransmitter function, and usually correlates with the duration of post-traumatic amnesia.[14] When these symptoms persist, the athlete should be evaluated with magnetic resonance imaging (MRI). Return to competition should be deferred until all symptoms have resolved and diagnostic studies are normal. Once symptoms have resolved, neuropsychiatric testing can be used for future comparison.

Individuals at increased risk for post-concussion syndrome include athletes with multiple concussions, those with concussions in close proximity to one another, and athletes sustaining a double hit, such as a direct helmet-to-helmet hit followed by hitting the head against the ground when falling. At even higher risk is the athlete that experiences additional head trauma when they are symptomatic from a prior concussion through the course of the same game. Post-concussion syndrome is typically quite debilitating, but the symptoms usually clear over a course of months. Although rare, there are reports where post-concussion symptoms have taken as long as 5 years to clear after head trauma; some cases have been reported where symptoms never cleared.[15] Many athletes that recover from post-concussion syndrome, especially those with shorter duration, are able to safely return to competitive sports. For those who do not recover, it is presently not possible to rule out incipient CTE.

Malignant brain oedema and second-impact syndrome

Malignant brain oedema syndrome is seen primarily in paediatric and adolescent athletes. The syndrome consists of rapid neurological deterioration from an alert, conscious state to coma and sometimes death, usually within minutes after head trauma.[16,17] Pathology studies show diffuse brain swelling often with little or no direct brain injury. The cerebral swelling results from hyperaemia or vascular engorgement.[18,19] Athletes with this syndrome require immediate medical intervention following advanced trauma life support (ATLS) protocols and transfer to a medical facility with neurosurgical capability. For those who survive this condition, the rate of permanent impairment is nearly 100%.

Saunders and Harbaugh[20] coined the term 'second impact syndrome of catastrophic head injury' in 1984. However, Schneider first described two cases matching the description in 1973.[21] Second-impact syndrome (SIS) occurs when an athlete who sustains a head injury, often a concussion or cerebral contusion, sustains a second head injury before symptoms associated with the first have cleared.[22–24] The symptoms may include visual, motor, or sensory changes, and difficulty with thought or memory. The second head injury may be relatively minor, perhaps only a blow to the chest that indirectly imparts accelerative forces to the brain. The athlete may appear stunned, but usually does not lose consciousness and often completes the play. The athlete may remain on the field or walk off under his own power. Within seconds to minutes, the athlete precipitously deteriorates, usually collapsing to the ground. The athlete quickly becomes unconscious with rapidly dilating pupils, loss of eye movement, and evidence of respiratory failure.

The pathophysiology of SIS is thought to involve a loss of autoregulation of the brain's blood supply. The loss of autoregulation leads to vascular engorgement within the cranium, which in turn markedly increases intracranial pressure and leads to herniation either of the medial surface (uncus) of the temporal lobe, lobes below the tentorium, or the cerebellar tonsils through the foramen magnum. Animal research has shown the vascular engorgement of the brain after a second mild head injury is difficult if not impossible to control.[25,26] The usual time from the second impact to brainstem failure is rapid, taking only 2–5 min. Once brain herniation and brain stem compromise occur, ocular involvement and respiratory failure precipitously ensue. Demise occurs far more rapidly than usually seen with an epidural hematoma.

Although some have questioned whether SIS is a real phenomenon, it is likely more common than previous reports have suggested.[27,28] Over a 13-year period (1980–1993) the National Center for Catastrophic Sports Injury Research in Chapel Hill, North Carolina, identified 35 probable cases among American football alone.[23] Seventeen of these cases were confirmed at the time of surgery or at autopsy, while 18 cases lacked sufficient documentation at autopsy, but most probably represented additional cases. Careful scrutiny excluded the diagnosis in 22 of the 57 cases originally suspected.

Second impact syndrome is not limited to American football. Fekete described a 16-year-old high-school hockey player who fell during a game, striking the back of his head on the ice.[29] He lost consciousness and afterward complained of unsteadiness and headaches. While playing in the next game 4 days later, he was checked forcibly and fell striking his left temple on the ice. His pupils rapidly became fixed and dilated and he died within 2 h while in transit to a neurosurgical facility. Autopsy revealed brain contusion of several days' duration, and oedematous brain with a thin layer of subdural and subarachnoid haemorrhage, and bilateral herniation of the cerebellar tonsils into the foramen magnum. Though Fekete did not use the label 'second impact syndrome', the clinical course and autopsy findings are consistent with it.

Other case reports of SIS exist. McQuillen *et al.*[24] described an 18-year-old downhill skier who suffered the syndrome and remained in a persistent vegetative state. Kelly *et al.*[30] reported on a 17-year-old football player who died as a result of the syndrome. Physicians who cover athletic events, especially those in which head trauma is likely, must understand SIS and be prepared to initiate emergency treatment.

Since SIS has a mortality rate of nearly 50% and a morbidity rate approaching 100%, prevention is of the utmost importance. An athlete who is symptomatic from a head injury *must not* participate in contact or collision sports. Return to play should be delayed until all cerebral symptoms have subsided, preferably for at least 1 week. Whether it takes days, weeks, or months to reach the asymptomatic state, the athlete *should not* be allowed to practice or compete while still suffering post-concussion symptoms. Team physicians and trainers must educate coaches, players, and their parents as to the significance of the problem. Files from the National Center for Catastrophic Sport Injury Research include cases of young athletes who did not report their cerebral symptoms, fearing they would not be allowed to compete. Unaware of the severity of these symptoms, the athletes played in an active post-concussive state, which resulted in the development of SIS.

Intracranial haemorrhage

The leading cause of death from athletic head injury is intracranial haemorrhage. There are four types of haemorrhage of which the examining trainer or physician should be aware. Because all four types of intracranial haemorrhage may be fatal, rapid and accurate initial assessment as well as appropriate follow-up is mandatory after an athletic head injury.

Epidural haematoma

An epidural or extradural hematoma is typically the most rapidly progressing intracranial haematoma (see Figure 46.1).

The mechanism of injury is usually a direct blow to the head or an acceleration-deceleration force. The energy transmitted to the skull results in a fracture of the temporal bone and classically causes a tear of the middle meningeal artery supplying the covering (dura) of the brain. Fracture bleeding can also contribute. The resulting haematoma accumulates inside the skull, but outside the covering of the brain. As the bleeding results from a torn artery, it may progress rapidly and reach a fatal size in 30–60 min. Due to the force transmitted to the skull and brain, there often is an initial loss of consciousness, which may be followed by a 'lucid interval', and then further loss of consciousness as the bleeding progresses. Alternatively, the athlete may not regain consciousness or may remain conscious initially before developing an increasing headache and progressive loss of consciousness. This deterioration occurs as the clot accumulates and the intracranial pressure increases. This lesion, if present, will almost always declare itself within an hour or two following the time of injury. Often the brain substance is free from direct injury; thus if the clot is promptly removed surgically, full recovery may be expected. Because the lesion is rapidly and almost universally fatal if missed, all athletes receiving a major head injury must be very closely and frequently observed during the ensuing several hours, preferably for a full 24 h. Observation should be done at a facility where full neurosurgical services are available.

Subdural haematoma

A subdural haematoma occurs directly on the brain and under the dura and is the most common cause of fatal athletic head injury (see Figure 46.2).

A subdural haematoma often results from a torn vein running on the surface of the brain to the dura. It may also result from a torn venous sinus or even a small artery on the surface of the brain. There is often associated injury to the brain tissue and the final outcome is usually most influenced by the extent of the brain injury rather than the haematoma collection itself. If a subdural haematoma necessitates surgery in the first 24 h, the mortality rate is high owing not to the clot itself, but to the associated brain damage from the initial impact. With a subdural that progresses rapidly, the athlete usually does not regain consciousness and the need for immediate neurosurgical evaluation is obvious.

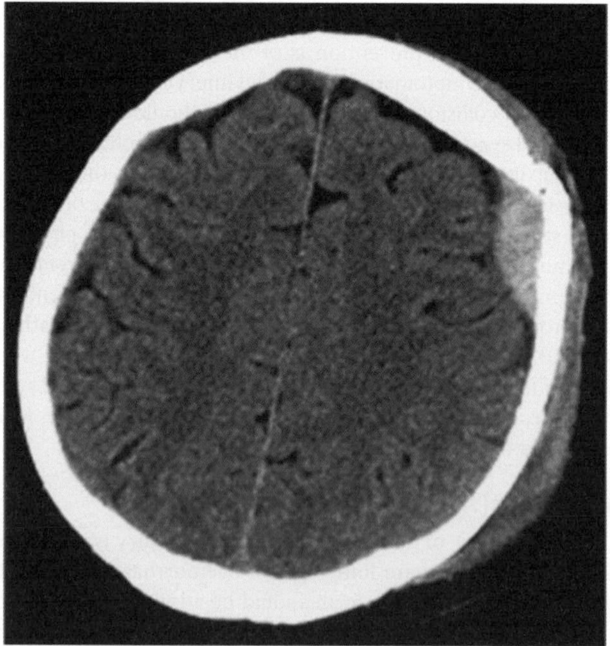

Figure 46.1 Classic lens shape of an epidural haematoma with associated temporal bone fracture.

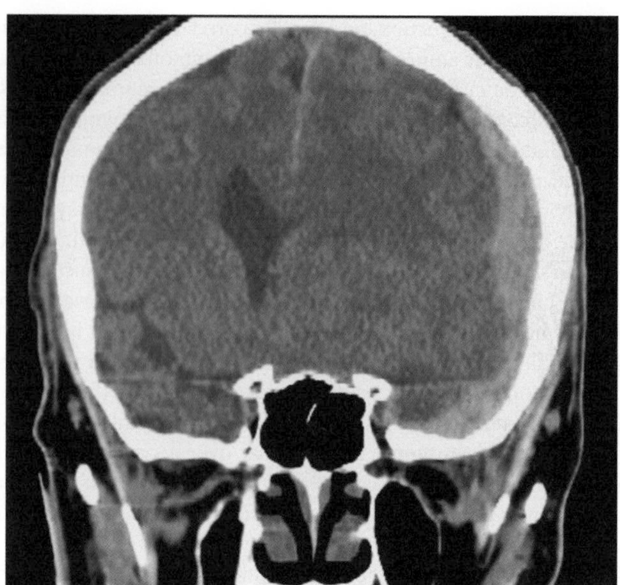

Figure 46.2 Subdural haematoma causing mass effect and midline shift.

Occasionally, the brain itself is not directly injured and a subdural haematoma develops slowly over a period of days to weeks. This chronic subdural haematoma, although often associated with headache, may initially cause a variety of mild, almost imperceptible mental, motor, and sensory signs and symptoms. After 1 week the subdural haematoma begins to form a surrounding membrane from infiltrating fibroblasts. The haematoma becomes encapsulated and dynamic fluid and protein shifts can occur across the membrane. Because recognition of a chronic subdural haematoma and removal will lead to a full recovery, it must always be suspected in an athlete who has previously sustained a head injury and who, days or weeks later, is 'not quite right'. A computerized axial tomography (CAT) scan of the head will show such a lesion.

Subarachnoid haemorrhage

In a subarachnoid haemorrhage, the bleeding is confined to the surface of the brain (see Figure 46.3).

The bleeding typically results from disruption of the tiny surface brain vessels and is analogous to a bruise, although haemorrhage can also result from a ruptured cerebral aneurysm or arteriovenous malformation. Because bleeding is superficial, surgery is not usually required unless a congenital vascular anomaly is present. Subarachnoid haemorrhage typically causes a severe headache and often an associated neurologic deficit is present, depending on the area of the brain involved. Bleeding can cause irritation to the brain and precipitate a seizure. If a seizure occurs it is important to logroll the patient onto his side, so that blood or saliva will roll out of the mouth and the tongue cannot fall back, obstructing the airway. If one

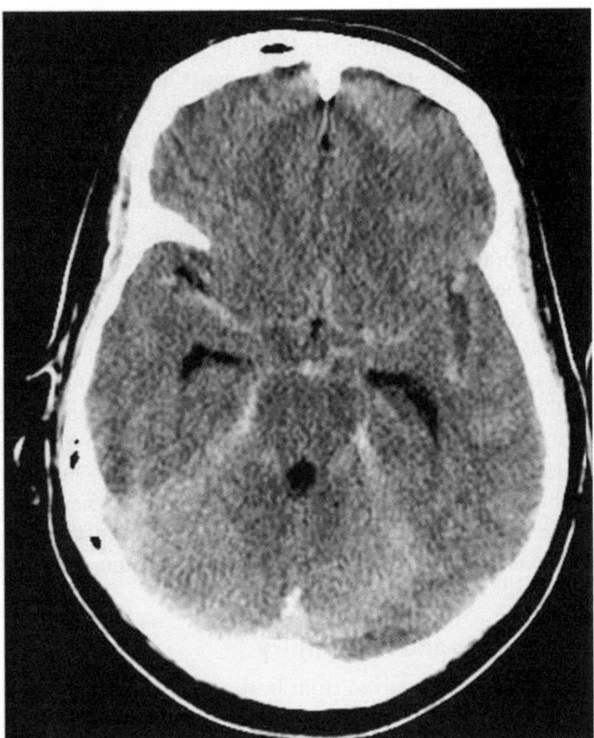

Figure 46.3 Diffuse subarachnoid haemorrhage fills the basal cisterns and adjacent Sylvian (lateral) fissures.

has a padded tongue depressor or an oral airway, it can be inserted between the teeth. However, under no circumstances should one insert their fingers into the mouth of an athlete who is having a seizure, as amputation can easily result. Usually such a traumatic seizure will last only for a minute or two. The athlete will then relax and should immediately be transported to the nearest medical facility.

Intracerebral haematoma

An intracerebral haematoma involves bleeding into the brain substance, usually from a torn artery. The mechanism of injury is usually a direct blow to the head. It can also occur from rupture of a congenital vascular lesion such as an aneurysm or arteriovenous malformation. Intracerebral haematomas are not typically associated with a lucid interval and may be rapidly progressive. If the athlete is conscious, they usually will display a focal neurologic deficit corresponding to the area of the brain involved. Neurologic deterioration can be rapid and death occasionally occurs before the injured athlete can be transported to a hospital. Because of the intense reaction such a tragic event precipitates among fellow athletes, family, students, and even the community at large, it is imperative to obtain a compete autopsy to clarify fully the causative factors. Often the autopsy will reveal a congenital lesion, which may indicate that the cause of death was other than presumed and potentially unavoidable.

A less-severe type of intracerebral haematoma can occur in the form of a cerebral contusion. The mechanism of injury is usually a direct blow to the skull causing an acceleration-deceleration force and inward deformation of the skull. Compression of brain tissue underlying the site of impact can lead to the contusion. Contusions can vary substantially in size due to factors including the amount of force imparted and the area of the skull involved. Contusions directly under the area of impact are termed the coup lesion. As the brain decelerates and then rebounds against the opposite side of the skull it can result in a contusion in this site, the so-called countercoup lesion (see Figure 46.4).

The clinical outcome of patients with a cerebral contusion depends on multiple factors such as the size, number, and location of the injury. Because the frontal and temporal lobes are often the site of contusions, they may result in behavioural or mental status changes. Both identification and resolution of contusions can be seen on CT scanning.

Diffuse axonal injury

Diffuse axonal injury (DAI) results from high energy shearing forces imparted to the brain that literally sever axonal connections and cause microscopic bleeding (see Figure 46.5).

The athlete is usually rendered unconscious with a low Glasgow Coma Scale (GCS).[7] Initial head CT scan may appear negative or show microscopic bleeding on susceptibility weighted images. Immediate neurosurgical triage for treatment of increased intracranial pressure is indicated.

Skull fracture

A skull fracture is simply a break in a skull bone (see Figure 46.6.). Skull fractures are grouped into four main types: linear, depressed, diastatic, and basilar. Linear skull fractures are the most common, accounting for about 70% of all skull fractures and virtually all fractures resulting from sports activities.

With a linear fracture there is a break in the bone, but the break does not result in any movement of the bone. With a depressed skull fracture, the area of the skull that is broken is pushed inward or sunken. This type of fracture has a higher risk of injury to the underlying brain. Diastatic skull fractures are fractures that occur along the growth plates or sutures of the skull. These fractures tend to occur in newborns and infants and are not typically seen after

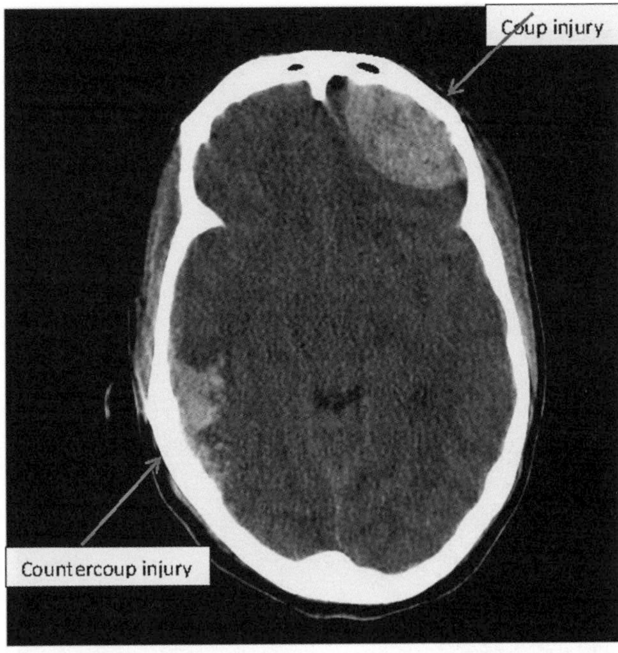

Figure 46.4 Left frontal coup epidural haematoma with countercoup parenchymal haemorrhage.

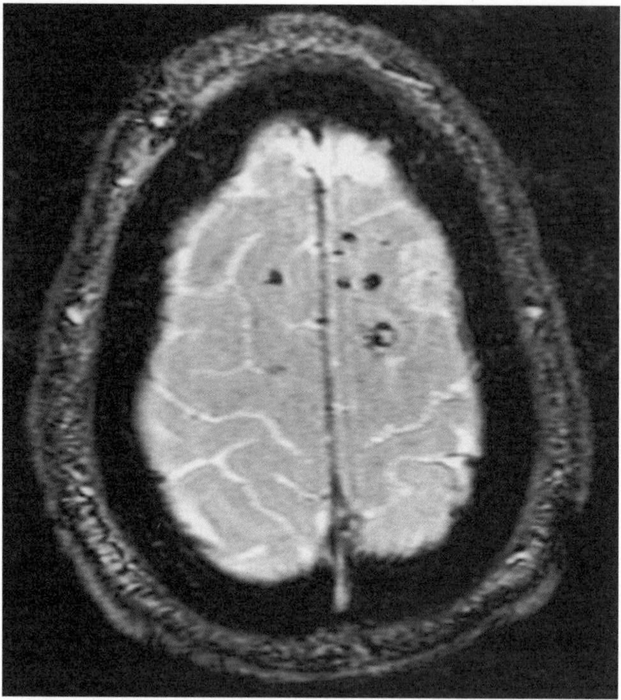

Figure 46.5 MRI example of diffuse axonal injury with multiple areas of small haemorrhagic lesions characterized by signal loss.

sporting activities. Basilar skull fractures are fractures that occur at the base of the skull or the portion underneath the brain. This type of fracture can occur even with helmet use in activities like motor vehicle racing, and injury occurs when a compressive force is imparted through brain to the base of the skull.

Diagnosis of a skull fracture begins with a history and physical examination. The history usually reveals a high-energy mechanism, especially if the athlete wears protective head gear, as in auto racing. Depressed and open skull fractures should be apparent on physical examination. However, linear skull fractures may not be obvious. In some cases, the headgear may not have functioned properly, e.g. a baseball player hit on the head by a pitch. In rare cases, the athlete may not wear head gear at all, such as soccer goalie who contacts the goal post with his head resulting in fracture. Most athletes who have sustained a skull fracture will be rendered unconscious from the initial impact to the skull and underlying brain. Although the neurologic injury and other associated injuries take precedence over the skull fracture in initial treatment, diagnosis of the skull fracture is important to minimize potential late complications.

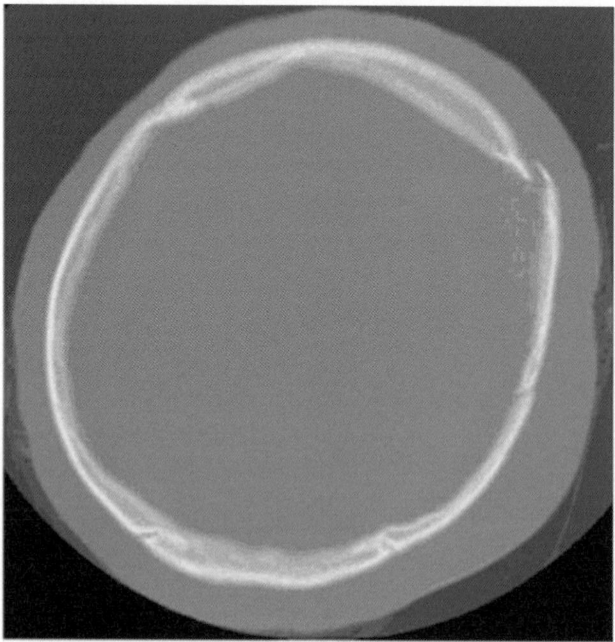

Figure 46.6 Bone window of same CT image seen in Figure 46.1. More clearly showing skull fracture overlying epidural haematoma.

Initial treatment for an athlete with a skull fracture focuses on the ABCs of advanced trauma life support (Airway, Breathing, and Circulation). The athlete's cervical spine should be immobilized with a rigid collar until spine injury can be ruled out. The athlete should be transported to a medical centre that provides neurosurgical services. In the rare event of an open skull fracture, the wound should be covered with sterile gauze and intravenous antibiotics administered.

Sports helmets and head injury

Sports helmets have evolved from leather head coverings to constructs made of multiple materials often including a soft inner liner, a middle impact energy-absorbing layer, and a hard outer shell. Helmets have proved quite effective at reducing the risk of skull fracture in sports and there is increasing evidence supporting the efficacy of helmets in reducing other moderate to severe brain injuries.[31] Mertz *et al.* showed that with a helmet the risk of skull fracture from a 180 gravities (g) impact was only 5%.[32] Helmets attenuate and disperse over a wider area the force transmitted to the skull and brain from a direct linear impact. Many blows to the head involve a tangential force, which result in a shearing force to the brain; helmets do not provide as much protection for these types of blows as with a direct blow. Additionally, brain tissue is more sensitive to shearing force than compression force. It has been estimated that the bulk modulus of brain tissue is approximately 10^5 greater than the shear modulus.[33] More investigation is needed to know how much protection, if any, helmets provide against rotational accelerations to the brain following impact.

Cervical spine injuries

Epidemiology

More than 30 million children participate in youth sports each year in the US and of the estimated 5.5 million children who participate in football an estimated 28% are injured each year.[34] A recent study found that nearly 40% of all life-threatening injuries in children age 6–18 years are a result of sporting activities.[35] The authors also found one in four cervical spine fractures in paediatric patients are sports related. Cervical spine injuries in younger children differ from those in adults due in part to anatomy. In children, the head is larger relative to the torso, resulting in a relatively higher centre of gravity and a larger moment arm acting on the cervical spine. Additionally, children have multiple open vertebral physes and generally more lax ligamentous structures. The combination of these factors results in a higher proportion of injuries involving the upper cervical spine than seen in adults. Mechanism of injury also plays a role in the location of cervical spine injuries. A recent study examining patterns of cervical spine injuries in children found very high forces, such as those seen in motor vehicle collisions, tended to result in a higher proportion of axial spine (C1–2) injuries, whereas lower-energy mechanisms as seen in most sporting or recreational activities tended to result in more subaxial (C3–7) injuries.[36] This study found that in children aged 2–7 years, motor vehicle collisions were the most common cause, accounting for 37% of all cervical spine injuries. In children 8 to 15 years, however, sports accounted for the same percentage of injuries as motor vehicle collisions, at 23%. Of those sports injuries, 53% were subaxial.

Initial assessment

On the field, management of an athlete who is down and suspected of having a cervical spine injury begins with the ABCs of acute trauma care. If the patient is prone and there is concern for the airway, the athlete should be carefully log rolled into the supine position with one person in charge of maintaining cervical alignment. In sports such as football or hockey where helmets and shoulder pads are worn, they should remain in place during the initial evaluation. This is provided the facemask can be quickly removed allowing access to the airway. A study by Swenson *et al.*[37] on ten healthy adult individuals showed that if the helmet is removed and the shoulder pads remain in place, an increase in cervical lordosis results. Although young children have an increased head to torso size, removing only the helmet still results in an increased lordosis.[38] For children 6 years of age or younger, however, a backboard with a cut-out for the helmet is recommended to maintain neutral alignment. Swartz *et al.*[39] looked at facemask versus helmet removal, and found removing the facemask took less time and resulted in less motion in all three planes. If the helmet has to be removed, then the shoulder pads should also be removed, following the generally accepted 'all or none' policy. A recent study has shown that some of the newer football helmets, with increased protection around the mandible, can make basic airway manoeuvres more difficult, such as chin lift[40] (see Figure 46.7).

Participants attempting to perform bag mask ventilation on 146 college athlete volunteers reported the helmet as a cause of difficulty in 10.4% of athletes wearing a modern hockey helmet, and in 79% of athletes wearing a football helmet.[40] If such a helmet prevents proper management of the airway, then both the helmet and shoulder pads should be removed while maintaining cervical alignment.

The athlete who returns to the sidelines complaining of neck pain requires careful assessment. Generally, any athlete with restricted or painful cervical motion, bony tenderness, or any motor sensory deficit that involves more than a single upper extremity and does not quickly resolve should be removed from competition and be placed on spinal precautions and referred for further evaluation. The athlete who complains of symptoms consistent with a stinger, i.e. unilateral upper extremity burning pain and or weakness typically in a C5–6 distribution, should be removed from competition until all symptoms have resolved and there is normal and painless cervical range of motion and strength.

Imaging

Imaging of the young athlete with suspected cervical spine injury typically begins with plain radiographs including AP, lateral, and open-mouth odontoid views. Interpreting cervical spine radiographs in children can be challenging due to the developing anatomy where pseudo-subluxation of C2 on C3, and occasionally C3 on C4, can occur. In one retrospective review of 138 paediatric trauma patients, a 22% incidence of pseudo-subluxation of C2 on

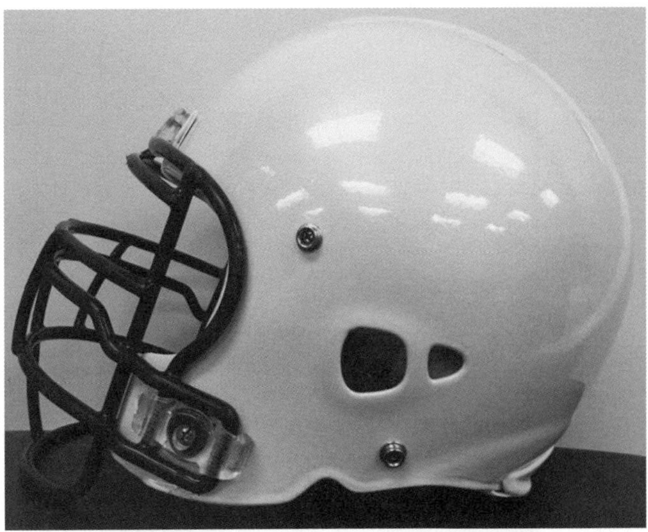

Figure 46.7 Example of a football helmet with increased protection around base of jaw, making airway manoeuvres such as chin lift more difficult.

C3 was found.[41] One way to differentiate pseudo-subluxation from true injury is to assess the spinolaminar (aka Swischuk's) line on the lateral C-spine X-ray. In cases of pseudo-subluxation, the spinolaminar line should pass within 1 mm of the anterior cortex of the posterior arch of C2 (see Figure 46.8). When this line passes >1.5 mm from the anterior cortex of the posterior arch of C2, acute injury is likely (see Figure 46.9).

The atlantodens interval, the distance from the anterior aspect of the dens to the posterior aspect of the anterior ring of the atlas, can show more variation in children than adults. The atlantodens interval in adults is usually ≤3 mm. However, in children younger than 8 years of age, an atlantodens interval of 3–5 mm is seen in about 20% of patients.[42] Understanding normal physes is another challenge unique to children. Unfused C1 ring apophyses, apical odontoid epiphysis, and secondary centres of ossification of the spinous processes can all be mistaken for fractures. Generally normal physes are smooth structures with sclerotic subchondral lines, whereas fractures are more irregular and lack sclerotic lines. In children under age 8 years, anterior wedging of the vertebral bodies up to 3 mm is within normal limits. Wedging can be most pronounced at C3 due to hypermobility of the paediatric cervical spine with increased motion especially at C2–C3.

Although multiple reports have recommended cervical spine CT scan as the preferred screening tool for adult trauma patients due to providing a quicker time to diagnosis and a shorter stay in the trauma resuscitation area compared to plain films, there remains some question with paediatric patients.[43–48] There is concern, especially in paediatric patients, regarding the radiation dose from CT scanning. A missed cervical spine injury, however, can have lifelong devastating consequences and therefore CT scan may be used when clinical suspicion for injury is high. A recent review of 1307 paediatric trauma patients compared CT scan to plain X-rays in diagnosing cervical spine fractures.[43] The study found CT scan had a sensitivity of 100% and a specificity of 98%, while X-rays had a sensitivity of 62%. The authors concluded that CT scans should be considered the primary modality when imaging possible paediatric cervical spine injury. The study also looked at flexion/extension views and the authors stated that 'flexion/extension views did not add to the decision making for C-spine clearance after CT

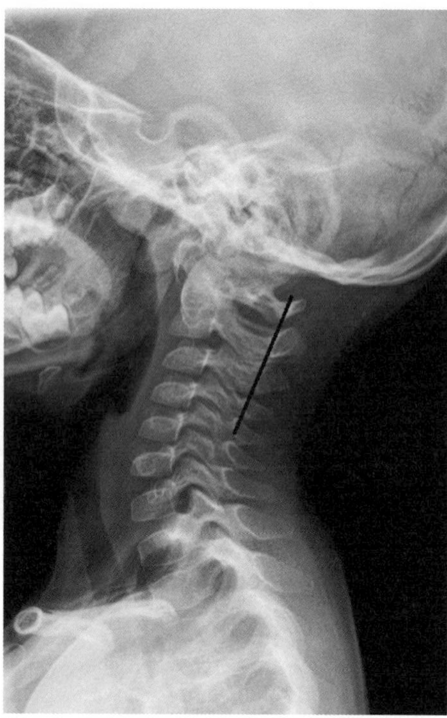

Figure 46.8 Lateral cervical spine radiograph demonstrating pseudosubluxation of C2–3 with Swischuk's (spinolaminar) line showing normal alignment.

evaluation and are probably not needed'.[43] A CT scan is likely most effective in older children and adolescents, where injury patterns are similar to adults. Younger children, however, are more prone to purely ligamentous or soft tissue injury, which may not be appreciated on CT scan. In these patients, MRI may be the modality of choice to identify injury. One study of MRI in 64 paediatric cervical spine patients found MRI demonstrated injury in 24% of patients where X-rays were normal and allowed for spine clearance in three children where CT scan was equivocal.[49]

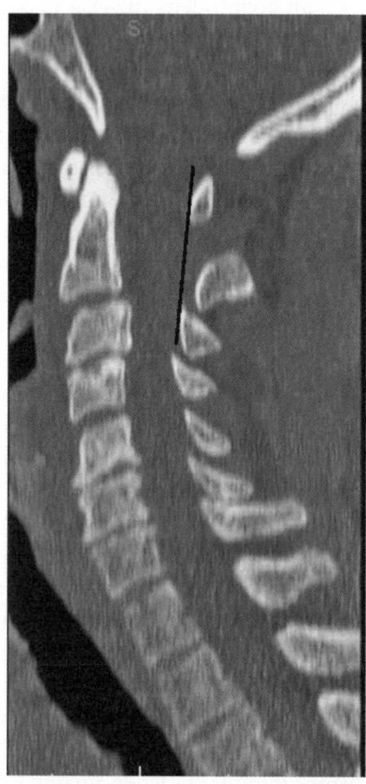

Figure 46.9 Sagittal image of CT scan showing abnormal spinolaminar line representing injury at C2–3.

The question of radiation exposure from CT scan in paediatric patients merits consideration. One study prospectively examined radiation exposure in paediatric patients undergoing CT versus conventional radiographs.[50] The authors found a 1.25 higher effective radiation dose with CT scan. Another study comparing CT scan to X-rays found a higher radiation dose with CT for patients with a GCS > 8, but for those with a GCS < 8 the doses were equivalent due to the higher need for repeated radiographs.[48] Although CT scans produce more radiation than plain radiographs, there are ways to shield patients. By following these protocols, CT exposure can be reduced by 30–50% in paediatric patients compared to adults with no loss in the quality of images.[51,52]

Fractures

Cervical spine fractures are relatively rare in athletic events, especially in younger children. In children 8 years or younger it is very uncommon to see a subaxial fracture from athletics. The atlantoaxial complex is most at risk in younger children, with the majority of serious injuries involving a ligamentous disruption rather than fracture. Axial compression with extension can potentially cause a fracture of the ring of C1, but the forces required to do so are rarely seen in youth sports. Similarly, odontoid fractures can occur, usually from a rapid deceleration with flexion mechanism, but again, the forces in youth sports rarely are high enough to cause such injury. When fractures of the odontoid occur, they tend to happen through the synchondrosis of C2 at the base of the odontoid. These fractures tend to displace anteriorly and reduction can usually be accomplished through immobilization of the cervical spine in extension. In adolescents, the cervical anatomy approaches that of adults and subaxial fractures are occasionally seen, with the most common being a compression fracture. More severe burst patterns can also occur in adolescents, usually between C5 and C7, which is a result of the increased forces on this portion of the spine as the anatomy matures.

Neuropraxias

Neuropraxias are more common than fractures in youth sports. A 'stinger' or 'burner injury' is the most common neurologic injury and involves a temporary burning sensation and/or weakness in a single upper extremity. Collision sports such as football and rugby pose the highest risk for stingers. In younger athletes a stinger most commonly results from a forced stretching of the head and neck away from the involved limb resulting in traction to the brachial plexus with the C5 and C6 roots most commonly affected. In older adolescents and adults, the stinger more commonly results from a forced compression of the head and neck towards the involved limb. The shoulder may simultaneously be forced upwards causing a momentary narrowing of the cervical foramen and resulting in a pinching or compression of the nerve root and transient radiculopathy. Some children have congenital narrowing of the cervical foramen, placing them at increased risk of sustaining a stinger.[53] Athletes who have sustained a stinger typically report immediate burning and weakness in the involved extremity and report a 'dead arm' sensation. The rule is that both sensory and motor function typically return to normal within seconds to minutes, with full recovery usually occurring by 10 min. With repetitive injury, permanent damage can occur; rarely with a severe cervical pinch mechanism, a nerve root(s) can be severed.

Cervical cord neuropraxias are important to differentiate from stingers. Stingers are limited to a single upper extremity, whereas cervical cord neuropraxias typically present with transient quadriplegia and either loss of sensation in all four extremities, or a burning or tingling sensation. Motor function usually recovers within minutes, but sensory changes can last longer. Athletes with a congenital narrowing or stenosis are thought to be at increased risk of cervical cord neuropraxias. Although the determination of cervical stenosis is an area of some controversy, general consensus holds that between C3 and C7 the anteroposterior (AP) spinal canal heights in adolescents and adults are normal above 15 mm and stenotic below 13 mm. Resnick *et al.*[54] have stated that CT and myelography are more sensitive than plain X-rays in determining spinal stenosis. They note that X-rays fail to appraise the width of the spinal cord and cannot detect when stenosis results from ligamentous hypertrophy or disc protrusion. Ladd and Scranton[55]state that the AP diameter of the spinal canal is 'unimportant' if there is total impedance of the contrast medium. For all these reasons spinal stenosis cannot be ruled out based only on bony measurements. 'Functional' spinal stenosis, defined as the loss of the cerebrospinal fluid around the cord or in more extreme cases deformation of the spinal cord, whether documented by contrast CT, myelography, or MRI, is a more accurate measure of stenosis.[56] The term functional is taken from the radiographic term 'functional reserve' as applied to the protective cushion of cerebrospinal fluid (CSF) around the spinal cord in a normal spinal canal.

Cervical spinal stenosis in the athlete may be a congenital/developmental condition or may be caused by acquired degenerative changes in the spine. For the athlete with severe stenosis and no CSF around the spinal cord on MRI, collision sports should be avoided. The athlete with spinal stenosis is at risk for neurologic injury during hyperextension of the cervical spine.[57] When the neck is hyperextended, the sagittal diameter of the spinal canal is further compromised by as much as 30% by in folding of the interlaminar ligaments. Matsuura *et al.* studied 42 athletes who sustained spinal cord injury and compared them to 100 controls. They found that 'the sagittal diameter of the spinal canals of the control group was significantly larger than those of the spinal cord injured group'.[58] Eismont *et al.* have stated that 'the sagittal diameter of the spinal canal in some individuals may be inherently smaller than normal, and this reduced size may be a predisposing risk factor for spinal cord injury'.[57] The idea that spinal stenosis predisposes to spinal cord injury is not new, with multiple authors as far back as the 1950s reaching the same conclusion including Wolfe *et al.*,[59] Penning,[60] Alexander *et al.*,[61] Mayfield,[62] Nugent,[63] and Ladd and Scranton, who stated that 'patients who have stenosis of the cervical spine should be advised to discontinue participation in contact sports'.[48] More recent support for this stand comes from the National Center for Catastrophic Sports Injury Research, where cases of quadriplegia have been seen in athletes with cervical stenosis but without fracture or dislocation. In athletes with a normal-sized canal, quadriplegia has not been seen without fracture/dislocation of the spine. And most importantly, full neurologic recovery has been observed in 21% of athletes who were rendered initially quadriplegic after fracture/dislocation with normal size cervical canals, while complete neurologic recovery has not been seen in any athlete after fracture/dislocation and quadriplegia when spinal stenosis was documented by MRI.[64]

Ligamentous injury

Cervical instability due to ligamentous disruption may prove challenging to diagnose immediately after injury in the youth or adolescent athlete. As mentioned, some degree of laxity can be normal in children and muscle spasm following injury may prevent initial subluxation of the cervical spine. Atlanto-occipital dislocation is a serious injury in children, with a mortality rate of approximately 50%.[65] Fortunately this injury is quite rare in sports and typically results from distraction forces more typically seen in high-speed motor vehicle collisions (see Figure 46.10).

The atlanto-occipital joint is less stable than the lower cervical joints, with the alar ligaments, joint capsule, and the tectorial membrane serving as the primary stabilizers. The basion dental interval (BDI), or distance from the basion to the tip of the odontoid as seen on a lateral radiograph, can be used to assess for atlanto-occipital dislocation (see Figure 46.11).

A BDI > 12.5 mm is indicative of injury, although this measurement is not as reliable in children less than 5 years of age.[66,67] Atlantoaxial injury can occur as the C1–C2 articulation is also relatively less stable than lower cervical joints. The transverse ligament runs posterior to the odontoid and limits anterior translation of C1. The apical and two alar ligaments serve to limit rotation around the odontoid. The atlanto-dens interval (ADI), i.e. the distance from the anterior aspect of the odontoid to the posterior cortex of the C1 anterior ring, should measure <5 mm in children <8 years of age, and <3 mm in older children and adolescents.[68] With injury to the transverse ligament, the ADI will increase, causing a decrease in the space available for the cord, but provided the apical and alar ligaments are intact, translation will usually be limited and spinal cord compression is rare.

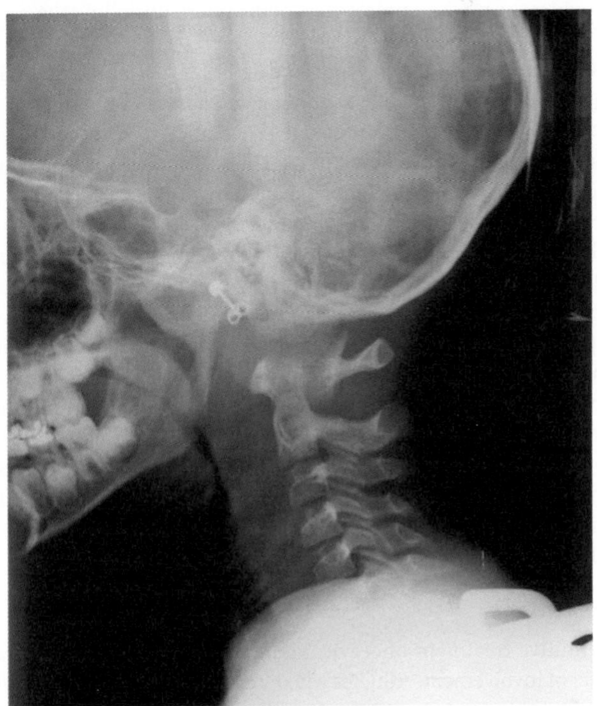

Figure 46.10 Lateral c-spine X-ray showing atlanto-occipital dislocation.

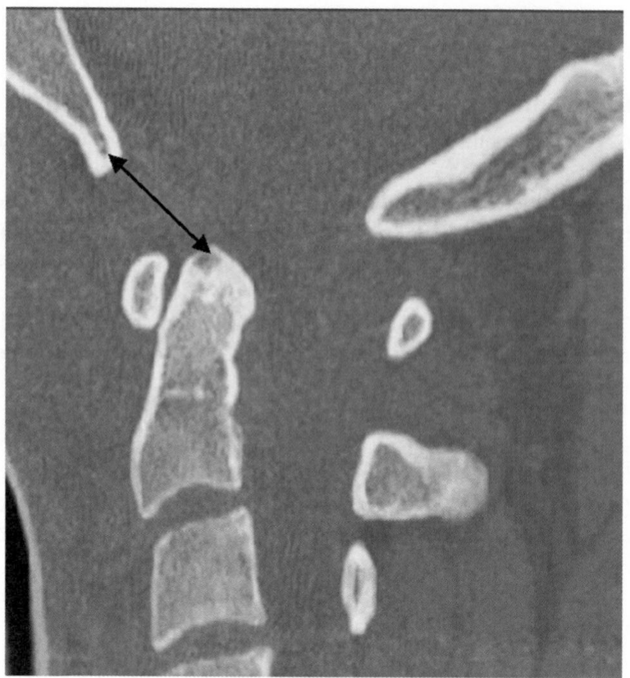

Figure 46.11 Representation of abnormal basion dens interval as seen on CT scan.

Atlanto-axial rotatory subluxation involves a rotational deformity of C1 on C2. This condition can be seen with trauma or secondary to infection, such as Grisel's syndrome. A young athlete with atlanto-axial subluxation will present with the neck flexed to one side and rotated towards the other. The odontoid view X-ray will show asymmetry of the lateral masses; the lateral mass that is more anterior will appear wider and closer to midline. CT scan usually provides the most complete view of the injury, including the degree of facet subluxation.

The athlete with Down syndrome deserves special consideration. Individuals with Down syndrome have increased mobility at the occipitocervical and atlantoaxial articulations. Whether to perform radiographic screening of the child or adolescent athlete with Down syndrome is a matter of debate. Many of the Special Olympic organizations require lateral flexion and extension radiographs for athletes in high risk sports such as diving, equestrian, and soccer.[69] Athletes with normal radiographs may participate without restrictions, but those with an increased atlantodens interval should avoid high risk sports. For athletes in low risk sports with normal neck and neurologic examination, radiographic screening is generally not recommended. As Herman has stated, 'for many of these special athletes, the value of participation in safe and well-supervised sports and recreational programs outweighs the potential risks of injury related to cervical hypermobility'.[69] Readers interested in a more in-depth discussion of athletes with Down syndrome are referred to Chapter 28.

Treatment

Definitive treatment of cervical injuries depends on the type and level of involvement. Athletes who have sustained a stinger can generally return to competition when all motor and sensory symptoms have cleared and they have full painless cervical range of motion. In rare cases, the motor and sensory symptoms of a stinger last more than a few minutes. In these cases, MRI of the spine should be considered to look for a herniated disc or other compressive pathology. If symptoms persist more than 2 weeks, then electromyography (EMG) can allow for an accurate assessment of the degree and extent of injury.

Transient quadriplegia or any bilateral motor or sensory symptoms after injury necessitate removal of the athlete from competition and further diagnostic evaluation. Computerized tomography scanning can identify subtle fractures or malalignment, but may not show ongoing extrinsic cord compression or intrinsic cord abnormalities; MRI is the most sensitive study to evaluate for these conditions. Somatosensory evoked potentials may prove useful in documenting physiological cord dysfunction. Definitive treatment depends on the pathology identified.

Treatment of cervical spine fractures also depends on the type and level of injury. Some bony injuries, such as spinous process fractures or unilateral laminar fractures, may require no treatment or only immobilization in a cervical collar. Others, such as the bilateral pars interarticularis fracture of C2 ('hangman's fracture') may be treated with a cervical collar or Halo vest immobilization. Unstable injuries such as fracture dislocations should initially be reduced and temporarily stabilized with cervical traction using Gardner-Wells tongs or a halo ring device. Surgical treatment may subsequently be required for severely comminuted vertebral body fractures, unstable posterior element fractures, type II odontoid fractures, incomplete spinal cord injuries with canal or cord compromise, and in those patients with progression of their neurologic deficit.[70]

Treatment of the spinal cord-injured patient depends on the underlying injury. Injury to the spinal cord involves an initial mechanical disruption of axons, blood vessels, and cell membranes, which is then followed by secondary injury involving further swelling and inflammation, ischaemia, free radical production, and cell death. Only prevention can limit the initial injury, and treatment is focused on preventing secondary damage. In a review of 57 adult rugby players who sustained an acute spinal cord injury, most commonly due to facet dislocations, five out of eight who underwent reduction of the injury within 4 h had compete neurologic recovery, whereas 0 out of 24 who were reduced beyond 4 h had complete recovery.[71]

Return to play

The return to play decision depends largely on the type and extent of injury.[64] The athlete with a cervical ligament sprain or muscle strain/contusion with no neurologic or osseous injury can return to competition when he/she is free of neck pain with and without axial compression, has full range of motion, and neck strength is normal. Cervical radiographs should show no subluxation or abnormal curvature. It is preferable that the athlete is asymptomatic and can perform at his/her pre-injury ability prior to returning to competition.

The athlete who has sustained a stinger-type injury should cease practising and competing until motor and sensory symptoms have resolved and there is full and painless cervical range of motion. If residual symptoms are present or if there is concern for neck injury, return to play should be deferred. Athletes with brachial plexus injuries may be considered healed and safe for return to play when their neurologic examination returns to normal and they are symptom free. An athlete with a permanent neurologic injury should be prohibited from further competition.

The athlete who has sustained transient motor or sensory symptoms (neuropraxia) bilaterally or in an arm and leg, must have a cervical spine MRI to rule out either a spinal cord injury or a condition that puts the spinal cord at risk. If the cervical MRI is normal, the athlete can return to competition when free of neurological symptoms, free of neck pain with and without axial compression, has full range of motion with normal neck strength, and the neurologic examination is normal. Even with complete resolution of symptoms and a normal examination, having had such an event would be considered by some a relative risk for return to play. Having had three such events should be considered an absolute contraindication to return.

For the athlete who has sustained a cervical spine fracture, return to play is deferred at least until the fracture has healed. Generally, stable fractures managed non-operatively, such as those involving a spinous process or a unilateral lamina, that have healed completely will allow the player to return to competition by the next season. Athletes with a healed fracture who have required halo vest or surgical stabilization as part of the treatment are considered to have insufficient spinal strength to safely return to contact sports unless formal testing demonstrates it has returned to normal. Even after the fracture has healed and strength has returned, the altered biomechanics in surrounding spinal segments may produce an increased risk of further sports-related injury. If there is a one-level anterior or posterior fusion for a fracture, athletes are usually allowed to return to play when neck pain is gone, the range of motion is complete, muscle strength of the neck is normal, and the fusion is solid. When there are multilevel fusions or a fusion involving C1–C2 or C2–C3, return to contact or collision sports is contraindicated. The athlete could return to non-contact sports with low risk of neck injury, such as golf or tennis.

Conclusions

Head and neck injuries in young athletes range from mild muscle contusions to life-threatening conditions. Given the potential for serious injury, when in doubt, it is better to hold the athlete out until all appropriate diagnostic testing is performed. Younger children have different anatomy than adults, with unfused apophyses and generally more lax ligamentous structures, which may make radiographic diagnosis of cervical spine injuries more challenging. Magnetic resonance imaging can prove useful to rule out ligamentous injury when plain radiographs are equivocal, and can also help to determine if there is any soft tissue compression of the spinal cord. Return to competition after a head or neck injury is an individual decision, but guidelines exist to aid in that decision. For either a head or neck injury it is important that all symptoms have resolved, neurologic examination is normal, and cervical motion and strength is normal. For athletes who have sustained a cervical spine injury, imaging should not show residual instability or functional stenosis.

Summary

- Athletic head and neck injuries in young athletes include a wide spectrum of injuries.
- Concussion is a common head injury in young athletes and can occur without loss of consciousness.
- The athlete with post-concussive symptoms should not return to play.
- Sport helmets are effective at preventing skull fracture but do not prevent concussion.
- Pseudo-subluxation at C2–3 may be a normal finding in the young athlete.
- The young athlete with a suspected cervical spine injury should initially be immobilized with both the helmet and shoulder pads on, unless the helmet needs to be removed for airway concerns, and then both helmet and shoulder pads should be removed.

References

1. Boden BP, Pasquina P, Johnson J, Mueller FO. Catastrophic injuries in pole-vaulters. *Am J Sports Med.* 2001; 29: 50–54.
2. Boden BP, Tacchetti R, Mueller FO. Catastrophic injuries in high school and college baseball players. *Am J Sports Med.* 2004; 32: 1189–1196.
3. Cantu RC. Recurrent athletic head injury: risks and when to retire. *Clin Sports Med.* 2003; 22: 593–603.
4. Cooper MT, McGee KM, Anderson DG. Epidemiology of athletic head and neck injuries. *Clin Sports Med.* 2003; 22: 427–443.
5. Zemper E. Analysis of cerebral concussion frequency with the most common models of football helmets. *J Athl Train* 1994; 29: 44–50.
6. Gerberich SG, Priest JD, Boen JR, Straub CP, Maxwell RE. Concussion incidences and severity in secondary school varsity football players. *Am J Pub Health* 1983; 73: 1370–1375.
7. Langlois JA, Rutland-Brown W, Wald MM. The epidemiology and impact of traumatic brain injury: a brief overview. *J Head Trauma Rehabil.* 2006; 21: 375–378.
8. Echemendia RJ, Cantu RC. Return to play following sports-related mild traumatic brain injury: The role of neuropsychology. *Appl Neuropsychol.* 2003; 10: 48–55.
9. Grindel SH. Epidemiology and pathophysiology of minor traumatic brain injury. *Curr Sports Med Rep.* 2003; 2: 18–23.
10. Martland HS. Punch drunk. *JAMA.* 1928; 91: 1103–1107.
11. Corsellis JAN, Bruton CJ, Freeman-Browne D. The aftermath of boxing. *Psychol Med.* 1973; 3: 270–303.
12. World Health Organization. *The ICD-10 Classification of mental and behavioural disorders: Clinical descriptions and diagnostic guidelines.* Available from: http://www.who.int/classifications/icd/en/bluebook.pdf. Geneva: World Health Organization; 1992.
13. American Psychiatric Association. *Diagnostic and statistical manual of mental disorders (DSM-IV).* Washington, DC: American Psychiatric Association; 1994.
14. Guthkelch AN. Post-traumatic amnesia, post-concussional symptoms and accident neurosis. *Acta Neurochir Suppl.* 1979; 29: 120–123.
15. Cantu RC, Guskiewicz K, Register-Mihalik JK. A retrospective clinical analysis of moderate to severe athletic concussions. *PMR.* 2010; 2: 1088–1093.
16. Pickles W. Acute general edema of the brain in children with head injuries. *N Engl J Med.* 1950; 242: 607–611.
17. Schnitker MT. Syndrome of cerebral concussion in children. *J Pediatr.* 1949; 35: 557–560.
18. Langfitt TW, Tannenbaum HM, Kassell NF. The etiology of acute brain swelling following experimental head injury. *J Neurosurg.* 1966; 24: 47–56.
19. Langfitt TW, Kassell NF. Cerebral vasodilatation produced by brain-stem stimulation: Neurogenic control vs. autoregulation. *Am J Physiol.* 1968; 215: 90–97.
20. Saunders RL, Harbaugh RE. Second impact in catastrophic contact-sports head trauma. *JAMA.* 1984; 252: 538–539.
21. Schneider RC. *Head and neck injuries in football.* Baltimore, MD: Williams and Wilkins; 1973.
22. Cantu RC. Second impact syndrome: Immediate management. *Phys Sports Med.* 1992; 20: 55–66.
23. Cantu RC, Voy R. Second impact syndrome a risk in any contact sport. *Phys Sports Med.* 1995; 23: 27–34.

24. McQuillen JB, McWuillen EN, Morrow P. Trauma, sports and malignant cerebral edema. *Am J Forensic Med Pathol*. 1988; 9: 12–15.
25. Moody RA, Raumsuke S, Mullan SF. An evaluation of decompression in experimental head injury. *J Neurosurgery*. 1968; 29: 586–590.
26. Langfitt TW, Weinstein JD, Kassell NF. Cerebral vasomotor paralysis produced by intracranial hypertension. *Neurology*. 1963; 13: 622–641.
27. McCrory P. Does second impact syndrome exist? *Clin J Sports Med*. 2001; 11: 144–149.
28. McCrory P, Davis G, Makdissi M. Second impact syndrome or cerebral swelling after sporting head injury. *Curr Sports Med Rep*. 2012; 11: 21–23.
29. Feket JF. Severe brain injury and death following rigid hockey accidents. The effectiveness of the 'safety helmets' of amateur hockey players. *J Can Med Assoc*. 1968; 99: 1234–1239.
30. Kelly JP, Nichols JS, Filley CM, Lillehei KO, Rubinstein D, Kleinschmidt-DeMasters BK. Concussion in sports: Guidelines for the prevention of catastrophic outcome. *JAMA*. 1991; 266: 2867–2869.
31. McIntosh AS, Andersen TE, Bahr R, Greenwald R, Kleiven S, Turner M, Varese M, McCrory P. Sports helmets now and in the future. *Br J Sports Med*. 2011; 45: 1258–1265.
32. Mertz HJ, Prasad P, Irwin AL. Injury risk curves for children and adults in frontal and rear collisions. *Proceedings of the 41st Stapp Car Crash Conference Society of Automotive Engineers*. Warrendale, PA: Society of Automotive Engineers; 1997.
33. McElhaney JH, Roberts VL, Hilyard JF. Properties of human tissues and components: nervous tissues. *Handbook of human tolerance*. Tokyo: Automobile Research Institute Inc; 1976.
34. Dompier TP, Powell JW, Barron MJ, Moore MT. Time-loss and non-time-loss injuries in youth football players. *J Athl Train*. 2007; 42: 395–402.
35. Meehan WP3rd, Mannix R. A substantial proportion of life-threatening injuries are sports related. *Pediatr Emerg Care*. 2013; 29: 624–627.
36. Leonard JR, Jaffe DM, Kuppermann N, Olsen CS, Leonard JC, for the Pediatric Emergency Care Applied Research Network (PECARN) Cervical Spine Study Group. Cervical spine injury patterns in children. *Pediatrics*. 2014; 133: e1179–88.
37. Swenson TM, Lauerman WC, Blanc RO, *et al*. Cervical spine alignment in the immobilized football player: radiographic analysis before and after helmet removal. *Am J Sports Med*. 1997; 25: 226–230.
38. Treme G, Diduch DR, Hart J, *et al*. Cervical spine alignment in the youth football athlete-recommendations for emergency transportation. *Am J Sports Med*. 2008; 36: 1582–1586.
39. Swartz EE, Mihalik JP, Beltz NM, Day MA, Decoster LC. Face mask removal is safer than helmet removal for emergent airway access in American football. *Spine J*. 2014; 14: 996–1004.
40. Delaney JS, Al-Kashmiri A, Baylis P, *et al*. The assessment of airway maneuvers and interventions in university Canadian football, ice hockey, and soccer players. *J Athl Train*. 2011; 46: 117–125.
41. Shaw M, Burnett H, Wilson A, Chan O. Pseudosubluxation of C2 on C3 in polytraumatized children: Prevalence and significance. *Clin Radiol*. 1999; 54: 377–380.
42. Eubanks JD, Gilmore A, Bess S, Cooperman DR. Clearing the pediatric cervical spine following injury. *J Am Acad Orthop Surg*. 2006; 14: 552–564.
43. Rana AR, Drongowski R, Breckner G, Ehrlich PF. Traumatic cervical spine injuries: characteristics of missed injuries. *J Pediatr Surg*. 2009; 44: 151–155.
44. Nunez D, Zuluaga A, Fuentes-Bernardo D, *et al*. Cervical spine trauma: how much more do we learn by routinely using helical CT. *Radiographics*. 1996; 16: 1307–1318.
45. Hoffman JR, Mower WR, Wolfson AB, *et al*. Validity of a set of clinical criteria to rule out injury to the cervical spine in patients with blunt trauma. *N Engl J Med*. 2000; 343: 94–99.
46. Gale SC, Gracias VH, Reilly PM, *et al*. The inefficiency of plain radiography to evaluate the cervical spine after blunt trauma. *J Trauma*. 2005; 59: 1121–1125.
47. Griffen MM, Frykberk ER, Kerwin AJ, *et al*. Radiographic clearance of blunt cervical spine injury: plain radiograph or computed tomography scan. *J Trauma*. 2003; 55: 222–227.
48. Keenan HT, Hollingshead MC, Chung CJ, *et al*. Using CT of the cervical spine for early evaluation of pediatric patients with head trauma. *Am J Roentgenol*. 2001; 177: 1405–1409.
49. Flynn JM, Closkey RF, Mahboubi S, *et al*. Role of magnetic resonance imaging in the assessment of pediatric cervical spine injuries. *J Pediatr Orthop*. 2002; 22: 573–577.
50. Adelgais KM, Grossman DC, Langer SG, *et al*. Use of helical computed tomography for imaging the pediatric cervical spine. *Acad Emerg Med*. 2004; 11: 228–236.
51. Kamel IR, Hernandez RJ, Martin JE, *et al*. Radiation dose reduction in CT of the pediatric pelvis. *Radiology*. 1994; 190: 683–687.
52. Chan CY, Wong YC, Chau LF, *et al*. Radiation dose reduction in paediatric cranial CT. *Pediatr Radiol*. 1999; 29: 770–775.
53. Kelly JD4th, Aliquo D, Sitler MR, *et al*. Association of burners with cervical canal and foraminal stenosis. *Am J Sports Med*. 2000; 28: 214–217.
54. Resnick D. Degenerative disease of the spine. In: *Diagnosis of Bone and Joint Disorders*. Philadelphia: WB Saunders; 1981. p. 1408–1415.
55. Ladd Al, Scranton PE. Congenital cervical stenosis presenting as transient quadriplegia in athletes. *J Bone Joint Surg*. 1986; 68: 1371–1374.
56. Cantu RC. Functional cervical spinal stenosis: a contraindication to participation in contact sports. *Med Sci Sports Exerc*. 1993; 25: 316–317.
57. Eismont FJ, Clifford S, Goldberg M, *et al*. Cervical sagittal spinal canal size in spinal injury. *Spine*. 1984; 9: 663–666.
58. Matsuura P, Waters RL, Adkins S, *et al*. Comparison of computed tomography parameters of the cervical spine in normal control subjects and spinal cord-injured patients. *J Bone Joint Surg*. 1989; 71: 183–188.
59. Wolfe BS, Khilnani M, Malis L. The sagittal diameter of the bony cervical spinal canal and its significance in cervical spondylosis. *J Mt Sinai Hosp*. 1956;23: 283.
60. Penning L. Some aspects of plain radiography of the cervical spine in chronic myelopathy. *Neurology*. 1962; 12: 513–519.
61. Alexander MM, Davis CH, Field CH. Hyerextension injuries of the cervical spine. *Arch Neurol Psychiatry*. 1958; 79: 146.
62. Mayfield FH. Neurosurgical aspects of cervical trauma. *Clinical Neurosurgery, Vol. II*. Baltimore: Williams and Wilkins; 1955.
63. Nugent GR. Clinicopathologic correlations in cervical spondylosis. *Neurology*. 1959; 9: 273.
64. Cantu RV, Cantu RC. Current thinking: return to play and transient quadriplegia. *Curr Sports Med Rep*. 2005; 4: 27–32.
65. McCall T, Fassett D, Brockmeyer D. Cervical spine trauma in children: a review. *Neurosurg Focus*. 2006; 20: E5.
66. Bulas DI, Fitz CR, Johnson DL. Traumatic atlanto-occipital dislocation in children. *Radiology*. 1993; 188: 155–158.
67. Jarris JH Jr, Carson GC, Wagner LK. Radiologic diagnosis of traumatic occipitovertebral dissociation: 1. Normal occipitovertebral relationships on lateral radiographs of supine subjects. *Am J Roentgenol*. 1994; 162: 881–886.
68. Jones TM, Anderson PA, Noonan KJ. Pediatric cervical spine trauma. *J Am Acad Orthop Surg*. 2011; 19: 600–611.
69. Herman MJ. Cervical spine injuries in the pediatric and adolescent athlete. *Instr Course Lect*. 2006; 55: 641–646.
70. Maroon JC, Bailes JE. Athletes with cervical spine injury. *Spine*. 1996; 21: 19.
71. Newton D, England M, Doll H, *et al*. The case for early treatment of dislocations of the cervical spine with cord involvement sustained playing rugby. *J Bone Joint Surg Br*. 2011; 93-B: 1646–1652.

CHAPTER 47

Nutrition and eating disorders

Christine Sundgot-Borgen and Jorunn Sundgot-Borgen

Introduction

Optimal energy and nutrient intake are important for the health and performance of adolescent athletes. Studies focusing on nutrition and adolescent athletes are limited and there are currently no specific nutrition guidelines for young athletes. However, it has been suggested that suboptimal intake of protein, calcium, iron, and zinc may be prevalent in young athletes, particularly during growth spurts or in those who have restricted energy intakes. In some young developing athletes, body dissatisfaction, dieting, and disordered eating (DE) are experienced. Therefore, healthcare professionals and those working with athletes must pay attention to the spectrum of abnormal eating in young athletes, and develop effective approaches for screening, identification, referral, treatment, and prevention. This chapter reviews energy and nutrient requirements and intake and the continuum of DE in adolescent athletes.

Energy and nutrient requirements for young athletes

Energy

To achieve energy balance, energy intake must equal energy expenditure. For athletes, meeting energy requirements is a nutritional priority, and is essential to maintain appropriate body weight and body composition while training for sport.[1] Large metabolic variability within and between individuals[2] and methodological difficulties in estimating both energy intake and expenditure[3,4] make it an almost impossible task to define the accurate energy intake required for young athletes. When dealing with young athletes, one must consider the variability in training load and nutrition-related culture between sports, athletic levels, seasonal and training session differences, and differences between competition requirements.[2] Also, young athletes might adapt to the athletic lifestyle by conserving energy through increased sedentary behaviour during time not spent on sporting activity.[2]

Adolescents are less metabolically efficient than adults during walking and running, which might also be the case in other activities,[5] and adolescents' $kcal \cdot kg^{-1}$ (or $kJ \cdot kg^{-1}$) requirement during activity might be up to 30% higher than for adults.[6,7]

When calculating energy requirements for adolescent athletes, the energy required for growth and development must be included in the calculation, together with energy deposited in growing tissue and the energy expended to synthesize those tissues.[8,9] Also, an essential factor in understanding the energy requirements for adolescent athletes is the energy demands associated with exercise or physical activity (PA), which might be even greater than the increase in energy requirement associated with growth. Estimated energy expended through exercise and PA must also be included in the calculation of energy requirements.[9] The suggested daily energy requirements for adolescents from light to heavy PA[9] are based on quadratic equations[10] to estimate total energy expenditure (TEE), adding the amount of energy needed to grow new tissue and PA level to the estimated energy needs. The energy deposited in growing tissue is estimated to be 2.1 $kcal \cdot g^{-1}$ (8.6 $kJ \cdot g^{-1}$) of daily weight gain.[11]

For the inclusion of energy expended during PA and exercise, METs are included into the calculation. A MET is defined as the resting metabolic rate, that is, the amount of oxygen consumed at rest, being inactive in a sitting position, approximately 3.5 mL $0_2 \cdot kg^{-1} \cdot min^{-1}$ (1.2 $kcal \cdot min^{-1}$ or 5.0 $kJ \cdot min^{-1}$ for a 70 kg person).[12] Light PA is defined as 2.2 METs for boys and girls age 10–19 years, moderate PA as 2.9 METs for boys and girls aged 10- to 14 years, and three METs for 15- to 19-year-olds. Heavy PA is defined as 3.6 and 3.3 METs in 10- to 14-year-old boys and girls, respectively, and 5 and 4.5 METs in 15- to 19-year-old boys and girls, respectively.[9] A table for proposed estimated energy requirements for adolescent boys and girls in different activity levels is presented in Torun *et al.*[9(p20)]

Adolescent athletes who maintain growth and development and thereby naturally gain weight are suggested to be in a positive energy balance.[13] Energy balance is, however, not the most precise estimate of adequate energy intake in young athletes.

In the case of young athletes, energy availability (EA) is the amount of energy remaining to support all other body functions after the energy expended in exercise (EEE) and sporting activities is removed from energy intake (EI). Energy availability can therefore be calculated from the equation EA = EI-EEE.[13,14] Low energy availability (LEA) occurs when an individual's dietary EI is insufficient to support the EE required for health, function, and daily living, once the cost of exercise and sporting activities is taken into account.[13–16] Relative Energy Deficiency (RED) connotes that LEA can occur even in the scenario where EI and total EE are balanced, (i.e. there is no overall energy deficit) by impairing physiological functioning.[15,16]

Recommended EA for adults is 45 $kcal \cdot kg^{-1}$ (188.3 $kJ \cdot kg^{-1}$) fat-free mass (FFM) and equated with energy balance.[17] For adolescents, Torun *et al.*[9] have suggested similar amounts of energy per kg body mass, with variations in suggested requirements in relation to age, gender, and PA level. When investigating adequate EI in adolescent athletes, estimated EI and EE should not be the only variables measured, but growth, body mass, and other anthropometric variables should be included to create a more comprehensive picture of the energy adequacy.[4] Young athletes who are at normal weight and body composition and restrict EI are of special concern when it comes to optimal nutrient intake.

Macronutrients

Carbohydrate

Adequate carbohydrate intake is the main fuel of brief or sustained high-intensity work, and is essential for optimal nervous function. With performance >90 min in prolonged intermittent, high-intensity activity, glycogen stores might be depleted, and the replenishment of these stores is regulated by daily carbohydrate intake and timing of this consumption.[18] The daily intake of carbohydrate should promote restoration of muscle and liver glycogen stores, and is a fundamental goal of recovery between training sessions and competitions.[18] The range in recommended daily intake (RDI) allows nutrient and energy intake to conform to the athlete's exercise commitment which will fluctuate between days and periods.[18] In the absence of specific recommendations for adolescent athletes, the recommendations for adult athletes should be used until further documentation is available. Still, recommendations for the individual adolescent athlete should be presented in the light of the actual training load, the characteristics of training and competition setting, and in light of other activities included in the athlete's schedule.[19]

Pre-exercise carbohydrate intake can optimize glycogen stores prior to exercise or competition, and has been found to increase endurance and exercise performance in adult athletes.[18] Therefore, it is assumed that adolescent athletes who meet for training or competition with fuelled muscles through appropriate carbohydrate consumption during the day and prior to exercise can work harder for a longer period, compared to those who have not replenished their glycogen stores.

During exercise glycogen stores might be depleted, depending on intensity and duration of the activity. Although more research is needed on the effect of exogenous carbohydrate intake during exercise in adolescent athletes, existing studies with adolescents have demonstrated a performance effect in various sports.[20–22] Consumption of carbohydrates through solid or fluid sources during exercise (see Table 47.1) presents an effective strategy to provide an exogenous source to the muscle and central nervous system.[18,20] Performance-enhancing effects by exogenous intake can spare muscle glycogen and is proposed to be an additional fuel source when the muscle glycogen becomes depleted and blood glucose concentration is reduced.[23] (Readers interested in carbohydrate supplementation during exercise are referred to Chapter 6 for further discussion).

In the absence of muscle damage, muscle glycogen can be restored within 24 h,[24] depending on the consumption of carbohydrates post exercise.[18] For one training session per day, carbohydrate intake should be consumed within 1–2 h post-exercise, but for days with <8 h recovery between exercise sessions or competition, intake within 30 min post exercise (see Table 47.1) is crucial to replete stores as optimally as possible prior to the next session.[18,25,26]

Existing data on adolescent athletes show a variation in reported carbohydrate intake among individuals, and sports. Nikic *et al.*[27] reported the mean carbohydrate intake of adolescent basketball players to be 6.3 ± 2.1 $g \cdot kg^{-1}$ (body weight, BW), while 5.6 $g \cdot kg^{-1}$ (BW) was found in 15-year-old soccer players and adolescent sprint athletes.[8,28] A somewhat lower intake of carbohydrates was reported for female sprint athletes (5.1–5.4 $g \cdot kg^{-1}$ [BW])[8] and rhythmic gymnasts.[29] In female swimmers, carbohydrate intake was 5.9 (range, 2.1–11.5) and 6.5 $g \cdot kg^{-1}$ (BW) in 11–14- and 15- to 19-year-olds, respectively.[30]

Based on existing data, one might suggest that male adolescent athletes have higher intakes of carbohydrates than females, and that males are more likely to meet recommended intakes.[31,32] This is in contrast to findings from female athletes who might reach recommended intakes for exercising only at or below light to moderate intensity.[18]

Protein

To obtain positive nitrogen balance and normal cellular function and synthesis of all bodily tissue, adequate energy and protein intake are required. In addition, in adolescents the protein intake should support growth.[4,8,33] Recommendations for protein intake in the general adolescent population have been set at 0.8–1.2 $g \cdot kg^{-1} \cdot day^{-1}$ for maintenance of health.[34] In addition to extra protein needs compared to adults, adolescent athletes need to meet the protein

Table 47.1 Summary of guidelines for carbohydrate intake by athletes.

	Activities and exercise intensity	Recommended intake
Daily carbohydrate needs for fuel and recovery	General PA, 30–60 min·day^{-1} 3–4 times·week^{-1}* and low intensity or skill-based activities	3–5 $g \cdot kg^{-1}$ BW
	Moderate exercise programme (e.g. ~1 h·day^{-1})	5–7 $g \cdot kg^{-1}$ BW
	Endurance programme (e.g. moderate-high intensity 1–3 h·day^{-1})	6–10 $g \cdot kg^{-1}$ BW
	Strength-trained athletes	4–7 $g \cdot kg^{-1}$ BW
	Very high training load (e.g. moderate-high intensity of >4–5 h·day^{-1})	8–12 $g \cdot kg^{-1}$ BW
Pre-event fuelling	For exercise >90 min	7–12 $g \cdot kg^{-1}$ BW per 24 h
	For exercise >60 min	1–4 $g \cdot kg^{-1}$ BW consumed 1–4 h prior to exercise
During exercise	Lasting <45 min	Not needed
	Endurance exercise including 'stop and start' sports lasting 1–2.5 h	30–60 $g \cdot h^{-1}$
	Ultra-endurance exercise lasting >2.5–3 h	Up to 90 $g \cdot h^{-1}$
Post-exercise	Speedy refuelling, <8 h recovery between two fuel-demanding sessions	1–1.2 $g \cdot kg^{-1}$ BW per hours for the first 4 h, then resume daily fuel needs

PA = physical activity; BW = body weight.

* ISSN Recommendations.

Source data from Kreider RB, Wilborn CD, Taylor L, *et al.* ISSN exercise and sport nutrition review: research and recommendations. J Int Soc Sports Nutr. 2010; 7: 1–43.

requirements for training and recovery; these requirements are slightly higher than those for the sedentary adolescent.[35] Studies in youth athletes indicate that a positive nitrogen balance is achieved by daily protein intakes between 1.35 and 1.6 $g \cdot kg^{-1} \cdot day^{-1}$.[36,37] Similar amounts have been recommended for adult athletes[38,39] and adolescent athletes.[19] For adolescent athletes, the timing of the protein intake might be more important than the amount, when trying to maximize adaptation to exercise. Spreading out the high-quality protein sources in a moderate amount into the different daily meals is recommended to increase protein synthesis rate.[26,29] It is important to note that intake above proposed recommendations does not have an additional benefit, but can promote amino-acid catabolism and protein oxidation.[39] Protein requirements should be met by normal diet. To enhance long-term health, consumption of lean protein sources should be promoted.[26]

Prior to exercise, the athlete should focus on spreading protein intake into each main meal, with a moderate but unspecified amount also in the pre-event meal.[26,39] Post-exercise, the main nutritional goal should be to provide sufficient energy, carbohydrate, fluid, and electrolytes, to replace muscle glycogen stores, and facilitate recovery. In adult athletes, the addition of protein is important, as it will provide amino acids for the maintenance and repair of muscle protein.[26] This strategy might also be important for the adolescent athlete. The consumption of ~20–25 g high quality protein within 30 min following a training session or competition has been recommended to enhance the acute protein synthetic response to the training stimulus and should be combined with the recommendations for carbohydrates (see Table 47.1).[38,40]

Adolescent athletes in general seem to achieve greater protein intakes than the RDI for the non-athletic adolescent population.[23] There is evidence that adolescent athletes have intakes of ~1.2–1.6 $g \cdot kg^{-1} \cdot day^{-1}$. However, suggested recommendations for adolescent athletes are set in the higher end of this range.[2,8,36,41,42]

Fat

Adequate intake of dietary fat is important to meet energy needs and to support growth and maturation in adolescent athletes.[43] Dietary lipids are essential for the absorption of fat-soluble vitamins (A, D, E, and K), to provide essential fatty acids, and are essential in the synthesis of cholesterol and other sex hormones.[2,44] Dietary fat is important during the transition from child to adult when there is an increase in adipose and lean tissue.[45] The adipose tissue and fat stored as triacylglycerol within the muscle is the main endogenous energy store for the adolescent athlete.[46] However, since the storage in the individual is generally large, replenishment of these stores after exercise has not been considered.[24] In addition, despite increased interest regarding the role of intramuscular triacylglycerol on exercise performance, the effect of strategies that are discussed for adult athletes remain unstudied in the adolescent population, leaving carbohydrate as the main energy substrate to focus on when it comes to promote exercise nutrition strategies.[19]

Adolescent athletes are recommended to follow public health guidelines for the general adolescent population, consuming 20–35% of total EI from dietary fat.[19] High-fat diets in adolescent athletes are not recommended, and intake above public health guidelines could contribute to excessive weight gain and is associated with the pathogenesis of cardiovascular disease.[10,26] However, dietary fat intake should not be below 20%.[47] Intake of unsaturated fat sources such as plant-based sources and fish should be encouraged, while intake of high concentrated saturated- and trans-fats sources such as fried food, processed food, and fat from animal products should be limited.[19]

Considering the increased total energy need in adolescent athletes compared to non-athletes, their total dietary fat intake is also higher.[22] Dietary surveys of adolescent athletes suggest that current dietary practices typically provide a fat intake of at least 30% of total EI, with saturated fat intakes somewhat above recommendations, seen in sprint,[8] female[48] and male[31] soccer players, and in female rhythmic gymnasts.[29] Therefore, based on assessment of dietary intake in adolescent athletes, there is a need to further investigate the long-term effects on health, body composition, and performance consequences of fat intake above recommendations in adolescent athletes.

Micronutrients

Calcium

Calcium is essential in the maintenance, growth, and repair of bone tissue and contributes to normal function in the nervous and muscle system, and to normal blood clotting. Calcium and vitamin D are key nutrients in bone synthesis. Inadequate intake of these nutrients increases the risk of low bone mineral density (BMD) and stress fractures.[26] Bone remodelling is at its highest level during the period of adolescence.[49] To achieve sufficiently high peak bone mass, and to reduce the subsequent risk of osteoporosis later in life, taking advantage of this period is critical.[50] Calcium requirements (see Table 47.2) are increased in adolescents compared to adults, due to significant bone growth during this period. Exercise interventions, particularly with high-impact PA, have demonstrated a positive influence of PA on bone accrual.[51,52] Weight-bearing PA is positively associated with bone stiffness.[53] However, the small additional bone mineral accretion due to regular exercise with weight-bearing PA most likely does not increase the calcium requirements for adolescent athletes.[19] Guidelines for the general adolescent population should therefore be followed. Intake beyond recommendations does not result in further bone retention or improvements in other calcium-related health or performance factors.[54] (Readers interested in PA and bone health are referred to Chapter 18).

Recommendations for calcium intake vary among countries. For specific national recommendations, see Table 47.2.

Calcium is one of the micronutrients found to be low in athletes' diets, with inadequate intake being more likely in female adolescent athletes. Low intake is often related to energy restriction or avoidance of animal products.[29,30,53,56] The severity of the deviation from the recommended intake depends on the nationality of athletes and the recommendations in their countries. It has been proposed that intervention strategies aiming to increase calcium intake are needed, especially in female adolescent athletes.[19]

Vitamin D

To obtain adequate calcium uptake, to regulate serum levels of calcium and phosphorus, and to promote bone health, an adequate vitamin D intake is necessary.[26] In addition, vitamin D regulates the development and the homeostasis of the skeleton, muscle, and nervous systems.[57] One vitamin D source is exposure to sunlight, meaning that those athletes who live in northern latitudes, or those who train indoors most of the year without adequate outdoor activities, are at risk of poor vitamin D status.[19] Another risk is inadequate consumption of foods naturally rich in, or fortified with,

Table 47.2 Australian, United States, United Kingdom, European, and Scandinavian recommendations for iron, vitamin D, calcium, and zinc per day.

	Australian*	US**	UK*****	European***	Scandinavian****
Boys					
Iron					
9–13 y	8 mg	8 mg	11.3 mg	10 mg (11–17 y)	11 mg
14–18 y	11 mg	11 mg	11.3 mg		11 mg†
Vitamin D					
9–13 y	5.0 μg	15 μg	–	15–25 μg	10 μg
14–18 y	5.0 μg	15 μg	–	15–25 μg	10 μg
Calcium					
	9–11 y: 1000 mg				
9–13 y	12–13 y: 1300 mg	1300 mg	1000 mg	1150 mg (11–17 y)	900 mg
14–18 y	14–18 y: 1300 mg	1300 mg	1000 mg		900 mg††
Zinc					
9–13 y	6 mg	8 mg	9.0 mg	10.7 mg (11–14 y)	11 mg (10–13 y)
14–18 y	7 mg	11 mg	9.5 mg	14.2 mg (15–17 y)	12 mg (14–17 y)
Girls					
Iron					
9–13 y	8 mg	8 mg	14.8 mg	13 mg (11–17 y)	15 mg
14–18 y	15 mg	15 mg	14.8 mg		15 mg
Vitamin D					
9–13 y	5.0 μg	15 μg	–	15–25 μg	10 μg
14–18 y	5.0 μg	15 μg	–	15–25 μg	10 μg
Calcium					
	9–11 y: 1000 mg				
9–13 y	12–13 y: 1300 mg	1300 mg	800 mg	1150 mg (11–17 y)	900 mg
14–18 y	14–18 y: 1300 mg	1300 mg	800 mg		900 mg††
Zinc					
9–13 y	6 mg	8 mg	9.0 mg	10.7 mg (11–14 y)	8 mg (10–13 y)
14–18 y	7 mg	9 mg	7.0 mg	11.9 mg (15–17 y)	9 mg (14–17 y)

* NHMRC[129]; ** USDA & HHA[130] (revised guidelines are presented later in 2015); *** EFSA[131]; **** Norwegian Directory of Health[132]; ***** Department of Health, HMSO, UK[133]; The Dietary Reference Values as defined in the 1991 COMA report do not set a Reference Nutrient Intake for vitamin D for adults or children over 4 years of age who receive adequate sunlight exposure; †18 years = 9 mg; ††18 years = 800 mg.

vitamin D. In addition to low exposure to sunlight, inadequate intake increases the risk of poor vitamin D status.[58] Individuals are exposed to sunlight in different amounts, making it problematic to establish dietary recommendations for vitamin D.[19] For specific recommendations, see Table 47.2. Regular monitoring of status should be undertaken in those adolescent athletes who are at high risk of vitamin D deficiency and insufficiency. This is important, since low vitamin D status in adolescent athletes has the potential to impair health and performance and to increase the risk of injury that could have long-term consequences for bone health. For those suffering from insufficiency or deficiency, correction through natural vitamin D sources or through supplementation should be considered to ensure health and performance.[19]

A review by Ogan and Pritchett[59] reported that different adult athletic populations have a high prevalence of vitamin D insufficiency and deficiency. Studies with adolescent populations have found a high prevalence of insufficiency in female gymnasts,[60] rhythmic gymnasts,[29] and soccer players.[31] In a study of adolescent male and female indoor and outdoor athletes, as many as 73% had vitamin D insufficiency.[61]

Iron

Iron is required for the formation of oxygen-carrying proteins (haemoglobin and myoglobin) and for enzymes involved in energy production. The oxygen-carrying capacity is especially essential for endurance exercise, as well as for normal function of the nervous, behavioural, and immune systems in which iron plays an important part.[57,58] Increases in haemoglobin production, blood volume, and muscle mass are normal characteristics of growth and maturation. These factors account for the majority of increased iron needs in developing adolescents. For girls, iron requirement increases at the onset of menses.[62] Although adolescent athletes might have a higher iron turnover than non-athletes, there is no evidence for requirement beyond the RDI values for the general adolescent population. The requirement for iron intake varies somewhat among different national guidelines, ranging from 8 to 15 mg·day^{-1}, where girls generally have higher requirements than boys, and adolescents have higher requirements than children (see Table 47.2). Differences in assumptions regarding the efficacy of iron absorbed and utilized give rise to different recommendations among countries.[63] Even a mild shortfall in tissue iron status might affect performance by reducing maximum oxygen uptake, aerobic efficiency, and endurance capacity.[64]

Suboptimal iron status results in adverse athletic performance in addition to negative effects on training adaptations,[65] where adverse effects most likely are due to reduction in oxygen transport, adenosine triphosphate (ATP) production, and deoxyribonucleic acid (DNA) synthesis.[19] Therefore, high rates of depleted iron stores, with and without anaemia, are of concern to athletes. In the female athlete specifically, suboptimal iron status can be a result of low iron intake and/or loss of iron in menstrual blood.[66,67]

When diagnosing iron status disorders, it is important to recognize the progression from depleted iron stores, early functional iron deficiency, and iron-deficiency anaemia.[64] Iron supplementation should be considered only if medically warranted.[19]

Depleted iron stores with clinical symptoms are observed frequently in studies conducted on adolescent athlete populations, particularly in endurance athletes.[65,66,68] Male athletes typically exceed dietary iron recommendations, and there are generally no concerns regarding iron intake in male adolescent athletes. Although average female adolescent athletes have intakes close to the recommended intake, individual intakes vary considerably.[29,30,42,55,56,69] Therefore, regular investigation of iron stores, along with interventions to optimize iron-rich food sources, should be considered with female adolescent athletes.

Zinc

Zinc plays a role in energy production, growth, building and repair of muscle tissue, and immune status.[58] Zinc status directly affects thyroid hormone levels, basal metabolic rate, and protein use, all factors that are important for health and exercise performance in the adolescent athlete.

Diets that are low in energy and animal products are associated with inadequate intake of zinc. Individuals who consume adequate energy with a variation in food choices are most likely to reach recommendations.[58] Studies reporting zinc intake show contradictory results. In two studies, both energy intake and intake of zinc were below recommended levels in female swimmers[30] and male basketball players.[27] On the other hand, adequate zinc intake was reported for rhythmic gymnasts,[29] male soccer players,[31] male cyclists, and runners.[32]

Disordered eating and eating disorders

The continuum of disordered eating

Both young male and female athletes are at risk of developing DE and eating disorders (EDs). Eating disorders are defined as a clinical mental disorder (the Diagnostic Statistical Manual of Mental Disorders [DSM-5]) and are characterized by abnormal eating behaviours, an irrational fear of gaining weight, and false beliefs about eating, weight, and body shape.[70] Disordered eating includes eating patterns of concern due to their subclinical anomaly, but they do not demonstrate severe psychopathology nor do they meet the DSM-5 criteria. There is a continuum of DE from normal to abnormal eating that ranges from a healthy body image, body weight, body composition, and energy balance, to abnormal eating, including anorexia nervosa (AN), bulimia nervosa (BN), and binge eating disorder (BED) (Figure 47.1).

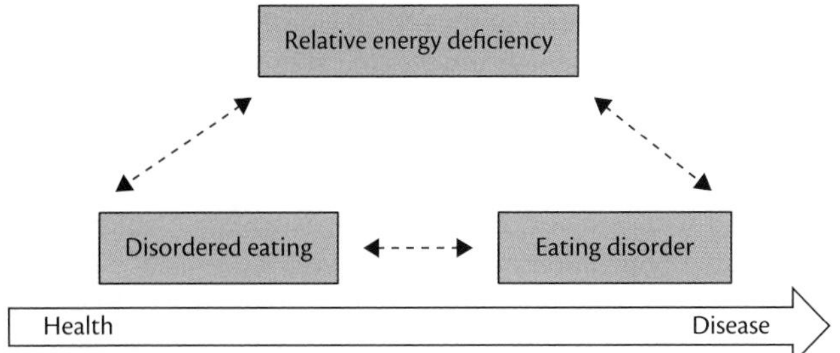

Figure 47.1 The disordered eating continuum.

As indicated in Figure 47.1, RED may be placed on this continuum and might lead to DE or ED, and athletes with DE and ED often have RED. Eating disorders are classified as clinical and subclinical. The clinical EDs include AN, BN, and BED. Binge eating disorder is defined as frequent binge-eating patterns, but without recurrent inappropriate compensatory methods such as purging.[71] Binge eating disorder is often associated with obesity and is expected not to be common in athletes. The continuum of DE also includes the subclinical 'other specified feeding or eating disorder' (OSFED). The term OSFED is used to classify patients with a DE or ED of concern, although the person does not meet all clinical criteria for AN, BN, or BED. Individuals with OSFED may also be described as having DE patterns, and these can be physical, psychological, and behavioural.

Disordered eating is common in athletes and includes abnormal eating behaviours such as restrictive eating, fasting, frequently skipping meals, and using diet pills, laxatives, diuretics, or enemas.[72] Young athletes who are at normal weight and body composition and reduce their EI to lose weight during the period of growth and development during which they actually should gain weight are of special concern. Dieting and rapid weight loss to lose weight and/or meet a specific weight class (e.g. wrestling, lightweight rowing, boxing, Taekwondo, judo, ski-jumping) or to meet the unwritten rule in aesthetic sports (e.g. diving, gymnastics, and figure skating) and endurance sports (e.g. cross-country skiing, running, and cycling) are of great risk, especially if using extreme energy restriction and dehydration methods. Weight cutting at an early age (12.6 ± 6.1 years) has been reported.[73] For some, DE behaviours start as early as 9 years of age[74] and track from adolescence to adulthood with rising rates of extreme weight control methods and binge eating episodes.[75]

The syndrome of Relative Energy Deficiency in Sport (RED-S) refers to impaired physiological functioning caused by RED.[15] It is important to emphasize that not all athletes with reduced or LEA have an ED or DE. When athletes suffer from LEA in the absence of an ED, they are usually unintentionally undereating, and it might be due to a sudden increase in training volume, appetite suppression, a high carbohydrate and fibre intake, or lack of time. Practical experience indicates that unintentional LEA typically most often occurs in sports with high energy demands.

Prevalence of disordered eating and eating disorders

It is difficult to provide accurate and precise estimates of prevalence data due to the fact that studies use various methodological approaches (e.g. screening tools, n-size, age, sports, performance level, and lack of control groups).[76–79] However, most data suggest that both male and female athletes are at greater risk for developing DE and ED than the general population, and that female athletes are at greater risk for developing EDs or DE than males.[80] However, it is important to differentiate data regarding symptoms associated with DE and EDs. A recent Norwegian study including the total population of young first-year students at Norwegian elite sport high schools reported that the prevalence of EDs (using clinical interview) is about 13% and 3% among adolescent female and male elite athletes, respectively, compared to 5% and 0% in female and male controls, respectively.[81] However, the results from the screening data (by questionnaire only) showed a significantly higher prevalence of reported symptoms associated with EDs and DE in non-athlete female and male controls.[82] Also, Hausenblas *et al.*[83] reported that female athletes had greater Drive for Thinness (DT) and Body Dissatisfaction (BD) symptoms and a higher prevalence of EDs than male athletes, non-athletes reported greater BD symptoms than athletes, and there were no sport-group differences (i.e. middle/long distance running, sprinting, and field events) for either ED symptoms or prevalence.

Due to the high prevalence of DE and EDs reported among young athletes, a need for education regarding risk factors, early identification, appropriate management, effective treatment, and preventive efforts for the special subpopulation of young athletes has been suggested.

Risk factors for the development of disordered eating and eating disorders

There are many factors predisposing individuals for DE and EDs, and the reason why athletes may develop DE and EDs is multifactorial, with environmental and social factors, psychological predisposition, low self-esteem, family dysfunction, abuse, biological factors, and genetics potentially all contributing.[72] Eating disorders occur due to a variety of general trigger factors.[71] For the purpose of this chapter, we will focus on sport-specific factors.

Dieting to be thin or to win is a common entry point for athletes. Sport-specific risk factors for EDs and DE have been reported by Sundgot-Borgen.[84] Athletes with EDs were found to start sport-specific training and dieting earlier than those without EDs. Sudden increases in training volume, overtraining, injuries, pressure to reduce body weight or change body composition, chronic dieting, and weight cycling were associated with greater risk. An interesting point is that certain personality traits in athletes are also those identified in individuals with EDs. These include perfectionism and over-compliance, which are traits generally desired by coaches.[79] A difficult aspect among those who are young competitive athletes is the fact that reducing body fat or body mass, maintaining low body fat or body mass, or not gaining body mass during growth may initially lead to improved performance due to an improved power-to-mass ratio. If this is encouraged by the coach and other athletes observe it, it may trigger energy restriction. Perhaps similar to social pressures for thinness in girls, leanness and muscularity appear to characterize at-risk male athletes.[85]

Consequences and complications

Disordered eating and EDs can manifest in nutrition-related complications that also may influence sport performance. In young athletes, DE and EDs can interfere with growth and development. The earlier the EDs begin, the longer the disorders might continue.[19] Low EI leads to insufficient macro- and micronutrient intakes with a potential risk for short and long-term nutrient deficiencies. In relation to the macronutrients, inadequate 24 h carbohydrate intake might negatively affect total EI and will reduce the ability to store glycogen in muscle and liver. This increases the risk of glycogen depletion during training or competition, leading to early fatigue and reduced cognitive function, and the ability to obtain optimal glycogen repletion post-exercise is reduced. There is also an increased risk of injury and since carbohydrates are essential for the immune cells, an inadequate intake might suppress the ability to stay healthy.[18,86,89]

Low EA will result in protein being used as a substrate for energy, potentially reducing its availability for its primary functions, affecting growth and development, and leading to muscle mass accretion and muscle wasting,[2,88] both of which can have a negative effect on health and performance.

Very low fat intakes fail to deliver adequate essential fatty acids and fat-soluble vitamins. Also, severe restriction of fat sources might limit the intake of protein-rich foods such as meat and dairy foods, along with the associated nutrients such as iron, zinc, and calcium.[2] Inadequate EI is also associated with inadequate micronutrient intake. Low intake of calcium and vitamin D are of special concern, possibly leading to compromised musculoskeletal and immune health at an early age, with continued complications during adulthood.[19]

Even a mild shortfall in tissue iron status might affect health[65] and performance by reducing maximum oxygen uptake, aerobic efficiency, and the body`s endurance capacity,[89] most likely due to the reduction in oxygen transport, ATP production, and DNA synthesis.[19] In addition, poor zinc status, most often found in athletes with inadequate EIs, is associated with a decrease in cardiorespiratory function, muscle strength, and muscle endurance.[90]

Health-related consequences of LEA involve overall impaired physiological function, integrating factors such as metabolic rate, menstrual function, bone health, immune function, protein synthesis, cardiovascular health, psychological health, and related performance issues.[15] Effects on physiological and psychological function vary by degree and duration of LEA, DE behaviour, and age of the athlete.[76]

Long-term suppression of reproductive function through LEA can negatively impact musculoskeletal[91] and cardiovascular health.[92] Low EA at <30 $kcal \cdot kgFFM^{-1} \cdot day^{-1}$ (<125.5 $kJ \cdot kgFFM^{-1} \cdot day^{-1}$) also leads to abrupt changes in markers of bone turnover and metabolic markers independent of oestradiol.[93] Low EA is recognized as the key link to both menstrual dysfunction and compromised bone mass.[72]

Osteoporosis presents a great risk for fragility fractures later in life. The International Society for Clinical Densitometry (ISCD) and others[15,91] recommend using age-specific Z-scores to evaluate bone health in pre-menopausal women, young men, adolescents, and children.[94] Low EA is related to BMD Z-scores. Barrack and colleagues[95] found that adolescent female runners who consumed less energy than recommended (LEA) had low BMD Z-scores (Z-scores were <−1 at the spine) compared with runners consuming more energy. They also had reduced bone turnover, lower body mass, lower BMI, lower 25 (OH) Vitamin D3, lower oestradiol levels, and reported fewer menstrual cycles in the past year.[95]

Studies have also shown that female athletes with menstrual dysfunction have lower BMD than athletes with normal menstrual function. While initially thought to be a female problem, similar links between EDs and DE, suppression of sex steroid hormones, and compromised BMD have recently been identified in male athletes,[96–98] especially endurance athletes.[99] Low EA can also affect other systems beyond menstrual function and bone, including thyroid hormone, which results in a decrease in resting metabolic rate.

Finally, compromised energy and nutrient intakes affect growing athletes. Especially visible in gymnasts, growth retardation and delayed puberty are side effects of high training volumes and inadequate nutrition.[100] While catch-up growth after periods of weight reduction in young athletes[101,102] is possible, some bone loss may be irreversible.[103]

Bingeing and purging can lead to gastric and oesophageal complications, some of which are irreversible.[104,105] While dehydration may be a common side effect of daily training, an additional loss of body water due to vomiting or laxatives, diuretics or enemas may cause potassium losses, leading to hypokalaemia and cardiac arrhythmias.[104] Electrolyte imbalances are especially of concern in high-intensity sports, where a blackout and fall could have severe consequences. Purging can alter pH levels and lead to metabolic alkalosis, while severe laxative abuse can result in metabolic acidosis.[104] Both metabolic alkalosis and acidosis are expected to interfere with the athlete's capacity to manage metabolic challenges during exercise. Dehydration can also occur due to rapid weight loss. This type of dehydration increases the risk of hyperthermia and exertional heat illness.[106] Athletes who lose weight rapidly over a short period of time (>5% body mass) with little time to refuel before competition, might suffer from performance declines due to dehydration, as well as due to glycogen depletion and low blood glucose levels with increased risk of injury, including heat illness.[107,108] Losing weight is generally not recommended in young athletes below 18 years of age.[47]

Prevention of eating disorders in athletes

Besides raising awareness and making guidelines available for how to identify and treat young athletes with DE and EDs, sport organizations should emphasize prevention through screening and education. Based on existing literature guidelines, educational highlights and recommendations are listed below.[15,79,109–112]

Healthcare providers need to:

- Continue to support efforts of DE and EDs prevention and recognize the need for coaches' and athletes' education.
- Be trained in the screening, identification, referral, and treatment approaches. (See RED-S CAT-risk assessment.[16])

Coaches, parents, and other support staff need to:

- Be educated and understand which sports are at greatest risk and why.
- Learn about trigger factors and the potential effect their comments and actions may have on an athlete.
- Be able to recognize the signs and symptoms of DE or EDs and understand short- and long-term medical and performance complications.
- Learn that a lower weight and body fat do not always lead to long-term performance enhancement. Weight and body composition should be de-emphasized and performance should be the centre of attention.
- Be aware of the scientific evidence of how nutrition and body composition relate to health and long-term success.
- Understand that body weight and body composition assessment should be the task of trained professionals (and not coaches), and that the rationale for assessment be communicated to the athlete, and methods chosen should be carefully considered.
- Need to understand that having DE or EDs is associated with increased risk for injuries and illness and that providing a supportive environment also promotes a safe and ethical playing field.
- Understand that coaches should refrain from approaching athletes about changes in body weight and body composition.

Athlete education should focus on performance nutrition, including the importance of energy balance and availability as they relate to health, growth, development, and performance. Examples include:

- The extra need for calories when training intensity and duration are higher. Education should also target the need to fuel performance before, during, and after exercise.
- While providing awareness of DE and EDs risks, signs and symptoms, and consequences, educational approaches should generally remain covert, positive, and focus on performance nutrition using theoretical and practical, hands-on approaches.
- Young athletes should feel comfortable discussing concerns about body weight and body composition with coaches, trainers, and staff, but this requires a de-stigmatization of DE and EDs.
- Young athletes should no longer need to hide eating problems but feel able to discuss concerns with coaches.

Although preventing DE and EDs among athletes is recommended,[15,72,109,112–114] only limited research exists aiming to prevent DE and EDs among elite young athletes. However, there are a few promising prevention programmes for young athletes available.[83,115,116] Due to the limited work on prevention of EDs in athletes, there is no consensus on best practice. However, focusing on health-promoting factors has been highlighted as essential.[107] The Health, Body and Sports Performance Intervention programme[82] is a sport-specific intervention built on the social-cognitive framework.[117] Its primary focus is to enhance self-esteem by strengthening the athlete's self-efficacy. The intervention is influenced by the elaboration-likelihood model[118] and the cognitive-dissonance theory.[119] Young athletes (especially elite) constitute a unique population as they are under pressure to improve performance and conform to the requirements of sport, in addition to being under socio-cultural pressure. On the other hand, if the information indicates that healthy eating can increase the likelihood of good sport performance (e.g. by focusing on the relationship between body composition, health, nutrition, and performance), young athletes will most likely pay more attention.[112] Although education is certainly an important part of ED prevention programmes, it is unlikely to be effective unless it is accompanied by preventive efforts designed to change the beliefs and behaviours of the participants.[113] Interestingly, Nowicka *et al.*[120] found by interviewing 18 Swedish elite coaches in high-risk sports, that those who did not have sufficient knowledge of ED symptoms easily questioned their own observations in the face of athletes' statement of denial. The researchers also found that knowledge of EDs per se did not automatically encourage the coaches to act. In fact, many of the coaches were uncomfortable and found it difficult to talk with their athletes when observing symptoms of EDs.[120] Thus, healthcare professionals should continue to support ED prevention and recognize the need for coaches' education, even in the face of initial resistance. While education can increase awareness and knowledge of the risks and consequences of DE and EDs in athletes, the culture of the sport may not allow for behaviour change. Thus, national and international sport governing bodies should focus on enforcing rules and regulations related to body mass and body composition.

Recovery from eating disorders

Recovery from an ED is variable. For some, the disease is of short duration, especially for DE, as energy restriction may only be temporary with full recovery after intervention.[121] The best prognosis for full recovery is seen in young individuals with a relatively short history of DE or EDs.[122] In newly diagnosed athletes, average recovery time spanned across a year, but varied greatly.[123] Relapse periods are a common issue in EDs and DE, especially in athletes. What helps athletes to recover from EDs seems to be the deep desire to regain health and energy to participate in their sport.[123]

Treatment of eating disorders in athletes

The first steps before treatment for DE and EDs is initiated are screening, identification, and diagnosis. The most valid and reliable screening approach is by clinical interview by a trained psychologist or during pre-participation examination by a physician. Short surveys or assessments can flag athletes for follow-up in order to confirm risk of an ED or DE. Other healthcare professionals who work with athletes directly (e.g., sports nutritionists, athletic trainers, physical therapists, strength and conditioning coaches), can act as 'eyes' in the identification process.

Once athletes are identified, they need to be referred to a treatment team experienced in DE and EDs. It is important to determine whether DE and EDs occur transiently, are associated with the specific demands of the sport,[121] or whether the symptoms are more consistent with an ED, as appropriate treatment will vary.

Re-establishment of sound eating practices

Reducing overall nutritional risk and clarifying myths through evidence-based education and hands-on training are critical to re-establishing sound eating practices. It is important to build a solid foundation of knowledge for the athlete to trust that increased and regular food intake will lead to performance enhancement (perceived as positive) as opposed to weight gain (perceived as negative), and which is often inaccurately equated with a performance loss. A small-step approach is best (e.g. adding 300–600 kcal $\cdot$ week^{-1} [1250–2500 kJ $\cdot$ week^{-1}] in underweight athletes and normalizing eating patterns in athletes with BN).

For athletes with low sex steroid hormones, increasing EA is the main goal. Female athletes can resume normal menstrual function within 6 months by adding dietary energy.[124–126] These studies used a post-exercise carbohydrate and protein drink, adding an average 350 kcal $\cdot$ day^{-1} (1464 kJ $\cdot$ day^{-1}).

Pharmacological treatment approaches (e.g. oral contraceptives) to regulate the menstrual cycle have not produced positive effects on bone mass and should be discouraged in young athletes. Bone is also regulated by nutritional means, and thus, failing to remedy nutritional deficits will likely affect bone mass independently from hypoestrogenism.

Role of the sports medicine physician

The treatment team also includes the sports medicine physician who should coordinate treatment after conducting a physical examination, including blood, urine, and bone parameters.[79] If a persistent ED exists, the athlete needs psychological care,[76] which may include the family, especially with young individuals.[127] Treatment guidelines are published in the *Practice Guidelines for Treatment of Patients with Eating Disorders*, 3rd edition.[70]

Treatment approaches vary greatly. Whether an athlete is 'unfit' to participate in training and competition should be determined on an individual basis among the treatment team members. The stop light system, published in the International Olympic Committee Consensus Statement,[15] is useful for both risk assessment and return to play.[16] Athletes with clinical EDs or practising extreme weight-loss methods should not be allowed to compete (they are classified as being the colour RED), while those with various indicators (e.g. prolonged low % body fat, substantial weight loss of 5–10%, attenuation of expected growth and development, menstrual dysfunction, abnormal hormone profile in men, reduced BMD, stress fractures, cardiovascular issues, or lack of progress from treatment) are classified as YELLOW. These athletes should be carefully monitored. While treatment is necessary for athletes to return to play, prevention is the best approach.[15]

Ethical and methodological considerations in sport and exercise medicine research

The limited knowledge related to energy and nutritional requirements and eating disorders in young athletes is partly explained by the special workload associated with appropriate research ethics. Limited access to children and adolescents for the purpose of research, as well as the need for informed consent from both the athletes and parents/guardians, make research more complicated than with adults.[128] Research in sport and exercise medicine with adults often involves muscle biopsies, exercise to failure, and exercise resulting in 'poor' physiological state. This type of request is considered inappropriate with children and adolescents as participants in research.[4,62] It has also been questioned whether asking questions or focusing on eating behaviour, body image problems, and DE behaviour in young athletes might increase the risk for eating disorders in young athletes. However, this has not been investigated.

Age categories are often used to group study samples, but such a categorization does not account for the developmental and maturational stages of young athletes. Participants in one age group might differ from each other both in cognitive and physiological development. Young athletes therefore cannot be placed into one homogenous group.[2] Also, most of the existing studies are cross sectional, have small sample sizes and do not use gold-standard methods and designs, and are therefore very limited when it comes to assessment of energy and nutrient intake and DE and ED. Furthermore, it is difficult to provide accurate and precise prevalence data of DE and EDs due to the fact that studies use various methodological approaches (e.g. screening tools, sample sizes, age, sports, performance level, and lack of control groups).[76–79] In addition, most of the screening questionnaires are developed for inpatients and/or adults. Therefore, there is a need for development and validation of age-, gender-, and sport-specific questionnaires.

Conclusions

The small number of studies and the lack of methodological quality make it difficult to draw conclusions on nutritional status and needs in the adolescent population. Thus, further research is needed. Young athletes consuming inadequate energy may end up with delayed maturation, attenuated growth, and poor sports performance. Suboptimal intake of protein, calcium, iron, and zinc may be prevalent in young athletes, particularly during growth spurts, or in those who have restricted energy intakes. Young athletes should be encouraged to be responsible for their own food choices and be educated on how to choose suitable food and optimize eating behaviour. A continued focus on the prevention of extreme dieting and eating disorders is important for all those working with young athletes. Healthcare professionals must educate coaches and those working with young athletes about how to identify DE and EDs, and how they can be important players in the continuous preventive work of DE and EDs in sports. Treatment interventions targeting young athletes with different ED diagnoses are required. By systematically identifying and validating existing prevention programmes and treatment interventions for young athletes with DE and EDs, and by exposing gaps in the current literature, the evidence obtained can inform exercise and sports medicine researchers, funding bodies, and policy makers, and create new opportunities for future research.

Summary

- Based on existing data, optimal energy and nutrient intake in adolescent athletes is not certain due to the methodological challenges and the limited number of studies.
- It seems reasonable to suggest that there might be some potential for nutritional improvement to promote health and performance, especially among female adolescent athletes.
- It is important to take into consideration the potential differences between the adult and the adolescent athlete that may affect the need for dietary carbohydrate, such as specific modifications in training and competition load, altered substrate utilization, and the ability to store carbohydrate.
- It is indicated that the risk of inadequate micronutrient intake, such as iron, calcium, and zinc, is associated with energy restriction and exclusion of certain food groups.
- Abnormal vitamin D status is reported for both genders, where lack of exposure to sunlight seems to produce the greatest risk.
- Since disordered eating (DE) and eating disorders (EDs) exist among young athletes, it is important to understand the risks and triggers of DE and EDs.
- Prevention is the best treatment and strategies should integrate education and screening for early identification.
- It is important that sports develop policies and procedures that can be used on a national and local level. Education should target athletes, parents, volunteers, coaches, officials, and healthcare providers.

References

1. American Dietetic Association; Dietitians of Canada; American College of Sports Medicine, Rodriguez NR, Di Marco NM, Langley S. American College of Sports Medicine position stand. Nutrition and athletic performance. *Med Sci Sports Exerc.* 2009; 41: 709–731.
2. Petrie HJ, Stover EA, Horswill CA. Nutritional concerns for the child and adolescent competitor. *Nutrition.* 2004; 20: 620–631.
3. Burke LM. Energy needs of athletes. *Can J Appl Physiol.* 2001; 26(Suppl): S202–S219.
4. Meyer F, O'Connor H, Shirreffs SM. International Association of Athletics Federations: Nutrition for the young athlete. *J Sports Sci.* 2007; 25(Suppl 1): S73–S82.
5. Bar-Or O. Nutritional considerations for the child athlete. *Can J Appl Physiol.* 2001; 26(Suppl): S186–S191.
6. Krahenbuhl GS, Williams TJ. Running economy: changes with age during childhood and adolescence. *Med Sci Sports Exerc.* 1992; 24: 462–466.
7. MacDougall JD, Bell RD, Howald H. Skeletal muscle ultrastructure and fiber types in prepubescent children. In: Nagle FJ, Montoye HJ (eds.) *Exercise in health and disease.* Springfield, IL: Thomas; 1982. p. 113–117.
8. Aerenhouts D, Deriemaeker P, Hebbelinck M, Clarys P. Energy and macronutrient intake in adolescent sprint athletes: a follow-up study. *J Sports Sci.* 2011; 29: 73–82.
9. Torun B. Energy requirements of children and adolescents. *Public Health Nutr.* 2005; 8: 968–993.
10. Foodand and Agriculture Organization of the United Nations. *Fats and fatty acids in human nutrition: report of an expert consultation.* Rome: Office of Knowledge Exchange, Research and Extension; 2010.
11. World Health Organization. *Measuring change in nutritional status.* Geneva: World Health Organization; 1983.
12. Jette M, Sidney K, Blumchen G. Metabolic equivalents (METS) in exercise testing, exercise prescription, and evaluation of functional capacity. *Clin Cardiol.* 1990; 13: 555–565.
13. Loucks AB, Kiens B, Wright HH. Energy availability in athletes. *J Sports Sci.* 2011; 29(Suppl 1): S7–S15.
14. Louks AB. Energy balance and energy availability. In: Maughan RJ (ed.) *Sports Nutrition. The Encyclopaedia of Sports Medicine: An IOC Medical Commission Publication, Volume XIX*, 2nd ed. Oxford: Wiley-Blackwell; 2013. p. 72–87.
15. Mountjoy M, Sundgot-Borgen J, Burke LM, *et al.* The IOC consensus statement: beyond the Female Athlete Triad--Relative Energy Deficiency in Sport (RED-S). *Br J Sports Med.* 2014; 48: 491–497.
16. Mountjoy M, Sundgot-Borgen J, Burke LM, *et al.* The ICO relative energy deficiency in sport clinical assessment tool (RED-S CAT). *Br J Sports Med.* 2015; 49: 421–423.
17. Loucks AB. Energy balance and body composition in sports and exercise. *J Sports Sci.* 2004; 22: 1–14.
18. Burke LM, Hawley JA, Wong SH, Jeukendrup AE. Carbohydrates for training and competition. *J Sports Sci.* 2011; 29(Suppl 1): S17–S27.
19. Desbrow B, McCormack J, Burke LM, *et al.* Sports Dietitians Australia position statement: sports nutrition for the adolescent athlete. *Int J Sport Nutr Exerc Metab.* 2014; 24: 570–584.
20. Batatinha HA, da Costa CE, de Franca E, *et al.* Carbohydrate use and reduction in number of balance beam falls: implications for mental and physical fatigue. *J Int Soc Sports Nutr.* 2013; 10: 2–6.
21. Dougherty KA, Baker LB, Chow M, Kenney WL. Two percent dehydration impairs and six percent carbohydrate drink improves boys basketball skills. *Med Sci Sports Exerc.* 2006; 38: 1650–1658.
22. Smith JW, Lee KA, Dobson JP, Roberts TJ, Jeukendrup AE. Fluid and carbohydrate ingestion improve performance in American football players. *Med Sci Sports Exerc.* 2013; 45: 545–555.
23. Jeukendrup A, Cronin L. Nutrition and elite young athletes. *Med Sport Sci.* 2011; 56: 47–58.
24. Burke LM, Kiens B, Ivy JL. Carbohydrates and fat for training and recovery. *J Sports Sci.* 2004; 22: 15–30.
25. Kreider RB, Wilborn CD, Taylor L, *et al.* ISSN exercise and sport nutrition review: research and recommendations. *J Int Soc Sports Nutr.* 2010; 7: 1–43.
26. Rodriguez NR, DiMarco NM, Langley S, *et al.* Position Statement of the American Dietetic Association, Dietitians of Canada, and the American

College of Sports Medicine: Nutrition and athletic performance. *J Am Diet Assoc.* 2009; 109: 509–527.
27. Nikic M, Pedisic Z, Satalic Z, Jakovljevic S, Venus D. Adequacy of nutrient intakes in elite junior basketball players. *Int J Sport Nutr Exerc Metab.* 2014; 24: 516–523.
28. Briggs MA, Cockburn E, Rumbold PL, Rae G, Stevenson EJ, Russell M. Assessment of energy intake and energy expenditure of male adolescent academy-level soccer players during a competitive week. *Nutrients.* 2015; 7 8392–8401.
29. Silva MR, Paiva T. Low energy availability and low body fat of female gymnasts before an international competition. *Eur J Sport Sci.* 2015; 15: 591–599.
30. da Costa NF, Schtscherbyna A, Soares EA, Ribeiro BG. Disordered eating among adolescent female swimmers: dietary, biochemical, and body composition factors. *Nutrition.* 2013; 29:172–177.
31. Hidalgo YTER, Bermudo FM, Penaloza MR, Berna Amoros G, Lara Padilla E, Berral de la Rosa FJ. Nutritional intake and nutritional status in elite Mexican teenage soccer players of different ages. *Nutr Hosp.* 2015; 32: 1735–1743.
32. Tong TK, Lin H, Lippi G, Nie J, Tian Y. Serum oxidant and antioxidant status in adolescents undergoing professional endurance sports training. *Oxid Med Cell Longev.* 2012; 2012: 741239.
33. Nemet D, Eliakim A. Pediatric sports nutrition: an update. *Curr Opin Clin Nutr Metab Care.* 2009; 12: 304–309.
34. Smit E, Nieto FJ, Crespo CJ, Mitchell P. Estimates of animal and plant protein intake in US adults: results from the Third National Health and Nutrition Examination Survey, 1988–1991. *J Am Diet Assoc.* 1999; 9: 813–820.
35. Tipton KD, Jeukendrup AE, Hespel P, International Association of Athletics Federations: Nutrition for the sprinter. *J Sports Sci.* 2007; 25(Suppl 1): S5–S15.
36. Aerenhouts D, Van Cauwenberg J, Poortmans JR, Hauspie R, Clarys P. Influence of growth rate on nitrogen balance in adolescent sprint athletes. *Int J Sport Nutr Exerc Metab.* 2013; 23: 409–417.
37. Boisseau N, Vermorel M, Rance M, Duche P, Patureau-Mirand P. Protein requirements in male adolescent soccer players. *Eur J Appl Physiol.* 2007; 100: 27–33.
38. Phillips SM, Van Loon LJ. Dietary protein for athletes: from requirements to optimum adaptation. *J Sports Sci.* 2011; 29(Suppl 1): S29–S38.
39. Slater G, Phillips SM. Nutrition guidelines for strength sports: sprinting, weightlifting, throwing events, and bodybuilding. *J Sports Sci.* 2011; 29(Suppl 1): S67–S77.
40. Hawley JA, Burke LM, Phillips SM, Spriet LL. Nutritional modulation of training-induced skeletal muscle adaptations. *J Appl Physiol.* 2011; 110: 834–845.
41. Gibson J, Mitchell A, Harries M, Reeve J. Nutritional and exercise-related determinants of bone density in elite female runners. *Osteoporosis Int.* 2004; 15: 611–618.
42. Heaney S, O'Connor H, Gifford J, Naughton G. Comparison of strategies for assessing nutritional adequacy in elite female athletes' dietary intake. *Int J Sport Nutr Exerc Metab.* 2010; 20: 245–256.
43. Bushman BA. Calorie requirements for young competitive female athletes. *ACSM's Health and Fitness Journal.* 2012; 16: 4–8.
44. Lichtenstein AH, Kennedy E, Barrier P, *et al.* Dietary fat consumption and health. *Nutr Rev.* 1998; 56(5 Pt 2): S3–S19; discussion S28.
45. Wahl R. Nutrition in the adolescent. *Pediatr Ann.* 1999; 28: 107–111.
46. Shaw CS, Clark J, Wagenmakers AJ. The effect of exercise and nutrition on intramuscular fat metabolism and insulin sensitivity. *Ann Rev Nutr.* 2010; 30: 13–34.
47. Sundgot-Borgen J, Garthe I. Elite athletes in aesthetic and Olympic weight-class sports and the challenge of body weight and body compositions. *J Sports Sci.* 2011; 29(Suppl 1): S101–S114.
48. Reed JL, De Souza MJ, Kindler JM, Williams NI. Nutritional practices associated with low energy availability in Division I female soccer players. *J Sports Sci.* 2014; 32: 1499–1509.
49. MacKelvie KJ, Khan KM, McKay HA. Is there a critical period for bone response to weight-bearing exercise in children and adolescents? a systematic review. *Br J Sports Med.* 2002; 36: 250–257.
50. Rizzoli R, Bianchi ML, Garabedian M, McKay HA, Moreno LA. Maximizing bone mineral mass gain during growth for the prevention of fractures in the adolescents and the elderly. *Bone.* 2010; 46: 294–305.
51. Herrmann D, Hebestreit A, Ahrens W. [Impact of physical activity and exercise on bone health in the life course: a review]. *Bundesgesundheitsblatt Gesundheitsforschung Gesundheitsschutz.* 2012; 55: 35–54.
52. Tan VP, Macdonald HM, Kim S, Nettlefold L, Gabel L, Ashe MC, *et al.* Influence of physical activity on bone strength in children and adolescents: a systematic review and narrative synthesis. *J Bone Miner Res.* 2014; 29: 2161–2181.
53. Herrmann D, Buck C, Sioen I, *et al.* Impact of physical activity, sedentary behaviour and muscle strength on bone stiffness in 2–10 year-old children-cross-sectional results from the IDEFICS study. *Int J Behav Nutr Phys Act.* 2015; 12: 1–12.
54. Kerr D, Khan, K, Bennell K. Bone, exercise and nutrition. In: Burke LM, Deakin V (eds.) *Clinical sports nutrition*, 4th ed. North Ryde: McGraw-Hill; 2010. p. 200–210.
55. Gibson JC, Stuart-Hill L, Martin S, Gaul C. Nutrition status of junior elite Canadian female soccer athletes. *Int J Sport Nutr Exerc Metab.* 2011; 21: 507–514.
56. Martinez S, Pasquarelli BN, Romaguera D, Arasa C, Tauler P, Aguilo A. Anthropometric characteristics and nutritional profile of young amateur swimmers. *J Strength Cond Res.* 2011; 25: 1126–1133.
57. Institute of Medicine (US) Standing Committee on the Scientific Evaluation of Dietary Reference Intakes. *Dietary Reference Intakes for Calcium, Phosphorus, Magnesium, Vitamin D, and Fluoride.* Washington, DC: National Academies Press; 1997.
58. Volpe SL. Vitamins, minerals and exercise. In: Dunfor M (ed.) *Sports nutrition: A practice manual for professionals.* Chicago: American Dietetic Association; 2006. p. 61–63.
59. Ogan D, Pritchett K. Vitamin D and the athlete: risks, recommendations, and benefits. *Nutrients.* 2013; 5: 1856–1868.
60. Lovell G. Vitamin D status of females in an elite gymnastics program. *Clin J Sport Med.* 2008; 18: 159–161.
61. Constantini NW, Arieli R, Chodick G, Dubnov-Raz G. High prevalence of vitamin D insufficiency in athletes and dancers. *Clin J Sport Med.* 2010; 20: 368–371.
62. Smith JW, Holmes ME, McAllister MJ. Nutritional considerations for performance in young athletes. *J Sports Med.* 2015; 2015: 734649.
63. Beck KL, Conlon CA, Kruger R, Coad J. Dietary determinants of and possible solutions to iron deficiency for young women living in industrialized countries: a review. *Nutrients.* 2014; 6: 3747–3776.
64. Deakin V. Prevention, detection and treatment of iron depletion and deficiency in athletes. In: Burke LM, Deakin V (eds.) *Clinical sports nutrition*, 4th ed. North Ryde: McGraw-Hill; 2010. p. 222–267.
65. Rodenberg RE, Gustafson, S. Iron as an ergogenic aid: ironclad evidence? *Curr Sports Med Rep.* 2007; 6: 258–264.
66. Gropper SS, Blessing D, Dunham K, Barksdale JM. Iron status of female collegiate athletes involved in different sports. *Biol Trace Elem Res.* 2006; 109: 1–14.
67. Koehler K, Braun H, Achtzehn S, *et al.* Iron status in elite young athletes: gender-dependent influences of diet and exercise. *Eur J Appl Physiol.* 2012; 112: 513–523.
68. Sandstrom G, Borjesson M, Rodjer S. Iron deficiency in adolescent female athletes—is iron status affected by regular sporting activity? *Clin J Sport Med.* 2012; 22: 495–500.
69. Juzwiak CR, Amancio OM, Vitalle MS, Pinheiro MM, Szejnfeld VL. Body composition and nutritional profile of male adolescent tennis players. *J Sports Sci.* 2008; 26: 1209–1217.
70. American Psychiatric Association. (2014). DSM-5 Implementation and Support 2014 [updated 2014; cited 2014]. Available from: http://www.dsm5.org/Pages/Default.aspx/5.
71. Treasure J, Claudino AM, Zucker N. Eating disorders. *Lancet.* 2010; 375(9714): 583–593.
72. Nattiv A, Loucks AB, Manore MM, *et al.* American College of Sports Medicine position stand. The female athlete triad. *Med Sci Sports Exerc.* 2007; 39: 1867–1882.

73. Artioli GG, Gualano B, Franchini E, *et al.* Prevalence, magnitude, and methods of rapid weight loss among judo competitors. *Med Sci Sports Exerc.* 2010; 42: 436–442.
74. Neumark-Sztainer D, Hannan PJ. Weight-related behaviors among adolescent girls and boys: results from a national survey. *Arch Pediatr Adolesc Med.* 2000; 154: 569–577.
75. Neumark-Sztainer D, Wall M, Larson NI, Eisenberg ME, Loth K. Dieting and disordered eating behaviors from adolescence to young adulthood: findings from a 10-year longitudinal study. *J Am Diet Assoc.* 2011; 111: 1004–1011.
76. Beals KA, Houtkooper L, Dalton B. Disordered eating in athletes. In: Burke LM, Deakin V (eds.) *Clinical sports nutrition*, 4th ed. North Ryde: McGraw-Hill; 2010. p. 184–185.
77. Rosendahl J, Bormann B, Aschenbrenner K, Aschenbrenner F, Strauss B. Dieting and disordered eating in German high school athletes and non-athletes. *Scand J Med Sci Sports.* 2009; 19: 731–739.
78. Sundgot-Borgen J, Torstveit MK. Prevalence of eating disorders in elite athletes is higher than in the general population. *Clin J Sport Med.* 2004; 14: 25–32.
79. Sundgot-Borgen J, Torstveit MK. Aspects of disordered eating continuum in elite high-intensity sports. *Scand J Med Sci Sports.* 2010; 20(Suppl 2): 112–121.
80. Bratland-Sanda S, Sundgot-Borgen J. Eating disorders in athletes: overview of prevalence, risk factors and recommendations for prevention and treatment. *Eur J Sport Sci.* 2013; 13: 499–508.
81. Martinsen M, Sundgot-Borgen J. Higher prevalence of eating disorders among adolescent elite athletes than controls. *Med Sci Sports Exerc.* 2013; 45: 1188–1197.
82. Martinsen M, Bahr R, Borresen R, Holme I, Pensgaard AM, Sundgot-Borgen J. Preventing eating disorders among young elite athletes: a randomized controlled trial. *Med Sci Sports Exerc.* 2014; 46: 435–447.
83. Hausenblas HA, Symons Downs D. Comparison of body image between athletes and nonathletes: A meta-analytic review. *J Appl Sport Psychol.* 2001; 13: 323–339.
84. Sundgot-Borgen J. Risk and trigger factors for the development of eating disorders in female elite athletes. *Med Sci Sports Exerc.* 1994; 26: 414–419.
85. Neumark-Sztainer D, Eisenberg ME. Body image concerns, muscle-enhancing behaviors, and eating disorders in males. *JAMA.* 2014; 312: 2156–2157.
86. Gleeson M, Bishop NC. Elite athlete immunology: importance of nutrition. *Int J Sports Med.* 2000; 21(Suppl 1): S44–S50.
87. Nieman DC. Immunonutrition support for athletes. *Nutr Rev.* 2008; 66: 310–320.
88. Campbell B, Kreider RB, Ziegenfuss T, *et al.* International Society of Sports Nutrition position stand: protein and exercise. *J Int Soc Sports Nutr.* 2007; 4: 1–7.
89. Burke LM, Deakin V (eds.) *Clinical sports nutrition*, 4th ed. North Ryde: McGraw-Hill; 2010.
90. Lukaski HC. Vitamin and mineral status: effects on physical performance. *Nutrition.* 2004; 20: 632–644.
91. De Souza MJ, Williams NI, Nattiv A, *et al.* Misunderstanding the female athlete triad: refuting the IOC consensus statement on Relative Energy Deficiency in Sport (RED-S). *Br J Sports Med.* 2014; 48: 1461–1465.
92. Rickenlund A, Eriksson MJ, Schenck-Gustafsson K, Hirschberg AL. Amenorrhea in female athletes is associated with endothelial dysfunction and unfavorable lipid profile. *J Clin Endocrinol Metab.* 2005; 90: 1354–1359.
93. Ihle R, Loucks AB. Dose-response relationships between energy availability and bone turnover in young exercising women. *J Bone Miner Res.* 2004; 19: 1231–1240.
94. Leib ES, Lewiecki EM, Binkley N, Hamdy RC, Official positions of the International Society for Clinical Densitometry. *J Clin Densitom.* 2004; 7: 1–6.
95. Barrack MT, Van Loan MD, Rauh MJ, Nichols JF. Body mass, training, menses, and bone in adolescent runners: a 3-yr follow-up. *Med Sci Sports Exerc.* 2011; 43: 959–966.
96. Castro J, Toro J, Lazaro L, Pons F, Halperin I. Bone mineral density in male adolescents with anorexia nervosa. *J Am Acad Child Adolesc Psychiatr.* 2002; 41: 613–618.
97. Hackney AC. Effects of endurance exercise on the reproductive system of men: the 'exercise-hypogonadal male condition'. *J Endocrinol Invest.* 2008; 31: 932–938.
98. Hind K, Truscott JG, Evans JA. Low lumbar spine bone mineral density in both male and female endurance runners. *Bone.* 2006; 39: 880–885.
99. Stewart AD, Hannan J. Total and regional bone density in male runners, cyclists, and controls. *Med Sci Sports Exerc.* 2000; 32: 1373–1377.
100. Weimann E, Witzel C, Schwidergall S, Bohles HJ. Peripubertal perturbations in elite gymnasts caused by sport specific training regimes and inadequate nutritional intake. *Int J Sports Med.* 2000; 21: 210–215.
101. Caine D, Lewis R, O'Connor P, Howe W, Bass S. Does gymnastics training inhibit growth of females? *Clin J Sport Med.* 2001; 11: 260–270.
102. Roemmich JN, Sinning WE. Weight loss and wrestling training: effects on growth-related hormones. *J Appl Physiol.* 1997; 82: 1760–1764.
103. Drinkwater BL, Nilson K, Ott S, Chesnut CH. Bone mineral density after resumption of menses in amenorrheic athletes. *JAMA.* 1986; 256: 380–382.
104. Carney CP, Andersen AE. Eating disorders. Guide to medical evaluation and complications. *Psychiatr Clin North Am.* 1996; 19: 657–679.
105. Pomeroy C, Mitchell JE. Medical issues in the eating disorders. In: Brownell K, Robin J, Wilmore JH (eds.) *Eating, body weight, and performance in athletes: disorders of modern society.* Philadelphia: Lea & Febiger; 1992. p. 202–221.
106. Oppliger RA, Case HS, Horswill CA, Landry GL, Shelter AC. American College of Sports Medicine position stand. Weight loss in wrestlers. *Med Sci Sports Exerc.* 1996; 28: ix-xii.
107. Tarnopolsky MA, Cipriano N, Woodcroft C, *et al.* Effects of rapid weight loss and wrestling on muscle glycogen concentration. *Clin J Sport Med.* 1996; 6: 78–84.
108. Viitasalo JT, Kyrolainen H, Bosco C, Alen M. Effects of rapid weight reduction on force production and vertical jumping height. *Int J Sports Med.* 1987; 8: 281–285.
109. Bonci CM, Bonci LJ, Granger LR, *et al.* National athletic trainers' association position statement: preventing, detecting, and managing disordered eating in athletes. *J Athl Train.* 2008; 43: 80–108.
110. Meyer NL, Sundgot-Borgen J, Lohman TG, *et al.* Body composition for health and performance: a survey of body composition assessment practice carried out by the Ad Hoc Research Working Group on Body Composition, Health and Performance under the auspices of the IOC Medical Commission. *Br J Sports Med.* 2013; 47: 1044–1053.
111. Sundgot-Borgen J, Meyer NL, Lohman TG, *et al.* How to minimise the health risks to athletes who compete in weight-sensitive sports review and position statement on behalf of the Ad Hoc Research Working Group on Body Composition, Health and Performance, under the auspices of the IOC Medical Commission. *Br J Sports Med.* 2013; 47: 1012–1022.
112. Thompson RA, Sherman, RT. *Eating disorders in sport.* New York: Routledge; 2010.
113. Beals KA. *Disordered eating among athletes: A comprehensive guide for health professionals.* Champaign, IL: Human Kinetics; 2004.
114. Sangenis P, Drinkwater B, Loucks A, Sherman R, Sundgot-Borgen J, Tompton R. *IOC Medical Commission Position Stand on The Female Athlete Triad.* Available at: http://www.femaleathletetriad.org/for-professionals/position-stands/#title3. 2005.
115. Becker CB, McDaniel L, Bull S, Powell M, McIntyre K. Can we reduce eating disorder risk factors in female college athletes? A randomized exploratory investigation of two peer-led interventions. *Body Image.* 2012; 9: 31–42.

116. Elliot DL, Goldberg L, Moe EL, Defrancesco CA, Durham MB, Hix-Small H. Preventing substance use and disordered eating: initial outcomes of the ATHENA (athletes targeting healthy exercise and nutrition alternatives) program. *Arch Pediatr Adolesc Med.* 2004; 158: 1043–1049.
117. Bandura A. *Social foundations of thought and action—A social cognitive theory.* Englewood Cliffs, NJ: Prentice-Hall; 1986.
118. Petty R, Cacioppo JT. *Communication and persuasion: central and peripheral routes to attitude change.* New York: Springer-Verlag; 1986.
119. Festinger L. *A theory of cognitive dissonance.* Stanford: Stanford University Press; 1957.
120. Nowicka P, Eli K, Ng J, Apitzsch E, Sundgot-Borgen J. Moving from knowledge to action: A qualitative study of elite coaches' capacity for early intervention in cases of eating disorders. *Int J Sports Sci Coach.* 2013; 8: 343–356.
121. Sundgot-Borgen J. Eating disorders, energy intake, training volume, and menstrual function in high-level modern rhythmic gymnasts. *Int J Sport Nutr.* 1996; 6: 100–109.
122. Fairburn CG, Harrison PJ. Eating disorders. *Lancet.* 2003; 361(9355): 407–416.
123. Arthur-Cameselle JN, Quatromoni PA. Eating disorders in collegiate female athletes: factors that assist recovery. *Eat Disord.* 2014; 22: 50–61.
124. Dueck CA, Matt KS, Manore MM, Skinner JS. Treatment of athletic amenorrhea with a diet and training intervention program. *Int J Sport Nutr.* 1996; 6: 24–40.
125. Guebels C, Cialdella-Kam L, Maddalozzo G, Manore MM. *REMEDY: Menstrual Status and Energy Availability in Active Women.* American College of Sports Medicine (ACSM) Annual Meeting, Denver, CO: 2011.
126. Kopp-Woodroffe SA, Manore MM, Dueck CA, Skinner JS, Matt KS. Energy and nutrient status of amenorrheic athletes participating in a diet and exercise training intervention program. *Int J Sport Nutr.* 1999; 9: 70–88.
127. Lock J, le Grange D, Forsberg S, Hewell K. Is family therapy useful for treating children with anorexia nervosa? Results of a case series. *J Am Acad Child Adolesc Psychiatr.* 2006; 45: 1323–1328.
128. Denhoff ER, Milliren CE, de Ferranti SD, Steltz SK, Osganian SK. Factors associated with clinical research recruitment in a pediatric academic medical center–a web-based survey. *PLOS One.* 2015; 10: e0140768.
129. National Health and Medical Research Council. *Nutrient reference values for Australia and New Zealand 2015* [20.11.2015]. Available from: https://www.nrv.gov.au/nutrients.
130. McGuire S. *US Department of Agriculture and US Department of Health and Human Services, dietary guidelines for Americans, 2010,* 7th ed. *Adv Nutr.* 2011; 2: 293–294.
131. European Food Safety Authority. Scientific opinion on dietary reference values for calcium. EFSA Panel on dietetic products, nutrition and allergies (NDA). *EFSA Journal.* 2015; 13: 1–82.
132. Norwegian Directory of Health. *Recommendations on diet, nutrition and physical activity.* Norwegian Directory of Health. [20.11.2015]. Available from: https://helsedirektoratet.no/Lists/Publikasjoner/Attachments/806/Anbefalinger-om-kosthold-ernering-og-fysisk-aktivitet-IS-2170.pdf.
133. Dietary reference values for food energy and nutrients for the United Kingdom. Report of the panel on dietary reference values of the Committee on Medical Aspects of Food Policy. *Rep Health Soc Subj (Lond).* 1991; 41: 1–210.

CHAPTER 48

Dietary supplements

Ronald J Maughan and Susan M Shirreffs

Introduction

In considering the use of dietary supplements by young athletes, account must be taken of the various factors that are unique to this population, and the differences between the child athlete and the mature adult athlete must be recognized. The spectrum of age and of physical, mental, and emotional development, as well as the diverse training and competition demands that apply to this group, also make generalizations difficult. Some children compete, and indeed compete with distinction, in sport at senior international level, while the majority lack the will and the physical attributes necessary for training and competition at this level. Younger children are very much reliant on others, whether parents or coaches, for most decision making, while many, but not all, beyond their mid-teens function autonomously. This applies very much in the case of supplements where decisions to use, and therefore to purchase, are contingent on access to the necessary financial resources.

Before discussing the use of supplements, it is important to define what is meant by the term 'dietary supplements' and to agree on what is included in this category and what is excluded. Various attempts have been made to define supplements and to establish what should, or should not, be included in this category. Such definitions are essential if we are to ensure that everyone refers to the same thing when discussing supplements, but there is no universal agreement. Comparing surveys of the prevalence of use is therefore problematic when the entities included or excluded have not been clearly defined. Some would include sports drinks, gels, energy bars, and herbal products as supplements, while others would exclude them. Such distinctions make an enormous difference to the interpretation of the prevalence statistics. Even the terminology can be confusing, with no clear appreciation of the implicit distinction between a dietary supplement and a nutritional supplement. The latter might be presumed to have some nutritional value, while the former may be anything added to the diet. The recent growth in awareness and consumption of functional foods has further confused the issue, with some specific foods being consumed to provide nutrients that would previously have been consumed in the form of supplements. Fortified foods might also be included in the same category, being consumed to add specific nutrients to the diet rather than for the other properties of the food.

Attempts to define supplements for legal or regulatory purposes have been no more successful and some such attempts have simply added further confusion. For example, according to the Dietary Supplements Health and Education Act 1994 (DSHEA) passed by the US Congress, a dietary supplement is 'a product, other than tobacco, which is used in conjunction with a healthy diet and contains one or more of the following dietary ingredients: a vitamin, mineral, herb or other botanical, an amino acid, a dietary substance for use by man to supplement the diet by increasing the total daily intake, or a concentrate, metabolite, constituent, extract, or combinations of these ingredients'. To define a supplement based on whether the diet of the consumer is deemed to be healthy or otherwise seems both futile and foolish.

Prevalence of supplement use

The use of dietary supplements is embedded deeply in modern sport at all levels of participation. This reflects in part the drive of those who engage in sport to reach their goals, but must also be seen in the context of the widespread use of supplements in the general population. Comparison between surveys is not straightforward. As well as differences in the categorization of supplements, some ask about lifetime history of use, while others ask about regular use or, more specifically, about use in the last week or month. Bailey *et al.*[1] reported the results of a survey of dietary supplement use based on the US National Health and Nutrition Examination Survey (NHANES) data for the period 2003–2006. Supplement use was measured through a questionnaire and about half of the US population (44% of males, 53% of females) reported the use of one or more supplements in the preceding month. Among children and adolescents, the estimated prevalence of use was lower, but was about 30–40% across all ages up to 18 years (Table 48.1). Another survey of 1280 US adolescents aged 14–19 years found that 79% of the sample had used complementary or alternative medicine products in their lifetime (49% in the previous month) and that 46% had used dietary supplements in their lifetime (29% in the previous month)[2].

Chen *et al.*[3] surveyed Chinese mothers with children under 5 years of age in Perth, Western Australia (n = 237) and in Chengdu and Wuhan, China (n = 2079): 23% and 32% of the Chinese children were taking dietary supplements in Australia and China, respectively. Other surveys[4,5] produce similar results, confirming that supplement use in children is universal and common.

Based on the NHANES survey of 2007–2010, Bailey *et al.*[6] reported that dietary supplements were used by 31% of children aged up to 19 years, and the reasons given for supplement use included to 'improve overall health' (41%), to 'maintain health' (37%), for 'supplementing the diet' (23%), to 'prevent health problems' (20%), and to 'boost immunity' (14%). From the same survey, it was reported, perhaps not surprisingly, that parents who use dietary supplements are more likely to have children who use them.[7] Against this background of widespread supplement use, it should be noted that an analysis of 9417 records from the US National Health Interview Survey (NHIS) 2007 data set suggested that less

Table 48.1 Prevalence of dietary supplement use in the past month among the US population aged ≥1 year by age

n	Age (y)	Any supplement (%)	MVMM*	Botanical
18,758	All ≥ 1	49 ± 0.9	33 ± 1	14 ± 1
1781	1–3	39 ± 1	26 ± 2	2 ± 0
1975	4–8	43 ± 2	32 ± 2	4 ± 1
2233	9–13	29 ± 2	20 ± 1	3 ± 1
2812	14–18	26 ± 2	16 ± 1	5 ± 1

*MVMM: multi-vitamin, multi-mineral supplement.

Data from the National Health and Nutrition Examination Survey (NHANES) survey 2003–2006 (Bailey RL, Gahche JJ, Lentino CV, et al. Dietary Supplement Use in the United States, 2003–2006. J Nutr. 2011; 141: 261–266.)

Table 48.2 Prevalence of supplement use among various groups of young athletes

Age	n	% users	Sample	Reference
11–13 years	110	97	Canada, multi-sport	Wiens *et al.*[10]
10–14 years	36	75	Germany, multi-sport	Braun *et al.*[11]
14–16 years	302	98	Canada, multi-sport	Wiens *et al.*[10]
15–16 years	62	75	Germany, multi-sport	Braun *et al.*[11]
<16 years	198	42	South Africa, Rugby	Duvenage *et al.*[12]
17–18 years	91	99	Canada, multi-sport	Wiens *et al.*[10]
17–18 years	32	75	Germany, multi-sport	Braun *et al.*[11]
<18 years	75	67	Japan, Youth Olympics team	Sato *et al.*[55]
18 years	32	62	UK, National track and field	Nieper[56]
19–25 years	34	98	Germany, multi-sport	Braun *et al.*[11]

than 2% of the US general population aged younger than 18 years were using supplements with the specific aim of enhancing sports performance.[8] Although this fraction seems small, it represents about 1.2 million individual children.

The previously cited reports relate to surveys of the general population, but there are numerous reports on the prevalence of supplement use among young athletes. The older literature has been reviewed and summarized by McDowall.[5] Comparisons between surveys are difficult due to differences in definitions of supplements, in study populations, in what constitutes a 'user' of supplements, and in sampling methodologies. Nevertheless, it is apparent that use is widespread: based on data from 7 different surveys, McDowall[5] reported a prevalence of use that varied from 22% to 71%. It is clear also that the prevalence and patterns of use vary between boys and girls, though not all surveys show consistent results. One study of US high-school athletes found that more boys (21%) than girls (3%) had used creatine.[9]

Some more recent surveys have reported almost universal use of supplements: Wiens *et al.*[10] found that 97–99% of young Canadian athletes from various sports were supplement users. Among elite young German athletes, Braun *et al.*[11] reported a prevalence of supplement use of about 75% in athletes aged from <15 up to 18 years, but among athletes aged 18–25 years, usage was close to 100%. Others, however, have reported findings that are more consistent with the picture revealed by McDowall.[5] Duvenage *et al.*[12] reported that 42% of young (under 16 years) male South African rugby players reported using at least one supplement. Other surveys from South African rugby players showed that 54–56% of rugby-playing school boys aged under 17 years and including under-13 s reported some form of supplement use[12]. Because of the differences between surveys, however, it is not possible to form a clear picture of whether the prevalence of supplement use has changed over time. Some of the available data are summarized in Table 48.2.

Ethical issues in supplement use

It is well recognized that decisions relating to supplement use among athletes are strongly influenced by the behaviours of peer athletes—especially the most successful ones—and by advice from those in positions of authority, including a parent and/or coach.[12] The child athlete is unlikely to make a spontaneous decision to use supplements. Whether overt or subtle, pressure from those in authority is likely to be the deciding factor. It is therefore important that these individuals recognize the potential for harm as well as for good, and consider carefully the balance between risks and benefits before recommending supplement use. As highlighted elsewhere, the evidence to allow a comprehensive risk-benefit analysis is lacking, but the possibility of harm to health must weigh heavily in any analysis. It should be stressed that most supplements are probably completely safe, but it is equally true that most have not been evaluated in children, nor at the high doses or in the combinations that are often used by athletes. It may be deemed irresponsible to recommend supplement use to children who are not in a position to evaluate the risk. Several organizations have published position statements.

Although it is common practice among sports dieticians and nutritionists to suggest that supplements should not be recommended to athletes aged younger than 18 years of age, this generalization fails to take account of individual differences in biological maturity. The use of a chronological age cut off is therefore somewhat arbitrary in biological terms, but the difficulties in assessing biological maturity prevent any other option. There are also, in many countries, legal issues relating to the age of consent that must be taken into consideration when advising young athletes.

Exceptions to the 'food first' approach may occur in a few—very few—specific situations. Where a diagnosed deficiency cannot be corrected promptly and effectively by implementation of an appropriate eating strategy, short-term use of supplements may be warranted. Such a situation may, for example, arise in the case of a diagnosed iron-deficiency anaemia. While this should be amenable to resolution by dietary change, this takes time and a supplement may be useful in the interim. In the case of athletes who follow a very restricted diet, either in the variety of foods they choose or in the amounts of food consumed, a low-dose, broad spectrum multivitamin, multi-mineral supplement (sourced from a reputable supplier) is likely to do more good than harm. This should not replace efforts to encourage good eating habits, but should be recognized as a reasonable precaution.

Supplements in a balanced diet

Athletes often cite the need to ensure an adequate intake of all essential nutrients as a reason for taking vitamin and mineral supplements. Several investigations, however, have found that users of micronutrient supplements generally have better nutrient intakes from food than those who do not use supplements.[13–15] In other words, those most in need of supplementation are less likely to take supplements, while those with least need for them are most likely to use them. If this is indeed true, it diminishes one of the most commonly cited reasons for supplement use, i.e. to compensate for dietary inadequacies or to ensure an adequate intake of specific nutrients.

With the recent increase in concerns over food allergies in children, the implications of the removal of some foods or food groups from the diet has raised concerns over the ability of the remaining foods to ensure an adequate intake of all essential nutrients. Foods that are eliminated from the diet often include milk, eggs, soya, wheat products, fish, and nuts, all of which would normally be expected to make significant contributions to dietary vitamin and mineral intake.[16] Low micronutrient intakes as a result of a dietary elimination have been reported in food allergic children, and sustained low intakes will increase the risk of vitamin and mineral deficiency and of the associated impairment of function and risk of illness.[17] This is not to suggest that routine supplementation with these nutrients is warranted, but it does suggest a need for thought before excluding any foods or food groups from the diet. Perry and Pesek[18] reported that, while the true prevalence of food allergy is unknown, up to 25% of the general population believes that they may be allergic to some food. However, the actual prevalence of food allergy diagnosed using appropriate procedures appears to be 1.5 to 2% of the adult population and approximately 6 to 8% of children. Thus, while small, the prevalence is not negligible, and the concern must be that only those who need to eliminate foods from the diet should do so.

The adequacy of the diet, in terms of meeting needs for all essential nutrients is defined by two main factors: the choice of foods and the amount of those foods eaten. The athlete who trains hard and who eats sufficient food to meet the energy demands of training should have a considerably higher intake of protein, vitamins, minerals, and other essential food components than his or her sedentary counterparts. Requirements for some nutrients will be increased by training, but this increase is generally less than the increase in energy demand. It should be recognized, though, that not all athletes have a high energy demand at all times of the training-competition cycle and not all consume a varied diet. Supplementation should not be seen as a compensation for poor dietary choices, though it is often perceived in that way by young athletes. In the surveys reported by Duvenage *et al.*[12] about 40–50% of respondents rated their diet as 'poor or very poor'. The first solution implemented ought to be better food choices rather than supplement use. Educating young athletes about appropriate food choices should take priority in this situation.

Assessing nutrient intake and status

There is an extensive published literature on the nutrient intakes of adults and children and the results of these dietary surveys are often used as evidence of inadequate dietary intakes of various nutrients in substantial fractions of the population under investigation. The inevitable, though often unspoken, conclusion of many of these reports is that supplementation is necessary to ensure an adequate intake of all essential nutrients. These reports are typified by that of Kaganov *et al.*[19], who reported that, 'The proportion of children living in Europe whose intake of at least some vitamins and trace elements are at or below the estimated average requirements is substantial'.[19(p3524)] They continued to say that, 'The most common deficiencies across age groups included vitamin D, vitamin E, and iodine'.[19(p3524)] This fails to understand the derivation and meaning of estimated average requirements and fails to recognize that a nutrient deficiency cannot be identified on the basis of an estimate of intake alone. The estimated average requirement (EAR) is set at a level that should meet the needs of half of the population: for half of the population, an intake of less than the EAR may still be sufficient to meet their needs. The obvious difficulty, of course, is that we do not know which half! Notwithstanding the fact that the lower an individual's intake of any specific nutrient, the greater the risk that the intake is insufficient, a dietary deficiency cannot be diagnosed on the basis of intake, and care needs to be taken when interpreting survey data.[20]

Supplements and health

Macronutrients

An adequate energy intake is necessary for growth, for activities of daily living and, for athletes, to sustain the daily training load. All athletes require that the residual energy in the diet, after meeting the energy demands of training or competition, is sufficient to meet the energy demands of all other activities. While an adequate level of energy availability for these activities has been discussed at length for adult female athletes,[21] there is limited information relating specifically to young athletes of either sex. In addition to total energy intake, however, the amounts of protein and carbohydrate are important, and while the main function of fat is to provide a compact source of energy in the diet, an adequate intake of essential fatty acids is important. The proportions of fat and carbohydrate in an energy-sufficient diet will also affect muscle substrate use at rest and during exercise, which has implications for exercise performance.[22] There are numerous studies on the effects of variations in dietary fat and carbohydrate intake on performance and on the adaptations that occur in response to training.[23] For obvious reasons, the overwhelming majority of these studies, especially those that require invasive measurements, have been carried out in adults. The metabolic response of young children to exercise is different from that of adults, but the same general principles apply. Therefore, it seems sensible to ensure that the diet contains adequate amounts of carbohydrate, especially during periods of intensive training or around competitions where carbohydrate availability might be a limiting factor. This can be achieved easily from normal foods without recourse to specific sport or other carbohydrate-containing supplements.

Recommended protein intakes for children, when expressed relative to body mass, are generally slightly higher than those for adults in order to ensure the availability of sufficient amino acids for growth. These recommendations also vary from country to country, reinforcing the idea that they are no more than approximations, and that they should not be taken as absolute guidelines. Australian recommendations for children are shown in Table 48.3.[24]

Young athletes who eat sufficient healthful food to meet the energy demands of training are very unlikely to fail to consume sufficient protein. It is increasingly recognized, though, that the distribution of protein intake over the day may be particularly important when there is a need to maintain a positive nitrogen balance.[25]

Table 48.3 Protein intake Estimated Average Requirement (EAR) and Recommended Dietary Intake (RDI) for children and adolescents.

Age	EAR	RDI
All		
1–3 y	12 g·day^{-1} (0.92 g·kg^{-1})	14 g·day^{-1} (1.08 g·kg^{-1})
4–8 y	16 g·day^{-1} (0.73 g·kg^{-1})	20 g·day^{-1} (0.91 g·kg^{-1})
Boys		
9–13 y	31 g·day^{-1} (0.78 g·kg^{-1})	40 g·day^{-1} (0.94 g·kg^{-1})
14–18 y	49 g·day^{-1} (0.76 g·kg^{-1})	65 g·day^{-1} (0.99 g·kg^{-1})
Girls		
9–13 y	24 g·day^{-1} (0.61 g·kg^{-1})	35 g·day^{-1} (0.87 g·kg^{-1})
14–18 y	35 g·day^{-1} (0.62 g·kg^{-1})	45 g·day^{-1} (0.77 g·kg^{-1})
Adult men		
19–70 y	52 g·day^{-1} (0.68 g·kg^{-1})	64 g·day^{-1} (0.84 g·kg^{-1})
Adult women		
19–70 y	37 g·day^{-1} (0.60 g·kg^{-1})	46 g·day^{-1} (0.75 g·kg^{-1})

Data from Australian Government Ministry of Health. Nutrient Reference Values for Australia and New Zealand: Protein. Available at: https://www.nrv.gov.au/nutrients/protein Accessed 15 December 2015.

Many children eat their evening meal relatively early and a long time may elapse until the next meal: breakfast often contains relatively little protein, so the elapsed time between successive protein intakes may approach 18 h (if dinner is consumed at 18.00 h and lunch at noon the next day).

Vitamins and minerals

As with macronutrient intakes, various recommendations are published for vitamin and mineral intakes for children. Data are lacking regarding specific different requirements in the child athlete compared to the general population. Nevertheless, there is no evidence that deficiencies are common in young athletes, or at least not more common than in the general population. Where health and performance are at stake, however, the temptation exists to assume that routine supplementation may prevent any deficiency symptoms. This should not be necessary for young athletes who eat a varied diet, and food is the preferred source of all essential nutrients. It is important to note that there may be situations where supplementation of iron and calcium/vitamin D may be warranted.

Iron

Iron-deficiency anaemia is the most common and widespread nutrient deficiency in the general population and affects adults, children, athletes, and non-athletes, with about 3% of the population affected.[26] It must be recognized, though, that iron plays many important biological roles other than its central role in oxygen transport, and modest depletion of iron stores may be a concern for the athlete even though it is without effect on the non-athlete.[27] High iron losses and impaired absorption, rather than an inadequate dietary intake, must also be considered as possible factors contributing to poor iron status. It has recently been reported that iron deficiency is a common finding in young women with heavy menstrual bleeding and that this is accompanied by symptoms of fatigue.[28] Sandstrom *et al.*,[29] however, reported that the prevalence of iron deficiency and iron-deficiency anaemia was similar in adolescent female athletes and non-athletes: this finding was despite factors that should favour a better iron status in the athlete group, such as higher iron intake and less menstrual bleeding. Notwithstanding the widespread concern over iron status, supplementation should be considered only if impaired status is diagnosed and if an effective food-based solution cannot be implemented.

Calcium and vitamin D

The key roles of calcium and vitamin D, which promote intestinal calcium absorption and regulate calcium metabolism in bone, muscle, and other tissues, are widely recognized. Bone growth and remodelling occur at high rates during the early adolescent years and are also stimulated by any exercise that imposes stress on the skeleton.[30] There is evidence from dietary surveys and from assessments of bone mineral content that calcium intake of many adolescent athletes is less than the recommended amount and that bone health may be compromised at this crucial stage of development.[31] This is perhaps because of the avoidance of dairy produce in this population, and should be addressed by an appropriate education programme to identify good food sources of calcium and encouragement to consume these products. In recent years, the focus of much research on Vitamin D in athletes has been on its roles in maintaining muscle function, and it has been suggested that supplementation may enhance performance, especially in athletes who train indoors or who may be exposed to little sunshine. It has been hypothesized that vitamin D insufficiency in athletes might negatively affect sport performance. A recent placebo-controlled study of the effect of vitamin D-3 supplementation on performance in adolescent swimmers who had been diagnosed to be suffering from vitamin D insufficiency[32] concluded that Vitamin D-3 supplementation was effective in raising the serum 25(OH)D concentrations, but had no effect on physical performance. Nevertheless, a review of the evidence by Sports Medicine Australia concluded that, 'Correction of any vitamin D deficiency or insufficiency through supplementation may be necessary to ensure optimal performance and bone health in adolescent athletes'.[31(p578)] As always, this should be an informed decision that takes account of the individual circumstances.

Supplements and performance

It is important to recognize that the available information relating to the efficacy of most dietary supplements is severely limited. There are a few supplements for which there is some evidence of efficacy, and for which the risks of adverse effects are sufficiently low that their use may be warranted in specific situations. This evidence, however, is derived almost entirely from adults. In large part this is because of the additional ethical considerations that apply when conducting research on children. It is also the case that most of the available evidence on efficacy is derived not from athletes but from recreationally active individuals. It might be argued that these individuals more closely represent child athletes in terms of their training loads and competition level than would a population of elite athletes, but nonetheless the distinction should be recognized. It is important to consider the implications for the translation of that research to young athletes. A further qualification is that most well-controlled investigations have used laboratory tests that may be said to resemble sporting events, but most often do not.

Assessing performance and supplement effects

Assessing performance using laboratory simulations may appear rather straightforward, at least for simple tasks such as cycling, running, or weightlifting. This is not the case,[33] because even with stringent standardization of prior diet, exercise, and lifestyle factors, and with careful control of test conditions in the laboratory, some residual variability in performance remains. This variability is large relative to the margin between success and failure in competitive sport. This means that performance effects meaningful to the athlete are difficult to identify, even with a relatively large study population. Small effects within the day-to-day variability will appear as no effect, leading to the conclusion that the *absence* of evidence of efficacy in the case of most supplements cannot be taken to be evidence of absence of efficacy.

In the case of outcomes where the end point is less well-defined, as in maintenance of a healthy immune system, repair to muscle after injury, and modulation of physique, it is unrealistic to expect clear evidence, even with the investment of much time and money.[33] A 2-year publicly-funded (at a cost of over US $12.5 million) investigation of the effects of glucosamine and chondroitin on knee pain (the GAIT study) concluded that, for the overall group of 1583 patients in the GAIT study neither glucosamine nor chondroitin sulphate, either individually or in combination, was effective in reducing pain.[34] Because the outcome may prove to be unfavourable, it is seldom in the interest of supplement manufacturers to make such an investment, so the absence of information is not surprising.

Supplements that may benefit performance

There is evidence that the use of some supplements can improve some aspects of performance in some individuals, and this has often led to ill-informed decisions regarding the use of these purported ergogenic aids.[35] Substances for which there is some positive evidence include:

Protein	Creatine
Caffeine	Alkalinizing and buffering agents
Nitrate	Carnitine

This is a short list from the many thousands of supplements on sale to athletes. The effects, both positive and negative, of these and other supplements have been extensively reviewed elsewhere and will not be reviewed in detail here. What will be emphasized is that even in the case of supplements where there is strong evidence for a performance benefit, such as creatine, there may be no benefit if:

- The exercise task is one where supplementation will have no effect on the factors that limit performance.
- Status is not affected by supplementation. This may be the case for an individual whose biological stores are at a maximum before supplementation, or if the dose is too small or the supplementation period is too short.
- The product used does not contain the active ingredient.

It is also the case that not everyone responds positively, even when there is a statistically significant benefit in the test group. This has led to suggestions that there may be 'responders' and 'non-responders' in any given group. This may, of course, just be random variation and repeated exposure is required to be sure that an athlete does or does not respond.

Risks of supplement use

Quality assurance issues in the supplement industry

The regulation of the food and dietary supplement industries varies greatly between countries, but athletes today travel extensively and the Internet has removed many of the national barriers that formerly existed regarding buying and selling. Consumers are therefore faced with an uncertain situation, and may find that the products they purchase and consume do not meet their expectations. Dietary supplements on sale in the US are not subject to premarket review for safety or efficacy by the Food and Drug Administration (FDA) unless they contain new dietary ingredients. Manufacturers are not required to secure FDA approval before producing or selling dietary supplements, thus limiting the checks on products that are offered for sale to the general public. Similar regulation (or lack thereof) applies in most countries, though local regulations do vary and some products that are classified as medicines in one country are classified as a dietary supplement in another country. Elite athletes, even those competing at junior level, are regular international travellers, whether for training camps or for competition, and many are well aware of the opportunities to purchase supplements that are not legally available in their home countries. Internet buying and selling has also eliminated many of the limitations on the supplements that an athlete can obtain and has removed most of the checks on the quality of supplements that are on sale by preventing opportunities for inspection of manufacturing, packaging, and storage premises.

Because dietary supplements are classified as foods rather than as drugs, the legal requirements that govern their production and distribution are less strict, and are less strictly enforced, than those related to pharmaceuticals. Government food inspectors publish regular reports of breaches of food safety regulations, often covering issues such as the presence of undeclared allergens, bacterial and fungal organisms, foreign objects (glass, metal, etc.), heavy metals, and other potentially hazardous substances. The websites of the US FDA and the UK Food Standards Agency (FSA) contain daily notices of food product recalls because of manufacturing issues. In a 14-day period in January 2013, the FDA issued recall notices for food products because of undeclared milk (two products from different companies), peanuts, and eggs, the presence of metal fragments (two products from different companies), and the presence of listeria (two products from different companies) and *E. coli*.[36] In the corresponding period, the UK Food Standards Agency notified recalls of products because of the presence of salmonella and *B. cereus* and because of inspections that revealed poor standards of hygiene in two separate factory premises[37].

It is not unusual to find cases of poor hygiene in the manufacture, storage, and provision of foodstuffs to the general public, so it should not be surprising that some dietary supplement manufacturers fail to follow good manufacturing practice. A 2012 report by the FDA revealed that violations of manufacturing rules were found in half of the nearly 450 dietary supplement firms it had inspected in the previous 4 years. In 2012, FDA inspectors found violations of good manufacturing practices during two-thirds of the 204 inspections they conducted in nearly 200 supplement firms' facilities, with 70 of these inspections resulting in the agency's most serious rating. Some supplement products have been shown to contain impurities (lead, broken glass, animal faeces, etc.) because of poor quality control during manufacture or storage. The risk of gastrointestinal upset because of poor hygiene during the production and storage of products is a concern to athletes. At best, this may be nothing more than a minor inconvenience, but it may cause the athlete to miss a crucial competition.

This same lax approach to quality assurance can lead to large variations in the content of the active ingredients in supplements. Some investigations have shown that some products do not contain any measurable amount of the substances identified on the label, while others may contain up to 150% of the stated dose.[38,39] Where relatively expensive ingredients are involved, it seems that some products contain little or none of these ingredients.[40] The consumer, of course, has no way of knowing this. In a survey of the caffeine content of supplements on sale in military bases, Cohen *et al.*[41] analysed the caffeine content of 31 products that are known to have added caffeine or herbal ingredients that naturally contain caffeine. Eleven of the supplements listed herbal ingredients: these products had no caffeine or only trace levels. Nine of the other 20 products had labels with accurate caffeine information. Another five had varying caffeine contents that were either much lower or higher than the amount listed on the label. The remaining six products did not have caffeine levels on their labels, but each of these had a high caffeine content of between 210 and 310 mg per serving. For the athlete who plans to use caffeine as part of a competition strategy, this variability is rather alarming.

A recent analysis of commercially available herbal products used deoxyribonucleic acid (DNA) analysis to assess the identity of herbal species present in those products.[42] More than half (59%) of the herbal products tested contained species of plants that were not listed on the label, and one-third (33%) of the authenticated herbal products also contained contaminants and/or fillers not listed on the label. They also found that several products contained materials from plants that are known to be toxic, to have adverse side effects, and/or to interact negatively with other herbs, supplements, or medications. This is clearly a public health issue rather than a specific problem for athletes, but all consumers are at risk of adverse reactions.

Adverse health effects

Most commonly consumed supplements have little effect on the consumer, whether positive or negative, but the potential for dietary supplements to adversely affect health is widely recognized. In some cases, this may be the result of toxic effects of the active ingredients, in some the result of an interaction between the ingredients and other supplements or drugs that are co-ingested, and in other cases this may be the result of the presence of undeclared ingredients that are known to be harmful.[43]

Where products are effective, it is likely that there is some risk of adverse outcomes as well as some possible benefit. Methylhexanamine, commonly known as 1,3-dimethylamylamine or DMAA, is a stimulant that has been marketed as the primary active ingredient of many popular dietary supplements, with claims that it can promote fat loss and increase energy levels during exercise. Both of these claims are attractive to many athletes, and perhaps especially to young athletes at a time when they experience the body composition changes that are normally associated with adolescence. The widespread use of methylhexanamine has attracted the attention of the regulatory authorities and it is now classified as a medicine in many, but not all, countries. Methylhexanamine has been linked in the popular media to a number of adverse events, including the deaths during military training of two soldiers who suffered fatal heart attacks during training in 2010.[44] A female marathon runner who collapsed and died near the finish of the 2012 London Marathon had been consuming a commercially available product during the race and the coroner's investigation concluded that it had likely contributed to her death.[45]

Elsewhere, there is growing evidence of adverse health effects resulting from inappropriate supplement use and in most cases these reports identify the presence of undeclared ingredients as the primary cause of harm. Several reports have documented cases of serious adverse effects on health resulting from the use of dietary supplements containing undeclared anabolic steroids. So it is clear that some products on the market remain unsafe.[46] A recent survey of liver injuries in hospital patients implicated the use of bodybuilding supplements as the most common cause of liver injury.[47] Using data from the Drug-Induced Liver Injury Network (DILIN), which was established in 2003 by the National Institute of Diabetes and Digestive and Kidney Diseases to collect and analyse cases, it was found that in the period from September 2004 to March 2013, 845 cases of liver injury were thought to be either 'definitely', 'highly likely', or 'probably' from an herbal or dietary supplement, or from the use of prescription drugs. In 2004–2005, 7% of all liver injuries were attributed to herbal and dietary supplements, but this figure increased to 20% in 2010–2012. Although the steroid prohormone 3β-hydroxy-5α-androst-1-en-17-one is classified as a prohibited substance by the World Anti-Doping Agency (WADA), it is marked as a supplement and is available without prescription in some parts of the world. A recent report shows that even a short period of use of this supplement in healthy resistance-trained men enhances resistance training gains relative to placebo, which inevitably makes it attractive to athletes; however, there was also clear evidence that markers of cardiovascular health and liver function were compromised.[48]

In a review of adverse events associated with the use of ephedra-containing supplements, Haller *et al.*[49] identified 140 adverse events that were reported to the FDA in the space of only 3 years (1997 to 1999): ten of these cases related to individuals who were younger than 18 years, and there were ten deaths and 13 cases of permanent disability.

The message from the accumulated evidence is clear that supplement use carries some risk, and that the risk cannot be readily quantified. No matter how small, the possibility of serious adverse health effects must weigh very heavily in any cost-benefit analysis, and particularly so in the case of young athletes. The fact that the consequences may not be apparent for months or even years, and that they may be irreversible, suggests very strongly that this is too high of a price to pay.

Positive doping outcomes for athletes

Athletes who are liable to testing for the use of drugs that are prohibited in sport—and those who advise these athletes—should be aware of the possibility that some supplements have been found to contain substances that will cause a positive doping test.[50] Only a very small number of individuals are tested for evidence of the use of doping agents, but these are invariably the most successful performers. For these athletes, a failed drugs test may mean the loss of medals won or records set, as well as temporary suspension from competition. It also leads to damage to the athlete's reputation and perhaps to permanent loss of employment and income.

For the young athlete, it may adversely affect a career before it has really begun.

Where there has been deliberate cheating, such penalties seem entirely appropriate, but it is undoubtedly true that some failed doping tests can be attributed to the innocent ingestion of dietary supplements. The strict liability principle that is applied by the WADA is based on the recognition that it is not always possible to distinguish between deliberate cheating and inadvertent doping, so athletes must accept personal responsibility for all supplements (and medications) that they use. Where the athlete can establish that a positive test was the result of inadvertent ingestion rather than deliberate doping, there may be some relaxation of the sanctions imposed, but the athlete will still be guilty of a doping offence.

Numerous published studies show that contamination of dietary supplements with prohibited substances is not uncommon.[43,46,48–50] A wide range of stimulants, steroids, anorectic drugs, and other agents that are included on the WADA prohibited list have been identified in otherwise innocuous supplements. These instances are quite distinct from the legitimate sale of some of these substances, as their presence is not declared on the product label: in some cases, these adulterated products are even labelled as being safe for use by athletes. In some, but not all, cases, the extraneous additions have actions that are linked to the intended use of the product. Thus, anabolic agents have been found in supplements sold as muscle growth promoters, stimulants in herbal tonics, and anorectic agents in herbal weight-loss supplements. These observations suggest that this is either a deliberate act to add active ingredients to otherwise ineffective products, or that the manufacturers have allowed some mixing of separate products at the manufacturing facility. This might occur in the preparation of the raw ingredients or in the formulation of the finished product. In some cases, the amount of supplement present may be high, even higher than the normal therapeutic dose. Geyer *et al.*[51] purchased a body-building supplement in England and upon analysis found it to contain methandieneone (commonly known as Dianabol) in an amount substantially higher than the therapeutic dose. This drug was present in amounts high enough to have a substantial and obvious anabolic effect, but high enough to also produce serious side effects, including liver toxicity and carcinogenicity. Unlike many of the earlier cases involving cases of steroids related to nandrolone and testosterone, these are not trivial levels of contamination. This raises the probability of deliberate adulteration of the product with the intention of producing a measurable effect on muscle strength and muscle mass.[52] The prospect of adverse health effects at these high doses also raises real concerns.

In many cases, though, the amounts of prohibited substances found in supplements are far too small to have any physiological effect but may be sufficient to result in a positive doping outcome.[53] In these cases, the athlete risks a severe penalty with no prospect of any benefit.

Conclusions

The use of dietary supplements does not compensate for poor food choices and an inadequate diet, but supplements that provide essential nutrients may be a short-term option when food intake or food choices are restricted due to travel or other factors. Of the many different dietary ergogenic aids available to athletes, a very small number may enhance performance for some athletes when used in accordance with current evidence under the guidance of a well-informed professional. Athletes contemplating the use of supplements and sports foods should consider their efficacy, their cost, the risk to health and performance, and the potential for a positive doping test.

The problems that may result from ill-informed or unrestrained use of supplements by young athletes are increasingly recognized and the decision by some responsible authorities to address these issues is welcome (e.g. the South African Institute for Drug Free Sport[54]).

Summary

- The oral consumption of nutrition/dietary supplements is widespread in the general population and among sports people. This is true for children as well as adults.
- Despite this, there is very little research on any aspect of dietary supplement consumption in child/youth athletes. Translation of information from adult populations must be undertaken with caution.
- Ethical considerations around the use of dietary supplements by child athletes are the same as those for the adult population, but with the additional aspect of consideration of effects on growth and development.
- It is likely that only a very small number of dietary supplements will have a beneficial effect on performance for child athletes who have no underlying nutritional deficiencies.
- Some supplements are known to be harmful and carry a risk of serious adverse health effects as well as the possibility of a failed doping test.

References

1. Bailey RL, Gahche JJ, Lentino CV, *et al.* Dietary supplement use in the United States, 2003–2006. *J Nutr.* 2011; 141: 261–266.
2. Wilson KM, Klein JD, Sesselberg TS, *et al.* Use of complementary medicine and dietary supplements among US adolescents. *J Adol Health.* 2006; 38: 385–394.
3. Chen S, Binns CW, Maycock B, Liu Y, Zhang Y. Prevalence of dietary supplement use in healthy pre-school Chinese children in Australia and China. *Nutrients.* 2014; 6: 815–828.
4. Chen SY, Lin JR, Kao MD, Hang CM, Cheng L, Pan WH. Dietary supplement usage among elementary school children in Taiwan: their school performance and emotional status. *Asia Pac J Clin Nutr.* 2007; 16(Suppl 2): 554–563.
5. McDowall JA. Supplement use by young athletes. *J Sports Sci Med.* 2007; 6: 337–342.
6. Bailey RL, Gahche JJ, Thomas PR, Dwyer JT. Why US children use dietary supplements. *Pediatr Res.* 2013; 74: 737–741.
7. Dwyer J, Nahin RL, Rogers GT, *et al.* Prevalence and predictors of children's dietary supplement use: the 2007 National Health Interview Survey. *Am J Clin Nutr.* 2013; 97: 1331–1337.
8. Evans MWJr, Ndetan H, Perko M, Williams R, Walker C. Dietary supplement use by children and adolescents in the United States to enhance sport performance: results of the National Health Interview Survey. *J Primary Prevent.* 2012; 33: 3–12.
9. Kayton S, Gullen RW, Memken JA, *et al.* Supplementation and ergogenic aid use by competitive male and female high school athletes. *Med Sci Sports Exerc.* 2002; 35: S193.
10. Wiens K, Erdman KA, Stadnyk M, Parnell JA. Dietary supplement usage, motivation, and education in young, Canadian athletes. *Int J Sport Nutr Exerc Metab.* 2014; 24: 613–622.

11. Braun H, Koehler K, Geyer H, Kleinert J, Mester J, Schänzer W. Dietary supplement sse among elite young German athletes. *Int J Sport Nutr Exerc Met.* 2009; 19: 97–109.
12. Duvenage KM, Meltzer ST, Chantler SA. Initial investigation of nutrition and supplement use, knowledge and attitudes of under-16 rugby players in South Africa. *S Afr J Sports Med.* 2015; 27: 67–71.
13. Reaves L, Steffen LM, Dwyer JT, Webber LS, Lytle LA, Feldman HA, *et al.* Vitamin supplement intake is related to dietary intake and physical activity: The Child and Adolescent Trial for Cardiovascular Health (CATCH). *J Am Diet Assoc.* 2006; 106: 2018–2023.
14. Rock CL. Multivitamin-multimineral supplements: who uses them? *Am J Clin Nutr.* 2007; 85; 277S–299S.
15. Gunther S, Patterson R, Kristal AR, Stratton KL, White E. Demographic and health-related correlates of herbal and specialty supplement use. *J Am Diet Assoc.* 2004; 104: 27–34.
16. Meyer R, De Koker C, Dziubak R *et al.* A practical approach to vitamin and mineral supplementation in food allergic children. *Clin Transl Allergy.* 2015; 5: 11.
17. Christie L, Hine RJ, Parker JG, Burks W. Food allergies in children affect nutrient intake and growth. *J Am Diet Assoc.* 2002; 102: 1648–1651.
18. Perry TT, Pesek RD. Clinical manifestations of food allergy. *Pediatr Ann.* 2013; 42: 96–101.
19. Kaganov B, Caroli M, Mazur A, Singha A, Vania A. Suboptimal micronutrient intake among children in Europe. *Nutrients.* 2015; 7: 3524–3535.
20. Gibson R. *Principles of Nutritional Assessment*, 2nd ed. Oxford: Oxford University Press: 2005.
21. Kim BY, Nattiv A. Health Considerations in Female Runners. *Physical Med Rehab Clin North Am.* 2016; 27: 151–178.
22. Krogh A, Lindhard JL. The relative values of fat and carbohydrate as sources of muscular energy. *Biochem J.* 1920; 14: 290–363.
23. Hawley JA, Leckey JJ. Carbohydrate dependence during prolonged, intense endurance exercise. *Sports Med.* 2015; 45: S5–S12.
24. Australian Government Ministry of Health. *Nutrient Reference Values for Australia and New Zealand: Protein.* Available at: https://www.nrv.gov.au/nutrients/protein [Accessed 15 December 2015].
25. Phillips SM, van Loon LJC. Dietary protein for athletes: From requirements to optimum adaptation. *J Sports Sci.* 2011; 29(Suppl 1): S29–S38.
26. Shaskey DJ, Green GA. Sports haematology. *Sports Med.* 2000; 29: 27–38.
27. Rodenberg RE Gustafson S. Iron as an ergogenic aid: ironclad evidence? *Curr Sports Med Rep.* 2007; 6: 258–264.
28. Wang W, Bourgeois T, Klima J, Berlan ED, Fischer AN, O'Brien SH. Iron deficiency and fatigue in adolescent females with heavy menstrual bleeding. *Haemophilia.* 2013; 19: 225–230.
29. Sandstrom G, Borjesson M, Rodjer S. Iron deficiency in adolescent female athletes–is iron status affected by regular sporting activity? *Clin J Sports Med.* 2012; 22: 495–500.
30. MacKelvie KJ, Khan KM, McKay HA. Is there a critical period for bone response to weight-bearing exercise in children and adolescents? A systematic review. *Br J Sports Med.* 2002; 36: 250–257.
31. Desbrow B, McCormack J, Burke LM, *et al.* Sports dieticians Australia position statement: Sports nutrition for the adolescent athlete. *Int J Sport Nutr Exerc Metab.* 2014; 24: 570–584.
32. Dubnov-Raz G, Livne N, Raz R, Cohen AH, Constantini NW. Vitamin D supplementation and physical performance in adolescent swimmers. *Int J Sport Nutr Exerc Metab.* 2015; 25: 317–325.
33. Saris WH, Antoine JM, Brouns F, *et al.* PASSCLAIM—Physical performance and fitness. *Eur J Nutr.* 2003; 42(Suppl 1): 150–195.
34. Clegg DO, Reda DJ, Harris CL, Klein MA, O'Dell JR, Hooper MM. Glucosamine, chondroitin sulfate, and the two in combination for painful knee osteoarthritis. *N Eng J Med.* 2006; 354: 795–808.
35. Maughan RJ, Greenhaff PL, Hespel P. Dietary supplements for athletes: Emerging trends and recurring themes. *J Sports Sci.* 2011; 29(Suppl 2): S57–S66.
36. USFDA. *Recalls, Market Withdrawals, & Safety Alerts.* Available from: http://www.fda.gov/Safety/Recalls/ucm2005683.htm. [Accessed 8 February 2016].
37. Food Standards Agency. *Food alerts news.* Available from: http://www.food.gov.uk/news-updates/recalls-news/. [Accessed 8 February 2016].
38. Parasrampuria J, Schwartz K, Petesch R. Quality control of dehydroepiandrosterone dietary supplement products. *JAMA.* 1998; 11; 280: 1565.
39. Gurley BJ, Gardner SF, Hubbard MA. Content versus label claims in ephedra-containing dietary supplements. *Am J Health Syst Pharm.* 2000; 57: 963–969.
40. Green GA, Catlin DH, Starcevic B. Analysis of over-the-counter dietary supplements. *Clin J Sport Med.* 2001; 11: 254–259.
41. Cohen PA, Attipoe S, Travis J, Stevens M, Deuster P. Caffeine content of dietary supplements consumed on military bases. *JAMA Intern Med.* 2013; 8;173: 592–594; discussion 594.
42. Newmaster SG, Grguric M, Shanmughanandhan D, Ramalingam S, Ragupathy S. DNA barcoding detects contamination and substitution in North American herbal products. *BMC Med.* 2013; 11: 222.
43. Maughan RJ. Dietary supplement (and food) safety for athletes. In: Rawson ES, Volpe SL (eds.) *Nutrition for elite athletes.* Boca Raton, FL: CRC Press; 2015. p. 193–204.
44. Lattman P, Singer N. Army Studies Workout Supplements after Deaths. *The New York Times* [newspaper on the Internet]. 2012 Feb 2. [cited 7 March 2016] Available from: http://www.nytimes.com/2012/02/03/business/army-studies-workout-supplements-after-2-deaths.html?_r=2.
45. Claire Squires inquest: DMAA was factor in marathon runner's death. BBC online. 2013 January 30 [cited 8 February 2016]. Available from: http://www.bbc.com/news/uk-england-london-21262717
46. Krishnan PV, Feng ZZ, Gordon SC. Prolonged intrahepatic cholestasis and renal failure secondary to anabolic androgenic steroid-enriched dietary supplements. *J Clin Gastroenterol.* 2009; 43:672–675.
47. Mechcatie E. Liver injury from herbal and dietary supplements on the rise. *Internal Medicine News.* 2013 November 5 [cited 8 February 2016]. Available from: http://www.internalmedicinenews.com/cme/click-for-credit-articles/single-article/liver-injury-from-herbal-and-dietary-supplements-on-the-rise/d4dfaf68b00193e60bf80ae86a9c97fa.html.
48. Granados J, Gillum TL, Christmas KM, Kuennen MR. Prohormone supplement 3β-hydroxy-5α-androst-1-en-17-one enhances resistance training gains but impairs user health. *J Appl Physiol.* 2014; 116: 560–569.
49. Haller CA, Benowitz NL. Adverse cardiovascular and central nervous system events associated with dietary supplements containing ephedra alkaloids. *N Eng J Med.* 2000; 343: 1833–1888.
50. Maughan, RJ. Contamination of dietary supplements and positive drugs tests in sport. *J Sports Sci.* 2005; 23: 883–889.
51. Geyer H, Bredehoft M, Marek U, Parr MK, Schanzer W. Hohe Dosen des Anabolikums Metandienon in Nahrungsergaenzungsmitteln gefunden. *Dtsch Apoth Zth.* 2002; 142: 29.
52. Geyer H, Parr MK, Koehler K, Mareck U, Schänzer W, Thevis M. Nutritional supplements cross-contaminated and faked with doping substances. *J Mass Spectrom.* 2008; 43: 892–902.
53. Watson P, Judkins C, Houghton E, Russell C, Maughan RJ. Supplement contamination: detection of nandrolone metabolites in urine after administration of small doses of a nandrolone precursor. *Med Sci Sports Exerc.* 2009; 41: 766–772.
54. South African Institute of Drug-Free Sport. (2011). Position Statement of the South African Institute of Drug-Free Sport (SAIDS) on the use of supplements in sport in school going youth. 2011 October [cited 2015 November 8]. Available from: http://www.sasma.org.za/articles/SAIDS%20Position%20Statement%20for%20YOUTH.pdf
55. Sato A, Kamei A, Kamihigashi E. Use of supplements by young elite Japanese athletes participating in the 2010 youth Olympic Games in Singapore. *Clin J Sport Med.* 2012; 22: 418–423.
56. Nieper A. Nutritional supplement practices in UK junior national track and field athletes. *Br J Sports Med.* 2005; 39: 645–649.

CHAPTER 49

Doping and anti-doping

Alan Vernec and David Gerrard

Introduction

Regular physical activity results in positive outcomes for musculoskeletal, cardiorespiratory, and neurological development. Similarly, social scientists describe enhanced socialization, teamwork, self-reliance, and dependability in children who engage in team games and organized sport. However, at an indeterminate point in their development, young athletes begin to take sport more seriously, signalling a phase of increased vulnerability to the use of performance-enhancing substances. Pressure from peers and parents, increased financial incentives, and the stress of competition are among the influential factors identified by young athletes in the context of contemporary elite sport.

The essence of doping in sport carries a connotation of harm to health, unethical practice, and disregard for the legitimate clinical use of medication. When these issues challenge duty of care to young athletes, there exists a moral and professional obligation to act. Medical care to young athletes should be delivered in a manner that respects both professional medical and anti-doping codes. This chapter reviews the history and development of anti-doping strategies for sport. In addition, it addresses the Prohibited List, specific responsibilities of physicians, current anti-doping educational strategies, and the ethics of contemporary elite sport.

A brief history of doping in sport

Early history

Doping, along with other forms of cheating in sport, is not a recent phenomenon. In the third century BC, Greek athletes were reported to be consuming varieties of psychedelic mushrooms to induce a state of euphoria that prepared them for competition, while Roman gladiators were described as using stimulants to overcome fatigue, and crushed ox testicles for the enhancement of performance.[1]

Doping in modern sport has been reported since the middle of the 19th century, and is notorious for the reported death of an English cyclist in 1896 as the result of using ephedrine during the Paris-Bordeaux cycle race. A dramatic increase in sport doping was registered from the 1960s and, despite an attempt by the International Olympic Committee (IOC) to introduce doping control to the Mexico Olympics of 1968, the first true controls were only introduced at the 1976 Montreal Olympic Games. In 1974, reliable testing methods were discovered for testosterone and anabolic steroids, which were added to the IOC's list of Prohibited Substances in 1976. In Montreal, two weightlifters were found guilty of doping and were required to return their gold medals.[2]

At the 1983 Pan-American Games in Caracas, Venezuela, many athletes withdrew after they learned that a new and more rigorous drug-testing regimen had been introduced. However, there were still strong suspicions of state-sponsored doping practices in some countries, such as the German Democratic Republic (GDR). The State-sanctioned operation of drug misuse in the GDR was ultimately revealed when, at the reunification of Germany in 1989, the secret reports of the Stasi were made public. The actions of the GDR government in sanctioning the use of potent ergogenic drugs, including anabolic androgenic steroids to young female athletes, remains as perhaps the most appalling act of doping in sport. This era in East German sport has been widely researched for its impact upon the lives of young athletes whose sporting talents had been identified through a network of specialized 'Sport Schools' (*Kinder und Jugendsportschulen*).[3]

It was at the 1988 Seoul Olympic Games where the world became acutely aware of doping problems in sport when Canadian sprinter Ben Johnson was stripped of his 100 m gold medal after testing positive for the use of stanozolol, a potent anabolic androgenic steroid. The subsequent Dubin Inquiry initiated by the Canadian Government highlighted, among other things, the significant contribution to sports doping of members of the 'athlete entourage'. Johnson's coach Charlie Francis and doctor Jamie Astaphan were both found to be complicit in this widely publicized act of sports doping.[4]

The 1990s saw a shift from the use of stimulants to blood 'boosting' through the use of autologous blood transfusions as well as the use of recombinant erythropoietin (EPO). It became apparent that the existing framework was inadequate to combat the scourge of doping, most notably following the 1998 Festina Scandal, during which French customs officials and the police discovered performance-enhancing drugs in a Tour de France team support vehicle.

The first World Conference on Doping in Sport was held in 1999, followed by a series of meetings with major input from International Sport Federations and the IOC, culminating in the creation of the World Anti-Doping Agency (WADA). This new agency's mission was, and remains today, to protect clean athletes by leading the fight against doping in sport.

Since the advent of the modern doping era, anti-doping organizations continue to be challenged. Cycling has had more than its share of notoriety, especially in the early 2000s, which resulted in numbers of sanctions, the most notable being Lance Armstrong. After his recovery from testicular cancer, Armstrong went on to win seven Tour de France titles, consistently proclaiming never to have used illegal, performance-enhancing substances. In 2012, however, he was ultimately sanctioned following a prolonged investigation by the United States Anti-Doping Agency (USADA). His very public fall from grace was a significant landmark in anti-doping.

Creation of the World Anti-Doping Agency and the World Anti-Doping Code

WADA began operations in 2002 and, with the input of key stakeholders including the IOC, International Federations, and Government agencies, developed the World Anti-Doping Code (the Code).[5] This key document harmonized the rules and regulations for all aspects of anti-doping. It was accompanied by a series of International Standards: i) Laboratories, ii) Prohibited List, iii) Therapeutic Use Exemption (TUE), iv) Testing and Investigations, and v) Results Management.[6,7,8,9] All subsequent reference to the Code, the List, and WADA Standards will be to those versions in force in 2016. The resultant international consistency with the processes and practices of anti-doping has been to the benefit of all athletes desirous of clean and fair competition. WADA is a unique organization funded equally by sport and by all the governments of the world.

As of July 2015, there were 677 signatories to the Code, including all Olympic sporting federations and the majority of international sports bodies, with the North American professional leagues of baseball, hockey, American football, and basketball as notable exceptions. Fundamental to the establishment of a single, overarching anti-doping document is its universality. The Code applies to all national and international level athletes, as defined by their relevant international federations (IFs) or national anti-doping organizations (NADOs). However, in each country, the reach of anti-doping may extend to lower levels within sports contingent upon many local factors.

Every athlete should be aware if they are subject to drug testing and anti-doping rules. Every elite athlete, irrespective of age, should have a general knowledge of their obligations under the Code. This important principle applies equally to every member of the whole athlete support team ('entourage'), including attending physicians, and is a matter of responsibility emphasized in the section on roles and responsibilities of physicians.

Young athletes in elite sport are subject to financial and competitive pressures

Elite sport is increasingly a domain of the young. Full-time (and sometimes highly paid) teen-aged athletes in sports such as swimming, tennis, and golf are commonplace, and young players are recruited early for team sports including soccer and rugby. For better or worse, many children specialize in specific sports at a younger age, frequently under the influence of zealous parents, enthusiastic coaches, national sport federations, and, on occasion, through government policy.[10] These young protégés frequently compete nationally, as well as in international youth and junior championships. In some disciplines, the pinnacle of success is often achieved during early adolescence. There is no blanket age limit for Olympic competitors,[11] although this issue has been an area of recent contention in gymnastics, where the Federation Internationale de Gymnastique raised the minimum competitive age from 14 to 15 and then to 16 years, in response to concerns about the well-being of preadolescent Olympic athletes.[12]

The youngest Olympic medallist was the Greek gymnast Dimitrios Loundras, who competed in the 1896 Athens Olympics at the age of 10 years, 218 days, winning a bronze medal in a team event. The youngest gold medallist was American swimmer Donna Elizabeth de Varona, who competed in the 4 × 100 m freestyle relay heats at the 1960 Olympics, and was presented with a gold medal at the age of 13 years and 129 days.[13] Preadolescent athletes still compete at the elite level, particularly in sports such as swimming, diving, gymnastics, and golf.

Over the past three decades, elite sport has transformed to a very lucrative profession for many young athletes. There is a significant investment in time and money in the early career of an athlete, with the costs of medical or sports science support, individualized coaching, and travel combining to create, in some cases, pressure by significant others to realize a 'return on investment'. By way of example, in a recent case, the father of a Canadian athlete argued that money invested in a limited partnership to assist his daughter's athletic career should be considered a business loss for taxation purposes.[14]

Sport has become a massive industry, with the highest earning athletes receiving hundreds of millions of dollars in annual gross earnings from salaries, bonuses, prize money, endorsements, appearances, and licensing income.[15] It is therefore not surprising that on rare occasions, the lure of financial return clouds the decision of those who seek performance enhancement at any cost, even where this implicates the use of prohibited drugs. Those with responsibility to guide, advise, and mentor athletes have an obligation to be aware of such pressures, and to remain alert to the vulnerability of young athletes during documented phases of their career.

Classes of prohibited substances

Evolution of the Prohibited List

The concern for fair play and the health of athletes gave rise to anti-doping measures. In 1928, the first international federation to specifically ban substances was the International Amateur Athletic Federation, then the IAAF.[16] At that time, no athletes underwent formal doping control and there was no capability for reliable sample analysis. By today's standards, it was an impractical situation based on little more than goodwill and honesty, with little, if any, capacity for consistent implementation, and even less punitive value. Today, a widespread programme of education leaves athletes in little doubt as to the stringency of doping control, the capabilities of accredited laboratories, and the personal consequences of a doping infraction. The contemporary concept of non-analytical sanctions has also evolved, whereby an athlete may be sanctioned without the evidence of any prohibited substance found in a biological sample, whether by the Athlete Biological Passport or by other means.

Until 1967, it remained the responsibility of each sport to develop its own list of prohibited substances. However, the newly formed IOC Medical Commission developed a 'universal' list that became applicable to traditional Olympic sports as well as others who began to recognize the growing influence of sports doping.[17] Originally there were four categories of Prohibited Substances: i) central nervous system stimulants, ii) psychomotor stimulants, iii) sympathomimetic amines, and iv) narcotic analgesics.[18,19]

Following instances of blood doping during the 1984 Olympics, the IOC Medical Commission added the act of autologous blood transfusion to the prohibited list category thereby establishing the additional concept of a 'Prohibited Method'.[20] Further methods have since been added, including the prohibition of intravenous fluids greater than 50 mL every 6 h, without clinical justification.

Shortly after the adoption of the Code in 2004, WADA assumed responsibility for maintaining, revising, and publishing the List of Prohibited Substances and Methods (the List).[6] The WADA Prohibited List Expert Group (EG), consisting of sport physicians, specialists, pharmacologists, toxicologists, and sport scientists was subsequently charged with the responsibility of producing the List following extensive stakeholder consultation.[21] The revised List ultimately comes into effect on 1 January each year.

Criteria for inclusion of substances and methods on the Prohibited List

To become considered for inclusion on the List, a substance or method is required to meet any two out of the three following criteria:

i) The potential to enhance sport performance.

ii) The potential or actual health risk to the athlete.

iii) Violation of the spirit of sport as defined in the Code.

Athletes are known to use doses that may sometimes far exceed recommended therapeutic dosages.[22] Ethical constraints make it near impossible to demonstrate unequivocal ergogenic effects or adverse health consequences through true, randomized, controlled studies using high doses of potentially harmful drugs. Nevertheless, a wealth of information exists that highlights a range of adverse findings associated with many drugs traditionally misused in sport. These include long-term psychological disorder, cardiovascular dysfunction, and a diverse range of endocrine consequences from the misuse of anabolic androgenic steroids.[23–25]

The Prohibited List is formulated following widespread stakeholder consultation and the inclusion or rejection of any substance is agreed upon after investigation of the literature, significant deliberation and repeated stakeholder input. Once a substance is added to the List, there is no potential for subsequent legal or clinical challenge of the ergogenic status of a particular listed substance.[6] Its simple presence in the urine of a tested athlete constitutes an anti-doping rule violation (ADRV) with attendant consequences. This means that an athlete (or third party) cannot argue against the performance-enhancing effects of any listed substance on the grounds of any unique circumstance. If the substance is prohibited, its use or attempted use would render the athlete liable to a sanction in the absence of an approved TUE.

Categories of the Prohibited List

Those responsible for a duty of therapeutic care to athletes are obligated to have an awareness of doping control and knowledge of the general content of the Prohibited List. Some physicians who work only peripherally in sport may be aware of the prohibited status of anabolic steroids, erythropoietin, or growth hormone, but may not realize that many common therapeutic agents are also prohibited, such as insulin and some beta-2 agonists. Despite the fact that the Prohibited List has expanded since its introduction, it is valid to expect that physicians responsible for elite athletes should know where to access the List and its accompanying standard of implementation. Elite athletes are well aware of the existence of a Prohibited List and must comply with a non-negotiable occupational framework no different to the medical requirements demanded of airline pilots or professional Scuba divers. The WADA List of Prohibited Substances and Methods appears in Box 49.1.

Box 49.1 Prohibited list substances and methods

Substances and methods prohibited in- and out-of-competition

S0—Non-approved substances (e.g. drugs under pre-clinical development or discontinued, designer drugs, substances approved only for veterinary use)

S1—Anabolic agents, anabolic androgenic steroids, other anabolic agents

S2—Peptide hormones, growth factors, and related substances and mimetics

S3—Beta-2 agonists

S4—Hormone and metabolic modulators

S5—Diuretics and other masking agents

Substances and methods prohibited in-competition only

S6—Stimulants

S7—Narcotics

S8—Cannabinoids

S9—Glucocorticoids

M1—Manipulation of blood and blood components

M2—Chemical and physical manipulation

M3—Gene doping

Substances prohibited in particular sports

P1—Alcohol

P2—Beta-blockers

WADA 2016 Prohibited List, https://www.wada-ama.org/

It is important to note that not all prohibited substances are individually named in the List. In many sections, there are footnotes stating that '... other substances with a similar chemical structure or similar biological effect(s)' are also prohibited.[6]

The principle of Strict Liability

The principle of 'Strict Liability' is a key element of the Code. It articulates the unequivocal responsibility the athlete has for any prohibited substance found in their sample of urine or blood. This principle exists because many athletes often state, upon testing positive, that the ingestion of a prohibited substance was 'unknowing' or, alternatively, that an analytical error of their sample must have occurred. This rule, articulated clearly in the Code, has withstood challenge in both the Court of Arbitration of Sport in Lausanne, as well as in civil courts.[26]

The anti-doping process and stringent annual accreditation of the WADA-approved analytical laboratories minimize false positive results and stamp these laboratories as among the most reliable in the analytical world.[27] It is important to realize that even the inadvertent ingestion of a prohibited substance may invoke an ergogenic response, resulting in an unfair competitive advantage. Furthermore, it is not an easy matter for anti-doping authorities to decide on what was intentional or inadvertent doping.

It is vitally important that athletes and their physicians always verify the current status of any prescribed medications. There are several reliable sources of drug status information, including the relevant National Anti-Doping Agency and centralized drug databases such as the Global Drug Reference Online (GlobalDRO).[28] The Global Drug Reference Online accepts both generic and proprietary name queries for drugs available in the US, Canada, the UK, and Japan, and returns an up-to-date status, indicating whether or not the drug is prohibited according to the current List.

Therapeutic Use Exemption

A brief history

By the late 1990s, a significant body of concern existed for the increasing advent of drug misuse in sport. The establishment of WADA removed responsibility for anti-doping matters from the IOC Medical Committee and harmonized an international approach to doping in sport. The Code and accompanying International Standards embody the spirit and regulations necessary to foster clean sport.

Where best practice principles dictated the use of 'prohibited drugs', many physicians struggled to match the exigencies of clinical practice and elite sport. The diseases and disorders affecting young athletes that most commonly challenged physicians were type-1 diabetes, attention-deficit hyperactivity disorder (ADHD), and chronic asthma. Prohibited substances were, in some instances, widely recommended as first-line therapy and there needed to be a process by which their appropriate use could be justified.

Historically, the IOC had developed a Medications Advisory Committee (MAC) that scrutinized all requests to use prohibited substances, particularly where these applied to the care of athletes at the time of Olympic Games. Since 1991, the work of the MAC overcame widely held prejudices against the therapeutic use of banned drugs in sport on the understanding that strict clinical criteria must be met. This stance served to respect both the athlete's health and the imperative for appropriate medical management, while acknowledging the sentiment of fair play in sport. The work of the MAC was an important precursor to the modern concept of TUE.[29]

In 2004, WADA formed an international advisory group of physicians subsequently designated as the Therapeutic Use Exemption Expert Group (TUE EG) and NADOs became empowered to establish Therapeutic Use Exemption Committees (TUECs), whose membership and responsibilities were clearly delineated in the International Standard for Therapeutic Use Exemptions (ISTUE).[9] Channels of inquiry were soon established and treating physician(s) were guided in a process that allowed appropriate application for TUE. The benefits to elite young athletes became measured in their receipt of an appropriate standard of care in the knowledge that their achievements in sport would remain untainted by accusations of drug misuse.

Fairness in sport and the Therapeutic Use Exemption process

An overarching responsibility for physicians managing the health of young athletes is the accurate documentation of the circumstances requiring the use of a prohibited substance. This is in their obligation to the Code and the ISTUE.[5,9] This process ensures that any athlete with a genuine medical condition is not denied access to competition. However, in submitting an application for exemption to use a prohibited substance, the attending physician must consider the mandatory criteria listed in Box 49.2.

The TUE process is a delicate balance between inclusion and fairness in sport. Most people, particularly physicians, are in favour of encouraging and allowing those with medical conditions to participate in sport. However, in order to take a prohibited substance, one must have a clearly documented medical condition, with a legitimate need for that substance without recourse to any permitted alternative. In the spirit of fair play and the concept of a level playing field, the athlete must also fulfil the criterion (b) mentioned in Box 49.2, which states that the medication may not produce any additional enhancement of performance. There are some, albeit rare, situations where the need for a medication in combination with this criterion results in the exclusion of an athlete from elite sport.[30]

While there is no finite list of medical conditions for which the TUE process applies, there are a few disorders that frequently come to the attention of TUE Committees. With particular relevance to young athletes, these conditions include ADHD, requiring the use of amphetamine-like substances such as methylphenidate; acute asthma or exercise-induced bronchial hyper-reactivity, requiring pulses of systemic glucocorticoids; and insulin-dependent diabetes and acute anaphylactic or hyper-allergenic reaction, necessitating the use of systemic glucocorticoids and/or adrenaline.

Another perspective of the TUE process is derived from the analysis of medications for which approval is sought. Figure 49.1 illustrates the range of prohibited substances drawn from WADA TUE files in the 2015 calendar year for athletes aged 18 years and younger in all sports in which participation is subject to the Code. These statistics align closely with the array of disorders commonly affecting young athletes described above and indicated first-line treatments.

Box 49.2 Criteria for granting a therapeutic use exemption

a. The *Prohibited Substance* or *Prohibited Method* in question is needed to treat an acute or chronic medical condition, such that the *Athlete* would experience a significant impairment to health if the *Prohibited Substance* or *Prohibited Method* were to be withheld.

b. The *Therapeutic Use* of the *Prohibited Substance* or *Prohibited Method* is highly unlikely to produce any additional enhancement of performance beyond what might be anticipated by a return to the *Athlete's* normal state of health following the treatment of the acute or chronic medical condition.

c. There is no reasonable *Therapeutic* alternative to the *Use* of the *Prohibited Substance* or *Prohibited Method*.

d. The necessity for the *Use* of the *Prohibited Substance* or *Prohibited Method* is not a consequence, wholly or in part, of the prior *Use* (without a *TUE*) of a substance or method which was prohibited at the time of such *Use*.

WADA 2016 International Standard on TUEs, https://www.wada-ama.org/

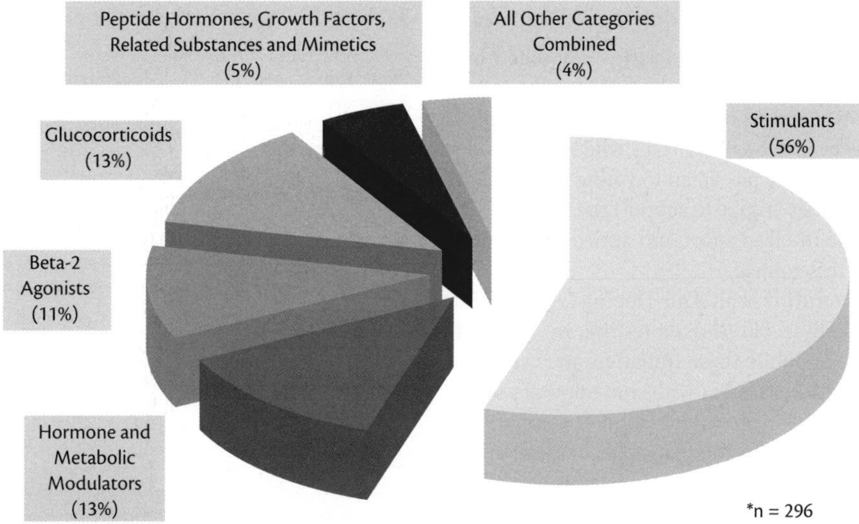

Figure 49.1 The 2015 World Anti-doping Agency young athlete Therapeutic Use Exemption experience.
Approved Therapeutic Use Exemptions by prohibited substance for athletes 18 years of age and under in all sports.
WADA ADAMS TUE Database, 2015.

Diagnostic criteria

For the assistance of physicians seeking to obtain TUE for their patients, the WADA website includes TUE Guidelines that clearly identify the diagnostic criteria to support such applications. These guidelines have been informed by current best practice, with contributions from a number of sources, including specialist physicians in the particular area. The principle underpinning these guideline documents is that athletes in any sport and in any part of the world should be assessed in accordance with a common set of criteria. Every effort is made by WADA to regularly review these documents to ensure that contemporary clinical practice is being observed. As of 2016, there are 19 such documents available through the WADA website. The existing list of conditions addressed by these Guidelines appears in Table 49.1.

Roles and responsibilities of physicians

Fundamental responsibilities

Fundamental responsibilities all physicians have in their duty of care are highlighted when these extend to the management of elite young athletes. Participation in competitive sport infers respect for the values of fair play, and attending physicians require knowledge of prohibited drugs, awareness of the process of TUE, recognition of doping practices, risks of inadvertent doping, drug side effects, and appreciation of the ethical standards by which clean athletes are bound.

Health and rights of young athletes

The protection of the health and rights of athletes to fairness in sport began as a responsibility of the IOC. However, with the establishment of WADA, the IOC entrusted the responsibility for clean sport and anti-doping to this new entity. Currently, the IOC Medical Commission specifically addresses issues relating to athlete health and well-being, demonstrated by position documents that focus upon the young athlete. These include statements on sexual harassment, fostering the young elite athlete, and surveillance of trends in injury and illness. A consensus statement on youth athletic development[31,32] addressed fundamental concerns for welfare and socialization from recreation to elite competition, providing a foundation for understanding musculoskeletal growth, psychological development, and the energy requirements of sport. These imperatives are identified as essential to developing '... *healthy, capable, resilient young athletes* ...' in pursuit of '... *enjoyable participation and success*.'[31(p843)] Encouragement for the young athlete to acquire skills from a menu of physical activities is regarded as the stimulus for sustained sport participation and lifelong activity, with attendant health benefits.

Table 49.1 World Anti-Doping Agency therapeutic use exemption physician guidelines.

WADA TUE Physician Guidelines **Medical information to support the decisions of TUEC**	
ADHD	*Infertility/polycystic ovarian syndrome*
Adrenal insufficiency	*Inflammatory bowel disease*
Anaphylaxis	*Intravenous infusion*
Androgen deficiency–male hypogonadism	*Intrinsic sleep disorders*
	Post-infectious cough
Asthma	*Musculoskeletal conditions*
Cardiovascular conditions	*Neuropathic pain*
Diabetes mellitus	*Renal transplantation*
Female-to-male transsexual athletes	*Sinusitis/rhinosinusitis*
Growth hormone deficiency (adults)	
Growth hormone deficiency (child & adolescents)	

WADA TUE Physician Guideline Documents, Medical Information to Support the Decisions of TUECs, https://www.wada-ama.org/

Supporting clean athletes and anti-doping initiatives

The relationship between athlete and physician is embodied in a statement of safety, ensuring that, '... *sport is practised without danger to the health of athletes and with respect for fair play and sports ethics.*'.[33] This principle is even more important when we consider the clinical responsibility of every physician to young athletes. The sport and medical communities engage to support the rights of athletes everywhere to engage in clean sport and anti-doping initiatives should be viewed in this context.

Every athlete under the scrutiny of an Anti-Doping Organization (ADO) is monitored and subjected to drug testing, in- and out-of-competitive sport. To the public these initiatives may seem an intrusion of privacy, but to those familiar with contemporary sport, doping control has become routine to a generation of competitors. This is clearly in mutual respect for the principles of clean sport. Contemporary high-profile cases provide stark reminder of the small yet concerning use of banned substances.[34]

Knowledge of prohibited substances in sport

A challenging area for some physicians is the prescribing of drugs that may be prohibited in sport, especially when many of these agents may be first-line treatment in the management of certain medical conditions. Some physicians initially object to the intervention of an external authority that restricts therapeutic options, when patient well-being is the doctor's primary responsibility.

However, informed sport physicians are aware that elite competitive sport carries non-negotiable decisions around the List of Prohibited Substances and Methods (the List), which was established to address the misuse of performance-enhancing drugs.[35] Each year, extensive anti-doping education of athletes and coaches is undertaken internationally and this greatly facilitates the understanding of responsibilities to the drug testing process. In some countries, e.g. New Zealand, athletes in the national drug-testing pool carry a small wallet card provided by their NADO providing relevant anti-doping information for their attending doctor.

Among the more innovative NADOs, USADA has an extensive website for the education of health professionals responsible for the management of elite athletes, including an online tutorial for physicians.[36] In other countries, desktop formularies contain updated, reliable information on prohibited substances. Additionally, the WADA website provides a menu of detailed information relating to the List. Educational information available to physicians and athletes alike includes websites and interactive platforms available through WADA and the major NADOs. A selected list of helpful anti-doping educational material appears in Table 49.2.

Awareness of the Therapeutic Use Exemption process

On justified occasions when there is no alternative but to treat an athlete using a prohibited substance, physicians may invoke the option of TUE.[37] The TUE process protects the athlete from a punitive sanction arising from the adverse finding of a banned substance in a sample of urine or blood. In the interests of consistency and integrity in sport, this process demands adequate diagnostic evidence and specialist endorsement meeting specified criteria. However, without a valid TUE, a positive test for a prohibited substance will likely result in a doping infraction, with a range of attendant consequences, including suspension from sport.

Table 49.2 Examples of anti-doping educational resources.

Anti-doping agency	Educational resources
Anti-Doping Authority the Netherlands	Print resources, anti-doping education for athlete entourage, fitness centre information, interactive E-learning
Australian Sports Anti-Doping Authority	E-Learning, YouTube channel, print resources, lesson plans
Canadian Centre for Ethics in Sport	E-Learning programmes, online education
Drug-Free Sport New Zealand	On-line seminars, questionnaires, handbooks, wallet cards
Japan Anti-Doping Agency	Mobile applications, printed resources, online educational material
South African Institute for Drug-Free Sport	Outreach programmes, online workshops and seminars, position statements
United States Anti-Doping Agency	Handbooks, interactive seminars
UK Anti-Doping	International standards, athlete entourage leaflet, sport toolkit
World Anti-Doping Agency	Physician Tool Kit, International Standards, TUE Guidelines, TUE Physician Guidelines for Medical Conditions

Understanding major doping side effects

Research has shown that young athletes are potentially vulnerable to drug misuse at identifiable phases in their competitive development, with parallels drawn between exposures to recreational drugs in the social context. In elite sport, a desire to win at any cost, body image, peer or parental pressure, and recovery from injury have been identified as significant influences.[38]

Every sports physician requires an understanding of anti-doping and in particular should present an honest, informed opinion on matters of drug side effects. As a common example, there is a substantial body of literature that addresses the dangers of the inappropriate use of anabolic androgenic steroids and their precursors.[39] These include inappropriate mood swings, uncharacteristic aggression, premature fusion of bony growth plates, and virilization effects in young females.[40] Young anabolic steroid users have also been shown to have an increase in the use of other illicit substances, including marijuana and alcohol.[41]

The misuse of stimulants such as ephedrine and other amphetamine-like substances carries the risk of wide ranging side effects, including arrhythmias, hypertension, anxiety, tremors, insomnia, seizures, and psychotic episodes.[42,43] Stimulants have found favour in events demanding rapid energy expenditure (sprinting) and also where weight loss is deemed part of the body image demanded by sports such as gymnastics, diving, and synchronized swimming. More recently there has been concern over the addition of ephedrine to certain dietary supplements, highlighting the risks of inadvertent doping by young, well-intentioned athletes.[42,44] It is not within the scope of this chapter to explore the area of dietary supplementation, and interested readers are referred to Chapter 48. However, the availability of a range of popular products founded on scant scientific evidence is a concern to many health professionals in sport.

Ethical responsibilities of physicians

The ethical role of the sports physician is frequently distinct from the normal patient relationship. Physicians must be aware of circumstances that are regularly challenged by the nature of the sporting environment and to have clear strategies in place to deal with these.

An outline of these considerations is provided in the WADA Toolkit for practising physicians, highlighting five responsibilities, informed by ethical norms central to the practice of sports medicine.[45] These responsibilities are as follows:

i) *Care*—Long-term well-being must always take precedence over performance goals and a physician must never favour personal interests above the health of the athlete-patient for any reason. While a mature athlete may decide to accept potential long-term health consequences, this demands very careful consideration of the risks. However, this is unacceptable in the care of a young athlete.

ii) *Confidentiality*—A sports physician may have conflicting interests when employed by a team franchise or national federation. While patient confidentiality is generally considered sacrosanct, it is not absolute. An athlete's injury or health problem may put others at risk or have grave consequences to a team, and it must be made clear to all parties that traditional confidentiality may not always apply. Details of the type of information, and under what circumstances this may be divulged, should be spelled out in an agreement.

iii) *Truth telling*—A physician must be clear and unequivocal with every athlete-patient, including explaining all risks and side effects of medications and treatments as well as needs to communicate to third parties.

iv) *Professional competence*—All sports physicians dealing with elite athletes are obligated to keep abreast of current developments in the anti-doping field as a reflection of medical competence.

v) *Professional distance*—Sports physicians must balance subjective, compassionate care with objective advice and treatment. Through demands of training and performance many athletes challenge accepted health norms, frequently blurring the traditional boundaries of clinical objectivity.

Box 49.3 Means of invoking an anti-doping rule violation pursuant to the code

2.1—Presence of a *Prohibited Substance* or its *Metabolites* or *Markers* in an *Athlete's Sample*

2.2—*Use* or *Attempted Use* by an *Athlete* of a *Prohibited Substance* or a *Prohibited Method*

2.3—Evading, Refusing or Failing to Submit to *Sample* Collection

2.4—Whereabouts Failures

2.5—*Tampering* or *Attempted Tampering* with any part of *Doping Control*

2.6—*Possession* of a *Prohibited Substance* or a *Prohibited Method*

2.7—*Trafficking* or *Attempted Trafficking* in any *Prohibited Substance* or *Prohibited Method*

2.8—Administration or *Attempted Administration* to any *Athlete In-Competition* of any *Prohibited Substance* or *Prohibited Method,* or *Administration* or *Attempted Administration* to any *Athlete Out-of-Competition* of any *Prohibited Substance* or any *Prohibited Method* that is prohibited *Out-of-Competition*

2.9—*Complicity*

2.10—*Prohibited Association*

WADA 2015 World Anti-Doping Code, https://www.wada-ama.org/

Current anti-doping strategies

Anti-doping rule violations

Discussion so far has focused on the use of prohibited substances and application of the principle of TUE. Those in the sporting community who equate a positive urine sample as the only proof of doping, demonstrate an incomplete knowledge of the full gamut of anti-doping rules embedded in the Code. However, the presence of a prohibited substance in a biological sample is only one of ten means to an ADRV described in Box 49.3.

Use or attempted use: The Athlete Biological Passport

Beginning in the 1990s, coinciding with the advent of erythropoietin (EPO) use in sport, some international federations, such as the ISU (International Skating Union), the UCI (Union Cycliste Internationale), and the IBU (International Biathlon Union), implemented a 'No-Start Rule' to deal with athletes competing with an unnaturally high haematocrit. Ironically some cyclists, frustrated by the fact that their own doctors were trying to unfairly restrict their haematocrit to a maximum of 55%, mockingly referred to Danish cyclist Bjarne Riis (the 1996 Tour de France winner) as 'Mr. 60%'. Once the No-Start Rule came into effect, the athlete would be prevented from competing for safety reasons if the haemoglobin concentration or haematocrit exceeded a certain number or percentage. There is still debate around what is a truly safe level upper haematocrit in healthy athletes,[46,47] and the No-Start Rule was considered a surreptitious means to deal with doping. Perhaps the issue of greatest concern was that some athletes felt challenged to dope until they could achieve a haematocrit just below the cut-off. The No-Start Rule, fraught with scientific and legal issues, was slowly phased out.

A Canadian cyclist and World Junior champion was 16 years old when she started using EPO in 1998. She was forced to sit out the 2003 Women's World Championship road race because her haematocrit exceeded the UCI threshold in place at that time.[48] This non-participation aroused suspicion and she eventually confessed to doping in 2007. The athlete was sanctioned for 10 years and both her manager and her physician (who prescribed the EPO) were banned from sport for life. The latter also had his medical license suspended by his provincial licensing board for 3 months.

Observations of fluctuating haematocrit levels noted with the No-Start Rule led to the development of the Athlete Biological Passport (ABP), one of the most significant tools introduced in anti-doping.[49] A group of experts were brought together in 2006 following discussions at the Torino Winter Olympics and by 2009 robust legal and scientific Athlete Biological Passport Guidelines and Technical Documents were published by WADA. The principles of the ABP are that one may detect use of a prohibited substance [Article 2.2 of the Code[5]] indirectly by serial measure of biomarkers, rather than direct detection of the prohibited substance or method. The haematological module of the ABP primarily applies haemoglobin and reticulocyte percentages to indirectly detect the use of Erythropoiesis Stimulating Agents or blood transfusions. A Bayesian type algorithm using the athlete's own reference values, rather than population values, was developed to detect deviations from normal physiological variation resulting in a notification of an atypical passport finding. The passport, or longitudinal profile, of the athlete, along with other information such as altitude training and competition period, would then be evaluated by experts (haematologists, sport physicians, physiologists) who would decide the likelihood of doping, atypical physiology, or pathology. The experts could suggest further testing, including specific analytical tests or, if three experts unanimously agreed that doping was most likely to have occurred, then the Anti-Doping Organization would proceed towards an ADRV based solely on the ABP.

In 2014, the steroidal module of the ABP was launched to detect steroidal doping, the use of androgenic anabolic steroids (AAS), and especially the abuse of endogenous substances such as testosterone that were harder to detect than exogenous AAS such as stanozolol; the Steroidal Module uses similar principles as the haematological module. The Steroidal Module of the ABP primarily considers the testosterone:epitestosterone (T:E) ratio, which is generally quite stable in any one individual. With the advent of the new steroidal module, one's own values are automatically compared to prior values, permitting anti-doping organizations to reliably further reduce the threshold for mass spectroscopy (IRMS) testing. One of the first successes of the steroidal module was to identify a Korean swimmer with an atypical (for him) T:E ratio of 2.4:1, far above his regular values, which had been quite steady at less than 1:1. The ABP algorithm directed the laboratories to perform IRMS, which confirmed the use of exogenous testosterone.

Further modules are being developed including an endocrine module, aimed at detecting the abuse of growth hormones and their analogues using specific biomarkers such as insulin-like growth factor 1 (IGF-I). It is known that human growth hormone (hGH) and other compounds modulating hGH signalling are being abused by athletes.[50] Although there is a direct analytical test for hGH, the detection window is limited by its short half-life. Therefore, the passport approach using more stable biomarkers of hGH should improve the ability to detect hGH abuse. On very rare occasions a young athlete may legitimately require the use of hGH for a genuine medical condition. This would invoke the process of TUE. Examples of such clinical conditions include isolated growth hormone or multiple pituitary deficiencies or idiopathic short stature. However, these conditions in elite young athletes are not common and it is stressed that very comprehensive medical justification for the use of therapeutic hGH would be required before TUE approval was granted. (Interested readers are referred to Chapter 5 for an analysis of hormone responses to exercise and to Chapter 33 for a discussion of hormone responses to training).

The burgeoning fields of proteomics and genomics are also providing opportunities for the discovery of new biomarkers of doping.[49,51] These are the focus of current research whereby the discovery and validation of new biomarkers will enhance the scope of the ABP to detect doping in sport.

Out-of-competition testing and whereabouts

Initially all anti-doping tests were conducted in-competition, but it became apparent that athletes could administer certain substances with significant ergogenic effect during training. Even a cursory knowledge of clearance times or pharmacokinetics meant that athletes could dope at will and not be caught during competition testing. This eventually gave rise to the concept of out-of-competition testing and, in 1989 the IAAF and other federations signed a declaration that included random out-of-competition testing.[52] It also became clear that some athletes could avoid drug tests by training in remote centres. To close this loophole a system of location referred to as 'athlete whereabouts' was created by which elite athletes who are part of a registered testing pool must provide their actual whereabouts through an online system linked to their ADO. Failure to provide the information as required, or failing to be located for testing based on the information provided, could constitute a doping infraction.[5] It is therefore important for young elite athletes and their support entourage to be familiar with this important facet of contemporary anti-doping administration.

Present anti-doping programmes promote the concept of strategic or 'intelligent' testing. This implies that athletes are carefully evaluated for their risk of doping rather than allocating tests on a random basis. Intelligent testing takes into account the anti-doping potential of specific athletes, as well as the profile of a particular sport and its association with doping substances. In other words, the aim is to know who to test, when to test, and what to test for, rather than adopt a random scattergun approach.

Investigations

Investigations now play a larger role in the ability to detect doping athletes. Information from sources such as customs officials, Interpol or even 'whistle-blowers' may lead to investigations and eventually, to anti-doping sanctions. The ABP may also influence the investigation of a group of athletes through the presence of distinct profiles. As an example, ABP monitoring demonstrated the unusually high haematological values in Russian athletes that formed part of the evidence in the doping scandal of 2015.[53] The Steroidal Module has also enabled the detection of unusually similar profiles in athletes, leading to deoxyribonucleic acid (DNA) testing that proved complicity by certain athletes in sample switching.[54,55] It is clear that investigations are an established, and increasingly important, part of anti-doping.

Possession, administration, complicity, and prohibited association

Simple possession of a prohibited substance without a TUE could lead to an ADRV for either the athlete or any member of their support entourage, including their doctor. However, there is allowance for physicians to carry medications and equipment with acceptable justification, deemed necessary for normal practice and in emergency situations.

Physicians have registered concern about intentional complicity, as they may be approached by or need to treat an athlete who has taken prohibited substances. The physician is not obliged to break confidentiality and would not be considered complicit if there was no specific intent to aid and abet doping behaviour or practices.

Prohibited Association is a new Code Article that directly deals with athlete support personnel and was added to the 2015 Code due to feedback from athletes, recognizing that athletes rarely engage in doping activities in isolation. Young athletes in particular are often under the sway of their entourage, yet they have historically suffered almost the totality of the resulting punishment, while the coaches and physicians who created and promulgated the doping environment were not prevented from adversely influencing the next generation of impressionable young athletes. This new article prohibits association by an athlete, in a professional or sport-related capacity, with any support person who is serving a period of doping-related ineligibility, or who has been criminally or professionally found guilty of an offence within the past 6 years for conduct that would have constituted an ADRV.

Anti-doping rule violations prevent athletes and their entourage from participating in sport, which can be particularly significant for athletes. However, the entourage, including physicians, may be subject to other sanctions outside of the anti-doping realm, which may have more serious consequences. In most countries medical licensing bodies consider doping athletes to be unethical behaviour contrary to the medical code. Deliberate doping, especially of youth, would constitute a serious ethical breach and physicians could be suspended from practising medicine. In some jurisdictions (e.g. Canada and New Zealand), doping is specifically mentioned in the medical codes.[56,57] There are a few countries (e.g. Italy and Germany) where involvement in doping is considered a criminal offence.

Advanced analytical techniques

Anti-doping analytical methods

Due to the escalating problem of doping in sport, WADA, since its inception, spearheaded an active scientific programme with the goal of elevating anti-doping science. With contributions from experts in the fields of science, medicine, and law, it has been possible to improve and develop advanced testing methods, anticipate and detect new drugs of abuse earlier in clinical development, and preserve samples for detection as testing methods evolve. By implementing proactive strategies such as these and by promoting innovative research, anti-doping organizations are anticipating and addressing future challenges threatening the integrity of sport.

Drug testing methods are largely dictated by the substance under detection and the analytical sensitivity required.[7] Most anti-doping detection methods are based upon gas and liquid chromatography methods coupled to mass spectrometric detection (GC/LC-MSn), due to the versatility, sensitivity, and high selectivity these techniques afford. Current chromatographic methods coupled to mass spectrometry can reach sensitivity levels in the femtogram $\cdot$ mL^{-1} (10^{-18} $kg \cdot L^{-1}$) range.

However, the detection of proteins and peptides with high sensitivity and selectivity requires antibody-based technology. Immunoassay is therefore the analytical method of choice for specific prohibited substances such as luteinizing hormone, chorionic gonadotropin, and hGH.

For other prohibited substances, physical separation of proteins may be required to distinguish endogenous from exogenous variants of a hormone. An example is the detection of recombinant human erythropoietin (rhEPO), a widely abused hormone for blood boosting in endurance sports. Development of an isoelectrofocusing detection method for rhEPO[58] is still considered a major breakthrough in anti-doping analysis. More recently, improved electrophoretic methods have permitted efficient detection of the recent generation of EPO-like substances.

Pharmaceutical industry collaboration with the World Anti-Doping Agency

The majority of doping cases relate to abuse of legitimate medicines, including drugs still in clinical development, to enhance performance. Collaborations between WADA and pharmaceutical companies have accelerated efforts to identify substances with doping potential and mobilize suitable testing methods even before clinical development is complete.[59]

One well-documented example involves Mircera™, a new generation Erythropoietin Stimulating Agent (ESA) developed by Roche to treat anaemia. The collaborative development of testing methodologies by Roche and WADA led to the detection of Mircera™ in the blood samples of a cyclist at the 2008 Tour de France and several athletes at the Beijing Olympic Games, only a few weeks after the drug was officially marketed.

More recently, the first cases of abuse of the Selective Androgen Receptor Modulator (SARM) Ostarine and the HIF-stabilizer FG-4592 (roxadustat) were detected while the substances were still in clinical development. GW501516, a cardioprotective and anti-diabetes compound abandoned during clinical development in 2007 due to concerns of serious adverse events, was detected in 2012 and 2013 in several athlete samples, highlighting the importance of industry/anti-doping agency collaboration to encourage fair play in sport and protect the long-term health of athletes.

Designer drugs

A designer drug is an illegal/unapproved drug developed to bypass existing rules including methods of detection. Such was the case in 2003, when the Bay Area Laboratory Co-Operative (BALCO) affair revealed that three designer anabolic steroids, norbolethone, tetrahydrogestrinone, and desoxymethyltestosterone, were provided to enhance the performance of a small number of elite athletes. The existence of these drugs came serendipitously from tip-offs and subsequent investigations, and not by the traditional anti-doping tests in laboratories.

Today, examples of designer drugs come primarily from the stimulant class. Tens of new designer drugs are released on an international scale every year.[59] Some of these stimulants find their way into dietary supplements creating a serious risk of inadvertent doping for athletes and a significant health risk for the general population. Youth are particularly vulnerable as some of these stimulants target social and musical events or are made available through open access on the Internet. Cannabinoid derivatives are also among the new psychoactive substances being widely released as street drugs, endangering youth and permeating the field of sports. Designer drugs are more challenging to identify due to their illegal nature, the absence of information and reference material to reliably detect them, and their high frequency of release on a worldwide scale.

Anti-doping authorities have now established collaboration with police and customs forces (Interpol and the World Customs Organization) and collaborate with world organizations specialized in the field of novel psychoactive drugs.[60] This collaboration will help to identify such drugs as early as possible and to rapidly inform the network of scientific and anti-doping experts.

Sample storage and re-analysis

An important deterrent in the fight against doping is the ability to store urine and blood samples for retesting when new or more sensitive methods of detection become available. A 10-year statute of limitation has been established in the World Anti-Doping Code, allowing all samples collected at an Olympics to be stored for future re-analysis. Re-testing of the 2004 summer Olympic Games in Athens, 8 years after collection, led to revelations of five doping cases and the sanctioning of several athletes, including the return of four Olympic medals. Since coming into force, sample storage from all Olympic Games and a few other major competitions has resulted in multiple doping infractions. To maximize the chances to identify and catch doped athletes, samples are classified for retesting based upon risk factor analysis and information gathering from anti-doping authorities.

Anti-doping research

Prior to the establishment of WADA there was no research activity specifically focused on anti-doping. Anti-doping initiatives have always been keen to integrate new technologies and improve on existing testing capabilities. Since 2001, a significant proportion of the WADA budget has been dedicated to anti-doping research. In addition, WADA was assigned the role of coordinating international research initiatives in order to prioritize efforts, minimize duplication, and optimize the use of resources. The research programme has resulted in major achievements, including the detection of rhGH, the refinement of rhEPO detection, the consolidation of detection of anti-doping substances, integration of new methodologies, and anticipation of doping trends.

Future research will need to address contemporary analytical challenges in sports anti-doping, serving to enhance and consolidate the Athlete Biological Passport, integrate new detection methods through a combination of biomarkers, and apply the cutting-edge use of proteomics to analytical science.

The ethics and values of sport

Why fight against doping?

Examination of the contemporary doping scene and the countervailing anti-doping movement begs some fundamental questions, including why doping has come into sport, why we should fight against it, if it is worth fighting for, and what it all means for the sports physician.

Physicians are not afforded the luxury of philosophising on the values of elite competitive sport. Instead they must deal directly with the effect of this milieu on their patients. For many this encompasses injury management and issues of return to play. However, unique nuances in clinical sport medicine require knowledge of ethical scenarios beyond the scope of routine medical practice.

One such example is the corruption of sporting values, precipitated by the mentality of winning at all costs; this belief is frequently engendered in young athletes by support personnel, whose profound influence can distort behaviour and attitude. This influence may extend to the physician whose relationship with a young athlete is borne of great trust. As the only professional who has sworn an oath to protect the well-being of the patient-athlete, the onus is on the physician to respect this obligation and remain independently objective. Relationships corrupted by a desire to win at all costs may be mediated through third parties, including a domineering coach with career prospects aligned to the success of their athletes, or a parent seeking to live vicariously through the prowess of a child. It therefore becomes essential for physicians to recognize these issues, maintain an ethical stance, and where possible, take the appropriate action. (The interested reader is referred to Chapter 50 for further discussion).

Values of sport

Very often, the values of sport are hijacked. While winning can become the overriding motivation for taking part, more subtle ways might directly affect physicians. For example, there is the fundamental concept of courage regarded as a virtue, promoted through sport, and valued for its potential to develop character in young people. However, when the promotion of courage endangers the health of an athlete, serious questions are raised. An athlete who plays through the pain barrier is often deemed courageous by putting the team ahead of their own health. Portrayed as a hero who battles adversity, that same athlete's values become less celebrated when medical consequences are measured in chronic pain, disability, and premature retirement from sport.

There are a number of positive values, which fall under the euphemism of 'the Spirit of Sport' or 'Olympism'. These are identified in the pursuit of excellence, identified by many international federations and encouraged by authorities as underpinning all sporting endeavours. These values are:

i) Fairness

ii) Inclusion

iii) Respect

iv) Equity

While they have unique characteristics, these values are complementary and are commonly promoted and reinforced from a young age by informed members of the athletic entourage. Children possess an innate sense of these values and even regulate themselves during simulated play. During spontaneous play, children will frequently implement their own system of peer regulation, having no problem identifying any transgressor. This sense of fairness and other positive values can be eroded by exposure to overriding vested interests from adults. This is proposed as an explanation for the many athletes who show reluctance to identify other athletes whom they know to be doping or, to vocally support clean sport.

In physical activity and organized sport, as in areas of health promotion, prevention through education is regarded as the primary focus for maintaining positive values. However, the reality is that the anti-doping movement employs a three-pronged model of detection, deterrence, and prevention, with most of the energy and budget focused on the first two areas. Underpinning prevention is the acceptance of values-based education as the most effective way to protect against doping. To be maximally effective, it must utilize a long-term strategy and target young people as they develop moral identity. Involvement of the athletic entourage is critical, particularly parents, teachers, coaches, and physicians. Those promoting the values, at the very least, must know what they are and why they are important.

What is values-based education?

Values-based education takes a person-centred, holistic approach, engaging participants in the moral and ethical arguments of fair play, the spirit of sport, and the reasons for having rules. This approach promotes positive attitudes toward clean sport and ultimately leads to athletes engaging in doping-free behaviour.

This type of programme involves a more comprehensive approach that goes beyond traditional anti-doping education which simply provides information. A values-based education programme seeks instead to develop decision-makers, resulting in athletes who choose to be clean rather, than be deterred for fear of detection.[61] Awareness and information are also essential components to ensure inadvertent doping does not occur.

The physician's role in relation to these initiatives is through awareness and by fostering an environment that promotes these common values. Although they are not directly responsible for educating athletes, physicians will operate in an environment where values-based education is taking place, and they should be aware and supportive of this process.

Vulnerability to doping

While the temptation to dope touches virtually all elite athletes, it is important for an entourage to be able to identify athletes who are particularly vulnerable. The entourage may then improve the likelihood of successful intervention or prevention. There are a number of scenarios where athletes may be especially vulnerable to the pressures of doping,[62] which include:

i) Return or recovery from injury.
ii) Change in club/environment.
iii) Change in sporting level (e.g. entering a high-performance centre) or a higher level of pressure.
iv) Failure in a competitive endeavour, or performance setback.
v) Overtraining or insufficient recovery time.
vi) Absence or weakness of deterrents (such as doping controls, severe sanctions, etc.).
vii) Engagement in certain types of sport (weight categories, endurance, pure speed, or strength).
viii) Lack of resources (poor access to competent professionals, training information, and technology).
ix) Degradation or loss of personal relationships (with parents, peers) or emotional instability caused by life transitions (puberty, graduation, dropping out, geographical moves).

Note that these scenarios represent occasions where an athlete is particularly vulnerable, although anti-doping education should not be limited to these circumstances.

Recognizing doping

Physicians are in a unique position to be able to detect likely doping behaviour with the opportunity to positively intervene before a young athlete suffers the myriad consequences of doping. Although a physician may not always be in regular contact with the athlete/patient, he or she should still be alert to the signs that an athlete may be doping.[62] Some personal characteristics and behaviours that may signal an athlete is engaging in doping behaviour are included in Box 49.4.

Box 49.4 Possible cues to doping behaviour in young athletes

Low self-esteem or depression

Body image dissatisfaction, concern about weight maintenance or rapid change in weight

Unruly, disrespectful of authority

Impatience with obtaining results

Propensity for cheating/bending the rules in other areas of life

Expressed belief that everyone else is doping

Disbelief in harmful effects of doping

History of substance abuse in family

Expressed admiration for achievements of known doped athletes

Thrill-seeking behaviour

Use of other substances, alcohol or tobacco

Non-discretionary use of dietary supplements

Source: WADA Doping and Related Issues—Anti-Doping Textbook http://antidopinglearninghub.org/en

Conclusions

Although the history of drug use by athletes is as old as sport itself, only in recent times has there been a development of regulations and codes to address the ethical and health issues that arise from doping. There are many examples in the literature of athletes and their entourage seeking performance enhancement through prohibited drugs, but it took the advent of drug-related deaths in sport in the mid-1960s for authorities to accelerate anti-doping policies and programmes. Despite innovation and progress in the field of anti-doping, escalating rewards from elite sport have continued to drive the desire to succeed at any cost, which includes the misuse of drugs.

In 1967, the IOC established the first list of drugs prohibited in sport as part of its mandate to safeguard athlete health. The effective administration of anti-doping analyses demands sophisticated methods of detection and for many years there was an acknowledged lag between the cheaters and the testers. The establishment of WADA, an organization with specialized responsibilities and enhanced capabilities in drug detection, represented a significant leap forward in the fight against doping. The international harmonization of anti-doping rules, the refinement of analytical techniques, and an array of expanded regulatory powers now function in complementary ways to alter the landscape of sport to favour the clean athlete.

Regular revision of the Prohibited List ensures that current trends in drug misuse are appropriately monitored and that this information is available to sports physicians, who have professional obligations to be familiar with this List. When athletes need genuine medical intervention requiring the use of prohibited substances, the process of TUE may be invoked to ensure that their health is appropriately balanced against the requirements of fairness in their sport. For young athletes with asthma, ADHD, and type-1 diabetes, for example, physician familiarity with the TUE process is extremely important to their routine medical care and continued participation in sport. Physicians with vested responsibilities to young athletes have always been bound by unequivocal codes of ethical practice. However, those who disregard this responsibility may now also be subjected to sanctions.

The modern advent of youth sport highlights the continuing need for educational strategies that are values-based, widely accessible, and readily implemented. Physicians should be aware of the phases and circumstances in an athlete's developing career where their vulnerability to drug misuse is predictably increased. Those involved in treating athletes need to recognize possible doping behaviour and side effects and to intervene appropriately to provide support to the athlete. Finally, we should all examine and reflect upon the fundamental ethical underpinnings that contribute to the value of sport.

Summary

- There is a long history of drug misuse in sport.
- Since its creation, the World Anti-Doping Agency (WADA) has assumed responsibility from the International Olympic Committee for all matters of anti-doping.
- The WADA administers an internationally agreed Code, harmonizing the list of prohibited substances and methods, laboratory standards, detection methodologies, sanctions, and educational strategies.
- Physicians responsible for the care of young athletes are obligated to be well acquainted with their responsibilities under the Code
- Athletes requiring the use of prohibited drugs for legitimate clinical reasons may invoke the process of Therapeutic Use Exemption.
- Evidence-based, complementary methods of drug detection are driven by science and research.
- Contemporary anti-doping strategies include out-of-competition testing, use of investigations, and the implementation of the Athlete Biological Passport.
- Education with the goal of prevention of doping behaviour is critical, particularly when focused on youth development in sport.
- The overarching goal of the WADA and the stakeholders in sport is protection of the clean athlete.

We acknowledge Andrew Slack, Olivier Rabin, and Tony Cunningham for their contributions to this chapter.

References

1. Yesalis CE, Bahrke MS. History of doping in sport. *Int Sports Studies.* 2002; 24: 42–76.
2. Butler M. Doping violations: Olympic Athletics. In: *IAAF World Championships Beijing 2015 Statistics Handbook.* Monaco: IAAF; 2015. p. 419–420.
3. Gerrard DF. Playing foreign policy games: States drugs and other Olympian vices. *Sport in society: Cultures, commerce, media, politics.* 2008; 11: 459–466.
4. Pipe A. Drugs, sport, and the new millennium. *Clin J Sport Med.* 2000; 10: 7–8.
5. World Anti-Doping Agency. *World Anti-Doping Code.* Montreal: World Anti-Doping Agency; 2015 [cited 2016 January]. Available from: https://www.wada-ama.org/en/resources/the-code/world-anti-doping-code
6. World Anti-Doping Agency. *Prohibited List.* Montreal: World Anti-Doping Agency; 2016 [cited 2016 January]. Available from: https://www.wada-ama.org/en/resources/science-medicine/prohibited-list
7. World Anti-Doping Agency. *International Standard for Laboratories (ISL).* Montreal: World Anti-Doping Agency; 2015 [cited 2016 January]. Available from: https://www.wada-ama.org/en/resources/laboratories/international-standard-for-laboratories-isl
8. World Anti-Doping Agency. *International Standard for Testing and Investigations.* Montreal: World Anti-Doping Agency; 2015 [cited 2016 January]. Available from: https://www.wada-ama.org/en/resources/world-anti-doping-program/international-standard-for-testing-and-investigations-isti-0
9. World Anti-Doping Agency. *International Standard for Therapeutic Use Exemptions.* Montreal: World Anti-Doping Agency; 2016 [cited 2016 January]. Available from: https://www.wada-ama.org/en/resources/therapeutic-use-exemption-tue/international-standard-for-therapeutic-use-exemptions-istue
10. Riordan J, Jones RE. *Sport and physical education in China.* New York: Taylor and Francis; 1999.
11. International Olympic Committee. Olympic Charter. Lausanne: International Olympic Committee; 2015 [cited 2016 January]. Available from: http://www. fig-gymnastics.com/ publicdir/rules/files/ main/TR%202016-e. pdf
12. Federation Internationale de Gymnastique. Technical regulations. Lausanne: Federation Internationale de Gymnastique; 2015 [cited 2016 January]. Available from: http://www.fig-gymnastics.com/publicdir/rules/files/main/TR%202015-e.pdf
13. Rob Wood. *Oldest and Youngest Olympians (Summer Games).* 2016 [cited 2016 January]. Available from: http://www.topendsports.com/events/summer/oldest-youngest.htm
14. Hains D. Behind the Bouchard family's double fault in tax court. *The Globe and Mail.* 2014 July 7. Available at: http://www.theglobeandmail.com/report-on-business/industry-news/the-law-page/behind-the-bouchard-familys-double-fault-in-tax-court/article19500417/
15. Arshad R. The world's 100 highest-paid athletes. *Forbes.* 2015 June 14.
16. Vettennieme E. Why was doping banned in 1928? The IAAF, stimulants and the impact of racial beliefs. *Linkunta & Tiede.* 2010; 47: 24–29.
17. Ljungqvist A. Half a century of challenges. *Bioanalysis.* 2012; 4: 1531–1533.
18. Mottram D. The evolution of doping and anti-doping in sport. In: *Drugs in sport.* Mottram D, Chester N (eds.) New York: Routledge; 2015. p. 24.
19. Muller RK. History of doping and doping control. *Handb Exp Pharmacol.* 2010; 195: 1–23.
20. Klein HG. Blood transfusion in athletes-games people play. *New Engl J Med.* 1985; 312: 854–856.
21. Mazzoni I, Barosso O, Rabin O. Structure and review process by the World Anti-Doping Agency. *J Anal Toxicol.* 2011; 35: 608–612.
22. Bahrke MS, Yesalis CE. Abuse of anabolic androgenic steroids and related substances in sport and exercise. *Curr Opin Pharmacol.* 2004; 4: 614–620.
23. Achar S, Rostamian A, Narayan SM. Cardiac and metabolic effects of anabolic androgenic steroid aubse on lipids, blood pressure, left ventricular dimension and rhythm. *Am J Cardiol.* 2010; 106: 893–901.
24. Lumia AR, McGinnis MY. Impact of anabolic androgenic steroids on adolescent males. *Physiol Behav.* 2010; 100: 199–204.
25. Kanayama G, Hudson JI, Pope HGJ. Long-term psychiatric and medical consequences of anabolic-androgenic steroid abuse: a looming public health concern? *Drug Alcohol Depend.* 2008; 98: 1–12.
26. World Anti-Doping Agency. Final arbitral decision, *ASADA v. O'Neill and ors*, CAS 2008/A/1591, 1592 & 1616. Montreal: World Anti-Doping Agency; 2009 [cited 2016 January]. Available from: https://www.wada-ama.org/en/resources/legal/cas-wada-v-oneill-ca-asada
27. Boghosian T, Barroso O, Ivanova V, Rabin O. Ensuring high quality in anti-doping laboratories. *Bioanalysis.* 2012; 4: 1591–1601.
28. GlobalDRO. Colorado Springs, London, Ottawa, Tokyo: GlobalDRO; 2016 [cited 2016 January]. Available from: http://globaldro.com/Home.
29. Fitch KD. Therapeutic use exemptions (TUEs) at the Olympic Games. *Br J Sports Med.* 2013; 47: 815–818.
30. World Anti-Doping Agency. Decision rendered by the Court of Arbitration for Sport, *International Shooting Sport Federation (ISSF) v. WADA*, CAS 2013/A/3437. Montreal: World Anti-Doping Agency; 2015 [cited 2016 January]. Available from: https://www.wada-ama.org/en/resources/cas-international-shooting-sport-federation-issf-v-wada
31. Bergeron M, Mountjoy M, Armstrong N, *et al.* International Olympic Committee consensus statement on youth athletic development. *Br J Sports Med.* 2015; 49: 843–851.
32. Pipe A, Best T. Drugs. *Sport Med Practice.* 2002; 12: 201–202.

33. International Olympic Committee. *Olympic Movement Medical Code*. Lausanne: International Olympic Committee; 2009 [cited 2016 January]. Available from: https://www.olympic.org/medical-and-scientific-commission
34. United States Anti-Doping Agency (USADA). Colorado Springs, CO: USADA; 2012 [cited 2013 May]. Available from: http://www.usada.org/
35. Gerrard DF. Drug misuse in modern sport: Are cheats still winning? *NZ Fam Phys*. 2005; 32: 7–10.
36. United States Anti-Doping Agency (USADA). HealthPro Advantage. Colorado Springs, CO: USADA; 2016 [cited 2016 January]. Available from: http://www.usada.org/resources/healthpro
37. Chan D, Hardcastle S, Lentillon-Kaestner V, *et al*. Athletes' beliefs about and attitudes towards taking banned performance-enhancing substances: A qualitative study. *Sport Exerc Perf Psych*. 2014; 3: 241–257.
38. World Anti-Doping Agency. *Doping and Related Issues—Anti-Doping Textbook*. Montreal: World Anti-Doping Agency; 2015 [cited 2016 January]. Available from: http://antidopinglearninghub.org/en
39. Bird SR, Goebel C, Burke LM, *et al*. Doping in sport and exercise: anabolic, ergogenic, health and clinical issues. *Ann Clin Biochem*. 2015; 53(Pt 2): 196–221.
40. Lamb DR. Anabolic Steroids in athletics: how well do they work and how dangerous are they? *Am J Sports Med*. 1984; 12: 31–83.
41. Onakomaiya MM, Henderson LP. Mad men, women and steroid cocktails: a review of the impact of sex and other factors on anabolic androgenic steroids effects on affective behaviors. *Psychopharmacology (Berl)*. 2016; 233: 549–569.
42. Casella M, Dello Russo A, Izzo G, *et al*. Ventricular arrhythmias induced by long-term use of ephedrine in two competitive athletes. *Heart Vessels*. 2015; 30: 280–283.
43. Berman JA, Setty A, Steiner MJ, *et al*. Complicated hypertension related to the abuse of ephedrine and caffeine alkaloids. *J Addict Dis*. 2006; 25: 45–48.
44. Schaefer M, Smith J, Dahm D, *et al*. Ephedra use in a select group of adolescent athletes. *J Sports Sci Med*. 2006; 5: 407–414.
45. World Anti-Doping Agency. Sport Physician's tool kit. Montreal: World Anti-Doping Agency; 2015 [cited 2016 January]. Available from: https://www.wada-ama.org/en/resources/education-and-awareness/sport-physicians-tool-kit-online-version
46. Shibata J, Hasegawa J, Siemens HJ, *et al*. Hemostasis and coagulation at a hematocrit level of 0.85: functional consequences of erythrocytosis. *Blood*. 2003; 101: 4416–4422.
47. Pearson TC, Wetherley-Mein G. Vascular occlusive episodes and venous haematocrit in primary proliferative polycythaemia. *Lancet*. 1978; 2: 1219–1222.
48. Frattini K. *Cycling community would welcome apology, returned titles from Jeanson, says Cycling Canada CEO*. London: Immediate Media Company; 2015 [cited 2016 January]. Available from: http://www.cyclingnews.com/news/cycling-community-would-welcome-apology-returned-titles-from-jeanson-says-cycling-canada-ceo/
49. Sottas PE, Vernec A. Current implementation and future of the Athlete Biological Passport. *Bioanalysis*. 2012; 4: 1645–1652.
50. Brennan BP, Kanayama G, Hudson JI, *et al*. Human growth hormone abuse in male weighlifters. *Am J Addict*. 2011; 20: 9–13.
51. Pitsiladis Y. The Athlome Project Consortium: A concerted effort to discover genomic and other 'OMIC' markers of athletic performance. *Physiol Genomics*. 2015; 48: 183–90.
52. International Association of Athletics Federations (IAAF). IAAF commitment to healthy and drug-free athletics. Monaco: IAAF; 2015 [cited January 2016]. Available from: http://www.iaaf.org/about-iaaf/medical-anti-doping
53. World Anti-Doping Agency. *The Independent Commission Review. Final Report*. Montreal: World Anti-Doping Agency; 2015 [cited 2016 January]. Available from: https://www.wada-ama.org/en/resources/world-anti-doping-program/independent-commission-report-1
54. Thevis M, Geyer H, Mareck U, *et al*. Individualization of urine samples in doping control by steroid profiling and PCR-based DNA analysis. *Anal Bioanal Chem*. 2007; 388: 1539–1543.
55. Thevis M, Geyer H, Sigmund G, *et al*. Sports drug testing: Analytical aspects of selected cases of suspected, purported, and proven urine manipulation. *J Pharm Biomed Anal*. 2012; 5: 26–32.
56. College of Physicians and Surgeons of Ontario (CPSO). *Anabolic Steroids, Substances and Methods Prohibited in Sport*. Toronto: CPSO; 2010 [cited 2015 December]. Available from: http://www.cpso.on.ca/CPSO/media/uploadedfiles/policies/policies/policyitems/anabolic_steroids.pdf?ext=.pdf
57. Medical Council of New Zealand (MCNZ). Wellington: MCNZ; 2015 [cited 2015 November] Available from: www.mcnz.org.nz
58. Lasne F, De Ceaurriz J. Recombinant erythropoietin in urine. *Nature*. 2000; 405: 635.
59. Rabin O. Involvement of the health industry in the fight against doping in sport. *Forensic Sci Int*. 2011; 213: 10–14.
60. United Nations Office on Drugs and Crime (UNODC). Early Warning Advisory on New Psychoactive Substances. New York: UNODC; 2015 [cited 2016 January]. Available from: https://www.unodc.org/LSS/Page/NPS
61. World Anti-Doping Agency. ADO Guide to the Code. Montreal: World Anti-Doping Agency; 2015 [cited 2016 January]. Available from: https://www.wada-ama.org/en/resources/the-code/ado-reference-guide-to-the-code
62. World Anti-Doping Agency. *Coach's Tool Kit*. Montreal: World Anti-Doping Agency; 2014 [cited 2016 January]. Available from: https://www.wada-ama.org/en/resources/education-and-awareness/coachs-tool-kit

CHAPTER 50

Protecting child athletes

Medical mismanagement and other forms of non-accidental violence

Margo Mountjoy, Sandi Kirby, and Anne Tiivas

Introduction

Participation in sport has many recognized benefits for children's physical, psychological, and social health and development. Despite these benefits, sport participation is not without inherent risks for sport-related injury or illnesses, and many chapters in this book eloquently summarize the well-established science base in these fields. Sport, as an institution within a larger cultural society, is not automatically protected from the risks of abuse and harassment, which are identified by the United Nations as 'non accidental violence'.

Young people have the right to live free from violence as outlined in the United Nations (UN) Convention on the Rights of the Child. Article 19 defines violence as, 'all forms of physical violence, injury and abuse, neglect or negligent treatment, maltreatment or exploitation, including sexual abuse while in the care of parent(s), legal guardian(s) or any other person who has care of the child'.[1] The UN Declaration of Human Rights applies these rights to the sporting context, where athletes have 'the right to enjoy a safe and supportive sport environment'.[2] The Olympic Charter supports this concept stating that 'the practice of sport is a human right. Every individual must have the possibility of practising sport, without discrimination of any kind .... with respect for universal fundamental ethical principles ... and the preservation of human dignity'.[3] The 2016 International Olympic Committee (IOC) Consensus Statement on Harassment and Abuse in Sport clearly outlines that athletes of all ages have the right to engage in 'safe sport': *... an athletic environment which is respectful, equitable and free from all forms of non-accidental violence to athletes.*[4]

The UN Conventions on the Rights of the Child defines child as 'every human being below the age of eighteen years unless under the law applicable to the child, majority is attained earlier'.[1] Children around the world play and participate in organized sport. When they participate in organized sport and are identified as having potential to be talented, they can be referred to as child athletes. Once a child acquires the label of 'athlete', it frequently overrides their identity as a child, and often their rights as children are eroded as well.

Child victimization exists in every community in any country. Sport is also present in every community. Despite sport being in the public domain and highly child populated, there remain gaps in the field of research on child well-being and on non-accidental violence against children in sport.[5] The child abuse research in sport has, however, grown over the last two decades, as has the global understanding of the infringements of children's rights in sport.[6–8]

Failure to protect child athletes from non-accidental violence has many consequences for the child victims, the victims' families and teammates, and for sport organizations in general. For the athlete, the experience of abuse and harassment in sport can result in serious and long-term effects, including physical, cognitive, emotional, behavioural, and mental health consequences. As well, victims can suffer from long-term impaired personal relationships in the family, workplace, and/or community.[9] For sport, the consequences of non-accidental violence are also significant resulting in reputational damage, a reduction in public confidence, athlete drop out, loss of fans, and sponsorship opportunities.

Box 50.1 Child Athlete Voices

'Yeah, there was definitely times when you could have someone [one of the coaches] really having a go at you, to the point that like you'd be crying.'

(Young man: district level rugby, national level athletics)

'I mean the whole training was like, if you do one thing wrong then suddenly like you are being screamed at in the middle of an entire gym whether there is 5 year olds in there, or just your team in there. You are pointed out, isolated out, whether it's sent out the gym or just like screamed at or laughed at in front of the entire club.'

(Young woman: international level gymnastics)

'She would just swear at you and go mental, and her face would go bright red and storm off, and just wouldn't accept any sort of argument or reasoning at all.'

(Young man: national level swimming, national level triathlon)

'We had a competition in training called ... we called it 'juice boy' basically, just a penalty shoot-out and the loser has to wear a pretty pink helmet the next time they go on the ice. There was one occasion where the goalies were told to let everybody score except this one kid.'

(Young man: district level ice-hockey, local level football)

To clearly describe the problem, this chapter reviews the underlying science base in the field of non-accidental violence in child athletes, with a particular focus on the unique vulnerabilities of the elite child athlete, the athlete with a disability, and the lesbian, gay, bisexual, and transgender (LGBT) population. The research findings outlining the area of medical mismanagement of child athletes as a form of non-accidental violence will be explored. To provide an action plan, the landscape of prevention measures for the protection of children in sport will be outlined.

Protecting child athletes from forms of non-accidental violence

Non-accidental violence: the science base

The accumulating research indicates that any non-accidental violence athletes experience in sport is not limited to adult athletes. Though much of the research focuses on athletes in general, this chapter highlights the research that is applicable to children in sport. The science base for the types of non-accidental violence in sport identified in the recent *IOC Consensus Statement: Harassment and Abuse in Sport* are defined and discussed.[10] These include psychological abuse, physical abuse, sexual abuse, and neglect. These forms of non-accidental violence are placed in the overall sport context in Figure 50.1.

Psychological abuse

Psychological abuse is a form of interpersonal violence experienced by athletes. It is sometimes referred to as emotional abuse. Reported forms of psychological abuse in athletes include denigrating, belittling, or humiliating an athlete, ignoring them, isolating them, shouting and/or swearing at them, denying them attention and support, and scapegoating them.[11–13] For the child athlete, the harm from these emotional forms of abuse is intensified when the source is a person who has perceived power over them, such as a coach, a medical officer, an athletic trainer, or a sport psychologist. Gervis and Dunn also report that as child athletes become elite performers (national and international athletes), the 'behaviour of their coaches changed and became more negative' and that 'if the potential of a child athlete is recognized externally, this elevated the position of the coach …' which may then lead coaches to develop an attitude of …' a win at all costs approach'.[9] Leahy[14] regards psychological abuse as the gateway to all other abuses that children (and adults) experience; this is a position endorsed in the IOC Consensus Statement.[10]

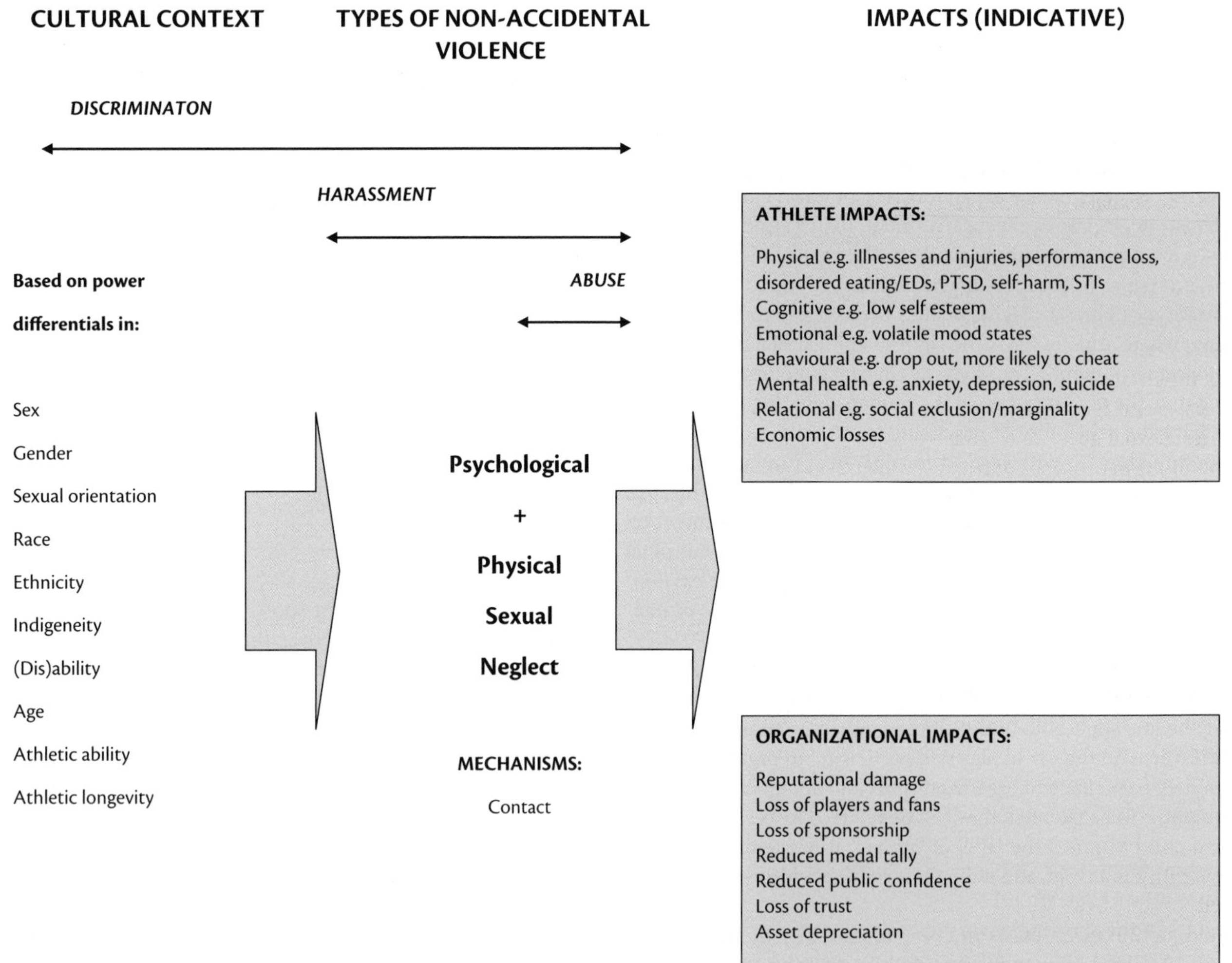

Figure 50.1 Non-accidental harms in the sport context.

Physical abuse and forced physical exertion

Physical abuse includes direct behaviours (e.g. hitting, slapping, kicking, pushing, shoving, beating, picking up and throwing a child down, and violent shaking) and maltreatment (e.g. overtraining, playing while injured, ill, or in pain, doping, forced ingestion of alcohol or noxious substances).[7,15] Physical abuse may happen on the field of play (e.g. excessive force during contact sports) or away from the field of play. In sport, forced physical exertion is the pushing of children beyond their safe physical limits. It may be exertion over a single time frame to the point where the child collapses or vomits from distress, or it may be repeated exertions over a training block of time that have a cumulative effect of wearing down the child's physical and mental resources. Another example of physical abuse in sport is where training programmes are carried out in extreme environmental conditions (heat, cold, wind) or where the child is unable to obtain sufficient recovery time, fluids, or food during the training or in-between training sessions. Physical punishment alternating with periods of kindness is a technique utilized by perpetrators to keep children uncertain and vulnerable.[16]

Sexual abuse

Sexual harassment is sexualized verbal, non-verbal, or physical behaviour, intended or unintended, legal, or illegal, based upon an abuse of power and trust and considered by the victim or a bystander to be unwanted. Sexual abuse is any sexual activity, with or without penetration, where consent is not or cannot be given, often involving manipulation by grooming and entrapment of the athlete, and sometimes involving aggressive coercion.[6] Sexual abuse may be but one of many expressions of 'coaches' abuse of their power'.[9] Sport is full of gendered power relations, that is, where most of those in power are male and older than less powerful athletes. Sexual harassment rates vary from 19 to 92% and sexual abuse from 2 to 49%.[6,17–19] For both male and female children in sport, the higher their performance level, the more sexual harassment and/or abuse they experience, although girls report this experience far more than boys.[20] Males are most often reported as perpetrators.[16]

It is important to note that sexual abuse can be perpetrated by both males and females from all socio-economic groups and in all societies. Sexual abuse and harassment by peers is as common as that by adults in positions of trust—both in the sports environment and in the general population.[7] Assumptions, often based on stereotypes, about the perceived level of risk posed by particular groups, can lead to children being unprotected.

Neglect

The child athlete is particularly vulnerable to the physical effects of neglect in the sporting context. For example, children are more vulnerable to the effects of under hydration, which can occur from exercising in the extreme heat relative to the adult athlete (see chapter 14). In addition, the child athlete is more vulnerable to nutrient and energy deprivation required for the additional nutritional demands of growth and development of the child athlete (see Chapter 47). Finally, the child athlete has a vulnerable musculoskeletal system that is susceptible to sport injury at growth plates and apophyses[2] (see Chapter 40).

Neglect in the sporting environment also includes the failure to prevent overuse injuries and overtraining (see Chapter 38). The failure to provide a safe sporting environment (equipment, refereeing, field of play) is another form of neglect in sport. These failures in oversight can lead to acute preventable injuries and/or recurrent injuries. In particular, sport concussion in the child athlete is an area of concern as the long-term effects of traumatic brain injury on the child brain are largely unknown. Finally, the denial of the child athlete to medical care when needed is another form of neglect.[13]

Conceptual framework

The various forms of non-accidental violence or threats to the child athlete can be organized into three categories, based on the relationships between the abuser and the victim. These categories are summarized in a conceptual model as depicted in Table 50.1. This model not only acts a resource to identify the various forms of threats to children, but also serves as a model to help focus prevention activities.

Delivery mechanisms of non-accidental violence

The methods or ways that non-accidental violence is expressed in sport are varied. Non-accidental violence can either be experienced by direct contact of the perpetrator to the victim, or non-contact in nature. Where physical proximity to children and youth is possible, physical or sexual abuse is possible. Even where there is no physical contact, verbal and sexual harassment, homophobic harassment, bullying, cyber-bullying, and neglect can occur[7,22,24] As the child athlete may experience more than one type of abuse concurrently and/or over time, they may also experience more than one mechanism of expression of that abuse.

The coach-athlete relationship

For the child athlete, the coach is a person in a position of trust, power, and authority. Although coaches are not the only ones who are in positions of power in relation to the athletes, they are the principal ones.[25] Other members in the child athlete entourage with power of the child include sport leaders, administration staff, team managers, sport scientists, team physicians, physiotherapists, nutritionists, chiropractors, psychologists, sport agents, and parents/caregivers. Even within sport teams or clubs, there is a power differential between the younger child athlete and his/her older peers or teammates who may be more senior team members, at a higher skill level, or in a more 'favoured position' on the team roster.

In sport culture globally, the coach has authority that allows him/her to dictate and control opportunities for the child athlete;

Table 50.1 Threats to child athletes.

Threats to child athletes		
Individual	**Relational**	**Organizational**
Injury Depression Self-harm Eating disorders Disordered eating	Sexual harassment Sexual abuse Physical abuse Forced physical exertion Emotional abuse Virtual maltreatment Neglect Bullying	Abuse from spectators Discrimination Cultures which normalize abuse Unhealthy training programmes Hazing Medical mismanagement Systematic doping Age-cheating

Mountjoy M, Rhind D, Tiivas A, *et al*. Safeguarding the child athletes in sport: a review, a framework and recommendations for the IOC youth athlete development model. Br J Sports Med. 2015; 49: 883-886.

for example, a coach may wish to protect and enhance the status of certain athletes, or subjectively provide rewards. They are adults who have direct and regular contact with child athletes and they may also integrate themselves into athletes' families and the athlete's private life.[16] Identifying behaviours that should signal risk factors for child safety include a coach/perpetrator who is a boundary challenger or who has a sense of entitlement in the coach-athlete relationship.[25] Examples of 'boundary challenging' behaviours are telling racist or sexist jokes, criticizing other coaches in front of athletes, touching athletes without cause, personal massaging, or counselling of athletes outside the realm of coaching, or engaging in ambiguous sexual behaviour.[16] Winning coaches may also behave with a sense of impunity and entitlement towards athletes and may seek to control everything around the athlete.[26] Public scrutiny of winning coaches is not the norm and can thus enable coaches to 'hide behind their record' if they are abusing athletes.

A coach or other person with sexual or violent motives who has access to child athletes may be able to take advantage of a single situation (opportunist abuser) or groom athletes into a prolonged period of sexual abuse. The motivations of adults who sexually abuse children are wide ranging. Not all abusers are conditioned paedophiles with a sexual attraction to a particular age group of children. For many adults, sexual abuse is one among many methods of exerting power over a child. Myths and stereotypes about the nature of sexual offending can contribute to children being unprotected. The grooming process for sexual harassment and abuse employed by a perpetrator follows a predictable pattern both inside and outside of sport. The steps utilized by a perpetrator in grooming the athlete victim are summarized in Box 50.2.

Box 50.2 The grooming process of child athletes

1. Targeting the victim

finding the vulnerable athlete

beginning a friendship and bond

2. Building trust and friendship

making the athlete feel special with gifts and rewards
developing the 'give/take' relationship, e.g. 'you have to do this, because I have done that for you'

3. Developing control and loyalty

refusing the athlete access to significant others, friends and supports

restricting access to parents and family

checking and testing the athlete's commitment

4. Building and securing secrecy

breaking of sexual boundaries silencing and disempowering the victim to speak out, e.g. 'you owe me', 'it's our little secret' 'no one will believe you'

From Brackenridge and Kirby[27].

Conditions for the continuation of violence and abuse include:

- if the perpetrator (coach or other person) is successful. For example: if the child athlete entourage tolerates harmful behaviours as the price to pay for winning;
- if silent bystanders do not act to protect the child athlete either because they are not suspicious, do not understand their responsibilities to report abuse, or are unwilling to raise any concerns;
- if there are no reporting procedures for complaints or concerns—or procedures are not well-publicized;
- if codes of ethics and behaviour are not established;
- if the sport culture enables the spending of considerable time with the child athlete away from scrutiny (e.g. exclusive coaching, late-night practices, extra help with finances or homework);
- if the sport culture is tolerant of discrimination and abuse of power; and
- if the child athlete cannot speak out.

Groups of children in sport vulnerable to non-accidental violence

The elite child athlete

Child athletes may be viewed as career athletes, that is, they are on a career path of training and performance with goals to be achieved and competitions to be won. They become elite athletes by virtue of their selection to national team rosters or because they compete as talented athletes 'on tour' (e.g. tennis or golf). They cope with the pressures of training and competing under the watchful, but not always altruistic, guidance of coaches and adult others. They often do this while away from traditional supports of children their age – social friends, school peers, family members, the home community, and other trusted adults in their social milieu.

Children as young as 5 years of age can be in formal training for competitive sport. Particularly in sports such as gymnastics, swimming, and diving, young athletes may be encouraged to start formal sport specialization training in early childhood. Concerns are identified in elite child sport about the pressures placed on a growing child by low minimum-age categories of competition in some sports, and the number of international competitions prior to going to the World Championships or the Olympic Games. In addition to the duration of training for elite child athletes, there is also concern about the intensity of the training, with the inherent risks of injury and illness in some sport disciplines. All of these factors can render the elite child athlete vulnerable and subject to intimidation.

Current sport talent systems and the use of sport terminology to describe children who participate in sport at talent and elite level can contribute to the diminution of the respect for their rights as 'children' first and 'athletes' second. As they progress through talent pathways young athletes are increasingly subject to the requirements and needs of others. Sport at elite level is big business and athletes are its commodities. Systems are largely developed for and by adults. The purpose of the athlete entourage at elite level is geared towards ensuring that the athlete is prepared to compete. Medical and other sport science support is often focused on the athlete's performance rather than a holistic approach to the athlete's well-being. Talent/high performance-development programmes need to place greater emphasis on young athlete's physical and mental development, well-being, and support needs than they do currently. Where safeguarding and protecting children is not seen as a central principle underpinning sports governance and administration, young athlete's well-being will continue to be compromised.

For the elite child athlete, sport participation can displace other academic, social, and family activities from their daily lives. They work under pressure often without the habitual social supports enjoyed by other children their own age. The nature of intensive training may require them to relocate from their home community, or to commute extensively. With frequent competitions to attend, better performance translates into increased travel. The child athlete, however, is still under the legal age to control their finances, drive, consume alcohol, travel unchaperoned; and importantly, give sexual consent.

Child athletes are also unable to render consent with respect to their participation in sports that have considerable risk for physical injury. i.e. sports where the level of physical contact is high (e.g. rugby or boxing), or where there is a substantial inherent risk due to the dangerous nature of the sport (e.g. ski jumping, bobsled). Trusted others must make the decisions about participation in contact or risky sport on behalf of the child athletes. Further, though sport is not inherently concerned with sex, sexual activity, or sexual harm, the social relations in sport, including sexual relations, is part of the fabric of sport. With child athletes, there is additional need to protect them from sexual activity they cannot legally consent to, and from sexual abuse or exploitation by persons in positions of trust, power or authority over them in sport, and from coercive sexual activity or sexual threats they may receive in the context of sport.[16,20]

Not all child athletes face the same issues and barriers. Some face distinct challenges based on one or more forms of discrimination while others face none. However, there are risks to child athletes unique to sport, including the coach-athlete relationship, the intensity of sport practice, the demands of competition, media interest in child athletes, athlete recruitment practices, practices requiring physical measurement, and biological passports, varied training locations and times, and sport initiation or hazing practices. Risks may also be increased simply by the nature of sport involvement. This can include exposure to a large number of adults in a wide variety of situations, the expectation to act in adult ways despite their young age, and travelling and lodging in relation to competition.

Sport research shows child athletes are made to be more vulnerable to violence if they:

- are female;
- participate in early-peaking sports;[27]
- have body-image concerns;
- import vulnerabilities from outside of sport;[16]
- are removed from parents (e.g. for the purpose of athletic training or coaching, for talent identification and 'camp' training programmes, for professional contracts);[20]
- are subject to loss of privacy and/or interference with her/his privacy, family, or home;
- are subject to negative, abusive attacks of her/his reputation through inappropriate exposure, and negative social media coverage;
- are subject to travel and hotel/billeting stays;
- are subject to violence by coaches and peer athletes through grooming and hazing/initiation practices;[15,28,29] and
- have coaches and other persons in authority over them who run 'closed practices' and express intolerance of open discussion of discrimination issues related to abuse but do tolerate the 'rule-breaking' or discriminatory behaviours in others.

Research with children is notoriously difficult to engage in and much of what we know about non-accidental violence of child athletes comes to us from those athletes long after the abuse and often only when they retire from sport.[20] There are relatively consistent data coming from the Caribbean, Australia, New Zealand, the UK, and some parts of Europe, Canada, and the USA. Data are now beginning to come in from Africa (Uganda, Nigeria, and Ethiopia) and from Asia (South Korea and Japan). There are negligible data from Central and South America and most of Asia. Future areas of research into the world of the child athlete should include the following areas: misuse/ harassment of child athletes; physical harm due to intensive training, over-training (and under-performing); physical and emotional harm through participation in aggressive sport; disrespectful and harmful treatment based on the child athlete's characteristics (perceived or actual); sexual harassment and abuse; deprivation (emotional and social isolation, disordered eating, disordered sleep/rest/recovery, isolation from 'normal' social relationships, including sexual relationships); self-harm; economic exploitation; and violence of various forms among children.

In sum, while sport can be a positive and nurturing experience for children, sport delivered with inadequate safeguards for athlete protection can lead to non-accidental violence to the child athlete.

The lesbian/gay/bisexual child athlete—and the transgender athlete

For sport to be safe and welcoming for all, sport must consider the needs of child athletes who are lesbian, gay, bisexual, or transgender. Such athletes often experience discrimination on the basis of their LGB identities. Homophobia is the 'irrational fear and misunderstanding about sexual orientation leading to harassment, uneasiness, anxiety, isolation, and violence '... behaviours and feelings of these kinds create unsafe environments that impede learning, adversely affect friendships, and hurt teams, athletes and coaches alike'.[30(p1)] Homophobia is expressed as antipathy, contempt, prejudice, aversion, or hatred on the basis of or due to negative perceptions about one's or a group's non-heterosexual orientation. Homosexuality is a crime in approximately 70 countries, 38 of them in Africa.

Seventy-three percent of the 9500 participants in a study by Denison and Kitchen[22] reported that sport was unwelcoming for LGB athletes. Further, they reported that for LGB athletes most stayed 'closeted' to avoid discrimination and cited fear of harassment as the reason. The two largest sources of homophobia were reported to be from the school physical education class (21%) and the spectator stands (41%). Seventy-nine percent of participants (younger than 22 years of age) reported they had witnessed or experienced homophobia in a sporting environment; 62% of gay men under 22 and 51% of lesbians reported being personally targeted; and 57% of bisexual men and 29% of bisexual females reported experiencing homophobia. The forms of homophobia and/or discrimination included cyber-bullying, physical assaults (pushing, hitting, punching, use of weapons, etc.), vandalizing property, verbal threats (threats to do harm), deliberate exclusion from social groups, bullying, verbal insults/slurs (use of derogatory words), phrases like 'that's so gay' or 'don't be so gay', and jokes/humour. Fear of rejection or fear of damaging team unity and spirit kept many young athletes in the closet. Suicide rates are problematic, for example, rates among Canadian homosexual teenagers are 10–12 times higher than the rate for heterosexual teenagers.[23] The research confirms that sport does not feel safe, nor is it actually safe, for the majority of LGB participants, including those who are under 22 years of age.

Sport uses chronological age and biological sex as co-requirements for event allocation. Trans-athletes can be seen by sport as complicating this picture. A transgendered person is one whose gender identity does not correspond to their biological sex. Gender is expressed in a variety of ways (dress, language, body language). For the child athlete, transgendered dress or behaviour might draw derision or discrimination from others in sport. Conflicts may arise in gender-prescribed sports such as rhythmic gymnastics, dance, and pairs skating in figure skating, and synchronized swimming.

A transsexual person is an individual who does not identify with their birth sex and may at some point seek sex reassignment. Although regulations vary between International Sport Federations, transsexuals who have completed sex re-assignment including surgery are generally welcome in sport in the chosen sex, but with various restrictions. There is very little research on transgendered and transsexual athletes in sport, although there are new policies being created for the acceptance of trans-athletes in local to international sport. When they are prepubescent, there appear to be no issues but for postpubescent athletes, conditions apply for permission to compete.

Lesbian, gay, bisexual, and trans-athletes may be subject to multiple or aggravated forms of discrimination on the basis of race, colour, sex, language, religion, political or other opinion, national, ethnic, indigenous or social origin, property, birth, age, or other status in addition to their sexual orientation or their trans identity.

The child athlete with a disability

The world of sport is rapidly expanding for persons with disabilities. Sport opportunities are available for children with various physical impairments, and to those who are visually impaired, deaf, and those with intellectual challenges. Children with physical or cognitive impairments may need additional supports and supervision to ensure they have equal and safe opportunities to participate in sport. Three streams of sport participation by those living with disabilities include the i) World Games for the Deaf, ii) the Special Olympics for those with intellectual disabilities, and iii) the Paralympic Games. Overall, the human rights approach to sport indicates that consideration be given to the age, the gender, and the disability of children in sport. (Interested readers are referred to Chapter 28 for further discussion).

Athletes with disabilities include 'those who have long-term physical, mental, intellectual, or sensory impairments which in interaction with certain barriers may hinder their full and effective participation in society on an equal basis with others'.[32(p3)] About 15% of the world's population live with disabilities, about 80% of whom live in developing countries with attendant concerns about inequities and exclusion. Experts conservatively estimate that people with disabilities are at least four times more likely to be victimized than people without disabilities:[33] those individuals with an intellectual impairment are at the highest risk of victimization.[34] For children, the number of victimized disabled children is estimated at 31% compared with 9% non-disabled children.[35] Recent data from sport confirm this increased risk of non-accidental violence.[36]

Emotional abuse, physical abuse, neglect, bullying (and cyberbullying), and sexual abuse occur in sport, though there is no comprehensive research on the nature and scope of these for child athletes with disabilities. Research in the field of violence in the population of children with disabilities is oriented towards prevalence rates and risk factors such as dependency, vulnerable living arrangements, social powerlessness, communication skill deficits, impaired judgment (the inability to detect who is safe to be around), learned compliance and the reluctance to challenge others, being viewed as a 'safe target for abuse', family isolation, and living in a system that has long rewarded compliant behaviours among those living with disabilities.[37] There is no published research about perpetrators of non-accidental violence of athletes with disabilities.

In sport, disability is an evolving concept, one, which results from interaction between those with impairments and the barriers to their full and effective sport participation.[38] As innovations in sport and physical activity expand, there is a pressing need to understand the nature of individual development and how participation can be enhanced or inhibited for persons with sensory, intellectual, or physical disabilities. These athletes need to be provided with age and gender appropriate assistance, and with information and education on non-accidental violence in sport.[39]

In addition to these general risks, specific vulnerabilities to non-accidental violence for child athletes with disabilities relate to:

- making uninformed assumptions about care needs of athletes;
- exploiting the athletes' dependence on personal care (e.g. communication requirements, travel requirements, and competition logistics); and
- blurring of the roles and responsibilities in the coach-athlete relationship[37] and, where present, the caregiver-athlete relationship[40].

Together, the rights of children of all ages, and in particular, the security from additional discriminations that may be experienced by LGBT children, female children, and/or children living with disabilities, suggest that a safe and welcoming sport environment for all children must take all into account.[29]

Medical mismanagement: a form of non-accidental violence in sport

As seen in Table 50.1, medical mismanagement is an organizational threat for the child athlete. Members of the support science team (physician, physiotherapist, nutritionist, psychologist, physiologist etc.), through unethical practice, lack of knowledge about child protection, and an abuse of power can also pose a threat to the child athlete. The Olympic Movement Medical Code provides clear behavioural expectations and guidelines for the appropriate and professional medical management of the athlete taking into consideration the sport culture and context. In particular, this ethical code explores the athlete/health care provider relationship reviewing the concepts of consent, confidentiality, and privacy, quality of care and treatment, as well as the special requirements of the child athlete. The Olympic Movement Medical Code also addresses the protection and promotion of athlete health during training and competition with respect to injury prevention, provision of field of play safety, and the ethical determination of the fitness to participate in sport and return to play following absence due to injury or illness.[41]

The Hippocratic Oath is pledged by all medical students upon graduation as they enter practice as a physician. This Oath outlines the ethical principles to guide medical practice and protect patients from harm. Sport culture however, can sometimes challenge the ethical principles outlined in the Hippocratic Oath by placing undue pressure on members of the athlete's medical support team to 'blur the boundaries', which may result in the provision of potentially unethical medical treatment for athletes. Specific factors that can negatively influence medical decision-making in the sport context include sponsorship pressures, competition qualification schedules, coach pressure, vicarious parental pressure for success, media attention, and the commodification of the athlete by members of the entourage.[42]

Examples of medical mismanagement of the child athlete include:[13]

- clearing the athlete to participate in sport despite medical contraindications for eligibility;
- encouraging return to play following injury or illness before recovery is complete;
- allowing the athlete to train or compete with injury, illness, and / or pain;
- failure to complete periodic health screening (prevention work) to identify injury or illness risks;
- failure to provide safe training and competition venues;
- failure to provide protection for exercising in extreme environments;
- failure to provide appropriately trained medical personnel for training and competition venues (relying on untrained coaches to monitor athlete health and provide primary care;
- practising in a field of medicine beyond the clinician's trained scope of practice;
- failure to recognize athlete risk factors such as injuries in child athletes to the growth plates, epiphyses, and apophyses; and
- failure to report child protection concerns to appropriate sport and statutory authorities.

Another form of medical mismanagement is the excessive and often systematic prescription of analgesic medication to athletes. In particular, in soccer, up to 25% of youth athletes report the utilization of prescription drugs including pain relief, stimulants, sleeping aids, and anti-anxiety. The over-prescription of these medications can lead to health consequences from side effects, and even dependency.[43] The actual need to prescribe these drugs in a youth population raises an important ethical question about the safety of the training and sport in general. Rather than relying on medication to train and perform, attention in the youth athlete population should be better focused on appropriate youth athlete development with balanced training and attention to lifestyle issues as outlined in the IOC Youth Athlete Development Consensus Statement.[21]

A final form of medical mismanagement is the systematic implementation of doping regimens under 'medical' supervision. Examples of this form of non-accidental violence have been reported in athletes at the elite level—in particular in child athletes during the 2010 Singapore Summer Youth Olympic Games (ages 14–18 years). In this instance there were two anti-doping rule violations (ADRV) for diuretics used to cut weight to make a weight category in wrestling.[44] In the 2014 Nanjing Summer Youth Olympic Games, one ADRV was reported also for a diuretic in the weight category sport of Taekwondo.[45] Finally, in the 2014 Glasgow Commonwealth Games, there was another diuretic ADRV for a 16-year-old weight lifter.[46] The abuse of athlete health through the utilization of prohibited doping substances and methods in addition to the unethical behaviour should never be condoned in sport.

Child athlete protection in sport

Given the available science base on non-accidental violence in youth sport, it is apparent that prevention is an urgent matter. Everyone in sport at all levels must act with a unified voice delivering the message of the importance of athlete protection and the preservation of 'safe sport' governance principles. Child athlete protection will have a different and unique focus depending on the type of organization, the cultural and political context within which it operates. Integration, collaboration, and coordination of all related groups is imperative for maximum preventative benefit.

Preventative action to ensure that children are safe from all forms of harm is typically described as 'safeguarding'. Child protection is action that is required to protect specific children who are suffering or at risk of suffering harm from any form of non-accidental violence. Not all countries have statutory instruments in place that are supported by structures, systems, and government guidance which enable the safeguarding and protection of children and young people. In some communities, statutory and law enforcement agencies may be seen as sources of violence and corruption to which they are unlikely to turn for protection. Consequently, the roles of organizations that have primary prevention and care roles, such as health care providers, schools, sports organizations, and NGOs need to take the initiative. Even in countries that have highly developed child protection systems, it is rare that sport is recognized as part of the multi-agency network that should contribute to a holistic approach to safeguarding and protecting children.

Reports into the circumstances surrounding child deaths and into institutional and organizational abuse have long recognized the importance of agencies and organizations working together in children's best interests. Mechanisms which support communication between sports bodies and statutory agencies to understand each other's roles and responsibilities in protecting children need to be developed.

Sport, particularly elite sport, has traditionally operated outside of the requirements on public bodies to ensure children's well-being and protection. It is only in the last 15–20 years, through the revelations of abuse by high-profile individuals in sport and the consequent bad publicity and loss of sponsorship, that sports bodies have recognized the need to take action to improve the quality of children's experience of sport.

Sports organizations generally do not have a long history of delivering child-centred practice as they have been developed and run by adults for adults. Sport coaching generally is only recently developing education and qualifications for coaching children, which recognize their different development needs from adults. The UK Coaching Framework (including its Coaching Children curriculum) and the Netherlands Master Coach programmes are positive developments in this area. While children in countries where children's rights are well established are aware of their rights and are used to their views being sought when they are in school or in receipt of other public services, sports bodies still lack confidence in how to communicate with children and involve them in decisions that affect them, including health care.

The International Safeguards for Children in Sport framework describes the key steps which sports organizations need to take based on the experiences of organizations which have implemented them.

Sports organizations and their staff and volunteers are not expected to be experts in child protection, but they do need to be provided with sufficient information and training in order to fulfil their roles and responsibilities in child protection. In addition, the child athlete's entourage needs context-specific training to recognize and respond to the different needs of talented and elite young athletes. This should include awareness of the reasons why this cohort of young people is made more vulnerable to abuse within sport and what actions need to be taken to prevent this and how to respond when they have concerns. Due to the traditionally closed nature of many elite sport establishments it is essential that athletes, their parents, and their entourage have access to independent sources of advice and support. Crucially, young athletes need to be able to make informed choices about their training, education, health care, and life choices.

Many young athletes will bring with them problems from home or from their community. The pressures of performance sport may exacerbate existing mental health problems, self-harm, suicidal ideation, eating disorders, or other health issues. Bullying may be exacerbated both in the real world and through cyber-bullying. Some children may be experiencing abuse in their families, including abuse that is tied to parental expectations of their performance. They may be pushed to cheat and risk disciplinary sanctions. Children who are dependent on education scholarships may feel pressured to exceed training and performance regulations. The athlete's entourage is not expected to be experts in all of these areas. In fact, there are dangers when professionals act outside of their competency areas and either seek to intervene or fail to intervene, based on only a little knowledge, or in misplaced faith in a professional's perceived power or status. It is essential that the child athlete's entourage understands the importance of a holistic approach to their well-being and knows where to turn for help when child protection concerns arise either within or outside of the sport environment. Every organization should have a designated role for child protection. The child athlete should have access to independent advice and support.

The current media attention on wider sport integrity issues such as financial corruption, doping, match-fixing, and illegal betting largely fails to address the well-being of athletes—particularly young and other vulnerable athletes. The image of sport and the potential impact on the income by vested interests appears to be the primary concern of the media and of the international bodies concerned. All those concerned with children's well-being need to contribute to raising the profile of athlete well-being and protection in order to secure the resources needed to address the scale of the problems faced by our young people.

Key organizations in child athlete protection

For all sports organizations, safeguarding and protecting children should form an integral part of good governance and be reflective of strong child athlete-centred leadership. However, sports organizations need help from leading sports bodies and child rights and protection agencies to achieve this. A multi-agency and multidisciplinary approach is required at all levels of sport delivery.

A summary of the key organizations active in sport in the area of child athlete protection can be found in Table 50.2. As the pinnacle of international sport, the IOC has been active in athlete protection through the development and promotion of best practice for and resources to support the protection of elite young athletes. For example, the IOC has published two Consensus statements in the field in 2008[47] and 2016,[10] and has established a Working Group on Harassment and Abuse in Sport consisting of representatives from the IOC Athletes Commission, Women and Sport Commission, IOC Medical Commission, IOC Entourage Commission, and the International Paralympic Commission. Other related activity of

Table 50.2 Organizations and institutions responsible for child athlete protection.

Institution/organization	Example
International sport organizations	International Olympic Committee International Sport Federations Commonwealth Games Continental Sport Organizations International Paralympic Committee
International governance/ sport integrity agencies	World Anti-Doping Agency International Centre for Ethics in Sport
National sport organizations	National Olympic Committees National Sport Organizations National Anti-Doping Agencies National Centres for Sport Ethics
Local sport organizations	Regional Sport Organizations Leagues Clubs
Child advocacy groups	United Nations International Children's Emergency Fund Commonwealth Advocacy Board International Safeguards for Children in Sport Founders group
Child rights organizations	Non-governmental organizations (NGOs) and specialist child/athlete protection agencies Canadian Centre for Child Protection (CCCP) National Centre for Missing and Exploited Children (NCMEC)
Non-governmental organizations	International Fair Play Movement
Sport medicine bodies	International Federation of Sport Medicine National Level Sport Medicine Organizations
Sport ethics bodies	Panathlon International
Sport research organizations	Brunel International Research Network for Athlete Welfare (BIRNAW)
Governments	Implementation of the United Nations Rights of the Child requirements into government funded sport programmes

the IOC includes the publication of related Consensus Statements on the Fitness and Health of Children,[48] the IOC Periodic Health Evaluation,[49] Exercise in Extreme Environments,[50] Age Determination,[51] and the IOC Youth Athlete Development Model.[21] The IOC has also developed a coach and athlete educational programme on Sexual Harassment and Abuse in Sport that forms an integral component of the educational programme during the Olympic and Youth Olympic Games. This educational tool is also available online at http://sha.olympic.org

Finally, the IOC can show leadership through ensuring athlete protection at all Olympic events as well as including athlete protection as a bidding criterion for the right of a country to host Olympic events. All international, regional, and national sport organizations have a duty of care to develop and implement policies and procedures to ensure the protection and well-being of their athletes. For example, the International Netball Federation and the International Sailing Federation are among 50 organizations to date that have adopted the International Safeguards for Children in Sport 2014.[52]

Non-Governmental Organizations who function within the realm of sport also have the responsibility to prevent non-accidental violence in sport through the implementation of safeguarding principles. An illustration of this principle is the International Fair Play Movement that has recognized the need to promote safeguarding practice as a key element of fair play principles.[53] In the realm of sport for development, there is also a need and role for athlete protection. For example, the United Nations International Children's Emergency Fund (UNICEF) and the Commonwealth Advisory Board for Sport have both embedded safeguarding requirements to their support for development programmes.

The most active international alliance in the field of safeguarding and protecting children in sport is the International Safeguards for Children in Sport Founders Group. This group was founded in 2012 by the National Society for the Protection of Cruelty to Children—Child Protection in Sport Unit (NSPCC-CPSU), UNICEF, Right to Play, the Commonwealth Secretariat, Keeping Children Safe, Beyond Sport, Women Win, UK Sport, and Comic Relief. Beyond Sport has supported and promoted the development of the International Safeguards for Children in Sport at its annual Summits, including a special inaugural award recognizing and honouring activity in safeguarding children in sport in 2015.[54] Implementation of the International Safeguards is being supported through a pilot project which combines virtual learning sets hosted by Founders Group members, resources hosted on the www.sportanddev.org platform, and a research programme co-ordinated by Brunel University (UK); these safeguards and implementation guidelines can be found online,[55] and include information covering all of the key types of sport contexts involved in the project—from international and national elite sport organizations to small development projects.

An example of a national level organization in the field is the UK's NSPCC-CPSU,[56] which is a specialist capacity-building organization created in 2001 initially in response to the growing concern about high-profile cases of child abuse in sport. It supports the implementation of its Standards for Safeguarding and Protecting Children in Sport for national governing bodies of sport, sports partnerships, and programmes for young people which are funded through the respective home country sports councils in England, Northern Ireland, and Wales, and by UK Sport for Olympic and Paralympic sports. It provides a comprehensive website www.thecpsu.org.uk for training, consultancy, and case-management support. It supports multi-agency strategic partnerships in England and Wales, which comprise sport and statutory agencies collaborating to address the key national issues for safeguarding and protecting children in and through sport. Other initiatives include the Australian Sport Commission's Play by the Rules[57] programme and the Netherlands Olympic Committee's programme.[58]

Governments have a key role to play in legislating to ensure the protection of children as well as other vulnerable groups both within and outside of sport. All governments that are signatories to the UN Convention on the Rights of the Child must reflect this in relevant laws. Government departments that have responsibilities for sport should ensure that national child protection guidance reflects sport's role in protecting young athletes. Some national sports councils set minimum child protection standards as criteria of funding to sports bodies and sports programmes.[59] Other government departments that have the responsibility for child protection should ensure that there is an integrated and collaborative approach between criminal justice, health, education, children's services, and sport. There should be systems and guidance to enable their agencies to work together to prevent non-accidental violence in sport medical mismanagement to ensure protection child athletes.

Existing key child athlete protection statutes

Table 50.3 outlines the many pivotal international statutes and declarations that provide the foundational principles underpinning child athlete protection prevention.

Table 50.3 International Statues and Declarations on Child Athlete Protection.

Organization	Statutes, statutory guidance, international declarations
Panathlon International	Panathlon Declaration of Ethics in Youth Sport (2004)
Safe Sport International	Declaration of Principles 2014
International Safeguards for Children in Sport Founders Group	International Safeguards for Children in Sport 2014—global framework.
United Nations	UN Convention on the Rights of the Child Universal Declaration of Human Rights UN Sport for Peace and Development project
United Nations International Children's Emergency Fund	Protecting Children from Violence in Sport—A Review (2010)
European Union programmes	International Centre for Ethics in Sport—Safeguarding Youth Sport—project focused on safeguarding talented and elite young athletes—final report 2015 Sport Respects Your Rights—Youth empowerment sexual harassment and abuse prevention project 2015 Gender Equality in Sport—Proposal for Strategic Actions (2014–20)
United Nations Educational, Scientific and Cultural Organization (UNESCO)	2013 UNESCO Declaration of Berlin

Implementation of child athlete prevention in sport

The International Safeguards for Children in Sport Founder's Group has developed a framework to assist sport organizations in the implementation of child athlete protection from non-accidental violence in sport. This framework is based on a review of the related research and was developed through consultation with over 50 organizations in several countries. The framework consists of eight Safeguards:[52]

1. Developing Your Policy
2. Procedures for Responding to Safeguarding Concerns
3. Advice and Support
4. Minimizing Risks to Children
5. Guidelines for Behaviour
6. Recruiting, Training and Communicating
7. Working with Partners
8. Monitoring and Evaluating

To facilitate successful implementation of these safeguarding principles, the International Safeguards for Children in Sport Founder's Group developed Pillars of implementation characterized by the acronym 'CHILDREN'. These Pillars are found in Table 50.4.[52]

In addition to the implementation of the Child Athlete Safeguarding Principles, sport organizations should ensure that they adopt and implement the WADA Anti-Doping Code[60] as well as the Olympic Movement Medical Code[41] to mitigate child athlete non-accidental violence through medical mismanagement.

Action Plan

The protection of child athletes requires a multi-disciplinary approach with the entire athlete entourage understanding each other's roles and responsibilities. To be effective, the Action Plan for all involved in children's sport must address:

- Prevention: the creation of a safe sporting environment through the implementation of the eight Safeguards.
- Investigation: the development of complaints reporting procedures, investigation, and disciplinary processes which link to relevant statutory agency processes, medical investigations, and possibly the criminal justice system.
- Treatment and recovery: the identification and integration of a multi-disciplinary treatment team to support the treatment and recovery of the child athlete victim, the victim's family, the victim's teammates, and other members of the entourage. This team should consist of the sport medicine team physician, a sport psychiatrist, sport psychologist, and other professionals as indicated by the particular situation on a case-by-case basis. For health professionals in sport who may be concerned about indicators of sexual abuse, it is essential that specialist advice is taken from statutory child protection agencies and staff with designated responsibility for child protection within their own agency. Where health professionals are operating within a sports context, these protocols may not be well established and lines of reporting should be clarified from the outset.

Conclusions

It is prudent to remember that the benefits of sport participation for children in a healthy and safe sport environment are numerous and far outweigh the health risks of physical inactivity. Coaches, sport physicians, sport administration staff, parents, and other members of the child athlete entourage should establish and implement best practices to ensure a safe, respectful, and welcoming sport experience for all participants.

Table 50.4 International Safeguards for Children in Sport Founder's Group–Pillars of Implementation for safeguarding principles

Pillar	Description
Cultural sensitivity	The Safeguards need to be tailored to the cultural and social norms of the context
Holistic	Safeguarding should be viewed as integrated into all aspects of an organization as opposed to being an additional element
Incentives	There needs to be a clear reason for individuals and an organization to work towards the Safeguards
Leadership	The Safeguards need to have strong support from those working in key leadership roles
Dynamic	Safeguarding systems need to be continually reviewed and adapted to maintain their relevance and effectiveness
Resources	The implementation of the Safeguards needs to be supported by appropriate resources (e.g. human, time and financial)
Engaging stakeholders	A democratic approach should be adopted which invites and listens to the voices of those in and around the sport (e.g. parents, coaches, community leaders)
Networks	An organization's progress towards the Safeguards will be strengthened by developing networks with other organizations

Box 50.3 Example of emotional abuse: child athlete narrative

'They (the coaches) just come from this world where anything and everything goes. She screamed at us, and it wasn't yelling, it was screaming. That was terrifying. Just hearing her voice now would terrify me. And it was mean. You know you can yell and say things like "you're doing it all wrong" and stuff like that. It was really hurtful. It seemed like she really tried to hurt you. And everything you did was wrong. Everything! You would do one thing wrong and she would come stomping over and stand over you and then physically manoeuvre your body and scream in your face. Sometimes she would smash CDs or whip CD cases at you. If you were practising and God forbid you messed up and something was in her range she would kick it so hard–it was like she was a soccer player! ...You didn't want to get too close to her at all. But on the other hand she was such a mother to all of us. Like we loved her–I loved her .... Because the way they treat you when you do so well, it's like I'm perfect, I could do no wrong. They are so proud of you and everyone is so happy, but then the second that it's not going so well you feel so insignificant, and small, and like nothing. It was always those two extremes. I think at a young age you know it's wrong, but at the same time you don't because you working towards competing and it feels so good when you do well, you just feel caught'.[61(p17)]

Anonymous child athlete voice of abuse

Summary

- Sport participation has health benefits for children.
- Non-accidental violence in sport (harassment and abuse) occurs in all sports and at all levels.
- The forms of non-accidental violence in sport include psychological, physical, sexual, and neglect.
- Psychological abuse is the gateway to all other forms of abuse.
- Medical mismanagement by members of the child athlete support team can be mitigated by the adoption and implementation of the Olympic Movement Medical Code and the World Anti-Doping Agency Code.
- Prevention of non-accidental violence in sport is based on the prevention framework consisting of eight Safeguarding principles implemented via the principles summarized by the CHILDREN acronym.
- The action plan should include: prevention, investigation, treatment, and recovery.

References

1. UNCRC 1989. United Nations Convention on the Rights of the Child. *UNCRC, 1989*. Article 1, adopted 1989, entered into force 2 September, 1990 in accordance with article 49. Available from: http://www.ohchr.org/en/professionalinterest/pages/crc.aspx [Accessed 16 Jan 2016].
2. UN Declaration of Human Rights adopted 10 Dec 1948, general assembly resolution 217. Available from: http://www.un.org/en/universal-declaration-human-rights/ [Accessed 16 Jan 2016].
3. The Olympic Charter, entered into force as from 2 August 2015. Available from: http://www.olympic.org/Documents/olympic_charter_en.pdf [Accessed 16 Jan 2016].
4. Ljungqvist A, Mountjoy M, Brackenridge CH, *et al.* IOC Consensus Statement on sexual harassment & abuse in sport. *Int J Sport Exer Psych.* 2008; 6: 442–449.
5. Stirling A, Kerr G. Sport psychology consultants as agents of child protection. *J App Sp Psych.* 2010; 22: 305–319.
6. Brackenridge CH, Fasting K. Sexual harassment and abuse in sport: The research context. *J Sexual Aggression.* 2002; 8: 3–15.
7. Brackenridge CH. Ending violence against athletes. *J Int Centre for Sport Security.* 2015; 2: 18–23.
8. Alexander K, Stafford A, Lewis R. *The experiences of children participating in organized sport in the UK.* London: NSPCC; 2011.
9. Gervis M., Dunn N. The emotional abuse of elite child athletes by their coaches. *Child Abuse Rev.* 2004; 13: 215–223.
10. Mountjoy M, Brackenridge C, Arrington M, *et al.* The IOC Consensus Statement: Harassment and abuse in sport. *Br J Sports Med.* 2016; 50: 1019–1029.
11. Leahy T, Pretty G, Tenenbaum GA. Perpetrator methodology as a predictor of traumatic symptomatology in adult survivors of childhood sexual abuse. *J Interpers Violence.* 2004; 19: 521–540.
12. Stafford A, Alexander K, Fry D. 'There was something that wasn't right because that was the only place I ever got treated like that': Children and young people's experiences of emotional harm. *Childhood.* 2015; 2: 121–137.
13. Mountjoy M, Rhind D, Tiivas A, *et al.* Safeguarding the child athletes in sport: a review, a framework and recommendations for the IOC youth athlete development model. *Br J Sports Med.* 2015; 49: 883–886.
14. Leahy T. Working with adult athlete survivors of sexual abuse. In: Hanrahan S, Andersen M (eds.) *Routledge handbook of applied sport psychology: A comprehensive guide for students and practitioners.* London: Routledge; 2010. p. 303–312.
15. Kirby SL, Wintrup G. Running the gauntlet: An examination of initiation/hazing and sexual abuse in sport. *J Sexual Aggression.* 2002; 8: 49–68.
16. Brackenridge CH. *Spoilsports: Understanding and preventing sexual exploitation in Sport.* London: Routledge; 2001.
17. Chroni S, Fasting, K. Prevalence of male sexual harassment among female sports participants in Greece. *Inq in Sport and Phys Educ.* 2009; 7: 288–296.
18. Baker TA, Byon, KK. Developing a scale of perception of sexual abuse in youth sports. (SPSAYS). *Meas in Phys Educ and Exerc Sci.* 2014; 18: 31–52.
19. Fasting K, Brackenridge CH, Knorre N. Performance level and sexual harassment prevalence among female athletes in the Czech Republic. *Women in Sport and Phys Act J.* 2010; 19: 26–32.
20. Kirby SL, Greaves L, Hankivsky O. *Dome of silence: Sexual harassment and abuse in sport.* London: Zed Books, Ltd; 2000.
21. Bergeron M, Mountjoy M, Armstrong N, *et al.* International Olympic Committee Consensus Statement on youth athletic development. *Br J Sport Med.* 2015; 49: 843–851.
22. Denison E and Kitchen A. *Out on the fields: The first international study on homophobia in sport.* Sydney: Repucom; 2015 May 10. Available from: http://www.outonthefields.com/
23. Goodyear S. Homophobia rampant in Canadian schools: Report. *Toronto Sun.* 2011 May 12 [cited 16 Jan 2016]. Available from: http://www.torontosun.com/2011/05/12/homophobia-rampant-in-canadian-schools-report
24. Kavanagh EJ, Jones I. '#cyberviolence: developing a typology for understanding virtual maltreatment in sport. In: Rhind D, Brackenridge CH (eds.) *Researching and enhancing Athlete Welfare.* London: Brunel University Press; 2014. p. 34–44.
25. Kirby SL, Demers G, Parent S. Vulnerability/prevention: considering the needs of disabled and gay athletes in the context of sexual harassment and abuse. *Int J Sport and Ex Psych.* 2008; 6: 407–426.
26. Fusco C, Kirby S. Are your kids safe? Media representations of sexual abuse in sport. In: Scraton S, Watson B, eds. *Sport, leisure and gendered spaces.* Vol. 67. Eastbourne: Leisure Studies Association; 2000. p. 43–72.
27. Brackenridge CH, Kirby S. Playing safe: assessing the risk of sexual abuse to elite child athletes. *Int Rev Sociol Sport.* 1997; 32: 407–418.
28. Brackenridge C, Fasting K, Kirby S, *et al.* Protecting children from violence in sport; a review from industrialized countries. Florence: UNICEF Innocenti Research Centre; 2010.
29. Johnson J, Holman M. *Making the team: Inside the world of sport initiations and hazing.* Toronto: Canadian Scholars' Press; 2004.
30. United Nations Committee on the Rights of the Child. *General Comment No. 13: The right of the child to freedom from all forms of violence.* Available from: http://www2.ohchr.org/english/bodies/crc/docs/CRC.C.GC.13_en.pdf [Accessed 16 Jan 2016].
31. Demers G. Homophobia in sport: Fact of life, taboo subject. *Can J Women and Coaching.* 2006; 2: 1–2.
32. United Nations Convention on the Rights of Persons with Disabilities. Resolution adopted by the General Assembly 24 January 2007. Article 2. Available from: http://www.un.org/disabilities/convention/conventionfull.shtml [Accessed 16 Jan 2016].
33. Sobsey D. *Violence and abuse in the lives of people with disabilities: The end of silent acceptance?* Baltimore: Paul H. Brook Publishers; 1994.
34. Sobsey D, Doe T. Patterns of sexual abuse and assault. *J Sex and Dis.* 1991; 9: 243–259.
35. Sullivan PM, Knutson JF. Maltreatment and disabilities: a population based epidemiological study. *Child Abuse and Neglect.* 2000; 24: 1257–1273.
36. Vertommen T, Schipper-van Veldhoven N, Wouters K, *et al.* Interpersonal violence against children in sport in the Netherlands and Belgium. *Child Abuse and Neglect.* 2015; 51: 223–36.
37. Valenti-Hein D, Schwartz L. *The sexual abuse interview for those with developmental difficulties.* Santa Barbara, CA: James Stanfield Company; 1995.

38. Rasmussen TJ, Bird MM, Dinesen C. *Different. Just like you: A psychosocial approach promoting the inclusion of persons with disabilities.* International Federation of Red Cross and Red Crescent Societies 2 Reference Centre for Psychosocial Support. 2015. Available from: http://assets.sportanddev.org/downloads/1.pdf [Accessed 16 Jan 2016].
39. United Nations Convention on the Rights of Persons with Disabilities. Resolution adopted by the General Assembly 24 January, 2007. Article 16. Available from: http://www.un.org/disabilities/convention/conventionfull.shtml [Accessed 16 Jan 2016].
40. Kerr A. *Protecting disabled children and adults in sport and recreation—The guide.* Leeds: National Coaching Foundation; 1999.
41. The International Olympic Committee (IOC). *The Olympic Movement Medical Code.* Lausanne: International Olympic Committee; 2009. Available from: https://stillmed.olympic.org/media/Document%20Library/OlympicOrg/IOC/Who-We-Are/Commissions/Medical-and-Scientific-Commission/Olympic-Movement-Medical-Code-01-10-2009.pdf#_ga=1.41250282.994748731.1473865375 [Accessed 16 Jan 2016].
42. Creighton D, Shrier I, Shultz R, *et al.* Return to play in sport: A decision-based model. *Clin J Sport Med.* 2010; 20: 379–385.
43. Tscholl P, Feddermann N, Junge A, *et al.* The use and abuse of painkillers in international soccer: data from 6 FIFA tournaments for female and youth players. *Am J Sports Med.* 2009; 37: 260–265.
44. International Olympic Committee (IOC). *2010 Singapore Youth Olympic Games Anti-Doping Rule Violation.* Lausanne: IOC; 2010. http://www.olympic.org/content/press-release/press-release-pr65-2010/. [Accessed 16 Jan 2016].
45. International Olympic Committee (IOC). *2014 Nanjing Youth Olympic Games Anti-Doping Rule Violation.* Lausanne: IOC; 2014. Available from: http://www.olympic.org/news/ioc-disqualifies-athlete-for-violating-anti-doping-rules-at-the-summer-youth-olympic-games/240150. [Accessed 16 Jan 2016].
46. Commonwealth Games. 2014 Glasgow Commonwealth Games Anti-Doping Rule Violation. Available from: http://www.bbc.com/sport/0/commonwealth-games/28541211 [Accessed 16 Jan 2016].
47. Ljungqvist A, Mountjoy M, Brackenridge CH, *et al.* IOC Consensus Statement on sexual harassment and abuse in sport. *Int J Sport Exer Psych.* 2008; 6: 442–449.
48. Mountjoy M, Anderson LB, Armstrong N, *et al.* IOC Consensus Statement on the health and fitness of children through sport. *Br J Sport Med.* 2011; 45: 839–848.
49. Ljungqvist A, Jenoure P, Engebretsen L, *et al.* The International Olympic Committee Consensus Statement on periodic health evaluation of elite athletes. *Clin J Sport Med.* 2009; 19: 347–365. *Br J Sports Med.* 2009; 43: 631–644.
50. Bergeron MF, Bahr R, Bartsch P, Bourdon L, *et al.* International Olympic Committee Consensus Statement on thermoregulatory and altitude challenges for the high-level athlete. *Br J Sports Med.* 2012; 46: 770–779.
51. Engebretsen L, Steffen K, Bahr R, *et al.* International Olympic Committee Consensus Statement on age determination in high level young athletes. *Br J Sports Med.* 2010; 44: 476–484.
52. International Safeguards for Children in Sport. Available from: http://www.righttoplay.com/moreinfo/newsevents/Documents/International%20Safeguards%20for%20Children%20in%20Sport_FINAL%202014.pdf. 2014 [Accessed 16 Jan 2016].
53. International Fair Play Movement. Budapest: International Fair Play Committee. Available from: http://www.fairplayinternational.org/mission-1 [Accessed 16 Jan 2016].
54. Beyond Sport 2015 Awards. Beyond Sport Awards 2015 winners announced. 2015 October 20. Available from: http://www.beyondsport.org/press-releases/beyond-sport-awards-2015-winners-announced/ [Accessed 16 Jan 2016].
55. Rhind D, Kay T, Hills L. *Developing the International Safeguards for Children in Sport.* London: Brunel University; 2016. Available from: http://www.brunel.ac.uk/environment/themes/welfare-health-wellbeing/research-projects/developing-the-international-safeguards-for-children-in-sport
56. United Kingdom, Child Protection in Sport Unit. London: National Society for the Prevention of Cruelty to Children; 2016. Available from: https://thecpsu.org.uk/ [Accessed 16 Jan 2016].
57. Australian Commission, Play by the Rules. Belconnen, Australian Capital Territory; 2016. Available from: http://www.playbytherules.net.au/ [Accessed 16 Jan 2016].
58. Netherlands Olympic Committee/ NSF. Arnhem: NOC*NSF International; 2016. Available from: http://www.nocnsf.nl/en [Accessed 16 Jan 2016].
59. UK Sports Coach. *Safeguarding and protecting children in sport.* London; 2016. Available from: http://uksport.gov.uk/ [Accessed 16 Jan 2016].
60. World Anti-Doping Agency (WADA). *World Anti-Doping Code.* Montreal: WADA; 2015. Available from: https://www.wada-ama.org/en/resources/the-code/world-anti-doping-code [Accessed 16 Jan 2016].
61. Stirling A. Elite child athlete narratives of emotional abuse. In: Brackenridge C, Rhind D (eds.) *Elite child athlete welfare: International perspectives.* London: Brunel University Press; 2010. p. 70–79.

Index